M.B.

# SURGERY

*Official Publication* SOCIETY OF UNIVERSITY SURGEONS
SOCIETY FOR VASCULAR SURGERY





Volume 50
July—December, 1961

St. Louis
The C. V. Mosby Company

VOLUME 50


Printed in the United States of America

Volume 50 Number 1

# SURGERY

JULY, 1961

## Society of University Surgeons

# Basic surgical education

H. WILLIAM SCOTT, JR., M.D.
NASHVILLE, TENN.
*From the Department of Surgery, Vanderbilt University School of Medicine*

One hundred years ago the cannonading of Fort Sumter in Charleston Harbor heralded the beginning of the War Between the States—the bloodiest 4 years of American history. Wounds sustained by our forebears in this period of unparalleled violence were associated with an extraordinarily high mortality rate. From accounts by surgeons such as Weir Mitchell of the Union Army and Hunter McGuire of the Confederacy it is quite clear that virtually every penetrating wound of a body cavity proved fatal. Wounds of the extremities, except of the most trivial type, were best treated by amputation and the men who survived the shock of the procedure and the dreaded hospital gangrene afterward were pitifully few in number, whether they wore blue uniforms or gray. The over-all fatality rate for wounded men who were treated in the forward surgical units of the United States Army in World War II has been estimated at 4.5 per cent and in Korea the same fatality rate was 2.5 per cent.

Presidential address read at the Twenty-second Annual Meeting of the Society of University Surgeons, Kansas City, Kan., Feb. 9-11, 1961.

The staggering difference in the results of surgical management of the war wounded in this hundred-year period, while most impressive, gives only a minute reflection of the enormous developments in the field of surgery in the time that has elapsed. To summarize or place in proper perspective the tremendous advances in human biology, in the understanding of the normal and abnormal responses of the human organism in health and disease, and in the development of seemingly sound principles of surgical care of the injured and the sick which have taken place in the 100 years since the first gun was fired at Fort Sumter fortunately exceeds the scope of this discussion. These extraordinary developments, however, present an enormous challenge to the members of a society such as ours, composed of men who are charged with the dual responsibility of transmitting this huge fund of information to their students and trainees and of developing new knowledge in their fields through individual effort and by providing stimulus and opportunity for younger men.

In the great surgical clinics of Germany in the late nineteenth century there evolved plans of prolonged postgraduate clinical and laboratory training in early recognition of this challenge. Modifications of these plans were most successfully introduced into this country in that period by William Osler in medicine and by William Stewart Halsted in surgery. The postdoctoral educational concepts of Osler and Halsted have largely established the basis of our present-day residency systems of training.

Much has been written concerning Dr. Halsted's residency plan of graduate surgical education. It has been the subject of excellent addresses before this and other surgical societies on numerous occasions in the last several decades. As Pearce[5] has pointed out, "Halsted was intensely interested in extending the knowledge of surgery and so attracted superior graduate students. He shared with them his enthusiasm for research and improved clinical care. All the resources of the laboratory and the clinic were at their disposal." The stimulating atmosphere of Halsted's residency provided an approach in breadth and in depth to the general field of surgery. The prolonged period of study, investigation, and progressively increasing clinical responsibility produced outstanding surgeons. However, Halsted's system of graduate surgical education was not immediately adopted by many institutions and, in fact, very few hospitals in the United States and Canada offered this form of training until the last 2 decades. When the Society of University Surgeons was founded in 1938, recognition of the value of the Halsted type of graduate surgical education was emphasized and established as a requisite for membership. There were, however, but 10 institutions represented in the founders' group. Recognition of the need for improving the quality of surgical training on a country-wide basis, with emphasis on the residency system, prompted the founding of the American Board of Surgery in 1937. The influence of the Board in elevating standards of surgical training in this country has been enormous, although at times bordering on the chaotic, as its critics will hasten to point out.

Halsted and others fostered the development of special fields of surgery. After becoming competent surgeons, certain of his residents were encouraged to concentrate on special areas of interest. This resulted in the contributions to the surgical specialties by individuals of the mold of Hugh Young in urology, Crowe in otolaryngology, Baer in orthopedics, Davis in plastic surgery, and Cushing and Dandy in neurosurgery. The development of specialization has been of incalculable value in contributions to present-day surgical knowledge and skills. The establishment of separate residency programs in the surgical specialties in university hospitals was given impetus by World War I and great stimulus to the growth of the specialties has been provided by the various specialty boards which, like the American Board of Surgery, have been established in the last 3 decades.

Since World War II there has been a staggering increase in the number of hospitals which offer residency training opportunities in surgery and the surgical specialties. Most of this increase has been the result of the development of residency programs in hospitals unrelated to universities. Among the multiple factors responsible for this tremendous increase in the number of residencies were (1) the influence of the various boards on both surgical aspirants and hospitals, (2) the American College of Surgeons and its efforts to upgrade surgical services and training programs, and (3) the activities of the Conference Committee on Graduate Training in Surgery which, since 1950, has been responsible for national approval of residency training programs. The fourth factor has been the desire on the part of many hospitals and their staffs to attract residents largely for purposes of improving service to patients. This factor, while commendable in one light, has in all too many instances made of Halsted's residency plan of graduate education as Mulholland[4] has said, "a modern mockery, wherein, instead of the resident being provided with facilities, he has become just another facility, an invaluable and rather inexpensive facility."

According to data assembled by Frank

Glenn[3] for a recent report, there are at the present time in the United States 2,267 programs in hospitals which offer 12,364 residency positions in general surgery and the surgical specialties. In general surgery 704 hospital programs approved by the Conference Committee offer a total of 5,837 positions. There are 1,563 approved programs in the 9 surgical specialties which offer 6,527 positions. The magnitude of graduate surgical education in the United States is illustrated by these almost astronomical figures. Concomitant with the quantitative growth of opportunities for such graduate education, the trend of specialization has resulted in an increasing separation of the surgical subspecialties from general surgery, both in residency programs and in practice. That this trend represents the progress of our times with productive benefits is undeniable and generally commendable. However, continuation of this trend in graduate surgical education in an unguided manner may lead to a ridiculous degree of overspecialization of interests with extremely narrow perspectives and premature acquisition of skills on a trade school basis. As Victor Bonney[1] has pointed out, "Too restricted attention to one subject cramps the outlook, narrows the mind, destroys the sense of proportion, deforms the specialty and tends in the end to transform it into a cult."

In his presidential address to this Society in 1948 Zollinger[7] discussed the manner in which the postwar trends in specialization were converting the field of general surgery into a narrow specialty. He also presented data at that time which indicated that the majority of teachers of surgery held the opinion that a broad training in general surgery is essential before intensive specialization. He concluded that a general surgical service has a twofold obligation—to supply the basic surgical training for the surgical specialties and to furnish the requisite experience for the general surgeon.

Thirteen years have now elapsed since Dr. Zollinger's presentation. During this period the trends of specialization have continued. Despite Pearce's suggestion that surgical education is rightfully a function of the medical schools, it has become increasingly apparent that the universities and their affiliated hospitals are inadequate numerically to supply all the demands of graduate surgical education. The influence of the various boards and reviewing agencies in graduate surgical education has become stronger. Although a joint conference of the surgical specialty boards is held annually, each of the boards is entirely autonomous and establishes its own criteria for qualification. With the exception of the Board of Thoracic Surgery, none of the specialty boards has a direct relationship to the American Board of Surgery. Perhaps this is as it should be in a democracy and probably there is no particular reason for the American Board of Surgery to stand *in loco parentis* to any of the specialty boards. I don't believe the members of the American Board of Surgery would wish to assume such an onerous paternal obligation even in the unthinkable event that such a relationship might be brought about. Nevertheless, it is important to realize that the various boards which have become so enormously powerful in the direction of the patterns of graduate surgical education are individually autonomous entities with a minimal degree of interdependence.

In the last several years various groups concerned with graduate education in surgery have become gravely concerned with the trends which are promoting premature and overly complete specialization and which seem to be making a "modern mockery" of Halsted's residency plan. Among others, these groups include the Regents and the Graduate Training Committee of the American College of Surgeons, the American Board of Surgery and the various specialty boards, and the Conference Committee on Graduate Training in Surgery. While the studies and discussions of these groups have brought out wide differences of opinion, most of them have indicated some degree of unanimity concerning the mutual interdependence and interlocking needs of general surgery and the surgical specialties in residency training. Data collected by the American College of Surgeons have indicated that there is considerable support among directors of surgical training programs for the idea of providing more general surgical training for specialty residents, but opinions are divided as to what this training should consist of, how long it should be, and when it should take place in relation to concentrated residency experience in the specialty. The majority of directors of general surgical programs seem to be of the opinion that basic residency experience in general surgery should precede concentrated experience in a surgical specialty. On the contrary, some of the directors of residency programs in surgical specialties have voiced the opinion that their preference is to have their trainees obtain general surgical experience after basic education in their particular surgical specialty. Many of the supporters of the latter opinion have stated that their reasons for this view are (1) that basic principles in surgical care are provided as well in specialty residencies as in general surgical programs, (2) that specialty residents assigned to general surgery are given a "better deal" if they have a more advanced training status, and (3) that instruction in certain technical aspects of general surgery is the desired aim of a general surgical assignment for a specialty resident, that is how to perform a bowel resection, how to perform a radical neck dissection, and so forth. Some of the directors of training programs in certain surgical specialties, notably ophthalmology, anesthesiology, and obstetrics and gynecology, have expressed the opinion that general surgical training is not necessary for trainees in their specialty.

A review of the current residency training requirements of the various specialty boards indicates that 1 year of residency training in general surgery is considered desirable by the boards of urology, otolaryngology, neurosurgery, and orthopedics. Three years of general surgical residency are required by the Boards of Plastic Surgery and Proctology, while the Board of Thoracic Surgery demands full general surgical training with certification by the American Board of Surgery prior to thoracic board examinations. On the other hand, 3 of the specialty boards, specifically ophthalmology, anesthesiology, and obstetrics and gynecology, require no general surgical training in the qualifications for their examinations. Thus, the various specialty boards vary greatly in their official concepts of graduate surgical education.

As a means of counteracting the adverse effects of premature specialization and of providing a broader base for the graduate education of both general surgeons and surgical specialists, it has been recently proposed to the Graduate Training Committee of the American College of Surgeons that a 2-year plan of basic residency in general surgery and the surgical specialties be developed to provide broad grounding in the fundamentals of surgical care prior to subsequent training either in general surgery or in the specialties. This proposal has evoked considerable discussion. The Society of University Surgeons has inherently a large stake in the patterns of residency training with interest in both undergraduate and graduate education in surgery. This Society has the potential of exerting great influence on developments in surgical education on both national and international levels. It occurred to me that an appraisal of the opinions of the heads of departments of surgery and a survey of the current patterns of graduate surgical education in the member institutions of the Society of University Surgeons would be helpful in determining the merit of this proposal and, if it seems desirable, in establishing what an optimal plan for basic surgical training might consist of. Concomitantly, I thought it would be interesting to ascertain what the various member institutions of this Society are actually doing in their own programs of graduate surgical education at the present time. Accordingly, I have assembled information concerning the current patterns of residency training in our member institutions. Thirty-seven overworked department heads have been kind enough to provide opinions and facts about their own programs and I am very grateful to them.

The facilities for graduate surgical education available to our member institutions are extensive. The majority of member hospitals in which university residencies are based have over 500 beds. Eighteen of the group are hospitals of over 700 beds with a maximum of 3,000 beds. In addition, all except 3 extremely large units among our Society's member institutions are affiliated with at least 1 or 2 other hospitals in their residency programs. Fourteen member institutions have 3 to 5 such affiliates and one institution has 6 affiliates with a total of 5,500 beds available for residency training in medicine, surgery, and the specialties. The hospitals affiliated with our member institutions include 31 privately and publicly supported general hospitals and 20 Veterans Administration hospitals in addition to 24 specialized units, most of which are concerned with tuberculosis, cancer, or pediatrics.

Most of the university hospitals offer straight surgical internships and this form of internship is preferred by 22 of the 37 department heads for their trainees. Eight chiefs prefer a rotating or mixed internship and 5 have no preference. Two chiefs prefer either a straight surgical or a straight medical internship.

The university hospital residencies in general surgery are all at least 4 years in length. In Fig. 1 it is seen that most of our programs actually provide at least 5 years of residency experience after the internship. The few 6- and 8-year residencies are specifically designed for academic aspirants. The university residencies are all dedicated to the theme of graduated, increasing clinical responsibility, culminating in the total responsibility of the senior resident. The latter part of each program is thus necessarily devoted to a concentrated period of experience in depth in general surgery. In most of our member institutions thoracic and cardiovascular surgery are included as a part of this senior experience. In addition to the period of senior responsibility, the university resident

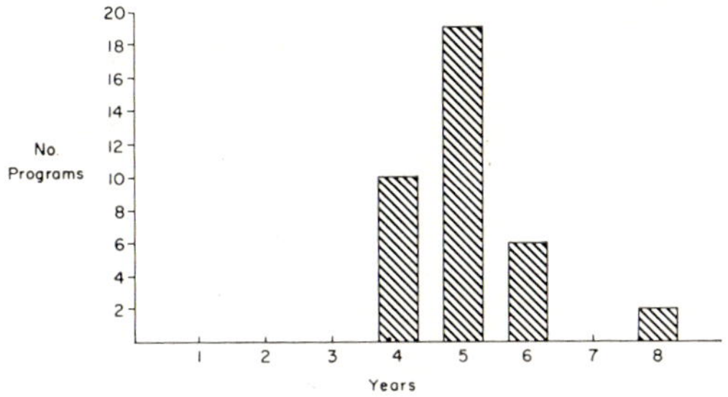


**Fig. 1.** University surgical residency programs. The usual number of years after internship.

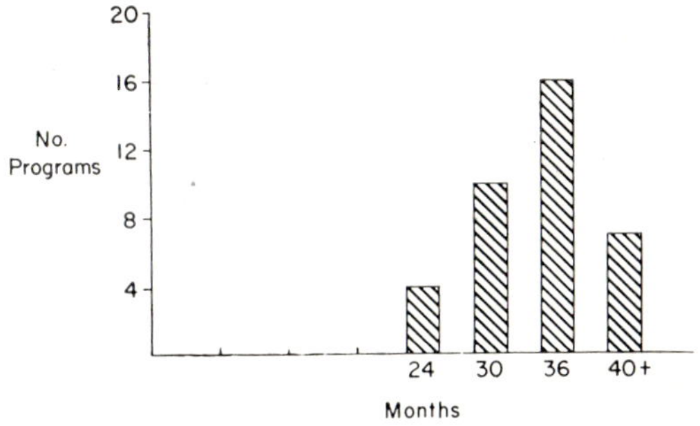


**Fig. 2.** Usual duration of clinical assignments in general surgery in university surgical residency programs.

is provided preliminary experience in general surgery, the various specialties, and in the laboratory during his period as assistant resident. Fig. 2 is a tabulation of data from our survey indicating the time each resident usually spends prior to and including his senior experience in our member institutions in general surgery, exclusive of the surgical specialty and laboratory assignments provided. The length of time varies from a minimum of 24 months to a maximum of 48 months.

Fig. 3 indicates the patterns of surgical specialty and laboratory assignments provided by our member hospitals in their general surgical residencies. There is, of course, flexible variation in these patterns in each of our residency programs and these tabulations can only summarize the dominant trends. It is interesting that only one institution apparently provides no experience

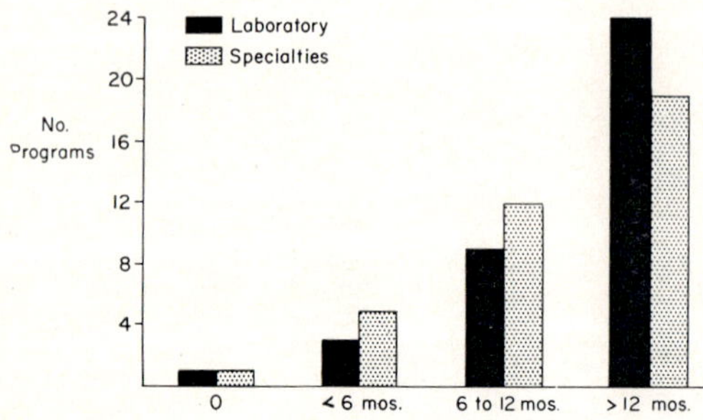


**Fig. 3.** Usual duration of assignments in laboratory and specialties in university surgical residency programs.

in the surgical specialties in its residency. Another program provides no specific time in laboratory experience, but this is available to the residents who may elect it.

From these simple tabulations it can be discerned that the current prototype of graduate education in general surgery among the member institutions of the Society of University Surgeons consists of a straight surgical internship followed by a 5-year residency program which provides 36 months of experience in general surgery, 12 months in specialty assignments, and 12 months in the laboratory.

A more detailed analysis of the content of the residency programs in general surgery in our member institutions is presented graphically in Fig. 4. From this it can be seen that in addition to or as a part of general surgery, our residencies provide educational opportunities in a wide variety of special fields. Pathology, with other basic disciplines, pediatric, thoracic, and cardiovascular surgery and proctology, are universal features of the university programs; the latter 3 are usually included in the general surgical services. With the exception of 1 or 2 residencies, experience is also routinely provided in plastic surgery, urology, experimental surgery, and orthopedics or fractures, or both. Half of the programs provide some experience in anesthesiology and gynecology, but only a few include otolaryngology.

These data reflect the majority opinions of the directors of residency programs in the member institutions of this Society concerning the value of the basic disciplines and the experimental laboratory work with a breadth of clinical experience in general surgery and the special fields in graduate surgical education. When these data are compared with the results of a similar analysis made by Zollinger in 1948 it is apparent that in the last 13 years there has been a definite trend to include more of the specialty fields in the university residencies in general surgery. The smallest increment of progress in this regard has been made with gynecology, which Zollinger noted in 1948 to represent "the most glaring discrepancy between the actual needs of the practitioner of surgery and what is offered in the [general surgical] training programs."

In Fig. 5 the usual patterns of the first 2 years of university surgical residency programs are summarized graphically. During this junior assistant residency period the majority of our university programs provide clinical experience in both general surgery and the specialties and, in many instances, some time in the laboratory is also provided. Programs which offer only clinical assignments in the first 2 years as a rule arrange laboratory opportunities during the third year of the residency.

It can be concluded that the period of the first 2 years of our university surgical

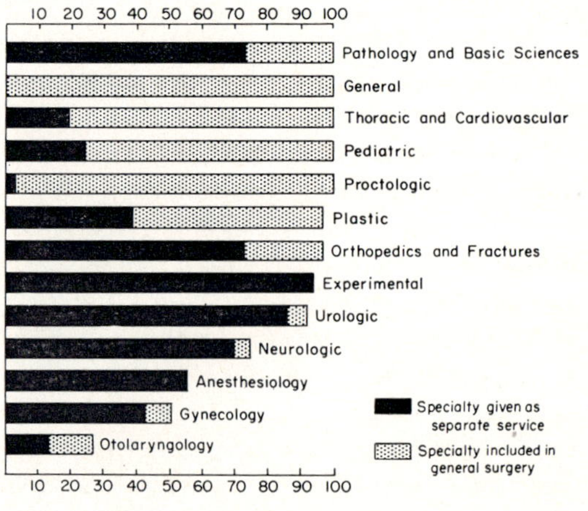


**Fig. 4.** Analysis of content of university surgical residency programs.

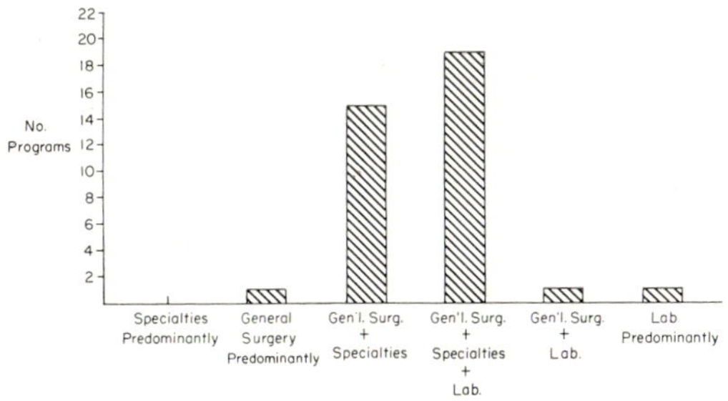


**Fig. 5.** The usual patterns of the first 2 years of university surgical residency programs.

residencies, designed primarily for the education of general surgeons, actually constitutes a basic program of education in the general field of surgery including the specialties.

It is the universal and firm conviction of the heads of our university departments of surgery that experience in general surgery is of paramount importance in the education of surgical specialists. This conviction is shared by the directors of educational programs in thoracic surgery, plastic surgery, proctology, and in the budding specialty of pediatric surgery. It is shared to a more limited degree by our orthopedists, urologists, otolaryngologists, and neurosurgeons and apparently not at all by many anesthesiologists, ophthalmologists, and gynecologists. There is no unanimity of opinion, however, among the specialists who recognize the value of general surgical training as to what this experience should be, or how it should be related to the specialty residency programs. Virtually all of our professors of surgery believe that experience in general surgery and experience in the specialties are inseparable components of the graduate education of both general surgeons and surgical specialists. Most of these teachers of surgery have the conviction that any individual destined toward a career in surgery or a special surgical field should have in his graduate education fundamental grounding in the principles of surgical care, including experience with a wide variety of problems in the general field of surgery, before he limits his learning activities to an anatomic, physiologic, or pathologic area of specialized interest. The majority of the heads of our departments of surgery thus tend to favor the proposal for a basic residency in surgery as a preliminary period of graduate education prior to more concentrated residency training in general surgery or the surgical specialties.

If a basic surgical residency is to provide grounding in fundamental principles of whole surgical care, it is logical that it must entail clinical opportunities to cope with a wide variety of the problems encountered on both general surgical and specialty services. Increasing clinical responsibility, including increasing operative experience under supervision, should be a part of these opportunities. It is obvious that there must be collaboration by general surgical and specialty divisions in implementing a basic residency, and to be successful it would appear mandatory that such a program be as valuable and desirable for men who go into the specialties as for trainees who continue in general surgery. It seems unlikely that these goals could be obtained in a single year of residency experience. They would probably require a minimal period of 2 years after the internship.

The details of structure and content of a basic surgical residency require careful consideration. The basic period should not be a rigid, stereotyped series of assignments which are imposed upon the junior resident as requirements, but should be flexible enough to allow the trainee some freedom of choice within the limitations of a given hospital's educational facilities. The patterns of the first 2 years of the majority of university hospital surgical residencies lend themselves admirably to such a plan. It is my suggestion that the basic residency include approximately 12 months of general surgical experience and approximately 12 months of experience in surgical specialties, including the possibility of a brief period in the laboratory as a substitute for one or more specialty assignments. During the period of assignments in general surgery the trainee would have the same learning opportunities as he has at present in general surgical residencies. He would serve as a junior assistant resident with responsibilities in the general surgical wards and in the operating rooms, with perhaps brief rotations to the outpatient department and/or the emergency service. In order to promote flexibility in the program and to permit increasing clinical responsibility with increasing operative experience in general surgery, it might be desirable to divide the general surgical assignments equally between the 2 years.

The content of the program in so far as the specialties are concerned poses a more difficult problem. Multiple brief rotations through all of the available organized specialties in a large institution might result in superficiality. We have seen previously in the analysis of university surgical residencies that certain of the special fields are commonly included in the activities of the general surgical service, specifically, proctology and pediatric, thoracic, cardiovascular, and plastic surgery. Therefore, it appears that the major needs for specific specialty assignments in a basic surgical residency would be provided by urology, orthopedics, gynecology, and neurosurgery. Furthermore, these are the specialties which have the greatest number of organized residency programs in the teaching hospitals. It is my suggestion that the trainee might elect, with the approval of the program director, one of 3 alternatives, (1) to rotate through each of the special assignments, (2) to substitute for one or more of them an equivalent period of time in the laboratory (surgical pathology, surgical research, physiology, and so forth), or (3) to substitute for one or more of them clinical assignments to other specialty services represented in the institution, such as plastic or thoracic surgery or otolaryngology, and so forth, which might be more contributory to the trainee's subsequent plan for specialization.

I suggest that the organization of the basic surgical residency be under the direction of the head of the department of surgery with the advice, collaboration, and assistance of a committee composed of the heads of the specialty departments or divisions with the head of the department of surgery as chairman. It seems logical to suggest that all appointments to the basic residency be made by this committee. Furthermore, to avoid any new complexities of nomenclature, it seems logical that these appointments be as "assistant resident surgeon," or the equivalent term in use by an individual hospital, and that the men so appointed be carried on the roster of trainees assigned to the hospital's general surgical service.

After the basic residency period the trainee would continue with more concentrated residency experience in the field of his choice, and with completion of his training should have the qualifications for examinations of a specific board. This plan does not in any way preclude the possibility or the desirability of gaining additional experience during the subsequent years of training, either in the laboratory or in clinical fields other than that of the specific residency which is elected. Neither does it preclude the possibility or desirability of any trainee's obtaining much more extensive laboratory or clinical research experience prior to or during the basic residency period by a leave of absence from the clinical program.

In Fig. 6 a schema is presented which indicates the manner in which the proposed basic residency would be related to more advanced and specialized surgical training. In this schema the possibility of a basic board examination is suggested. This might be developed by collaboration of the various specialty boards with the American Board of Surgery to serve as a qualifying examination in basic science and in the fundamentals of surgical care.

Both ophthalmology and anesthesiology have been omitted from this schema and from the bulk of the preceding discussion on the basis of features unique to these specialties and the statements made previously by their representatives to the effect that a basic surgical residency would be of little value to their trainees.

What would be the specific effects on the current patterns of graduate surgical educa-

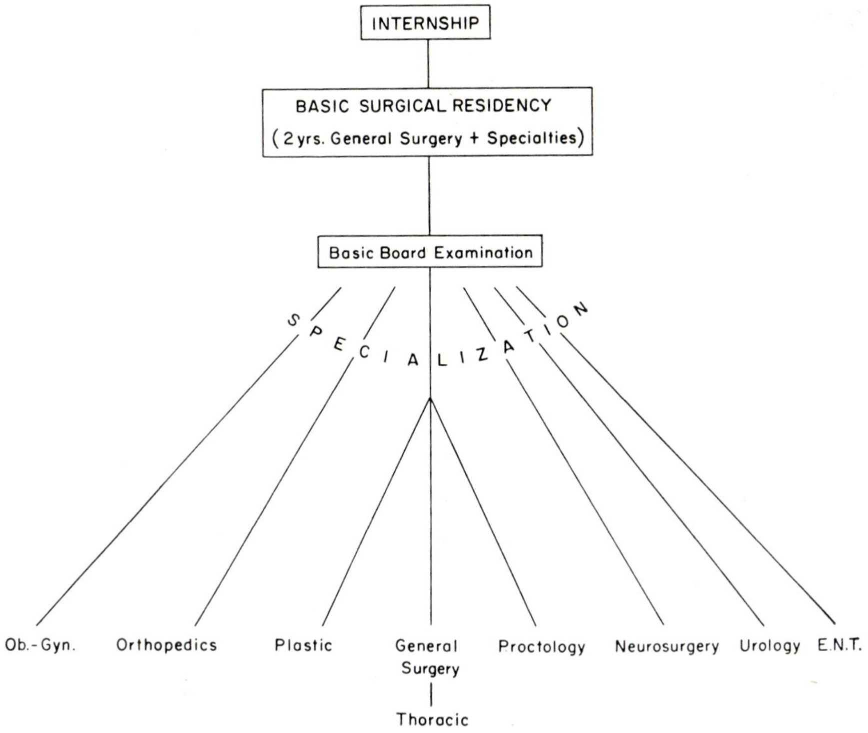


**Fig. 6.** Schema which indicates the relationship of the proposed basic surgical residency to more advanced and specialized training.

tion if such a proposal were to be generally adopted? In the majority of general surgical programs, especially those in university hospitals, relatively little change would be necessary in the present patterns of assignment and rotation. As we have seen, most university surgical residencies and, indeed, most of the approved residencies in general surgery in nonuniversity hospitals already provide the essentials of this proposal in the patterns of their first 2 years. There would be no need for increasing the over-all length of residency programs above the current provisions which lead to board qualifications in proctology in plastic, thoracic, and cardiovascular surgery, or in general surgery. The more intensive interest and collaboration of the specialistics in a basic residency plan, however, should add considerable strength to the preliminary education of individuals who complete their training in general surgery or the aforementioned specialties which currently require 3 or more years of general surgical training as a part of their graduate educational plans.

The greatest changes which would result from general adoption of the basic residency proposal would be in the current patterns of graduate education of orthopedists, urologists, otolaryngologists, neurosurgeons, and gynecologists. At present, even in many of our university hospitals, most of these specialty programs accept their trainees directly from the internship. Except for gynecology, each of these specialties encourages or requires 1 year of general surgical residency training as a part of its respective board qualifications. However, there is in general no specific plan as to how this year of general surgery is related to the remainder of the specialty residency or as to what it is to provide. In many instances this "general surgical" year has been a source of great discontent both to directors of specialty programs and their trainees. In the survey made by the American College of Surgeons recently the complaint was frequently registered that the specialty trainee who rotated to a general surgical service was not given the same clinical opportunities or as much to do as the equivalent trainee in general surgery. This source of discontent and intramural disharmony in our teaching hospitals would be eliminated by the general adoption of the basic residency proposal.

This proposal would at first glance have the effect of increasing by 1 year the current residency training requirements in orthopedics, neurosurgery, otolaryngology, and urology and by 2 years the requirements for board qualifications in obstetrics and gynecology. In this regard it should be noted that a few of our university residencies in these specialties already require 2 or 3 years of general surgical training prior to the specialty residency. If the basic surgical residency provides an adequate grounding in fundamentals (which currently must be provided by the specialty program) with a breadth of clinical experience in general surgery and the special fields it is possible that the length of time a resident must now spend in the concentrated experience of his elected specialty could be reduced accordingly. This would have to be decided by the directors of the respective specialty residencies in collaboration with their representative boards. That an additional period of time would result from adoption of the basic residency plan for the resident in the specialty of obstetrics and gynecology would appear to be unavoidable. However, I can think of no special field of medicine which would profit more by the adoption of the basic residency proposal.

Currently the popular 3-year residencies which lead to board qualification in obstetrics and gynecology provide only an 18-month period in which surgical principles and their concentrated application to gynecology are learned by the trainee—the remainder of the residency is devoted to obstetrics. The board-certified specialist in this field thus has usually a total of a year and one-half of limited surgical residency experience to equip him in his subsequent management of the pelvic problems of our mothers, wives, and daughters.

In his presidential address to the Southern Surgical Association in 1954, an eminent gynecologist, Dr. John Burch,[2] decried the deficiencies of the residency programs in obstetrics and gynecology, as well as those in general surgery, in providing adequate experience for the man who is to deal with the surgical problems of the female pelvis. He summarized the dilemma by indicating that the general surgical residencies provided the surgical "know-how" but without adequate knowledge of gynecology, while in the residencies in obstetrics and gynecology the reverse was the case. A basic surgical residency prior to concentrated training in gynecology would be a logical solution.

In conclusion it is my conviction that the acceptance and development of the basic surgical residency plan would improve graduate surgical education on a country-wide basis, both in general surgery and the surgical specialties. Implementation of the plan with direction which would insure that it provide basic surgical education and not simply a series of stereotyped training assignments would be ideally initiated by university hospitals and especially by the member institutions of the Society of University Surgeons.

To summarize this discussion concisely I can do no better than to quote from the address given by Dr. Isidor Ravdin[6] a few years ago at the dedication of the Mayo Memorial Building at the University of Minnesota. Among other things, Dr. Ravdin said, "Halsted founded a new concept in the training of young surgeons. . . . In this age of specialization there is a lack of appreciation of the necessity for rigorous training in general surgery as the cornerstone upon which all surgical achievement is founded. Even though the young surgeon should finally select a relatively narrow field his preliminary training should be as broad as it is possible to make it."

## REFERENCES

1. Bonney, V.: The forces behind specialism in surgery, Lancet **1:** 69, 1943.

2. Burch, J. C.: What's wrong with pelvic surgery? Ann. Surg. **141:** 573, 1955.
3. Glenn, F.: Basic surgical training, Bull. Am. Coll. Surgeons. In press.
4. Mulholland, J. H.: Learning to be a surgeon, Ann. Surg. **148:** 297, 1958.
5. Pearce, H. E.: The effect of specialization on graduate education in surgery, J. A. M. A. **170:** 301, 1959.
6. Ravdin, I. S.: A surgeon takes a second look at surgery, J. A. M. A. **158:** 532, 1955.
7. Zollinger, R. M.: The postwar trends in the training of the general surgeon, SURGERY **24:** 161, 1948.

# The use of low molecular weight dextran and serum albumin as plasma expanders in extracorporeal circulation

DAVID M. LONG, JR., M.D.*
LUIS SANCHEZ, M.D.
RICHARD L. VARCO, M.D.
C. WALTON LILLEHEI, M.D.
MINNEAPOLIS, MINN.
*From the Department of Surgery and Variety Club Heart Hospital, University of Minnesota Medical School*

The quest for blood substitutes and plasma expanders is a principal concern for investigators in many surgical fields. Because of the large quantities of blood generally used to prime extracorporeal circuits and artificial oxygenators, the problem of a safe, effective plasma expander is of particular interest to groups engaged in open-heart surgery. Ideally, substitution of a plasma expander for donor blood can decrease the likelihood of blood incompatibility reaction and the incidence of viral hepatitis. In addition, the problems of acidosis and trauma to vital corpuscles and plasma proteins may be lessened. Practically speaking, the work and expense of securing and cross-matching donor blood are also lessened.

Our interest in the investigation of low molecular weight dextran as a plasma expander was stimulated by the work of Gelin[13] and his colleagues[11, 19, 20, 31] and Thorsen and Hint.[27] Gelin described the occurrence of intravascular aggregation after injury and during hypothermia and the reversal of these effects by the use of low molecular weight dextran. Others[2, 10, 17] had observed the phenomenon of intravascular aggregation or sludging of blood corpuscles in a great number and variety of stressful conditions. It is difficult to envision how the decrease in the capillary blood flow and plugging of venules and arterioles by sludged blood cells and thrombi could be anything but deleterious. Nevertheless, we had not considered intravascular aggregation to be of any real consequence in extracorporeal circulation before the report by Gelin. His work demonstrated that the anemia of injury was due primarily to the loss of red blood corpuscles from the circulation by the process of intravascular aggregation. The decrease in circulating hemoglobin in traumatized animals and human beings could be largely prevented by the daily administration of low molecular weight dextran. Even more intriguing was the finding that multiple microscopic infarcts in vital organs can be caused by the aggregation of blood corpuscles.

After open-heart operations we noted that patients developed an anemia similar in degree and duration to that seen in patients after fractures, burns, myocardial infarction, and other forms of injury.[9] It was assumed generally that the anemia after extracorporeal circulation was due to a combination

Supported by grants from the Graduate School, University of Minnesota; Minnesota Heart Association; Life Insurance Medical Research Fund; United States Public Health Service; National Heart Institute Grant No. H-830; and Cardiovascular Surgical Research Fund.

Read at the Twenty-second Annual Meeting of the Society of University Surgeons, Kansas City, Kan., Feb. 9-11, 1961.

*Special Research Fellow, National Heart Institute, National Institutes of Health, United States Public Health Service.

of the shortened life expectancy of transfused erythrocytes and mechanical injury of the blood cells by pumps and oxygenating apparatuses.

Open-heart operations are unquestionably a significant form of trauma, as is any major surgical procedure. The moderate anemia seen in most patients is in itself of no real concern to the patient or the physician. However, if even a part of this postoperative anemia is indicative of widespread arteriolar and venular occlusion and thrombosis, there may be adequate explanation for the puzzling and indefinable morbidity and death seen occasionally in some of these patients. Thus, for these reasons, we were stimulated to examine the microcirculation during extracorporeal circulation. Our initial attitude was one of skepticism. Moreover, during the initial phases of the study, no clear-cut changes in small-vessel blood flow were discerned. However, accurate appraisal of the microcirculation requires some experience, skill, and training, as do other microscopic techniques. With additional experience in the microscopic examination of the blood flow in small vessels, the changes due to intravascular aggregation became apparent, and it became evident that the restoration of normal small-vessel circulation could be accomplished by the administration of Rheomacrodex.* In addition, the development of microinfarcts in the liver, kidney, and myocardium, as observed after prolonged periods of extracorporeal circulation in dogs, could be prevented or minimized by Rheomacrodex.

These observations in dogs raised certain questions as to whether there might be any undesirable effects from use of low molecular weight dextran and whether other plasma expanders such as serum albumin might have beneficial effects. Moreover, the question has been raised as to whether 5 per cent dextrose in water or normal saline solution might also have antisludging properties when added to blood, simply because of the dilutional effect.

When properly prepared, normal human serum albumin is a safe and effective plasma expander. The principal disadvantage with its use is the limited supply and relatively high expense of the processing required for separation of albumin from human plasma. Synthetic materials such as dextran may be prepared in large quantities so that the expense can be decreased. The fact that Rheomacrodex also prevented intravascular aggregation made this substance particularly attractive. However, past experience with previously available dextran preparations demonstrated that the administration of quantities in excess of 1,000 to 1,500 ml. resulted in serious bleeding problems.[4, 6, 16, 23, 25, 26] The work of a number of investigators in this country,[24] in Sweden,[14, 18] and in the armed forces[1] during the Korean conflict indicated that the bleeding was due to the large molecular fraction of dextran preparations. The safe upper limit of molecular weight in this consideration is probably approximately 80,000.

Careful studies on dogs in this laboratory indicated that Rheomacrodex had no effect on coagulation mechanisms in the normal anesthetized dog or in the dog subjected to cardiopulmonary bypass. However, coagulation defects did develop from time to time after extracorporeal circulation in human subjects for various reasons related either to basic coagulation defects or technical problems, and the postoperative blood loss from chest tubes was sometimes far greater than that encountered with the ordinary thoracotomy. The purpose of this study was therefore twofold. First, an attempt was made to quantitate the physiologic effects of the use of plasma expanders. Second, we were interested in evaluating the effect of Rheomacrodex and normal human serum albumin* on coagulation mechanisms and blood loss in patients with many varying types and

*Rheomacrodex refers to the low molecular weight dextran used in this study which was supplied by Pharmacia Laboratories, New York, N. Y. The average molecular weight of this substance is 41,000 and the intrinsic viscosity is 0.19. The low fraction has an average molecular weight of 14,500 and is 11.4 per cent of the total, and the high fraction has a molecular weight of 68,000 and is 10.6 per cent of the total. A solution of 10 per cent Rheomacrodex in 0.9 per cent saline solution has a buffer capacity of 1.5 ml. of 0.1 N sodium hydroxide per liter and a pH of 5.1.

*Supplied by Merck Sharp & Dohme, West Point, Pa.

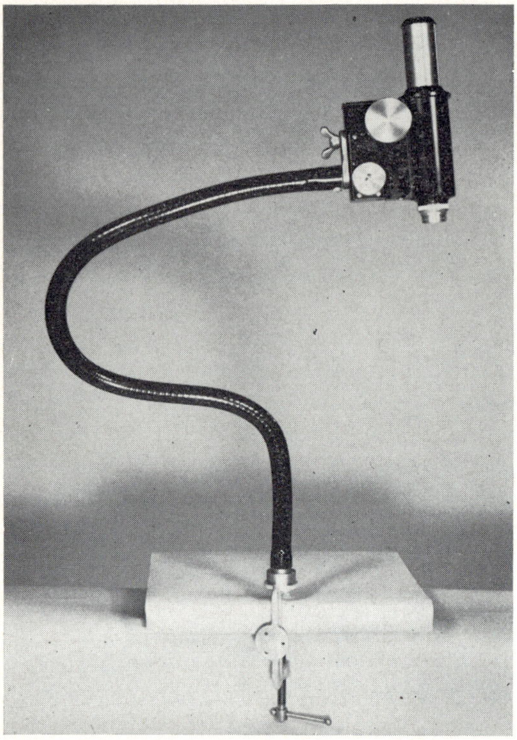

**Fig. 1.** This dissecting microscope has a magnification system of ×50 and is used to examine the microcirculation of the ocular conjunctiva of patients. The microscope is mounted on a semirigid arm taken from a desk lamp. This system provides sufficient stability for accurate examination of the blood flow and flexibility for positioning in crowded areas.

stages of heart disease after extracorporeal circulation.

## METHODS

The microcirculation was observed in the ocular conjunctiva of 40 patients before, during, and after extracorporeal circulation. In addition, the microcirculation was observed in a larger number of patients in the recovery rooms after operation and during periods of complicated convalescence. The technique used was similar to that of Gelin[13] and of necessity much less complicated than that used by Knisely[17] and others. A monocular microscope (Fig. 1) with a magnification of ×50 was attached to one end of a flexible arm and a C clamp was attached to the other end. The arm was attached to the operating table or the patient's bed and the microscope was positioned over the eye of the patient. The light source consisted of a common flashlight of sufficient intensity but with little heat emission. Ophthalmic ointment or an ophthalmic solution of methylcellulose was used to prevent drying of the conjunctiva in unconscious patients during periods of long examination. With training and a cooperative patient, surprisingly thorough appraisals of the microcirculation were made with this simple technique.

The equipment used in the extracorporeal circulation consisted of the helix reservoir bubble oxygenator and the Sigmamotor pump.[8] Donor blood was collected within 24 hours of operation in siliconized bottles with 2,000 U.S.P. units (20 mg.) of sodium heparin in 20 ml. of 0.9 per cent saline solution. The patients were divided into 3 series. Selection of patients for any given series was made by a single blind control method. Three sets of 200 cards marked "control," "albumin," or "dextran" were randomly mixed in a sealed box. The technician in charge of the oxygenator drew a card from the box just before priming the oxygenator. If a control card was drawn, no albumin or Rheomacrodex was added to the priming volume. Albumin or Rheomacrodex were added as indicated according to the formulas (1) normal human serum albumin, 5 per cent solution, 20 ml. per kilogram of body weight (1.0 Gm. per kilogram); and (2) Rheomacrodex, 10 per cent solution in 0.9 per cent saline solution, 20 ml. per kilogram of body weight (2.0 Gm. per kilogram). An additional 150 ml. of plasma expander was added to the oxygenator for each additional 1,000 ml. of blood added during cardiopulmonary bypass. In the last 12 patients in this study, the quantity of plasma expander used in priming was increased to 25 ml. per kilogram of body weight.

Purposeful deviations from this completely blind control system occurred in some cases. When the patient had one of the more difficult types of acquired multivalvular disease or severe tetralogy of Fallot which might necessitate a prolonged perfusion and a control card was drawn, Rheomacrodex was added to the oxygenator. In addition, in several cases there were difficulties in securing a sufficient volume of blood because of an unusual blood type and a plasma expander was then used. Cross matching of blood was performed with Rheomacrodex when unusual antibodies were detected in the patient's blood and Rheomacrodex was used in the oxygenator circuit. The alterations were considered justifiable in view of the clinical nature of the experiment. However, for these reasons, the distribution of more difficult cases in which longer periods of extracorporeal circulation were needed was weighted toward the 2 plasma expanders. Patients who died in the operating room are not included in this report since no postoperative data were available for comparison.

Hemoglobin levels, platelet counts, venous clotting time, prothrombin time, clot retraction, and plasma electrolyte levels were determined preoperatively and postoperatively as soon as the patient arrived in the postanesthesia recovery room in as many instances as possible according to the limits of the laboratory facilities. Plasma fibrinogen determinations were made by the Kjell-Jacobson technique. Serum proteins were measured by paper electrophoresis with the Spinco apparatus.

Total carbon dioxide content, oxygen content, and oxygen capacity in arterial blood were measured manometrically with the Thomas-Van Slyke apparatus in approximately one-half of the patients according to the limits of laboratory facilities. The Beckman G pH meter was used to determine pH on all patients. Arterial blood samples for these determinations were drawn anaerobically at 4 different intervals, (1) preoperative (arterial blood was drawn from the patient approximately one-half hour before the onset of extracorporeal circulation), (2) control (arterialized blood sample was drawn from the oxygenator reservoir before the start of extracorporeal circulation), (3) pump off (arterialized blood sample was drawn from the oxygenator reservoir at the conclusion of extracorporeal circulation), and (4), postoperative (arterialized blood sample was drawn from the patient approximately 90 minutes after the finish of extracorporeal circulation).

Plasma bicarbonate $(HCO^-_3)p$ corrected to pH 7.4 was calculated from this data by means of the Henderson-Hasselbalch equation and rearrangements thereof according to Brown.[5] The plasma bicarbonate $(HCO^-_3)p$ corrected to pH 7.4 was subtracted from 24.0 mM. per liter, the normal value for $(HCO^-_3)p$ for human beings, to obtain the value for bicarbonate deficit. Free plasma hemoglobin, $Hb_p$, was determined at 3 different time intervals, (1) preoperative (arterialized blood was drawn from the oxygenator reservoir before start of extracorporeal circulation), (2) pump off (arterialized blood was drawn from the oxygenator reservoir at the finish of extracorporeal circulation), and (3) final (arterialized blood was drawn from the patient approximately 90 minutes after the finish of extracorporeal circulation). Dextran levels in serum were determined according to the anthrone method of Wallenius.[29]

The volume of urine output was measured for the first 4 12-hour intervals after the patient returned to the postanesthesia recovery room. The volume of chest drainage was also tabulated for the first 12-hour intervals immediately after operation to determine the effect of the plasma expanders on postoperative bleeding.

## RESULTS

**Microcirculation studies.** Examination of the blood vessels of the ocular conjunctiva in human patients revealed both similarities and dissimilarities with the observations made in dogs during cardiopulmonary bypass.[21] In healthy dogs, intravascular aggregation and changes in the microcirculation were rarely seen before the onset of cardiopulmonary bypass. During the first 10 or 15 minutes, inconsistent alterations, such as decreased velocity and venous distention, were seen frequently. The passage of blood through the small vessels then returned to normal. However, after 45 to 60 minutes of

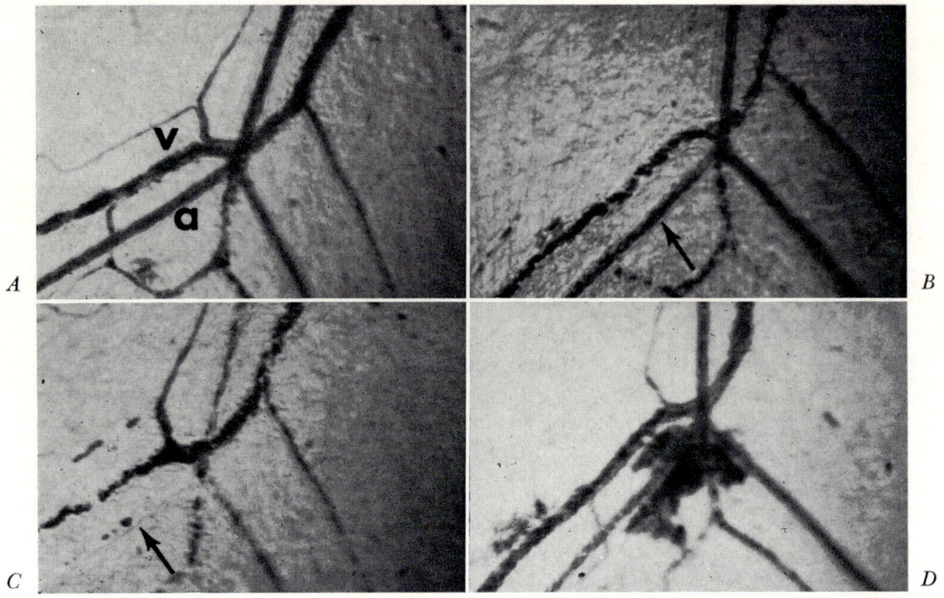


**Fig. 2.** These photographs illustrate the changes which occur in the microcirculation of the mesentery of the dog during prolonged extracorporeal circulation. The dog was normothermic and the perfusion rate was maintained at 100 ml. per kilogram per minute. Only small fluctuations occurred in the mean blood pressure. *A,* Control shows essentially normal circulation. The venule in this area is marked *v* and the arteriole *a*. *B,* The same area 25 minutes after the beginning of extracorporeal circulation shows the early granular appearance of the corpuscular suspension in the venule. Tip of arrow rests exactly on outside of wall of arteriole. Note the exaggerated axial accumulation of cells and thickening of the peripheral layer of plasma in this arteriole due to the intravascular aggregation in the central portions. *C,* After 2 hours of extracorporeal circulation, the velocity of blood flow in the vessels is greatly diminished and large aggregates of corpuscles are present in the small vessels. Arrow points to wall of arteriole. The size of this arteriole had not decreased, but the fluid circulating through the arteriole is plasma with only a few aggregated cells. *D,* After 3 hours and 10 minutes of extracorporeal circulation and 10 minutes after addition of Rheomacrodex, 1.5 Gm. per kilogram body weight. The suspension of the corpuscles has improved and most of the aggregates have disappeared. Some of the venules are thrombosed, however. Velocity of blood flow is increased in all vessels. The mass of red blood cells at the bifurcation is due to a collection of blood between the mesentery and the light source and not due to hemorrhage into the mesentery. (×200; reduced ⅕.)

extracorporeal circulation small clumps of red and white corpuscles and platelets formed, and there was an exaggeration of axial streaming and an increase in the layer of plasma on the periphery of the vessels (Figs. 2 through 7). To the naked eye and at low magnifications, exaggerated axial accumulation may be misinterpreted as vasospasm or decrease in the bore size of the vessels. The number and size of the aggregates gradually increased. After 2 hours of extracorporeal circulation the velocity of blood flow in the arterioles and venules was decreased. Corpuscular movement through capillaries was frequently absent in large fields of examination. Aggregates of cells began to adhere to the walls of veins and temporary occlusion of both arterioles and venules was observed frequently. Eventually thrombosis of vessels occurred. Pinkish-yellow fluid, presumably plasma, sometimes accumulated around the areas of microinfarction. Out of over 100 dogs studied during prolonged extracorporeal circulation, only one showed no evidence of impairment in the microcirculation. In fact, the blood flow seemed to improve with time in this one dog.

All of these same alterations in microcirculation were observed in the studies on human subjects. However, many of the patients demonstrated large numbers of intravascular aggregates before the onset of extracorporeal circulation. In some instances, the observation of intravascular aggregation correlated with preoperative elevations of the erythrocyte sedimentation rate. In patients who received no Rheomacrodex or albumin, impairment of the microcirculation occurred much earlier in the course of extracorporeal circulation than was observed in dogs. Within 20 to 30 minutes, there was decrease in the velocity of blood flow and increase in the number of aggregates with occlusion of small vessels. Small arteriovenous shunts became more apparent by contrast. When intravascular aggregation was present before extracorporeal circulation, it became more severe during bypass and never improved even at perfusion rates as high as 110 ml. per kilogram per minute. In good-risk patients, such as those with simple atrial septal defects or uncomplicated ventricular septal defects, the duration of extracorporeal circulation was short and intravascular aggregation was not found until 3 to 5 days postoperatively. In 1 patient with a tetralogy of Fallot lesion, no impairment of the microcirculation was observed during 1 hour and 42 minutes of extracorporeal circulation. It is of interest that this patient had an excellent urine output postoperatively but had elevation of circulating fibrinolysins and bled excessively during the postoperative period.

Patients who received Rheomacrodex as a part of this study demonstrated no evidence of intravascular aggregation. Patients who received albumin demonstrated little or no evidence of intravascular aggregation. When the period after extracorporeal circulation was uncomplicated, the microcirculation remained normal until the third to fifth postoperative day. However, if blood loss from the thoracotomy necessitated replacement with additional blood in the operating room, the serum levels of dextran dropped to very low values immediately and intravascular aggregation appeared. Dextran was excreted rapidly in the early postoperative period and serum albumin levels also dropped. Patients with chronic heart failure or the more severe forms of heart disease then developed intravascular aggregation within 6 hours postoperatively. In patients without complications, just as in the control groups, intravascular aggregation did not appear until the third to fifth day postoperatively. Severe intravascular aggregation was seen regularly when infection or oliguria complicated the postoperative convalescence.

**Distribution of patients.** The age and sex distribution and the mean weight for the 124 patients studied are listed in Table I. From this table it can be seen that the average age and the average weight of the patients in the dextran and albumin series were greater than those of the controls. The distribution of the patients according to cardiac lesion is presented in Table II. Although not reflected directly in this table, the older patients with

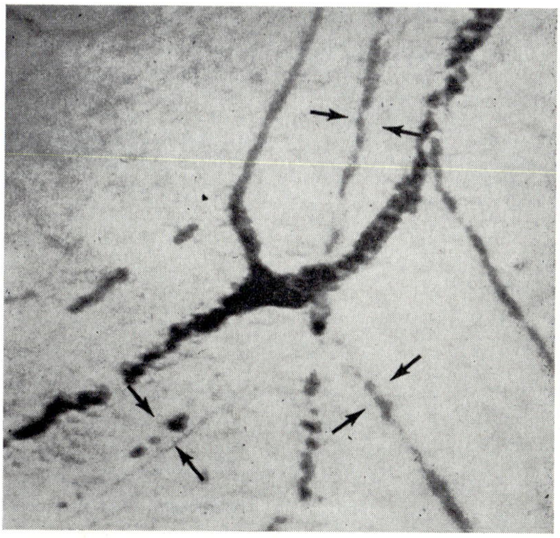

**Fig. 3.** Enlargement of Fig. 2, *C*, illustrates the plasma-skimming effect in the arteriole. Arrows point to walls of arteriole. The lumen of the arteriole has not changed in size. At lower magnifications or when visualized by the naked eye, this type of change in the arteriolar blood flow is sometimes misinterpreted as vasoconstriction, since the arteriole cannot be seen.

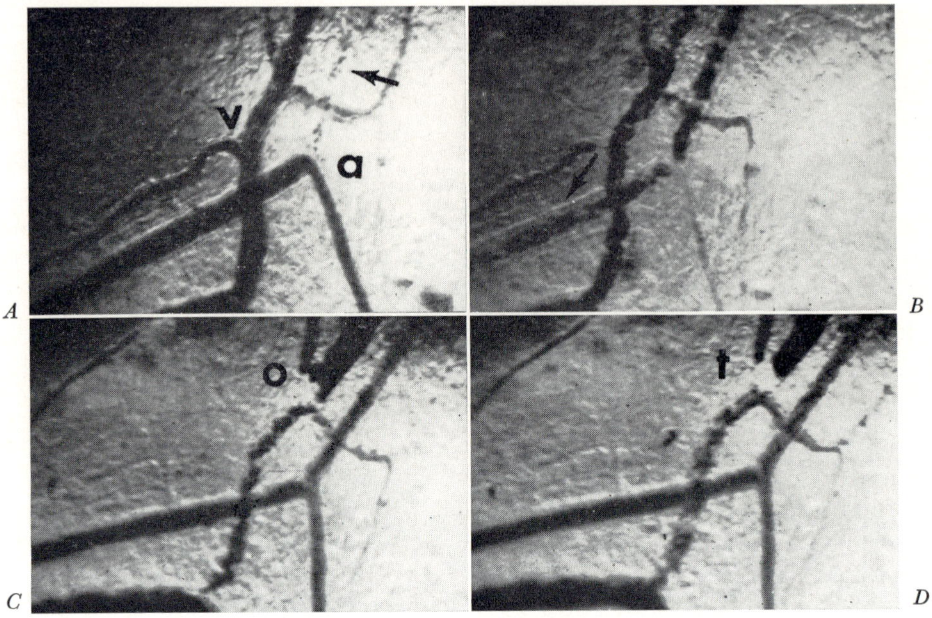


**Fig. 4.** Another set of vessels in the mesentery of the dog during extracorporeal circulation at a flow rate of 100 ml. per kilogram per minute. *A,* Control area illustrates a normal variation in circulation. Note that the branch of the arteriole *(a)* in the upper right *(arrow)* contains primarily plasma with a few corpuscles. The individual corpuscles are well separated, however, and are not aggregated. *B,* Thirty minutes after the onset of extracorporeal circulation. Beginning aggregation in the venule and exaggerated axial accumulation of corpuscles with plasma skimming in the arteriole *(arrow)*. *C,* Two hours and 30 minutes after onset of extracorporeal circulation. Occlusion *(o)* of the venule with clumps of corpuscles. *D,* Three hours and 5 minutes of extracorporeal circulation and 15 minutes after the administration of Rheomacrodex. Velocity of blood flow has improved and aggregates are disappearing. However, by this time the venule has become thrombosed (t). (×200; reduced ⅙.)

tetralogy of Fallot lesion and with the farther advanced acquired valvular heart disease were generally given plasma expanders, either by blind selection or by purposeful deviation from this system.

**Hematologic and biochemical changes.** The patients were analyzed according to the increase in plasma hemoglobin during the period of extracorporeal circulation and this information is presented in Table III. The mean increase in plasma hemoglobin per minute of extracorporeal circulation in the dextran series was 42 per cent less than that of the control series. This figure was statistically significant with a p value $< 0.001$. The increase in plasma hemoglobin in the albumin series was 19.6 per cent less than in the control series, but this change was not statistically significant.

During the first 90 minutes after extracorporeal circulation, there was a decrease in the plasma hemoglobin. The mean decreases and standard errors of the means were control 26.5 ± 6.6 mg. per cent, dextran 33.5 ± 5.1 mg. per cent, and albumin 26.4 ± 10.6 mg. per cent. Analysis of the differences between the dextran and albumin experimental groups and the control group showed that the differences were not statistically significant. Therefore, there was no evidence that the excretion or clearance of free plasma hemoglobin from the circulation was significantly different in the 3 groups.

An attempt was made to quantitate changes in plasma bicarbonate deficits during the period of extracorporeal circulation in order to estimate the effects of the plasma expanders on the development of metabolic

**Table I.** *Age, sex distribution, and weight*

| *Age (yr.)* | *Control group* | *Dextran group* | *Albumin group* |
|---|---|---|---|
| 0- 2 | 0 | 0 | 1 |
| 3-10 | 23 | 14 | 13 |
| 11-20 | 15 | 12 | 13 |
| 21-30 | 2 | 6 | 4 |
| 31-40 | 2 | 3 | 4 |
| 41-50 | 3 | 2 | 2 |
| Over 50 | 0 | 4 | 1 |
| Average age | 13.5 | 21 | 17.5 |
| Male | 20 | 27 | 17 |
| Female | 25 | 14 | 21 |
| Average weight (Kg.) | 32.7 | 46.1 | 43.3 |

acidosis. The plasma bicarbonate deficit was calculated in the patient's blood before extracorporeal circulation $(\Delta HCO^-_3)_1$ and in the priming blood $(\Delta HCO^-_3)_2$ in the oxygenator reservoir. Since the priming volume of the oxygenator was usually approximately equal to the patient's blood volume, the average bicarbonate deficit before extracorporeal circulation was calculated:

$$\frac{(\Delta HCO^-_3)_1 + (\Delta HCO^-_3)_2}{2}$$

The value for this initial bicarbonate deficit was then subtracted from the bicarbonate deficit calculated at the end of extracorporeal circulation. We recognized that there were unavoidable errors in the calculation of bicarbonate deficit, particularly because of difficulties in securing representative samples of blood. However, it was assumed that the errors would be reproduced in each group. Experimental studies have proved that the metabolic acidosis acquired during extracorporeal circulation is directly proportional to the volume and age of the priming blood and the duration of the extracorporeal circulation at comparable rates of perfusion. The mean increases in bicarbonate deficit and the standard errors of the means in the 3 groups were control, 0.063 ± 0.011 mM. per liter per minute; dextran, 0.062 ± 0.011 mM. per liter per minute; and albumin, 0.073 ± 0.009 mM. per liter per minute. The differences in these 3 groups were not statistically significant.

Changes in platelet count were calculated by measuring the difference between the preoperative platelet count and the postoperative platelet count which was carried out immediately after the patient reached the postanesthesia recovery room. In Table IV it can be seen that the decrease in platelet count was significantly less in the dextran series than in the control series, and there was no significant difference between the albumin series and the control series. It may be noted, however, that the preoperative platelet counts were significantly less in the dextran series than in the control and the albumin series. In order to ascertain whether there may have been larger decreases in platelet counts in patients with higher preoperative values, 2 additional assessments were also made. Patients with preoperative levels between 200,000 and 300,000 platelets per cubic millimeter were selected from each group. In Table IV it can be seen that the decrease in platelets in these selected patients also was significantly less in the dextran series than in the control series, and again

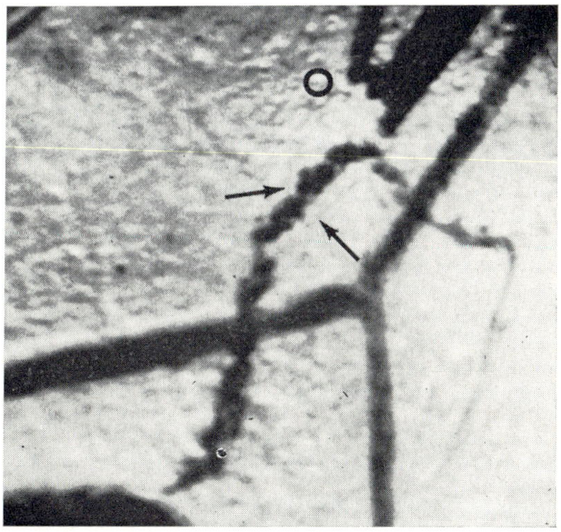


**Fig. 5.** Higher magnification of Fig. 4, *C.* The area of occlusion of the venule is marked *o.* Arrows rest on walls of venule. Arrow on left points to an area where cellular aggregates are adhering momentarily to the venular wall and then tumbling along the periphery of the venule. Arrow on right points to an area of plasma skimming.

**Table II.** *Lesion distribution*

| *Lesion* | *Control group* | *Dextran group* | *Albumin group* |
|---|---|---|---|
| *Congenital* | | | |
| Atrial septal defect | 12 | 5 | 6 |
| Atrial septal defect, patent ductus arteriosus | 2 | 0 | 1 |
| Atrial septal defect, pulmonary stenosis | 0 | 1 | 0 |
| Atrial septal defect, anomalous pulmonary venous return | 0 | 1 | 1 |
| Atrial septal defect, mitral stenosis | 0 | 1 | 0 |
| Ventricular septal defect | 12 | 13 | 9 |
| Ventricular septal defect, pulmonary stenosis | 1 | 1 | 3 |
| Ventricular septal defect, atrial septal defect | 1 | 0 | 0 |
| Ventricular septal defect, atrial septal defect, pulmonary stenosis | 0 | 2 | 0 |
| Atrioventricular canal | 2 | 0 | 5 |
| Atrioventricular canal, anomalous pulmonary venous return | 0 | 0 | 1 |
| Pulmonary stenosis | 2 | 2 | 1 |
| Tetralogy of Fallot | 6 | 7 | 4 |
| Left ventricular—right atrial shunt | 1 | 1 | 0 |
| Aortic valvular stenosis | 1 | 0 | 0 |
| *Acquired* | | | |
| Left ventricular aneurysm | 0 | 1 | 0 |
| Aortic valvular stenosis | 0 | 2 | 1 |
| Aortic valvular insufficiency | 2 | 2 | 2 |
| Mitral valvular stenosis | 0 | 0 | 1 |
| Mitral valvular insufficiency | 3 | 1 | 2 |
| Mitral valvular stenosis, mitral valvular insufficiency | 0 | 0 | 1 |
| Aortic valvular stenosis, mitral valvular insufficiency, mitral valvular stenosis | 0 | 1 | 0 |
| Totals | 45 | 41 | 38 |

**Table III.** *Plasma hemoglobin increase during extracorporeal circulation*

| | *Control group* | *Dextran group* | *Albumin group* |
|---|---|---|---|
| No. of patients | 42 | 41 | 36 |
| Mean duration of extracorporeal circulation (min.) | 47.3 | 65.0 | 54.8 |
| Preoperative plasma hemoglobin (mg. %) | 25 | 28.4 | 26.9 |
| Increase in plasma hemoglobin | 98.0 | 77.9 | 91.6 |
| Ratio $\frac{\text{Increase}}{\text{Duration}}$ (mg. %/min.) | 2.07 ± 0.026 | 1.20 ± 0.026 ($p < 0.001$) | 1.67 ± 0.176 ($p = 0.124$) |

Values given as mean ± the standard error of the mean.

there was no significant difference between the albumin and control series. The ratios of decrease in platelet count to preoperative platelet count were also analyzed, and again there was significantly less decrease in the dextran series.

The bleeding time, venous clotting time, prothrombin time, and fibrinogen levels were measured preoperatively and postoperatively in unselected patients (Table V). Bleeding time increased in all 3 groups of patients and venous clotting time decreased. The mean prothrombin time was slightly elevated preoperatively in the control and albumin series and moderately elevated in the dextran series. Large increases in the mean prothrombin time were observed in all 3 groups postoperatively. The upper limit for a normal prothrombin time in this laboratory was considered to be 14.5 seconds. Fibrinogen levels decreased in all 3 groups of patients, with a greater decrease in the dextran and albumin series. However, analysis of these studies and studies on a larger group of patients showed that the decrease in plasma fibrinogen was proportional to the preoperative fibrinogen value, that is, patients with higher initial fibrinogen levels showed larger decreases after extracorporeal circulation and those with low fibrinogen levels showed smaller decreases, no change, or slight increases. The lowest postoperative fibrinogen level observed in this study was 0.13 Gm. per cent, so that no significant hypofibrinogenemia was encountered.

The preoperative and postoperative hemoglobin levels were also tabulated (Table V). In the control series there was a mean decrease in hemoglobin of 1.1 Gm. per cent. The mean decrease in hemoglobin was 1.3 Gm. per cent in both the dextran and albumin series.

Changes in plasma proteins (Table VI) followed a consistent pattern between the 3 groups, although the changes varied widely from patient to patient. Serum albumin levels decreased in all 3 series with the largest decrease in the dextran series due probably to an additional dilution effect. There was also a decrease in alpha 1, alpha 2, beta, and gamma globulins, although the mean values were within the normal range for these serum proteins. The changes in alpha 1, alpha 2, and gamma globulins were least in the patients who received Rheomacrodex.

Plasma electrolytes (Table VII) showed a consistent change in all 3 groups. Potassium levels decreased postoperatively, probably because of the respiratory alkalosis reflected in the low arterial carbon dioxide tension seen early in all patients in the recovery room. The carbon dioxide combining power and plasma chloride levels were decreased, which reflected a metabolic acidosis.

Serum dextran levels were measured in the blood from the oxygenator reservoir at the conclusion of extracorporeal circulation. At this time, the serum level of Rheomacrodex was found to range between 1,200 and 2,000 mg. per cent. The minimal effective level of Rheomacrodex was estimated to be approximately 1,400 to 1,600 mg. per cent. Ninety minutes after the conclusion of extracorporeal circulation the serum dextran level was measured in a sample of arterial blood from the patient. At this time, the serum levels of Rheomacrodex ranged from 500 to 1,200 mg. per cent.

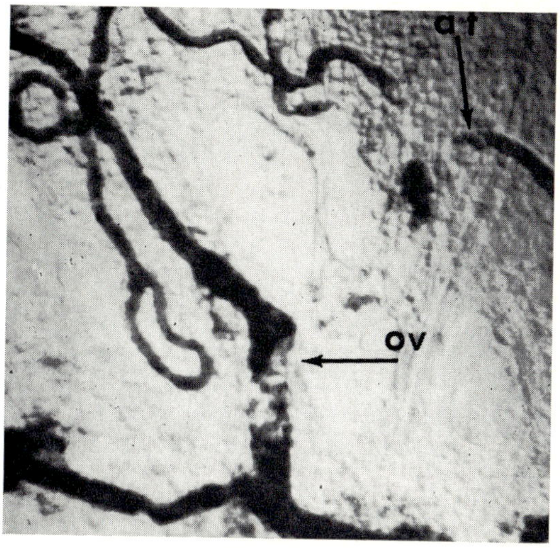


**Fig. 6.** Photograph of small vessels of the mesentery of the dog after 1½ hours of extracorporeal circulation which shows an area of arteriolar thrombosis *(at)* and an area of temporary occlusion of a venule by a large aggregate of red blood cells *(ov)*.

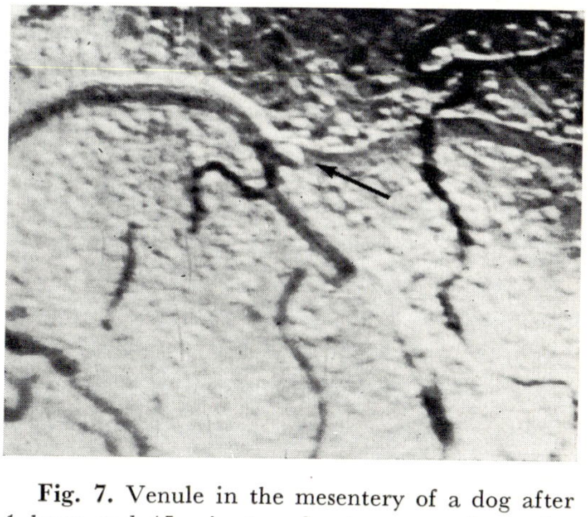

**Fig. 7.** Venule in the mesentery of a dog after 1 hour and 45 minutes of extracorporeal circulation. Arrow points to an occlusion of a venule by a translucent mass that probably represents an aggregate of platelets, an aggregate of white blood cells, or a chylomicron. The velocity of blood flow was very slow in the vessels in this area, and there were several large clumps of corpuscles.

**Table IV.** *Comparison of platelet count change*

| | *Control group* | *Dextran group* | *Albumin group* |
|---|---|---|---|
| *All patients* | | | |
| No. of patients | 26 | 23 | 19 |
| Pre-operative | 257 ± 19.0 | 214 ± 6.7 | 242 ± 12.7 |
| Change | -111 ± 17.2 | -65 ± 8.3 | -103 ± 13.6 |
| | | ($p = 0.018$) | ($p > 0.65$) |
| *Patients with preoperative level 200,000 to 300,000* | | | |
| No. of patients | 12 | 14 | 14 |
| Pre-operative | 248 | 244 | 252 |
| Change | -113 ± 9.8 | -75 ± 11.2 | -103 ± 14.3 |
| | | ($p = 0.018$) | ($p > 0.65$) |

Platelet counts presented in thousands per cubic millimeter and values given as mean and standard error of the mean.

**Chest drainage postoperatively.** The chest drainage was calculated for each 12-hour period during the first 48 hours postoperatively. The chest drainage during the first 12 hours postoperatively more accurately reflected the influence of plasma expanders on the coagulation mechanisms. After the first 12 hours there was a rapid decline in the quantity and the hemoglobin level of the chest drainage. The mean values and the standard errors of the means for the chest drainage in the initial 12 hours were as given in Table VIII. The small differences between the 3 groups were not statistically significant. The mean values for the late postoperative period were second 12-hour period, control 7.7 ml. per kilogram, dextran 8.0 ml. per kilogram, and albumin 7.8 ml. per kilogram; third 12-hour period, control 3.4 ml. per kilogram, dextran 5.4 ml. per kilogram, and albumin 4.8 ml. per kilogram; and fourth 12-hour period, control 2.3 ml. per kilogram, dextran 2.7 ml. per kilogram, and albumin 4.5 ml. per kilogram.

**Urine output.** The quantity of urine output during the first 48 hours postoperatively was tabulated in Table IX. As can be seen in this table, the mean urine outputs varied little from group to group. Periods of oliguria in individual patients were correlated with episodes of hypotension or hypovolemia. In at least 2 patients in the control series, anuria was correlated with severe intravascular aggregation. After the rapid administration of Rheomacrodex, 1.5 Gm. per kilogram (15 per cent solution of Rheomacrodex in 5 per cent dextrose), the intravascular aggregation disappeared and the patients began to excrete normal quantities of urine. In these 2 patients, vital signs also improved, the patients became alert, and clinical evidence of pulmonary edema disappeared.

## COMMENT

Clowes,[7] in his recent extensive review of extracorporeal circulation, concluded, ". . . it now appears that the single greatest factor in tissue damage during perfusion of the whole organism is no longer one of metabolic homeostasis, but rather, one of damage to blood elements which adversely affects the circulation and function of the various organs of the body." The studies of Gelin[13] suggested to us this same concept. Gelin showed a causal relationship between the loss of blood corpuscles by the mechanism of intravascular aggregation and the production of microinfarcts in vital organs by occlusion of small blood vessels with the cellular aggregates. Our earlier experimental studies on dogs[21] demonstrated that intravascular aggregation and microinfarctions of the kidney, liver, and myocardium occurred during prolonged periods of extracorporeal circulation. In addition, the intravascular aggregation and the microinfarcts could be prevented or minimized by the administration of low molecular weight dextran.

In this present clinical study a host of variables were encountered related to varying types and stages of heart disease, age of the patients, magnitude of the surgical procedure, and differing technical problems. By use of a blind control method of selection, an attempt was made to equalize these variables in the control series and the series of patients who received plasma expanders. Ordinarily, clinical observations do not possess the exactness of laboratory experiments. The use of Rheomacrodex in experimental extracor-

**Table V**

| Determination | Control group | | | Dextran group | | | Albumin group | | |
|---|---|---|---|---|---|---|---|---|---|
| | *No. of patients* | *Pre-operative* | *Post-operative* | *No. of patients* | *Pre-operative* | *Post-operative* | *No. of patients* | *Pre-operative* | *Post-operative* |
| Bleeding time (min.) | 20 | 4.4 | 6.6 | 17 | 4.4 | 7.0 | 16 | 4.4 | 6.1 |
| Venous clotting time (min.) | 14 | 16.5 | 14.2 | 9 | 16.8 | 14.2 | 11 | 13.7 | 13.3 |
| Prothrombin time (sec., patients/control) | 20 | 14.8/13.2 | 17.6/13.2 | 16 | 15.7/13.1 | 17.5/13.4 | 17 | 14.8/13.0 | 17.5/13.3 |
| Fibrinogen (Gm. %) | 10 | 0.28 | 0.25 | 8 | 0.33 | 0.23 | 10 | 0.29 | 0.20 |
| Hemoglobin (Gm. %) | 43 | 14.6 | 13.5 | 41 | 14.4 | 13.1 | 38 | 14.0 | 12.7 |

**Table VI.** *Serum protein changes (Gm. %)*

| | *No. of patients* | *Albumin* | *Globulin* | | | | | *Total proteins* |
|---|---|---|---|---|---|---|---|---|
| | | | *Alpha 1* | *Alpha 2* | *Beta* | *Gamma* | *Total* | |
| *Control group* | 14 | | | | | | | |
| Preoperative | | 3.6 | 0.32 | 0.72 | 0.96 | 1.20 | 3.20 | 6.83 |
| Postoperative | | 3.4 | 0.28 | 0.51 | 0.90 | 1.01 | 2.72 | 6.16 |
| *Dextran group* | 9 | | | | | | | |
| Preoperative | | 3.7 | 0.29 | 0.64 | 1.10 | 1.13 | 3.16 | 6.88 |
| Postoperative | | 3.2 | 0.29 | 0.51 | 0.90 | 1.01 | 2.71 | 5.89 |
| *Albumin group* | 13 | | | | | | | |
| Preoperative | | 3.5 | 0.33 | 0.76 | 1.13 | 1.24 | 3.47 | 7.02 |
| Postoperative | | 3.3 | 0.28 | 0.50 | 0.90 | 0.95 | 2.65 | 5.99 |

**Table VII.** *Plasma electrolytes*

| | *No. of patients* | *Na (mEq./L.)* | *K (mEq./L.)* | *Cl (mEq./L.)* | *$CO_2$ combining power (mM./L.)* | *BUN (mg. %)* |
|---|---|---|---|---|---|---|
| *Control group* | 29 | | | | | |
| Preoperative | | 141 | 4.6 | 105 | 23.3 | 13.2 |
| Postoperative | | 143 | 3.8 | 100.5 | 22.0 | |
| *Dextran group* | 29 | | | | | |
| Preoperative | | 141 | 4.7 | 103 | 26 | 15.0 |
| Postoperative | | 142.2 | 3.8 | 100.4 | 22.2 | |
| *Albumin group* | 27 | | | | | |
| Preoperative | | 141.2 | 4.4 | 104.3 | 25 | 13.8 |
| Postoperative | | 141.8 | 3.7 | 100.1 | 22 | |

poreal circulation had very significant advantages. Proof of the same advantages for man and lack of deleterious effects of Rheomacrodex in human usage could be achieved best by creation of a valid system of blind control administration of the drug such as outlined in this study.

The administration of Rheomacrodex was accompanied by a reduction in the destruction of red blood cells, as indicated by the significantly decreased plasma hemoglobin levels, and a decreased destruction of platelets, as reflected in the higher postoperative platelet count. These changes were the im-

**Table VIII.** *Chest drainage in first 12 hours postoperatively*

| | *No. of patients* | *Chest drainage* (ml./Kg.)* |
|---|---|---|
| Control group | 45 | 21.2 ± 2.0 |
| Dextran group | 41 | 23.2 ± 2.0 |
| Albumin group | 38 | 24.6 ± 4.0 |

*Mean values with the standard error of the mean.

**Table IX.** *Urine output*

| | *First 24 hr. (ml./Kg.)* | *Second 24 hr. (ml./Kg.)* |
|---|---|---|
| Control group | 22.6 | 24.0 |
| Dextran group | 20.0 | 21.6 |
| Albumin group | 24.6 | 19.1 |

portant differences that could be documented statistically between the patients in the control and albumin series and those in the dextran series. The importance of these highly significant differences lay not so much in the actual decrease in plasma hemoglobin and platelet destruction, but rather in their reflection of the decreased intravascular aggregation and intravascular destruction of corpuscles and thereby improvement in the quality of the microcirculation in vital organs.

The phenomenon of intravascular aggregation was also found to occur in patients during extracorporeal circulation as determined by actual observation of the conjunctival circulation. Whereas intravascular aggregation was observed infrequently in dogs prior to actual bypass, moderate intravascular aggregation was observed in many patients after anesthesia and during thoracotomy but before the institution of extracorporeal circulation. In some patients, especially those with chronic congestive heart failure and serious disability, intravascular aggregation was present even when they were examined preoperatively on the wards. The presence of intravascular aggregation in these patients also was reflected to some degree by the elevation of the preoperative erythrocyte sedimentation rates. When present before extracorporeal circulation, intravascular aggregation always became more severe during the cardiopulmonary bypass. Intravascular aggregation severe enough to cause death was estimated to occur in at least 5 per cent of patients in the control series. In these patients, the intravascular aggregation was reversed by the administration of Rheomacrodex and the patients recovered from what was thought to have been a moribund condition.

The serum levels of Rheomacrodex fell rapidly by renal excretion during the first 6 hours postoperatively so that there was no longer any protection against intravascular aggregation. This finding accounts in part for the persistence of a mild postoperative drop in hemoglobin concentration and the elevation of the erythrocyte sedimentation rate during the third to fifth day postoperatively. For these reasons we recently have begun to use Rheomacrodex to replace part of the fluid requirements during the early postoperative course, particularly when the recovery period was complicated for any reason. It might be emphasized in this regard that the use of Rheomacrodex to replace part or all of the immediate postoperative fluid requirements is less likely to precipitate pulmonary edema in a patient with impaired myocardial reserve than would the use of a similar quantity of normal saline or glucose in water. Because of the size of the dextran molecules, the colloidal osmotic pressure of the blood is increased and thereby helps to counterbalance any increase in hydrostatic pressure in the pulmonary veins.

The administration of Rheomacrodex or albumin did not alter the development of a mild to moderate metabolic acidosis in the patients studied. It also may be mentioned that in these clinical perfusions, when generally physiologic flow rates were used, the priming blood in the oxygenator contributed a major share of the metabolic acidosis. These findings confirmed the observations made in canine perfusions[21] in which the rate of increase in metabolic acidosis was identical in dogs which received Rheomacrodex and in control animals. In these experimental studies, the rate of increase of metabolic acidosis was greatly accentuated by the administration of norepinephrine or epinephrine and decreased by the administration of hexamethonium chloride. This observation suggested that redistribution of blood flow due to sympathetic nervous system activity accounted for much of the metabolic acidosis seen with extracorporeal circulation. In his studies on intravascular aggregation during hypothermia, Lofstrom[20] was able to demonstrate an oxygen deficit in the body by the administration of low molecular weight dextran at a critical point during the rewarming period. This study was interpreted as an indication that the oxygen deficit and probably also the metabolic acidosis of some tissues was not reflected adequately in the peripheral blood because of intravascular aggregation and poor tissue perfusion resulting in a delayed release of the acid metabolites from these areas.

The dilution of the oxygen capacity of the blood due to addition of plasma expanders was detectable but minimal. Dilution of the corpuscular elements during moderate hypothermia may actually be highly advantageous in that the velocity of blood flow through small vessels is increased by the decreased viscosity.

Decreases in serum protein levels were measured consistently. With the exception of serum albumin, the changes in serum protein levels were no greater in the dextran series in spite of a 10 to 15 per cent additional dilution factor. Whether or not the Rheomacrodex has an effect in stabilization of the solution of serum proteins in addition to the stabilization of suspension of corpuscles is a problem now under study. Changes in plasma electrolyte levels were consistent in all 3 series and followed well-established patterns.

Of particular concern to us was the effect of the plasma expanders on the bleeding and coagulation mechanisms and the quantity of postoperative bleeding. High molecular weight dextran and even Macrodex (average molecular weight 80,000), when given in large quantities, will produce serious problems with bleeding.[4, 16, 21, 25, 26] Gelin[14] encountered no problems with bleeding when low molecular weight dextran was used. In an instructive single experiment, Bromwell and associates[4] were able to demonstrate that a patient who bled after administration of commercial dextran did not bleed when given a low molecular weight dextran. The same patient subsequently bled excessively when commercial dextran was infused at a third skin grafting operation. Swank[24] also reported that changes in platelet count, fibrinogen levels, and prothrombin time were associated with the high molecular weight dextrans only. In experiments on dogs, we produced prolongation of bleeding times with high molecular weight dextran. Administration of low molecular weight dextran resulted in no change in the bleeding time and a slight decrease in venous clotting time. Nevertheless, there remained considerable doubt in the minds of many investigators in this country and in Sweden concerning the safety of low molecular weight dextran. This doubt was the principal reason for the reluctance to accept this drug and probably accounted for the indifference and relative obscurity relegated to the brilliant work of Gelin,[13] Lofstrom,[19] Zederfeldt,[31] and Thorsen and Hint.[27]

Abnormalities in bleeding and clotting after extracorporeal circulation have been reported by several investigators.[15, 22, 28] Therefore, the administration of Rheomacrodex in this situation was a critical test. The experimental studies conducted in our laboratory convinced us that this drug was not only safe but also produced many highly advantageous effects. The analyses we have reported confirm the experimental observations that the Rheomacrodex did not cause any detectable increase in operative or postoperative bleeding in patients who underwent extracorporeal circulation.

These findings concerning the effects of Rheomacrodex on blood coagulation reflect a need for a re-evaluation and expansion of generally accepted concepts. On the one hand, the Rheomacrodex prevented intravascular clotting by preventing the development of adhesive properties on the surfaces of the corpuscles. The cells then did not adhere to each other or to the walls of the blood vessels. The administration of heparin in dosages of up to 5 mg. per kilogram did not alter this form of intravascular thrombosis significantly. This stage of intravascular clotting was found to be important in large blood vessels also, as demonstrated by the use of Rheomacrodex in preventing large-vein thrombosis[3] and thrombosis after endarterectomy.[14] On the other hand, Rheomacrodex did not interfere with clotting mechanisms involved in coagulation of blood at the ends of severed blood vessels or in extravascular clotting.

The effect of Rheomacrodex on renal blood flow and urine output was studied[12, 21] and is being studied in this laboratory. No differences in mean urine output were found in this clinical study. However, in individual patients, when urine output was low, infusion of Rheomacrodex in adequate quantities brought about a return to normal urine output. In patients with renal shutdown of several days' duration, there was no significant change with Rheomacrodex except when it was given during the diuretic phase. The experimental studies indicated that Rheomacrodex influenced the rate and distribution of renal blood flow. Since the largest molecule of this dextran preparation was capable of crossing the glomerular membrane,[29] the Rheomacrodex also acted as an osmotic diuretic. As is well known, an osmotic diuresis exerts a significant protective influence against nephrotoxic agents. Urine and serum concentrations of Rheomacrodex have been measured at a ratio of 6 to 1, respectively, in patients after open-heart operations. This rapid excretion of dextran elevates urinary specific gravity to 1045 and above.

Allergic reactions were reported with some of the earlier dextran preparations.[30] No evidence of allergic reactions with the presently available Rheomacrodex were observed by us after administration of large quantities to over 200 dogs and approximately 200 human patients since September, 1958.

The absence of any significant advantages attributable to normal human serum albumin was difficult to explain. There appeared to be a qualitative improvement in blood flow in the small vessels in patients in the albumin series. However, in animal experiments, the quantity of albumin necessary to prevent intravascular aggregation was generally in the range of 2.5 to 3.0 Gm. per kilogram of body weight, compared to 1.0 to 1.5 Gm. per kilogram of body weight for Rheomacrodex. As noted, the dosage of albumin used in this clinical study was 1.0 Gm. per kilogram. At this dose level, the effects of albumin appeared to be only those of dilution with no significant decrease in corpuscular destruction due to prevention of intravascular aggregation.

## CONCLUSIONS

1. The use of low molecular weight dextran (Rheomacrodex) during extracorporeal circulation in patients resulted in a statistically significant decrease in the destruction of red blood cells and platelets.
2. This lessened reduction of platelets and decreased destruction of erythrocytes was interpreted as being indicative of a better microcirculation during extracorporeal circulation.
3. Rheomacrodex prevented or minimized intravascular aggregation and thrombosis during extracorporeal circulation as judged by direct observation of the conjunctival vasculature.
4. Serum albumin did not produce any significantly beneficial effects in the dosage studied.
5. Compared to a control series of patients, patients given Rheomacrodex and normal human serum albumin demonstrated no deleterious effects upon the coagulation mechanism. The use of Rheomacrodex and normal human serum albumin in large quantities did not produce any increase in postoperative bleeding.

The microphotographs were made by Maurice Meyer, D.D.S., Ph.D., Department of Physiology, University of Minnesota. The authors also wish to express their gratitude to Dr. John Haglin, Mr. Fred Emmings, Mrs. Mildred Jones, Miss Bernice

Luckwaldt, and Miss Alice Beiersdorf for assistance in preparation and tabulation of this material and also to Miss Ann McHale for her technical assistance.

## REFERENCES

1. Artz, C.P., Howard, J. M., and Frawley, J.: The Clinical observations of dextran and modified fluid gelatin in combat casualties. Report of the surgical research team of Korea, Army Medical Service Graduate School, Washington, D. C., 1954.
2. Bigelow, W. G., Heimbecker, R. O., and Harrison, R. C.: Intravascular agglutination (sludged blood) vascular stasis and sedimentation rate of blood in trauma, Arch. Surg. **59:** 667, 1949.
3. Borgstrom, S., Gelin, L. E., and Zederfeldt, B.: The formation of vein thrombi following tissue injury, Acta chir. scandinav., suppl. 247, 1959.
4. Bromwell, A. W., Artz, C. P., and Sako, Y.: Evaluation of blood loss from a standardized wound after dextran, S. Forum **5:** 809, 1954.
5. Brown, E. B.: Plasma electrolyte composition in dogs breathing high $CO_2$ mixtures, U. S. Air Force Report No. 57, p. 115, 1957.
6. Carbone, J. V., Furth, F. W., Scott, E., Jr., and Crosley, W. H.: An hemostatic defect associated with dextran infusion, Proc. Soc. Exper. Biol. & Med. **81:** 101, 1954.
7. Clowes, G. H. A., Jr.: Extracorporeal maintenance of circulation and respiration, Physiol. Rev. **40:** 826, 1960.
8. DeWall, R. A., and Lillehei, C. W.: Design and clinical application of the helix reservoir pump-oxygenator system for extracorporeal circulation, Postgrad. Med. **23:** 561, 1958.
9. DeWall, R. A., Long, D. M., Jr., Gemmill, S. J., and Lillehei, C. W.: Certain blood changes in patients undergoing extracorporeal circulation, J. Thoracic Surg. **37:** 325, 1959.
10. Fahraeus, R.: Der Stromungswilderstand des Blutes in verschiedenen Teilen des Gefassystem, Uppsala Universitats Araskrift, 1932.
11. Fajers, C. M., and Gelin, L. E.: Kidney, liver, and heart damage from trauma and from induced intravascular aggregation of blood cells: An Experimental study, Acta path. et microbol. scandinav. **46:** 97, 1959.
12. Finsterbusch, W., Long, D. M., Jr., Sellers, R. D., Amplatz, K., and Lillehei, C. W.: Renal arteriography during extracorporeal circulation in dogs with a preliminary report upon the effects of low molecular weight dextran, J. Thoracic Surg. **41:** 252, 1961.
13. Gelin, L. E.: Studies in anemia of injury, Acta chir. scandinav., suppl. 210, 1956.
14. Gelin, L. E.: Personal communication, 1960.
15. Hocksema, T., Mustard, J. F., and Mustard, W. T.: Study of some coagulation factor changes occurring in blood during extracorporeal circulation, Trans. Am. Soc. Artificial Int. Organs **5:** 225, 1959.
16. Howard, J. M., Teng, C. T., and Loeffler, R. K.: Studies of dextrans of various molecular sizes, Ann. Surg. **143:** 369, 1956.
17. Knisely, M. H., Eliot, T. S., and Block, E. H.: Sludged blood in traumatic shock, Arch. Surg. **51:** 220, 1945.
18. Lofstrom, B.: Personal communication, 1960.
19. Lofstrom, B.: Induced hypothermia and intravascular aggregation, Acta anaesth. scandinav., suppl. III, 1959.
20. Lofstrom, B.: Intravascular aggregation and oxygen consumption, Acta anaesth. scandinav. **3:** 41, 1959.
21. Long, D. M., Jr., Varco, R. L., and Lillehei, C. W.: Measurements of hepatic and renal function during extracorporeal circulation and the effect of low molecular weight dextran. In press.
22. Nilsson, I. M., and Swedeberg, J.: Coagulation studies in cardiac surgery with extracorporeal circulation using a bubble oxygenator, Acta chir. scandinav. **117:** 47, 1959.
23. Ricketts, C. R.: Interaction of dextran and fibrinogen, Nature **169:** 970, 1952.
24. Swank, R. L.: Personal communication, 1960.
25. Swank, R. L.: Suspension stability of the blood after injections of dextran, J. Appl. Physiol. **12:** 125, 1958.
26. Seegars, W. H., Levine, W. G., and Johnston, S. A.: Inhibition of prothrombin activation with dextran, J. Appl. Physiol. **7:** 617, 1955.
27. Thorsen, G., and Hint, H.: Aggregation, sedimentation and intravascular sludging of erythrocytes, Act chir. scandinav. suppl. 154, 1950.
28. Von Kaulla, K. N., and Swan, H.: Clotting deviations in man during cardiac bypass; fibrinolysis and circulating anticoagulant, J. Thoracic Surg. **36:** 519, 1958.
29. Wallenius, G.: Renal clearance of dextran as a measure of glomerular permeability, Acta Soc. med. upsal., suppl. 4, 1954.
30. Wilkerson, A. W.: Dextran without reactions, Lancet **2:** 604, 1956.
31. Zederfeldt, B.: Studies on wound healing and trauma, with special reference to intravascular aggregation of erythrocytes, Acta chir. scandinav., suppl. 224, 1957.

## ADDENDUM

Low molecular weight dextran is now utilized routinely as a plasma expander for patients undergoing open-heart operations in this clinic. For all but a few of the most complex procedures, this has made it possible to eliminate completely the need for drawing heparinized blood for open-heart operations. Ordinary citrated bank blood is utilized entirely to replace losses.

The helix reservoir bubble oxygenator is primed only with dextran (10 per cent in 0.9 per cent saline or 15 per cent in 5 per cent dextrose) in a quantity equal to one-third of the estimated total fluid requirements for 24 hours. In practice this priming volume in cubic centimeters may be approximated by multiplying the body weight (kilograms) by 16. At the conclusion of the bypass, the oxygenator contents are returned to the patient. Moderate total body hypothermia (25 to 30° C. rectal) with the Zuhdi helical coil heat exchanger (Arch. Surg. 82: 320, 1961) permits very adequate oxygenation at flow rates of 20 to 30 ml. per kilogram of body weight. This in turn permits a very simple low volume extracorporeal circuit.

In addition to the specific effects of low molecular weight dextran in improving tissue perfusion, such a technique has been found to yield increased patient safety with wider application of heart-lung bypass procedures.

Specifically, much less blood is utilized for these operations, which means improved acid-base balance and better blood coagulation since the patient is not filled with large quantities of acid foreign blood. Likewise, a decreased risk from incompatibility reactions and serum hepatitis is evident. Finally, the greatly lessened load on the blood bank for donor procurement means open-heart procedures can be scheduled with the same ease and frequency as other thoracotomy procedures.

*(For discussion, see page 47.)*

# Denaturation of plasma proteins as a cause of morbidity and death after intracardiac operations

WILLIAM H. LEE, JR., M.D.
DIETER KRUMHAAR, M.D.
ERIC W. FONKALSRUD, M.D.
OLE A. SCHJEIDE, PH.D.
JAMES V. MALONEY, JR., M.D.
LOS ANGELES, CALIF.
*From the Department of Surgery, The Laboratory of Nuclear Medicine and Radiation Biology of the Department of Biophysics and Nuclear Medicine, and the Department of Radiology, University of California Medical Center*

For the past several years, there has been apparent general satisfaction with the safety and utility of pump-oxygenators currently in clinical use. Several factors are now recognized, however, which promote distrust of these oxygenators, (1) an inherent, unexplained mortality rate of several per cent associated with cardiopulmonary bypass operations, which increases with prolonged pump-oxygenator perfusion, (2) "sludging" of blood during bypass,[22] (3) a 100 per cent incidence of cerebral fat embolism in clinical cases,[23] and (4) neurological complications after cardiac operations with pump-oxygenator perfusion which vary in incidence from 6 to 20 per cent.[11, 14]

This report provides evidence which relates these phenomena to interface denaturation of plasma proteins by intermolecular energies known to exist at the surface film interface between blood and gas in the 3 oxygenators studied (disc, bubble, and screen). The investigation is divided into 2 phases to facilitate presentation; Part I, biochemical and biophysical evaluation of interface denaturation of plasma proteins by the pump-oxygenators; and Part II, biologic effects of the oxygenator-denatured proteins.

For more than 20 years, the denaturation of protein molecules by contact with an interface between a gas phase (such as air) and a water phase (such as blood) has been recognized.[8, 26] A review of the voluminous literature which has accumulated regarding this subject in the journals of protein chemistry is far beyond the scope of this report. For convenience, however, the salient points which seem to be generally accepted by leading investigators in this field will be briefly reviewed. The details can be found in the articles of Anson,[2] Cheesman and Davies,[9] Kauzmann,[17] Putnam,[27] and Waugh.[31]

Fig. 1 illustrates schematically a simplified version of the theory which explains surface film denaturation of protein molecules. A globular protein molecule moves into the interface between gas and liquid. Strong surface forces (electrostatic), operating over a depth of from 10 to 40 Å, exert a polarizing effect which results in the orientation of a monomolecular layer in the interface. Because of the molecular configuration of

Supported in part by United States Public Health Service grants-in-aid HTS-5357 and H-2812, Blalock Foundation, and The John and Mary R. Markle Foundation (Dr. Maloney).

Read at the Twenty-second Annual Meeting of the Society of University Surgeons, Kansas City, Kan., Feb. 9-11, 1961.

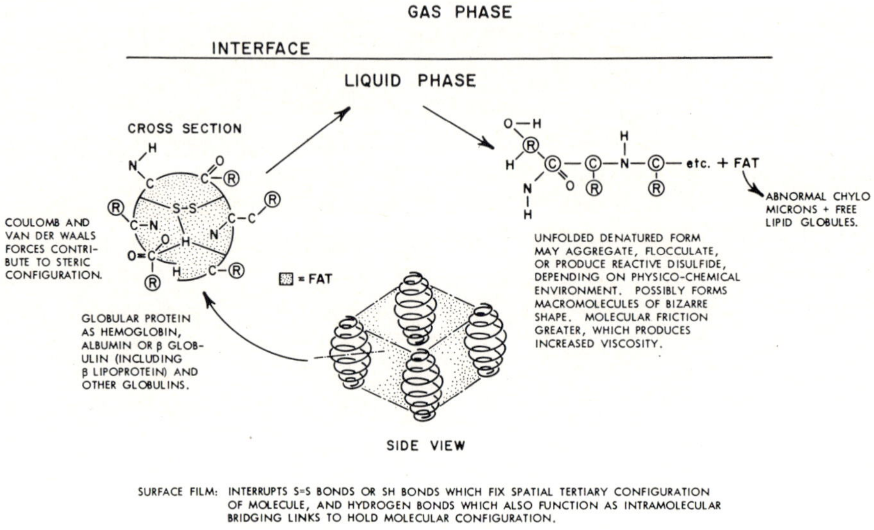


**Fig. 1.** Schema of protein denaturation at gas-liquid interface.

the protein molecule (polar groups, largely external; nonpolar groups, internal), response to the stress of the surface polarizing forces results in disruption of intramolecular sulfhydryl and/or hydrogen bonds which stabilize secondary and tertiary structure of the protein molecule. The net result is an unfolding of the globular molecule into a linear or randomly coiled chainlike molecule which allows orientation of its constituent polar groups in the interface. If the protein molecule transports lipids, these may be released in a "free" state. The physical and chemical results of this alteration in molecular configuration are multiple and complex, and vary according to pH, temperature, salt concentration of the solution, and the specific protein involved. In general, however, 4 physicochemical changes may occur (and may be measured as an index of denaturation): (1) Unfolding of the molecule may expose so-called "masked" chemical groups from within the molecule and increase the chemical reactivity of the molecular constituents (especially sulfhydryl and disulfide groups).[24, 31] (2) The unfolded, linear, or randomly coiled molecule is much more asymmetrical in shape, and thus creates many changes in the physical properties[17] (such as an increase in viscosity due to an increase in intermolecular friction).[7] (3) The changes in symmetry, chemical reactivity, and steric configuration may result in aggregation to form macromolecules which may (a) flocculate, precipitate, or develop a gelation potential,[13, 26] (b) have altered solubility characteristics in salt solutions,[25] (c) have altered mobility in an electrophoretic field,[1, 16] or (d) have an increased affinity for nonaqueous phases due to the exposed nonpolar (hydrophobic) groups.[9] This can result in adsorption onto surfaces which have lipid components, such as erythrocytes or chylomicrons. (4) The unfolded molecule, if concerned with lipid transport (as are alpha or beta globulins and some albumin subfractions), may lose its associated lipid component to the plasma as "free" lipid.

## METHODS

The methods used to evaluate the physicochemical aspects of oxygenator denaturation of plasma proteins in this study were selected on the basis of the considerations described.

**Part I. Biochemical and biophysical evalu-**

**ation.** In order to study the degree and nature of alteration of plasma proteins caused by the oxygenators, plasma of freshly drawn anticoagulated blood (dog and human) was separated from the cells by centrifugation at 1,200 r.p.m. for 1 hour, then oxygenated in a disc, bubble, or screen oxygenator (standard clinical models) for from 3 to 20 hours. Control aliquots and oxygenated aliquots from each batch were subjected to identical analyses.

*Viscosimetry.* A standard Ostwald viscosimeter was used to determine specific viscosity of the plasma. Plasma concentration (2 to 8 per cent) was plotted against viscosity in 34 experiments.[8] Each viscosity determination was made in triplicate.

*Solubility analysis.* Control and oxygenated samples were centrifuged (2,000 r.p.m. for 20 minutes), and relative amounts of precipitate estimated. Any "cream" which floated to the top was noted and examined microscopically. The precipitate was qualitatively identified by the ninhydrin and xanthoproteic tests. The samples were then subjected to differential salt fractionation ($NH_4SO_4$) to estimate changes in "salting out" potential after oxygenation.

*Sulfhydryl and disulfide estimation.* Reactivity of constituent sulfhydryl and disulfide groups of control and oxygenated plasma was estimated by the nitroprusside test.[15]

*Electrophoresis.* Standard paper electrophoresis was carried out on control and oxygenated plasma for protein-fraction estimation and for evidence of change in electromobility of the fractions.

*Turbidity analysis.* Estimation of turbidity in control and oxygenated specimens (after centrifugation at 2,000 r.p.m. for 20 minutes) was carried out by reading per cent transmission in a Beckman spectrophotometer, model B, at 500 and 700 m$\mu$. The samples were then cleared by ether extraction before and after staining with sudan IV and estimations of turbidity repeated with notation of the distribution of sudan through the plasma and ether phases after repeat centrifugation. The nature of the particles which caused turbidity was also studied microscopically by means of fat stains (oil red O and sudan IV).

*Ultracentrifugation.* Samples of control and oxygenated (only bubble and disc oxygenators used) plasma were subjected to ultracentrifugation at 30,000 r.p.m. for 30 minutes. Plasma samples from different levels were studied microscopically and by chemical lipid fractionation for the presence and character of chylomicrons (morphologic) and lipids, oil red O uptake method.

In addition, aliquots of the low-level (high-density) control plasma were oxygenated, then recentrifuged and examined by turbidometry, ether extraction, and fat staining for alterations in the status and distribution of lipids.

**Part II. Biologic evaluation.** Three general types of experiments were carried out.

*First experiment.* Plasma obtained by centrifugation of freshly drawn blood as described in Part I (with aseptic precautions observed throughout the procedure) was oxygenated for 3, 12, or 20 hours, then reinfused into 20 healthy dogs via a femoral venous cannula (dosage range 10 to 15 ml. per kilogram of body weight). Saline cross-matches were performed on control plasma and oxygenated plasma to assure blood type compatibility between donor and recipient animals prior to oxygenation of plasma.

*Second experiment.* Compatible whole blood was oxygenated in a disc oxygenator for from 2 to 20 hours in 5 experiments, then reinfused into the animals via a femoral vein–femoral artery bypass perfusion.

*Third experiment.* Standard cardiopulmonary bypass was carried out on 5 animals for 3 hours with the disc oxygenator at a flow rate of 100 ml. per kilogram per minute.

In all 3 types of experiments, 5 physiologic parameters were studied before, during, and after the infusions; (1) in vitro microscopic hemagglutination of erythrocytes, with a standard saline cross-match procedure (cells diluted 1 to 5 with 0.85 per cent sodium chloride); (2) sedimentation rate; (3) in vivo observation (continuous) of microcirculation in the conjunctiva or mesentery, or

**Table I.** *Criteria for recording alterations in suspension stability*

| | |
|---|---|
| *Factor A. Erythrocyte aggregates* | |
| + | visible in vessels 20 μ or less |
| ++ | visible in vessels 50 μ or less |
| +++ | plugging vessels 10-15 μ |
| ++++ | plugging vessels 50 μ or more |
| *Factor B. "White" aggregates* | |
| + | visible at all |
| ++ | more than 2 per field or 1 per min. (flow) |
| +++ | more than 5 per field or 1 per 15 sec. |
| ++++ | more than 2 flowing in vessel |
| *Factor C. Erythrocyte transudation* | |
| + | microscopic single red blood cell leaks |
| ++ | rapid leaking of single cells to result in diffuse perivascular hemorrhage |
| +++ | microscopic "flame" hemorrhage |
| ++++ | gross "flame" hemorrhage |
| *Factor D. Stasis (indicate approximate size of vessels and whether venous or arterial)* | |
| + | detectable decreased velocity of flow in any vessel |
| ++ | decreased flow, with occasional temporary cessation of movement in vessel |
| +++ | effective flow ceased; intermittent, sluggish, "locomotive" chugging flow occasional |
| ++++ | no movement of aggregates, possibly with settling of cells and spillage down gravitation slopes |
| *Factor E. Thrombosis (dark color, solid cast, frequently highly refringent)* | |
| + | capillaries |
| ++ | vessels to 20 μ (per cent of each) |
| +++ | vessels to 50 μ |
| ++++ | larger vessels |

both, with an apparatus and a technique previously described[18, 21, 28] (criteria for recording alterations in suspension stability are tabulated in Table I); (4) blood pressure, as measured with a Statham pressure transducer from a femoral artery cannula and recorded on a Sanborn oscillograph; and (5) assessment of general biologic deterioration, that is, loss of spontaneous respiration, signs of decerebration, survival, and reaction from anesthesia.

## RESULTS

### Part I. Biochemical and biophysical evaluation.

*Viscosity.* In 33 of the 34 analyses, oxygenated plasma displayed an increase in viscosity characteristic of protein denaturation (Fig. 2). In the other analysis, the control plasma demonstrated the typical viscosity curve of denaturation, as did the oxygenated plasma. This was attributed to inadequate rinsing of detergent-cleaned glassware in the early phase of the investigation. There was no correlation between the increment of viscosity and length of oxygenation from 3 to 20 hours.

*Solubility.* Immediately after the plasma oxygenation there was always a small amount of precipitate which reacted positively to ninhydrin and xanthoproteic tests and indicated denatured protein (Fig. 3). In addition, much larger amounts of soluble denatured proteins were present in the oxygenated plasma as demonstrated by salt fractionation of crude globulin and albumin groups (Fig. 4) in the control and oxygenated plasmas.

*Sulfhydryl and disulfide estimation.* Table II summarizes the results of these analyses. The nitroprusside color reaction was transient and the evaluation of the test subjective. Therefore the estimation was crude. The test was ultimately abandoned, although the data indicated a slight increase in sulfhydryl reactivity after oxygenation. Plasma proteins, such as serum albumin, contain relatively few (17) sulfhydryl groups per mole compared to other proteins, such as egg albumin, which have been used in most of the basic work covering intramolecular sulfhydryl linkages. Amperometric titration methods, such as that of Benesch and associates,[3] should give more sensitive results concerning sulfhydryl reactivity.

*Electrophoresis.* Paper-strip electrophoresis was performed on control plasma and plasma oxygenated for 10 and 20 hours. In general, all demonstrated some change in electromo-

**Table II.** *Disulfide/sulfhydryl tests (nitroprusside, 0 to ++++): summary of 10 experiments with disc, screen, and bubble oxygenators*

| | |
|---|---|
| Control | 0-trace |
| 10-hr. oxygenation | trace − + |
| 20-hr. oxygenation | trace − ++ |

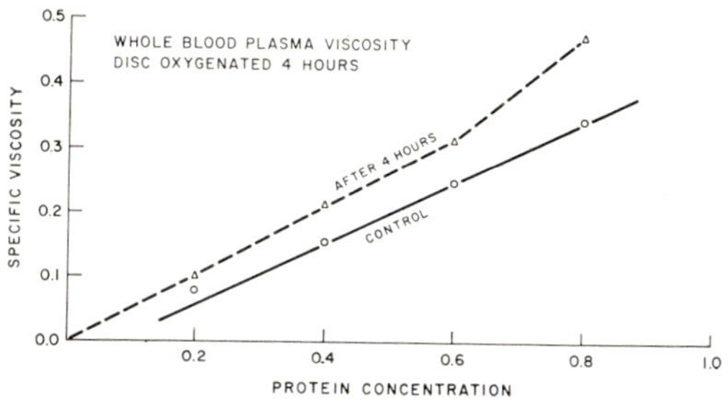


**Fig. 2.** Viscosity change in plasma after oxygenation. The curve is characteristically deviated upward, with most marked increments in the higher concentrations.

bility as manifested by (1) condensation of component in the beta-gamma region to form a dense abnormal band or (2) a decrease in albumin peak by about 10 per cent with a corresponding rise in $alpha_2$ globulin, beta globulin, and gamma globulin totaling approximately 10 per cent (Fig. 5). These changes progressively increased with oxygenation of 10 to 20 hours in the same plasma batches.

*Turbidity.* Oxygenated plasma always developed a marked turbidity (Fig. 6). The bubble oxygenator produced the most marked turbidity (reduction of light transmission to about 10 per cent of the control after 1 hour oxygenation). The disc and screen oxygenators produced approximately 80 per cent transmission in 1 hour, and 40 per cent (of control) in 12 hours.

The turbidity was found to be largely (70 to 90 per cent) due to alterations in the lipid phase of the plasma, since extraction of the turbid plasma with ether restored light transmission to 80 to 90 per cent of the control and selectively removed sudan IV dye from the plasma phase to the ether phase.

Microscopic examination of the turbid plasmas showed the presence of abnormally high concentrations (100 to 1,000 times control) of particles morphologically resembling chylomicron aggregates (Fig. 7) or free lipid globules varying in size from 4 to 30 $\mu$. The globules took up oil red O stain.

*Ultracentrifugation.* After ultracentrifugation, a white disc of creamy material formed on the top of the oxygenated plasma but not on the control plasma. Microscopically this material was composed of lipid globules and chylomicron aggregates. Results of chemical analysis of material taken from the top few lambda of frozen ultracentrifuged human plasma are given in Table III. Other similar analyses of dog plasma consistently showed higher lipid content in the top level of the oxygenated aliquot after 1 hour of oxygenation, with the increase predominantly in the sterol ester and unesterified sterol groups.

Frequently, the creamy material separated in plasma which had been oxygenated for from 12 to 20 hours after standard centrifugation at 2,000 r.p.m. for 20 minutes.

When low-level, high density fractions of

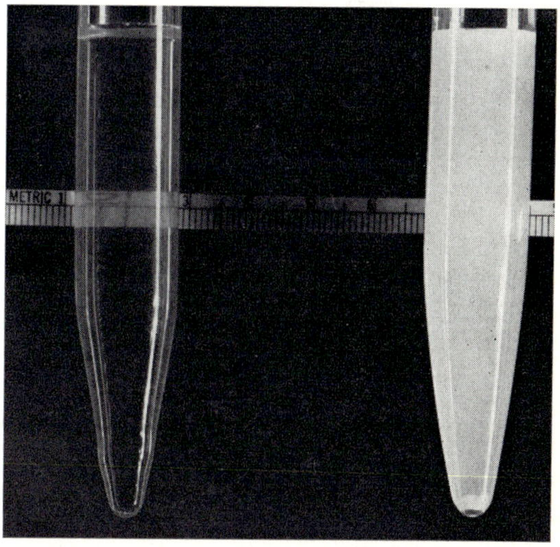

**Fig. 3.** Note precipitate at bottom of the turbid plasma which had been oxygenated for 1 hour.

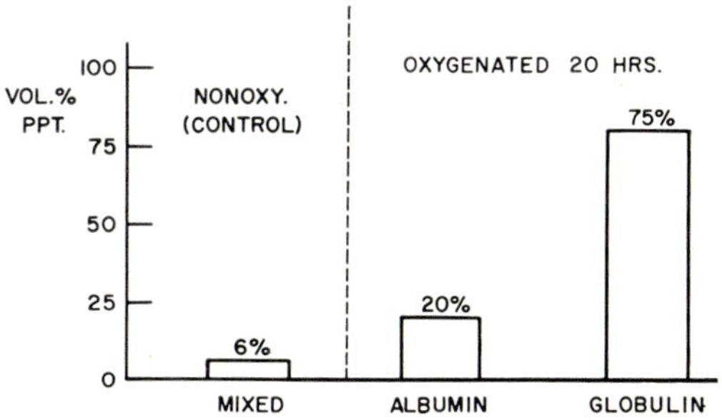


**Fig. 4.** "Salting out" of soluble denatured protein (plasma).

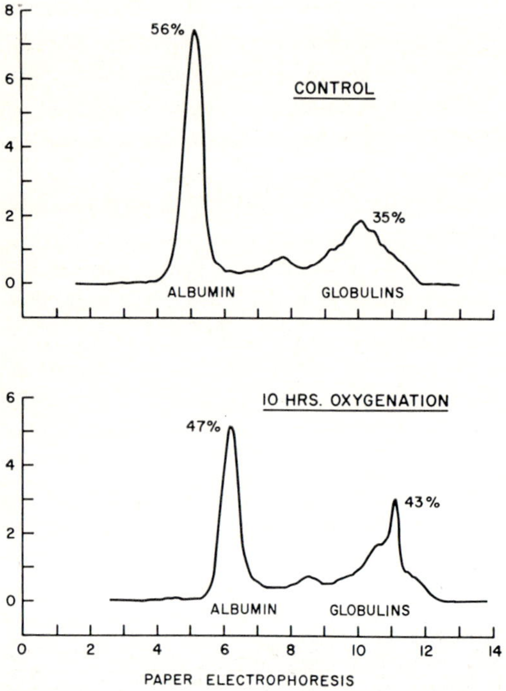


**Fig. 5.** Ten-hour oxygenation of plasma produces 9 per cent decrease in albumin peak and 8 per cent increase in globulin peak.

ultracentrifuged fresh plasma were oxygenated and then examined for turbidity and lipid globules, the results demonstrated that oxygenator-denaturation elaborated free lipid from the alpha globulin and/or albumin fraction, as well as from the beta globulin fraction of plasma proteins.

**Part II. Biologic evaluation.**

*First experiment.* When compatible, nonoxygenated control plasma was infused into the dogs (5 control experiments), there were no significant alterations in the parameters studied. Infusion (10 to 15 ml. per kilogram of body weight) of plasma which had been oxygenated for from 2 to 6 hours consistently produced transient moderate intravascular agglutination of erythrocytes, which was well tolerated by the animals (no arteriolar occlusion, no change in arterial blood pressure, and no signs of general deterioration). However, infusion of plasma which had been oxygenated for from 10 to 20 hours produced marked biologic changes which are summarized in Table IV. The sludging in this group included progressive occlusion of arteriolar and capillary channels.

*Second experiment.* Oxygenation of fresh, compatible whole blood in a disc oxygenator for 2, 5, 10, 12, and 20 hours, with subsequent reinfusion into dogs by means of a femoral vein–femoral artery bypass perfusion (with oxygenator) resulted in marked occlusive sludging and death within 30 minutes to 4 hours. No attempt was made to provide supportive measures to these dogs to achieve survival. Death was preceded by hypotension and respiratory failure.

*Third experiment.* Five dogs subjected to standard cardiopulmonary bypass on the disc oxygenator at 100 ml. per kilogram per minute for 3 hours demonstrated progressive sludging (arteriolar, capillary, and venular) after 20 minutes and microcirculatory occlusion after 1 hour, with an initial rise in blood pressure (10 to 30 per cent). One to 6 hours after the procedure, however, these animals developed hypotension and failed to recover from anesthesia.

In all of these groups, there was no correlation between sedimentation rate and hemagglutination (in vivo or in vitro). The corrected sedimentation rates were almost always reduced after oxygenated blood or plasma was introduced into the dogs.

In 15 of the experiments (and in 2 cases in which fresh heparanized human blood and plasma were used), saline cross-matches between donor plasma and recipient cells were compared on control and oxygenated plasmas. Nine showed marked hemagglutination with oxygenated plasma, but not with control plasma (Figs. 8 and 9); 3 showed slight hemagglutination after the

**Table III**

| | *Control plasma* | *Oxygenated plasma* |
|---|---|---|
| Total lipids (mg./ml.) | 71.3 | 103.3 |
| Triglyceride (%) | 59.8 | 61.6 |
| Phospholipid (%) | 22.6 | 18.3 |
| Sterol ester (%) | 14.4 | 13.7 |
| Unesterified sterols (%) | 3.0 | 6.3 |

**Table IV.** *Reinfusion experiments with plasma oxygenated 20 hours (10-15 ml./Kg. body weight, 24 dogs)*

| | % |
|---|---|
| Delayed anesthetic recovery | 90 |
| Signs of decerebration | 40 |
| Prolonged hypotension | 25 |
| Death | 16 |

Sludging occurred in 100 per cent but was minimal in the 10 per cent which escaped all of the above syndromes.

plasma was oxygenated; 5 were inconclusive or negative on saline, but positive on direct undiluted matching. The matching was carried out after incubation at 37° C. to avoid cold hemagglutination.[20] The saline dilution factor of 1 to 5 was used to exclude simple rouleaux formation.[30]

Erythrocytes from the blood of 6 dogs were examined by electron microscopy before and after infusion of oxygenator-denatured compatible plasma, or before and after a 3-hour pump-oxygenator perfusion. This pilot study demonstrated a definite gelatinous coating which encapsulated clumps of cells in the blood after perfusion or infusion (Fig. 10). This coating was distinct when blood was diluted in nonsaline isotonic fluid (such as glucose), and was reduced to an indistinct haze in saline diluents, again suggesting a globulin-like colloid as the adsorbed material.

Random sections of liver, kidney, heart, lungs, and spleen from dogs infused with plasma oxygenated for 20 hours, when stained by the oil red O technique, demonstrated free lipid diffusely scattered in all these tissues, especially in the perivascular spaces in liver, lung, heart, and spleen, and heavily throughout the renal tubules.

## COMMENT

From the theoretical considerations sifted from the literature of protein chemistry and the results obtained in Part I of this report, the hypothesis that plasma proteins are significantly denatured by clinical pump-oxygenators now in use is confirmed. It is further apparent from the results in Part II of this report that significant alterations of physiologic parameters (especially of the circulatory system) may result from introduction of oxygenator-denatured proteins into an organism. Whether or not the organism can tolerate this insult and survive depends upon a variety of factors, many of which remain undefined at the present. However, in order to attempt to devise means of preventing or reversing the pathologic effects of oxygenator-denaturation of plasma proteins (or of preventing denaturation per se), it is worthwhile to hypothesize the events or mechanisms by which denaturation produces physiologic aberrations.

There seem to be 2 basic factors which result from the protein denaturation and which can give rise to diffuse obstruction

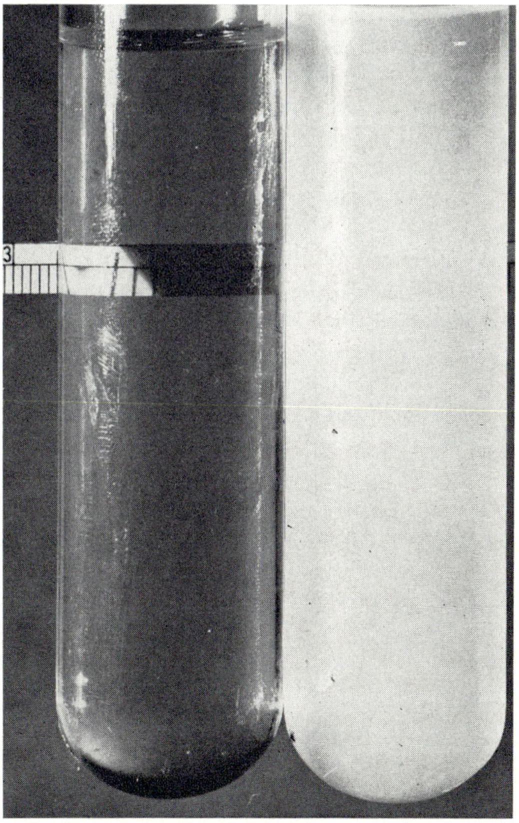


**Fig. 6.** The marked turbidity of the tube containing oxygenated plasma was produced by 1 hour in a bubble oxygenator. The control tube contains an aliquot of the same plasma prior to oxygenation.

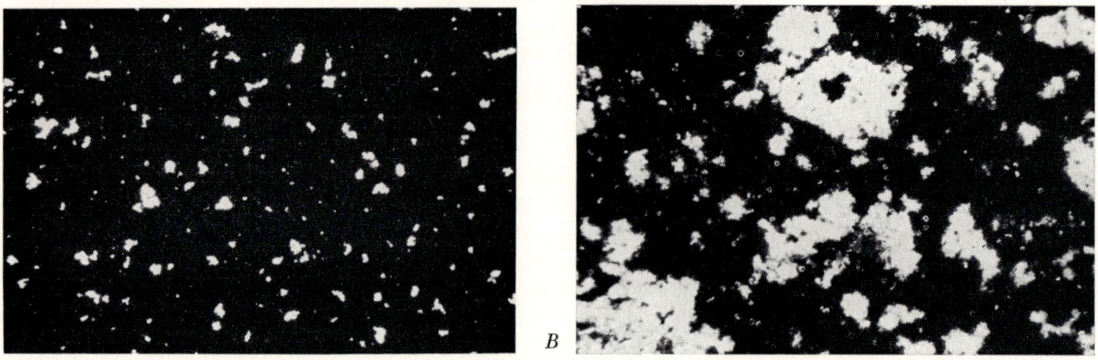

*A* *B*

**Fig. 7.** *A,* Chylomicrons before oxygenation. *B,* Chylomicron aggregates after 1-hour oxygenation. (Dark field; ×970.)

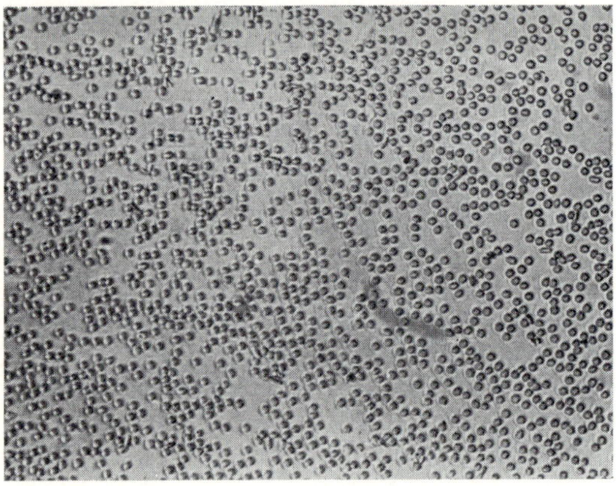

**Fig. 8.** Control plasma on saline cross-match. No hemagglutination.

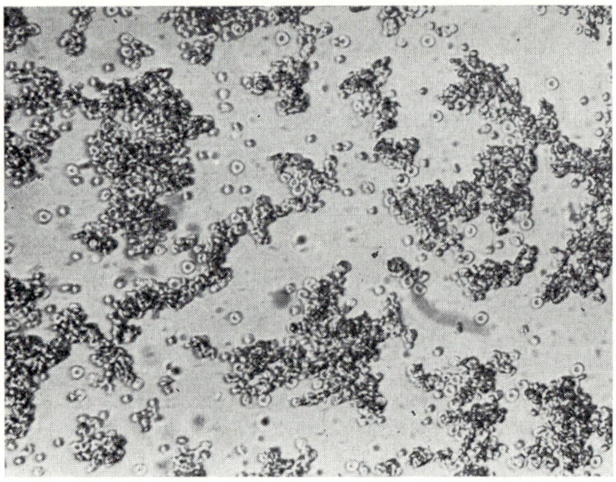

**Fig. 9.** Hemagglutination after oxygenation of plasma on saline cross-match.

of the microcirculation, (1) the release of free lipids, which can (but do not always) produce fat emboli, and (2) a rigid intravascular hemagglutination (sludging) which (to a variable extent) results in plugging of arterioles, capillaries, and venules. Other sequellae of sludging have been discussed in detail elsewhere [4, 5, 10, 19] but remain controversial as causes of death and will not be considered here.

There are at least 2 possible sources of the "released" lipids, (1) deconjugation of the lipid and protein complexes of lipoproteins by interface denaturation, and (2) progressive denaturation, aggregation, and deterioration of the protein capsules of chylomicrons, resulting in eventual "release" of the lipid nucleus which then coalesces with other denuded chylomicrons to form larger globules capable of plugging small vessels.

The hemagglutination phenomena are probably more complex. The studies of Fähraeus[12] and Thorsen[29] indicate that highly asymmetrical, high molecular weight colloids cause a decreased suspension stability of erythrocytes and sludging. The degree of hemagglutination increases with the concentration and molecular weight of the colloids. Thorsen also maintains that the phenomenon is a result of adsorption of the colloid onto the erythrocytes and subsequent molecular aggregation of these coatings. Ditzel[10] has demonstrated that abnormal globulin adsorption onto erythrocytes (in diabetic sludging) is associated with more severe degrees of sludging. Bloch[6] has reported evidence which strongly suggests that there is a coating on sludged blood cells. These data, coupled with those described in this report, lead us to believe that unfolded denatured globulin molecules are adsorbed onto erythrocyte membranes, and there they aggregate with other coated cells to produce hemagglutination. The rigidity of the sludged blood cell masses (which determines the degree of plugging) probably depends upon the gelation potential of the denatured globulins, and this may vary with several factors,[13] such as salt concentrations, pH, temperature, duration of the state of gel, and the introduction of other low molecular weight colloids which can reduce average colloid molecular weight (such as low molecular weight dextran[29]) or reduce molecular asymmetry.

The membrane oxygenator was not included in this evaluation because a clinical model was not available at our institution. One of the obvious approaches to the solution of clinical problems caused by plasma protein denaturation in an oxygenator is to interpose a membrane between the blood-gas phases of an oxygenator and thus prevent interface denaturation. However, should the membrane be made of a hydrophobic (nonwettable) material with low dielectric constant, such as polyethylene, Teflon, or nylon, surface-polarizing forces at the plastic-blood interface should theoretically denature proteins (perhaps to a lesser degree) just as in the case of gas-water or oil-water interfaces.

The ideal membranes should be hydrophilic and of high dielectric constant, in addition to possessing the other known desirable attributes of membranes for oxygenators. Thus, oxygen exchange would occur between a gas phase (outside) and an aqueous filtrate phase *within* the hydrated membrane. Any denatured proteins would be trapped in the membrane and their escape into the circulating blood prevented. Certain nitrocellulose compounds may fulfill the desired specifications, but the engineering and design problems encountered in the practical assembly of such an oxygenator have yet to be mastered.

There were no qualitative differences in the denaturation of proteins by the 3 oxygenators studied in this report (disc, bubble, and screen), and no statistically significant quantitative differences, except as noted in the results.

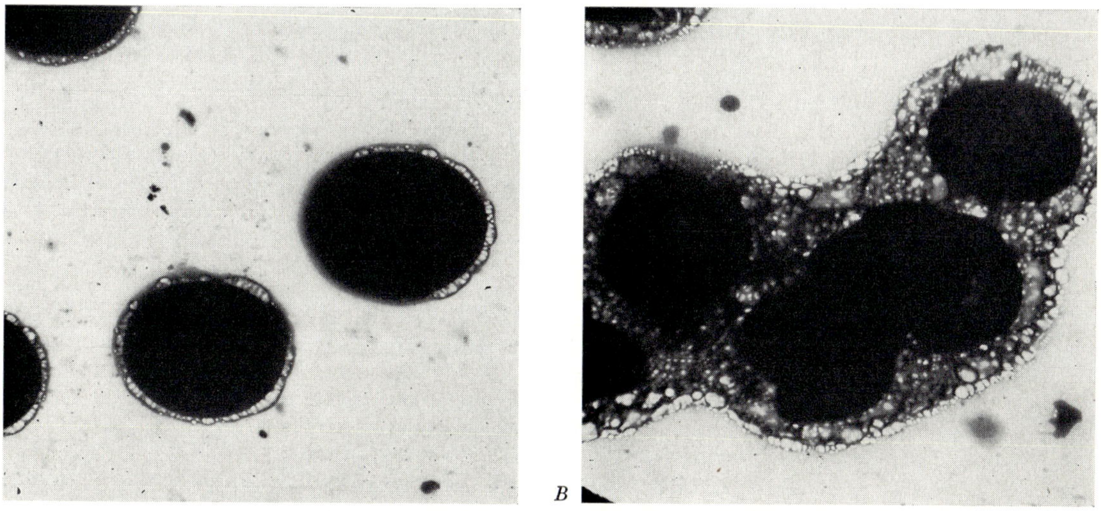

*A* *B*

**Fig. 10.** *A,* Electron micrograph of erythrocytes, dog blood diluted in isotonic glucose (1 to 10), before perfusion. *B,* Electron micrograph of same experiment at same dilution, but after perfusion. Note the coating which encapsulates the clumped erythrocytes.

## SUMMARY AND CONCLUSIONS

Plasma proteins are denatured by contact with surface-polarizing forces at the blood-gas interface in currently used disc, bubble, and screen oxygenators.

The introduction of blood containing such denatured proteins into an organism can produce morbidity or death by 2 mechanisms, fat emboli and rigid blood "sludge" which occludes microcirculation.

This study thus demonstrates a cause for morbidity and death associated with pump-oxygenator perfusions in cardiac operations, emphasizes the remarkable tolerance of the body for insults to its physiologic mechanisms, and calls for the development of entirely new principles of design or maneuver in the use of pump-oxygenators for prolonged extracorporeal circulation.

The authors wish to acknowledge Drs. Gerald L. Hassler, S. H. Lawrence, David H. Mosier, and Daniel C. Pease for their advice and assistance. We are also grateful to Mr. Clifton Davenport, Mrs. Gloria Baltes, and Mrs. Genevieve Armstrong for their technical assistance in this project.

### REFERENCES

1. Al-Shamma, A., Pfaff, W. W., Stemmer, E. A., and Allen, J. G.: Changes in human citrated plasma produced by 60° C. heat exposure for 10 hours, and the protective action of formaldehyde and dextrose, S. Forum **9:** 91, 1958.
2. Anson, M. L.: Protein denaturation and the properties of protein groups, Advance. Protein Chem. **2:** 361, 1945.
3. Benesch, R. E., Lardy, H. A., and Benesch, R.: Sulfhydryl groups of crystalline proteins, J. Biol. Chem. **216:** 663, 1955.
4. Best, C. H., and Taylor, N. B.: The physiological basis of medical practice, Baltimore, 1955, Williams & Wilkins Company, ed. 6, p. 10.
5. Bloch, E. H.: Microscopic observations of the circulating blood in the bulbar conjunctiva in man in health and disease, Ergebn. Anat. **35:** 1, 1956.
6. Bloch, E. H., Rowell, A., Meryman, H. T., Warner, L., and Kafig, E.: A comparison of the surfaces of human erythrocytes from health and disease by *in vivo* light microscopy and *in vitro* electron microscopy, Angiology **7:** 479, 1956.
7. Bull, H. B.: Viscosity of solutions of denatured and of native egg albumin, J. Biol. Chem. **133:** 39, 1940.
8. Bull, H. B., and Neurath, H.: The denaturation and hydration of proteins. II. Surface denaturation of egg albumin, J. Biol. Chem. **118:** 163, 1937.
9. Cheesman, D. F., and Davies, J. T.: Physicochemical and biological aspects of proteins at interfaces, Advance. Protein Chem. **9:** 439, 1954.
10. Ditzel, J.: Relationships of blood protein composition to intravascular erythrocyte aggregation (sludged blood), Acta med. scandinav., suppl. 343, 1959.
11. Ehrenhaft, J. L.: Cerebral complications of open heart surgery. Read at the Annual Meeting of the Pan-Pacific Surgical Association, Honolulu, Hawaii, Sept. 28–Oct. 5, 1960.
12. Fåhraeus, R.: The suspension stability of the blood, Acta med. scandinav. **55:** 1, 1921.
13. Ferry, J. D.: Protein gels, Advance. Protein Chem. **4:** 1, 1948.
14. Fowler, W., Kavan, E. M., and Walter, R. D.: Neurologic and electroencephalographic findings during and after open heart surgery with the cardiopulmonary bypass. In press.
15. Grunert, R. R., and Phillips, P. H.: A modification of the nitroprusside method of analysis for glutathione, Arch. Biochem. **30:** 217, 1951.
16. Hamit, H. F.: Status of human plasma as a plasma volume expander, J. A. M. A. **174:** 1617, Nov. 1960.
17. Kauzmann, W.: Some factors in the interpretation of protein denaturation, Advance. Protein Chem. **14:** 1, 1959.
18. Knisely, M. H.: An improved fused quartz-rod living tissue illuminator, Anat. Rec. **71:** 503, 1958.
19. Knisely, M. H., Warner, L., and Harding, F.: Ante-mortem settling. Microscopic observations and analyses of the settling of agglutinated blood cell masses to the lower sides of vessels during life, Angiology **11:** 535, 1960.
20. Landsteiner, K., and Levine, P.: On the cold agglutinins in human serum, J. Immunol. **11-12:** 441, 1926.
21. Lee, W. H., Jr., Bradham, R. R., Threat, B., and Davenport, C.: Evaluation of the dissolution effect of fibrinolysin on induced vascular microthrombi. A direct approach. SURGERY, in press.
22. Long, D. M., and Lillehei, C. W.: Effect of low molecular weight dextran upon physiologic changes introduced by total body perfusion from a pump-oxygenator. In press.
23. Miller, J. A., Fonkalsrud, E. W., Latta, H. L.,

and Maloney, J. V., Jr.: Fat embolism associated with extracorporeal circulation and blood transfusion. Unpublished data.
24. Mirsky, A. E., and Anson, M. L.: Sulfhydryl and disulphide groups of proteins, J. Gen. Physiol. **18:** 307, 1935.
25. Mirsky, A. E., and Anson, M. L.: Sulfhydryl and disulphide groups of proteins, J. Gen. Physiol. **19:** 427, 1936.
26. Neurath, H., Greenstein, J. P., Putnam, F. W., and Erickson, J. O.: The chemistry of protein denaturation, Chem. Rev. **34:** 157, 1944.
27. Putnam, F. W.: Plasma Proteins, New York, 1960, Academic Press, Inc., vol. 1.
28. Stallworth, J. M., Lee, W. H., Jr., and Jeffords, J. V.: Methods used to evaluate vasodilator drugs, Angiology **9:** 366, 1958.
29. Thorsen, G., and Hint, H.: Aggregation, sedimentation, and intravascular sludging of erythrocytes. Interrelation between suspension stability and colloids in suspension fluid, Acta chir. scandinav. **154:** 1, 1950.
30. Walther, G.: Auto-hemagglutination, rouleaux formation, and sedimentation rate, Folia haemat. **38:** 281, 1929.
31. Waugh, D. F.: Protein-protein interactions, Advance. Protein Chem. **9:** 325, 1954.

*(For discussion, see page 47.)*

# Effects of total circulatory standstill in profound hypothermia

BENJAMIN F. RUSH, JR., M.D.
ROBERT J. WILDER, M.D.
RONALD FISHBEIN, M.D.*
MARK M. RAVITCH, M.D.
BALTIMORE, MD.
*From the departments of surgery of The Johns Hopkins Hospital, the Baltimore City Hospitals, and The Johns Hopkins University School of Medicine*

This study was designed as an investigation of the effects of 2 hours of total circulatory arrest, at a temperature of 4° C. (rectal), upon morbidity, mortality rate, blood oxygen changes, serum electrolyte shifts, and histologic changes in dogs. The phrase "circulatory arrest" refers to the maintenance of dogs at 4° C. with cardiac standstill, and with the pump-oxygenator and the respirator used in these experiments turned off.

## MATERIALS AND METHODS

A total of 16 male and female mongrel dogs which weighed 15 to 20 kilograms were used. Three of the dogs were sacrified for various studies immediately after rewarming. In the 13 remaining animals, every attempt was made to achieve resuscitation and long-term survival.

Hypothermia was produced by means of "core cooling" with De Bakey pumps and a disc oxygenator combined with a double Brown-Harrison heat exchanger. The chest cavity was not opened so that the effects of cooling and circulatory arrest alone could be evaluated. A partial bypass was used with 2, or sometimes 3 venous catheters from a femoral and a jugular vein or veins. Venous return to the pump-oxygenator was by gravity drainage. The arterial catheter was inserted into the femoral artery. While the animal was being prepared for hypothermia, the trachea was intubated with a cuffed tube connected to a Harvard piston respirator through a Douglas bag containing 95 per cent oxygen and 5 per cent carbon dioxide. At the end of 1 hour of this type of respiration the animal's blood and tissue had become "denitrogenized." The partial pressure of nitrogen had been replaced by that of the oxygen—carbon dioxide mixture. This increased somewhat the amount of oxygen available to tissues during the period of cardiac arrest, and also fixed the animal's carbon dioxide level at approximately 27 mEq. per liter before the start of the experiment.

To prevent the upward drift in temperature which occurs after the onset of circulatory arrest, the animals were packed in ice and were thus maintained at 4° ± 1° C. (rectal) over this period. Quinidine, 40 mg. per kilogram of body weight, and low molecular weight dextran,* 2 Gm. per kilogram of body weight in a solution of 10 per

Supported by the National Institutes of Health Grants H-5245, H-2825, and A-2029.

Read at the Twenty-second Annual Meeting of the Society of University Surgeons, Kansas City, Kan., Feb. 9-11, 1961.

*This work was done during the tenure of a Research Fellowship of the Heart Association of Maryland.

*Courtesy of Baxter Laboratories, Inc.

cent glucose, were mixed into the priming blood of the pump-oxygenator prior to the start of perfusion. The pump-oxygenator was primed with 2,500 ml. of heparinized dog's blood, which had been drawn the night before and stored with 50 ml. of 5 per cent glucose per 500 ml.

The blood in the pump-oxygenator was cooled to 4° C. prior to the start of perfusion. Induction of hypothermia was carried out as rapidly as possible. Average flow rates ranged from 40 to 47 ml. per kilogram per minute during cooling. Temperatures of 3.5° to 4.0° C. (rectal) and 1.5° to 2.5° C. (esophageal) were usually achieved in from 40 to 60 minutes. The pump-oxygenator and the piston respirator were then turned off for 2 hours.

Immediately before rewarming, the blood in the pump-oxygenator was warmed to 25° C. Circulation in the dog was then rapidly established. The average flow rates during rewarming were 43 to 48 ml. per kilogram per minute. The attempt was made to raise body temperature as rapidly as possible to normal.

Esophageal and rectal temperatures were recorded in all animals during the course of induction of hypothermia, during circulatory standstill, and during rewarming. Brain, muscle, skin, small intestinal, and bronchiolar temperatures were also recorded in some of the animals. Samples of femoral artery blood were drawn for the determinations of sodium, potassium, carbon dioxide, chloride, pH, osmolality, blood urea nitrogen, calcium, phosphorus, and hematocrit at intervals throughout the experiment.

With the circulation arrested, changes in metabolites and electrolytes resulting from cellular activity are reflected only in the extracellular fluids. Certainly few changes would be expected in blood lying in the major vessels. Samples drawn repeatedly from the aorta, for instance, at the end of circulatory arrest showed no change in concentration of blood constituents. In order to obtain an indication of the extracellular fluid changes, blood was circulated through the dog for 5 minutes at the end of circulatory arrest before a sample was drawn. To avoid dilution of this sample by the large volume of blood in the various components of the oxygenator and heat exchanger, these units were cut out of the circuit during the recirculation period. In 3 animals blood was recirculated through the bypass for 5 minutes every 30 minutes during the period of circulatory arrest and blood samples were taken. Since these animals were not strictly in complete circulatory arrest during the 2-hour period, they were sacrificed on rewarming and not considered in the studies of survival. The changes observed would undoubtedly be greater if, by recirculation, complete perfusion of the tissues were possible at these temperatures and samples could be secured which fully reflected the composition of the peripheral fluids.

Animals in which long-term survival was attempted were attended almost constantly by a physician during the first 24 hours after resuscitation. Complete formal autopsy was performed on animals which died after attempted resuscitation, or which were deliberately sacrificed. All organs, including the brain, were examined grossly and microscopically.

## RESULTS

**Flow rates.** Flow rates in the hypothermic animal tend to fall with decreasing temperature when pump speed is kept constant. Dextran has been reported to help maintain flow rates at higher levels.[2, 7] In Table I the flow rates in the surviving animals in the experiments in which dextran was utilized are compared with the average flow rates in animals in a previous series of experiments in which no dextran was used, but in which the same degree of hypothermia was achieved. In both circumstances flow tended to decrease with progressive lowering of body temperature. This decrease in flow rate was much more marked in animals which did not receive dextran. While dextran improved flow rates, it did not prevent the problem of blood sequestration. Observation with a dissecting microscope of the capillary blood flow in the conjunctiva and the

**Table I.** *Flow rates (ml./Kg./min.) in dogs which survived hypothermia*

| | Cooling (C.) | | | | Warming (C.) | | | |
|---|---|---|---|---|---|---|---|---|
| *Dextran* | *30°* | *20°* | *10°* | *5°* | *5°* | *10°* | *20°* | *30°* |
| Without | 34 | 29.74 | 24.4 | 19.4 | 15.3 | 25.5 | 24.5 | 29.3 |
| With (2 Gm./Kg.) | 44.7 | 46.8 | 40.8 | 40.1 | 43.0 | 44.2 | 46.8 | 48.3 |

omentum in several animals showed a cessation of flow in some of the capillaries in all as temperature fell. During rewarming, after 2 hours of circulatory arrest, there was absence of flow in many of the capillaries, and red blood cells could be seen clumped and trapped in these inactive vessels. Additional evidence of this phenomenon was the negative balance of blood which existed at the completion of rewarming and resuscitation. There was always a negative balance of blood ranging from 200 to 1,000 ml. which remained in the animal and did not return to the pump.

**Temperature changes.** Temperature changes varied considerably, depending on the region measured (Fig. 1). The esophageal temperatures were always lowest during cooling and reflected the nearness of the esophagus to the aorta, the inflow channel for cold blood from the heat exchanger. Of the various tissues recorded, the brain cooled most slowly. At some points during cooling the disparity between various areas was quite great. After 30 minutes of cooling the esophageal temperature had reached 5° C., while the brain temperature was still above 20° C. During the 2 hours of circulatory arrest, with the animal packed in ice, all temperatures tended to converge to a common mean of approximately 4° C. During the rewarming, the relation of temperatures was reversed, with the brain temperature rising most slowly and the esophageal temperatures rising most rapidly. Additional temperatures, recorded but not shown in Table I, are skin temperatures (which paralleled closely those for muscle), pulmonary-bronchial temperatures (which closely paralleled the rectal temperatures), and small bowel temperature (which fell more rapidly than brain temperature, but less rapidly than the rectal temperature). Because rectal temperature appeared to represent a reasonable mean of the various areas measured, we have used it throughout as a common reference point for the changes in electrolytes and other parameters measured.

**Electrolytes and hematocrit.** The most prominent electrolyte changes observed occurred in the serum potassium and phosphorus levels. Serum potassium levels increased in all of the animals as temperature fell from normal to the 4° C. level. During the 2-hour period of circulatory arrest there was a further and more marked increase in the serum potassium level. On rewarming of the animals, the serum potassium levels dropped very promptly to, and

**Table II.** *Electrolyte changes (mEq./L.) during 2-hour circulatory arrest at 4° C.*

| | *Start* | *End* | *Difference* | *p* |
|---|---|---|---|---|
| Sodium | 140.7 | 138.9 | –1.9 | >0.10 |
| Potassium | 3.7 | 4.9 | +1.2 | <0.01 |
| Chloride | 95.2 | 97.0 | +1.8 | <0.05 |
| Carbon dioxide | 27.6 | 29.3 | +1.5 | <0.10 |

**Table III.** *Blood and serum changes during 2-hour circulatory arrest at 4° C.*

| | *Start* | *End* | *Difference* | *p* |
|---|---|---|---|---|
| Serum urea nitrogen (mg. %) | 16.3 | 17.7 | +1.4 | >0.10 |
| Inorganic phosphorus (mEq./L.) | 5.2 | 6.6 | +1.4 | * |
| Hematocrit (mm.) | 35.6 | 39.6 | +4.0 | <0.01 |
| Serum osmolality (mOsm./L.) | 339 | 345 | +6.0 | <0.05 |

*P value was not calculated because phosphorus level was determined in only 3 animals.

usually below, the original control levels (Fig. 2).

Serum phosphorus levels showed a marked rise through the period of cooling and during the period of circulatory arrest. However, on rewarming of the animals the serum phosphorus continued to rise rather than return toward normal levels, so that at the end of rewarming the serum phosphorus levels had reached more than double the normal serum levels. Hematocrit and serum chloride rose slightly, but significantly, during circulatory arrest. Serum sodium levels remained unchanged. Average serum carbon dioxide and serum osmolality rose significantly over the period of circulatory arrest. Serum calcium and urea nitrogen levels showed no significant change (Tables II and III).

Blood pH, recorded in the instrument at the same temperature as in the dog, fell from an average of 7.37 at normothermia to 7.19 at the beginning of circulatory arrest, remained almost unchanged during the 2 hours of circulatory arrest, and returned to levels slightly below normal during rewarming.

**Oxygen consumption.** Oxygen content of the blood increased to a maximum average level of 22 vol. per cent with supersaturation and denitrogenization of the blood at the 4° C. level, just prior to circulatory arrest. During circulatory arrest the oxygen content fell persistently to a minimal average level of 6 vol. per cent at the end of 1½ hours. This minimal level was then maintained until circulatory arrest was ended, and, with rewarming, oxygenation was resumed (Fig. 3). Oxygen consumption over the first 90 minutes was 0.31 ml. per kilogram per minute.

**Deaths and morbidity.** All of the animals were successfully resuscitated and taken off the pump-oxygenator with apparently normal blood pressures at the end of the experiment. All of the animals showed some degree of return to consciousness in the subsequent hours, with contraction of pupils, return of corneal reflex, and spontaneous respiration. However, 6 of the animals died without

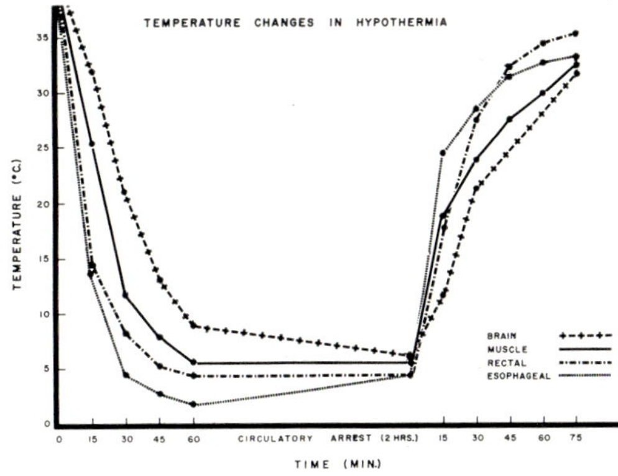


**Fig. 1.** Esophageal temperatures fell most rapidly to an average of 2° C. in 60 minutes. Brain temperatures fell most slowly and when the esophagus was at 5° C. the brain temperature registered at 25° C. During circulatory arrest with external cooling all temperatures tended to converge to a common mean of from 4° to 7° C.

completely regaining consciousness, from 6 to 16 hours after the end of the period of hypothermia (Table IV). Of the remaining 7 animals, all recovered consciousness and appeared to react like normal dogs, took food or water by mouth, and responded to whistles and calls. Three of the animals demonstrated moderate weakness of the hind legs, which cleared spontaneously. Of these 7 animals, 1 died in 28 hours of hemorrhage from the large and small bowel; 2 died at the end of 5 days, 1 from hemorrhage from a gastric "stress" ulcer and 1 from an ileoileal intussusception; and 1 died on the seventh postoperative day from inferior vena cava thrombosis (Table V). Three animals are alive and apparently well at the present time.

**Pathology.** Autopsies of the 10 animals which died of various causes after the experiment and those of 3 animals which were deliberately sacrificed at the end of the experiment showed the presence of 2 definite lesions in almost every instance. One was a necrosis of varying degree of the mucosa of the small and large bowel. In some instances necroses were small and scattered, while in others long segments of the small bowel were involved. In 8 of the animals an area of subendocardial hemorrhage was found

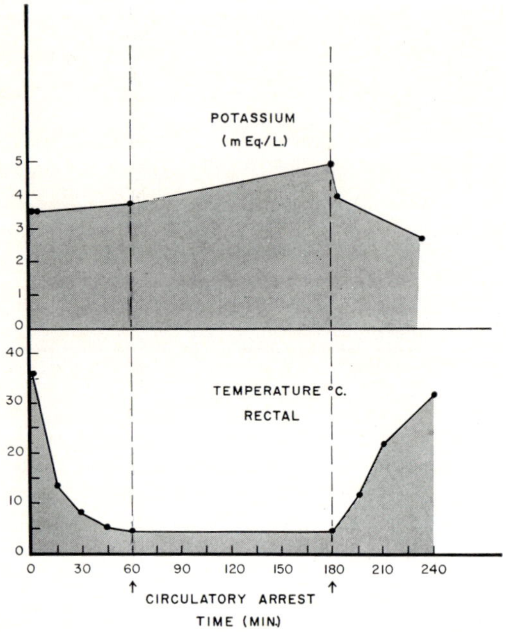


**Fig. 2.** Serum potassium changes are plotted against time and temperature. During cooling the potassium level rose significantly from a mean of 3.55 to 3.72 mEq./L. ($p = <0.01$). During circulatory arrest the potassium level increased again to 4.90 mEq./L. ($p = <0.01$). On rewarming the serum potassium fell 2.88 mEq./L. which was significantly below the control level.

on the left ventricular septum adjacent to the outflow tract.

## COMMENT

These studies have demonstrated a number of consistent physiologic changes in the course of circulatory arrest which are associated with profound hypothermia. Sealy and associates,[10] Neville and his colleagues,[9] and Björk[1] have shown that metabolism is decreased but continues with the utilization of oxygen at temperatures of approximately 10° C. In our experiments this was also true at 4° C. Despite the presence of maximum amounts of available oxygen in the blood and tissue at the beginning of circulatory standstill, all or nearly all utilizable oxygen was extracted from the body fluids at the end of 90 minutes of standstill. During the last 30 minutes of standstill any metabolic process was on an essentially anaerobic basis.

The changes in electrolytes and hematocrit during circulatory arrest and profound hypothermia are undoubtedly due to multiple factors. Three major factors occur to us; first, a shift of water out of capillaries due to increased capillary permeability; second, a shift of substances out of and into cells due to a loss of the ability of cell membranes to maintain the normal partitioning of intra- and extracellular electrolytes; and, finally, the gradual accumulation of substances due to the continuing metabolism.

In the first instance the rise in hematocrit over the period of circulatory arrest is evidence of a loss of water from the vascular compartment with hemoconcentration. In the second instance, the rise of the serum potassium level is evidence of a shift of electrolytes out of cells. The increase of potassium is too great to be accounted for by hemoconcentration alone, and cannot be blamed upon hemolysis because the dog's red blood cell is a "sodium" cell and contains almost the same concentrations of potassium as does serum. In the last instance, the slight but definite rise in the serum carbon dioxide level can be attributed to the continuing metabolism of oxygen over the period of circulatory arrest.

It is believed that the alterations in serum electrolytes observed represent a balance of changes which may be working in the same or in different directions. For instance, hemoconcentration would increase the concentration of serum sodium, while a shift of sodium into cells would lower serum levels. Serum potassium changes, on the other hand, would be additive, with hemoconcentration and shift of potassium out of cells both contributing to the increase noted. None of the changes observed were large enough to be a cause of death in themselves, and the

**Table IV.** *Mortality rate after 2-hour circulatory arrest at 4° C.*

| | *No.* | % |
|---|---|---|
| Early deaths | 6 | 46 |
| Late deaths | 4 | 31 |
| Survivals | 3 | 23 |
| | 13 | 100 |

**Table V.** *Cause of death*

| | No. |
|---|---|
| *Early deaths* | |
| Pulmonary edema | 4 |
| Unknown | 2 |
| *Late deaths* | |
| Bleeding small and large bowel (28 hr.) | 1 |
| "Stress" ulcer with hemorrhage (5 days) | 1 |
| Ileoileal intussusception (5 days) | 1 |
| Inferior vena cava thrombosis (7 days) | 1 |

changes were important only as they reflected the presence of other physiologic alterations.

To our knowledge there have not to date been any studies reported of biochemical changes at the level of temperature or the lengths of circulatory arrest employed in these experiments. Boyd and Webb[3] observed electrolytic shifts in dogs held at 5° C. for 1 hour, and reported a rise in potassium and chloride levels. They also noted a rise in serum sodium concentration which we have not observed. Cooling of animal tissues in vitro is known to induce a shift of sodium into cells and potassium out of cells.[5, 8] Anoxia induces a similar shift.[4] Electrolyte and hematocrit alterations noted in our studies may be due to the effects of cold or of anoxia, and probably are due to both.

The deaths and morbidity seen in these dogs established the fact that by the methods employed, 2 hours of circulatory arrest at 4° C. exceeds the $L.D._{50}$ for dogs, and suggest that by the technique employed, 1 to 1½ hours of arrest is the longest period that can be tolerated by dogs and still allow a majority to survive. On the other hand, it is interesting that some dogs tolerated even this long period of circulatory arrest with resuscitation and indefinite survival.

None of the animals showed evidence of brain damage, either on the basis of microscopic examination of the brains of the animals which died or the behavior of those which survived. Björk[1, 2] and Lesage and his group[6] have reported evidence of brain damage in dogs and human beings after 1 hour of hypothermia and circulatory arrest. However, in those series the lowest temperature reached was approximately 10° C. measured in the esophagus. Moreover, the dogs or human beings were not packed in ice, and temperatures tended to drift upward a considerable distance during circulatory arrest. Since brain temperature may be 10 to 20 degrees above the esophageal temperature, it is possible that the brains of the subjects may not have been well protected by cold.

The endocardial hemorrhage often noted in the left ventricle was an unexplained lesion and seemed too superficial to cause any functional change in the heart. This lesion has also been noted by Neville and associates.[9] The mucosal necrosis of the small bowel was often extensive and led to symptoms and even death in some of the animals. This change may arise from a maximum degree of sequestration of blood in the small bowel, with a failure of proper oxygenation of the bowel during rewarming which results in tissue anoxia and cell death.

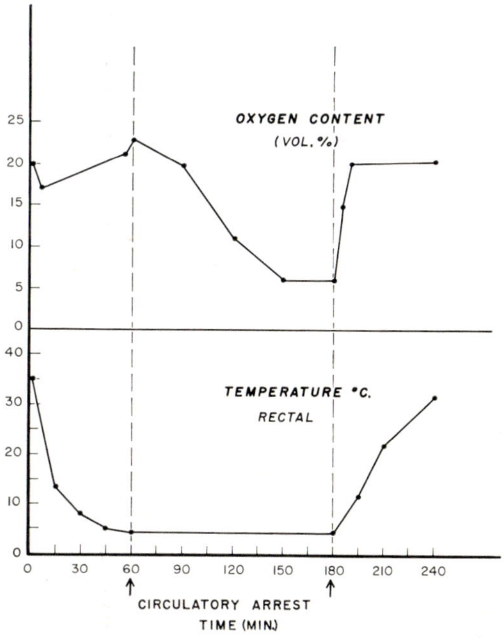


**Fig. 3.** The oxygen content fell from a high of 22 vol. per cent at the beginning of cardiac arrest to a low of 6 vol. per cent at 1½ hours of arrest. No additional uptake of oxygen occurred in the next half hour, and in this final period it is assumed that metabolism proceeds on an anaerobic basis.

## SUMMARY AND CONCLUSIONS

Sixteen dogs were cooled to a rectal temperature of 4° C. by "core cooling" with a pump-oxygenator and heat exchanger through a venoarterial bypass. Dextran was added to the blood in the pump-oxygenator. All circulation was arrested for 2 hours. Rectal temperatures of 4° C. were maintained during circulatory arrest by external cooling with an ice pack. The dog was then rewarmed. Thirteen animals were maintained and supported for observation of the morbidity and deaths which resulted from the technique. Observations of blood flow, temperature changes, changes in electrolyte concentration and hematocrit, oxygen consumption, and the gross and microscopic pathologic pictures were made.

Blood flow during induction of hypothermia and rewarming was increased by the addition of low molecular weight dextran to the system, but sequestration was not prevented. Temperature fell most rapidly in the esophagus and least rapidly in the brain. The disparity of temperatures between these two areas during cooling and rewarming was at times as much as 20° C. During the 2 hours of circulatory arrest and external cooling temperatures at all sites tended to converge to a common mean of approximately 4° C.

Oxygen utilization by body tissues continued at 4° C. at the average rate of 0.31 ml. per kilogram per minute for the first hour and a half of circulatory arrest and arterial oxygen content fell to 6 vol. per cent. During the last half hour of circulatory arrest no further oxygen uptake occurred and it is presumed that metabolism continued on an anaerobic basis.

During the period of circulatory arrest serum potassium, chloride, and carbon dioxide levels increased slightly, but significantly. Sodium calcium and blood nitrogen concentrations remained unchanged. Hematocrit and serum phosphorus levels increased.

All of the animals were successfully resuscitated and disconnected from the pump-oxygenator with a stable blood pressure after rewarming. Six animals died in 6 to 16 hours after the procedure, 4 of pulmonary edema and 2 of unknown causes. Four animals died 1 to 7 days after the procedure of various causes and 3 animals have survived 3 to 6 months.

Histologic examination of tissues of the dogs which died or were sacrificed after the procedure showed, among other changes, mucosal necrosis of small to large areas of the small and large bowel in all dogs. No evidence of central nervous system damage was found.

It is believed that during the long period of circulatory arrest there was impairment of normal electrolyte partitioning between intra- and extracellular fluids and increased capillary permeability with loss of water from the vascular compartment and hemoconcentration. It appears that 2 hours of circulatory arrest by the methods employed is the upper limit tolerated by the dog with any significant number of permanent survivals.

The authors express their thanks to the following technicians: John Hsiehi, John Penser, Barbara Broadway, Lucille Borgen, and Dorothy Frankel.

### REFERENCES

1. Björk, V. O.: An effective blood heat exchanger for deep hypothermia in association with extracorporeal circulation, but excluding the oxygenator, J. Thoracic Surg. **40:** 237, 1960.
2. Björk, V. O., and Hultquist, G.: Brain damage in children after deep hypothermia for open heart surgery, Thorax **15:** 284, 1960.
3. Boyd, J. W., and Webb, W. R.: Alterations in tissue and serum electrolytes during hypothermic circulatory arrest, Clin. Res. **9:** 35, 1961.
4. Coffman, J. D., and Gregg, D. E.: Ventricular fibrillation during uniform myocardial anoxia due to asphyxia, Am. J. Physiol. **198:** 955, 1960.
5. Conway, E. J.: Nature and significance of concentration relations of potassium and sodium ions in skeletal muscle, Physiol. Rev. **37:** 84, 1957.
6. Lesage, A. M., Freese, J. W., Sealy, W. C., and Young, W. G.: Studies of the effects of complete circulatory arrest in the profoundly hypothermic dog, S. Forum **11:** 188, 1960.
7. Lofstrom, B.: Induced hypothermia and intra-

vascular aggregation, Acta anaesth. scandinav., suppl. 3, 1959.

8. Mudge, G. H.: Electrolyte and water metabolism of rabbit kidney slices: effect of metabolic inhibition, Am. J. Physiol. **167:** 206, 1951.
9. Neville, W. F., Kameya, S., Oz, M., Bloor, B., and Clowes, G. H. A.: Profound hypothermia and complete circulation interruption, A. M. A. Arch. Surg. **82:** 108, 1961.
10. Sealy, W. C., Young, W. G., Brown, I. W., Smith, W. W., and LeSage, A. M.: Profound hypothermia combined with extracorporeal circulation for open-heart surgery, SURGERY **48:** 432, 1960.
11. Wilder, R. J., Rush, B. F., Yaycioglu, Y., and Ravitch, M. M.: Survival and physiologic studies with profound hypothermia (0° to 8° C.) and a pump-oxygenator in dogs, SURGERY **49:** 629, 1961.

## DISCUSSION

**Dr. George H. A. Clowes, Jr.** (Cleveland, Ohio). Dr. Long, Dr. Lillehei, and their associates have made an important contribution in drawing attention to the problem of red blood cell clumping during artificial perfusion of the whole body. This is similar to the phenomenon in shock described by Geline and may well account for certain of the untoward reactions which occur after the use of a pump-oxygenator. We are convinced that the greatest problem still existing in this field is the damage inflicted upon blood elements. Certain of the protein changes induced by oxygenation and pumping of blood have been quantitated by Drs. Lee and Maloney. I sincerely hope that work of the type they are doing may give us the ultimate answer to the ideal apparatus as well as an answer to the question of why there appears to be a limit to the time a perfusion may be continued.

For example, we believe that the lungs in roughly 30 per cent of patients are subject to a type of inflammatory reaction after perfusions of more than 1 hour's duration. This we have studied in dogs with the preliminary conclusion that a similar pattern of response can be produced by either mismatched donor blood or by severe blood trauma.

Although we have worked with dextran of low molecular weight, I cannot say that I think this material, valuable as it appears to be, is the ultimate answer. Rather, it appears that apparatus and techniques of perfusion must be developed which produce the least possible blood damage as measured by methods like those of Drs. Lee and Maloney.

I compliment Dr. Rush on his carefully conducted experiments and ask that he say a word about the degree of metabolic acidosis present during and after rewarming. Our information suggests that acidosis may be quite severe at this phase of perfusion under profound hypothermia in animals.

**Dr. Ray Heimbecker** (Toronto, Canada). Our studies were performed with the quartz-rod technique with transillumination of the capillary bed of the mesenteric vessels both before, during, and after cardiac bypass. The quartz rod provides an intense atraumatic illumination of the vascular tree.

The film shows the normal capillary bed at about 300 diopters. You can see rapidly flowing blood in all parts of the tree and now, after 1 hour of cardiac bypass, we see slow sludgelike flow. Here is a venule, here is an arteriole, and here is the sludgelike flow of agglutinated red blood cells leaving the capillary bed of the mesentery. After 1½ hours of bypass the agglutination of red blood cells is even more pronounced. Here is the slow, porridgelike flow of clumped red blood cells. Here is another area in which there is marked red blood cell agglutination. Here is still another area under even higher magnification and a few discrete cells are coming down, but red blood cell clumps fill this venule. Antisludge drugs have been sought with little success. Heparin itself seems to have a transient antisludge effect, and so may offer all patients who undergo cardiac bypass some protection.

**William E. Neville** (Cleveland, Ohio). In the main, we have found 2 factors which militate against success in profound hypothermia. One is the hypoxic acidosis which can occur even at 10° C. and another is the decay in oxygen tension in the brain during complete circulatory arrest. The slide depicts the pH values corrected for temperature in different groups of dogs which were cooled to 10° C. and rewarmed. In Group I, the animals were cooled to 10° C. by extracorporeal perfusion and immediately rewarmed. All of these animals survived and the pH values did not change during the perfusion. The dogs in Group II were subjected to 15 to 30 minutes of circulatory arrest at 10° C. Again in this group the pH values did not materially change and the animals did not become acidotic. In contrast, in the Group III in which circulatory arrest was maintained for 30 to 78 minutes the animals became markedly acidotic during the rewarming phase. This is a direct reflection of the hypoxic acidosis which originates during the long period of arrest at 10° C.

The majority of these dogs died, as did the animals in Group IV which we maintained on

*Discussion of papers by Long, Sanchez, Varco, and Lillehei; Lee, Krumhaar, Fonkalsrud, Schjeide, and Maloney; and Rush, Wilder, Fishbein, and Ravitch.

an extremely low perfusion of 10 to 20 ml. per kilogram at 10° C. before rewarming.

This slide depicts the decay in oxygen tension in the cerebrospinal fluid, which we believe reflects the oxygen tension of the brain, during circulatory arrest. This was measured in conjunction with Dr. B. M. Bloor, our neurosurgeon, and at 10° C. within 18.5 minutes there was very little oxygen left in the cerebrospinal fluid, although it actually took, on the average, 41 minutes to reach zero. From these data it appears that it is unsafe to completely interrupt the circulation for longer than one-half hour.

**Dr. Ben Eiseman** (Denver, Colo.). As you know, the viscosity of blood increases markedly during hypothermia, both because of the effect of cold and, more particularly, because of hemoconcentration. Dr. W. A. Anderson of Aberdeen, Scotland, and I reasoned that cardiac irregularities characteristic of deep hypothermia might be due in part to the increased work of the heart in pumping such high viscosity blood. We therefore investigated the efficacy of several substances that might change the flow characteristics of blood, as they might promote a greater tolerance to deep hypothermia in the splenectomized dog. The end point in these experiments was ventricular fibrillation or standstill and, as the slide shows, we tried a number of surface-tension depressants as well as low molecular weight dextran. There was wide individual variation but statistical analysis showed that neither low molecular weight dextran nor the surface-tension depressants were effective in increasing the dog's tolerance to hypothermia. Whatever the benefits of low molecular weight dextran, surface-tension depression is not among them.

**Dr. Wendell B. Thrower** (Charleston, S. C.). I would like to compliment Dr. Lee and the authors on the fine presentation and very excellent piece of work. We have long been interested in sludging at South Carolina. When Dr. Lee was with us he did some very good work in this area. Two things occurred to me while I listened. First, I wonder what effect hypothermia has on this denaturation and if it will decrease it or increase it, if we might pursue studies along this line, and if work has already been started along this line. The other question I would like to ask Dr. Lee concerns the hyperpyrexia that we see after open-heart operations. Is the denaturation of proteins related to hyperpyrexia?

**Dr. David M. Long** (closing). I want to thank the discussers for their remarks. It has been stimulating to hear these reports today. The studies by Dr. Lee on the etiology of intravascular aggregation are particularly interesting. The suspension stability of proteins may be as important as the suspension stability of the formed elements of the blood, and this is a problem that we are now studying. As for low molecular weight dextran being the answer to all the problems of extracorporeal circulation, it certainly is not. However, Rheomacrodex appears to be one of the answers. In about 5 per cent of our control series, we believed that the degree of intravascular aggregation was sufficiently severe to cause death. These few patients, who had severe intravascular aggregation and were in an apparently moribund state, were resuscitated by the rapid administration of appropriate quantities of a concentrated solution of Rheomacrodex with return to normal of the microcirculation.

Intravascular aggregation is a conspicuous finding in hypothermia as demonstrated by Dr. Bertil Lofstrom of Stockholm. However, in profound hypothermia the intravascular aggregation does not appear to be the cause of the neurological damage and unexplained morbidity and death. Rheomacrodex will prevent the intravascular aggregation in profound hypothermia and improve the circulatory dynamic as pointed out by Dr. Rush in his excellent study. However, the circulation through the small blood vessels is still far from normal. Obviously, there are a number of very difficult problems to be solved in the application of profound hypothermia.

**William H. Lee, Jr.** (closing). I would like to thank the discussers very much. In regard to Dr. Heimbecker's comments about sludging, I think we must keep in mind the fact that this phenomenon also occurs in many minor, as well as serious, diseases, as described by Dr. Edward Bloch in 1956 in some 3,000 cases of various diseases. Large sludge masses can be seen in the conjunctivae of individuals with nothing more serious than hangovers or minor respiratory disease, but these masses are visualized usually in small venules, and they appear to be elastic, deforming to pass through smaller vessels or fragmenting in small arterioles to reform after having passed through the capillary bed into the venules. I think that in an evaluation of this phenomenon in extracorporeal circulation the factor of greatest importance to circulation physiology is visible vascular occlusion, rather than the presence or size of sludge masses per se. The rigidity of the sludge mass is of prime importance in determining whether a sludge mass of a given size will obstruct the vascular tree or deform and pass through it. At present we would presume this factor to depend upon the rigidity of the gelled coating of denatured protein which we believe has adsorbed onto the red blood cell surface. The dextran effect upon sludging has been extensively discussed in the Scandinavian literature. The classical studies of Robin Fahraeus have been continued and elaborated by Thorsen, Gelin, and others concerning the influence of colloidal molecular weight on the suspension stability of the blood. These studies have contributed greatly to the understanding of the complex biophysics of blood and provide a fertile field for further investigation.

Time does not permit a theoretical discussion in answer to Dr. Thrower's question regarding hypothermia, and I have no factual data to offer him on this subject.

**Benjamin F. Rush, Jr.** (closing). I would like to thank the discussers. The measurement of pH in hypothermia is beset by a number of variables. The technique of measurement is most important. In our experiment the glass electrode was cooled, and the temperature in the pH meter maintained at the blood temperature of the hypothermic animal. With this method, a moderate acidosis was noted during cooling, with a drop from pH 7.38 at 37° C. to 7.15 at 5° C. No change in pH occurred during the 2 hours of cardiac arrest. During rewarming, pH rose again, but did not return to normal immediately. In animals that died, pH usually had begun to fall again subsequently. In surviving animals pH gradually rose and returned to normal in the next several hours. If the measurement of pH was carried out with the glass electrode at room or at body temperature, regardless of the experimental temperature of the blood, and "correction" factors were applied, gross overcorrection occurred.

If animals were kept at 4° C. for longer periods than reported here, that is, 4, 8, or 21 hours, electrolyte changes occurred in the same direction as at 2 hours, but were much more exaggerated. The potassium level rose as high as 11 mEq. per liter and the sodium level dropped as low as 120 mEq. per liter. Although these animals did not survive for more than 1 to 12 hours, the electrolytes still shifted toward normal on rewarming.

# The identification of the conduction system of the heart by audiofrequency conductimetry

WILLIAM A. BORMES, M.D.
WILLIAM C. GORMAN, M.D.
KENNETH L. KAYSER, B.E.E.
DERWARD LEPLEY, JR., M.D.
MILWAUKEE, WIS.
*From the Section of Thoracic and Cardiovascular Surgery, Division of Surgery, Marquette University School of Medicine; Surgical Service, Wood Veterans Administration Hospital; and Department of Electrical Engineering, Marquette University College of Engineering*

Many methods of identification of the conduction system of the heart have been described since the beginning of open-heart surgery. These have included bipolar electrocardiography,[13] iodine staining,[1, 2, 15] and plotting anatomic position.[3, 11] All of these methods have been unsatisfactory, either because of trauma, inconsistent results, or impracticality in clinical use.

The clinical importance of a simple and reliable method of locating the conduction system of the heart during repair of congenital defects cannot be overemphasized. The incidence of surgically induced heart block has been reported to be 10 per cent in patients with ventricular defects.[6] Permanent heart block in these individuals may result either in death by cardiac arrest or in a crippling reduced cardiac output.

This report describes a method for locating the conduction system of the dog heart by means of audiofrequency conductimetry. Lewis[5] first described a difference in conduction times between the myocardium and conduction system which has been confirmed by Sodi-Pallares[12] and Schaufer.[9] This observation suggested a greater resistance to the flow of electric current in the myocardium than in the conduction system of the heart. It was reasoned that if this were true, a relative difference in impedance between these two tissues should exist which could possibly be detected.

One of us (W. B.) suggested that on the basis of this principle an electronic device might be developed which would be capable of measuring the anticipated difference in impedance.

## MEASUREMENT OF RELATIVE DIFFERENCES IN IMPEDANCE IN THE DOG HEART

A Wheatstone bridge was connected to an oscillator with a frequency of 1 kc. (Fig. 1). The current at the tip of a bipolar detector probe was 0.3 Ma. at 0.3 v., assuming a resistance of 1,000 ohms across the heart.

The detector probe in its original form consisted of two 22 gauge copper wires insulated except at their tips. The wires were encased in a plastic insulating cylinder with their tips spaced 1.0 mm. apart. A speaker was provided to emit an audible signal which changed in volume with variation in impedance as encountered by the probe. Preliminary experimentation indicated that im-

Supported by United States Public Health Service Research Grant H-4475 (C2) and Department of Research, United States Veterans Administration Hospital, Wood, Wis.
Read at the Twenty-second Annual Meeting of the Society of University Surgeons, Kansas City, Kan., Feb. 9-11, 1961.

pedance differences could be easily detected in the right ventricle of the bypassed, arrested dog heart.

A transistorized unit with a frequency of 1 kc. and an output of 0.3 Ma. at the tip of the probe was then devised which is shown in Fig. 2. A null meter and bridge balance controls permitted absolute balance of the bridge. The speaker was activated by a contact which was closed when the bridge became extremely unbalanced. The null meter scale was divided into arbitrary units which indicated decreasing impedance from left to right. After the bridge had been balanced with the detector probe on an area of myocardium with high impedance, the cardiac septum was scanned with the probe. When an area of low impedance was encountered, a pronounced imbalance of the bridge occurred, the null meter hand moved to the right and struck a contact which activated the speaker, and an audible sound was produced.

In each instance, this area of low impedance corresponded anatomically with the usual site of the right bundle branch of the conduction system in the dog heart.

Our experiments were then devised to determine whether or not the areas of low impedance corresponded to the conduction system in the heart.

## METHODS AND RESULTS

In each of the 52 experiments to be described, a mongrel dog was placed on complete cardiopulmonary bypass with a disposable plastic oxygenator and a Sigmamotor pump. A right ventriculotomy or atriotomy was performed and the heart arrested by ischemia or cold blood. The detector probe was placed on the myocardium in the upper anterior portion of the ventricular septum or in the right ventricular epicardium and the bridge was balanced. Areas of low impedance designated by an audible signal from the speaker were then sought by passing the tip of the detector probe across the surface of the ventricular septum or annulus fibrosis. A summary of all experiments is shown in Table I.

**Detection and division of the right bundle branch.** In 14 animals, with the bridge balanced as described and with use of a right ventriculotomy incision, the right ventricular septum was scanned with the detector probe until an audible alarm announced an

**Table I.** *A summary of reported experiments*

| *No. of experiments* | *Procedure* | *EKG normal* | *EKG block* | *Lugol's stain** | *Dissection and histology* |
|---|---|---|---|---|---|
| 14 | Detection and incision of right bundle branch (2 mm.) | 0 | Right bundle, 14 | Bundle divided in all | |
| 14 | Detection and placement of sutures on each side of right bundle (2 mm.) | 9 | Right bundle, 5 | Bundle encroachment in 5, within 2 mm. in 9 | |
| 6 | Placement of sutures around atrioventricular node | 4 | Nodal rhythm, 2 | — | Sutures included in nodal tissue in 3 |
| 6 | Detection and incision of bundle of His (3 mm. incision) | 3 | Atrioventricular dissociation, 3 | Divided in 3, within 2 mm. in 3 | |
| 12 | Stimulation of atrioventricular node and right bundle branch, 2 to 4 min. | 11 | Right bundle, 1 | — | Minimal epicardial scarring in all, conduction tissue unaffected |

*Lugol's staining of tissues is routinely useful only in demonstrating the right bundle branch and bundle of His.

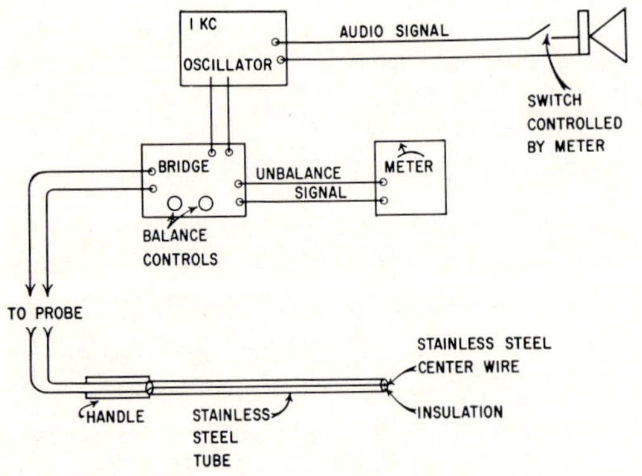


**Fig. 1.** Diagrammatic representation of the circuit used in measurement of impedance. The frequency of 1 kc. was arbitrarily selected. The probe design is that used in the described experiments.

area of low impedance. With successive passes of the probe, the limits of this area were located and a 2 mm. incision was made with a No. 11 scalpel blade (Fig. 3). The heart was then closed, bypass discontinued, and electrocardiographic tracings compared to those obtained preoperatively. Either immediately or during the next 5 days, the animals were sacrificed and the septum of the heart painted with Lugol's solution to demonstrate the right bundle branch of the conducting system. The relationship of the incision to the right branch was recorded and histologic sections were obtained from the area.

Each of the 14 animals showed complete right bundle branch block after the stab wound incision of the area of low impedance found on the right ventricular septum. Lugol's staining demonstrated division of the right bundle branch and histologic examination confirmed this finding after staining with Masson's trichrome.

**Detection of right bundle branch and placement of sutures on each side.** A similar procedure was used in a second group of 14 dogs except that in this group, instead of incising the area of lowest impedance detected by the probe, we placed sutures parallel to it, 2 mm. apart (Fig. 4). Once again, pre- and postoperative electrocardiographic tracings were obtained. The animal was sacrificed immediately after the procedure or within the next 2 weeks. The septum was painted with Lugol's solution to determine the location of the right bundle branch and histologic sections from the area of the sutures were prepared.

Right bundle branch block resulted in 5 of the animals. Nine showed no altered conduction as evidenced by comparative electrocardiographic tracings. Lugol's staining showed the sutures to be in close proximity in all experiments (Fig. 5, *A*), but the bundle fibers were partially encompassed by the sutures in the dogs which showed right bundle branch block. The results of the histologic study of sections again confirmed the findings.

**Location of the atrioventricular node.** A right atriotomy was performed after complete heart-lung bypass had been accomplished in 6 animals. An area of low impedance in the region of the atrioventricular node was found with the detector probe. While monitoring with the probe, we placed sutures completely about this site except in a narrow area thought to represent the origin of the bundle of His (Fig. 6). Electrocardiographic tracings were recorded before and after the experiment and histologic sections through the area surrounded by su-

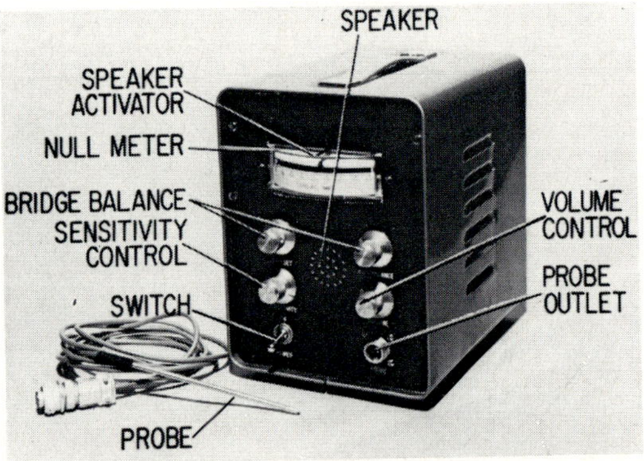


**Fig. 2.** The transistorized unit and detection probe. The connecting cord is coated with plastic and may be autoclaved. Frequency, 1 kc. The output at the tip of the probe is 3.0 ma. of current at 0.3 v. The null meter indicator is at the balanced position. The speaker activator may be moved to meet changing sensitivity.

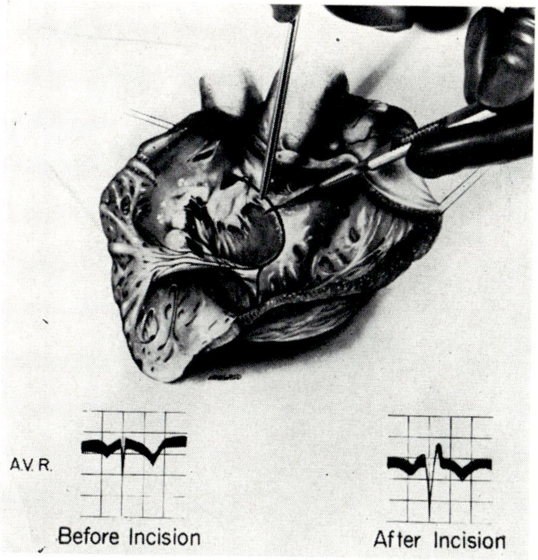


**Fig. 3.** Detection and division of the right bundle branch. The right bundle branch has been found and divided with a 2 mm. incision. Lugol's solution has been used after sacrifice of the animal to confirm division of the right bundle branch. Electrocardiogram showed right bundle branch block in all 14 animals.

tures were studied after the animal had been sacrificed.

In the 6 experiments performed, electrocardiographic tracings showed nodal rhythm in 2 animals postoperatively and normal rhythm in 4 others. Histologic sections were inconclusive in 3 experiments, but in the 2 in which altered conduction was produced, nodal tissue was demonstrated within the confines of the sutures. Fig. 5, *B,* shows a suture placed within 0.5 mm. of conduction tissue. Failure to accurately identify the atrioventricular node, which lies at a variable depth within the annulus fibrosis, was attributed to depth limitations of the detector probe available for study.

**Location of the bundle of His.** In 6 dogs a right ventriculotomy was performed, the chordae tendineae of the septal leaflet were divided, and the leaflet reflected. An area of low impedance thought to be consistent with the common bundle of His was found at the level of the atrioventricular ring and a 3 mm. incision was made with a No. 11 scalpel blade. Once again, electrocardiographic tracings were obtained before and after the experiment. Histologic sections of the area were made upon completion of the experiment or when the animal was sacrificed.

In 3 of the 6 experiments, the incision in the area determined by the detector probe produced complete atrioventricular dissociation on electrocardiogram and histologic sections confirmed division of the conduction tissue in these animals. Dissection of the bundle after iodine staining in the remaining animals showed the incision to be within 1 to 2 mm. of the conduction bundle. Here again, variable anatomic depth of the bundle and depth limitations of the probe prevented absolute identification.

**Studies to determine the effect of constant stimulation upon the conduction system.** The experiment to be described was devised to determine the effect, if any, on the myocardium and conduction system of a current of 0.3 Ma. at 0.3 v.

In 6 animals the area of the atrioventricular node was exposed and identified through a right atriotomy and in 6 others the right bundle branch was identified through a right ventriculotomy. In both groups these structures were stimulated constantly for

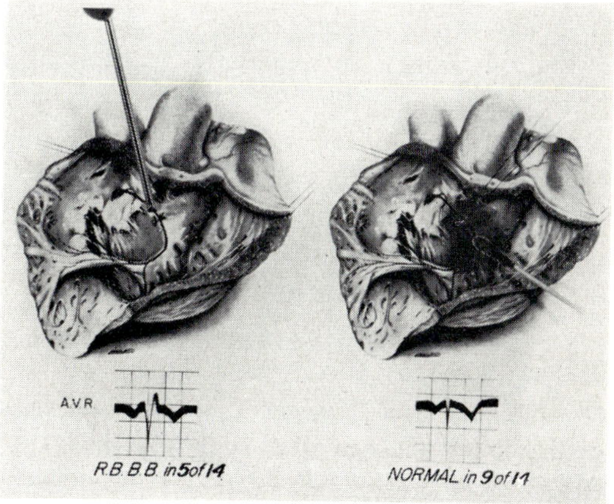


**Fig. 4.** Detection of right bundle branch and placement of sutures on each side. Sutures have been placed 2 mm. apart and include the identified right bundle branch between them. Electrocardiogram showed right bundle branch block in 5 dogs and was normal in 9. Painting with Lugol's solution demonstrated close proximity of sutures to the right bundle branch.

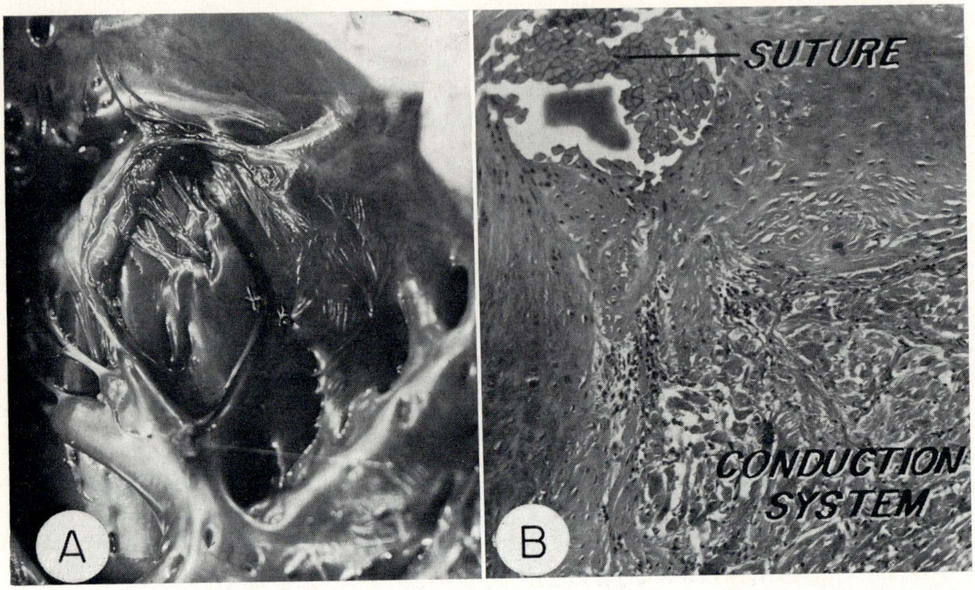


**Fig. 5.** *A,* Photograph of dog heart after sacrifice and application of Lugol's solution to the right ventricular septum. Note the close proximity of the sutures to the iodine-stained right bundle branch. *B,* Photomicrograph of section through atrioventricular node after detection and placement of sutures around it. Note the close proximity (0.5 mm.) of suture material to conduction tissue in upper right. (×130.)

from 2 to 4 minutes with the detector probe. The incisions were closed, bypass discontinued, and the animals allowed to survive for from 7 days to 4 months. All were followed by serial electrocardiograms and on sacrifice histologic sections were studied from the area of stimulation.

Only 1 animal in which the right bundle branch was stimulated for 4 minutes showed electrocardiographic evidence of bundle branch block. The remaining 5 animals showed no alteration of electrocardiogram during the observation period of from 1 week to 4 months. Chronic stimulation of the atrioventricular node in 6 animals produced no conduction change. Histologic sections of the area stimulated showed minimal evidence of endocardial scarring in all 12 dogs, but these changes did not involve the conduction system. The 1 animal which demonstrated right bundle branch block was sacrificed after 5 days because of empyema and showed no abnormality of the conduction tissue in the area stimulated. Seven of the 12 animals were observed for from 1 to 4 months with weekly electrocardiographic tracings and no alterations were noted.

## COMMENT

Numerous measurements of electrical impedance of myocardium and conduction tissue have shown conduction tissue impedance to average 30 to 50 per cent less than that of myocardium. With this consistent difference, the relative change in impedance can be rapidly determined with the electronic tools described. The wide variance in the impedance of any one tissue (that is, lung, liver, or muscle) noted by Schwan[10] has not limited the method, because the percentage of relative difference of impedance within the heart remains constant.

Consistent, concise, rapid location of the right bundle branch of the conduction system in the dog has been made possible. The location of the bundle of His in the dog, however, has been hampered by its anatomy. This structure lies within the annulus fibrosis of the right atrioventricular ring, is extremely short, and is high beneath the septal leaflet of the tricuspid valve. Identification requires division of the attachments of the septal leaflet, which is incompatible with life in the dog and does not provide good access to the probe.

Identification of the atrioventricular node has not been satisfactory in the normal dog heart because the node lies at a variable depth within the annulus fibrosis. It may be immediately subendocardial or at a depth of 3 or 4 mm.

Analogue studies in this laboratory (Fig. 7) have shown that the present probe design limits the detection depth to 1 mm. In an attempt to overcome this limitation, extensive studies including use of gold and platinum electrodes with varied spacing and frequencies ranging from 10 cycles per second to 3 megacycles were undertaken. Impedance stability of a given tissue was greatest at 50 kc. Frequencies above 1 megacycle contributed many problems not found at lower frequencies and have been abandoned. The polarization of the electrodes in electrolyte solutions such as blood is also being studied.

Studies of impedance in all areas of the heart have consistently shown a very low impedance in the septal leaflet of the tricuspid valve compared to that of the other 2 leaflets. The impedance of the septal leaflet has been found to be 25 per cent lower than that of the remaining 2 leaflets in most instances. In fact, its impedance approaches that found in the conduction system when a frequency of 1 kc. is used. The atrioventricular node is partially covered by the septal leaflet. In view of this finding, we conclude that the experiments directed at identification of the atrioventricular node in the dog by these methods are inconclusive.

Preliminary studies by continuous electrocardiographic monitoring have shown delayed conduction in the right ventricle after serial division of the chordae tendineae of the septal leaflet (Fig. 7). This, of course, suggests the possibility that some of the right bundle conduction fibers pass through this leaflet, but more study will be required to confirm or disprove this suggestion.

Projected application of these studies is directed toward detection of the bundle of His in operations for congenital heart disease. It is commonly accepted that surgically induced heart block is always a danger in 2 groups of patients—those with large ventricular septal defects and those with endocardial cushion defects. Reemtsma[7, 8] and

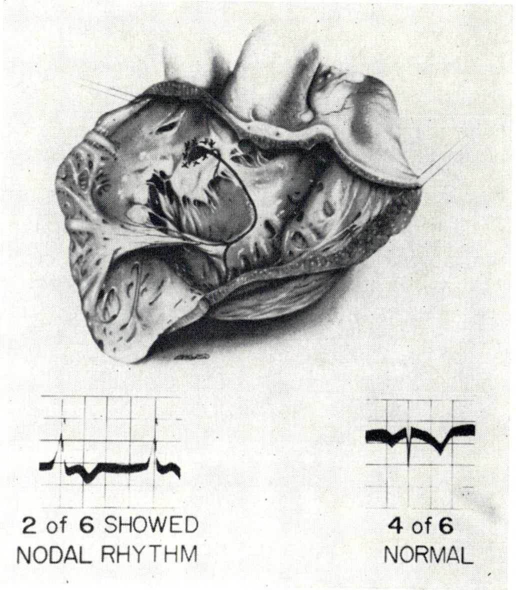


Fig. 6. Detection and placement of sutures around atrioventricular node. Electrocardiogram showed nodal rhythm in 2 of 6 animals. Histologic sections showed nodal tissue within the confines of the sutures in 3.

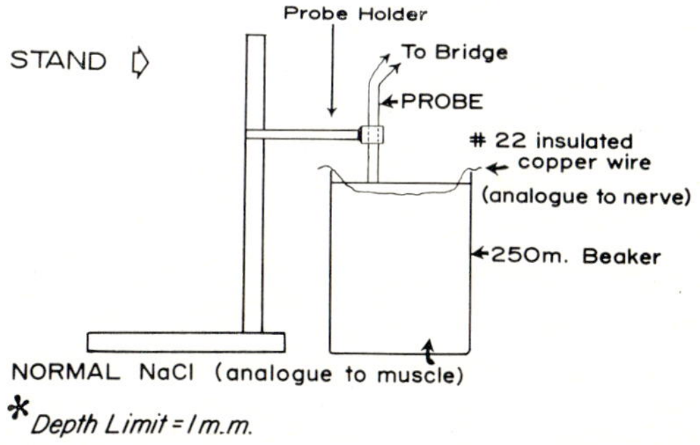


Fig. 7. Analogue study developed to investigate different probe designs and the effect of different frequencies. The copper wire represents an area of low impedance (conduction system) and the saline bath an area of high impedance (the myocardium). Raising or lowering the copper wire in the saline bath will determine depth of detection.

Lev,[4, 14] after extensive dissection and histologic studies of the conduction system of the hearts of patients who died with ventricular septal defects, have pointed out that this structure usually lies immediately subendocardially at the posterior inferior rim of a ventricular septal defect. In this instance, on the basis of experience in the dog heart, the conduction system lying within 1 mm. of the surface in human beings could be accurately and safely detected by the method described. Recently a somewhat different principle has been utilized and further modification of the design of the detection probe has been undertaken. Preliminary analogue studies and field plots suggest that with these changes detection depth can be increased threefold. In vivo studies are now in progress. It is anticipated that with continuing study, many practical applications of this electronic tool may result.

The finding of significant and persistent percentage differences in impedance in the tissues of one organ or one anatomic area should permit accurate differentiation between these tissues. In this event, more accurate identification of peripheral or cranial nerves to avoid injury during difficult dissection seems likely, and reconstructive procedures may be aided. The technique may also be useful in neurolysis, either by chemical or electrocoagulation techniques, of a variety of neural structures, that is, dorsolateral nucleus, trigeminal or sympathetic ganglia, the spinothalamic tracts, and so forth.

## SUMMARY

1. An electronic instrument has been devised which audibly signals impedance differences in adjacent areas of the dog heart.

2. The right bundle branch of the conduction system in the dog can be concisely and safely identified.

3. This method has proved inadequate in its present stage of development for precise location of the atrioventricular node and common bundle of His in the dog because of anatomic structure and depth limitations of the equipment.

4. The principle described may have widespread applications in modern surgery.

The authors are grateful to Medtronic Incorporated, Minneapolis, Minn., for their assistance in the development of the transistorized unit used in this study.

## REFERENCES

1. Allen, P., Lederman, J. J., and Pearl, G. J.: Prevention of surgical heart block by the use of a supravital stain, J. Thoracic Surg. **38:** 57, 1959.
2. Bittencourt, D., Long, J., Lee, Y. K., Lillehei, C. W.: Intravital staining of the atrioventricular bundle with iodine compounds during cardiopulmonary by-pass, Circulation Res. **5:** 5, 753, 1959.
3. Kirklin, J. W., Harshbarger, H. B., Donald, E. E., and Edwards, J. E.: Surgical correction of a ventricular septal defect. Anatomic and technical considerations, J. Thoracic Surg. **33:** 45, 1957.
4. Lev, M.: The architecture of the conduction system in congenital heart disease, A. M. A. Arch. Path. **65:** 174-191, 1958.
5. Lewis, T.: Excitatory process in dog's heart: ventricles, Phil. Tr. Lond. **B206:** 181, 1915.
6. Lillehei, C. W., Gott, V. L., Hodges, P. C., Jr., Long, D. M., and Bakken, E. E.: Transistor pacemaker for treatment of complete atrio-ventricular dissociation, J. A. M. A. **172:** 18, 2006, 1960.
7. Reemtsma, K., Copenhaver, W. M., and Creech, O., Jr.: The cardiac conduction system in congenital anomalies of the heart, SURGERY **44:** 1, 99, 1958.
8. Reemtsma, K., Delgado, J. P., and Creech, O., Jr.: Heart block following intracardiac surgery: localization of conduction tissue injury, J. Thoracic Surg. **39:** 5, 688, 1960.
9. Schaufer, H.: The general order of excitation and of recovery, Ann. New York Acad. Sc. **65:** 6, 743, 1957.
10. Schwan, H. P., and Kay, C. F.: The conductivity of living tissues, Ann. New York Acad. Sc. **65:** 6, 1007, 1957.
11. Sirak, H. D., Meckstroth, C. V., Ryan, J. M., Claasen, L. G., and Hosier, D. M.: The prevention of heart block in the surgical repair of interventricular septal defect, J. Thoracic Surg. **39:** 2, 229, 1960.
12. Sodi-Pallares, D., Medrano, G. A., Bisteni, A., and De Michelli, A.: The electrocardiograms of the conductive tissue in the normal dog's heart, Am. J. Cardiol. **4:** 4, 459, 1959.
13. Stuckey, J. H., Hoffman, B. F., Amer, N. S., Cranefield, P. F., Cappelletti, R. R., and

Domingo, R. T.: Localization of the bundle of His with a surface electrode during cardiotomy, S. Forum **10:** 551, 1959.

14. Widren, J., and Lev, M.: Dissection of atrioventricular node, bundle, and bundle branches in human heart, Circulation **4:** 863, 1951.
15. Winnemark, J. R., Benvenuto, P., and Lewis, J. F.: Destruction of the specialized conduction tissue in the live canine heart with iodine, J. Thoracic Surg. **39:** 2, 137, 1960.

## DISCUSSION

**Dr. M. A. Chiechi** (Newark, N. J.). Our approach to the problem of identifying the atrioventricular conduction system has been a different and, perhaps, a simpler one. The ideal method of detecting the atrioventricular conduction system should be simple and practical, should not produce ill effect or injury on conduction pathways, and should be short in duration with complete reversibility to normal sinus rhythm. At the University of Minnesota and at St. Michael's Hospital, Newark, New Jersey, we have successfully detected the atrioventricular node and bundle of the dog by means of pin-point cooling. The instrument is a stainless steel probe about 20 cm. in length and 3 mm. in internal diameter. The tip is sealed and polished smooth. Through a sidearm arrangement, a refrigerant solution, Freon 114, circulates into the probe and cools the tip down to 4° C. After touching the area of the atrioventricular conduction system for a period of about 5 to 7 seconds, we obtained atrioventricular dissociation. This lasted only 10 to 15 seconds and promptly reverted to normal sinus rhythm. The conduction system was examined 4 weeks after the experiment in several dogs. The slide shows the normal appearance of the tissue with glycogen bunched in one of the poles of the cells, the nuclei containing chromatin, and no evidence of fibrosis.

**Dr. C. Walton Lillehei** (Minneapolis, Minn.). I compliment Dr. Lepley and associates on a fine piece of work. The detection of the conduction pathways, even in the arrested heart, by their difference in electrical conductivity from adjacent myocardium is a brilliant solution to the problem of prevention of heart block. As Dr. Lepley well appreciated during the year he spent working with us, injury to the myocardial conduction system has heretofore been unavoidable in a certain percentage of patients with large ventricular defects. A general knowledge of the usual location of the main pathways is helpful, but in no way has it been a guarantee against their injury due to the variabilities encountered. Dr. Lepley has recently placed his apparatus at our disposal and we have tested it experimentally and are now utilizing it routinely in our patients.

We have had considerable interest in the past in finding a vital stain to outline these pathways. Iodine (Lugol's solution) locally was effective, but caused permanent damage (Circulation Res. 7: 753, 1959) and thus was of no clinical value. Fluorescein (with Wood's lamp) was very promising in the experimental laboratory and we utilized it clinically for a period about 18 months ago, but found that the tricuspid valve tissue and chordae fluoresced almost as well as the conduction tissue so that this lack of complete specificity made fluorescein less helpful than had been hoped. The discovery of a promising vital stain for this purpose still seems feasible.

Dr. Chiechi has just described another effective approach which he developed last year while working with us, but local cold does have the distinct disadvantage that it will not work in the arrested heart.

The concept of direct pacemaking via a myocardial electrode has been a significant advance in therapy especially for the two-thirds or three-fourths of patients who revert to sinus rhythm in the immediate days after corrective operations. However, even in this favorable group it should be remembered that the efficiency of the heart is impaired by at least 15 to 20 per cent even with an adequate ventricular rate due to asynchrony of atrial and ventricular contractions, and this can be an important factor in failure to survive in marginal patients (for example, those with very high pulmonary resistance).

The prognosis, however, for patients who remain in chronic block is more serious and it is here that the preventive methods will have their most important impact.

We have had 21 patients who remained in chronic complete block after intracardiac operations. All were treated initially with the electrical pacemaker for 3 to 4 weeks. In the follow-up period of 6 months to 4½ years after removal of pacemaker stimulation, 12 remain essentially well, but 9 have died sudden late deaths. In this group, patients with ventricular defects and severe pulmonary hypertension or severe tetralogies have done less well than their counterparts with less severe anatomic lesions and less well than those with atrioventricularis communis without severe pulmonary hypertension. We believe that the former patients remaining in chronic block should have a permanent pacemaker implanted.

**Derward Lepley, Jr.** (closing). I wish to thank the discussers. We have modified our probe design innumerable times. Very recently, using a different design of a probe and a slightly different principle, we have been able to erase surface resistance or impedance and measure accurately to a depth of 3 mm. in in vitro studies. We have performed preliminary in vivo studies in the dog and if additional in vivo studies confirm our finding, I believe we will have an effective clinical tool.

# Open intracardiac repair for transposition of the great vessels: 11 cases

JOHN W. KIRKLIN, M.D.
ROBERT A. DEVLOO, M.D.
WILLIAM H. WEIDMAN, M.D.
ROCHESTER, MINN.
*From the sections of surgery, anesthesiology, and pediatrics, Mayo Clinic and Mayo Foundation*

Eleven severely cyanotic patients have been operated on for repair of transposition of the great vessels. Nine were infants in intractable congestive heart failure and 2 were young children with profound disability. Three infants and 1 of the older children survived. One infant died later at home of apparently unrelated causes. The other 3 patients are well.

Associated lesions have been repaired, and the Senning[8] operation, based on the early concepts of Albert, has been performed for the transposition (Fig. 1). Profound hypothermia induced with perfusion by a pump-oxygenator has allowed most of the procedure to be carried out during total circulatory arrest.

## CASE REPORTS

Some pertinent facts concerning the patients operated on are presented in Table I. Additional details concerning patients who survived operation illustrate the types of cases encountered (Table II).

**Case 1.** A 1-year-old boy with cyanosis and a heart murmur noted at birth had failed to thrive and his motor development had been slow. Digitalis had been given when he was 4 months of age and its use was continued. Cyanosis, fatigue, and dyspnea gradually increased over the next month with considerable limitation of activity.

Examination showed the patient to be a thin boy, 28 inches long and weighing 14½ pounds. Cyanosis was advanced and generalized. The heart was overactive. A harsh systolic murmur, grade 3 (on the basis of 1 to 6, in which 1 is the least and 6 the loudest murmur), was heard best in the left third and fourth intercostal spaces and transmitted to the apex. The edge of the liver was palpable 3 cm. below the costal margin. The lungs were clear and the peripheral arterial pulses were normal.

The electrocardiogram showed a mean QRS axis of +170 degrees. There was evidence of atrial enlargement and overwork of the right ventricle. The left ventricular components were normal. A roentgenogram of the thorax showed evidence of cardiac enlargement with an increase of the pulmonary vascular markings.

**Case 2.** A 3-month-old boy had had dyspnea on exertion and cyanosis since birth. These conditions had gradually increased in severity and a heart murmur had been described when he was 2 months of age.

On examination, the infant was found to be severely dyspneic and extremely ill. Moderate cyanosis of the fingers and toes was evident and râles were heard throughout both lungs. The heart was overactive with a loud holosystolic murmur, grade 4, heard best in the left third and fourth intercostal spaces and transmitted to the apex. An apical diastolic murmur was present. The edge of the liver was palpable at the costal margin and the femoral pulses were normal. The electrocardiogram showed a mean QRS axis of +120 degrees with evidence of overwork of the left ventricle. The right ventricular components were normal. A roentgenogram of the thorax showed evidence of a large heart with increased vascular markings (Fig. 2).

The patient was hospitalized and all usual anticongestive measures were instituted. Despite a strict medical regimen of adequate doses of Lanoxin and diuretics, the patient continued to be desperately ill in congestive heart failure. Angiocardiography confirmed the clinical diagnosis of transposition of the great arteries with ventricular spetal defect (Fig. 3).

Read at the Twenty-second Annual Meeting of the Society of University Surgeons, Kansas City, Kan., Feb. 9-11, 1961.

**Table I.** *Intracardiac repair (including Senning operation) for complete transposition of great vessels*

| Case No. | Age (years) | Associated defects* | Ventricular pressures† after repair (mm. Hg) Right ventricle (systemic) | Left ventricle (pulmonary) | Outcome | Presumed cause of death |
|---|---|---|---|---|---|---|
| 1 | 1 | Ventricular septal defect | 80/10 | 50/10 | Survived | — |
| 2 | 3/12 | Ventricular septal defect | 91/3 | 35/2 | Survived | — |
| 3 | 13/12 | Ventricular septal defect, patent ductus arteriosus | 82/4 | 50/8 | Survived | — |
| 4 | 4/12 | Ventricular septal defect | 61/11 | 40/5 | Died 12 hr. after operation | Cardiac failure, right and left atrial pressure 23 mm. Hg with very low arterial pressure |
| 5 | 6 | Atrial septal defect | — | — | Survived | — |
| 6 | 4 | Ventricular septal defect | 56/15 | 60/10 | Died 48 hr. after operation | Irreducible pulmonary hypertension |
| 7 | 15/12 | Ventricular septal defect | 80/? | 105/? | Died 8 hr. after operation | Irreducible pulmonary hypertension |
| 8 | 16/12 | Ventricular septal defect, patent ductus arteriosus | 80/? | 45/? | Died 4 hr. after operation | Massive intra-abdominal hemorrhage (questionable source) |
| 9 | 2/12 | Patent ductus arteriosus | 77/11 | 65/7 | Died 30 min. after operation | Low cardiac output (questionable hypovolemia, questionable cardiac failure) |
| 10 | 11/12 | Ventricular septal defect | 85/? | 40/? | Died 28 hr. after operation | Respiratory insufficiency, pulmonary edema |
| 11 | 5/12 | Ventricular septal defect, patent ductus arteriosus | 75/? | 45/? | Died 12 hr. after operation | Low cardiac output (cardiac failure), respiratory insufficiency, pulmonary consolidation |

*Two patients (Cases 2 and 10) also had large persistent emptying of the left superior vena cava into the coronary sinus. Five patients had a probe-patent foramen ovale.
†All patients except one (Case 5) had equal pressures in the right and left ventricles before repair.

**Table II.** *Hemodynamic data in transposition of great vessels**

| Case No. | Oxygen saturation (%) Mixed venous | Right atrium | Right ventricle | Brachial artery | Pressures (mm. Hg) Right ventricle | Left ventricle |
|---|---|---|---|---|---|---|
| 1 | 35 | 35 | 50 | 50 | 82/4 | 80/6 |
| 2 | 33 | 28 | 42 | 50 | 90/6 | 75/2 |
| 3 | 33 | 34 | 36 | 47 | 90/9 | 90/6 |
| 5 | 49 | 60 | 68 | 68 | 72/10 | 31/8 |

*Dye-dilution curves in all cases showed dissociation of pulmonary and systemic circulations. Selective angiocardiograms demonstrated transposition of the great vessels in all patients. Ventricular septal defect was demonstrated in all patients except one (Case 5).

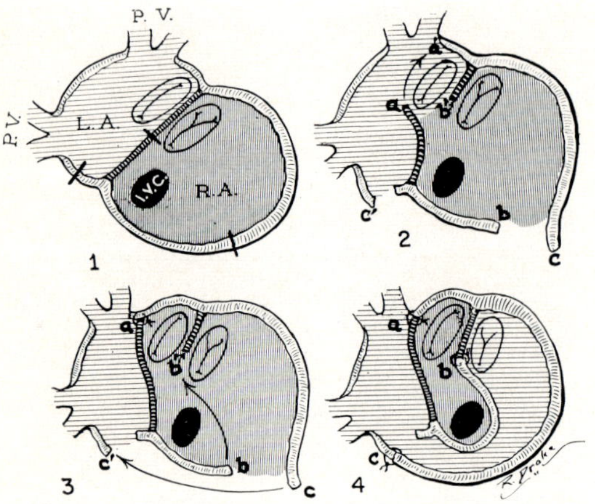


**Fig. 1.** Diagrammatic representation of surgical transposition of venous return (Senning operation) which corrects the circulatory abnormality in cases of complete transposition of the great vessels. *1,* The preoperative status. Pulmonary veins *(P.V.)* drain into left atrium *(L.A.)* and mitral valve. The inferior vena cava *(I.V.C.)* and superior vena cava (not shown) drain into right atrium *(R.A.)* and tricuspid valve. Points of incision into left atrium, right atrium, and atrial septum are indicated. *2,* Atrial septum *(a)* will be sutured anterior to left pulmonary vein ostia *(a'),* and posterior flap of free wall of right atrium *(b)* will be sutured to anterior septal remnant *(b'). 3,* This has been accomplished in part and *4,* completely. Systemic venous blood (vertical hatching) now drains into an atrium connected to mitral valve. This blood now goes to left ventricle and pulmonary artery. The right anterior wall of left atrium *(c')* is sutured to anterior flap of free wall of right atrium *(c)* to complete formation of an atrium draining pulmonary venous blood (horizontal hatching) to tricuspid valve. This blood goes then to right ventricle and aorta.

**Case 3.** A full-term infant, born after an uneventful pregnancy, was examined at the Mayo Clinic when he was 3 months of age. Cyanosis and a heart murmur had been discovered at birth. Cardiac failure had developed when he was 5 days of age and the patient had been treated with Lanoxin and a low sodium diet. Clinically, he improved, but the cyanosis continued. At 3 months of age, he weighed 11 pounds, which represented a 2½-pound gain in weight since birth.

Examination showed moderate generalized cyanosis. The heart was quiet with a soft grade 2 systolic murmur heard over the lower left sternal border. No diastolic murmurs were heard. The lungs were clear and the edge of the liver was palpable 2 cm. below the costal margin.

During the next 7 months the cyanosis increased gradually with mild clubbing of the fingers and toes. Fatigue and dyspnea with exertion increased. Gain in weight was slow, and motor development was retarded. During this time the infant had 2 severe attacks of bronchitis. At 1 year of age, he was inactive; he rarely rolled over and was unable to sit alone. A roentgenogram of the thorax taken at that time showed evidence of cardiac enlargement with an increase in pulmonary vascular markings. The electrocardiogram showed a mean QRS axis to the right, atrial enlargement, overwork of the right ventricle, and a normal left ventricle. The hemoglobin concentration measured 18.6 Gm.

The clinical impression was that of transposition of the great vessels with ventricular septal defect.

**Case 5.** On first examination at the Mayo Clinic, a 3-year-old child had a history of cyanosis at birth and a heart murmur first documented when he was 1 year of age. The cyanosis had increased gradually and muscular weakness and motor retardation were so severe that the patient, although 3 years of age, had not walked.

Examination showed him to be a severely cyanotic, small 3-year-old child who was 35½ inches tall and weighed 29 pounds. A grade 1 soft systolic murmur was heard in the third left intercostal space. The edge of the liver was palpable at the costal margin and the lungs were clear.

A roentgenogram of the thorax showed evidence of a large heart with increased pulmonary vascular markings. The electrocardiogram showed a mean QRS axis of −170 degrees with evidence of overwork of the right ventricle and depressed left ventricular factors (Fig. 4).

The clinical diagnosis was transposition of the great vessels and this was confirmed by selective angiocardiography into the right ventricle (Fig. 5).

The patient's activity increased somewhat, but the cyanosis increased with clubbing and by 6 years of age the child was able to walk only a block without extreme fatigue.

## TECHNIQUE OF OPERATION

The technique and management of anesthesia were essentially those described by Dawson and associates[2] for children who undergo open-heart operations. Anesthesia was induced by inhalation and induction was characteristically prolonged by 2 factors, (1) the relative isolation of central blood volume that results from the circulatory pattern in transposition, and (2) the decrease in cerebral blood flow secondary to polycythemia[4] which usually is present in these patients. With the surgical correction of the cardiac defect, normal recovery from anesthesia occurred.

A median sternotomy incision was made. The right common iliac artery, exposed extraperitoneally, was cannulated for arterial input. A Tygon tube with a three-sixteenth inch internal diameter was placed in the right atrium through the auricular appendage for venous drainage. Perfusion was established at a flow rate of approximately 2.5 L. per minute per square meter. When a patent ductus arteriosus was present it was ligated. Body temperature was reduced to approximately 12° C. (53.6° F.) by perfusion.[5] Total circulatory arrest was established and the aorta was cross-clamped. Systemic and pulmonary veins were transposed by Senning's technique (Fig. 1). The ventricular septal defect was repaired. In the first 9 cases circulatory arrest lasted an average of 58 minutes; in the last 2, 36 minutes. The venous cannula was placed in the left atrium through its appendage and perfusion was re-established. Warming by means of perfusion returned the body temperature to approximately 37° C. (98.6° F.). Defibrillation occurred spontaneously or was produced electrically. Perfusion was discontinued and decannulation was effected.

Postperfusion and postoperative care were accomplished as for other sick cyanotic patients with congenital heart disease.[6, 7]

## RESULTS

The outcome for each patient operated on is indicated in Table I. In cases of death the presumed cause is indicated.

Atrioventricular dissociation occurred in Case 3 only, and reverted to sinus rhythm in 48 hours. Technical failures in the Senning repair were not identified. Neither observation of pressures in the 2 venous systems and in the atria during the operation nor examination at necropsy disclosed evidence that the repair had obstructed pulmonary or systemic venous return. Healing had been good after this complex procedure in the specimen from the patient in Case 1, although the child had died at home 2½ months after having been dismissed from the hospital.

One patient (Case 8) died 4 hours after operation, probably as a result of massive

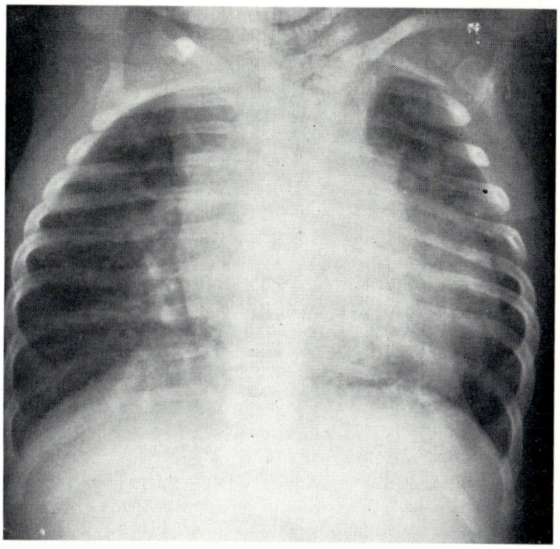

**Fig. 2.** Roentgenogram of the thorax of a 3-month-old child. The heart is enlarged and pulmonary vascular markings are definitely increased. Note the absence of a clear-cut shadow of the main pulmonary artery.

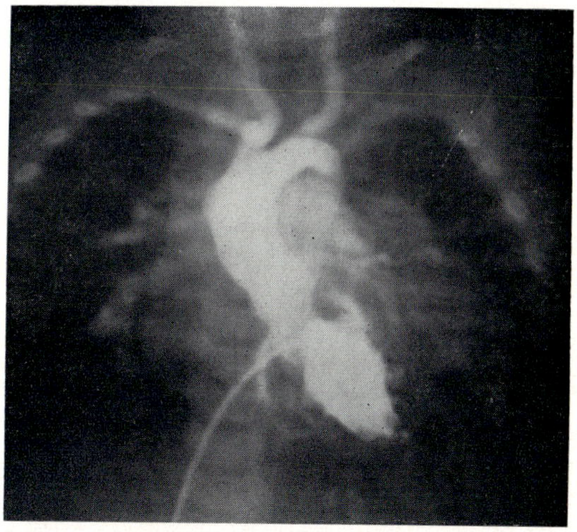

**Fig. 3.** Selective angiocardiogram into the right ventricle in a 3-month-old child, which demonstrates the origin of the aorta from the right ventricle. Medium has passed into the left ventricle through a ventricular septal defect and the pulmonary artery is seen arising from this chamber.

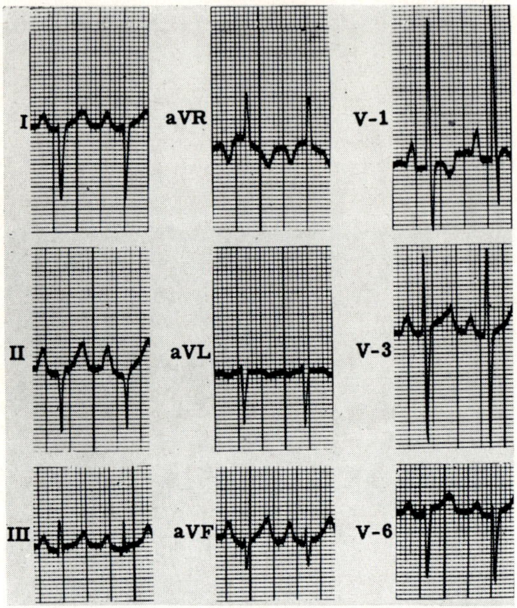


**Fig. 4.** Electrocardiogram of a 6-year-old child. Atrial enlargement is evident, and the tall R waves (33 mm.) in lead $V_1$ indicate right ventricular hypertrophy. The left ventricular complexes are depressed.

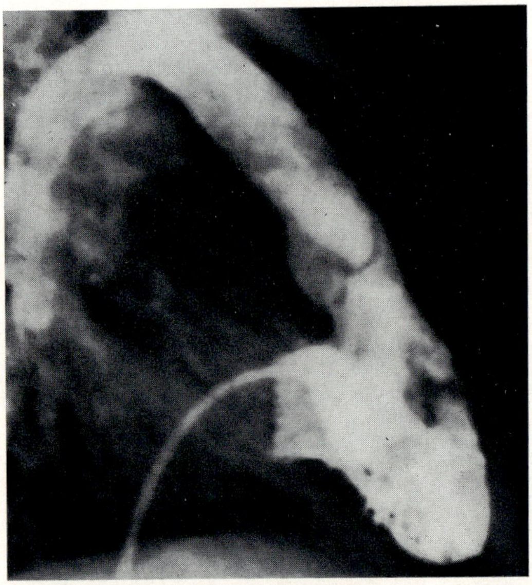

**Fig. 5.** Selective angiocardiogram into the right ventricle in a 6-year-old child, which demonstrates the origin of the aorta from the right ventricle. A ventricular septal defect is not visualized.

intraperitoneal and retroperitoneal hemorrhages which developed after the surgical procedure. Although the source could not be demonstrated at necropsy, the point of cannulation of the common iliac artery is suspected.

In 2 patients (Cases 4 and 11), high atrial pressure and low systemic arterial pressure indicated the presence of cardiac failure. Death seemed related, at least in part, to this condition in both babies. In Case 9, venous pressure was not measured after the patient's chest was closed, and the cause of the subsequent low cardiac output cannot be identified.

In 2 patients (Cases 10 and 11) respiratory insufficiency was evident clinically. At necropsy pulmonary edema was demonstrated in Case 10 and hemorrhagic pulmonary congestion in Case 11.

Surviving patients are pink and without evident neurological damage. The reduction in the size of the heart after operation in 1 patient (Case 3) is shown in Fig. 6.

## COMMENT

This experience indicates that complete repair is possible in the sick, small, cyanotic infant with transposition of the great vessels. It indicates also that many obstacles to survival exist in these patients, and that additional knowledge and refinements in technique are necessary if a lower mortality rate is to be achieved. Some of these refinements have been made and have been incorporated into the present method of care of these babies at the time of this report.

**Preoperative evaluation.** In cases of uncomplicated ventricular septal defect, atrial septal defect, and patent ductus arteriosus, irreducible pulmonary hypertension and an inoperable state are thought to exist when the pulmonary-systemic flow ratio is 1 or less.[3] The same appears to be true in cases of transposition of the great vessels.

The systolic pressure ratios of pulmonary ventricle to systemic ventricle were larger in 2 patients (Cases 6 and 7) after operation than before, which indicates that before operation the pulmonary-systemic blood flow ratio was less than 1. In Case 9, the 2-month-old baby showed only a small reduction in systolic pressure ratio of pulmonary ventricle to systemic ventricle after repair.

The pulmonary-systemic blood flow ratio in these infants must be assessed carefully in the preoperative period. If clear evidence of pulmonary plethora is noted on the roentgenogram of the thorax, operability is indicated. Otherwise, hemodynamic data must be obtained for calculation of pulmonary and systemic blood flow.

**Anesthesia.** Induction of anesthesia with cyclopropane and its maintenance with Fluothane have not caused discernible problems in the postoperative period and use of these agents is being continued. Use of muscle relaxants during maintenance of anesthesia is avoided because of their possible deleterious effect on ventilation in the postoperative period.

Knowledge of systemic venous pressure is essential during operation and the first 24 hours thereafter. A plastic needle inserted percutaneously into the external jugular vein serves well for this purpose, but if this is not possible the needle must be inserted into the femoral vein via the saphenous vein at the groin.

**Operation.** It is now believed[5] that circulatory arrest probably should not be prolonged beyond 30 minutes. Thus, in recent cases only a part of the procedure has been carried out during total circulatory arrest. Left atrial and pulmonary venous distention occurred in 1 patient during cooling. This led to the practice of opening the left atrium as cooling begins. An open ductus arteriosus must always be suspected and sought. Suture lines must be made with great precision, for even moderate bleeding after repair is highly disadvantageous in these sick small babies.

As soon as the field is exposed, the ductus arteriosus is isolated. It is found in the same general area as in patients without transposition. If patent, a ligature is placed around it and tied immediately after perfusion is started.

After cannulation, perfusion at 2.5 L. per minute per square meter is begun and cooling is started in the conservative manner previously described.[5] The vertical incision into the right anterior aspect of the left atrium is made (Fig. 7) and the intracardiac sucker is inserted for decompression of that chamber during cooling.

Body temperature is reduced to approximately 12° C. The level is judged by midesophageal temperature and by the tempera-

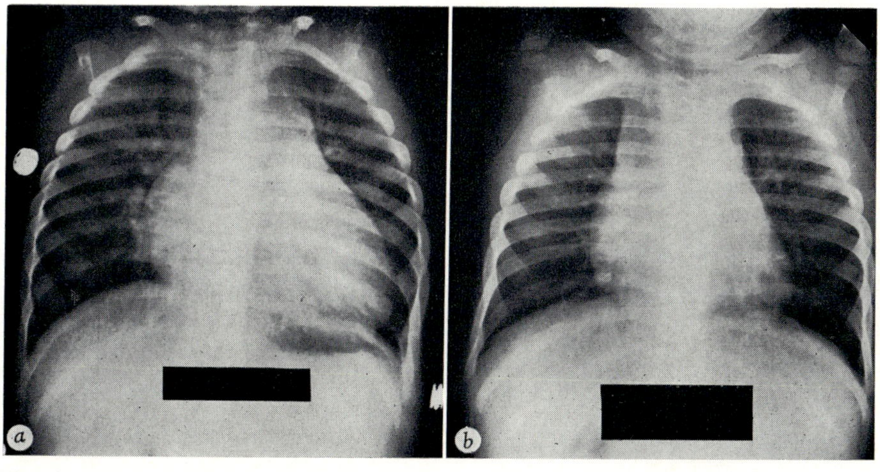


**Fig. 6.** Case 3. *a,* Before operation. *b,* Four months after operation. The reduction in heart size is evident.

ture of mixed venous blood. The aorta is cross-clamped. Perfusion is discontinued, the baby exsanguinated into the pump-oxygenator, and the right atrial cannula is removed. The right ventricle is opened by an incision paralleling the major coronary artery branches. The ventricular septal defect is repaired with interrupted silk sutures. The incision is made into the right atrium (Fig. 7), and the atrial septum is incised (Figs. 8 and 9) and resutured anterior to the orifices of the left pulmonary veins (Fig. 10). The posterior flap of right atrium is sutured anteriorly to the septal remnant (Fig. 11), completing the creation of a systemic venous atrium communicating with the mitral valve and left auricular appendage. This can all be accomplished in approximately 30 minutes. The venous cannula is inserted through the *left* auricular appendage and perfusion

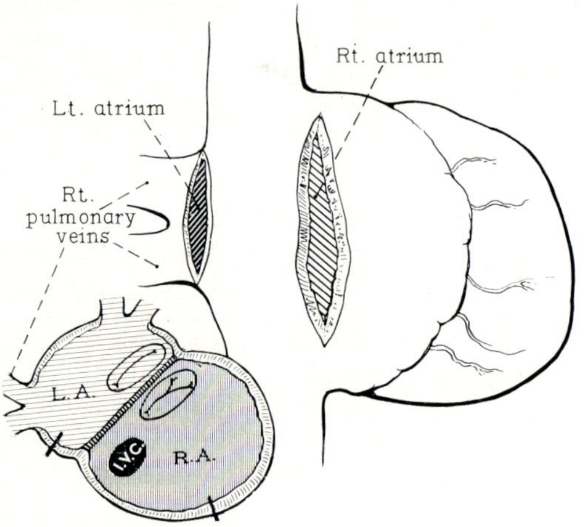


**Fig. 7.** Vertical incisions in right anterior aspect of left atrium and in right atrium. Insert shows incisions diagrammatically.

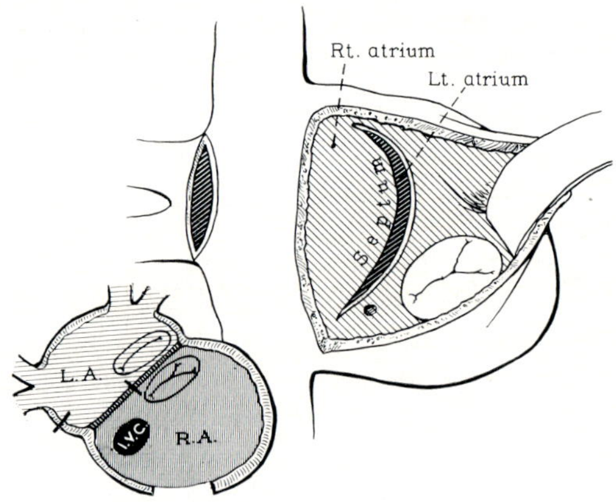


**Fig. 8.** Retraction exposes interior of right atrium, tricuspid valve, and coronary sinus. A long incision is made in atrial septum, anterior to fossa ovalis.

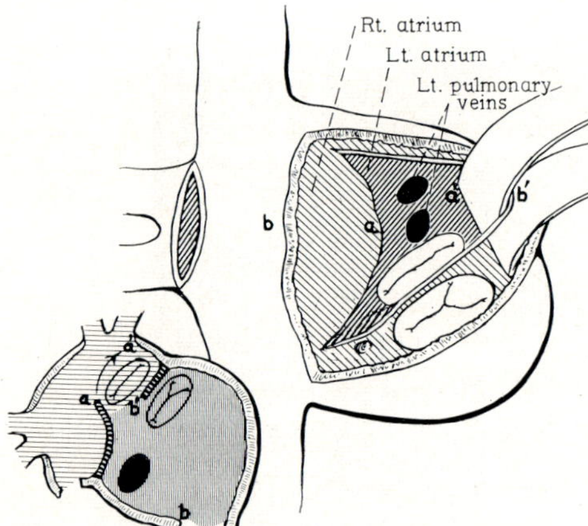


**Fig. 9.** Exposure of structures within left and right atria. *a,* Posterior septal flap; *a′*, left atrial wall; *b,* posterior right atrial flap; and *b′*, anterior septal remnant.

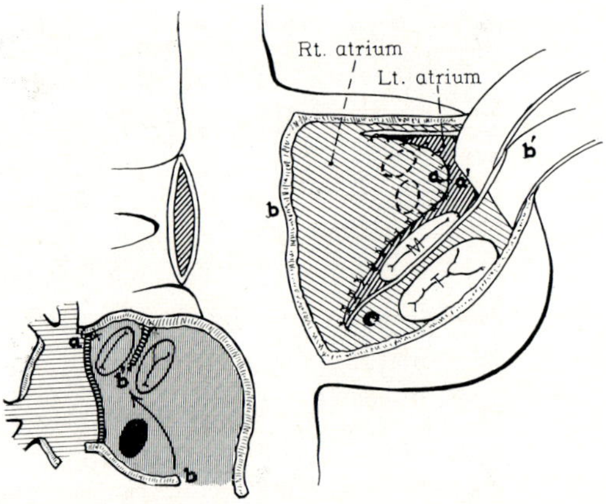


**Fig. 10.** Posterior septal flap *(a)* is sutured to left atrial wall *(a′)* just anterior to orifices of left pulmonary veins. This begins the construction of the pulmonary venous atrium.

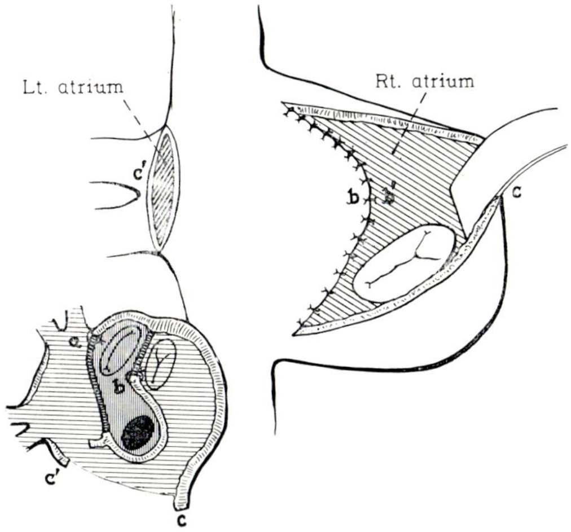


**Fig. 11.** Posterior right atrial flap *(b)* is sutured to anterior septal remnant *(b')*, creating a systemic and coronary venous atrium draining blood to mitral valve. At each end of this suture line flaps must be aligned so that there is no narrowing of caval orifices. Since this chamber is now complete, perfusion can again be established. Venous cannulation is through *left* auricular appendage.

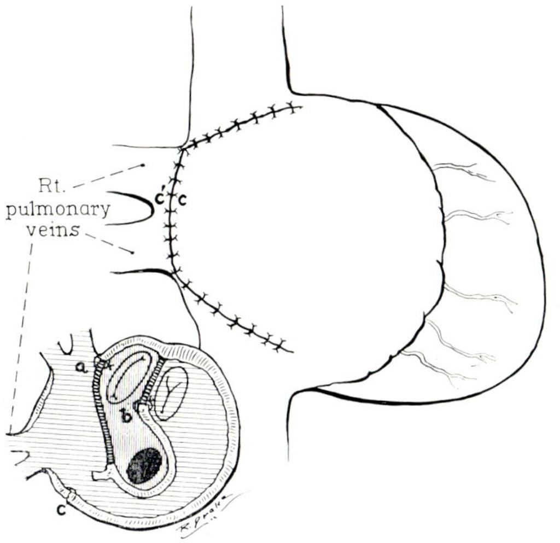


**Fig. 12.** The completion of the repair by suturing the anterior right atrial flap *(c)* to the posterior left atrial flap *(c')*. Pulmonary venous blood now drains to the tricuspid valve. This suture line in the thin-walled atria must be accurately placed throughout in order to prevent troublesome hemorrhage.

is begun at approximately 1 L. per minute per square meter with the perfusate at 18° C. The right ventricle is closed. Completion of the pulmonary venous chamber which communicates with the tricuspid valve and right auricular appendage is accomplished (Fig. 12). The intracardiac sucker is inserted into the right auricular appendage. The aortic clamp is removed. In the latter stages of the construction of the pulmonary venous chamber, flow rate is increased to 2.5 L. per minute per square meter and warming is begun. When the body temperature reaches 36° to 37° C., perfusion is discontinued.

**Supportive and postoperative care.** The need for administration of blood is determined by the venous and arterial pressures. Evidence for metabolic acidosis is sought and treatment is instituted. Digitalis is employed in therapeutic doses when indicated. In spite of these efforts, some infants may not survive because of cardiac failure (Cases 4 and 11). Respiratory complications were prominent in 2 patients (Cases 10 and 11); they pose a serious therapeutic challenge.

## SUMMARY

An experience with corrective surgical procedures for 11 patients with transposition of the great vessels is presented and the methods employed are described. Four patients survived, although 1 died 2½ months after dismissal from hospital of apparently unrelated interstitial pneumonia. The results in the other 3 patients appear to be excellent. A reduction of operative mortality rate demands additional knowledge and experience. When these are acquired, it is possible that the procedure can be accomplished in such critically ill infants at a more acceptable risk.

### REFERENCES

1. Albert, H. M.: Surgical correction of transposition of the great vessels, S. Forum **5:** 74-77, 1955.
2. Dawson, B., Theye, R. A., and Kirklin, J. W.: Halothane in open cardiac operations: a technic for use with extracorporeal circulation, Anesth. & Analg. **39:** 59-63, 1960.
3. DuShane, J. W., and Kirklin, J. W.: Selection for surgery of patients with ventricular septal defect and pulmonary hypertension, Circulation **21:** 13-20, 1960.

4. Kety, S. S.: Circulation and metabolism of the human brain in health and disease, Am. J. Med. **8:** 205-217, 1950.
5. Kirklin, J. W., Dawson, B., Devloo, R. A., and Theye, R. A.: Open intracardiac operations: use of circulatory arrest during hypothermia induced by blood cooling, Ann. Surg. In press.
6. Kirklin, J. W., and Payne, W. S.: Tetralogy of Fallot *in* Pediatric surgery, Chicago, The Year Book Publishers, Inc., in press.
7. Kirklin, J. W., Payne, W. S., Theye, R. A., and DuShane, J. W.: Factors affecting survival after open operation for tetralogy of Fallot, Ann. Surg. **152:** 485-493, 1960.
8. Senning, Å.: Surgical correction of transposition of the great vessels, SURGERY **45:** 966-980, 1959.

## DISCUSSION

**Dr. Denton A. Cooley** (Houston, Texas). Dr. Kirklin's presentation is significant since survival after total repair of complete transposition of the great vessels has been so rare. We have attempted to use the Senning technique 3 times without a survivor. Associated defects were present in each of the patients. Each had ventricular septal defects, one had a reversed shunt through a patent ductus arteriosus, and one 19-year-old boy had tight valvular pulmonic stenosis.

Again this year I would like to report our results with palliative therapy of transposition by means of the Blalock-Hanlon technique of creation of an atrial septal defect. During the past 6 years we have used this method in 45 patients with 30 survivors. In the recent group of 28 patients operated upon in a 2-year period, 23, or 82 per cent, survived operation. More than 40 per cent of our patients were less than 3 months of age. The improvement in the infants is particularly impressive, and we are satisfied with these results. Perhaps a two-stage procedure may ultimately be feasible in such patients. It would consist of creation of an atrial septal defect during infancy and subsequent total correction by the Senning procedure after the child had reached 3 to 5 years of age.

**Dr. John W. Kirklin** (closing). I think Dr. Cooley has raised a very important point, namely, whether one should perform an initial palliative operation in some of the infants prior to complete repair. I think it is extremely important to emphasize, as he has done, the fact that creation of an atrial septal defect does not compromise the possibility of performing a Senning procedure later. I suppose it will take considerably more time to know whether, in a 3-month-old baby for example, a preliminary palliative procedure or a primary complete repair should be carried out. I suppose it will depend ultimately on the risks involved in the 2 procedures.

# The surgical treatment of mitral insufficiency and combined mitral stenosis and insufficiency with use of the heart-lung machine

JEROME HAROLD KAY, M.D.
WILLIAM S. EGERTON, M.B.
PABLO ZUBIATE, M.D.
LOS ANGELES, CALIF.
*From the Department of Surgery of the University of Southern California School of Medicine, The Saint Vincent's Hospital, and The Los Angeles County General Hospital*

On Nov. 8, 1957, Gott and associates[2] presented a method for the open-heart correction of mitral insufficiency. This was an important milestone in the surgical treatment of rheumatic valvular heart disease and since then there have been other reports concerning open-heart operations for mitral insufficiency.

Thirty-four patients have been operated upon at The Saint Vincent's Hospital for mitral insufficiency or combined mitral stenosis and insufficiency in the past 2½ years.

## TECHNIQUE

The first 3 patients were operated upon by means of a right anterolateral approach. In the remaining 31 cases a median sternotomy incision was employed. Prior to the institution of cardiopulmonary bypass, the groove between the left and right atrium was dissected for a distance of approximately 1 cm. After bypass was begun, but before the left atrium was opened, a vent was placed in the left ventricle. This was accomplished by insertion of a trocar into the left ventricle near the apex of the heart. Care was taken to avoid cutting the descending branch of the left coronary artery. The trocar was removed and the vent was inserted into the ventricle. This vent prevented air from being ejected from the left ventricle into the aorta during ventricular contractions. It was kept in place until the mitral valve had been repaired and the left atrial incision had been closed. Before it was removed and the incision in the left ventricle closed, the apex of the heart was elevated and all the air from the left atrium and the left ventricle allowed to escape. After insertion of the left ventricular vent, the left atrium was opened posterior to the right atrium. The right atrium and anterior portion of the left atrium were retracted with a small Deaver retractor (Fig. 1). If there was fusion of the commissures, interrupted sutures of No. 2-0 silk were placed in the leaflets of the mitral valve. Traction was placed on these in order to better visualize the chordae tendineae while the commissurotomy was being performed.

Five types of insufficient valves have been encountered during repair. In the first type there was a stenosis of the anterolateral commissure with insufficiency at the posteromedial commissure (Fig. 2). In this condition an anterolateral commissurotomy was performed and the insufficiency at the posteromedial commissure corrected. A second type seen was a variation of this condition and consisted of a fusion of both the anterolateral and posteromedial commissures with insufficiency at or near the center of the

Aided by a grant from the United States Public Health Service and the Los Angeles County Heart Association.
Read at the Twenty-second Annual Meeting of the Society of University Surgeons, Kansas City, Kan., Feb. 9-11, 1961.

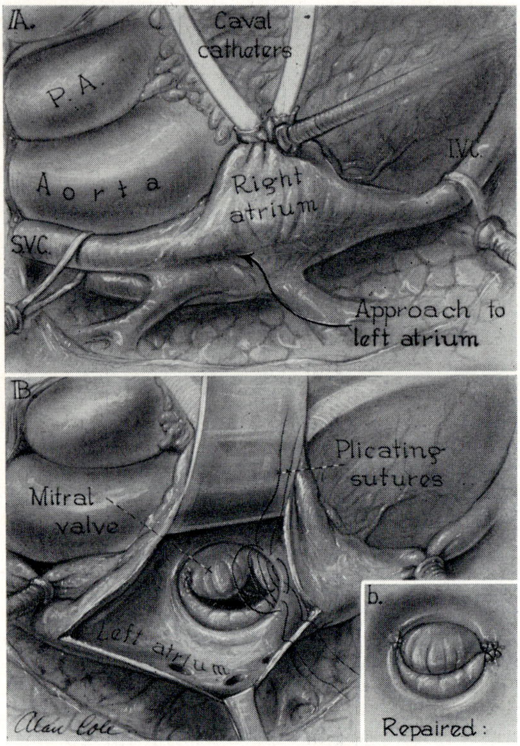


**Fig. 1.** Median sternotomy approach to the left atrium. The groove between the atria was dissected for 1 to 2 cm. Left atrium was opened posterior to the right atrium. Insufficiency was corrected after anterolateral commissurotomy had been performed.

mitral orifice. The opening in this valve prior to valvoplasty was usually about 1 to 1½ fingerbreadths wide. At times, with gentle or moderate pressure exerted by 1 or 2 fingers, the anterolateral or posteromedial area of fusion split in the anatomic position. If slight to moderate pressure did not produce a split, the commissure was opened with the use of a knife. Care was taken to avoid cutting the chordae tendineae. After the performance of the commissurotomy the function of the mitral valve could be evaluated by observation of the function of the heart as it beat in a dry field. Any insufficiency present could usually be corrected by foreshortening the annulus of the mural leaflet and preserving all of the annulus of the aortic leaflet. Usually a figure-of-eight suture of No. 2 silk was taken from the apex of the annulus at the posteromedial commissure to an area of the mural annulus about one-fourth of the distance from the apex of the annulus at the posteromedial commissure (Fig. 3). This suture could then be pulled tight and the function of the valve again assessed. Usually this was sufficient to correct the insufficiency and a second, similar reinforcing suture was taken at approximately the same area. The 2 sutures were then tied. The incision in the left atrium was closed with 2 rows of continuous No. 2-0 silk sutures. The left vent was removed and the incision in the left ventricle closed with interrupted figure-of-eight sutures of No. 2 silk. Case 1 concerns a patient with the second type of insufficient valve.

**Case 1.** A 46-year-old man had arthritis and chorea at the age of 9 years. He had been rejected from military service in 1942 because of a heart murmur. In 1953 there was an embolus to one kidney. Rapid palpitation had been present for 6 years before digitalis therapy was begun in 1953. In 1958 he had suffered a bout of severe chest pain with difficulty in breathing and 10 days later he noticed numbness of his left leg and foot which persisted for several hours. In 1958, a closed-heart operation was performed at another hospital. At the time of operation it was noted that the valve orifice was three-quarters of an inch in length and there was calcium in the aortic leaflet of the mitral valve. There was 3+ regurgitation through the mitral valve. The surgeon did not perform a commissurotomy for fear of increasing the insufficiency. The patient had no further emboli that could be detected until Feb. 23, 1960, at which time he had a pulmonary embolus and congestive failure. He was hospitalized until March 8, 1960, and lost 15 pounds while on a program of diuretic therapy. Anticoagulant therapy was begun. He remained fairly well while on a strict medical regimen which included a low-salt diet and administration of anticoagulants and digitalis. Prior to the present operation the patient's blood pressure was 100/58. There was enlargement of the heart with the apex at the left fifth intercostal space at the anterior axillary line. A grade III apical systolic murmur and a grade I apical diastolic murmur were present. There was an opening snap and an accentuated first mitral sound. The lungs were clear to percussion and auscultation. There were no râles. The liver was not palpable and no leg edema or ascites were present. On July 13, 1960, by means of a median sternotomy incision and open-heart operation with the heart-lung machine, the mitral valve was repaired. Although pressures were not measured at the time of operation it was believed that the left atrial pressure was nearly the same as the pulmonary artery pressure, approximately 60 mm. Hg. Examination of the mitral valve showed that there was an opening in the center approximately 1½ fingerbreadths wide. There was pronounced calcification of the posteromedial commissure. The anterolateral commissure was fused but the fusion was of a fibrous nature. There were pronounced rolled edges noted at the mural leaflet of the mitral valve. The aortic leaflet appeared to be fairly normal. With finger-fracture technique the posteromedial commissure was separated quite easily out to the annulus. However, in order to open the anterolateral commissure it was necessary to use a knife (Fig. 3). The anterolateral portion of the mitral valve was then competent, but there was still pronounced insufficiency at the posteromedial commissure. This was the same as it had been prior to the commissurotomy. The opening in the mitral valve was now 3½ fingerbreadths. The medial one-fifth of the mural annulus was foreshortened, as seen in Fig. 3. After closure of all of the incisions the patient was taken off cardiopulmonary bypass and it was noted that the pulmonary artery pressure was then only about one-third of the aortic pressure and the left atrial pressure appeared to be about one-third of what it had been prior to cardiopulmonary bypass. The patient made an uneventful recovery and 6 months after the operation he was able to play 18 holes of golf. No murmur was found on physical examination. The man was no longer on a salt-free diet and was maintained only on digitalis. The preoperative and postoperative roentgenograms can be seen in Fig. 4. There has been diminution in the size of the heart as well as in the size of the left atrial appendage.

In the third type of incompetent valve there was gross dilatation of the mitral annulus. No other abnormality was noted and except for the dilatation of the annulus the valve appeared quite normal. Occasionally there was slight thickening of the valve and as in the first type the insufficiency was usually present at the posteromedial commissure. The annulus in these patients was sometimes as large as 4 or 5 fingerbreadths. The correction of the insufficiency was essentially the same as for the first type and consisted of shortening the mural annulus at the posteromedial commissure with heavy sutures. It was also sometimes necessary to decrease slightly the size of the annulus of the mural leaflet at the anterolateral commissure with a figure-of-eight heavy silk suture (Fig. 5).

**Case 2.** A 42-year-old farmer was 6 feet, 4 inches tall and weighed 220 pounds. He had suffered frequent sore throats between the ages of 10 and 11. There was no history of rheumatic fever. A heart murmur had been first discovered when he was 26 years old. He felt well until 2 years prior to operation, at which time he developed episodes of atrial fibrillation. He was given digitalis, a low-salt diet, and quinidine therapy. During this period of time he was extremely fatigued and unable to work. He noticed exertional dyspnea, but there was no orthopnea, hemoptysis, or edema. At the time of physical ex-

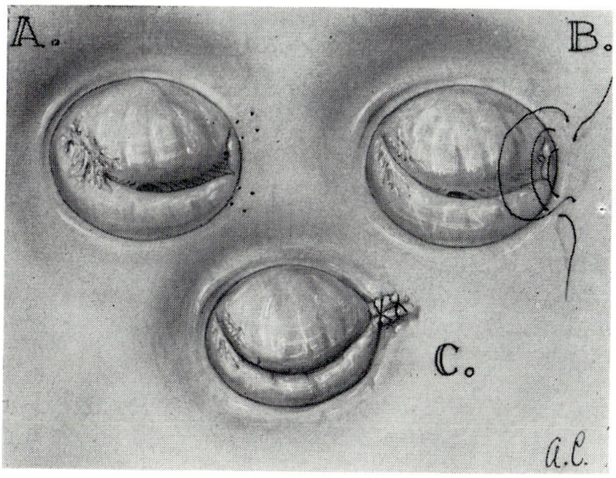


**Fig. 2.** Type 1. Insufficiency with stenosis of anterolateral commissure and insufficiency of posteromedial commissure. Commissurotomy was performed at anterolateral commissure and insufficiency corrected at posteromedial commissure.

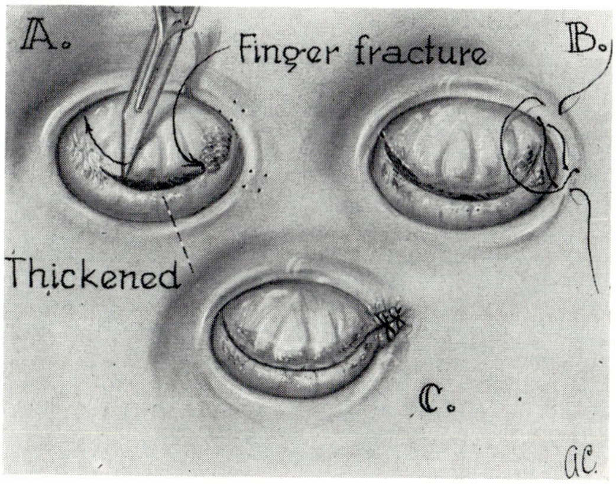


**Fig. 3.** Type 2. Stenosis caused by fusion of both commissures. Insufficiency was present at the center of the valve. Commissurotomy was performed at both commissures and insufficiency corrected at posteromedial commissure.

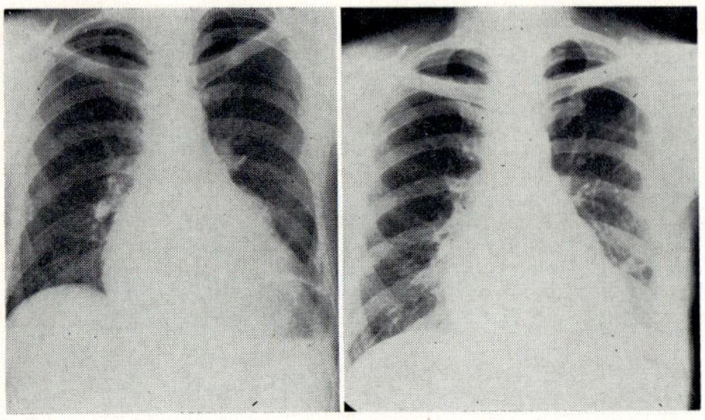

**Fig. 4.** Case 1. Preoperative chest roentgenogram and film taken 3 months after operation.

amination blood pressure was 140/70. The heart was slightly enlarged. There was a grade III to IV systolic murmur heard at the apex and referred into the axilla. Atrial fibrillation was present and no diastolic murmurs could be heard. Operation was performed on June 28, 1960. There was marked dilatation of the mitral annulus, which was at least 9 to 10 cm. in diameter. The aortic and mural leaflets appeared to be slightly thickened but of fairly normal consistency. The insufficiency was located at the posteromedial portion of the valve and was completely corrected by closure of only the posteromedial 4 cm. of the mural annulus. The aortic leaflet of the mitral valve then coapted perfectly against the mural leaflet. There was no evidence of mitral insufficiency. The mitral annulus was still 3 fingerbreadths in size. The patient made an uneventful recovery and 5 months after operation he was back at work with no detectable heart murmur.

In the fourth type of mitral insufficiency the abnormality was due to ruptured chordae tendineae with secondary dilatation of the annulus. In this lesion the portion of the leaflet of the mitral valve with the torn chordae tendineae was sutured with interrupted figure-of-eight sutures of No. 3-0 silk to the nearer papillary muscle. It was then usually necessary to narrow the annulus at the posteromedial commissure.

**Case 3.** A 50-year-old man had noticed shortness of breath on exertion for the previous 3 years. He had suffered 3 bouts of congestive failure and had been treated with bed rest and digitalis. He had noticed leg edema on occasion, but there was no history of orthopnea or hemoptysis. He tired quite easily. Physical examination showed a blood pressure of 120/80. The cardiac apex was at the left sixth intercostal space at the anterior axillary line, with a moderate left apical thrust and a grade IV apical systolic murmur referred into the axilla. This murmur was also referred into the right second intercostal space and over the entire precordium. The second pulmonary sound did not appear to be accentuated. The liver was palpable 2 fingerbreadths below the costal margin. There was no edema or ascites. On June 29, 1960, an operation was performed. The pulmonary artery was enlarged and the pulmonary artery pressure was noted to be approximately two-thirds of the aortic pressure. There was a grade IV to V systolic thrill over the left atrium and the left atrial pressure was approximately 35 or 40 mm. Hg. The left atrium was opened and the mitral annulus was found to be tremendous. It readily admitted 5 fingers. Three chordae tendineae at the medial portion of the aortic leaflet were found to be torn and were thought to be the primary source of the mitral insufficiency with secondary dilatation of the annulus. With 4 interrupted figure-of-eight sutures of No. 3-0 silk, the area of the aortic leaflet of the mitral valve where the chordae tendineae had been torn was sutured to the anterolateral papillary muscle. After this 2 interrupted figure-of-eight sutures of No. 2 silk were placed at the posteromedial commissure to exclude one-third of the mural annulus. This allowed better approximation of the mural and aortic leaflet during systole. However, there was still a slight amount of insufficiency present. This was corrected by placement of a figure-of-eight suture of No. 2-0 silk at the anterolateral commissure (Fig. 6). The patient had a complicated postoperative course and it was necessary to perform a tracheotomy. He gradually became better and was back at work 6 months after operation with no murmur audible. A section of lung removed at the time of operation showed severe pulmonary arteriosclerosis and hemosiderosis. Fig. 7 shows the improvement in the heart seen roentgenographically 3 months after operation.

The fifth type of valve with mitral insufficiency followed closed mitral commissurotomy. The insufficiency was usually due to a cut in the mural leaflet near the anterolateral commissure.

**Case 4.** In 1951 a 45-year-old woman had first noticed palpitation and a diagnosis of mitral stenosis was made. There was no history of rheumatic fever. Digitalis therapy was instituted in 1952 and at that time she had a cough, leg edema, and exertional dyspnea. An opening snap and a loud first sound as well as a systolic murmur were heard. Mitral commissurotomy was performed in 1954. She made an uneventful postoperative recovery but immediately after operation a loud systolic murmur was heard. In the year prior to the open-heart operation she had noted progressive dysnea which was pronounced on walking one-half flight of stairs or walking up a slight incline. There was no history of orthopnea, paroxysmal nocturnal dyspnea, or hemoptysis. On physical examination the blood pressure was 120/80. Rapid atrial fibrillation was present. The area of cardiac dullness was noted at the left fifth intercostal space midway between the midclavicular line and the anterior axillary line. There was a grade V apical systolic murmur referred to the axilla and back. $P_2$ was 3 times louder than $A_2$. The liver was not palpable. There was 2+ pitting leg edema. The lungs were clear to percussion and auscultation and no râles were present. Right-heart catheterization was performed. The right ventricular pressure was 60/7 simultaneously with a brachial artery pressure of 88/50. After 7 minutes of leg exercise the pulmonary artery pressure rose to 104/38. The patient was operated upon on July 21, 1960. There was a grade V systolic thrill over the left atrium and the left atrial pressure appeared to be at least 3 or 4 times normal. The pulmonary artery pressure was felt to be equal to the aortic pressure. On opening the left atrium it was apparent that at the previous operation the mural leaflet of the mitral valve had been cut approximately 4 mm. from the anterolateral commissure and the central 4 chordae tendineae of the aortic leaflet were torn. With 2 interrupted figure-of-eight sutures of No. 2-0 silk, the portion of the aortic leaflet of the mitral valve where the chordae tendineae were torn was sutured to the anterolateral papillary muscle. The previously made cut in the mural leaflet was also closed with 2 interrupted figure-of-eight sutures of No. 2-0 silk. The posteromedial aspect of the annulus was closed and the mitral annulus now easily admitted 2 fingers (Fig. 8). The opening had been 3½ fingerbreadths wide prior to annuloplasty. The patient made an uneventful postoperative recovery. At present she is engaging in full activity. There is a grade I apical systolic murmur present and the heart has decreased in size.

## COMMENT

In 1957, Lillehei and his co-workers[2] reported the cases of 5 patients operated upon with a right posterolateral incision through the bed of the fifth rib. The left atrium was opened posterior to the right atrium. All 5 of their patients survived the procedure and were much improved. In 4 patients mitral annuloplasty was performed. In the fifth patient an Ivalon prosthesis was sutured in place under the mural cusp in order to correct the insufficiency. In 1957, Merendino and Bruce[5] reported their results with the surgical treatment of mitral insufficiency by means of the open-heart technique in 2 patients. In 1958, Effler and associates[1] reported their technique of open-heart correction of mitral insufficiency. Their approach was somewhat different than Lillehei's in that the mitral valve was approached through a right anterolateral incision through the fourth intercostal space. The entry into the left atrium was then ac-

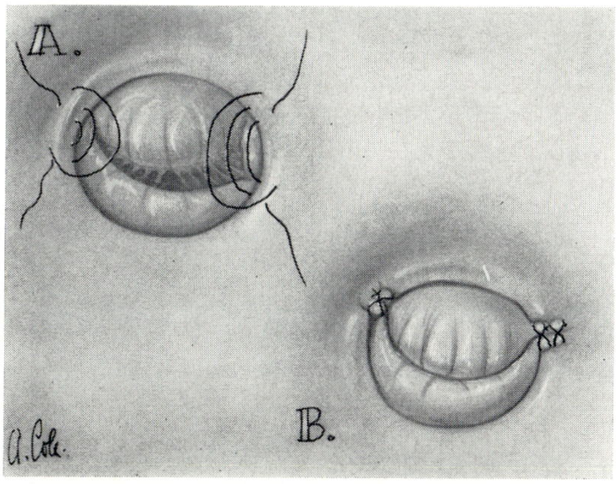


**Fig. 5.** Type 3. Insufficiency with only annular dilatation present. This type was usually corrected by shortening the annulus of mural leaflet at posteromedial commissure. Secondary similar suture may be necessary at anterolateral commissure.

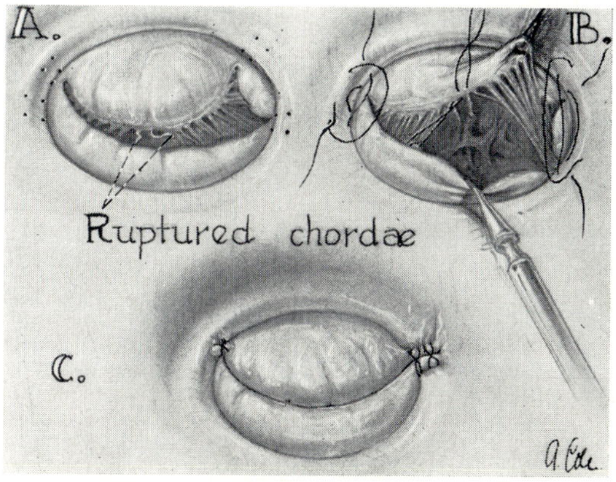


**Fig. 6.** Type 4. Mitral insufficiency due to torn chordae tendineae of the aortic leaflet repaired by suturing the involved area of the aortic leaflet to the anterolateral papillary muscle and then decreasing the size of the annulus.

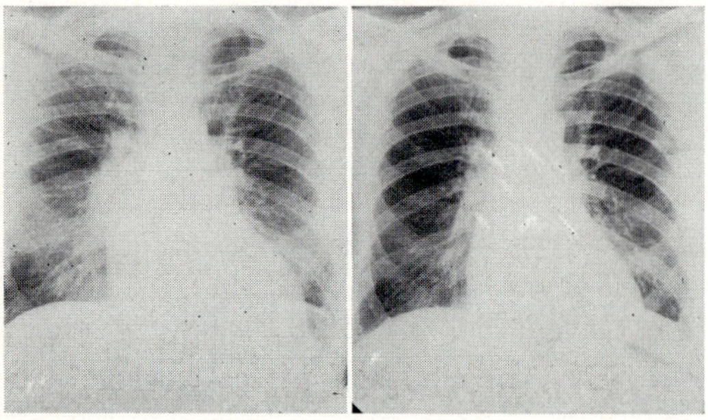

**Fig. 7.** Case 3. Preoperative roentgenogram and postoperative roentgenogram taken 4 months later which shows decrease in heart size.

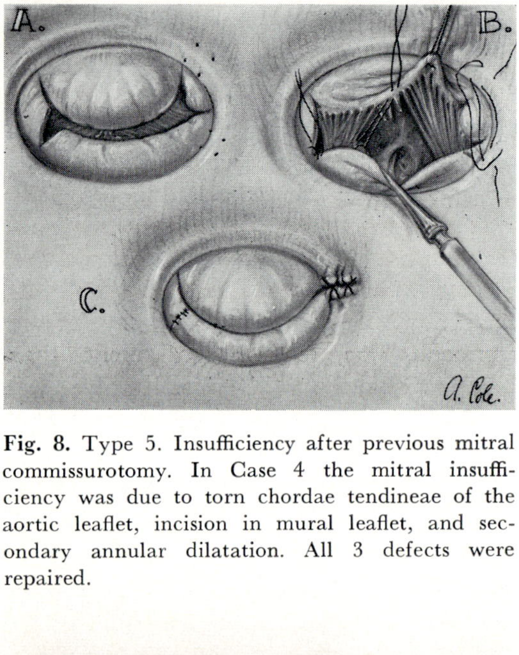


**Fig. 8.** Type 5. Insufficiency after previous mitral commissurotomy. In Case 4 the mitral insufficiency was due to torn chordae tendineae of the aortic leaflet, incision in mural leaflet, and secondary annular dilatation. All 3 defects were repaired.

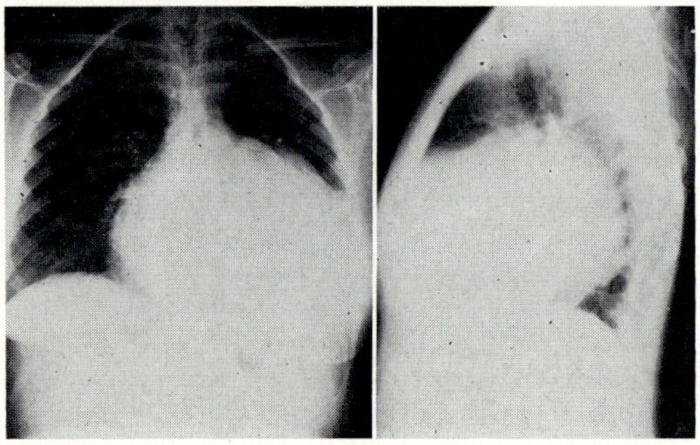

**Fig. 9.** Hypodynamic heart in patient with severe mitral insufficiency and secondary tricuspid insufficiency with pulsating liver. Patient died 24 hours after operation despite complete repair of mitral and tricuspid insufficiency.

complished either through the left atrium posterior to the right atrium on the right side or through a transsternal incision with the approach to the mitral valve made through the left atrial appendage. In still other cases they approached the mitral valve through the right anterior thoracotomy incision and then opened the right atrium and entered the left atrium through an incision in the foramen ovale. Effler stressed the importance of left-heart decompression through the left atrium. It was his belief that the left atrial vent prevented pulmonary damage by preventing high left-heart pressures which would be transmitted to the pulmonary vascular bed. The indwelling cannula in the left atrium also permitted the withdrawal of air from this chamber. In 1959, Helmsworth and his group[3] described the use of a left ventricular vent along with the use of a left atrial vent. Effler believed that the best treatment for ruptured chordae tendineae consisted of the approximation of the leaflets over the involved area by direct suture and buttressing of the atrial side by a crescent-shaped Ivalon prosthesis. For mitral insufficiency due to dilatation of the annulus it was his opinion that plication of the annulus over the anterolateral commissure would offer the best palliation. In 1958 Effler and co-workers were not enthusiastic about the surgical treatment of mitral insufficiency and believed that the ideal operation would consist of prosthetic valve replacement which would have to await the development of a satisfactory artificial valve. In 1958 Kay and his colleagues[4] described their method of correcting mitral insufficiency. They used the right anterolateral approach. They considered their results to be exceedingly satisfactory with methods similar to those of Lillehei. In 1961 Nichols and associates[6] described their open-heart technique for the surgical correction of mitral insufficiency. This was similar to other methods described, but the mitral valve was approached through a left posterolateral thoracotomy in the fifth intercostal space.

The present paper reports the cases of 34 patients operated upon for mitral insufficiency or combined mitral insufficiency and mitral stenosis. Although authors have preferred other approaches, the median sternotomy incision has been found to give adequate exposure. In order to avoid aortic air embolism a vent is placed in the left ventricle near the apex. This is removed as the last step in the procedure just prior to discontinuation of bypass. The first type of lesion discussed in this paper includes stenosis of the anterolateral commissure and insufficiency of the posteromedial commissure. In the second type there is associated stenosis of the posteromedial commissure with insufficiency at the center of the valve. A third type of valve was seen with gross dilatation of the annulus and no other abnormality. In the fourth type there were ruptured chordae tendineae with secondary dilatation of the annulus. In the fifth type the mitral insufficiency followed attempted closed-heart correction of mitral stenosis.

In 34 patients operated upon by the open-heart technique the most common method of treating the insufficiency consisted of decreasing the posteromedial portion of the annulus of the mural leaflet. The use of a plastic material has not been found necessary in any of these cases. Seven of the patients had undergone previous mitral commissurotomies and there have been 5 deaths in the entire series. There have been only 2 deaths among the last 28 patients treated. These deaths were usually in patients with tremendous hearts in whom there was not only a very hypodynamic heart associated with the mitral valve disease, but also secondary tricuspid insufficiency with chronic congestive failure and an enlarged, pulsating liver (Fig. 9).

## SUMMARY

The surgical treatment of mitral insufficiency has been described. The over-all mortality rate was 15 per cent. The results with this method have been most encouraging.

### REFERENCES

1. Effler, D. B., Groves, L. K., Martinez, W. V., and Kolff, W. J.: Open-heart surgery for mitral insufficiency, J. Thoracic Surg. **36:** 665-676, 1958.
2. Gott, V. L., DeWall, R. A., Gonzales, J. L., Hodges, P. C., Varco, R. L., and Lillehei, C. W.: The direct vision surgical correction of pure mitral insufficiency by use of annuloplasty or a valvular prosthesis, Univ. Minnesota M. Bull. **29:** 69-79, 1957.
3. Helmsworth, J. A., Kaplan, S., Clark, L. C., McAdams, A. J., Mathews, E. C., Edwards, F. K.: Myocardial injury associated with a systole induced with potassium citrate, Ann. Surg. **149:** 200-206, 1959.
4. Kay, E. B., Nogueira, C., Head, L. R., Coenen, J. P., Zimmerman, H. A.: Surgical treatment of mitral insufficiency, J. Thoracic Surg. **36:** 677-696, 1958.
5. Merendine, K. A., and Bruce, R. A.: One hundred and seventeen surgically treated cases of valvular rheumatic heart disease with preliminary report of two cases of mitral regurgitation treated under direct vision with the aid of a pump-oxygenator, J. A. M. A. **164:** 749, 1957.
6. Nichols, H. T., Blanco, G., Uricchio, J. F., and Likoff, W.: Open heart surgery for mitral regurgitation and stenosis, A. M. A. Arch. Surg. **82:** 128-138, 1961.

## DISCUSSION

**Dr. George H. A. Clowes, Jr.** (Cleveland, Ohio). We have operated upon 30 patients with mitral insufficiency now, 20 from the left side, 10 from the right side, and none through the midsternal incision. I think Dr. Kay has said the important things. After one has done whatever is necessary to free up the major valve leaflet, plication of the annulus is the most important feature of the repair. Our maneuvers have included removal of calcium from the leaflet, and repair of chordae tendineae that have been either fused or broken, but we have not put any prostheses into the mitral valve. Satisfactory results have been obtained in 65 to 70 per cent of the patients.

Dr. Kay mentioned another important matter. People who have had long-standing mitral valvular disease may have seriously damaged lungs with hypertrophied vessels secondary to long-standing pulmonary hypertension. If particular attention is not given to the respiratory activity immediately after the operation, inadequate gas exchange may take place. If pneumonitis is superimposed, the consequences of hypoxia or respiratory acidosis may be fatal. Under these conditions we have seen remarkable improvement brought about by the use of cortisone in addition to the usual steps taken to keep the lungs clear and aerating. We do not recommend the general use of corticoids, but they may be of great value in limiting postoperative pulmonary inflammation in patients of this sort.

**Dr. Osler A. Abbott** (Atlanta, Ga.). I would like to mention 2 aspects of this problem with which we have been concerned in a very limited series of patients who had surgical correction of mitral insufficiency by annular plication. First is the situation of a patient with a large dilated annulus associated with a significant decrease in the size of the valve leaflets. In one such instance the placement of annulus sutures in the usual areas (over the area of the posteromedial area and, to a lesser degree, the anterolateral commissural area) only narrowed the annulus without decreasing the insufficiency of the mitral valve. The leaflets seemed to be displaced downward without being brought into approximation. We decided to place the sutures through the annulus but, rather than bringing them out of the annulus above the valve substance, we continued the suture under the aortic or septal leaflet and entered the opposing area of annulus from below the leaflet. This suture was then brought around the annulus and re-entry made with the needle above the annulus. Then the suture was carried from the undersurface of the annulus along below the surface of the aortic or septal leaflet to emerge behind the opposing area of annulus within a few millimeters of the initial entry site of the suture. Thus, we have placed a mattress suture incorporating the annulus on each side of the aortic leaflet near the midpoint of its attachment, but the suture lay entirely below the leaflet without incorporating papillary muscles or chordae tendineae. Placing 3 or 4 such sutures and then drawing them snug not only narrows the annulus but advances the important septal leaflet toward the mural leaflet. In one such instance a gratifying result has been obtained by this method for a period of 8 months to date. Severe shortening of the chordae may increase the chance of needle injury of the leaflet during this maneuver. Such sutures may be placed and tested for their usefulness either in the annulus area near the dome of the septal leaflet or the usual zone of the annulus about the posteromedial commissure.

A second aspect of the problem has been the employment of continuous negative pressure within the primary pulmonary artery to aid in decompression of the pulmonary vascular bed during bypass. This can produce such sufficient reversal of blood flow within the lung that it can act as a good method for keeping the left atrium dry during direct-vision reconstruction procedures on the mitral valve.

**Dr. K. Alvin Merendino** (Seattle, Wash.). I appreciate very much the opportunity of hearing this excellent presentation by Dr. Kay, and I cannot resist saying a few things which I think should be said about this problem. First, I think that some have avoided this operation because of a fear that such sutures placed in the annulus will not hold securely. If the annulus is missed, there is no real strength in the adjacent tissues. However, our experience indicates that the sutures will certainly hold if they are in the annulus. We have not varied our original technique of the direct application of interrupted sutures approximating the posteromedial annulus. Our recent work-up of patients, some of which have now survived over 4 years, indicates that the initial good results have held up and remain excellent. As far as I am concerned, posteromedial annuloplasty has a tremendous value, not only in the patient with the dilated annulus, but often in patients who have an annulus of normal size. In the latter situation, merely a suture or two will frequently control the entire regurgitation. If one has posteromedial annuloplasty available, then the only time when one needs an artificial valve, in my opinion, is in cases of pure calcific mitral stenosis and mixed stenosis and insufficiency with calcification. The latter is the valve in which posteromedial annuloplasty has very little to offer in the control of regurgitation, and if one could excise and replace this valve, he would be way ahead of the situation. There are 2 other points that I think should be made with regard to mortality rate. Our biggest mortality rate has occurred in the patients with associated aortic insufficiency. The only way in our experience to control this is by cross-clamping the aorta. An aortic tourniquet does not control it as most of you well know. If one avoids the patient with the calcific valve and the patient with aortic insufficiency known to be present before operation, certainly the results are going to be good with posteromedial annuloplasty. If, however, functional aortic insufficiency occurs during operation, we have found that by elevation of the pericardium one can correct functional aortic insufficiency. In other words, when the heart becomes empty, the distortion or clockwise rotation of the myocardium by its sheer weight seems to distort the aortic annulus with resultant functional aortic insufficiency. If it is not recognized, one can have a very difficult time, indeed.

**Dr. Jerome H. Kay** (closing). I would like to thank the discussers. As Dr. Merendino stated, I also clamp the aorta whenever there is a fair amount of aortic insufficiency. However, I believe it is important in the patients with rheumatic heart disease not to clamp the aorta for more than 3 or 4 minutes at any one time. The heart-lung machine is also equipped with 4 coronary sinus suckers to keep the left atrium dry of blood during the repair. I think that actually we will need a plastic valve in only about 5 per cent of the patients and I think these will be the patients who have severely calcified valves.

# Myocardial response to prolonged acute oligemic hypotension

M. G. WEIDNER, JR., M.D.
LOREN ROTH*
F. A. SIMEONE, M.D.
CLEVELAND, OHIO
*From the Department of Surgery, Western Reserve University School of Medicine at Cleveland Metropolitan General Hospital*

Walton and his associates[3] have described the changes which take place in the force of myocardial contraction in dogs during hypotension produced by the repeated withdrawal of small increments of blood over a period of time. They described variable changes in heart force under the conditions of their experiment. More than half the dogs showed a pronounced decrease, some were not affected, and some showed an increase. Our experiments were undertaken to define the response of the heart to severe acute oligemic hypotension, with use of the data obtained with the Walton-Brodie strain gauge arch as well as from the usual techniques for hemodynamic studies.

## METHODS

Twenty-seven mongrel dogs which weighed 9.5 to 16.8 kilograms were anesthetized intravenously with pentobarbital sodium (27 mg. per kilogram). Artificial respiration was maintained by endotracheal tube and a mechanical respirator. The left side of the chest was opened through the fifth intercostal space. The pericardium was opened widely and fixed with sutures to form a cradle for the heart. A Walton-Brodie strain gauge arch was sutured to the left ventricle. The arms were then extended, as recommended by Boniface and associates,[1] so that the myocardium was stretched approximately 50 per cent beyond the diastolic length. Four cannulas were placed, (1) a polyethylene cannula (internal diameter 0.085 inch, length 8 inches) through a femoral artery into the aorta for rapid bleeding of the animal, (2) one in the other femoral artery for recording arterial pressures, (3) one through a femoral vein into the vena cava to a level above the renal veins for recording venous pressures, and (4) one through the left atrial appendage into the atrium for recording the left atrial pressures. In animals in which measurements of the cardiac output were made, a cannula was inserted through a jugular vein into the superior vena cava for injection of indocyanine green dye and one through a carotid artery into the aortic arch for withdrawal of blood. After all surgical procedures were completed, the animals were given heparin in the dosage of 5 mg. per kilogram of body weight.

The arterial, venous, and atrial pressures were recorded on a Grass polygraph by means of Statham pressure transducers. Electrical signals from the Walton-Brodie force gauge were led into the polygraph and recorded. The height of the control responses obtained before bleeding was assigned the value of 100. All other heights were expressed in

Supported by the Department of Army Grant No. DA-49-193-MD-2022.

Read at the Twenty-second Annual Meeting of the Society of University Surgeons, Kansas City, Kan., Feb. 9-11, 1961.

*Student Fellow of the Cleveland Area Heart Society.

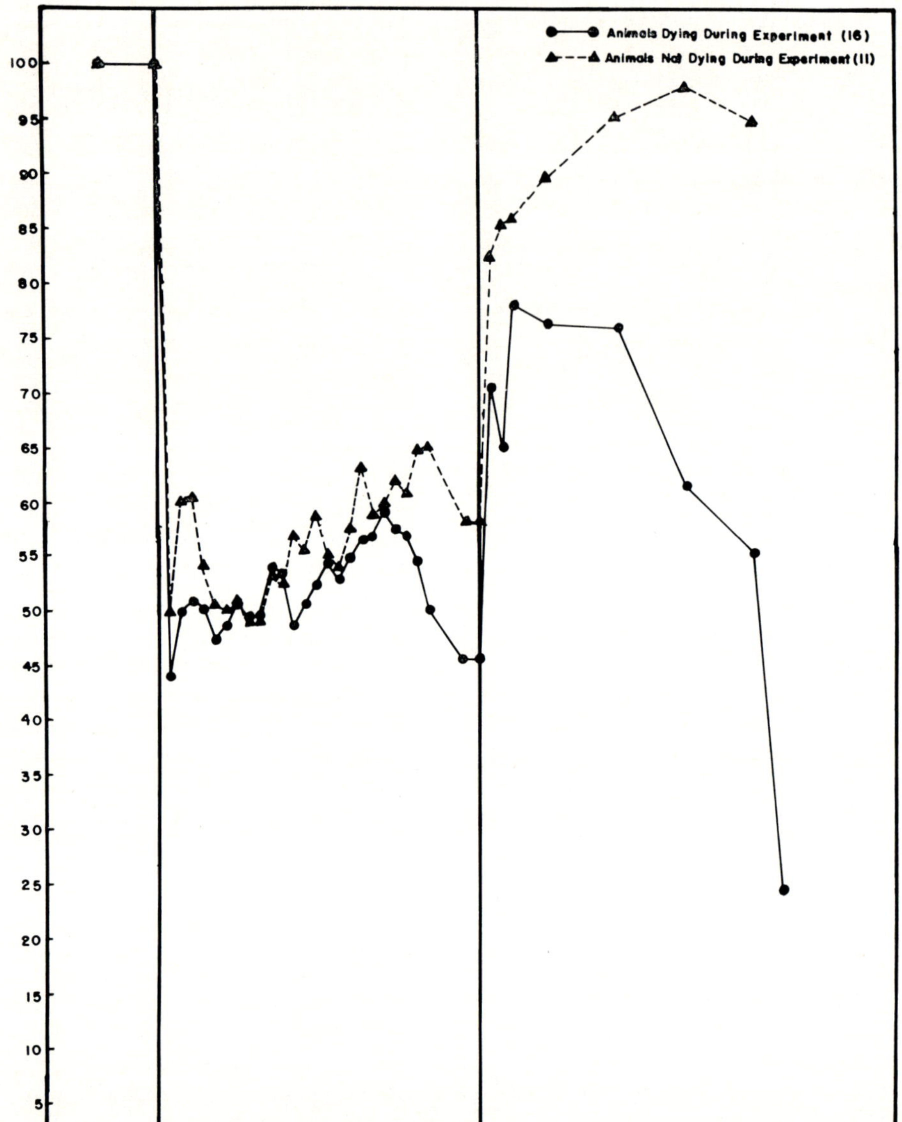


**Fig. 1.** The effect of acute prolonged oligemic hypotension upon myocardial contractile force is shown. The first vertical line represents the onset of bleeding, the second one represents the return of the blood to the animal.

percentages of this base line value. Cardiac outputs were measured by the dye dilution technique after injection of 2.5 mg. of indocyanine green dye into a jugular vein. Blood was drawn from the aortic arch through a Waters oximeter cuvette. The infrared output of the oximeter cuvette was recorded by the Grass polygraph. Lead II of the electrocardiogram was recorded.

After the initial measurements were recorded the animals were rapidly made hypotensive by bleeding into a siliconized bottle until a mean arterial pressure of 25 to 30 mm. Hg was reached. The initial bleeding time was from 1 to 3 minutes. The height of the reservoir was then adjusted to maintain this mean pressure. All animals were kept hypotensive until they began to reinfuse themselves from the reservoir without a rise in the mean arterial pressure. The animals were then reinfused and followed until death, or for 2 to 6 hours and then sacrificed.

## RESULTS

**Mortality rate.** Sixteen animals died during the experimental period. Five of these died either during or immediately after reinfusion. The remainder died before the end of the experiment. Observations on the 11 survivors continued for at least 2 hours after reinfusion.

**Bleeding.** Bleeding was performed rapidly in all animals. One to 3 minutes (average 2.2 minutes) was the time required to produce hypotension of the degree desired. In this series of experiments, the bleeding volume required to produce the desired levels of hypotension averaged 2.18 per cent of the body weight in all animals. The initial bleeding volume was 2.30 per cent of body weight in animals that lived and 2.04 per cent of body weight in those that died. The maximal volume bled averaged 3.53 per cent body weight in all animals, 3.76 per cent in the animals that survived, and 3.04 per cent body weight in those that died. The volume of blood in the reservoir just prior to reinfusion (final bleeding volume) averaged 3.05 per cent body weight in all animals, 3.43 per cent body weight in the survivors, and 2.62 per cent body weight in the nonsurvivors. These differences were not significant.

**Myocardial force.** With the rapid onset of oligemic hypotension, the force of the ventricular contractions fell to 45 to 50 per cent of the prebleeding value (Figs. 1 and 2). During the next 10 minutes, the contractions showed a more forceful pattern, but the change was not significant. After this burst of more forceful activity, the contractions again approached 50 per cent of the base line. There was then a general tendency for ventricular force to increase during the remainder of the period of hypotension. In the 11 animals that survived the experimental period, this degree of elevation was maintained (Figs. 1 and 3). In the 16 animals that died during the experiment, there was another decrease in force of contractions after approximately 90 minutes of oligemic hypotension (Figs. 1 and 4). During this time, the animals spontaneously infused themselves with blood from the reservoir.

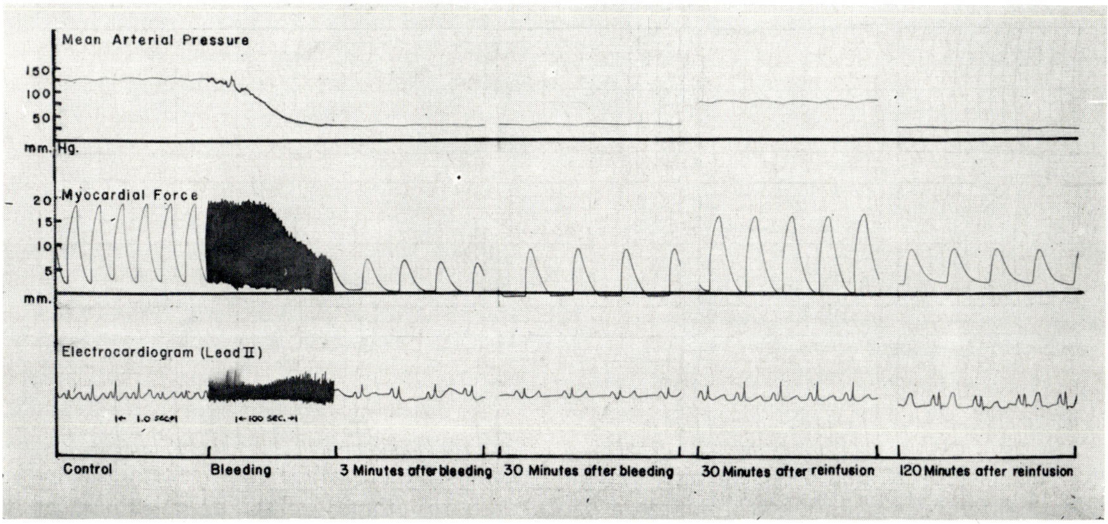


**Fig. 2.** Tracings from a typical experiment show recordings of mean arterial pressure, myocardial force, and electrocardiogram at the indicated times.

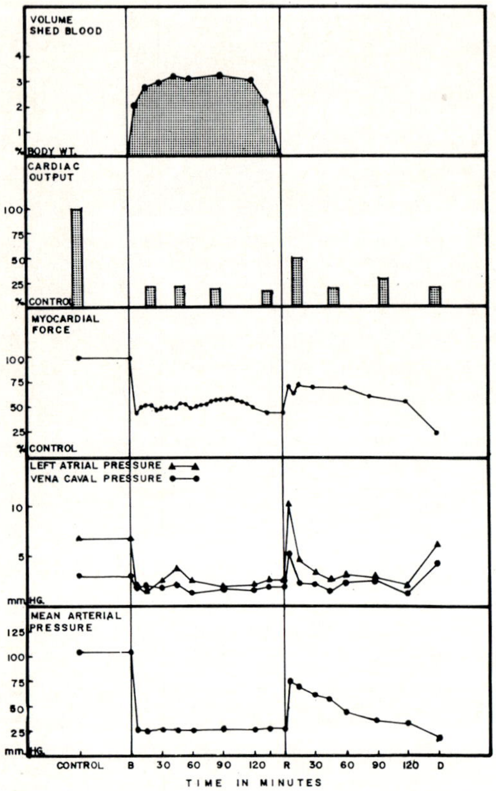


**Fig. 3.** The effect of oligemic hypotension upon myocardial force, cardiac output, and vena caval, left atrial, and mean arterial pressures is shown. These results are average values taken from the 11 animals which survived the experiment.

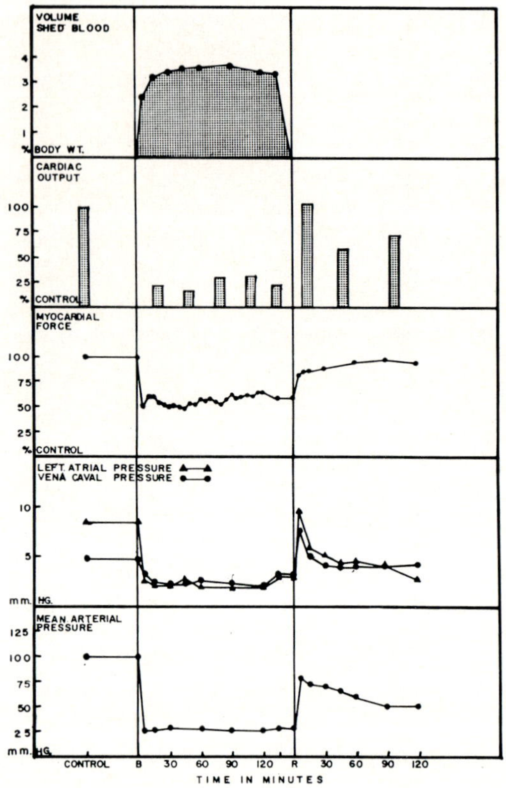


**Fig. 4.** The effect of oligemic hypotension upon myocardial force, cardiac output, and vena caval, left atrial, and mean arterial pressures is shown. These results are average values taken from the 16 animals that died during the experiment.

Upon mechanical reinfusion, myocardial force increased both in dogs that lived and those that died. In the 11 animals that survived after reinfusion, the force gradually approached the prebleeding value and remained at that level until the experiment was ended. In the 16 animals that died, the force approached prebleeding values and remained at that level for varying periods of time despite a progressively falling blood pressure. Finally, however, the myocardial force decreased until death.

**Vena caval and left atrial pressures.** During the period of hypotension the vena caval and left atrial pressures fell to very low values (Figs. 3 and 4). Generally, these pressures were maintained at the low levels. In an occasional animal there was a tendency for a slight increase in pressures, but never back to prebleeding values. Immediately after mechanical intra-arterial infusion over a period of 5 to 15 minutes, both pressures increased to slightly above prebleeding levels, but were not usually abnormally high. The pressures fell within 15 minutes to levels below normal which approximated the levels maintained during hypotension. In the animals that died during the experiment, there was a terminal increase in left atrial and vena caval pressures just prior to death (Fig. 4). However, these pressures were not abnormally high. Of particular importance is the fact that in all nonsurviving animals, the myocardial force remained high for at least 1 hour while the systemic arterial pressure progressively fell and the venous and left atrial pressures remained low (Fig. 4).

**Cardiac output.** Cardiac output fell to remarkably low values during oligemic hypotension, averaging 20 to 30 per cent of the prebleeding values (Figs. 3 and 4). Reinfusion in the animals that survived brought an increase in the cardiac output to approximately the prebleeding level. During the follow-up period the cardiac outputs in these animals fell slightly, but usually remained at 60 to 75 per cent of the prebleeding values until the experiment was discontinued (Fig. 3). In the animals that did not survive, the cardiac output increased to 50 per cent of the prebleeding value when the blood from the reservoir was rapidly infused. After 30 to 45 minutes the cardiac output in these animals rapidly fell to approximately 25 per cent of the prebleeding value and remained at this level until death (Fig. 4).

**Arterial pressure.** The arterial pressure was maintained at 25 to 30 mm. Hg by adjustment of the level of the reservoir. After reinfusion, the mean arterial pressure rose again to levels averaging 75 mm. Hg. In the animals that survived, the mean arterial pressure fell slightly and then remained at this lower level (Fig. 3). In the animals followed until death the arterial pressure failed to maintain itself for more than 15 to 30 minutes (Fig. 4).

**Electrocardiogram.** Electrocardiograms showed immediate depression of the ST segment and inversion of the T wave. Premature ventricular extrasystoles and ventricular tachycardia appeared late and were usually a warning that death was imminent. Extreme bradycardia usually followed the tachycardia and preceded ventricular fibrillation and death. All of these occurrences except ventricular fibrillation could be reversed with reinfusion of the blood.

**Heart rate.** The heart rate in the anesthetized animals was calculated from the electrocardiogram. The heart rate before bleeding averaged 160 beats per minute. Within 5 minutes of the onset of bleeding, the average heart rate was 133. The heart rate then continued to decrease through the experimental period. There were never any periods of tachycardia. There was no significant difference in heart rate between animals that survived and those that did not survive (Fig. 5).

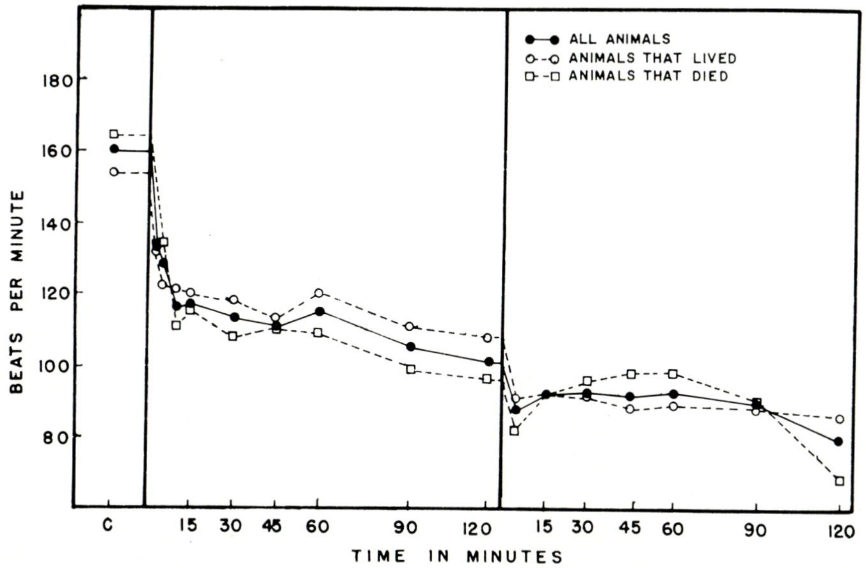


**Fig. 5.** This chart shows the effect of oligemic hypotension on the heart rate of animals anesthetized with pentobarbital. The first vertical line represents the onset of hemorrhage and the second represents the return of blood to the animal.

## COMMENT

One of the complicating factors in the study of shock has been the variety of methods utilized for the experimental model. While the present method presents yet another variation, it seemed preferable to produce the desired level of hypotension rapidly and to maintain it for an easily determined period of time. By this means, both early and late effects of oligemia could be studied with some precision with regard to level and duration of hypotension. Short periods of severe oligemia and hypertension can produce metabolic changes,[2] and it was believed, therefore, that the results from slower methods of producing the irreversible changes of oligemic hypotension would be difficult to interpret in terms of duration and severity of the stress. The present method was standardized in earlier studies and is a useful model for these specific variables.

The mortality rate during the experimental period was 60 per cent. However, it is probable that most of the other animals would have died had they been followed for longer periods. In the animals that survived, the blood pressure maintained itself at a level adequate to sustain life, though it was somewhat lower than the prebleeding level. In those that did not survive, the outcome could be foretold by a steadily decreasing arterial blood pressure after reinfusion.

The blood deficit necessary to produce the desired degree of hypotension was less in this series of animals than in those previously studied.[4] The blood loss during the preparation was not adequate to explain this difference. The deleterious additive effect of trauma on hemorrhagic shock is well known. The injury to tissue and other possible effects of trauma, aside from hemorrhage, could account for the somewhat decreased bleeding volumes because in the previous preparations there was essentially no operative trauma. The nonsurvivors exhibited insignificantly less bleeding volume than the survivors. The final bled volume of the nonsurvivors came close to being significant ($p = 0.1$) and indicates that these animals had taken back more of their blood prior to reinfusion.

The heart rates in these animals, anesthetized with Nembutal, were abnormally rapid prior to bleeding. Immediately after bleeding there was a relative bradycardia, which persisted throughout the experiment. Relative bradycardia has not been found in unanesthetized animals.[4]

The rapid production of oligemic hypotension shows immediate effects upon the heart, as reflected in force of ventricular contraction, electrocardiogram, cardiac output, heart rate, and venous pressure. The force of myocardial contraction, as measured by the Walton-Brodie strain gauge arch, decreases immediately to 50 per cent of the prebleeding value. This corresponds to an initial blood loss of 20 per cent of the estimated blood volume. The small increase in force seen throughout the hypotensive period could indicate that the myocardium can contract better if given the opportunity to do so. In fact, the force of myocardial contraction seems out of proportion to the very low cardiac output. A reasonable explanation for the slowly increasing force of contraction may be the progressive restoration of blood volume. During this prolonged period of time there will be hemodilution, which is detectable within 5 to 10 minutes of the onset of oligemia.

It was noted that in almost all animals there was a rather sharp increase in the force of ventricular contraction above the initial drop during the first 15 minutes after establishment of hypotension. In most animals it was noted also that small increments in bleeding after the establishment of hypotension would cause small increases in force. Walton and colleagues[3] also noted these changes and believed that they were the effects of sympathetic stimulation. These findings indicate the ability of the heart to compensate for acute blood loss by increased force of contraction.

It is known that after prolonged periods of oligemic hypotension metabolic changes have taken place in the myocardium, but the heart maintains the ability to contract with normal or nearly normal force until the very end. In fact, even though the blood pressure began to decrease shortly after reinfusion in the nonsurvivors, the myocardial force was maintained at or near the postinfusion level until a very low cardiac output was reached. The ventricular contractile force then fell off rapidly as death supervened.

There was no evidence that this terminal failure of ventricular contraction is the heart failure described clinically as right ventricular failure. These experiments demonstrate that the circulation, as manifested by arterial pressure, deteriorates after prolonged oligemic hypotension while the myocardial contractile force and the atrial and venous pressures remain near normal except during the terminal events.

The reason for the decrease in cardiac output and decreasing arterial pressure after reinfusion is a matter for speculation. Data from isotope studies indicate that after prolonged periods of oligemic hypotension there is selective pooling of blood in the splanchnic bed.[4]

The electrocardiograms of the animals showed immediate evidence of dysfunction, probably related to ischemia. This ischemia can be demonstrated also by polarographic studies made during oligemic hypotension.[2] However, the ability of the myocardium to recover is remarkable. Even after prolonged periods of hypotension, the electrocardiogram would return almost to normal after the return of blood.

While these studies do not define the cause of death from prolonged oligemic hypotension, they do suggest that the normal heart is not the weak link in the homeostatic chain. The myocardium can contract with normal force so long as it has an adequate volume of blood to propel. The primary cause of death in severe acute oligemic hypotension in previously normal dogs is not failure of the myocardium. It seems to be failure of adequate venous return secondary to accommodation of blood in other vascular beds.

## SUMMARY AND CONCLUSIONS

1. Experimental data are presented on the hemodynamic effects of severe acute oligemic hypotension. Parameters studied included myocardial force, arterial pressure, vena caval pressure, left atrial pressure, cardiac output, heart rate, and electrocardiogram.

2. The data indicate that the contractile force of the myocardium remains normal or nearly normal despite a progressive decrease in arterial pressure as the animal dies. The left atrial and vena caval pressures remain normal except for a terminal rise.

3. Failure of previously normal myocardium does not seem to be the cause of deterioration of the circulation and death in prolonged acute oligemic hypotension.

### REFERENCES

1. Boniface, K. J., Brodie, O. J., and Walton, R. P.: Resistance strain gauge arches for direct measurement of heart contractile force in animals, Proc. Soc. Exper. Biol. & Med. **84:** 263, 1953.
2. Simeone, F. A., Husni, E. A., and Weidner, M. G., Jr.: The effect of l-norepinephrine upon the myocardial oxygen tension and survival in acute hemorrhagic hypotension, SURGERY **44:** 168, 1958.
3. Walton, R. P., Richardson, J. A., Walton, R. P., Jr., and Thompson, W. L.: Sympathetic influences during hemorrhagic hypotension, Am. J. Physiol. **197:** 223, 1959.
4. Weidner, M. G., Jr., and Simeone, F. A. Unpublished data.

*(For discussion, see page 89.)*

# Dynamics of coronary arterial flow: flow alterations resulting from certain surgical procedures and drugs of surgical importance

ALBERT D. MENNO, M.D.
WORTHINGTON G. SCHENK, JR., M.D.*
BUFFALO, N. Y.
*From the Department of Surgery, University of Buffalo School of Medicine, and the Edward J. Meyer Memorial Hospital*

Measurement of coronary arterial blood flow is of considerable interest and importance for many reasons, not the least of which is the great need for quantitation of coronary blood flow in the evaluation of procedures aimed at myocardial revascularization for coronary arterial occlusive disease. The direct effects of various surgical manipulations and drugs on coronary arterial flow could not be studied previously because of inadequate instrumentation. This report presents data obtained in a study of coronary arterial pressure—flow alterations in a variety of experimental situations performed by means of new electronic techniques.

## METHODS

Young adult mongrel dogs ranging in weight from 20 to 32 kilograms were lightly anesthetized intravenously with pentobarbital sodium, intubated, and ventilated with a piston-type respirator. Leads were attached to the limbs to record the electrocardiogram and to trigger certain portions of the electronic recording equipment. Left ventricular pressure was recorded via a large-bore polyethylene catheter inserted into a carotid vessel and passed retrograde into the left ventricle. A second polyethylene catheter was inserted into a femoral artery and threaded retrograde to record aortic arch pressure. The single-ended inductance type of pressure transducers were employed. Through a left thoracotomy, a 2 cm. length of the proximal portion of the circumflex branch of the left coronary artery was isolated to allow placement of the flow transducer as shown in Fig. 1. Both pulsatile and mean flow through the intact coronary artery could then be recorded by use of the noncannulating square-wave electromagnetic flowmeter* described by Denison.[2]

An analogue computer integrator unit (K3-J†) was used to obtain the total flow during each individual cardiac cycle (the time integral, which measures the area under the instantaneous coronary arterial flow curve). This computer unit was "clamped" back to the zero base line just before each ventricular contraction by a pulse derived from the electrocardiogram R wave, suitably amplified (Philbrick UPA—2) and capacitatively coupled to a clamping relay. This arrangement permitted recording of both instantaneous coronary arterial flow wave form and total coronary flow per cardiac cycle.

Supported by grants-in-aid from the United States Public Health Service (H-3181) and the Erie County Heart Association.

Read at the Twenty-second Annual Meeting of the Society of University Sugeons, Kansas City, Kan., Feb. 9-11, 1961.

*Buswell Fellow in Surgical Research.

*Made by Carolina Medical Electronics, Winston-Salem, N. C.

†Philbrick Researches, Inc., Boston, Mass.

All the parameters were recorded simultaneously on a multichannel direct-writing recorder.

## RESULTS

**Normal coronary arterial dynamics.** Simultaneous recordings of aortic arch pressure and circumflex coronary artery pressure are seen in Fig. 2. It will be noted that the pressure wave forms were virtually identical in both excursion and phase. Hence, it was permissible to record the more easily obtainable aortic arch pressure in lieu of coronary artery pressure.

Pulsatile and mean pressure-flow data from a normal animal are shown in Fig. 3. It is apparent from comparison of arch pressure and coronary flow tracings that coronary flow and coronary pressure vary reciprocally, with the seeming paradox that peak coronary flow occurs with minimal coronary arterial pressure. The coronary flow pattern was found to be almost a mirror image of the left ventricular pressure curve, with most of coronary flow occurring when ventricular pressure was minimal. The normal systolic to diastolic flow ratio is approximately 1 to 6. If one compares the ventricular pressure curve and coronary flow curve, it can be seen that coronary flow dropped suddenly when ventricular pressure rose above a value which averaged 32 mm. Hg in this group of experiments. Similarly, coronary flow increased rapidly when ventricular pressure dropped again below a value which averaged 84 mm. Hg. The difference was probably a reflection of a difference in coronary artery pressure which was higher in the latter instance. The total coronary flow per stroke was indicated by the height to which the integrator curve rose above the base line before it was returned to that base line by the electrocardiogram-clamp circuit.

Flow values obtained by this method in 12 experiments are shown in Table I. Mean flow through this coronary vessel was 52 ± 5.6 ml. per minute per 100 Gm. of left ventricle. Response of coronary flow to momentary occlusion is illustrated in Fig. 4. After the fall to zero flow there was a marked "overshoot" of flow, which often amounted to a temporary threefold increment over the preocclusion value.

**Table I.** *Control values of left circumflex coronary artery flow (12 experiments)*

| | *Mean* | *Range* |
|---|---|---|
| Coronary flow (ml./min.) | 73 | 57-83 |
| Heart weight (Gm.) | 224 | 153-275 |
| Flow/100 Gm. of heart (ml./min.) | 33 | 27-41 |
| Flow/100 Gm. of left ventricle (ml./min.) | 52* | 41-64 |
| Mean blood pressure (mm. Hg) | 120 | 100-147 |

*Standard deviation ± 5.6.

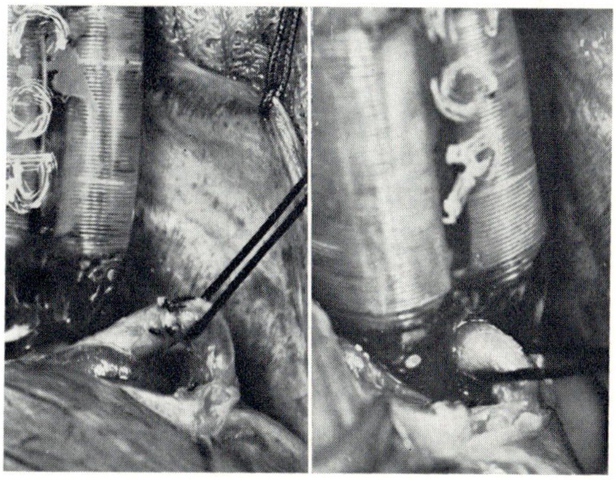

A B

**Fig. 1.** *A,* Coronary artery exposed for flow measurement. *B,* Flow probe in place.

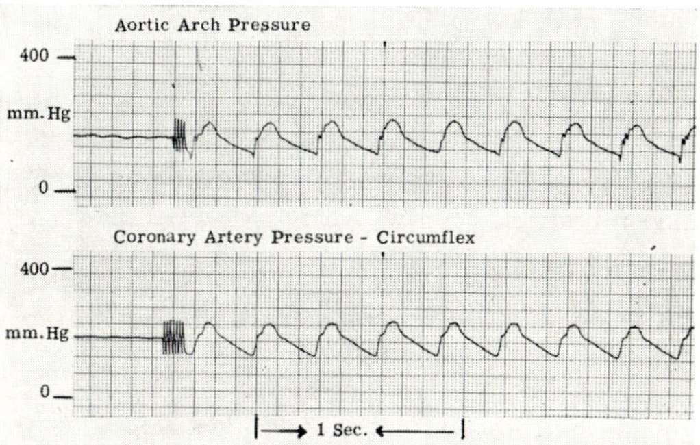


**Fig. 2.** Simultaneous recordings of coronary artery and aortic arch pressures.

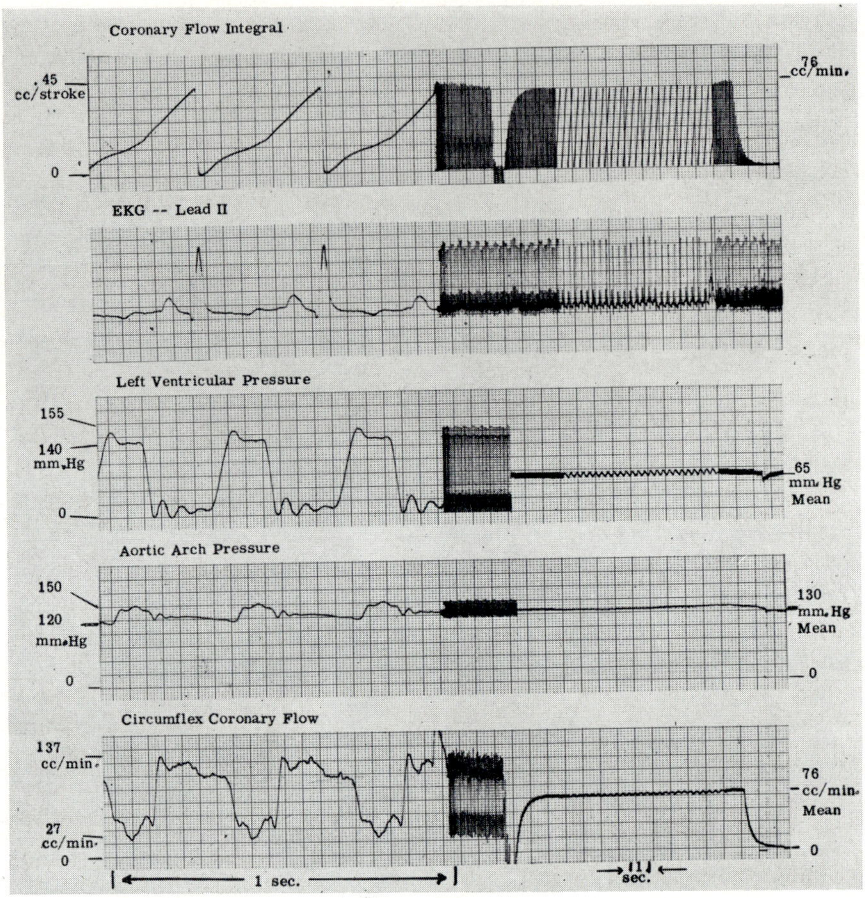


**Fig. 3. Simultaneous** recordings of coronary arterial flow, aortic arch pressure, left ventricular pressure, electrocardiogram, and coronary flow integral.

**Augmentation of coronary flow.**

*Mechanical.* An often used clinical expedient "to increase coronary blood flow" is the temporary occlusion of some aortic branch in an attempt to compensate for sudden hypotension or cardiac arrhythmia. The influence of this maneuver upon coronary arterial flow was evaluated quantitatively.

Occlusion of an aortic arch branch, the brachiocephalic artery, produced the alterations seen in Fig. 5. It will be noted that both arch pressure and coronary flow increased. Relative increases in arch pressure as compared with coronary flow are seen in Fig. 6. In 5 of the 7 experiments arch pressure increased proportionately more than coronary arterial flow.

Occlusion of the descending aorta also produced increases in both arch pressure and coronary flow as seen in Fig. 7, but with a reversal in relative changes from those in the previous experimental group. Fig. 8 illustrates the alterations observed in 9 ex-

**Table II.** *Effect of epinephrine on coronary blood flow*

| Experiment No. | Dose (mg.) | Coronary arterial flow (ml.) Control | Coronary arterial flow (ml.) Maximum after epinephrine | % rise in coronary flow |
|---|---|---|---|---|
| 3 | 0.4 | 25 | 154 | 516 |
| 6 | 0.4 | 90 | 390 | 334 |
| 10 | 0.1 | 63 | 399 | 533 |
| 13 | 0.3 | 84 | 420 | 400 |
| 14 | 0.4 | 63 | 350 | 455 |

periments and shows a greater increase in coronary flow than in arch pressure for 7 of the 9 animals.

*Pharmacologic.* The place of vasoconstrictor agents in the surgeon's armamentarium is still debatable. The influence of 2 such agents on coronary arterial blood flow has been studied, with the effects of epinephrine illustrated in Fig. 9. Shortly after intravenous injection of epinephrine, coronary flow showed approximately equal increase in its systolic and diastolic components so that the flow excursion was little altered. This was followed by a brief phase during which flow excursion was greatly widened, with reverse flow exhibited during a portion of each cycle. The third phase was reached when both systolic and diastolic portions of the coronary flow curve were greatly increased above the control values. The effect terminated with gradual fall in flow back to control values. The maximum response in coronary arterial flow to the intravenous administration of epinephrine is illustrated in Table II. A three- to fivefold increase in mean coronary flow is shown by these data.

L-norepinephrine (Levophed) produced a somewhat different response, as shown in Fig. 10, so that the reversal of coronary flow during each cycle continued throughout the early response to the agent.

*Hypoxia.* Because of a variety of causes, anesthetized patients occasionally become hypoxic, although this is never part of the surgeon's plan. Hence, the effect of this metabolic disturbance interests the surgeon. The response of coronary arterial blood flow to inhalation of a mixture of 10 per cent oxygen and 90 per cent nitrogen is shown in Fig. 11. Oxygen saturation of arterial blood was recorded continuously by use of a cuvette densitometer oximeter calibrated against the Van Slyke manometric apparatus. Coronary arterial flow increased in response to the hypoxia (+41 per cent) but not in exact proportion to the reduction in arterial oxygen saturation (–55 per cent). After coronary occlusion, "overshoot" still occurred which indicated further potential arterial vasomotor activity.

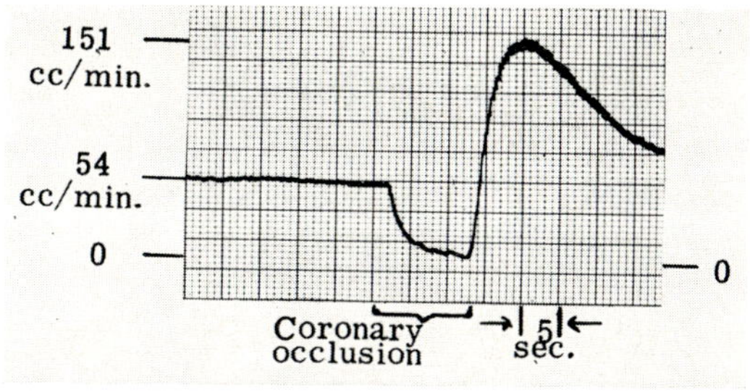


**Fig. 4.** Effect on coronary arterial flow of momentary occlusion of coronary artery. Overshoot is marked after fall to zero.

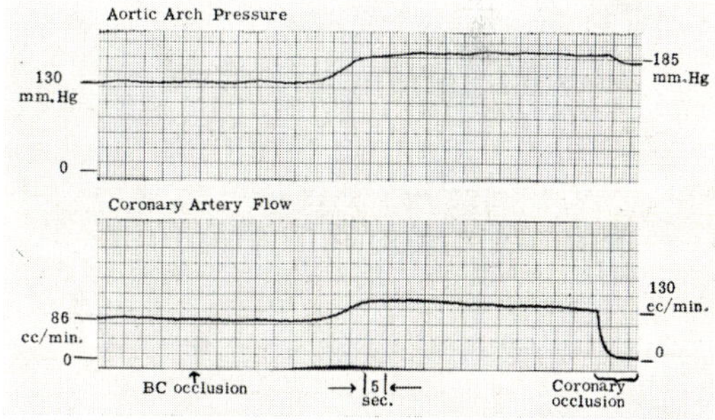


**Fig. 5.** Response of coronary arterial flow and aortic arch pressure to occlusion of brachiocephalic artery.

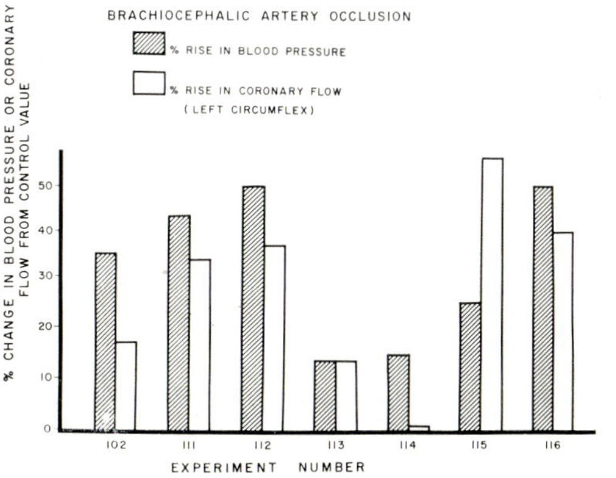


**Fig. 6.** Relative alterations of arterial pressure and coronary flow which result from brachiocephalic artery occlusion.

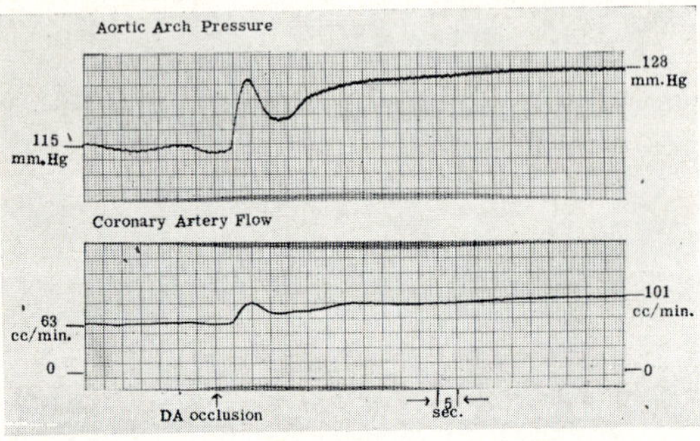


**Fig. 7.** Response of coronary arterial flow and aortic arch pressure to occlusion of descending aorta.

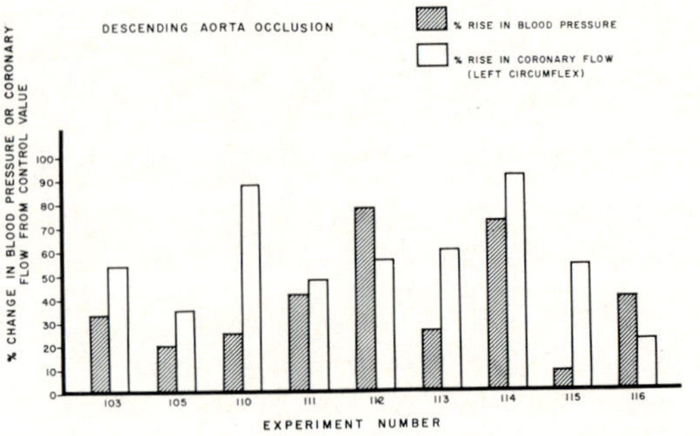


**Fig. 8.** Relative alterations of arterial pressure and coronary flow which result from occlusion of descending aorta.

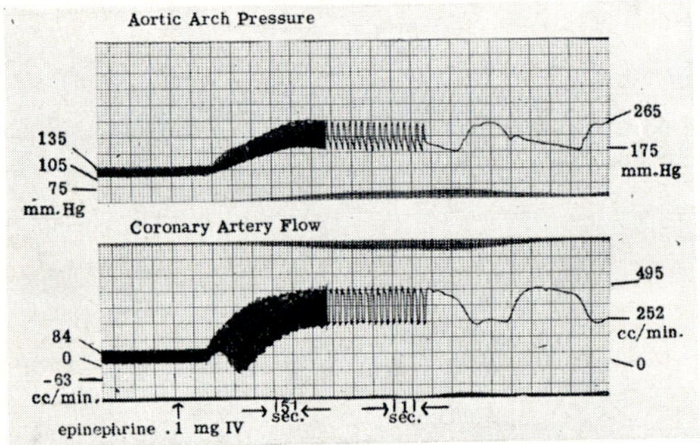


**Fig. 9.** Response of coronary flow and arterial pressure to intravenous administration of epinephrine.

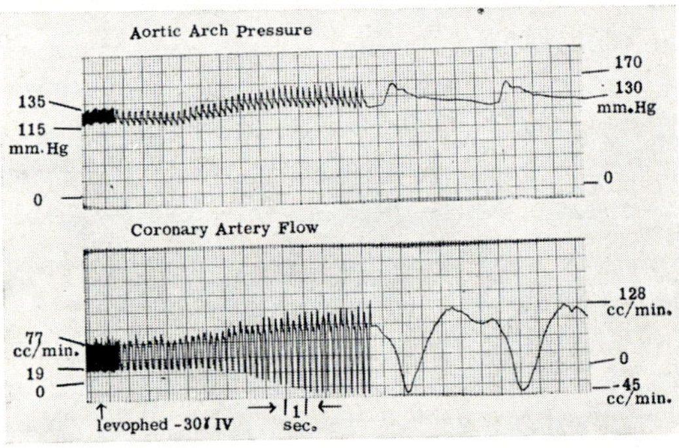


**Fig. 10.** Response of coronary flow and arterial pressure to intravenous administration of 1-norepinephrine.

**Induced hypotension.** Elective reduction of arterial pressure would have much wider surgical application if this procedure could be shown to be physiologically safe. The response of coronary arterial flow and aortic arch pressure to intravenous Arfonad administration is seen in Fig. 12. Profound reduction in aortic arch mean pressure was accompanied by only a small reduction in coronary flow.

**Aortic insufficiency.** Alteration in coronary arterial flow shortly after creation of aortic insufficiency by transventricular valvulotomy of the noncoronary cusp is seen in Fig. 13. Of greatest interest is the fact that coronary arterial flow peaks coincide with ventricular pressure peaks under these conditions. This is a direct reversal of the findings in the normal animal, for the systolic to diastolic flow ration was approximately 2.5 to 1 in this experiment. This observation has been confirmed in 3 animals to date.

## COMMENT

The methods used for flow measurement in this study were the same as those described by Marston and associates,[4] without whose assistance this work would not have been possible.

Our findings in regard to the phasic flow pattern in the left coronary arteries of normal dogs differ somewhat from those of Gregg and Green,[3] who used a differential manometric method. Their records show a small backflow phase to be present in the normal animal. This has never been seen in our experiments on the normal animal but did appear in response to vasoconstrictors.

While we have not included the fact as part of our data, the anterior descending branch of the left coronary artery has carried about 50 per cent as much flow as the circumflex branch in our experimental animals.

The estimate for total left coronary flow by this method would thus be 78 ml. per minute per 100 Gm. of ventricle, which is in the same range as the findings of Gregg and Green.

The phenomenon of "overshoot" in flow after arterial occlusion has been regularly observed in our work with other vessels, but has never been as pronounced as that exhibited by the coronary arteries. An astute observation which aids in the interpretation of this phenomenon was made by Dr. William M. Chardack[1] and the evidence shown in Fig. 14 is included with his permission. This illustration includes simultaneous recordings of aortic arch blood pressure (bottom), left circumflex coronary arterial flow (center), and electrocardiogram (top). Heart block had been produced experimentally in this animal and cardiac rate was determined by a pacemaker. Cardiac rate as set by the pacemaker is indicated beneath each electrocardiographic tracing. At frequent intervals coronary flow was brought to zero as a result of asystole after temporary cessation of the pacemaker impulse as shown at points *3, 4,* and *5.* This phenomenon is confirmed by the absence of any electrocardiogram and the abrupt fall in aortic arch blood pressure to zero. As systole resumed there was no "overshoot" in coronary flow. At points *7* and *10* coronary artery occlusion was performed and this was followed by prompt "overshoot" on release. This information supports the concept that "overshoot" is a result of vasodilatation which is possibly due to accumulation of metabolites. Point *6* in this recording is an "electronic zero" obtained by turning off the electromagnet supply voltage.

Another point of some interest gained from this tracing is the finding that coronary flow increases with increase in rate up

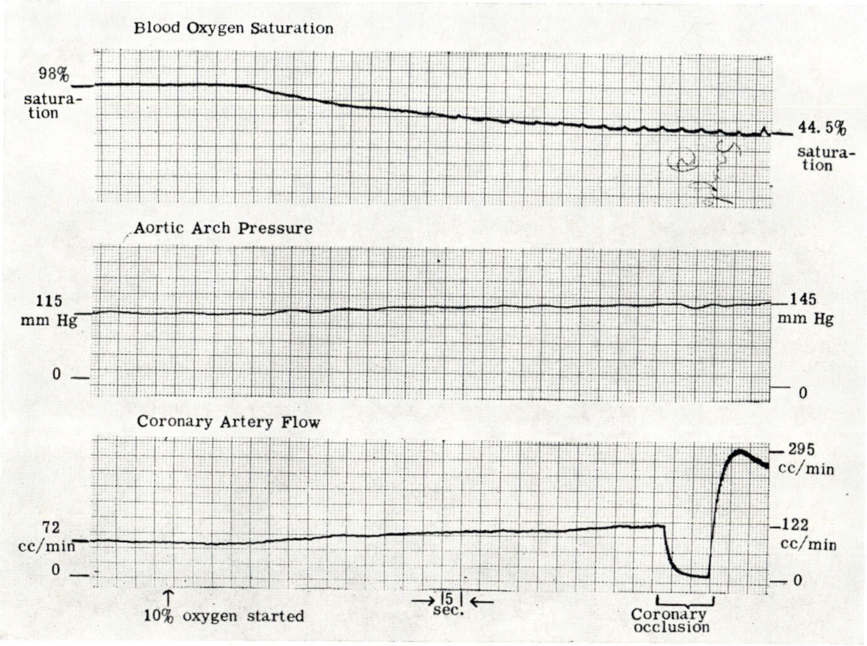


**Fig. 11.** Effect of hypoxia on coronary blood flow.

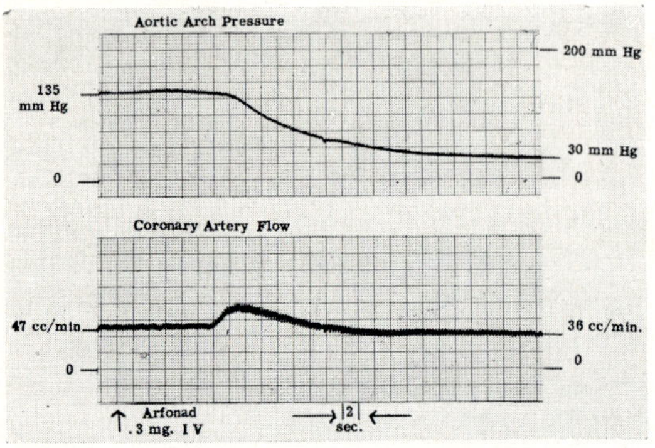


**Fig. 12.** Effect of intravenous Arfonad administration upon arterial pressure and coronary blood flow. Profound reduction in aortic arch mean pressure was accompanied by only a small reduction in coronary flow.

to 140 beats per minute, then decreases as rate is further increased.

The difference in response of coronary flow and arch pressure produced by occlusion of the brachiocephalic artery and descending aorta is perplexing and has served to demonstrate that there is another determinant, or determinants, for coronary flow which have not been delineated.

It is possible that the differences seen are the result of differences in activity of the carotid body, since with brachiocephalic artery occlusion it "perceives" a low pressure, and with descending aorta occlusion it "perceives" a high pressure. However, the mode of mediation of the coronary flow responses in the two situations remains unsettled.

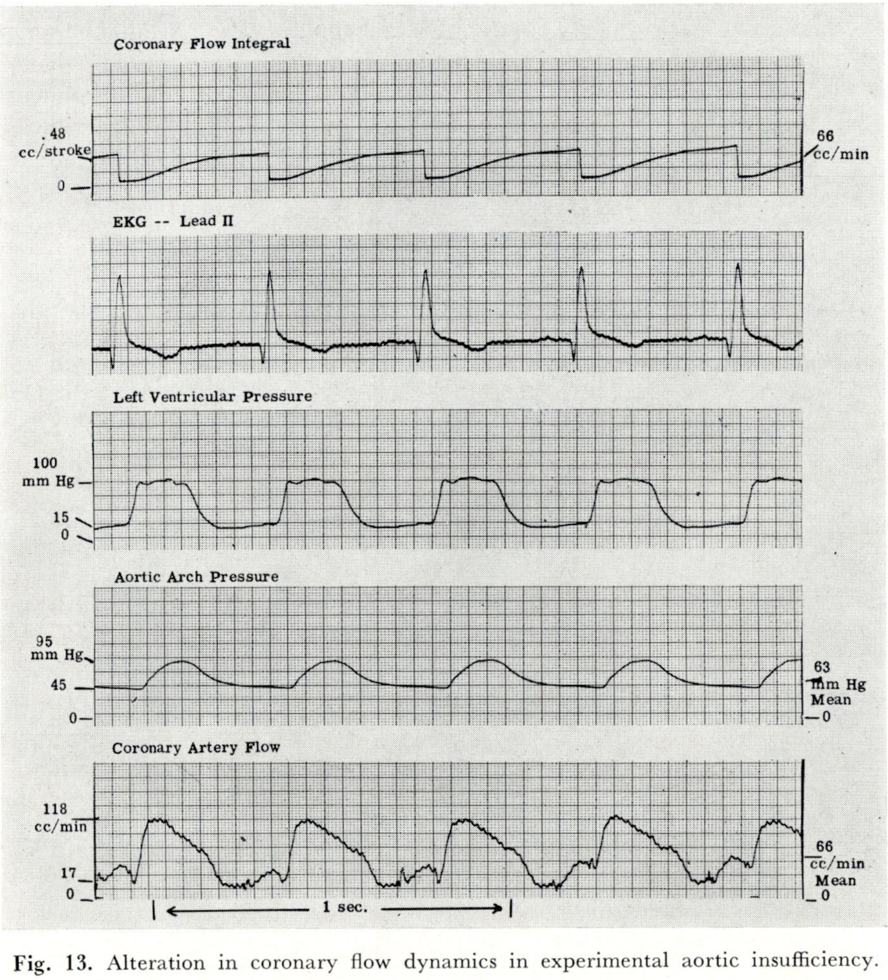


**Fig. 13.** Alteration in coronary flow dynamics in experimental aortic insufficiency.

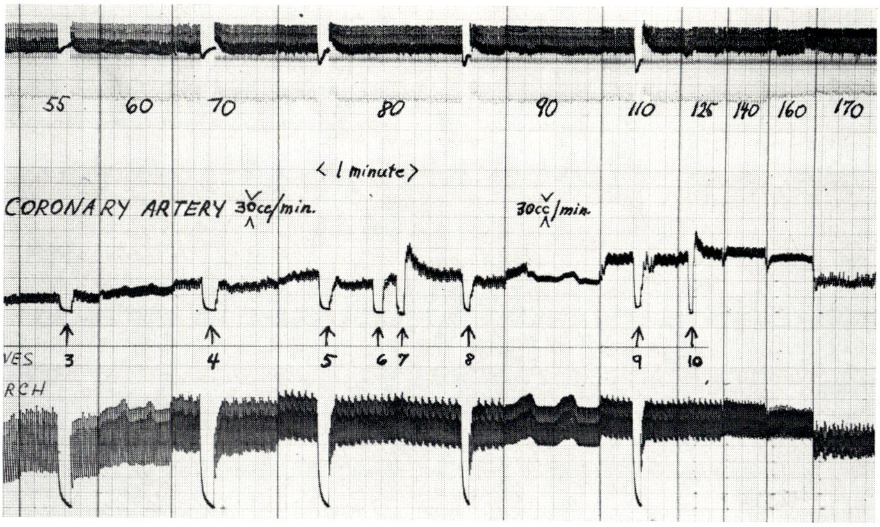


**Fig. 14.** Coronary flow study in animal with heart block. Cardiac rate was maintained by pacemaker. Top, electrocardiogram with cardiac rate indicated beneath. Center, coronary arterial flow. Bottom, arterial pressure. Points *3, 4, 5, 8,* and *9* indicate asystole produced by disconnection of pacemaker. At points *7* and *10* coronary artery was occluded. At point *6* the electrical supply to the flow probe magnet was disconnected.

The remaining findings here reported are in the nature of pilot surveys. They do show that the methods are adequate for the detection and registration of both instantaneous and mean alterations in coronary blood flow.

We believe that the method of flow measurement is sufficiently safe, as demonstrated by our experience in animals, to be applicable to human measurement whenever operative exposure is planned.

## SUMMARY AND CONCLUSIONS

1. A newer technique for the measurement of coronary arterial mean and instantaneous phasic flow in which a square-wave electromagnetic flowmeter is utilized is described.

2. A description of the instantaneous phasic characteristics of coronary arterial flow and the time relationships of these characteristics to electrocardiogram, ventricular pressure, arch pressure, and coronary artery pressure is included.

3. A series of observations on alterations of coronary mean flow and pulsatile characteristics produced by mechanical means, hypoxia, epinephrine, l-norepinephrine and Arfonad are described.

4. The applicability of this method to the measurement of coronary blood flow in patients is suggested.

### REFERENCES

1. Chardack, W. M.: Unpublished observations.
2. Denison, A. B., Jr., and Spencer, M. P.: Square-wave electromagnetic flowmeter design, Rev. Scient. Instruments **27:** 707, 1956.
3. Gregg, D. E., and Green, H. D.: Registration and interpretation of normal phasic inflow into a left coronary artery by an improved differential manometric method, Am. J. Physiol. **130:** 114, 1940.
4. Marston, E. L., Barefoot, C. A., and Spencer, M. P.: Noncannulating measurement of coronary blood flow, S. Forum **10:** 636, 1959.

## DISCUSSION*

**Dr. John E. Connolly** (Palo Alto, Calif.). I want to compliment Drs. Menno and Schenk on the work that they presented this morning. We, too, have been impressed with the desirability of studying the coronary blood flow under varying

*Discussion of papers by Weidner, Roth, and Simeone; and Menno and Schenk.

conditions and we have devised a radioactive technique which we think provides a simple quantitative measurement of coronary blood flow either with an open or closed chest. This is a modification of Kety's technique of estimating blood flow in skeletal muscles. $Na^{22}Cl$ is injected into the myocardium and its disappearance rate is measured with a scintillation counter placed over the heart. The relative coronary blood flow is then expressed in per cent per minute calculated from the logarithmic plots of the turnover rates. Thus, by injecting $Na^{22}Cl$ through a percutaneous needle into the myocardium, we can obtain a measure of coronary blood flow with a closed chest and by this simple technique we have been able to show, as Drs. Menno and Schenk have, that there is an augmentation of coronary blood flow with mechanical assistance in acute heart failure, with cross-clamping of the descending aorta, and also after the administration of pharmacologic agents.

**Dr. Worthington G. Schenk, Jr.** (closing). The findings which we have reported must be regarded as pilot studies which show what can happen under various experimental conditions. Only further study with larger groups of animals will determine what is most likely to happen under such conditions.

This technique for measurement of coronary blood flow is not an easy one; consequently, every experimental effort has not met with complete success.

# Porosity: primary determinant of ultimate fate of synthetic vascular grafts

SIGMUND A. WESOLOWSKI,* M.D.
CHARLES C. FRIES, M.D.
KARL E. KARLSON, M.D.
MICHAEL DE BAKEY, M.D.
PHILIP N. SAWYER,** M.D.
BROOKLYN, N. Y., AND HOUSTON, TEXAS
*From the Vascular Surgical Service, Department of Surgery, State University of New York Downstate Medical Center; and The Cora and Webb Mading Department of Surgery, Baylor University College of Medicine*

A 3-year study involving over 350 growing pigs and dogs,[2] selected human subjects, and 37 different synthetic fabrics was organized in the attempt to establish the specifications for the ideal synthetic vascular material.

It was found that the physical property of porosity correlated well with the biological fate of grafts implanted into the thoracic aorta of the growing pig. In order to measure the water porosity, a special machine was devised and built. This machine allowed excellent reproducibility of the test for water porosity (Fig. 1).

In Table I the fabrics tested are listed. These include Vinyon-N, nylon, Orlon, Dacron, Teflon, Ivalon, glass, and lead. The materials in this group produce a wide range of biological reactivity, yet the ultimate fate of grafts composed of these various materials correlated not with the material, but with the porosity. We are all familiar with photographs of good-looking grafts of Vinyon-N, Orlon, nylon, Dacron, Teflon, and even Ivalon. Fig. 2 shows the unique finding of a good-looking graft of glass after 1 year of implantation in the thoracic aorta of a growing pig. The fate of the glass graft is contrasted with that of a tightly woven Teflon graft shown after 7 months implantation in a growing pig in Fig. 3. In the Teflon graft there is massive calcification (seen through the inner capsule which has been laid down by the host) in a site immediately within the lumen of a graft material itself. Fig. 4 is an aortogram in a dog taken 7 months after implantation of a graft made of perforated metallic lead. Although the lead material has fractured and allowed aneurysm formation, there is an adequate lumen for blood flow. This graft did not thrombose.

**Table I.** *Synthetic materials tested*

| *Material* | *Cloth sheet* | *Woven tube* | *Braided tube* | *Knitted tube* | *Total* |
|---|---|---|---|---|---|
| Vinyon-N | 1 | — | — | — | 1 |
| Nylon | 1 | — | 1 | — | 2 |
| Orlon | 2 | — | — | — | 2 |
| Dacron | 4 | 5 | 3 | 3 | 15 |
| Teflon | 2 | 7 | — | 2 | 11 |
| Ivalon | 1 | (1) | — | — | 2 |
| Glass | 2 | — | — | — | 2 |
| Lead | 1 | (1) | — | — | 2 |
| Totals | 14 | 14 | 4 | 5 | 37 |

Each integer refers to a different material with different yarn, fabric, or fabrication characteristics.

Supported in part by United States Public Health Service Grants H-3286, H-3286 (C1), H-3286 (C2), and H-3286 (C3), and grants from The New York Heart Association, Johnson and Johnson Research Laboratories and the Special Research Fund of Dr. Clarence Dennis.

Read at the Twenty-second Annual Meeting of the Society of University Surgeons, Kansas City, Kan., Feb. 9-11, 1961.

*Third Research Scholar, American College of Surgeons.

**Markle Scholar.

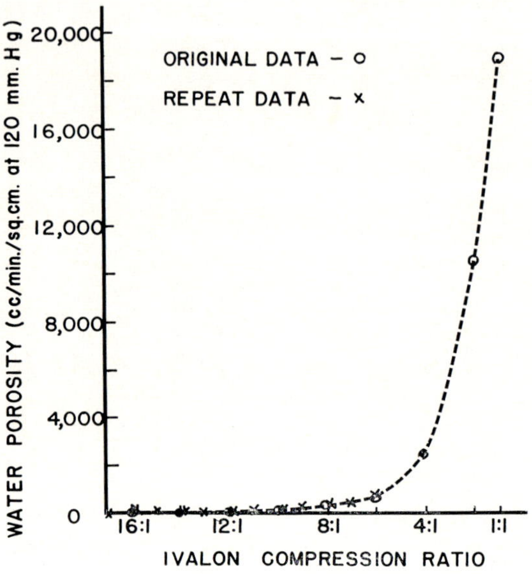


**Fig. 1.** Graph demonstrates excellent reproducibility of water porosity determinations. Test material was 2 separate lots of American Ivalon of varying compression ratio tested 1 year apart. Note the superimposition of the 2 curves, one plotted with circles and the other with crosses. (From S. A. Wesolowski.[2])

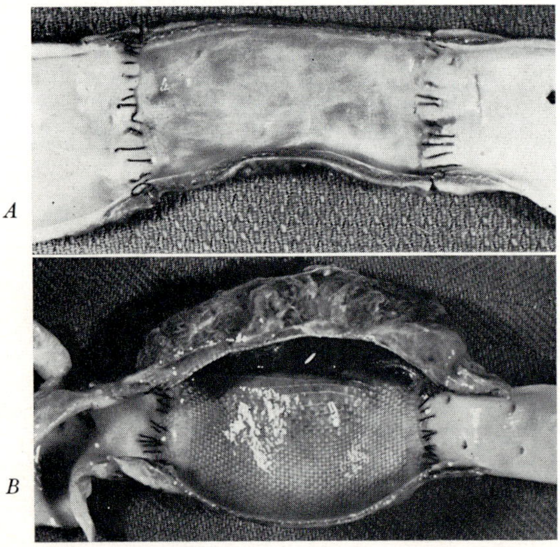


**Fig. 2.** Grafts of hand-fabricated fiber glass cloth. *A,* Implantation into thoracic aorta of growing pig for 1 year shows acceptable result. *B,* Graft after implantation into thoracic aorta of mature dog for 17 months. Although longitudinal seam separated and allowed saccular aneurysm formation and severe turbulence, all surfaces of inner aspect of specimen containing fiber glass are lined with ideal type of inner capsule (thin, transparent, and viable). (From S. A. Wesolowski.[2])

The results of these and all other implantations in this study[2] have demonstrated that the fate of the vascular graft is not primarily determined by the reactivity of the material which makes up its wall.

It has been possible to outline the method of formation of the new inner fibrous capsule of the implanted synthetic vascular graft. The synthetic graft is a foreign body which the host tends to encapsulate completely. The photomicrographs of Figs. 5, 6, and 7 demonstrate the method of formation of the inner fibrous capsule and the 2 major complications of inner capsular degeneration–calcification and septum formation. In each photomicrograph the lumen of the graft faces up. Fig. 5, *A,* is a photomicrograph of an Edwards-Tapp braided nylon graft 10 days after implantation into the thoracic aorta of a growing pig. A compact inner layer of fibrin has been formed. After 10 days this layer of fibrin shows the earliest signs of organization by fibrous tissue growing through the interstices of the synthetic wall. Fig. 5, *B,* demonstrates that new blood vessels grow through the interstices of the synthetic graft from the outer capsule into the inner fibrous capsule. The latter is termed by some workers "neointima" or "pseudointima." We prefer the term "inner fibrous capsule" because this layer is composed of scar tissue. With time and maturation of this scar, the capillaries growing through the interstices of the synthetic graft become choked off, which leads to degeneration of the inner fibrous capsule. This is the normal pathogenesis of maturing cicatrix throughout the body, with the exception that in the blood vessel wall, absorption of dead and dying tissue of the inner fibrous capsule is difficult. Such tissue therefore accumulates and undergoes hyaline degeneration and frank necrosis as demonstrated in Fig. 5, *C.* At this stage 2 layers of inner fibrous capsule are definitely formed, a basal layer of degenerate fibrous tissue and an inner layer adjacent to the lumen which is often not necrotic because of a longitudinal network of blood vessels supplied by adjacent intact areas of inner capsule. Fig. 5,

*D,* demonstrates what happens in a graft of a very low porosity material in which reorganization through the interstices of the synthetic material is delayed because of the tightness of the mesh. This degenerate fibrous tissue does not readily become absorbed, but precipitates calcium salts which are deposited within the lumen of the graft material. This particular graft was constructed of a fine-mesh Teflon.

When degeneration of the inner fibrous capsule occurs over a significantly wide area, full-thickness necrosis results (Fig. 6). This can lead to slough with distal embolization of the inner capsule as well as to production of injury currents[1] with the accumulation of mural thrombus on the inner surface of the graft. Such thrombus can become pedunculated or embolize, but most often it forms a stenosing septum which shows progression to complete obstruction.

Fig. 7, *A,* demonstrates what occurs in a graft of very high porosity. This is a graft of fiber glass in which degeneration and reorganization through the large interstices of the graft material occurred so rapidly that calcification was prevented. An inner fibrous capsule is shown with scattered patches of degeneration and new granulation tissue which replaces these patches. None of the glass grafts showed calcification. Fig. 7, *B,* however, shows that full-thickness necrosis of the inner capsule is not necessary to produce mural thrombosis and septum formation. A local patch of degeneration close to the graft material induces injury currents[1] which are transmitted, apparently by a condensor effect, to the luminal surface of the graft with the accumulation of mural thrombus and septum formation. Fig. 7, *C,* is a photomicrograph of a graft constructed of metallic lead from the thoracic aorta of a dog in the region of an interstice. In this area it can be seen that the inner capsule is calcifying and that in the adjacent outer capsule there is an intense inflammatory reaction composed of foreign-body giant cells. Fig. 7, *D,* is a photomicrograph in another location of the same graft constructed of metallic lead in an area where there is no inner fibrous capsule. It apparently had sloughed. It is to be noted that the outer fibrous capsule in this location does not contain any inflammatory foreign-body giant-cell reaction, which demonstrates that it is not the biological reactivity of the material per se that governs the inflammatory response in the host, but rather the degener-

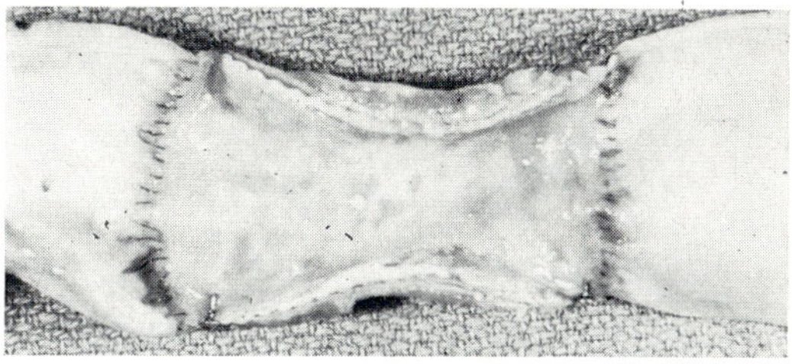

**Fig. 3.** Graft of narrow-loom crimped Teflon tube 285 days after implantation into the thoracic aorta of a growing pig. Note the marked accumulation of calcium salts in the inner capsule adjacent to the graft material. (From S. A. Wesolowski.[2])

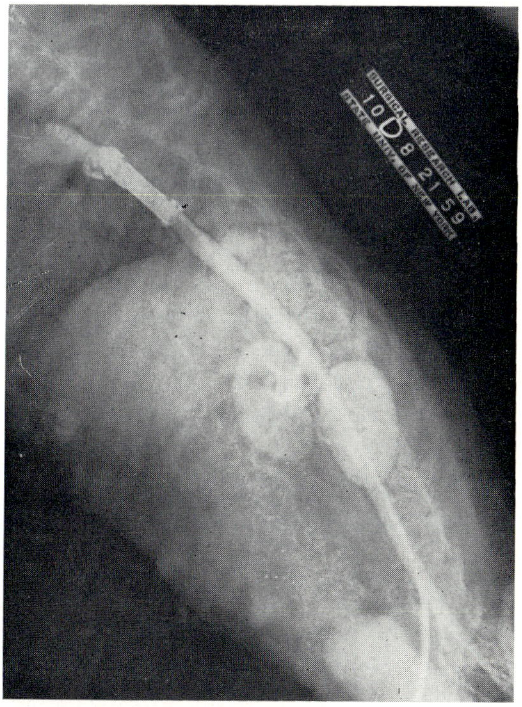

**Fig. 4.** Aortogram of a dog which had a metallic lead graft in the thoracic aorta for 7 months. (From S. A. Wesolowski.[2])

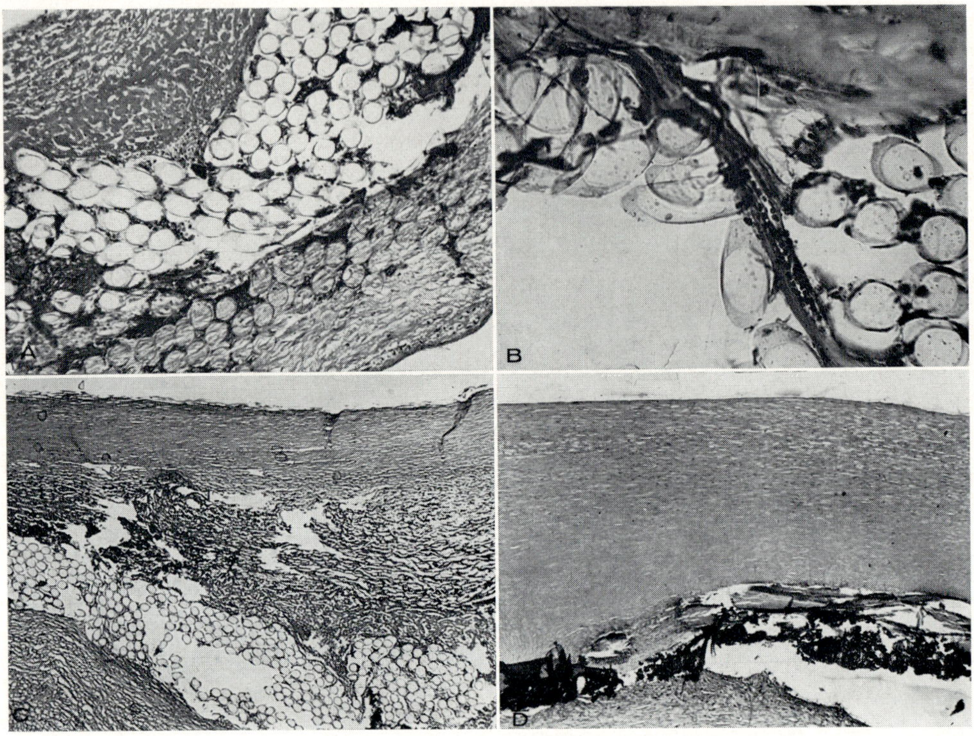


**Fig. 5.** *A,* Edwards-Tapp nylon grafts which were in pig thoracic aorta for *A,* 10 days (×100); *B,* 33 days (×250); and *C,* 75 days (×40). *D,* Brown Teflon graft (Hufnagel) which was in pig thoracic aorta for 200 days (×33). (Hematoxylin and eosin; reduced 4/11.) (From S. A. Wesolowski.[2])

ative changes in the scar tissue produced by the host itself.

Fig. 8 is a graph which correlates the physical porosity of the material with calcification. Each point of the plot is a letter which is the initial of the graft material of the particular series represented by each point. It is to be noted that the T's (Teflon) and D's (Dacron) are interspersed and fall very close to a curve line which represents an inverse relationship. At the zero calcification end of the scale the materials are very porous, whereas on the maximal calcification end of the scale the materials are only slightly porous. Extrapolation of this curve back to the zero calcification line demonstrates that the corrected porosity figures for the glass grafts, which exhibited no calcification, plot close to the extrapolated intersect at a water porosity of approximately 5,000 ml. of filtered water per minute per square centimeter of fabric at a pressure head of 120 mm. Hg. This is a water porosity greater than that of any of the graft materials used clinically.

As a result of this study we have formu-

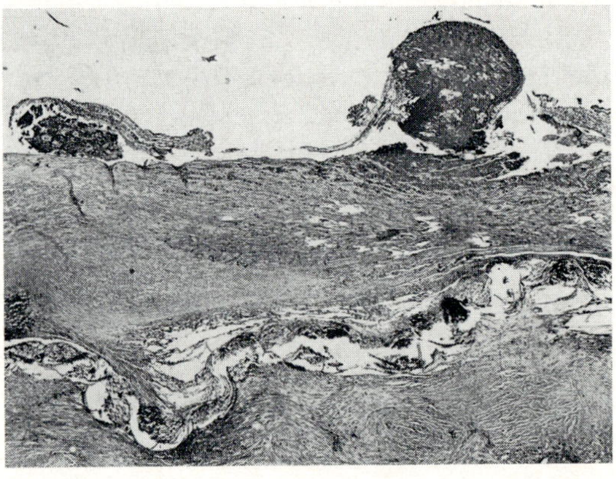

**Fig. 6.** Hand-sewn Vinyon-N graft (Karlson) which was in pig thoracic aorta for 7 months. (Hematoxylin and eosin; ×20; reduced 1/3.) (From S. A. Wesolowski.[2])

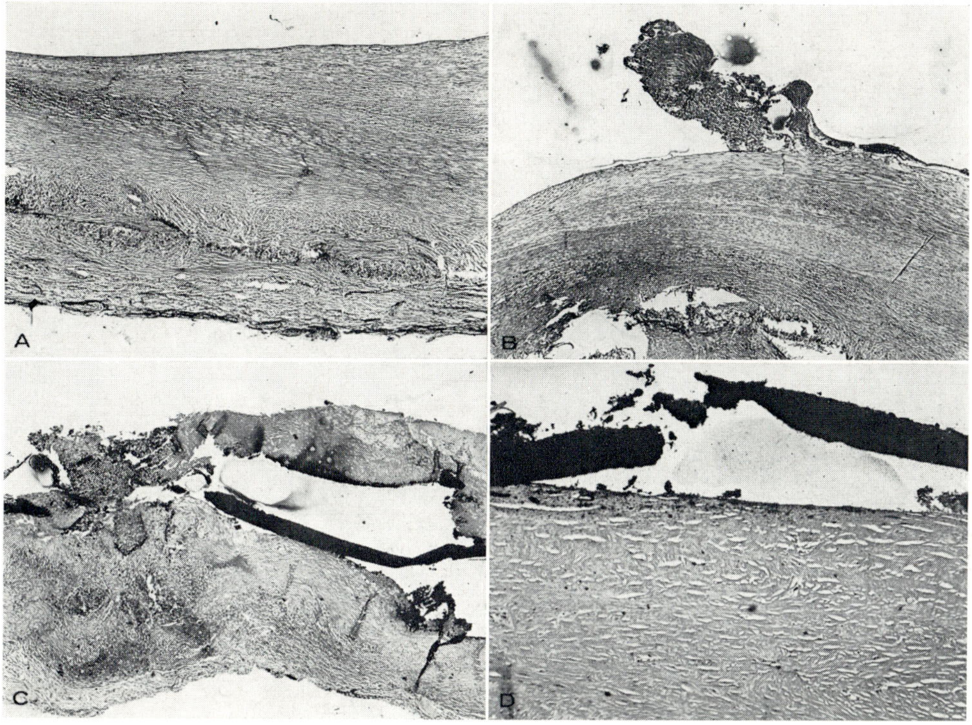


**Fig. 7.** *A*, Hand-sewn fiber glass graft (Meadox) which was in pig thoracic aorta for *A*, 1 year (×25), and *B*, 7 months (×20). *C*, Multiperforated metallic lead graft which was in thoracic aorta of dog for 7 months (×20). *D*, Same as *C* in another area. (Hematoxylin and eosin; reduced 4⁄11.) (From S. A. Wesolowski.[2])

lated 5 specifications for the ideal synthetic vascular graft material. (1) The graft material should be nontoxic and nonallergenic. (2) The material should be durable and should have no significant deterioration upon biologic implantation for prolonged periods of time. (3) The implantation porosity should be less than 50 ml. of water per minute per square centimeter of graft wall at a pressure equivalent to 120 mm. Hg; below this porosity the material can be implanted into a heparinized patient. (4) The biologic permeability should be equivalent to a water porosity in excess of 5,000 ml. water per minute per square centimeter of graft wall at a pressure head of 120 mm. Hg. (5) The graft material should have certain other desirable physical properties for ease of mechanical handling. The graft should be pliable so that diameter discrepancies can be easily handled during the performance of anastomoses. The graft

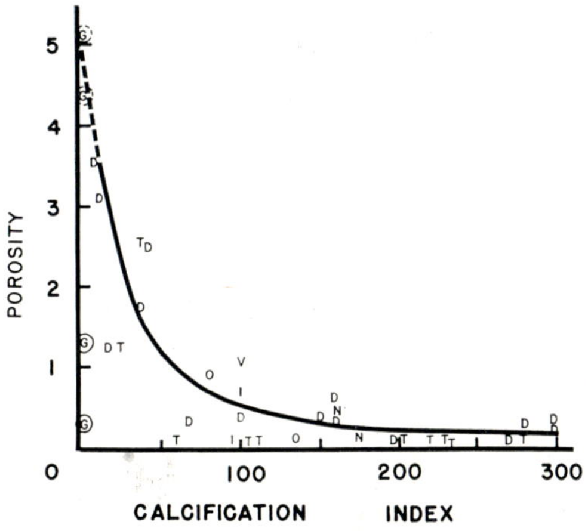


**Fig. 8.** Graph correlates physical porosity with calcification of graft. Each letter point shows average values for a series of graft implants. Ordinate scale is water porosity of graft material in thousands of milliliters of filtered water per minute per square centimeter of fabric at a pressure head of 120 mm. Hg. Calcification index is product of average degree of calcification for a particular series (0 to 4 scale) and percentage of grafts in series demonstrating calcification. (From S. A. Wesolowski.[2])

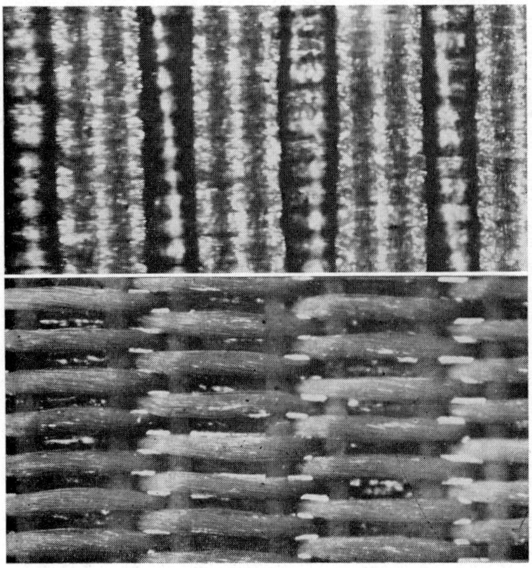


**Fig. 9.** Photomicrograph of a compound graft material of nonabsorbable Dacron alternated with an absorbable collagen derivative fiber in 2 to 1 ratio in the warp and all-Dacron filling. *A,* Before removal of absorbable fiber, with a porosity of 37. *B,* After removal of absorbable fiber, with a porosity of 5,460 ml. water per minute per square centimeter at 120 Hg. (×22; reduced ⅛.) (From S. A. Wesolowski.[2])

should also be crimped and twistable to minimize the occurrence of kinks and graft obstructions during implantation through subfascial or subcutaneous tunnels.

Fig. 9 illustrates a new concept for a synthetic vascular graft material which allows a low porosity on implantation and a high porosity upon biological healing. We have accomplished this by the use of a compound fabric which consists of alternating strands of a nonabsorbable fiber of polyester (Dacron) and an absorbable fiber. We are now in the process of testing these compound fabrics with collagen derivatives as the absorbable fiber and will report subsequently on these results. There is an obvious difference in porosity of the compound fabric at the time of implantation, when the absorbable material is still in place, and after removal of the absorbable material, when the porosity is greater than 5,000 ml. per minute per square centimeter of fabric.

## SUMMARY

1. The porosity of synthetic graft materials can be determined with adequate reproducibility in the laboratory with a constant head of filtered tap water.

2. Arterial grafts of all the presently available synthetic materials exhibit degenerative changes within the inner fibrous capsule which are independent of the material and its biologic reactivity.

3. Degeneration of the inner fibrous capsule leads to calcification and/or septum formation with graft stenosis.

4. Calcification can be avoided if the porosity of the material is greater than 5,000 ml. of water per minute per square centimeter of fabric with a pressure head of 120 ml. of mercury.

5. New specifications for the ideal synthetic vascular graft material have been enumerated.

6. The concept of the use of a compound fabric which consists of permanent and absorbable fibers to produce a graft material of initial low implant porosity and a final high porosity for high fibroblastic permeability has been described.

## REFERENCES

1. Sawyer, P. N., and Wesolowski, S. A.: The electric current of injured tissue and vascular occlusion, Ann. Surg. **153:** 34-42, 1961.
2. Wesolowski, S. A.: Evaluation of tissue and prosthetic vascular grafts, Springfield, Ill., 1961, Charles C Thomas, Publisher.

*(For discussion, see page 105.)*

# Experimental vein grafting in the portal venous system

P. N. SYMBAS, M.D.
J. H. FOSTER, M.D.
H. W. SCOTT, JR., M.D.
NASHVILLE, TENN.
*From the S. Rudolph Light Laboratory for Surgical Research, Vanderbilt University School of Medicine*

Vein grafts have been the subject of numerous experimental studies in the past decade[1, 2, 4, 8, 10-12, 15] Regardless of the substitute employed, most grafts placed in the abdominal vena cava have thrombosed.[4] In contrast, grafts in the thoracic vena cava have remained patent more frequently.[8, 11] The reason for this difference is uncertain. Thrombosis of vein grafts has usually been attributed to the relatively low pressure and low flow rate in the venous system.

A dual consideration prompted an experimental study of vein grafting in the portal system. The basic consideration was to assess the influence of the portal venous pressure, which is slightly higher than systemic venous pressure, on the results of vein replacement. Secondarily, we believed successful vein grafting in the portal system might have useful clinical implications.

## MATERIALS AND METHODS

Healthy adult mongrel dogs which weighed 12 to 14 kilograms were used. Anesthesia was induced intravenously with thiopental or pentobarbital, and an endotracheal tube and mechanical respirator were utilized. The grafting procedures were performed with aseptic technique through a right thoracoabdominal incision. Two types of grafting procedures were performed, (1) interpolation of a graft into the portal vein, and (2) placement of a shunt graft between the portal vein and inferior vena cava. A continuous everting suture, interrupted in 3 or 4 places, of No. 5.0 arterial silk was used in all the anastomoses. Postoperatively the animals were fed standard kennel rations and water ad libitum. Portal pressure was measured and portography performed at 1 week and 1, 2, 3, 7, and 14 months. An autopsy was performed on each animal which died or was sacrificed.

**Group I. Portal vein grafts.** In 31 animals the portal vein was divided and a 4 cm. graft interpolated (Fig. 1). At operation, heparin sodium (15 mg.) was injected into the splanchnic extremity of the portal vein immediately after application of the occluding clamp. Three types of grafts were utilized, (1) fresh autologous jugular vein, (2) fresh homologous thoracic inferior vena cava, and (3) crimped woven Teflon,* one-fourth to three-eighths of an inch in diameter. After operation each animal received 500 ml. of normal saline solution intravenously and lost blood was replaced quantitatively. Each animal received penicillin and streptomycin for 1 week. The animals were divided into 2 subgroups.

*Subgroup IA. Homologous and autologous portal vein grafts.* Fifteen homologous and 4 autologous vein grafts were implanted in the portal veins of 19 dogs. Seven animals

Read at the Twenty-second Annual Meeting of the Society of University Surgeons, Kansas City, Kan., Feb. 9-11, 1961.

*Procured from C. R. Bard, Inc., Summit, N. J.

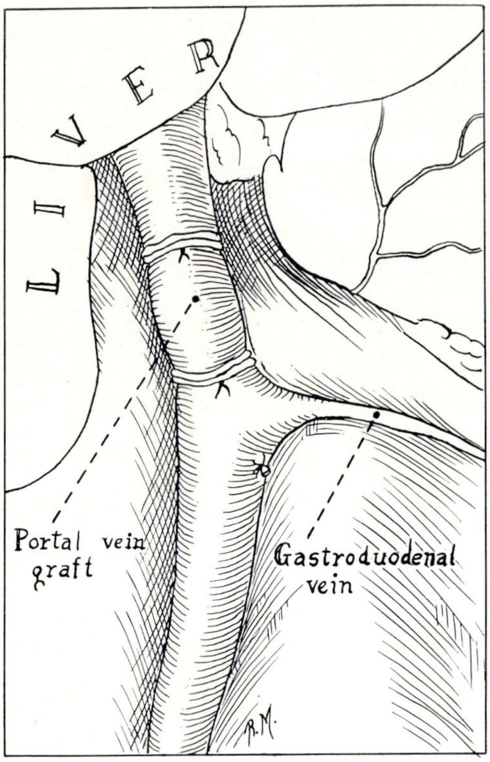


**Fig. 1.** Sketch of a graft implanted in the portal vein.

with homologous grafts served as controls and received no treatment in addition to that outlined above. Twelve animals, 4 with autografts and 8 with homografts, were given heparin sodium (3 mg. per kilogram of body weight) in the postoperative saline infusion. Clotting time was determined every 4 hours during the next 24 hours, and sufficient heparin sodium was injected by the deep subcutaneous route to keep the clotting time above 30 minutes. Thereafter, heparin sodium (2 mg. per kilogram of body weight) was administered every 8 hours for 1 week.

*Subgroup IB. Teflon prosthetic portal vein grafts.* By the technique outlined, a three-eighths inch woven Teflon prosthesis was implanted in the portal vein of 12 animals. Six animals served as controls and the other 6 received the heparin regimen outlined for Subgroup IA.

**Group II. Portacaval shunt grafts.** In 13 animals portacaval shunts were constructed by insertion of a homologous vein graft or Teflon prosthesis between the side of the portal vein and inferior vena cava (Fig. 2). The grafts, 4 cm. in length, were homologous thoracic vena cava in 8 animals and woven crimped Teflon (three-eighths inch) in 4 animals. Partial-occlusion clamps were applied to the portal vein and inferior vena cava during construction of the anastomoses. After completion of the shunt the portal vein was doubly ligated and divided at the level of the hilum of the liver. Pressures were measured in the inferior vena cava and portal vein before, during, and after the procedure. No special postoperative care was given any of the animals (specifically, heparin, antibiotics, and intravenous fluids were not administered).

## RESULTS

**Group I. Portal vein grafts.** This group was composed of 31 dogs in which a graft was interpositioned end-to-end into the portal vein.

*Subgroup IA. Homologous and autologous vein grafts.* Table I shows the results obtained with the vein grafts. One operative death occurred as the result of bleeding secondary to technical difficulties. All of the other animals survived the operative procedure. In the heparin-treated animals all grafts, both homologous and autologous vein, remained patent throughout the period of observation. In contrast, 5 of the 7 control animals died within 18 hours from thrombosis of the grafts. There were 2 survivors with patent grafts in the control group.

In the 13 surviving animals, portal pressure measurements were within normal limits throughout the follow-up period. The serial portograms showed no evidence of thrombosis or stenosis of the grafted segment (Fig. 3). In some animals portography showed a slight indentation at a suture line, which demonstrated no evidence of progression on subsequent portograms (Fig. 3). A few animals were sacrificed at varying time intervals. Photographs and pertinent tissue studies were obtained. These examinations showed patent grafts with a smooth intimal lining and no

**Table I.** *Homologous and autologous vein grafts*

| *Dog. No.* | *Date of operation (1959)* | *Portal vein occlusion time (min.)* | *Portal pressure* (range)* | *Roentgenographic and autopsy findings** | *Survival time* |
|---|---|---|---|---|---|
| *Homograft: heparin therapy* | | | | | |
| 171D | Aug. 31 | 48 | 130-200 | Patent | 12 mo. |
| 204D | Sept. 10 | 40 | 140-290 | Patent | Living |
| 267D | Oct. 6 | 43 | 200-290 | Patent | 47 days |
| 278D | Oct. 12 | — | — | — | Died† |
| 284D | Oct. 14 | 40 | 120-200 | Patent | 10 mo. |
| 300D | Oct. 20 | 58 | 140-190 | Patent | Living |
| 316D | Oct. 23 | 36 | 140-230 | Patent | Living |
| 335D | Oct. 28 | 46 | 150-200 | Patent | Living |
| *Autograft: heparin therapy* | | | | | |
| 144D | Aug. 17 | 58 | 140-280 | Patent | 12 mo. |
| 854C | Nov. 30 | 56 | 140-280 | Patent | Living |
| 382D | Dec. 1 | 52 | 140-180 | Patent | 9 mo. |
| 384D | Dec. 2 | 58 | 150-170 | Patent | 9 mo. |
| *Control group—homograft: no heparin* | | | | | |
| 280D | Oct. 13 | 36 | — | Thrombosed | 10 hr. |
| 393D | Oct. 19 | 50 | — | Thrombosed | 5 hr. |
| 324D | Oct. 26 | 35 | — | Thrombosed | 10 hr. |
| 848C | Oct. 30 | 35 | 130-300 | Patent | Living |
| 339D | Nov. 2 | 40 | 120-200 | Patent | 72 days |
| 349D | Nov. 4 | 36 | — | Thrombosed | 12 hr. |
| 274D | Oct. 7 | 46 | — | Thrombosed | 18 hr. |

*Portography and portal pressures at approximately 1, 3, 7, and 14 months.

†Operative death due to bleeding.

evidence of stenosis or thrombosis of the graft (Figs. 4 and 5). Elastic tissue stains revealed a substantial elastic tissue layer in the grafts, and in the autografts the muscular layer persisted.

The 6 remaining animals have now been observed for from 14 to 16 months. The grafts in these animals remain patent without evidence of stenotic occlusion or degeneration as judged by portography (Fig. 3).

*Subgroup IB. Teflon prosthetic portal vein grafts.* The results obtained with implantation of synthetic prosthesis into the portal veins are summarized in Table II. The grafts in the control animals (no heparin therapy) uniformly failed. In each of these 6 animals thrombosis of the graft and death occurred in less than 18 hours. In the 6 animals treated with heparin, the prosthesis thrombosed in 3 and remained patent in 3. However, 2 of the animals with patent prosthesis died within 1 week, one with bronchopneumonia on the fourth postoperative day and the second with anesthesia at the time

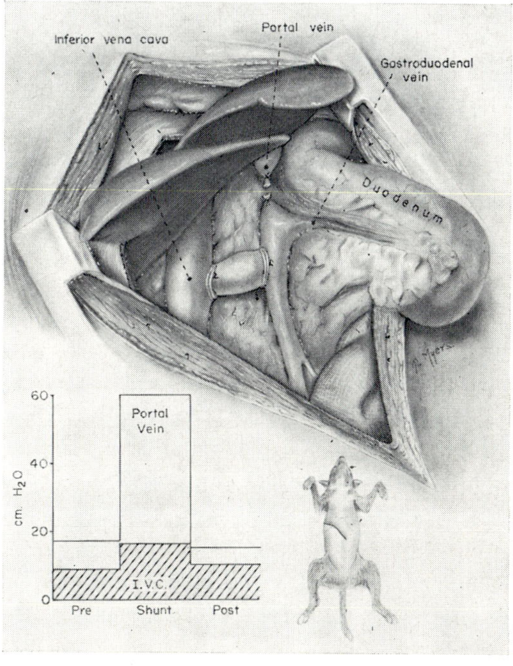


**Fig. 2.** Sketch of a portacaval shunt graft and a graphic representation of the portal and inferior vena caval *(I.V.C.)* pressures before, during, and after the shunting procedure.

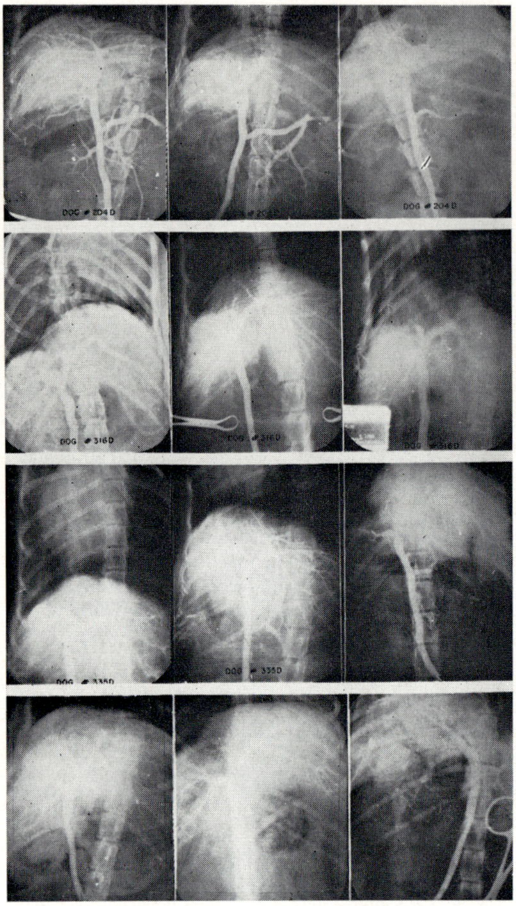


A

B

C

D

**Fig. 3.** Portograms made approximately 1, 7, and 14 months after implantation of 3 homologous vein grafts (*A, B,* and *C*) and a Teflon prosthesis (*D*) in the portal vein. Note that mild changes at the suture lines remain fairly constant.

of the first portogram. Each graft was patent. The remaining animal with a patent portal vein prosthesis has now been observed for 14 months. The periodic portograms have shown continued patency without evidence of progressive stenosis or narrowing (Fig. 3). Mild narrowing at the proximal suture line was noted on the first portogram and it remained constant on subsequent examinations. Portal pressure has remained in the range of normal.

**Group II. Portacaval shunt grafts.** Eight of the 9 homologous vein shunts remained patent throughout the period of observation (Fig. 6). The single instance of thrombosis occurred sometime after the first portogram. All 4 of the Teflon shunts remained patent (Fig. 7). The pressure difference between the portal vein and inferior vena cava ranged from 40 to 140 ml. of water. Postoperative portal venous pressures and other findings are summarized in Table III. In the postoperative period these animals became anorexic and lethargic and began losing weight. Progressive wasting and inanition culminated in death 32 to 70 days later. Survival time averaged 50 days. At autopsy the liver was found to be small and of brownish color. All the shunt grafts except one were patent, had a smooth intimal lining, and showed no evidence of thrombus formation or suture-line stenosis (Figs. 8 and 9). Histologic studies showed varying stages of hepatic parenchymal deterioration ranging from acute fatty infiltration to fibrosis. The homologous vein grafts contained a well-preserved elastic tissue layer and smooth intima. Each prosthetic graft had a fibrous layer surrounding it and a complete, smooth "intimal" lining. The lungs of most of the animals showed pathologic changes ranging from bronchopneumonia to pulmonary edema.

## COMMENT

In the past decade numerous studies of experimental vein grafting have been reported, and from these studies a general pattern of results has emerged. Grafts placed in the abdominal vena cava or jugular or femoral veins have usually become thrombosed.[1, 2, 4, 7, 9] An exception has been the venous autograft with which conflicting results have been obtained. Bryant,[2] Bower,[1] and Schauble[15] and their associates have reported a high incidence of patency (75 to 80 per cent) with autogenous vein replacements of the abdominal vena cava or jugular vein, while Jones,[9] Deterling,[7] and Collins[4] and their co-workers found that thrombosis usually occurred in autogenous veins placed in the inferior and superior venae cavae if the period of observation was sufficiently long. Replacement of the thoracic vena cava has yielded quite different results. A high incidence of continued patency has been reported with fresh aortic homografts and with Teflon prosthesis.[8, 11] Grafts of these types implanted in the abdominal vena cava have invariably thrombosed.

For the purposes of discussion, failure of vein grafts may result from either early thrombosis or late fibrous tissue occlusion. Early intraluminal thrombosis is usually attributed to operative trauma, low pressure, low flow rate, and host reaction to the graft. Late occlusion is generally due to gradual and progressive constriction by scar tissue at the suture lines. Lack of rigidity of the graft, low flow rate, low pressure, and host reaction are often cited as playing a role in this progressive stenosis.

A single previous study of interpolation of grafts into the portal vein has been found. In 1952 Daniel[6] reported on a series of dogs with Lucite tubes and fresh venous autografts implanted in the portal vein. The Lucite tubes invariably became thrombosed but approximately 25 per cent of the venous autografts remained patent.

In the present study of portal vein graft-

**Table II.** *Synthetic prosthesis grafts*

| *Dog No.* | *Date of operation (1959)* | *Portal vein occlusion time (min.)* | *Roentgenographic and autopsy findings* | *Survival time* |
|---|---|---|---|---|
| *Heparin therapy group* | | | | |
| 371D | Nov. 16 | 35 | Patent | 7 days |
| 375D | Nov. 17 | 35 | Patent | Living |
| 377D | Nov. 18 | 34 | Patent | 4 days |
| 379D | Nov. 18 | 34 | Thrombosed | 10 hr. |
| 917C | Nov. 23 | 38 | Thrombosed | 8 hr. |
| 671C | Nov. 25 | 35 | Thrombosed | Living |
| *Control group: no heparin* | | | | |
| 354D | Nov. 5 | 34 | Thrombosed | 12 hr. |
| 358D | Nov. 6 | 26 | Thrombosed | 10 hr. |
| 359D | Nov. 9 | 35 | Thrombosed | 6 hr. |
| 387D | Dec. 3 | 38 | Thrombosed | 8 hr. |
| 918C | Nov. 23 | 32 | Thrombosed | 9 hr. |
| 978C | Nov. 24 | 30 | Thrombosed | 9 hr. |

**Table III.** *Portacaval shunt grafts*

| *Dog No.* | *Date of operation (1959)* | *Preshunt pressures (mm./$H_2O$)* | | *Postshunt portal pressures (range)* | *Roentgenographic findings** | *Survival time (days)* | *Status at autopsy* |
|---|---|---|---|---|---|---|---|
| | | *Inferior vena cava* | *Portal vein* | | | | |
| *Homologous vein graft group* | | | | | | | |
| 393D | Dec. 7 | 120 | 200 | 110-250 | Patent | 42 | Patent |
| 394D | Dec. 9 | 110 | 150 | 180-240 | Patent | 46 | Patent |
| 397D | Dec. 10 | 115 | 180 | 140-260 | Thrombosed† | 35 | Thrombosed |
| 400D | Dec. 11 | 110 | 160 | 115-190 | Patent | 45 | Patent |
| 405D | Dec. 14 | 100 | 150 | 130-200 | Patent | 32 | Patent |
| 412D | Dec. 15 | 90 | 230 | 220-240 | Patent | 45 | Patent |
| 413D | Dec. 15 | 100 | 150 | 130-240 | Patent | 63 | Patent |
| 415D | Dec. 18 | 110 | 240 | 140-175 | Patent | 70 | Patent |
| 928C | Dec. 16 | 90 | 150 | 130-230 | Patent | 38 | Patent |
| *Prosthetic graft group* | | | | | | | |
| 417D | Dec. 21 | 100 | 150 | 100-160 | Patent | 56 | Patent |
| 420D | Dec. 22 | 190 | 230 | 95-200 | Patent | 42 | Patent |
| 421D | Dec. 23 | 130 | 180 | 140-240 | Patent | 63 | Patent |
| 938C | Dec. 18 | 100 | 170 | 130-230 | Patent | 70 | Patent |

*Portography at 1 and 5 weeks.

†Patent at 1 week, found thrombosed at final portography.

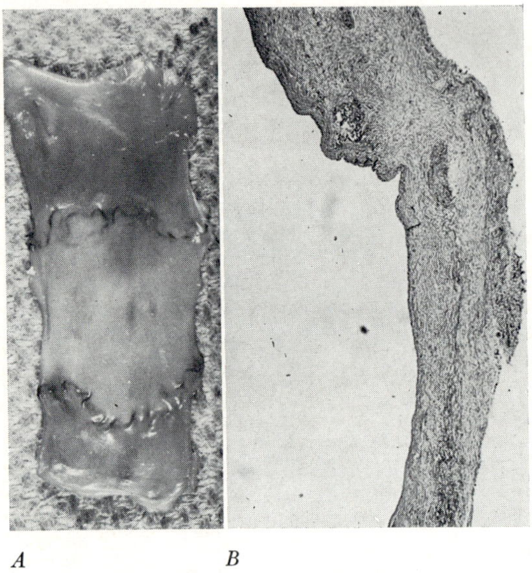

Fig. 4. Gross specimen (*A*) and photomicrograph (*B*) of an autologous vein graft 9 months after implantation in the portal vein. Muscular and elastic layers of the autogenous vein graft are clearly visible. Suture line is visible near top, immediately beneath intima.

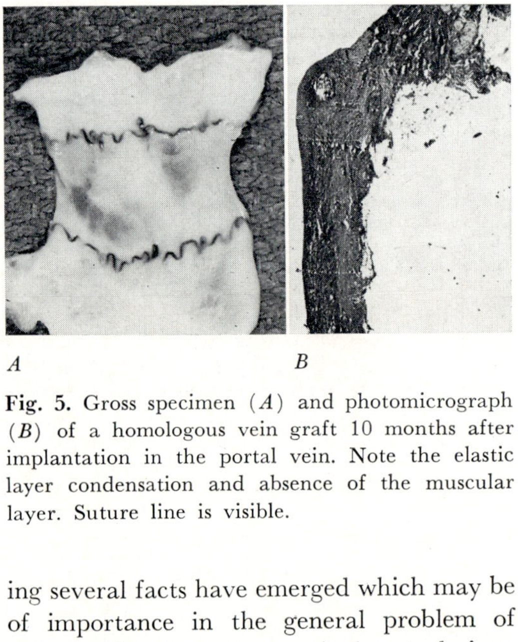

Fig. 5. Gross specimen (*A*) and photomicrograph (*B*) of a homologous vein graft 10 months after implantation in the portal vein. Note the elastic layer condensation and absence of the muscular layer. Suture line is visible.

ing several facts have emerged which may be of importance in the general problem of vein grafting. Despite a meticulous technique of implantation, venous homografts and Teflon prosthesis placed in the portal vein usually became thrombosed in a few hours unless a vigorous anticoagulant regimen was provided. This observation differs from the experience reported with vena caval grafts, in which a significant percentage of the grafts, even though they ultimately failed, remained patent for a few weeks or even months without anticoagulant therapy.[1, 2, 4] This raises the question proposed by Dale[5] of whether or not most vein grafts initially thrombose and then recanalize. This question could only be answered by repeated, frequent phlebography. However, the portal system is not really suitable for testing the thrombosis-recanalization hypothesis because acute thrombosis of the canine portal vein is almost invariably lethal and an opportunity for recanalization does not exist. The possibility that thrombosis and recanalization set the stage for late scar-tissue occlusion of vein grafts in the systemic venous system deserves consideration.

The heparin regimen employed in the present study was vigorous and would cause concern if used clinically. However, the purpose was to counteract any local clotting tendency which might accompany vein grafting, and meticulous hemostasis obviated postoperative bleeding as a problem. After 1 week no additional heparin was given. The results of this plan support the belief that a critical time period exists beyond which anticoagulant protection is not required. Every graft, regardless of type, that was patent at 1 week remained patent for the balance of the study. This includes 12 long-term observations of from 9 to 16 months.

These long-term results are strikingly different from the results reported with grafts in the systemic venous system in which a high incidence of delayed stenotic occlusion has been observed.[4, 7, 9, 11, 15] The only apparent environmental and technical differences in the present study are the slightly higher venous pressure (average 66 mm. $H_2O$) which exists in the portal system, and the use of anticoagulant therapy. It might be reasonable to assume that the heparin therapy provides protection during the time required for a smooth lining to cover any raw or rough areas in a grafted segment. Furthermore, this protection may have both immediate and long-range beneficial effects. It would be of interest to test this concept in a series of systemic venous grafts with the same intensive heparin regimen.

A previous experimental study of portacaval shunt grafts was reported by Southwick[17] in 1950. He described the use of preserved arterial homografts in the creation of portacaval shunts in dogs. All the grafts followed more than 6 weeks became thrombosed. There have been 3 clinical reports of the use of autogenous vein grafts in the construction of portal-systemic venous shunts. Six portacaval shunts and 7 splenorenal shunts were described.[13, 14, 18] There were 2 deaths in the early postoperative period; at autopsy the grafts were patent. Two patients had recurrent esophageal bleeding in less than 1 year. The other 9 patients remained well during a maximum follow-up period of 15 months. However, only 2 grafts had been assessed by portography; they were patent.

The most striking single feature of the present study consisted of the comparative results obtained with portal vein grafts and portacaval shunt grafts. Successful portal vein grafting required intensive postoperative anticoagulant therapy. Furthermore, this success was limited to the autologous and homologous vein grafts; 50 per cent of the synthetic prostheses became thrombosed. In sharp contrast, almost uniform success (93 per cent) was obtained with homologous veins and synthetic prostheses as portacaval shunt grafts without postoperative anticoagulant treatment. The gradient of pressure (average 66 mm. $H_2O$) between the portal vein and the inferior vena cava seems to be the only explanation for this difference. Portal pressure remained essentially unchanged during the follow-up period. The pressure differences undoubtedly reflect variations in blood flow. Actually the creation of a portacaval shunt diverts blood from a relatively high-resistance system to a relatively low-resistance system. Blood flow rates and vascular resistance undoubtedly played important roles in the results of this study; however, we have no data on these factors.

There seems to be a conflict between data obtained in this study and work of Bryant[2] with vein grafts placed adjacent to an induced arteriovenous fistula. Bryant ingeniously demonstrated that if an arteriovenous fistula was created proximal to a synthetic vein graft placed in the canine femoral vein,

*A*
*B*

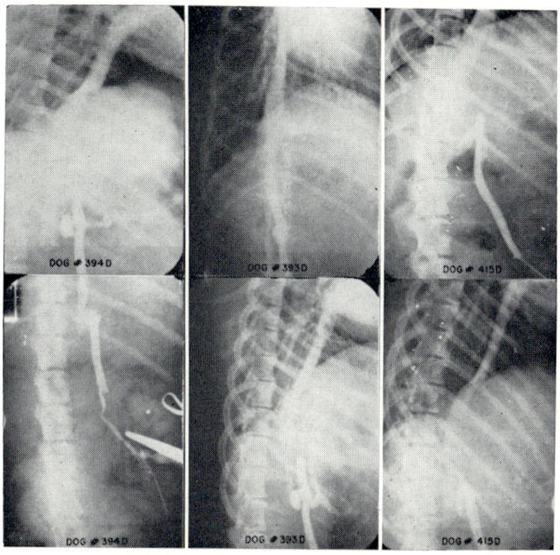

**Fig. 6.** Portograms in 3 animals made 1 *(A)* and 5 *(B)* weeks after creation of a homologous vein portacaval shunt.

*A*
*B*

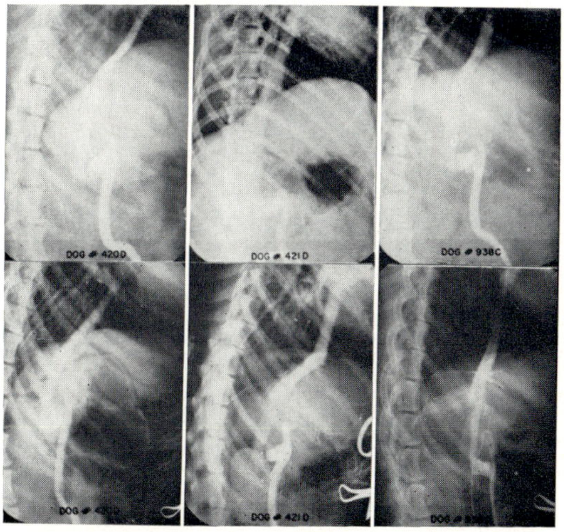

**Fig. 7.** Portograms in 3 animals made 1 *(A)* and 5 *(B)* weeks after creation of a Teflon prosthetic portacaval shunt.

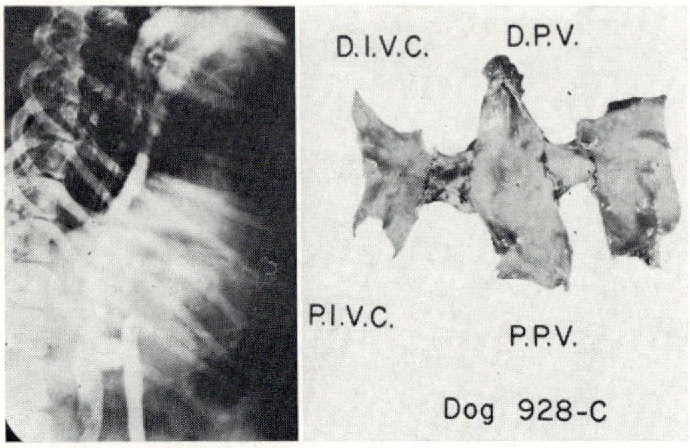


*A* *B*

**Fig. 8.** Portogram (*A*) and photograph of gross specimen (*B*) which show homologous vein portacaval shunt. *D.P.V.*, Portal vein at the level of ligation; *P.P.V.*, splanchnic limb of portal vein; *P.I.V.C.*, caudal inferior vena cava; and *D.I.V.C.*, cephalad inferior vena cava. Cava and graft have been divided sagittally.

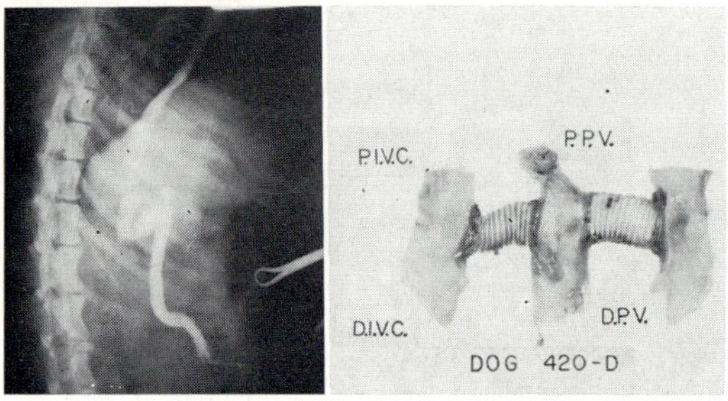


*A* *B*

**Fig. 9.** Portogram (*A*) and photograph of gross specimen (*B*) which show Teflon prosthesis portacaval shunt. *P.I.V.C.*, Cephalad inferior vena cava; *D.I.V.C.*, caudad inferior vena cava; *P.P.V.*, portal vein at level of ligation; and *D.P.V.*, splanchnic limb of portal vein. Cava and graft have been divided sagittally.

the graft remained patent. However, if the arteriovenous fistula was created distal to the synthetic vein graft, thrombosis invariably occurred. With the fistula proximal to the graft the pressure in the grafted segment measured 500 to 600 mm. $H_2O$, while with the fistula distally located the pressure was 150 to 200 mm. $H_2O$. The present study indicated that a pressure gradient of only 66 mm. $H_2O$ was sufficient to maintain patency of portacaval shunt grafts. The conflicting results may be explained by the relative diameter of the vessels involved and the grafting material used.

It is unfortunate that a long period of observation was not possible for the portacaval shunt grafts. Six to 10 weeks after the creation of the shunt the animals all died. This steady wasting of dogs with an Eck fistula has been noted previously on many occasions.[3, 16] If one can extrapolate the experience with the portal vein grafts, then continued, long-term patency of the shunt grafts might be expected if a normally functioning liver could be maintained. Further investigation will be required to determine whether or not this assumption is justified.

Many questions concerning portal vein grafts, portacaval shunt grafts, and vein grafts in general remain to be answered. Long-term observations on portacaval shunt grafts are needed. A study of relatively long-segment grafts, 10 to 15 cm. in length, placed in the portal vein or used as shunt grafts would be of interest. Heparin therapy in conjunction with systemic vein grafting deserves consideration. These and other questions are the subject of continuing study.

## SUMMARY

The feasibility of successful autologous or homologous vein grafting in the canine portal vein has been demonstrated. An intensive regimen of heparin therapy was required to prevent early thrombosis. Late stenosis or occlusion of the graft was not encountered in the 9- to 16-month follow-up period.

Almost uniform success (93 per cent) was obtained with homologous vein and woven Teflon prosthesis grafts used in the construction of portacaval shunts. Heparin therapy was not required in these animals.

The relatively higher venous pressure in the portal vein is presumed to be the essential factor in the superior performance of the long-term portal vein grafts.

The pressure gradient between the portal vein and abdominal vena cava is thought to be responsible for the excellent results obtained with portacaval shunt grafts.

**REFERENCES**

1. Bower, R., Federicci, V., and Howard, J. M.: Continuing studies of replacement of segments of the venous system, SURGERY **47:** 132-139, 1960.
2. Bryant, M. E., Jr., Lazenby, W. D., and Howard, J. M.: Experimental replacement of short segments of veins, A. M. A. Arch. Surg. **76:** 289-293, 1958.
3. Child, G. C., III.: The hepatic circulation and portal hypertension, Philadelphia, 1954, W. B. Saunders Company.
4. Collins, H. A., Burrus, G., and De Bakey, M. E.: Experimental evaluation of grafts in the canine inferior vena cava, Am. J. Surg. **99:** 40-44, 1960.
5. Dale, W. A.: Discussion of Bower, R., Federicci, V., and Howard, J. M.[1]
6. Daniel, W. W.: Bridging defects in the canine portal and superior mesenteric veins with plastic and vascular grafts, Cancer **5:** 1041-1048, 1952.
7. Deterling, R. A., and Bhonslay, S. B.: Use of vessel grafts and plastic prostheses for relief of superior vena cava obstruction, SURGERY **38:** 1008, 1955.
8. East, W. M., and Muller, H. W., Jr.: An experimental study of resection and replacement of superior vena cava, Am. J. Surg. **99:** 6-10, 1960.
9. Jones, T. W., Stevenson, J. K., Jesseph, J. E., and Harkins, H. N.: A critical evaluation of polyvinyl sponge (Ivalon) as a vascular and tissue substitute, Am. Surgeon **24:** 401-414, 1958.
10. McLean, L. D., Phibbs, C. M., Flom, R. S., and Brainard, J. B.: Replacement of vital veins. A comparative experimental study, Ann. Surg. **149:** 549-554, 1959.
11. Moore, T. C., and Riberi, A.: Superior vena cava replacement. III. Successful use of fresh autogenous aorta, SURGERY **44:** 898-993, 1958.
12. Ohara, I., and Sakai, T.: Transplantation of the large venous system with various blood vessel substitutes, SURGERY **42:** 928-935, 1957.
13. Reynolds, J. T., and Southwick, H. W.: Portal hypertension: use of venous grafts when side-to-side anastomosis is impossible, A. M. A. Arch. Surg. **62:** 789-800, 1951.
14. Rousselot, L. M.: Autogenous vein grafts in splenorenal anastomosis, SURGERY **31:** 403-410, 1952.
15. Schauble, J. F., Anlyan, W. G., and Postlethwait, R. W.: A study of grafts in the venous system, A. M. A. Arch Surg. **78:** 288-292, 1959.
16. Silen, W., Mawdsley, D. L., Weirich, W. L., and Harper, H. A.: Studies of hepatic function in dogs with Eck fistula or porto caval transposition. A. M. A. Arch. Surg. **74:** 964-970, 1957.
17. Southwick, H. W.: Experimental use of preserved arterial grafts in portal anastomosis, Arch. Surg. **61:** 667-673, 1950.
18. Theron, P.: Portal caval operation with special reference to use of vein grafts, South African M. J. **27:** 73-76, 1953.

## DISCUSSION*

**Dr. William Blakemore** (Philadelphia, Pa.). We are indebted again to this group for presenting the characteristics of the cloth mesh prostheses, which reminds me that Dr. Sawyer provided the data that we used in setting up a bank for homografts about 9 years ago. Their report also emphasizes the fact that we should state in detail the characteristics of cloth mesh prostheses in our clinical reports. When we went back to report our first 250 cases of homografts, it was difficult to find out from the literature the methods of processing the grafts and to evaluate the results for these procedures. I am sure it is going to be even more difficult to evaluate the long-term follow-up results from reports of the use of cloth mesh prostheses which do not always provide details of the material used. The results in this report give us some of the criteria for what should be included in publications of clinical experience in order to permit evaluation of results reported from various centers where there is particular interest in these problems.

**Dr. William G. Anlyan** (Durham, N. C.). I want to compliment Dr. Foster and his colleagues on their excellent results. We have been interested in the problem of vein grafts also and some of our work has been published previously. Our results with venous autografts inserted into the femoral and jugular veins of mongrel dogs showed better than 85 per cent patency. However, with prosthetics (nylon, Dacron, Teflon, and Merselene), none of 66 grafts inserted in the jugular and femoral veins were patent. We did not use anticoagulant or fibrinolytic agents. We should explore further the more favorable conditions outlined by Dr. Foster.

**Dr. George L. Jordan, Jr.** (Houston, Texas). Dr. Wesolowski is to be congratulated for his extensive work on this subject. As many of you know, he is publishing a monograph which will document his observations in more detail. In his monograph he takes a strong stand for the use of the growing pig as the best experimental animal and presents data to indicate its advantages in comparison to the dog. As a result we are now

*Discussion of papers by Wesolowski, Fries, Karlson, De Bakey, and Sawyer; and Symbas, Foster, and Scott.

using some of these squealing beasts in our laboratory, although in the past we have preferred the dog as an experimental animal. We have studied many of the materials reported by Dr. Wesolowski and we have independently arrived at some of the same conclusions concerning the desirability of proper porosity. Tightly woven Teflon grafts may develop ulceration and separation of the neointima or "inner capsule," whereas more porous grafts demonstrate ingrowth of fibrous tissue between interstices which allows good adherence of the inner and outer fibrous capsules.

**Dr. Thomas C. Moore** (Muncie, Ind.). I want to compliment Dr. Foster and his associates on their interesting study. We have been interested in this problem of venous replacement with synthetic grafts for some time and have had very encouraging results in superior vena caval replacement. In the last 50 consecutive animals we have had a patency of 86 per cent. The replacements included Teflon grafts of all sizes, large and small, ranging from five-sixteenths of an inch to three-fourths of an inch in diameter. We found that the grafts which remained patent beyond the early days after operation had a tendency to remain patent thereafter.

We also had good results in replacement of the pulmonary artery. Our attempts to create a shunt between the inferior vena cava and the right pulmonary artery were uniformly unsuccessful. Apparently, the pressure gradient was too great and these grafts uniformly became occluded. We also have attempted to make some experimental shunts between the portal system and the systemic. We had hoped that a more rigid type of graft might be more successful in this area. However, of 8 very rigid and relatively long Teflon grafts from the portal vein to the right atrium, through the diaphragm, we found that only 1 remained patent.

**Dr. Sigmund A. Wesolowski** (closing). First, I would like to comment about grafts into the venous system. In a previous study, conducted by Lester Sauvage at Walter Reed Army Medical Center, we noted that in the preparation of the growing pig the most successful graft to replace defects in the thoracic inferior vena cava was the autologous vein, which proved superior to homologous vein, homologous aorta, and Orlon tubes.

I would like to thank Drs. Blakemore and Jordan for their comments and would like to emphasize that we are of the opinion that for the screening of the biological fate of vascular graft materials, the use of the dog is archaic. The dog is a readily available animal for screening the mechanical problems of graft implantation and the short-term fates of grafts. However, we strongly recommend the use of the growing pig for the rapid assessment of the equivalent long-term biological fate of any vascular graft material.

**Dr. John H. Foster** (closing). We wish to thank Dr. Anlyan and Dr. Moore for their discussion and remarks. We have followed the work of both of these investigators in the field of vein grafting with interest and appreciation. I should like to record the fact that although I presented this paper, Dr. Symbas is deservedly the first author. Low molecular weight dextran has been referred to in presentations given earlier this morning. The Swedish workers, especially Dr. Lars-Erik Gelin, have stimulated our interest in the influence of this substance on blood viscosity and vascular thrombosis. Current work indicates that low viscosity dextran is helpful in the prevention of thrombosis after vein grafting.

# Ischemic gangrene without major organic vascular occlusion: an enlarging concept

JAMES D. HARDY, M.D.
FIKRI ALICAN, M.D.
JACKSON, MISS.
*From the Department of Surgery and University Hospital, University of Mississippi Medical Center*

Ischemic gangrene is usually due to organic vascular occlusion. Nevertheless, it has become increasingly apparent that ischemic necrosis of tissue can occur in the absence of actual organic occlusion of the arterial supply. The mechanisms by which the blood supply to the tissue in question may be reduced below the critical level necessary to sustain viability are multiple. The purpose of this report is to emphasize conditions under which gangrene may be produced in the absence of actual organic occlusion of the major nutrient arteries. Without question, additional groups of etiologic circumstances will be described in the future. The case reports to be presented include those of 3 patients who sustained shock of varied etiology and that of 1 patient who probably had ischemia of the bowel after resection of coarctation of the aorta. The possible synergistic effects between endotoxin and the catecholamines in the production of tissue necrosis will be considered.

## CASE REPORTS

**Case 1. Incipient bowel necrosis after resection of coarctation of the aorta.** An 11-year-old minister's son was admitted to the University Hospital on July 4, 1956, with the diagnosis of coarctation of the aorta. The parents had been told years before that the boy had a heart murmur, and his mother had noted from birth that the heartbeat was quite forceful. He often had throbbing headaches and cramps in the leg muscles after running. He complained that his feet often "went to sleep" and he slept with socks on. The family physician had recommended an aortic operation, but this had been declined by the parents until an episode of coma occurred, probably due to hypertensive encephalopathy after hard exercise on a hot day.

*Physical examination.* The presence of moderate hypertension in the arms with hypotension and weak pulses in the legs was confirmed. The chest radiograph showed notching of the ribs as well as an aortic shadow compatible with coarctation.

*Operation.* A left thoracotomy was performed on July 6, 1956, and the coarcted segment of the aorta was resected. This was followed by primary end-to-end anastomosis. Bounding foot pulses were present immediately thereafter.

*Postoperative course.* The postoperative course was remarkable because of excessive tachycardia associated with a febrile response. The pulse rate promptly rose to 140 from the preoperative rate of 80, and this level persisted for 2 days. The normal rate was not regained for almost 4 days. During this time the patient exhibited increased hypertension, an anxious expression, circumoral pallor, and excessive sweating. A prominent complaint was of abdominal pain, tenderness, and distention, the cause of which was not clear. Gradually these symptoms, reminiscent of those of epinephrine intoxication, subsided. The blood pressure in the arms declined to a normal level and that in the legs rose to exceed the pressure in the upper extremities, as measured with the sphygmomanometer.

*Comment.* At the time this patient was operated upon we were not familiar with the so-called postcoarctation syndrome. However, in 1954 Lober and Lillehei[16] had described panarteritis after repair of coarctation of the aorta. Sealy and his associates[23] later offered information which suggested that paradoxical postcoarctation hypertension associated with necrotizing arteritis[2] might

Supported by Army Contract No. DA-49-007-MD-627. Read at the Twenty-second Annual Meeting of the Society of University Surgeons, Kansas City, Kan., Feb. 9-11, 1961.

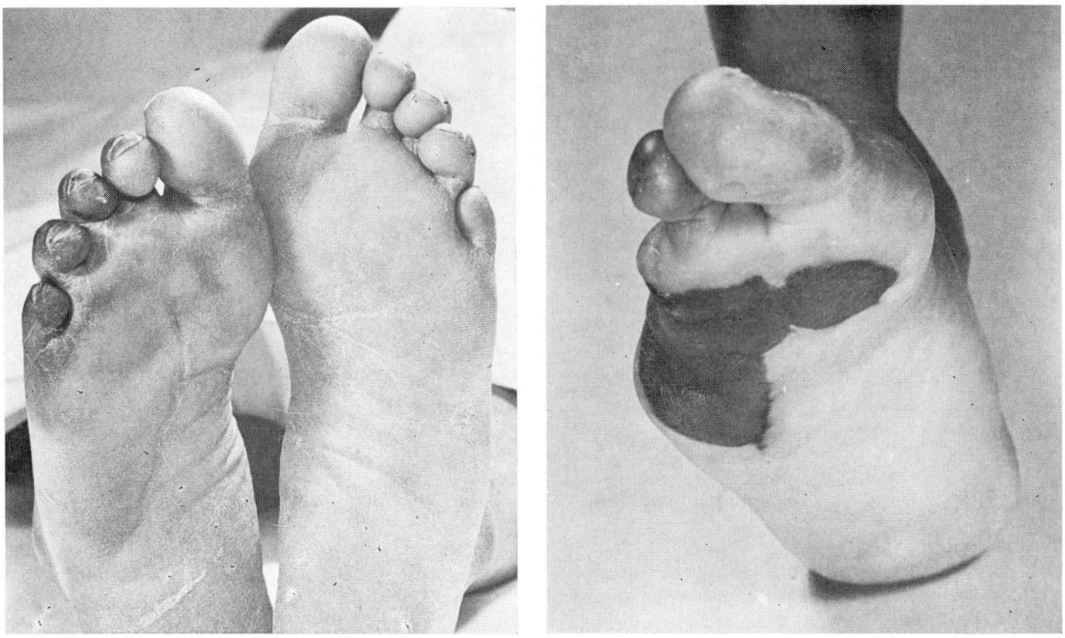

**Fig. 1.** Gangrene of the third, fourth, and fifth toes secondary to shock during diabetic coma. Superimposed vasospasm due to arterial and venous trauma may have accounted for the selective involvement of the right foot. Peripheral gangrene secondary to shock is usually bilateral and symmetrical.

be due to an increase in norepinephrine elaboration. They reported a case of gangrene of the bowel after resection of coarctation of the aorta, and suggested that this gangrene might be secondary to severe vasospasm produced by elevated catecholamine levels. Similar cases were reported by others.[18 20, 22, 24] In describing a particularly striking case, Cooley[8] concluded that the arterial changes were most probably secondary to a sudden increase in the blood pressure distal to the site of the previous coarctation. He pointed out that the arteries proximal to the level of coarctation were little affected, and that the relatively poor support of the walls of the mesenteric arteries rendered these vessels particularly vulnerable to the sudden increase in intraluminal pressure after repair of the coarctation.

There can be little doubt that the arteritis, however produced, is often associated with varying degrees of arteriospasm. Thus, the postcoarctation syndrome represents a circumstance in which arteriospasm may contribute significantly to the development of ischemia.

**Case 2. Gangrene secondary to prolonged shock in diabetic coma.** A 9-year-old girl was admitted to the University Hospital on Dec. 15, 1959, in diabetic coma. She was severely dehydrated and the blood pressure had been unobtainable for hours. A blood specimen was drawn from the right femoral artery, and a blood transfusion was started through the right saphenous vein by means of a cut-down at the ankle. After several additional hours of hypotension an adequate blood pressure was restored by the intravenous therapy and correction of the metabolic acidosis. The patient had received no vasopressor drug.

Two days after admission the patient complained of pain in the right foot. It was then noted for the first time that there was marked discoloration of the skin overlying the third, fourth, and fifth toes as well as a portion of the plantar surface (Fig. 1). Although the dorsalis pedis and posterior tibial pulses were still present bilaterally, as they had been on admission, therapy was ineffectual in preventing gangrene and these digits eventually had to be amputated.

*Comment.* Prolonged shock has resulted in symmetrical gangrene of the lower extremities on numerous occasions.[1, 6, 9, 25] In the present case, however, only the right leg was involved. Careful investigation showed only 2 likely causes for different degrees of perfusion of the 2 feet. It will be recalled that the cut-down was performed on the saphenous vein at the right ankle and that the right femoral artery was punctured for a blood specimen. The toenails had been deeply cyanotic at the time of admission, when the patient had been in shock for hours. One may speculate that these usually innocuous measures, performed on the vasculature of the right leg at a time when blood flow was at a critical level, could have produced just that amount of additional vasospasm required to cause gangrene. Of course, this was a juvenile diabetic patient and it is possible that some degree of arteriosclerosis existed. Even so, foot pulses were present, the wound healing and graft "take" were excellent (Fig. 1), and the blood supply of the remaining portion of the right foot appeared to be satisfactory. Thus, the factor of increased arteriospasm during shock, when the oxygenation of the low volume of blood actually reaching the foot may have been poor, must be given serious consideration as a major factor in the gangrene which developed.

**Case 3. Incipient gangrene of the small bowel associated with prolonged norepinephrine therapy for shock.** A 35-year-old man was admitted to the Veterans Administration Hospital on Jan. 14, 1961, in an acute psychotic state. The history obtained from relatives was incomplete, but it was known that the patient had been on a drinking bout for at least 2 days. At one time he had complained of abdominal pain, but thereafter his psychiatric condition had deteriorated to resemble what one observer considered to represent schizophrenia, catatonic type.

The laboratory data were not particularly remarkable. The white blood cell count was 8,800 with a normal differential. The patient was admitted to the neuropsychiatric ward where the blood pressure was found to be 200/120. Promazine therapy was started, but after 3 doses the blood pressure had fallen to 60/30 and the man's condition appeared to be critical. A Neo-Synephrine drip did not produce a satisfactory rise in the blood pressure and norepinephrine administration was begun. Such support had to be continued for 39 hours before a stable blood pressure above 100 mm. Hg could be maintained without vasopressor drug.

On Jan. 16, 1961, the patient was transferred to the medical ward, where he vomited approximately 500 ml. of straw-colored fluid. The abdomen was distended and surgical consultation was requested on January 17. Additional radiographs showed findings compatible with small bowel obstruction and, after a period of further observation and treatment, exploratory laparotomy was performed on January 18. Aside from generalized bowel distention, the most striking finding consisted of multiple, dark, ecchymotic areas along the antimesenteric border of the small bowel. Although the general appearance of the antimesenteric border improved somewhat after decompression of the bowel by means of enterotomy, it was the belief of the surgeon that the changes in the wall of the small bowel were not due entirely to distention secondary to adynamic ileus. The condition of the patient slowly improved over subsequent days.

*Comment.* It was not clear why this patient sustained such a markedly prolonged hypertensive reaction to promazine therapy, but such episodes are known to occur. It was believed likely that the patchy areas of discoloration along the antimesenteric border of the bowel were due to the combined effects of norepinephrine therapy and increased intraluminal pressure due to distention. Certainly spasm of the small vessels which supply the antimesenteric surface of the bowel would further jeopardize the viability of a tissue which has blood vessels already peculiarly vulnerable to the effects of distention, though paralytic ileus alone rarely produces a sufficient degree of distention to cause bowel necrosis.

There is ample record of the fact that excessive amounts of vasoconstrictor drugs can result in bowel necrosis, as they may in necrosis of the liver[5] and other tissues, such as skin. Brown and associates[4] reported the case of a 61-year-old man who received Neo-Synephrine for hypotension associated with postoperative myocardial infarction. At postmortem examination there was infarction and ulceration of the small bowel with an associated proliferative arteritis of the intramural vessels. None of the major vessels supplying this bowel were occluded. In another case, in which malignant pheochromocytoma with liver metastases was producing tremendous plasma l-norepinephrine levels, there was extensive gangrene of the bowel in the absence of major vascular occlusion.[3]

**Case 4. Perforated ulcer, shock, and incipient bowel necrosis.** A 73-year-old woman was admitted to the University Hospital on Dec. 14, 1959, with the chief complaint of pain in the abdomen of 5 days' duration and recent hematemesis. She had a long history of peptic ulceration, and an episode of gastrointestinal hemorrhage had occurred in 1959 for which she had been hospitalized in her community hospital and had received 2 blood transfusions. The present difficulty had begun 5 days prior to admission with cramping abdominal pain in the epigastrium associated with occasional vomiting. Nevertheless, she had not considered herself seriously ill until the last 24 hours, when she had vomited an estimated teacupful of blood. The abdominal pain and distention had increased progressively thereafter.

*Physical examination.* The blood pressure was not audible by stethoscope but was palpated at 80 mm. Hg systolic. The abdomen was distended 3 or 4 cm. above the xiphopubic line and tympanitic to percussion, with virtually absent bowel sounds. There were no palpable organs or masses and rigidity was not marked. Digital examination of the rectum yielded negative results, but when

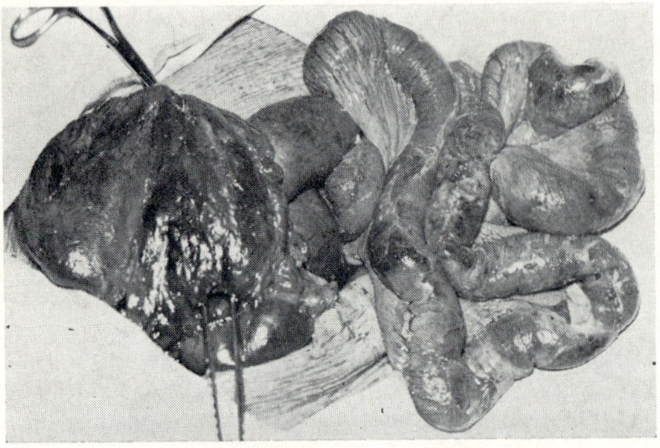

**Fig. 2.** Perforated gastric ulcer, peritonitis, and prolonged shock. There was patchy, incomplete necrosis of the antimesenteric surface of the bowel wall.

the proctoscope was introduced to a distance of 10 cm. the rectal mucosa was found to appear gangrenous. Roentgenograms of the abdomen disclosed distention of the bowel and free air in the peritoneal cavity. The apparently necrotic colonic mucosa and the large amount of free air in the peritoneal cavity were suggestive of volvulus of the sigmoid colon with perforation, although perforated peptic ulcer was statistically the more likely diagnosis, especially in view of the long history of peptic ulcer.

*Exploratory laparotomy.* Laparotomy was performed as soon as it was apparent that the blood pressure would not be substantially elevated by additional intravenous fluid therapy. Actually, the blood pressure remained at a shock level. As soon as the abdomen had been opened a tremendous amount of foul-smelling gas escaped, along with a brownish liquid exudate. The primary lesion was a 1 cm. perforated gastric ulcer just proximal to the pylorus (Fig. 2). There was no evidence of an attempt on the part of the omentum to seal the defect. A most remarkable additional finding was the presence of many areas of patchy "necrosis" along the antimesenteric border of the small bowel and colon. Inasmuch as it could not be determined clinically whether or not these areas involved the full thickness of the bowel wall, and since almost the entire length of the gut was intermittently involved, no surgical attack was made upon these lesions. The patient died immediately after operation.

*Autopsy.* A minimum of atherosclerosis of the aorta and its branches was found. In fact, the pathologist commented that the vessels were surprisingly elastic for a patient 73 years of age. There was marked distention of the stomach and small bowel, and the peritoneal covering was found to be granular with the exudate described at the time of operation. The stomach contained a small amount of dark reddish-black blood, as did the small bowel. The colon contained a small amount of brownish feces. The mucosa of the entire bowel, except for small areas of the colon, was dark maroon in color. The mucosa of the mediastinal esophagus exhibited the same changes. In the prepyloric area of the stomach was noted the remainder of an ulcer crater, 1.5 cm. in diameter, a portion of which had been excised for biopsy at the time the ulcer had been closed during operation. The microscopic studies showed that the changes in the bowel wall consisted largely of the focal areas of hemorrhage and impending necrosis previously outlined.

*Comment.* The extensive changes in the wall of the large and small bowel observed were very probably due to the prolonged shock which was caused by perforation of the gastric ulcer and aggravated by distention due to ileus. The bowel was not perforated at any point, and the apparently necrotic spots did not involve the full thickness of the wall. Nevertheless, these changes were certainly of critical degree and might well have permitted escape of endotoxins from the bowel lumen to the peritoneal cavity.

Severe shock due to various causes may be associated with hemorrhage into, and even slough of, the bowel mucosa. It is of interest to consider why the bowel mucosa may be especially vulnerable to ischemia.

For one thing, the organism reacts to hypotension by reducing blood flow to noncritical regions of the body, and these noncritical tissues include the bowel and the extremities. The arteries and arterioles of these organs, as well as of the kidneys, are considered to be particularly sensitive to the vasoconstrictor effects of the endogenous catecholamines produced to combat shock. Thus, it is perhaps not surprising that erythema, hemorrhage, and even slough of the intestinal mucosa are not rare after prolonged shock—unless the bowel is protected by perfusion of the superior mesenteric artery with oxygenated blood.[14] Moreover, in recent years an additional factor has been introduced. Thomas and associates[26] published evidence that endotoxin so sensitizes certain tissues to the vasospastic effects of epinephrine (and presumably norepinephrine) that local necrosis occurs. These workers also found that similar necrosis could be produced by the injection of a mixture of serotonin and epinephrine into the skin of rats. Yet neither serotonin nor epinephrine alone produced hemorrhagic necrosis. These observations are also supported by reports that the deleterious effects of injected endotoxin are lessened by the use of sympathetic ganglionic blocking agents such as Dibenzyline.[15]

In substance, therefore, the presence of endotoxin-forming bacteria in the lumen of the bowel could conceivably render the intestinal mucosa especially susceptible to the possible potentiating vasospastic effects of endotoxin and norepinephrine in shock. The frequency with which mucosal erythema, hemorrhage, and slough are found after prolonged shock renders attractive the hypothesis that endotoxin-norepinephrine synergism is a possible cause of tissue necrosis under appropriate circumstances.

## LABORATORY OBSERVATIONS

Although circulating endotoxin might have a vasospastic effect in the presence of normal or even reduced norepinephrine levels, the possibility of such effects should be increased if the injection of endotoxin were found to increase the plasma norepinephrine levels experimentally. This does occur, and illustrative data from our studies are presented in Table I. The plasma catecholamine levels[21, 27] were determined in more than 50 dogs in which profound shock was produced by lethal doses of *E. coli* endotoxin. In substance, the majority of the animals exhibited a rise in the plasma norepinephrine level but little or no rise in the epinephrine level. Furthermore, an occasional dog experienced rises in the plasma norepinephrine level which approached those found during hypertensive crises due to pheochromocytoma (Table I). The more frequently blood samples were drawn after injection of the endotoxin, the more informative was the resulting curve which reflected alterations in plasma norepinephrine values. At autopsy the dogs exhibited bloody fluid in the bowel lumen as well as extensive hemorrhages into the mucosa.

Clearly, the patient with bacteremia might be subjected to markedly elevated levels of endogenous norepinephrine. As yet we have not had an opportunity to measure plasma catecholamine levels in patients with septicemia, but it is known that such patients may exhibit ecchymotic hemorrhages in the alimentary mucosa.

**Table I.** *Plasma catecholamine levels in endotoxin shock: Dog No. 15 (gamma/L.)*

| *Samples* | *Epinephrine* | *Norepinephrine* |
|---|---|---|
| Control | 0.85 | 0.32 |
| 1 (5 min.) | 0.14 | 3.83 |
| 2 (24 min.) | 0 | 17.35 |
| 3 (45 min.) | 0 | 0.32 |

## COMMENT

The ultimate cause of acute tissue necrosis is hypoxia. It logically follows that many different pathologic mechanisms may contribute to the hypoxia affecting a given tissue. While the most common and dramatic cause of acute gangrene is organic arterial occlusion, other potential factors favoring the development of hypoxia at the cellular level must be acknowledged. Certain of these are presented in Fig. 3.

**Heart disease (defective cardiac output without shock).**

*Congestive failure.* It is not difficult to appreciate the fact that an excessively low cardiac output, such as may be associated with a ventricular aneurysm, for example, can contribute to defective tissue perfusion.[10] The patient with severe paradoxical motion of a major segment of the ventricular wall may have a cardiac output of less than one-half the normal value. If the peripheral vessels of such a patient were then to be subjected to excessive spasm, the distal tissues might well be rendered critically hypoxic.[19] These effects might be rendered even more harmful in the presence of anasarca.

*Aortic insufficiency.* For years it has been appreciated that patients with aortic regurgitation often have abdominal pain which need not be associated with congestive failure,[7, 12] and recently cases of intestinal infarction secondary to aortic insufficiency have been reported with increasing frequency.[13] Most, but not all, of these patients had had congestive heart failure as well as aortic valvular incompetence. Nevertheless, it appears to be well established that severe aortic insufficiency can result in bowel necrosis in the absence of congestive heart failure, shock, or occlusion of the mesenteric arteries. Furthermore, the bowel infarction associated with aortic insufficiency is usually related to the distribution of either the superior or the inferior mesenteric artery, or

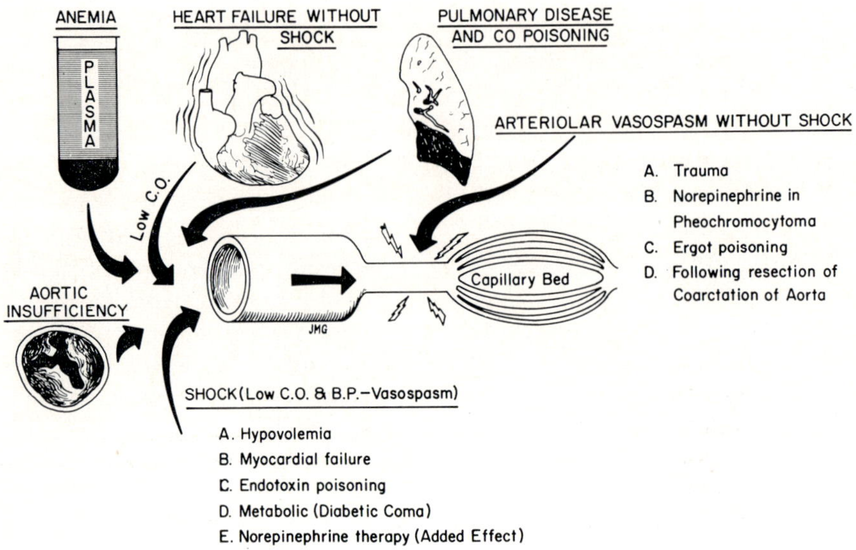


**Fig. 3.** Causes of tissue hypoxia without organic vascular occlusion. Although there is much overlapping, the diagram illustrates various mechanisms, the net effect of which is to reduce the amount of oxygen available at the tissue level.

both, in sharp contrast to instances of bowel gangrene not due to aortic insufficiency or mesenteric arterial occlusion.[10]

Although the hemodynamics of aortic valvular disease have been studied by various investigators,[11] the physiologic basis for the intestinal ischemia associated with aortic regurgitation is not settled. It is possible that filling of the mesenteric arteries in aortic insufficiency is analogous to that of the coronary arteries, and that perfusion of the extremities is thus superior to that of the bowel.[13] However, a perhaps more plausible explanation invokes the relationship of arteriolar tone and cross-sectional dimensions to the inherent stability of these vessels.[13] Nichol and his associates[17] pointed out that, because of vasomotor tone, the small blood vessels can have only limited stability. Thus, abrupt and marked reduction in aortic pressure, as during diastole in the patient with severe aortic insufficiency, is transmitted through the larger mesenteric artery to the mesenteric arteriole, the point of maximum resistance because of high tonus and small cross-sectional diameter. With the intraluminal pressure suddenly decreased markedly to below the critical level required to distend the arteriole, flow in the arteriole could actually be reversed. Such a pathophysiologic circumstance could result in edema, hemorrhage, hypoxia, and eventual necrosis of the tissue supplied. Although stagnation of blood frequently leads to thrombosis, thrombotic occlusion of major mesenteric vessels need not be present for intestinal infarction to occur.

**Defective blood oxygenation.**

*Pulmonary disease.* Peripheral gangrene has been described in association with various lung diseases, but certain of the patients may have been in shock, a special circumstance which will be discussed separately. Nevertheless, defective pulmonary ventilation, diffusion, or perfusion can certainly reduce the oxygen supply delivered to peripheral tissues. This would render such tissues unusually susceptible to vasospasm (Fig. 3). We have found no reported instances of peripheral gangrene secondary to emphysema, pulmonary arteriovenous fistula, or pulmonary arterial occlusion, but we did observe profound cyanosis of the hands and feet in a young woman dying of pulmonary arterial occlusion secondary to mediastinal collaginosis.

*Carbon monoxide poisoning.* It has been suggested that chronic carbon monoxide poisoning may contribute to the development of peripheral gangrene, though we have not found a report of such a case.

*Anemia.* Although theoretically the presence of severe anemia should markedly increase the probability of peripheral gangrene in the otherwise susceptible patient, it is remarkable how few such patients are encountered if those with ulcers associated with sickle-cell disease are excluded. And yet, perhaps this is not too surprising after all, for the tissues of the patient in whom anemia develops gradually become adjusted to the relative hypoxia. Vasospasm is not a prominent finding in these patients as it is in the subject rendered abruptly anemic (oligemic) by massive blood loss.

**The peripheral vascular bed.**

*Vasospasm without shock.* In Fig. 3 are presented illustrative circumstances under which gangrene may follow severe vasoconstriction in the absence of generalized systemic hypotension or shock. They include the reaction to trauma, malignant pheochromocytoma with metastases producing large amounts of vasoconstrictor material, ergot poisoning, and vasospasm arteriolitis after resection of coarctation of the aorta. To these might be added the phenomena grouped loosely as "Raynaud's disease" and "Raynaud's phenomenon" associated with partial organic vascular occlusion.

*Traumatic arteriospasm* producing gangrene has been reported for a great many years, but close scrutiny of many of these cases suggests that the diagnosis may have been at least partially in error. Arterial thrombosis or subintimal hemorrhage is readily confused with arteriospasm and, in fact, prolonged arteriospasm may lead to arterial thrombosis and distal gangrene. In any event, severe arteriospasm can unquestionably produce ischemia that may result in tissue necrosis under appropriate collateral circumstances.

**Shock.** The great common denominator of by far the majority of reported cases of gangrene without organic vascular occlusion has been shock. This has been true whether the necrosis was associated with severe heart disease, diabetic coma, infection, or hypovolemia. It is well known that an already ischemic tissue—leg, bowel, kidney, heart, or brain—tolerates a prolonged period of hypotension poorly. The patient in shock may present 3 important factors which favor the development of peripheral gangrene—reduced cardiac output, defective oxygenation of the blood, and severe differential vasoconstriction which occurs in an effort to preserve vital organs. Apparently the lower extremities have become gangrenous most often under these circumstances, with the bowel next in frequency. Melena is not rare after either prolonged shock or bowel ischemia due to other causes.

It is too soon to assess accurately the role of endogenous endotoxins and catecholamines, separately or synergistically, with respect to the production of tissue necrosis. However, the evidence suggests that these factors may prove to be important ones.

## SUMMARY AND CONCLUSIONS

1. The phenomenon of ischemic gangrene developing in the absence of major organic vascular occlusion has received increased attention in recent years.

2. Four cases of incipient or overt tissue necrosis unassociated with major organic vascular occlusion have been presented.

3. Pathophysiologic circumstances which may predispose to the development of gangrene include chronic heart failure with reduced cardiac output, derangements in one or more of the 3 major components of pulmonary function, and prolonged arteriospasm from any cause. Aortic insufficiency, a special form of heart disease, apparently may result in bowel infarction in the absence of congestive failure. Shock due to any cause may adversely affect peripheral blood flow in a variety of ways, and it is the most common predisposing cause of gangrene in the absence of major arterial occlusion.

4. The special problem of possible synergistic effects of endotoxin and endogenous norepinephrine in producing tissue necrosis

has been considered. Data are presented which demonstrate sharply elevated norepinephrine levels in dogs subjected to lethal endotoxin shock. The possible importance of the endotoxin-norepinephrine factor in producing the bowel changes found in one of our patients with peritonitis and shock has been reviewed.

5. Hypoxia is the ultimate cause of acute tissue necrosis in most instances. Any disease condition which interferes with the delivery of an adequate oxygen supply at the cellular level may predispose to gangrene, whether or not major arterial occlusion is an additional contributing factor.

## REFERENCES


1. Abrahams, D. G.: Incipient symmetrical peripheral gangrene complicating paroxysmal tachycardia, Brit. Heart J. **10:** 191, 1948.
2. Benson, W. R., and Sealy, W. C.: Arterial necrosis following resection of coarctation of the aorta, Lab. Investig. **5:** 359, 1956.
3. Brown, R. B., and Barowsky, M.: Further observations on intestinal lesions associated with pheochromocytomas, Ann. Surg. **151:** 683, 1960.
4. Brown, R. B., Rice, B. H., and Szakacs, J. E.: Intestinal bleeding and perforation complicating treatment with vasoconstrictors, Ann. Surg. **150:** 790, 1959.
5. Brunson, J. G., Eckman, P. L., and Campbell, J. B.: The increasing prevalence of unexplained liver necrosis, New England J. Med. **257:** 52, 1957.
6. Chatterjee, S. C.: Symmetrical peripheral gangrene in lobar pneumonia, Calcutta M. J. **37:** 221, 1940.
7. Clinico-pathologic conference: Aortic insufficiency with cardiac failure and recurrent abdominal pain, Am. J. Med. **11:** 507, 1951.
8. Cooley, D. A.: Complications of procedures on the thoracic aorta. *In* Complications in surgery and their management, Philadelphia, 1960, W. B. Saunders Company, p. 511.
9. Cotton, R. T., and Bedford, D. R.: Symmetrical peripheral gangrene complicating acute myocardial infarction, Am. J. Med. **20:** 301, 1956.
10. Ende, N.: Infarction of bowel in cardiac failure, New England J. Med. **258:** 879, 1958.
11. Gorlin, R., McMillan, I. K. R., Medd, W. E., Matthews, M. B., and Daley, R.: Dynamics of the circulation in aortic valvular disease, Am. J. Med. **18:** 855, 1955.
12. Harvey, W. P., Segal, J. P., and Hufnagel, C. A.: Unusual clinical features associated with severe aortic insufficiency, Ann. Int. Med. **47:** 27, 1957.
13. Hoffman, F. G., Zimmerman, S. L., and Cardwell, E. S., Jr.: Massive intestinal infarction without vascular occlusion associated with aortic insufficiency, New England J. Med. **263:** 436, 1960.
14. Lillehei, R. C.: Intestinal factor in irreversible hemorrhagic shock, SURGERY **42:** 1043, 1957.
15. Lillehei, R. C., and MacLean, L. D.: The intestinal factor in irreversible endotoxin shock, Ann. Surg. **148:** 513, 1958.
16. Lober, P. H., and Lillehei, C. W.: Necrotizing panarteritis following repair of coarctation of aorta, SURGERY **35:** 950, 1954.
17. Nichol, J., Girling, F., Jerrard, W., Claxton, E. B., and Burton, A. C.: Fundamental instability of small blood vessels and critical closing pressures in vascular beds, Am. J. Physiol. **164:** 330, 1951.
18. Perez-Alvarez, P. P., and Oudkerk, S.: Necrotizing arteriolitis of the abdominal organs as a postoperative complication following correction of coarctation of the aorta, SURGERY **37:** 833, 1955.
19. Perry, C. B., and Davie, T. B.: Symmetrical peripheral gangrene in cardiac failure, Brit. M. J. **1:** 15, 1939.
20. Reid, H. C., and Dallechy, R.: Infarction of ileus following resection of coarctation of aorta, Brit. J. Surg. **45:** 625, 1958.
21. Richardson, J. A., Richardson, A. J., and Brodie, O. J.: Fluorimetric determination of epinephrine and norepinephrine in plasma, J. Lab. & Clin. Med. **47:** 832, 1956.
22. Ring, D. M., and Lewis, F. J.: Abdominal pain following surgical correction of coarctation of the aorta: a syndrome, J. Thoracic Surg. **31:** 718, 1956.
23. Sealy, W. C., Harris, J. S., Young, W. G., Jr., and Callaway, H. A., Jr.: Paradoxical hypertension following resection of coarctation of aorta, SURGERY **42:** 135, 1957.
24. Singleton, A. O., Jr., McGinnis, L. M. S., and Eason, H. R.: Arteritis following correction of coarctation of the aorta, SURGERY **45:** 665, 1959.
25. Swan, W. G. A., and Henderson, C. B.: Peripheral gangrene in myocardial infarction, Brit. Heart J. **13:** 68, 1951.
26. Thomas, L., Zweifach, B. W., and Benacerraf, B.: Mechanisms in the production of tissue damage and shock by endotoxins, Tr. A. Am. Physicians **60:** 54, 1957.
27. Weil-Malherbe, H., and Bone, A. D.: The chemical estimation of adrenaline-like substances in blood, Biochem. J. **51:** 311, 1952.


*(For discussion, see page 125.)*

# Influence of l-norepinephrine on renal blood flow, renal vascular resistance, and urine flow in hemorrhagic shock

RUSSELL M. NELSON, M.D., Ph.D.
JAMES W. HENRY, B.A.
JAMES H. LYMAN, B.A.
SALT LAKE CITY, UTAH
*From the Departments of Surgery, Salt Lake Clinic, Latter-day Saints Hospital, and the University of Utah College of Medicine*

Controversy continues regarding the possible beneficial use of vasopressor agents in the clinical management of hemorrhagic shock. Some investigators have demonstrated an increase in mortality rate[5, 15, 16, 19] and others have demonstrated reduction of mortality rates with the use of l-norepinephrine.[7]

Van Slyke[17] and others have emphasized the role of the kidney in shock and many investigators have attempted to assess the effects of vasopressors on renal hemodynamics and function. Moyer and Handley,[13] utilizing renal function tests for the measurement of renal blood flow, found that epinephrine and norepinephrine, when administered by continuous infusion, caused a marked reduction in renal blood flow, renal plasma flow, and glomerular filtration rate. On the other hand, Morris and associates[12] observed improved renal blood flow with the use of vasopressors in hemorrhagic shock. Varying results have also been reported with regard to rate of urine formation in animals subjected to bleeding and subsequent vasopressor therapy.[8, 10, 18, 20]

The recent development of electromagnetic flowmeters has made possible the estimation of blood flow without cannulation or dependence upon the integrity of renal function. Such a flowmeter was employed in this experiment in order to estimate renal blood flow and to permit calculation of renal vascular resistance in dogs subjected to arterial hemorrhage and subsequent continuous infusion of l-norepinephrine. For comparison, the femoral artery was employed in 1 group instead of the renal artery.

## METHODS

Twenty-eight mongrel dogs averaging 20 kilograms body weight were employed in this study. The animals were anesthetized intravenously with Nembutal (30 mg. per kilogram) and intermittent positive-pressure insufflation of oxygen was given via an endotracheal tube. Surgical incisions were made in the femoral regions and in the right flank for exposure of the femoral vessels and right renal pedicle.

Arterial pressure was determined by insertion of a catheter into the distal aorta via an arteriotomy in the right femoral artery. A Statham strain gauge transducer was employed to permit electronic monitoring and recording.*

Renal (or femoral) blood flow was determined by encircling the right renal (or right femoral) artery with a probe which fit the artery. The current generated from the probe was then fed into the electromagnetic flowmeter† and thence to the oscilloscope

Supported by grants from the United States Public Health Service (No. H-5677), Utah Heart Association, and the American Heart Association.

Read at the Twenty-second Annual Meeting of the Society of University Surgeons, Kansas City, Kan., Feb. 9-11, 1961.

*Electronics for Medicine, White Plains, N. Y.

†Square-wave electromagnetic flowmeter with built-in integrator, Avionics Research Products Corp., Venice, Calif.

and photographic recorder. The flowmeter was calibrated after each experiment by allowing known volumes of blood removed from the dog to pass through the flowmeter in known increments of time. Zero flows were obtained in the dog by temporary clamping of the vessel.

Renal (or femoral) vascular resistance was calculated by dividing the pressure value by the value for blood flow.

Urine flow was measured by cannulation of the right ureter with a polyethylene catheter. The tip of the catheter was placed in the pelvis of the right kidney and connected to an electronic drop counter. The signal from the counter was also fed into the oscilloscope and recorder. The results are reported in urine drops per minute (53 drops of urine equals 1 ml.).

Rectal temperature was determined by a thermistor probe inserted into the rectum and connected to a telethermometer. Temperatures ranged between 98° and 102° F. with no apparent correlation with results observed.

The 28 animals studied were divided into 3 groups. Protocols for each group were divided into several periods of 30 minutes each. In Group 1 (7 dogs) these periods were (A) no infusion, (B) rapid arterial hemorrhage of 25 ml. per kilogram followed by observation without infusion, (C) control intravenous infusion of 0.9 per cent normal saline solution (1 ml. per minute for 30 minutes), (D) infusion of l-norepinephrine (4 mg. per 250 ml. of 0.9 per cent saline solution) by continuous intravenous drip (30 minutes) to bring the arterial pressure back to the control value (this was gauged to simulate the clinical use of l-norepinephrine; therefore, the infusion rate was not precisely constant but as close as one can get with the use of standard intravenous regulating screw clamps), and (E) no infusion.

In Group 2 (11 dogs), the protocol was designed to assess the effects of l-norepinephrine prior to hemorrhage as well as after hemorrhage. The 30-minute periods were (A) no infusion, (B) control intravenous infusion of 0.9 per cent saline solution (1 ml. per minute for 30 minutes), (C) continuous infusion of l-norepinephrine to produce an elevation of arterial pressure of approximately 25 per cent for 30 minutes, (D) no infusion, (E) rapid arterial hemorrhage (25 ml. per kilogram) followed by observation to the conclusion of the period, (F) control infusion 0.9 per cent saline (1 ml. per minute for 30 minutes), (G) continuous intravenous infusion of l-norepinephrine at a rate required to hold the arterial pressure at the control value, and (H) no infusion.

In Group 3 (10 dogs), in order to observe the changes in another vascular bed, blood flow was measured in the femoral artery instead of the renal artery. For technical reasons, it was not possible to measure renal and femoral blood flows in the same dogs. Five dogs were subjected to the protocol followed for Group 1 and 5 dogs were subjected to the protocol followed for Group 2.

Recordings during each of the 30-minute periods were essentially continuous. Calculations were made at each minute and the results reported represent the mean values obtained for each period of 30 minutes.

## RESULTS

**Group 1.** During the period of hemorrhage, there was a decline in arterial blood pressure, renal blood flow, and urine flow with a rise in renal vascular resistance. This was followed by a trend toward normal during the recovery. The infusion of l-norepinephrine, which restored the blood pressure to the range of control values, was associated with a reduction in renal arterial blood flow and urine flow, with a marked rise in renal vascular resistance. After the infusion of l-norepinephrine had been discontinued, there was again a rise in the volume of urine and a fall in the arterial pressure and the renal vascular resistance. The mean values for each period and the mean change in per cent of control values for each period are tabulated in Table I.

These results are demonstrated graphically in Fig. 1. On the abscissa, time is expressed as periods of observation and on the ordi-

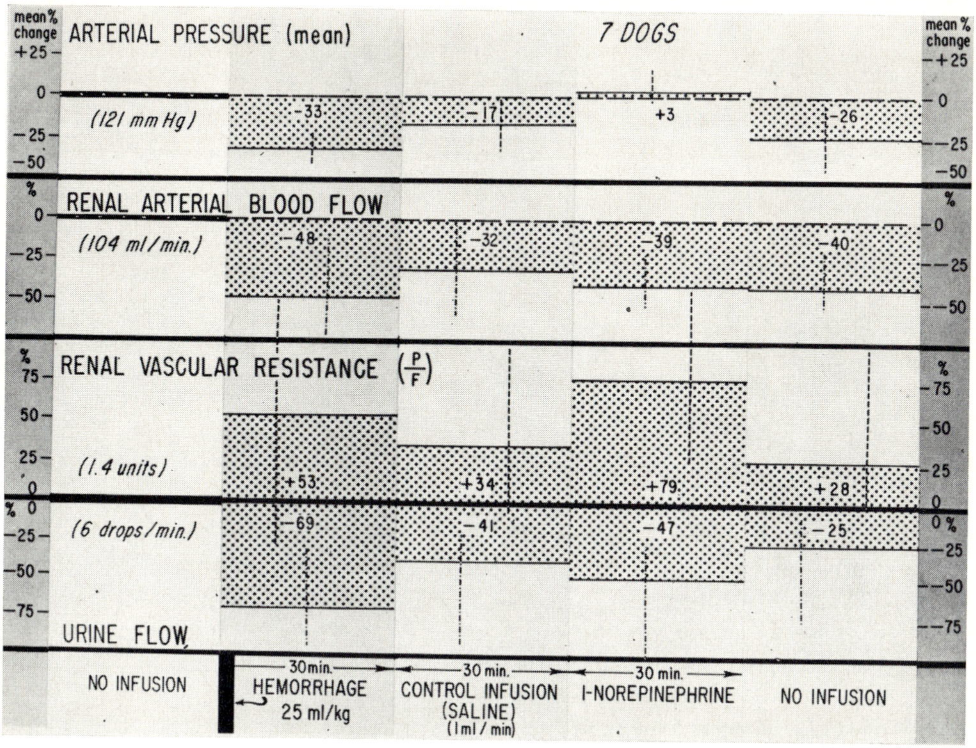


**Fig. 1.** Results in Group 1.

nate, the mean values for arterial pressure, renal blood flow, renal vascular resistance, and urine flow are expressed as per cent of the control values. The ranges of values are indicated by the vertical lines.

**Group 2.** Prior to hemorrhage, the infusion of l-norepinephrine at a rate sufficient to maintain the arterial pressure approximately 25 per cent above the control pressure was associated with a mean rise in the rate of urine flow to 32 per cent above the control level. During this period, there was a moderate rise in renal vascular resistance and no significant change in renal arterial blood flow.

During the period of hemorrhage, there was a marked rise in renal vascular resistance associated with the fall in arterial pressure, renal blood flow, and urine flow. After the hemorrhage, there was a trend for each of these values to return toward the control.

During the infusion of l-norepinephrine after hemorrhage, there was a marked rise in renal vascular resistance with a diminution in renal blood flow and in urine flow. After the l-norepinephrine was discontinued, the arterial pressure and renal vascular resistance again fell but renal blood flow and urine flow increased. These results are tabulated in Tables II, III, and IV. The data from these tables are represented graphically in Fig. 2. Values are expressed as in Fig. 1 for the control period and the mean change in per cent of the control values for each period of observation.

**Group 3.** The results in this series were similar to those observed in Groups 1 and 2 with 2 interesting variations. First, in the period of l-norepinephrine infusion after hemorrhage, urine flow increased in one dog to 33 per cent above the control value. Second, the femoral vascular resistance did not rise as high during the period of hemorrhage as did the renal vascular resistance in the first 2 groups. The results are tabulated in Tables V, VI, and VII.

The results from Group 3 are depicted

**Table I.** *Effects of hemorrhage and subsequent infusions on blood pressure, renal blood flow, renal vascular resistance, and urine flow (Group 1)*

| Dog | | Period A, no infusion | | | | Period B, hemorrhage (25 ml./Kg.) | | | | | | | | Period C, control (1 ml. | | | |
|---|---|---|---|---|---|---|---|---|---|---|---|---|---|---|---|---|---|
| | | BP (mean) | RBF | RVR | UF | BP (mean) | | RBF | | RVR | | UF | | BP (mean) | | RBF | |
| No. | Weight (Kg.) | mm. Hg | ml./min. | Units | Drops/min. | mm. Hg | % Δ | ml./min. | % Δ | Units | % Δ | Drops/min. | % Δ | mm. Hg | % Δ | ml./min. | % Δ |
| 1 | 22.7 | 117 | 186 | 0.6 | 4.1 | 88 | -25 | 100 | -46 | 0.9 | + 50 | 0.3 | -93 | 91 | -22 | 127 | -32 |
| 2 | 19.1 | 113 | 62 | 1.8 | 5.9 | 67 | -41 | 17 | -73 | 4.0 | +122 | 2.1 | -64 | 87 | -25 | 27 | -56 |
| 3 | 15.9 | 115 | 80 | 1.4 | 2.6 | 91 | -21 | 60 | -25 | 1.5 | + 7 | 1.0 | -62 | 96 | -17 | 78 | - 3 |
| 4 | 20.9 | | | | 8.0 | | | | | | | 1.5 | -81 | | | | |
| 5 | 23.6 | 105 | 67 | 1.6 | 3.5 | 64 | -39 | 26 | -61 | 2.3 | + 67 | 0.2 | -95 | 105 | 0 | 49 | -27 |
| 6 | 18.2 | 130 | 67 | 1.9 | 4.1 | 74 | -43 | 20 | -70 | 3.7 | + 95 | 2.8 | -32 | 99 | -24 | 27 | -60 |
| 7 | 17.3 | 145 | 161 | 0.9 | 14.0 | 103 | -29 | 139 | -14 | 0.7 | - 22 | 6.5 | -54 | 125 | -14 | 140 | -13 |
| Mean | 19.6 | 121 | 104 | 1.4 | 6.0 | | -33 | | -48 | | + 53 | | -69 | | -17 | | -32 |

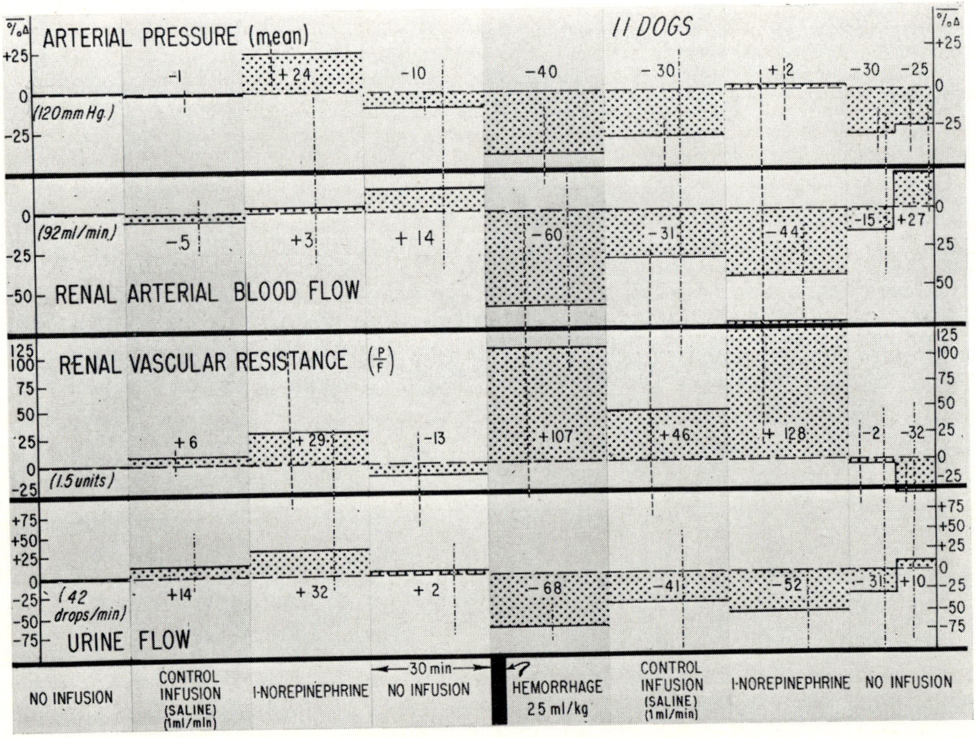


**Fig. 2.** Results in Group 2.

graphically in Fig. 3. Again, the ordinate represents mean values expressed as change in per cent of the control, with the ranges being indicated by vertical lines.

The mean values over a period of observation (as reported) do not illustrate the moment-to-moment changes that were observed on the records. Three sample tracings are reproduced to demonstrate some of these transient effects of l-norepinephrine. The top tracing in Fig. 4 demonstrates the effect of l-norepinephrine on renal blood flow before hemorrhage. It shows a temporary rise in renal blood flow followed by return

| *infusion, saline /min.)* | | | | *Period D, l-norepinephrine infusion* | | | | | | | | *Period E, no infusion* | | | | | | | |
|---|---|---|---|---|---|---|---|---|---|---|---|---|---|---|---|---|---|---|---|
| *RVR* | | *UF* | | *BP (mean)* | | *RBF* | | *RVR* | | *UF* | | *BP (mean)* | | *RBF* | | *RVR* | | *UF* | |
| *Units* | *% Δ* | *Drops /min.* | *% Δ* | *mm. Hg* | *% Δ* | *ml./ min.* | *% Δ* | *Units* | *% Δ* | *Drops /min.* | *% Δ* | *mm. Hg* | *% Δ* | *ml./ min.* | *% Δ* | *Units* | *% Δ* | *Drops /min.* | *% Δ* |
| 0.7 | +17 | 1.6 | -61 | 109 | - 7 | 121 | -35 | 0.9 | + 50 | 2.5 | - 39 | 80 | -32 | 108 | -42 | 0.7 | +17 | 1.0 | -76 |
| 3.2 | +78 | 4.5 | -24 | 128 | +13 | 31 | -50 | 4.1 | +128 | 3.4 | - 42 | 107 | - 5 | 31 | -50 | 3.5 | +94 | 5.2 | -12 |
| 1.2 | -14 | 2.1 | -19 | 118 | + 3 | 36 | -55 | 3.3 | +136 | 1.7 | - 35 | 63 | -45 | 35 | -56 | 1.8 | +28 | 1.9 | -27 |
| | | 0.5 | -94 | | | | | | | 0.0 | -100 | | | | | | | | |
| 2.1 | +31 | 2.0 | -43 | 120 | +14 | 38 | -43 | 3.2 | +100 | 1.9 | - 46 | 89 | -15 | 54 | -19 | 1.6 | 0 | 3.4 | - 3 |
| 3.7 | +95 | 3.2 | -22 | 122 | - 6 | 51 | -24 | 2.4 | + 26 | 3.0 | - 27 | 85 | -35 | 44 | -34 | 1.9 | 0 | 3.9 | - 5 |
| 0.9 | 0 | 11.0 | -21 | 144 | - 1 | 117 | -27 | 1.2 | + 33 | 8.3 | - 40 | | | | | | | | |
| | +34 | | -41 | | + 3 | | -39 | | + 79 | | - 47 | | -26 | | -40 | | +28 | | -25 |

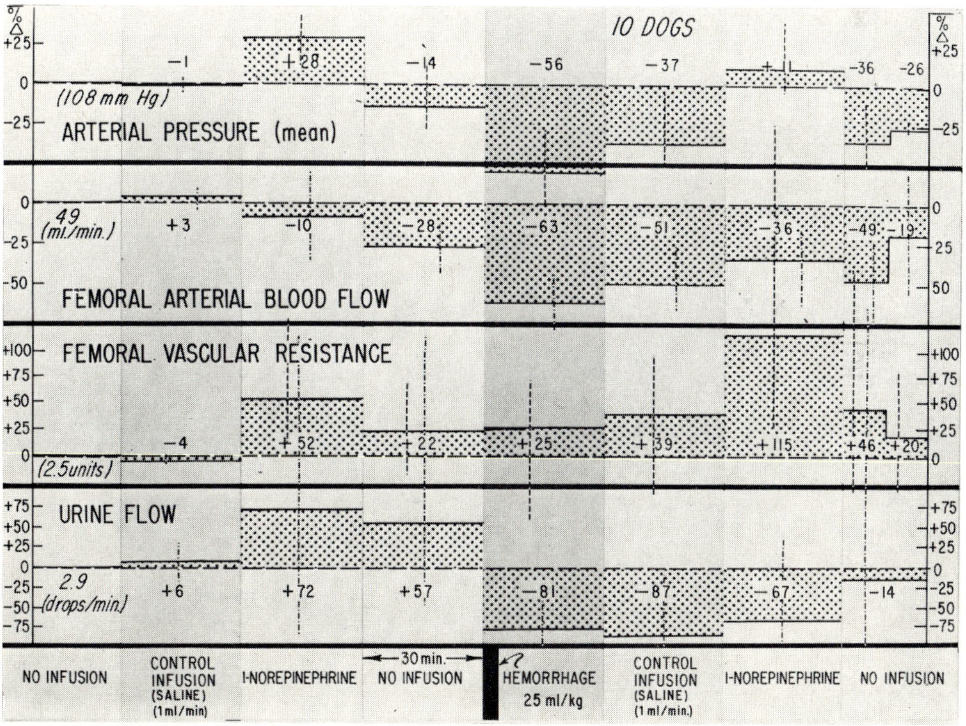


**Fig. 3.** Results in Group 3.

toward normal. The lower tracing, from a different animal which received l-norepinephrine after hemorrhage, shows a depression of renal blood flow associated with the rise in arterial pressure. (Time lines are at 1 second intervals.)

The transient effects of the start of the infusion of l-norepinephrine on femoral blood flow are shown in Fig. 5. This demonstrates that the rising blood pressure is accompanied by an initial rise in femoral arterial flow followed shortly by a return of the femoral flow toward and then below normal. This tracing also records the increase in rate of

**Table II.** *Effects of l-norepinephrine on blood pressure, renal blood flow, renal vascular resistance, and urine flow before and after hemorrhage (Group 2, periods A, B, and C)*

| Dog | | Period A, no infusion | | | | Period B, control infusion, saline (1 ml./min.) | | | | | | | | Period C, l-norepinephrine infusion before hemorrhage | | | | | | | |
|---|---|---|---|---|---|---|---|---|---|---|---|---|---|---|---|---|---|---|---|---|---|
| | | BP (mean) | RBF | RVR | UF | BP (mean) | | RBF | | RVR | | UF | | BP (mean) | | RBF | | RVR | | UF | |
| No. | Weight (Kg.) | mm. Hg | ml./min. | Units | Drops/min. | mm. Hg | % Δ | ml./min. | % Δ | Units | % Δ | Drops/min. | % Δ | mm. Hg | % Δ | ml./min. | % Δ | Units | % Δ | Drops/min. | % Δ |
| 8 | 20.9 | | | | 8.0 | | | | | | | | | | | | | | | | |
| 9 | 15.4 | 116 | 97 | 1.2 | 1.4 | 102 | -12 | 73 | -25 | 1.4 | +17 | 2.0 | +43 | 142 | +22 | 101 | + 4 | 1.4 | + 17 | 2.7 | + 93 |
| 10 | 16.8 | 120 | 100 | 1.2 | 2.9 | 116 | - 3 | 110 | +10 | 1.1 | - 8 | 3.3 | +14 | 158 | +31 | 77 | -23 | 2.1 | + 75 | 3.7 | + 28 |
| 11 | 18 | 100 | 113 | 0.9 | 5.0 | 100 | 0 | 113 | 0 | 0.9 | 0 | 5.9 | +18 | 132 | +32 | 119 | + 5 | 1.1 | + 22 | 7.7 | + 54 |
| 12 | 20 | 110 | 55 | 2 | 10 | 112 | + 2 | 49 | -11 | 2.3 | +15 | 12.2 | +22 | 130 | +20 | 69 | +25 | 1.9 | - 5 | 7.8 | - 22 |
| 13 | 15 | 92 | 154 | 0.6 | 2.3 | 92 | 0 | 156 | + 1 | 0.6 | 0 | 1.9 | -17 | 122 | +33 | 132 | -14 | 0.9 | + 50 | 0.9 | - 61 |
| 14 | 21.8 | 122 | 55 | 2.2 | 3.0 | 125 | + 2 | 53 | - 4 | 2.4 | + 9 | 2.5 | -17 | 162 | +33 | 63 | + 7 | 2.6 | + 18 | 8.5 | +184 |
| 15 | 26 | 155 | 138 | 1.1 | 2.5 | 158 | + 2 | 135 | - 2 | 1.2 | + 9 | 3.7 | +48 | 163 | + 5 | 120 | -13 | 1.4 | + 27 | 2.0 | - 20 |
| 16 | 29.5 | 123 | 52 | 2.4 | 2.3 | 125 | + 2 | 47 | -13 | 2.7 | +12 | 2.0 | -13 | 161 | +31 | 33 | -37 | 4.9 | +104 | 1.9 | - 17 |
| 17 | 26.4 | | | | 5.8 | | | | | | | 5.4 | - 7 | | | | | | | | + 12 |
| 18 | 17.7 | 144 | 66 | 2.2 | 2.3 | 144 | 0 | 66 | 0 | 2.2 | 0 | 2.3 | +53 | 151 | + 5 | 113 | +71 | 1.3 | - 41 | 6.5 | + 73 |
| Mean | 20.4 | 120 | 92 | 1.5 | 4.2 | | - 1 | | - 5 | | + 6 | | +14 | | +24 | | + 3 | | + 29 | 2.6 | + 32 |

**Table III.** *Effects of l-norepinephrine on blood pressure, renal blood flow, renal vascular resistance, and urine flow before and after hemorrhage (Group 2, periods D, E, and F)*

| | Period D, no infusion | | | | | | | | Period E, hemorrhage (25 ml./Kg.) | | | | | | | | Period F, control infusion, saline (1 ml./min.) | | | | | | | |
|---|---|---|---|---|---|---|---|---|---|---|---|---|---|---|---|---|---|---|---|---|---|---|---|---|
| | BP (mean) | | RBF | | RVR | | UF | | BP (mean) | | RBF | | RVR | | UF | | BP (mean) | | RBF | | RVR | | UF | |
| Dog No. | mm. Hg | % Δ | ml./min. | % Δ | Units | % Δ | Drops/min. | % Δ | mm. Hg | % Δ | ml./min. | % Δ | Units | % Δ | Drops/min. | % Δ | mm. Hg | % Δ | ml./min. | % Δ | Units | % Δ | Drops/min. | % Δ |
| 8 | | | | | | | | | | | | | | | 1.5 | -76 | | | | | | | 0.5 | - 94 |
| 9 | 98 | -16 | 73 | -25 | 1.3 | + 8 | 1.9 | +36 | 58 | -50 | 16 | - 84 | 3.6 | +200 | 0.2 | -86 | 80 | -31 | 44 | - 55 | 1.8 | + 50 | 1.5 | + 7 |
| 10 | 115 | - 4 | 110 | +10 | 1.0 | -16 | 3.4 | +17 | 48 | -60 | 15 | - 85 | 3.2 | +160 | 0.6 | -79 | 89 | -26 | 24 | - 76 | 3.7 | +210 | 0.7 | - 76 |
| 11 | 95 | - 5 | 118 | + 4 | 0.8 | -11 | 4.8 | - 4 | 64 | -36 | 40 | - 65 | 1.6 | + 78 | 0.9 | -82 | 76 | -24 | 79 | - 30 | 1.0 | + 11 | 1.9 | - 62 |
| 12 | 99 | -10 | 106 | +93 | 0.9 | -55 | 13.8 | +38 | 98 | -11 | 69 | + 25 | 1.4 | - 30 | 5.6 | -44 | 87 | -21 | 113 | +105 | 0.8 | - 60 | 8.8 | - 12 |
| 13 | 80 | -13 | 100 | -35 | 0.8 | +33 | 0.5 | -78 | 56 | -39 | 29 | - 81 | 2.0 | +230 | 0.8 | -65 | 61 | -34 | 51 | - 67 | 1.2 | +100 | 3.5 | + 52 |
| 14 | 115 | - 6 | 92 | +67 | 1.3 | -41 | 3.2 | + 7 | 59 | -52 | 0 | -100 | | | 0.7 | -77 | 84 | -31 | 5 | - 90 | | | 0.5 | - 83 |
| 15 | 135 | -13 | 138 | 0 | 1.0 | - 9 | 2.0 | -20 | | | | | | | 0.9 | -64 | 81 | -48 | 48 | - 65 | 1.7 | + 55 | 0.5 | - 80 |
| 16 | | | | | | | 2.8 | +22 | | | | | | | 1.4 | -39 | | | | | | | 0 | -100 |
| 17 | | | | | | | 4.1 | -29 | | | | | | | 2.4 | -59 | | | | | | | 5.4 | - 7 |
| 18 | 130 | -10 | 64 | - 3 | 2.0 | -10 | 1.9 | +27 | 100 | -31 | 44 | - 33 | 2.3 | + 5 | 0.4 | -73 | 114 | -21 | 85 | + 29 | 1.3 | - 41 | 1.5 | 0 |
| Mean | | -10 | | +14 | | -13 | | + 2 | | -40 | | - 60 | | +107 | | -68 | | -30 | | - 31 | | + 46 | | - 41 |

**Table IV.** *Effects of l-norepinephrine on blood pressure, renal blood flow, renal vascular resistance, and urine flow before and after hemorrhage (Group 2, periods G, H, and I)*

| Dog No. | Period G, l-norepinephrine infusion after hemorrhage | | | | | | | | Period H, no infusion | | | | | | | | Period I, terminal 15 minutes (no infusion) | | | | | | | |
|---|---|---|---|---|---|---|---|---|---|---|---|---|---|---|---|---|---|---|---|---|---|---|---|---|
| | BP (mean) | | RBF | | RVR | | UF | | BP (mean) | | RBF | | RVR | | UF | | BP (mean) | | RBF | | RVR | | UF | |
| | mm. Hg | % Δ | ml./min. | % Δ | Units | % Δ | Drops/min. | % Δ | mm. Hg | % Δ | ml./min. | % Δ | Units | % Δ | Drops/min. | % Δ | mm. Hg | % Δ | ml./min. | % Δ | Units | % Δ | Drops/min. | % Δ |
| 8 | | | | | | | 0.0 | -100 | | | | | | | | | | | | | | | | |
| 9 | 124 | + 7 | 42 | -58 | 3.0 | +150 | 0.3 | - 79 | 82 | -29 | 51 | -47 | 1.6 | +33 | 4.3 | +207 | | | | | | | 4.4 | +214 |
| 10 | 122 | + 2 | 43 | -57 | 2.9 | +140 | 1.6 | - 45 | 110 | - 8 | | | | | 2.1 | - 28 | 110 | - 8 | | | | | 2.2 | - 24 |
| 11 | 116 | +16 | 72 | -36 | 1.6 | + 78 | 2.7 | - 46 | 67 | -33 | 121 | + 7 | 0.6 | -33 | 1.3 | - 74 | 67 | -33 | 121 | + 7 | 0.6 | -33 | 2.0 | - 60 |
| 12 | 114 | + 4 | 50 | -11 | 2.3 | + 15 | 8.5 | - 15 | 100 | - 9 | 53 | - 4 | 1.9 | - 5 | 8.4 | - 16 | 100 | - 9 | 53 | - 4 | 1.9 | - 5 | 10.8 | + 8 |
| 13 | 104 | + 9 | 37 | -76 | 2.8 | +367 | 1.3 | - 43 | 40 | -57 | | | | | 0.1 | - 96 | | | | | | | | |
| 14 | 131 | + 7 | 25 | -55 | 5.2 | +136 | 1.3 | - 57 | 85 | -30 | | | | | 0.1 | - 97 | 85 | -30 | | | | | 0.4 | - 87 |
| 15 | 120 | -23 | | | | | 0.5 | - 80 | 92 | -41 | | | | | 1.0 | - 60 | 92 | -41 | | | | | 0.1 | - 96 |
| 16 | | | | | | | 0.1 | - 96 | | | | | | | 0.11 | - 95 | | | | | | | | |
| 17 | | | | | | | 5.4 | - 7 | | | | | | | 4.4 | - 24 | | | | | | | | |
| 18 | 134 | - 7 | 57 | -14 | 2.4 | + 10 | 1.4 | - 7 | | | | | | | | | 100 | -31 | 108 | +64 | 0.9 | -59 | 5.0 | +118 |
| Mean | | + 2 | | -44 | | +128 | | - 52 | | -30 | | -15 | | - 2 | | - 31 | | -25 | | +22 | | -32 | | + 10 |

**Table V.** *Effects of l-norepinephrine on blood pressure, femoral blood flow femoral vascular resistance, and urine flow before and after hemorrhage (Group 3, periods A, B, and C)*

| Dog | | Period A, no infusion | | | | Period B, control infusion of saline (1 ml./min.) | | | | | | | | Period C, l-norepinephrine infusion before hemorrhage | | | | | | | |
|---|---|---|---|---|---|---|---|---|---|---|---|---|---|---|---|---|---|---|---|---|---|
| | | BP (mean) | RBF | RVR | UF | BP (mean) | | RBF | | RVR | | UF | | BP (mean) | | RBF | | RVR | | UF | |
| No. | Weight (Kg.) | mm. Hg | ml./min. | Units | Drops/min. | mm. Hg | % Δ | ml./min. | % Δ | Units | % Δ | Drops/min. | % Δ | mm. Hg | % Δ | ml./min. | % Δ | Units | % Δ | Drops/min. | % Δ |
| 19 | 15.4 | 115 | 35 | 3.3 | 2.0 | 118 | +3 | 37 | +6 | 3.2 | - 3 | 2.4 | +20 | 150 | +32 | 42 | +20 | 3.6 | + 10 | 0.3 | - 85 |
| 20 | 26.0 | | | | 4.0 | | | | | | | 4.4 | +10 | | | | | | | 9.5 | +137 |
| 21 | 12.7 | 110 | 69 | 1.6 | 1.1 | 108 | -2 | 69 | 0 | 1.6 | 0 | 1.4 | +27 | 150 | +36 | 55 | -20 | 2.7 | + 69 | 4.4 | +300 |
| 22 | 21.8 | 88 | 73 | 1.2 | 3.2 | 87 | 0 | 76 | +4 | 1.1 | - 8 | 3.3 | + 3 | 127 | +44 | 46 | -37 | 2.8 | +133 | 3.2 | 0 |
| 23 | 15.0 | 135 | 47 | 2.9 | 4.2 | 135 | 0 | 51 | +9 | 2.6 | -10 | 3.5 | -17 | 161 | +19 | 40 | -15 | 4.0 | + 38 | 4.6 | + 10 |
| 24 | 14.1 | 123 | 44 | 2.8 | 2.1 | 117 | -5 | 42 | -5 | 2.8 | 0 | 2.0 | - 5 | 136 | +11 | 44 | 0 | 3.1 | + 11 | 3.5 | + 67 |
| 25 | 15.5 | 98 | 35 | 2.8 | 2.1 | | | | | | | | | | | | | | | | |
| 26 | 18.2 | 78 | 28 | 2.8 | 2.9 | | | | | | | | | | | | | | | | |
| 27 | 23.2 | 120 | 83 | 1.4 | 4.2 | | | | | | | | | | | | | | | | |
| 28 | 14.1 | 105 | 31 | 3.4 | 3.3 | | | | | | | | | | | | | | | | |
| Mean | | 108 | 49 | 2.5 | 2.9 | | -1 | | +3 | | - 4 | | + 6 | | +28 | | -10 | | + 52 | | + 72 |

**Table VI.** *Effects of l-norepinephrine on blood pressure, femoral blood flow, femoral vascular resistance, and urine flow before and after hemorrhage (Group 3, periods D, E, and F)*

| Dog No. | Period D, no infusion | | | | | | | | Period E, hemorrhage (25 ml./Kg.) | | | | | | | | Period F, control infusion, saline (1 ml./min.) | | | | | | | |
|---|---|---|---|---|---|---|---|---|---|---|---|---|---|---|---|---|---|---|---|---|---|---|---|---|
| | BP (mean) | | RBF | | RVR | | UF | | BP (mean) | | RBF | | RVR | | UF | | BP (mean) | | RBF | | RVR | | UF | |
| | mm. Hg | % Δ | ml./min. | % Δ | Units | % Δ | Drops/min. | % Δ | mm. Hg | % Δ | ml./min. | % Δ | Units | % Δ | Drops/min. | % Δ | mm. Hg | % Δ | ml./min. | % Δ | Units | % Δ | Drops/min. | % Δ |
| 19 | 82 | -29 | 30 | -14 | 2.7 | -18 | | | 54 | -53 | 19 | -46 | 2.8 | -15 | 0.0 | -100 | 60 | -48 | 24 | -31 | 2.5 | -24 | 0.2 | -90 |
| 20 | | | | | | | 6.0 | +50 | | | | | | | 0.5 | -87 | | | | | | | 0.0 | -100 |
| 21 | 83 | -25 | 38 | -45 | 2.2 | +37 | 4.6 | +318 | 28 | -75 | 13 | -81 | 2.1 | +31 | 0.2 | -82 | 55 | -50 | 23 | -67 | 2.4 | +50 | 0.0 | -100 |
| 22 | 80 | -9 | 53 | +27 | 1.5 | +25 | 3.2 | 0 | 35 | -60 | 26 | -64 | 1.3 | +8 | 2.1 | -34 | 53 | -40 | 29 | -60 | 1.8 | +48 | 0.6 | -81 |
| 23 | 150 | +11 | 31 | -34 | 4.8 | +66 | 2.8 | -33 | 96 | -29 | 20 | -57 | 4.8 | +66 | 0.2 | -95 | 91 | -33 | 20 | -57 | 4.5 | +55 | 0.2 | -95 |
| 24 | 100 | -19 | 36 | -18 | 2.8 | 0 | 1.1 | -48 | 29 | -76 | 24 | -45 | 1.2 | -57 | 0.2 | -90 | 60 | -51 | 32 | -27 | 1.9 | -32 | 0.0 | -100 |
| 25 | | | | | | | | | 42 | -57 | 10 | -72 | 4.2 | +50 | 0.1 | -95 | 63 | -36 | 13 | -63 | 4.8 | +71 | 0.0 | -100 |
| 26 | | | | | | | | | 24 | -69 | 7 | -75 | 3.2 | +14 | 0.0 | -100 | 48 | -38 | 12 | -57 | 4.0 | +43 | 0.0 | -100 |
| 27 | | | | | | | | | 77 | -36 | 34 | -59 | 2.3 | +64 | 2.7 | -36 | 113 | -6 | 57 | -31 | 2.0 | +43 | 3.8 | -10 |
| 28 | | | | | | | | | 57 | -46 | 10 | -68 | 5.7 | +68 | 0.2 | -94 | 69 | -34 | 10 | -68 | 6.9 | +100 | 0.0 | -100 |
| Mean | | -14 | | -28 | | +22 | | +57 | | -56 | | -63 | | +25 | | -81 | | -37 | | -51 | | +39 | | -87 |

**Table VII.** *Effects of l-norepinephrine on blood pressure, femoral blood flow, femoral vascular resistance, and urine flow before and after hemorrhage (Group 3, periods G and H)*

| Dog No. | Period G, l-norepinephrine infusion after hemorrhage | | | | | | | | Period H, terminal 15 minutes (no infusion) | | | | | | | |
|---|---|---|---|---|---|---|---|---|---|---|---|---|---|---|---|---|
| | BP (mean) | | RBF | | RVR | | UF | | BP (mean) | | RBF | | RVR | | UF | |
| | mm. Hg | % Δ | ml./min. | % Δ | Units | % Δ | Drops/min. | % Δ | mm. Hg | % Δ | ml./min. | % Δ | Units | % Δ | Drops/min. | % Δ |
| 19 | 120 | +4 | 29 | -17 | 4.1 | +24 | 0.1 | -98 | 67 | -42 | 26 | -26 | 2.6 | -21 | 1.4 | -30 |
| 20 | | | | | | | 1.1 | -73 | | | | | | | 0.3 | -92 |
| 21 | 121 | +10 | 25 | -64 | 4.8 | +300 | 0.1 | -91 | 60 | -45 | 25 | -64 | 2.4 | +50 | 5.0 | +355 |
| 22 | 101 | +15 | 28 | -61 | 3.6 | +300 | 1.6 | -50 | 65 | -26 | 32 | -56 | 2.0 | +67 | 3.1 | -3 |
| 23 | 138 | +2 | 21 | -55 | 6.6 | +128 | 1.2 | -71 | 120 | -11 | 24 | -49 | 5.0 | +72 | 1.8 | -57 |
| 24 | 115 | -7 | 32 | -27 | 3.6 | +29 | 0.1 | -95 | 68 | -45 | 34 | -23 | 2.0 | -29 | 0.0 | -100 |
| 25 | 139 | +40 | 28 | -20 | 5.0 | +79 | 1.6 | -24 | | | | | | | | |
| 26 | 90 | +15 | 24 | -14 | 3.8 | +36 | 0.0 | -100 | 38 | -51 | 13 | -54 | 2.9 | +4 | 0.0 | -100 |
| 27 | 145 | +21 | 63 | -24 | 2.3 | +64 | 5.6 | +33 | | | | | | | | |
| 28 | 107 | +2 | 18 | -42 | 5.9 | +74 | 0.0 | -100 | 75 | -29 | 8 | -74 | 9.4 | +177 | 0.5 | -85 |
| Mean | | +11 | | -36 | | +115 | | -67 | | -36 | | -49 | | +46 | | -14 |

urine flow upon infusion of l-norepinephrine prior to hemorrhage.

The summary of the urine flow studies in all 28 dogs showed that after the reduction caused by hemorrhage (mean equals –72.5 per cent of control), urine flow tended to increase in the period of the control infusion (mean equals –58 per cent of control). The infusion of l-norepinephrine stopped this trend toward increase in urine output (mean equals –56 per cent), which was again resumed after the l-norepinephrine was discontinued (mean equals –26 per cent). In 12 dogs, urine output was decreased during administration of l-norepinephrine after hemorrhage, and in 11 dogs there was an increase. The 5 remaining dogs showed no change. The wide variations in values obtained from one dog to the next are not surprising in view of the complex nature of the relationship between arterial pressure and urine flow.

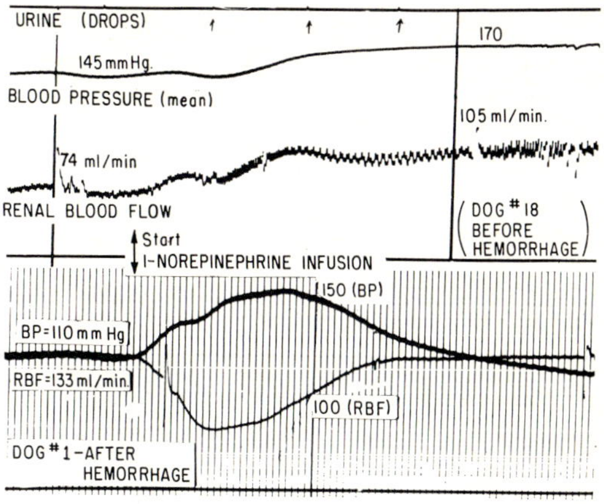


**Fig. 4.** Blood pressure and renal blood flow during l-norepinephrine infusion (1.5 minutes).

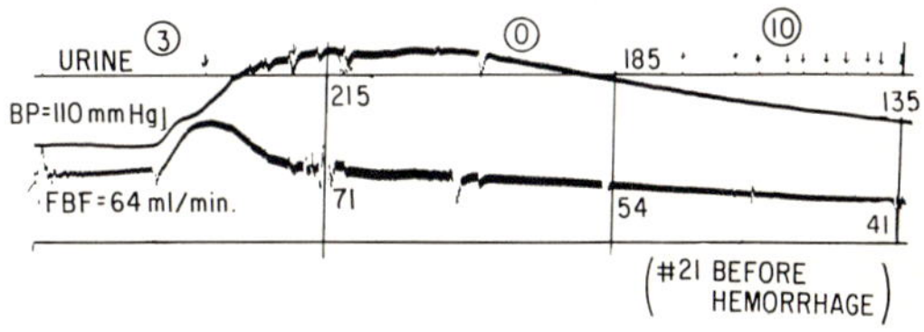


**Fig. 5.** Blood pressure and femoral arterial blood flow during l-norepinephrine infusion (3 minutes).

## COMMENT

It is realized that the entire physiologic response to hemorrhagic shock and to its treatment must be considered rather than the effect on simply one organ. Nonetheless, specific organ blood flow and function must be studied in order to understand the whole. King and associates[9] have found that norepinephrine produced a marked increase in cerebral vascular resistance and a decrease in cerebral blood flow despite a substantial increase in mean arterial pressure. Lansing and Stevenson[11] reported that the prolonged infusion of a small dose of l-norepinephrine exerts a beneficial effect in hemorrhagic shock by maintaining cardiac output. Berne,[1] however, found that the action of the vasopressors on the heart is primarily one of a stimulating effect on myocardial metabolism with the coronary vasodilatation coming secondarily due in large part to the hypoxia of the heart induced by these drugs. Unpublished data from our laboratory[14] indicate that after the increase in force of myocardial contraction with the infusion of l-norepinephrine, there is a rebound characterized by a reduction in the force of myocardial contraction below that of the control. Recently, Corday and Williams,[6] utilizing the techniques of photoelectric drop meter estimation of blood flow, determined that there was an increased blood flow to the brain and heart but a decreased flow to the intestines and kidney in hemorrhagic shock treated with vasopressors.

The property of kidney for autoregulation[2-4] suggests that it may be unlike other vital organs. Langston and Guyton[10] believed that 2 factors were involved in the renal response to vasopressor administration in hemorrhagic shock—the elevation of the blood pressure which has a tendency to increase the production of urine, and the direct effect of vasopressors on the kidney which causes a reduced rate of urine flow. They concluded that the effects of l-norepinephrine and epinephrine were the same. Recently Wulsin and Altemeier[20] reported that small doses of epinephrine in hemorrhagic shock reduced urine flow moderately while large doses of vasopressors reduced urine flow markedly. On the other hand, Webb and Jackson[8, 18] found that small doses of norepinephrine gave increased output while large doses depressed urine flow.

The results of our experiments show that blood volume is a factor in the renal response to vasopressors. The apparent increase in urine flow produced by l-norepinephrine in normovolemic dogs was associated with a rise in renal or femoral vascular resistance which paralleled the rise in blood pressure. This suggests that there was a constriction of the efferent arterioles of the kidney. This is in marked contrast to the effects seen after hemorrhage when the infusion of l-norepinephrine tended to depress the rate of urine flow. These findings may serve to elucidate the diphasic response to l-norepinephrine described by Webb and Jackson.[18] It is well known that the reserve volume of blood held in the spleen of a dog is quite variable. This may account not only for the varying degree of fall in blood pressure which is known to follow an arterial hemorrhage calculated on the basis of body weight, but it may also account for the great range of variation in urine flow in response to vasopressor infusions.

Little difference was observed in these experiments between renal artery and femoral artery data except that there was a higher rise in resistance in the renal vascular bed with hemorrhage. This may be due to the fact that, under anesthesia, there is still an active circulation in the renal vascular bed, while in the femoral vascular bed there is an inactive one, relatively speaking. Results might have been quite different if the dog could have been exercising his hind limbs.

## CONCLUSIONS

1. Arterial hemorrhage (25 ml. per kilogram) is associated with a reduction in blood pressure, renal blood flow, femoral blood flow, and urine flow. Renal vascular resistance rises, but there is little change in femoral vascular resistance.

2. In the recovery period after hemorrhage, renal blood flow, femoral blood flow, urine flow, and blood pressure tend to return toward normal.

3. The subsequent infusion of l-norepinephrine to restore blood pressure to control values is associated with a marked rise in renal vascular resistance and femoral vascular resistance with supression of renal blood flow and urine flow.

4. In contrast, elevation of arterial pressure by infusion of l-norepinephrine to dogs with normal blood volume results in an increase in the rate of urine flow, at which time there is no significant changes in renal blood flow.

5. Total blood volume has been found to be an important variable in the renal response to the infusion of a vasopressor agent.

We are grateful to Drs. Homer R. Warner and Rodney B. Harvey for help in reviewing the data, and to C. Gordon Frank, Robert Crist, Fred K. Christensen, and Harper Pearse for their assistance in the performance of these studies.

## REFERENCES

1. Berne, R. M.: Effect of epinephrine and norepinephrine on coronary circulation, Circulation Res. **6:** 644, 1958.
2. Bounous, G., Onnis, M., Nash, F., and Shumacker, H. B., Jr.: Renal autoregulation, Surg. Gynec. & Obst. **111:** 540, 1960.
3. Bounous, G., Onnis, M., and Shumacker, H. B., Jr.: The abolition of renal autoregulation by renal decapsulation, Surg. Gynec. & Obst. **111:** 682, 1960.
4. Bounous, G., Shumacker, H. B., Jr., and King, H.: Studies in renal blood flow. I. Some general considerations, Ann. Surg. **151:** 47, 1960.
5. Close, S. A., Wagner, J. A., Kloehn, R. A., and Kory, R. C.: The effect of norepinephrine on survival in experimental acute hemorrhagic hypotension, S. Forum **8:** 22, 1957.
6. Corday, E., and Williams, J. H., Jr.: Effect of shock and of vasopressor drugs on the regional circulation of the brain, heart, kidney and liver, Am. J. Med. **29:** 228, 1960.
7. Griffin, J. C., Jr., Webb, W. R., Lee, S. S., Hardy, J. D., and McRae, J. M., Jr.: The effect of norepinephrine (Levophed) on survival in standard oligemic shock, S. Forum **9:** 4, 1958.
8. Jackson, J., and Webb, W. R.: Influence of increments of a vasopressor on the rate of

urine formation in graded hemorrhage, S. Forum **11:** 125, 1960.
9. King, B. D., Sokoloff, L., and Wechsler, R. L.: The effects of l-epinephrine and l-norepinephrine upon cerebral circulation and metabolism in man, J. Clin. Invest. **31:** 273, 1952.
10. Langston, J. B., and Guyton, A. C.: Effect of epinephrine on the rate of urine formation, Am. J. Physiol. **192:** 131, 1958.
11. Lansing, A. M., and Stevenson, J. A. F.: Mechanism of action of norepinephrine in hemorrhagic shock, Am. J. Physiol. **193:** 289, 1958.
12. Morris, G. C., Jr., Moyer, J. H., and Beazley, H. L.: Renal function response to vasopressor agents in shock, S. Forum **5:** 798, 1954.
13. Moyer, J. H., and Handley, C. A.: Norepinephrine and epinephrine effect on renal hemodynamics, Circulation **5:** 91, 1952.
14. Nelson, R. M.: Rebound effect of l-norepinephrine on myocardial contractility. Unpublished data.
15. Remington, J. W., Hamilton, W. F., Boyd, G. H., Jr., Hamilton, W. F., Jr., and Caddell, H. H.: Role of vasoconstriction in the response of the dog to hemorrhage, Am. J. Physiol. **161:** 116, 1950.
16. Remington, J. W., Hamilton, W. F., Caddell, H. M., Boyd, G. H., Jr., Wheeler, N. C., and Pickering, R. W.: Vasoconstriction as a precipitating factor in traumatic shock in the dog, Am. J. Physiol. **161:** 125, 1950.
17. Van Slyke, D. D.: The effects of shock on the kidney, Ann. Int. Med. **28:** 701, 1948.
18. Webb, W. R., and Jackson, J.: Urinary responses to increments of norepinephrine in sequential hypovolemia, Clin. Res. **9:** 58, 1961.
19. Wiggers, H. C., Ingraham, R. C., Roemhild, R., and Goldberg, H.: Vasoconstriction and the development of irreversible hemorrhage shock, Am. J. Physiol. **153:** 511, 1948.
20. Wulsin, J. H., and Altemeier, W. A.: The effect of norepinephrine and blood transfusion on urine flow following arterial hemorrhage in dogs, S. Forum **11:** 123, 1960.

## DISCUSSION*

**Dr. Wendell B. Thrower** (Charleston, S. C.). First, I want to compliment Dr. Hardy on a very important study and report the case of a patient whom we operated on for aortic insufficiency about 6 months ago. The correction of the aortic insufficiency was thought to be excellent and actually the bypass was very uneventful. The patient did very well for about 16 hours and then suddenly developed upper abdominal pain which was thought, wrongly, to be due to referred pain from the thoracotomy. He developed a shock-like syndrome and died about 1 day later. At autopsy, although this patient had mild atherosclerosis, no evidence of thrombosis or embolus was found. We later went into his past history and, through his family, found that he had had intermittent upper abdominal pain for some years. This may have been related to ischemic bowel. I might point out that he never received any catecholamines and did not have any other significant pathologic process.

*Discussion of papers by Hardy and Alican; and Nelson, Henry, and Lyman.

# Pancreatic influences on gastric secretions

DAN W. ELLIOTT, M.D.
DAVID A. TAFT, M.D.
EDWARD PASSARO, JR., M.D.
ROBERT M. ZOLLINGER, M.D.
COLUMBUS, OHIO
*From the Department of Surgery, The Ohio State University College of Medicine, University Hospital*

The recognition of a pancreatic islet adenoma with profound ulcerogenic properties has renewed interest in the possibility that the pancreas normally influences gastric secretion. A pancreatic hormone could do this, but there is very little objective laboratory evidence that such a hormone exists. For instance, extraction of an ulcerogenic tumor has yielded an unidentified protein which stimulates gastric secretion,[9] but this protein has not been found in the normal pancreas.[5] Animal experiments also provide only meager and conflicting evidence of a pancreatic influence on the stomach. Hypersecretion of gastric acid has been found after total pancreatectomy[2] and after formation of an external fistula,[7] but not an internal fistula.[11] Therefore, we have repeated these experiments and added 3 new procedures with dogs under similar conditions in the same laboratory to determine whether or not the normal pancreas can exercise an endocrine influence on the stomach.

The acid production from denervated Heidenhain pouches was measured under standard conditions of diet and nutrition. Seven different operative procedures were then performed on the pancreas, and the subsequent changes in gastric acid secretion compared. All of the operative procedures completely excluded pancreatic juice from the duodenum. Only 1 of the 7, total pancreatectomy, removed islet function as well.

Denervated Heidenhain pouches were chosen for this study because they respond primarily to hormonal influences. The full 24-hour gastric secretions may be collected and measured quantitatively. However, the principal output of the pouch is elicited by food in the antrum of the stomach proper. For valid acid collections, the same diet must be taken each day. This is pointed out here because animals with pancreatic fistulas develop isotonic dehydration, lose weight rapidly, and quickly refuse to eat.[6, 7, 11] Adequate amounts of water and electrolytes can be given intravenously to replace losses from both external and internal fistulas. These fluids prevent dehydration, keep weight loss at a reasonable rate (4 to 5 per cent per week), prevent ulcers,[6] and do not falsely elevate pouch secretions.[7] In the experiments reported here, intravenous infusions have been given systematically. Acid collections have been reported only if they were taken from animals which ate normally.

## METHODS

Mongrel dogs of both sexes which weighed between 20 and 35 pounds were observed in the laboratory until a good food intake and a stable body weight seemed to be assured. Denervated gastric pouches were then con-

Supported by Research Grant A-2362, National Institutes of Health, Bethesda 14, Md.

Read at the Twenty-second Annual Meeting of the Society of University Surgeons, Kansas City, Kan., Feb. 9-11, 1961.

structed from the body of the stomach along its greater curvature, with care taken to exclude antral tissue. The diet was kept constant, and consisted of 30 ounces of canned dog food containing 3 per cent fat and 12 per cent protein by weight. A daily record was carefully maintained of each animal's actual consumption of food. If gastric drainage amounted to more than 100 ml. a day, 1 slightly rounded teaspoon of salt was added to the daily meal.

Acid was collected in toy rubber balloons and its volume was measured. A sample of each collection was titrated against 1/20 N sodium hydroxide to a color change in Töpfer's reagent. The results were expressed as milliequivalents of free acid per unit of time (usually 24 hours). On selected days, the full 24-hour production of acid was collected as a mixed sample and pepsin output determined by the method of Anson and Mirsky.[1]

After the daily production of gastric acid had appeared stable for a period of at least 3 weeks, 1 of the 7 pancreatic procedures was performed. In all of the procedures, one or more accessory pancreatic ducts was divided.

External pancreatic fistulas were constructed by the method of Greenlee and associates.[7] Internal fistulas to the urinary bladder were constructed by exclusion of the major pancreatic duct in a 2-inch segment of duodenum. The proximal end of this segment was closed and its distal end anastomosed to the dome of the bladder, usually without undue tension. Internal fistulas to the distal bowel were constructed by moving the major pancreatic duct on a button of duodenum into the terminal ileum or the midtransverse colon.

Six animals were subjected to immediate total pancreatectomy by an unusual technique. The head of the pancreas was carefully dissected free of the superior pancreaticoduodenal artery and vein, which were left undisturbed to supply blood to the duodenum. Meticulous dissection was required with a fine-silk technique, but this was thought desirable to preserve the normal innervation, motility, and endocrine function of the duodenum. Pancreatic duct ligation was usually accomplished by the same dissection, with complete separation of the pancreas from the duodenum. In 3 animals, 90 per cent of the pancreas was removed. A portion of the uncinate process, about the size of a 50 cent piece, was left behind with its duct completely obstructed.

Postoperatively, all animals were weighed at least twice a week. Animals with fistulas of any type were weighed daily and given intravenous infusions composed of one-half normal saline solution and one-half sodium lactate, with 30 mEq. of potassium added. The volume administered to each animal each day was regulated to prevent weight loss at a rate greater than the average observed in animals with pancreatic ductal obstruction—4 per cent of the preoperative weight per week.[6] Usually 500 to 1,000 ml. was required each day. No edema appeared in any of these animals. Serum sodium, potassium, chloride, carbon dioxide, and urea nitrogen concentrations were determined once or twice a week and remained within normal limits during the period of the study.

All the animals subjected to 90 per cent or total pancreatectomy had fasting blood sugar measurements once or twice a week. Insulin was given after total pancreatectomy only. Four to 10 units of NPH insulin each day maintained the fasting blood sugar level at between 100 and 200 mg. per cent. Four of the 6 animals subjected to total pancreatectomy had pancreatic enzymes added to their food. For this, Viokase (Viobin Corporation), a powder of whole lyophilized hog pancreas, was mixed with the daily meal in large doses, first 20 Gm. a day for 14 days, and then 30 Gm. a day for 14 or more days. Viokase was also given in the same manner to 3 animals with duct ligation, beginning 6 weeks or more postoperatively.

Selected dogs had the pouch secretions collected 6 times within each 24-hour period for 14 or more consecutive days. This established the pattern of acid secretion within the day, and determined its relationship to food intake. The daily meal was given at a

**Table I.** *Gastric acid production in pancreatic fistula*

| Dog No. | *Type of fistula* | *Treatment given* | *Weight loss per week (% preoperative weight)* | *Change in gastric acid* Started (postoperative day) | No. of collections | Change (% of base line) |
|---|---|---|---|---|---|---|
| 1 | External | Intravenous infusions daily | 5.1 | 5 | 15 | +140 |
| 2* | External | Intravenous infusions daily | 6.7 | 3 | 11 | + 65 |
| 3* | External | Intravenous infusions daily | 5.6 | 6 | 10 | − 43 |
| 4* | Bladder | Intravenous infusions daily | 4.9 | 5 | 17 | + 85 |
| 5 | Bladder | Intravenous infusions daily | 4.1 | 6 | 32 | + 60 |
| 6 | Bladder | Intravenous infusions daily | 4.7 | 4 | 29 | + 53 |
| 7* | Distal ileum | Intravenous infusions q.i.d. | 4.0 | 6 | 37 | + 78 |
| 8* | Transverse colon | Intravenous infusions q.i.d. | 3.2 | 7 | 28 | + 12 |
| 9 | Transverse colon | Intravenous infusions q.i.d. | 3.5 | 8 | 86 | + 91 |
| 10 | Transverse colon | Intravenous infusions q.i.d. | 4.2 | 6 | 56 | − 36 |

*Antral and duodenal ulcers were found at autopsy.

**Table II.** *Gastric acid production after total pancreatectomy*

| Dog No. | *Treatment given* | *Weight loss per week (% preoperative weight)* | *Change in gastric acid* Started (postoperative day) | No. of collections | Change (% of base line) |
|---|---|---|---|---|---|
| 11 | Viokase and insulin | 0 | 6 | 26 | + 39 |
| 12 | Viokase and insulin | 0 | 4 | 33 | 0 |
| 13 | Insulin only | 7.5 | 4 | 47 | − 16 |
| | Viokase begun on day 51 | 0 | — | 25 | + 45 |
| 14 | Insulin only | 7 | 6 | 49 | ±182 |
| | Viokase begun on day 55 | 0 | — | 19 | +192 |
| 15 | Insulin only | 7.0 | 4 | 40 | +140 |
| 16 | Insulin only | 10 | 7 | 16 | + 20 |

regular time and uneaten residue was withdrawn within 3 hours. Acid output was then measured at 3, 6, 9, 12, 18, and 24 hours after the food was eaten.

After all of the pancreatic procedures, stools were observed closely for the first appearance of the foamy, bulky, "oatmeal" stools of steatorrhea. After pancreatic duct ligation or 90 per cent pancreatectomy, fat absorption was measured in certain animals with radioactive triolein as reported by Baylin.[3]

Gastrointestinal motility was examined roentgenographically in representative animals. For this procedure, 8 ounces of the usual diet was mixed with 2 ounces of barium sulfate. After this meal, exposures of the abdomen were made in 2 planes at 30 minutes and at 1, 2, 3, 5, and 7 hours.

## RESULTS

All 4 types of pancreatic fistulas produced a modest increase in gastric acid secretion. First, a few days of acid suppression appeared in the immediate postoperative period. With resumption of a normal diet on the third to the sixth postoperative day, gastric hypersecretion became evident in 7 of the 10 dogs. Of the remaining 3, 1 showed little change (+12 per cent), and 2 showed a modest fall from base line output (Table I). For all the animals with fistulas the increases were small and ranged from 53 to 140 per cent of the individual base line collections, with an average increase of 73 per cent. Within a few days after the resumption of an oral diet and the appearance of gastric hypersecretion, the watery, foamy, "oatmeal" stools of steatorrhea were uniformly evident.

As long as adequate amounts of fluids could be given intravenously, all of the animals ate well and appeared to be in good health. However, in those with the external fistulas, weight loss averaged 6 per cent of the preoperative weight per week. Despite our best efforts, these animals lost weight somewhat faster than animals with duct obstruction, and the period in which accurate gastric collections were possible was relatively short.

It was somewhat easier to maintain fluid balance in animals with fistulas to the lower gastrointestinal tract. Weight loss was held to a desirable 4 per cent per week. Observations on gastric acid were carried out for from 37 to 80 days. There was no late change in gastric secretion after the first few days of oral diet. No peptic ulceration was observed while hydration was maintained, but 5 of the 10 animals developed ulcers after withdrawal of intravenous fluids.

Total pancreatectomy produced an increase in acid secretion in 5 of 6 animals. In only 2 were the increases marked (+182 and +140 per cent). In 2 they were very modest (+39 and +20 per cent) and in 2 there was essentially no change (Table II). One of the latter animals, however, developed an increase later (+45 per cent) after Viokase was added to the diet. All 6 of these animals had the usual temporary postoperative suppression of acid production. Upon resumption of the preoperative diet, acid production promptly assumed its new postoperative levels and became stabilized. Except for the 1 animal which received Viokase, none exhibited subsequent changes in the amounts of acid collections up to 49 days.

Viokase was fed immediately after operation to 2 of the 6 animals and was added to the diet of 2 additional animals after the fiftieth postoperative day. This prevented or halted weight loss and gross steatorrhea. It did not, however, seem to make any important difference in acid production. If these supplemental enzymes were not fed after total pancreatectomy, weight loss was exceedingly rapid, averaging 7.8 per cent per week.

After complete pancreatic obstruction, marked hypersecretion of gastric acid appeared in all 8 animals. The pattern of onset and the increase in amount of acid were strikingly different from those observed in all the other groups. With the omission of food in the first few postoperative days, the usual temporary suppression of acid was observed. Upon resumption of the preoperative diet, acid secretion returned to exactly the base line levels and remained there unchanged for from 20 to 30 postoperative days. Weight loss began with the operation and averaged 4 per cent of the preoperative weight per week for the entire group. The stools remained unchanged at first, although no enzymes were given by mouth. After the onset of steatorrhea, and at some time between the twentieth and the thirtieth postoperative day,

**Table III.** *Gastric acid production after complete pancreatic ductal obstruction*

| Dog No. | Weight loss per week (% preoperative weight) | Change in gastric acid | | |
|---|---|---|---|---|
| | | Started (postoperative day) | No. of collections | Change (% of base line) |
| 17 | 2.5 | 30 | 42 | +560 |
| 18* | 2.3 | 30 | 43 | +200 |
| 19 | 5.5 | 30 | 43 | +252 |
| 20* | 2.9 | 25 | 93 | +205 |
| 21 | 4.5 | 27 | 52 | +420 |
| 22 | 7.7 | 20 | 31 | +172 |
| 23 | 5.1 | 21 | 37 | +172 |
| 24* | 3.7 | 25 | 48 | +225 |

*Antral and duodenal ulcers were found at autopsy.

**Table IV.** *Gastric acid production after 90 per cent pancreatectomy with preservation of obstructed uncinate process*

| Dog No. | Weight loss per week (% preoperative weight) | Change in gastric acid | | |
|---|---|---|---|---|
| | | Started (postoperative day) | No. of collections | Change (% of base line) |
| 25 | 5.1 | 3 | 24 | +142 |
| 26 | 3.8 | 6 | 39 | +100 |
| 27 | 3.2 | 4 | 21 | + 30* |

*Fasting blood sugars ranged near 200 mg. per cent. No insulin was given.

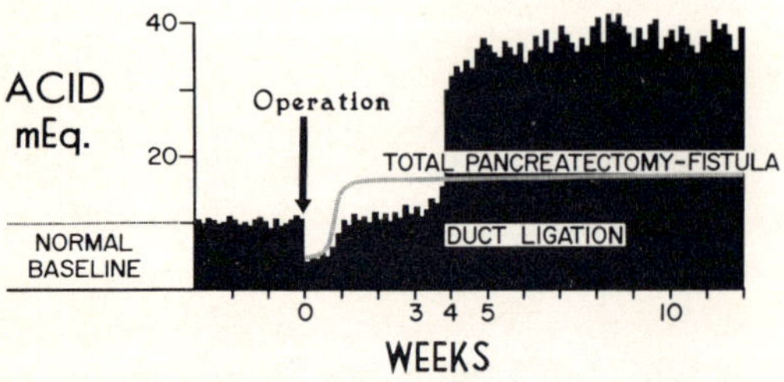


**Fig. 1.** The course of gastric hypersecretion after pancreatic duct ligation is compared with that found after total pancreatectomy or pancreatic fistula construction of any type.

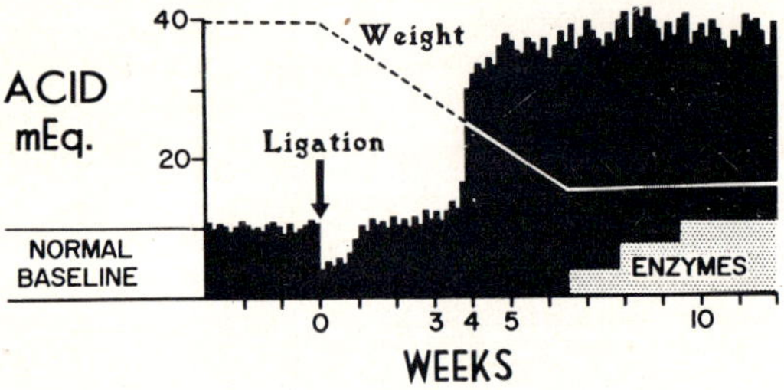


**Fig. 2.** Weight loss starts with pancreatic duct ligation and is promptly halted when pancreatic enzymes are mixed with the diet. However, gastric hypersecretion, once established, is not affected.

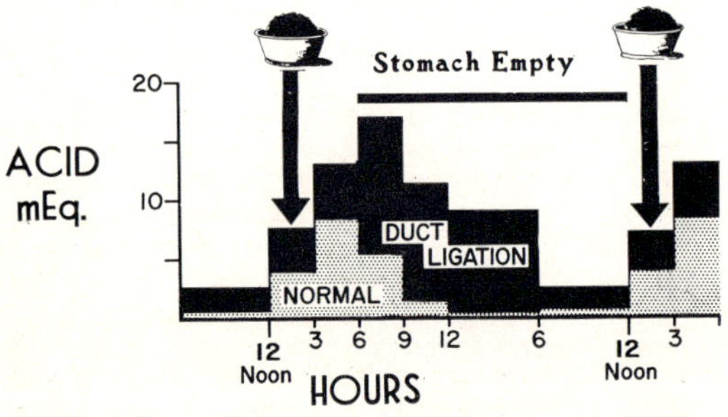


**Fig. 3.** Duct ligation produces a slight delay in the gastric response to food intake, but prolonged high levels of gastric secretion for up to 15 hours after the daily meal.

gastric acid output rose precipitously to a new high level which was maintained thereafter. The increases in acid production ranged from 172 to 560 per cent of the normal base line collections. The average increase for the group was 270 per cent. This average level of hypersecretion is 3½ times the normal base line (Table III). The secretory levels achieved in this group of animals were impressive and uniformly greater than those observed after any other pancreatic procedure. A comparison of the onset and the average levels of hypersecretion between animals with pancreatic duct obstruction, fistulas, and total pancreatectomy is illustrated in Fig. 1.

Triolein absorption was measured in 3 animals after hypersecretion had become well established, and in all 3 a low, flat curve of plasma radioactivity indicated marked impairment in fat absorption.

After hypersecretion had become well established in 3 of these animals, Viokase was mixed with their food. In all 3, the established steady loss of weight was promptly halted and steatorrhea was noticeably less. The enzyme dosage was increased to as much as 30 Gm. per day, or 3 times the recommended dose for human subjects, but this failed to produce a weight gain. There was, however, no noticeable change in gastric acid production as the result of enzyme administration (Fig. 2).

Early in the course of the experiment, we were puzzled by the failure of 2 animals to hypersecrete. Secondary laparotomies were performed, and minimal acinar atrophy was noted. In both cases, a small accessory duct was located and divided and hypersecretion followed after the usual delay.

Data on 2 animals were not included in the table because abscesses were found between the pancreas and duodenum accompanied by incomplete acinar atrophy. Both animals developed gastric hypersecretion of approximately 75 per cent above base line levels. Apparently acinar atrophy must be relatively complete to result in marked hypersecretion. However, partial compromise of acinar tissue may elevate acid secretion modestly.

After hypersecretion had become established in 2 animals, the entire atrophic pancreas was resected. Microscopic examination of the resected pancreas demonstrated nearly complete acinar destruction. Both animals were rendered diabetic and had insulin requirements similar to those of animals which had undergone total pancreatectomy at their first operation. Gastric acid formation was temporarily decreased, but did not fall as low as base line levels. Within 10 days after resection of the atrophic pancreas, hypersecretion was re-established at exactly the same level as before.

Resection of 90 per cent of the pancreas was performed in 3 animals and an obstructed segment of the most distal uncinate process was left. Within 3 to 6 days, gastric secretion rose to levels 142, 100, and 30 per cent above the respective base-line levels (Table IV). This gastric response resembled that found after total pancreatectomy in both onset and level of secretion. In 2 other respects, however, these animals responded as if they had duct obstruction. They did not require insulin (one had a mild rise in blood sugar level), and they lost weight without oral enzymes at an average rate of 4 per cent per week.

This procedure was performed to produce ductal obstruction while simultaneously removing most of the islet alpha cells. The obstructed uncinate process was retained, because in the dog it has been reported to contain no alpha cells.[4] If this were true, the removal of these cells prevented the marked gastric hypersecretion regularly produced by ductal obstruction. However, biopsy specimens were subsequently obtained from the retained uncinate process in each of these 3 animals and were examined by electron microscopy. Alpha cells were demonstrated in slightly diminished numbers in all three. Apparently, these animals had ductal obstruction, but had only a small quantity of acinar tissue to undergo atrophy.

Collections of gastric acid were made 6 times each 24 hours to learn whether or not hypersecretion occurs in the basal state between meals. These frequent collections were made from 4 animals after complete pancreatic obstruction and from 4 normal animals for comparison. In the normal animals, 70 per cent or more of the daily acid production took place within 6 hours after a meal, as is expected in denervated gastric pouches.[8] In all 4 animals, after duct obstruction, peak acid production was reached more slowly but hypersecretion persisted for 15 hours after food intake. A representative curve of daily acid production for a normal animal and for an animal with pancreatic obstruction has been superimposed in Fig. 3. The difference between these two curves is striking. Animals with pancreatic duct obstruction appear to be secreting acid at an accelerated rate for 18 of the 24 hours each day.

The delay and prolongation of the gastric response to food intake in animals with pancreatic acinar damage suggests an exaggerated intestinal phase of gastric secretion. However, very similar results could be produced by delays in gastrointestinal motility, which might result from operative dissection or adhesions. Therefore, gastrointestinal motility was studied by roentgenogram in 3 animals after total pancreatectomy, in 3 after duct obstruction, and in 5 normal dogs for comparison. The films taken during the first hour after either total pancreatectomy or duct obstruction actually suggested a slightly more rapid emptying of the stomach and filling of the upper small bowel (Fig. 4). In later films, the barium-tagged meal progressed through the lower small bowel and into the colon at about the same time in all

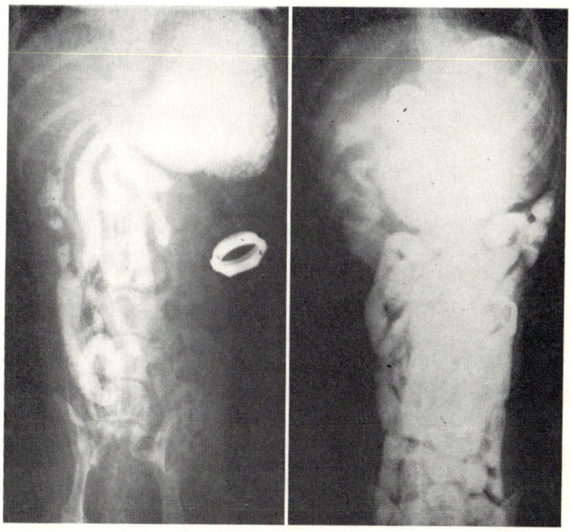

*A* *B*

**Fig. 4.** Roentgenograms taken 1 hour after a meal mixed with barium. *A,* Normal gastric emptying, and *B,* an animal with pancreatic obstruction and increased gastric emptying.

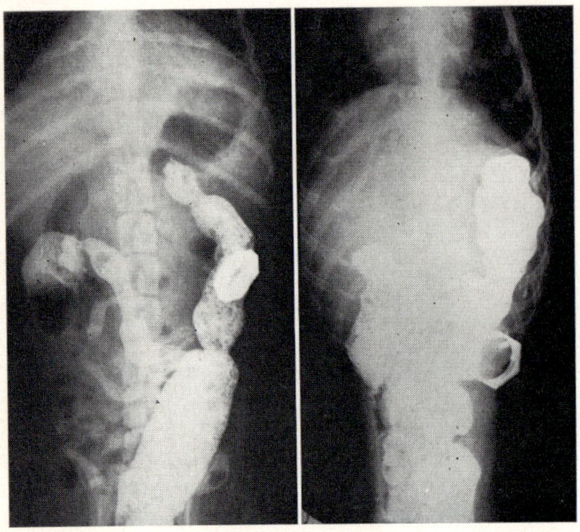

*A* *B*

**Fig. 5.** Roentgenograms taken 5 hours after a meal mixed with barium. *A,* Normal dog, and *B,* the animal with pancreatic obstruction. The stomach is empty in both animals, and there is no important difference in bowel motility.

3 groups of animals (Fig. 5). There were no important differences in gastrointestinal motility, regardless of the nature of the pancreatic procedure performed. These studies show that the stomach is completely empty at the end of 5 hours after food intake. Long after the stomach has emptied, animals with pancreatic acinar damage produce their principal secretion of gastric acid.

## COMMENT

Endocrine-stimulated gastric acid secretion increases almost uniformly whenever pancreatic juice is excluded from the upper small bowel. The modest increases seen after fistula construction and after total pancreatectomy are comparable. In these cases, no special endocrine mechanism arises from the pancreas. This hyperacidity may result from impaired digestion of fat. Normally, gastric acid is inhibited by fat in the small bowel, provided that both bile and lipase are present. Without lipase, inhibition of acid falls to one-half of normal, according to Menguy.[10] Accordingly, the exclusion of pancreatic juice from the duodenum can be expected to remove this normal "brake" on acid production.

Unlike all the other procedures, complete ductal obstruction is followed by normal gastric secretion for from 20 to 30 days. This is surprising, but may be explained by the observations of Frazer, Anlyan, and Isley, who found that after ductal obstruction, fat absorption is preserved for a similar period through pancreatic endocrine function.[12] Fat absorption falls to very low levels only after total pancreatectomy or advanced acinar atrophy. In a striking parallel, gastric secretion remains normal for from 20 to 30 days, until acinar destruction is advanced, before hypersecretion occurs.

Only a very potent blood-borne hormone could cause these denervated gastric pouches to secrete for 15 hours after a meal and to triple or quadruple their daily output. They do this only in the presence of both acinar destruction and intact islets. It is disappointing that complete removal of the damaged pancreas fails to halt this hypersecretion once it is established. Two possible explanations are apparent. Acinar destruction may cause a persistent hyperplasia of the parietal cells like that seen after repeated injections of histamine,[13] or it may trigger an extrapancreatic endocrine response not yet identified.

## SUMMARY

Pancreatic juice has been excluded from the duodenum by 7 different procedures in dogs with denervated gastric pouches. All of the methods produced gastric hypersecretion. The increase in acid secretion was prompt and modest after the formation of pancreatic fistulas or total pancreatectomy. Gastric secretion remained normal however, for from 20 to 30 days after ductal obstruction, until acinar atrophy was advanced. Then acid output rose sharply and reaching levels 3 or 4 times the normal base line.

The acid response to food intake persisted for 15 hours after the daily meal, long after the stomach had emptied. Gastrointestinal motility was not disturbed, as seen by roentgenograms. Neither oral administration of enzymes nor resection of the atrophic pancreas halted this hypersecretion once it had become established.

Hypersecretion from denervated gastric pouches was marked only in the presence of damaged acinar tissue and intact islets. This provides additional evidence of a potent pancreatic hormone capable of profound gastric stimulation.

**REFERENCES**

1. Anson, M. L., and Mirsky, A. E.: The estimation of pepsin with hemoglobin, J. Gen. Physiol. **16:** 59, 1932.
2. Barcena, J., Bravo, J. L., Baugh, C. M., Mountain, C. F., and Dragstedt, L. R.: Effects of total pancreatectomy on gastric secretion, S. Forum **7:** 380, 1956.
3. Baylin, G. J., Sanders, A. P., Isley, J. K., Shingleton, W. W., Hymans, J. C., Johnston, D. H., and Ruffin, J. M.: $I^{131}$ blood levels correlated with gastric emptying determined radiographically. II. Fat test meal, Proc. Soc. Exper. Biol. & Med. **89:** 54, 1955.
4. Bencosme, S., Maritz, S., and Frei, J.: Changes in dogs devoid of alpha cells, Endocrinology **61:** 1, 1957.
5. Code, C. F.: Personal communication, Nov. 14, 1960.
6. Elliott, D. W., Passaro, E., and Elliott, W. S.: Fluid balance in peptic ulceration induced by pancreatic fistulas, S. Forum **11:** 332, 1960.
7. Greenlee, H., Nelsen, T., and Dragstedt, L. R.: The effect of pancreatic fistula on gastric secretion, A.M.A. Arch. Surg. **79:** 1004, 1959.
8. Gregory, R. A., and Tracy, H. J.: Secretory responses of denervated gastric pouches, Am. J. Digest. Dis. **5:** 308, 1960.
9. Gregory, R. H., Tracy, H. J., French, J. M., and Sircus, W.: Extraction of a gastrin-like substance from a pancreatic tumor in a case of Zollinger-Ellison syndrome, Lancet **1:** 1045, 1960.
10. Menguy, R.: Studies on the role of pancreatic and biliary secretions in mechanism of gastric inhibition by fat, SURGERY **48:** 195, 1960.
11. Okinaka, A., Moody, F., Dineen, J., Beal, J., and Marten, K.: Experimental production of peptic ulcers without increased secretion of acid, SURGERY **46:** 70, 1959.
12. Tongen, L. A.: The quantitative relationship between parietal cells and gastric acidity, SURGERY **28:** 1009, 1950.

*(For discussion, see page 148.)*

# The occurrence of pancreatic antibodies and the experimental production of pancreatitis with pancreatic antiserum

ERIC W. FONKALSRUD, M.D.
WILLIAM P. LONGMIRE, JR., M.D.
LOS ANGELES, CALIF.
*From the Department of Surgery,*
*University of California Medical Center*

Autoimmunization has been cited as a possible etiologic factor in the development of unexplained chronic disease in certain specific organ systems. Investigations on the abnormalities of serum proteins in human thyroid diseases by Roitt and associates[19, 20] led to the discovery of thyroglobulin autoantibodies in the serum of patients with Hashimoto's thyroiditis. More recently, organ-specific circulating autoantibodies have been found in patients with ulcerative colitis,[1] lupus erythematosus,[5, 18] hepatitis,[7, 13] glomerulonephritis,[12] pancreatitis,[24] the postcardiotomy syndrome,[10] and certain hemolytic anemias.[6] Thal and associates[22] have demonstrated that specific antibodies to an antigen derived from the pancreas develop during naturally occurring pancreatitis in the human being and after chronic pancreatic damage or immunization with pancreatic extracts in the experimental animal.

Witebsky and Rose[21, 26] have demonstrated that direct immunization of animals with extracts containing organ-specific antigens incorporated into Freund-type adjuvants leads to histologic lesions in these organs and to the appearance of circulating antibodies directed against the specific antigens. Similarly, Masugi[15] produced glomerulonephritis in rabbits by passively injecting duck antiserum to rabbit kidney homogenate into normal rabbits. In cases in which kidney transplantation had been performed for glomerulonephritis, the normal transplanted kidney developed glomerulonephritis even though a simultaneous skin graft was not rejected, which suggested that antibodies to kidney were circulating even in cases of inactive glomerulonephritis.[16] More recently, LeVeen and his associates[11] have produced lesions resembling ulcerative colitis in dogs by means of the same technique.

The present report summarizes our experience with the detection of circulating pancreatic autoantibodies and antigens in patients with pancreatitis, and demonstrates that elevations in serum amylase (amylasemia) may be produced in normal dogs by passive transfer of antiserum to homologous pancreas.

## MATERIALS AND METHODS

Human pancreatic antigen was prepared by homogenizing and pooling histologically normal human pancreas obtained from the body of the gland from 3 fresh postmortem specimens. All extraneous blood and adipose and connective tissue were carefully removed from each specimen. The tissue was thoroughly homogenized in sterile normal saline solution in a ratio of 1 Gm. of tissue to 10 ml. of saline. The homogenate was filtered through gauze to remove large particles, and then centrifuged at 2,000 r.p.m. at 5° C. for 1 hour. The supernatant was removed as the antigen and frozen in small aliquots.

Supported by the Blalock Foundation.

Read at the Twenty-second Annual Meeting of the Society of University Surgeons, Kansas City, Kan., Feb. 9-11, 1961.

Human pancreatic antibody was obtained by the subcutaneous injection of 2 ml. of pancreatic antigen suspended in 1 ml. of Freund's adjuvant into each of 4 rabbits at weekly intervals for a total of 4 injections. The rabbits were exsanguinated 1 week after the last injection, and the serum was pooled. Antibodies to normal human serum were adsorbed and the remaining serum frozen in small aliquots.

Gel-diffusion studies, by the technique described by Ouchterlony,[17] were carried out at room temperature. Petri dishes were filled to a depth of 2 mm. with 1.5 per cent agar which contained a few drops of 0.1 per cent tincture of Merthiolate. Wells were created in the gel plates approximately 2 cm. apart and were filled twice during the first 24 hours of the diffusion study.

A clinical study was carried out in which the sera from 45 patients were tested against both pancreatic antigen and antibody by the gel-diffusion technique. Undiluted sera from 16 patients with acute or chronic relapsing pancreatitis, 3 patients with carcinoma of the pancreas, 19 unselected medical and surgical hospital patients, and 7 presumably healthy blood donors were examined. Each gel-diffusion reaction was carried out in triplicate, and the precipitation curves were recorded 1 week after the initial inoculation of the wells on the gel plates. The diffusion reactions were measured on the basis of intensity of precipitation lines between wells and recorded as 1 to 4 plus. The number of detectable antigen-antibody systems present in each case, as measured by the number of lines of precipitation on the diffusion plates, was also recorded. Serum amylase determinations were obtained within 7 days of the time blood was drawn for the diffusion studies.

## RESULTS

Circulating pancreatic antibodies were detected in 15 of the 16 patients with pancreatitis (Table I). Six of these patients had the diagnosis verified by laparotomy or autopsy. In most instances, at least 2 or more distinct antigen-antibody systems were detected, and these were of 2 to 3 plus intensity (Fig. 1). As many as 4 separate lines of precipitation were recorded in some cases; however, 1 or 2 systems were always considerably more prominent, and the additional lines were generally faintly visible. The sera from 7 patients with pancreatitis contained circulating antigens which gave a positive precipitin reaction with antiserum to human pancreas. Sera from each of 3 patients with histologically diagnosed carcinoma of the pancreas contained circulating antibodies and 2 of the patients had detectable antigens.

Pancreatic antibodies were detected in 5 of the 19 unselected medical and surgical patients, and circulating pancreatic antigen was found in 3 patients from this group. Four of the patients with detectable antibodies or antigens had marked inflammatory disease about the pancreas as a result of peptic ulcer, peritonitis, or carcinoma of the duodenum. One patient with lupus erythematosus had a single circulating pancreatic antibody, whereas the sera from another patient with the same disease contained neither antigen nor antibody. A patient with persistent gastroenteritis who required laparotomy was found to have 2 distinct circulating antigens, and a patient with carcinoma of the stomach had a single faintly detectable antigen. Two lightly detectable pancreatic antibodies were recorded in a patient with cirrhosis of the liver with esophageal varices. The serum from 1 of the 7 presumably healthy blood donors contained a very faintly visible single pancreatic antibody.

## EXPERIMENTAL DATA

Canine pancreatic antigen and rabbit serum containing antibodies to dog pancreas were prepared and stored in the same manner as that described previously for the human antigen and antibody. Sera obtained from 10 immunized and 4 normal rabbits were frozen and stored. Samples of antiserum from each of the immunized rabbits were individually tested against the pooled pancreatic antigen on the gel-diffusion plates. Sera from each of the rabbits contained at

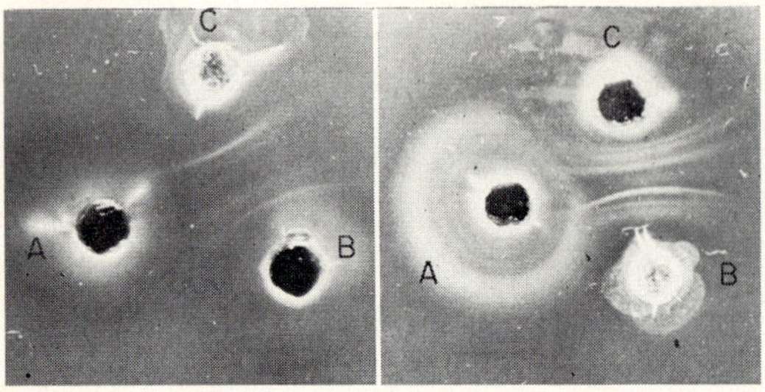


*1* *2*

**Fig. 1.** Photograph of gel-diffusion reactions in agar which demonstrates lines of precipitation between human pancreatic homogenate (*C*), and serum from patient with chronic relapsing pancreatitis (*B*). No precipitin curves are seen migrating to the sera from a blood donor (*A*).

**Fig. 2.** Photograph of gel-diffusion study which illustrates precipitin migration curves between canine pancreatic homogenate (*B*) and rabbit antiserum to dog pancreas (*C*). Normal dog serum (*A*) shows 2 faint lines of precipitation to antiserum to dog pancreas.

least 5 distinct antibody systems to dog pancreas, and almost all were of 3 to 4 plus intensity (Fig. 2). The rabbit antisera were then pooled and stored.

Six normal adult mongrel dogs which weighed from 10 to 15 kilograms were given intravenous injections of rabbit antiserum to dog pancreas. Blood was drawn immediately prior to and at frequent intervals after the antiserum injection, and serum amylase and lipase values determined. The serum amylase was measured in units by a modification of the Somogyi method.[8] The serum lipase was recorded in units and determined by the olive oil method.[9]

Three dogs were given infusions of the pooled rabbit antiserum in a dosage of 3 ml. per kilogram of body weight. A fourth dog received normal rabbit serum in the same dosage. In the experimental animals circulating antibodies were detected within 1 week of the antiserum infusion. Elevations in the serum amylase values were recorded within 4 days; they were noted to decrease only slightly during the first 2 postinfusion weeks, with a gradual return to normal levels within 1 month (Fig. 3). The control animal showed minimal changes in serum amylase values. A similar but less pronounced change was recorded in serum lipase determinations (Fig. 4). Emesis and diarrhea occurred sporadically in each of the animals including the control dog. At autopsy 1 month after the antiserum infusion, the histologic appearance of the pancreas of each animal was normal.

In a second group, 3 dogs were infused with rabbit antiserum, 2.5 ml. per kilogram, and then given a second infusion of 2 ml. per kilogram 12 days later. A control animal received normal rabbit serum on the same dosage schedule. Elevation of both serum amylase and lipase levels was again recorded, with a second slight increase in both enzyme determinations observed after the second antiserum infusion (Figs. 5 and 6). The amylasemia was more prolonged in the experimental animals, and the clinical symptoms were more prominent in each of the dogs in this group. These animals have been preserved for long-term follow-up studies.

## COMMENT

The etiology of chronic relapsing pancreatitis in human beings has not been clearly defined. Pancreatitis has been produced in animals by various investigators with a multitude of techniques which, in general, involved reflux or injection of materials into the pancreatic ducts, direct trauma to the gland, infection of the gland or ducts, and disturbance of the vascular supply of the pancreas. These factors are undoubtedly of significance in the production of pancreatitis; however, the recurrent nature of the disease in many instances suggests the presence of a hypersensitive state. Delayed hypersensitivity combined with the patient's ability to produce and maintain a high level of antibodies against his own pancreas for a protracted period may be of significance in the production of tissue damage.

The clinical results in the present study demonstrate that the sera of patients with recurrent pancreatitis and carcinoma of the pancreas contain one or more precipitating

**Table I.** *Clinical patients examined for circulating pancreatic antibodies and antigens*

| Patient No. | Age, race, and sex | Disease | Serum amylase | Serum contains circulating: Antibody | Serum contains circulating: Antigen | No. of systems detected: Antibody | No. of systems detected: Antigen |
|---|---|---|---|---|---|---|---|
| *Patients with acute or chronic relapsing pancreatitis* | | | | | | | |
| 1 | 39 WF | Chronic relapsing pancreatitis | 395 | 1+ | 3+ | 1 | 1 |
| 2 | 44 WF | Chronic relapsing pancreatitis | 510 | 2+ | 2+ | 2 | 2 |
| 3 | 38 WM | Chronic relapsing pancreatitis | 450 | 3+ | 0 | 4 | – |
| 4 | 40 NM | Pancreatitis with pancreatic pseudocyst | 495 | 2+ | 1+ | 2 | 2 |
| 5 | 46 WM | Recurrent alcoholic pancreatitis | 455 | 2+ | 0 | 2 | – |
| 6 | 41 NM | Chronic relapsing pancreatitis | 480 | 2+ | 0 | 1 | – |
| 7 | 38 WM | Recurrent alcoholic pancreatitis | 28 | 0 | 0 | – | – |
| 8 | 64 WM | Chronic pancreatitis | 264 | 3+ | 0 | 2 | – |
| 9 | 46 WM | Chronic relapsing pancreatitis | 66 | 3+ | 0 | 2 | – |
| 10 | 39 WM | Acute pancreatitis | 1,200 | 2+ | 0 | 2 | – |
| 11 | 46 WM | Chronic pancreatitis, diabetes | 340 | 2+ | 0 | 3 | – |
| 12 | 41 NM | Recurrent alcoholic pancreatitis | 576 | 2+ | 0 | 2 | – |
| 13 | 40 NM | Chronic relapsing pancreatitis | 480 | 2+ | 1+ | 1 | 1 |
| 14 | 25 CM | Chronic relapsing pancreatitis | 500 | 3+ | 2+ | 2 | 1 |
| 15 | 46 NM | Recurrent alcoholic pancreatitis | 700 | 3+ | 2+ | 4 | 1 |
| 16 | 67 WM | Relapsing pancreatitis, diabetes | 152 | 3+ | 0 | 1 | – |
| *Patients with other pancreatic disease* | | | | | | | |
| 17 | 57 WF | Carcinoma of pancreas | — | 2+ | 0 | 3 | – |
| 18 | 45 WM | Carcinoma of pancreas | — | 1+ | 1+ | 1 | 1 |
| 19 | 61 WM | Carcinoma of pancreas | — | 1+ | 2+ | 1 | 2 |
| *Unselected medical and surgical patients* | | | | | | | |
| 20 | — | Gastroenteritis | — | 0 | 2+ | – | 2 |
| 21 | — | Gastrointestinal bleeder, duodenal ulcer | — | 2+ | 0 | 3 | – |
| 22 | — | Bowel obstruction with peritonitis | — | 2+ | 1+ | 3 | 1 |
| 23 | — | Carcinoma of duodenum | — | 2+ | 0 | 1 | – |
| 24 | — | Carcinoma of stomach | — | 0 | 1+ | – | 1 |
| 25 | — | Cirrhosis with varices | — | 1+ | 0 | 2 | – |
| 26 | — | Lupus erythematosus | — | 2+ | 0 | 1 | – |
| 27 | — | Lupus erythematosus | — | 0 | 0 | – | – |
| 28 | — | Benign gastric ulcer | — | 0 | 0 | – | – |
| 29 | — | Benign gastric ulcer | — | 0 | 0 | – | – |
| 30 | — | Acquired aortic and mitral insufficiency | — | 0 | 0 | – | – |
| 31 | — | Arteriosclerosis with peripheral arterial occlusion | — | 0 | 0 | – | – |
| 32 | — | Cholecystitis and cholelithiasis | — | 0 | 0 | – | – |
| 33 | — | Acute lymphatic leukemia | — | 0 | 0 | – | – |
| 34 | — | Carcinoma of bladder | — | 0 | 0 | – | – |
| 35 | — | Carcinoma of rectum | — | 0 | 0 | – | – |
| 36 | — | Carcinoma of lung | — | 0 | 0 | – | – |
| 37 | — | Carcinoma of colon | — | 0 | 0 | – | – |
| 38 | — | Carcinoma of breast | — | 0 | 0 | – | – |
| *Control group of blood donors* | | | | | | | |
| 39 | — | — | — | 1+ | 0 | 1 | – |
| 40 | — | — | — | 0 | 0 | – | – |
| 41 | — | — | — | 0 | 0 | – | – |
| 42 | — | — | — | 0 | 0 | – | – |
| 43 | — | — | — | 0 | 0 | – | – |
| 44 | — | — | — | 0 | 0 | – | – |
| 45 | — | — | — | 0 | 0 | – | – |

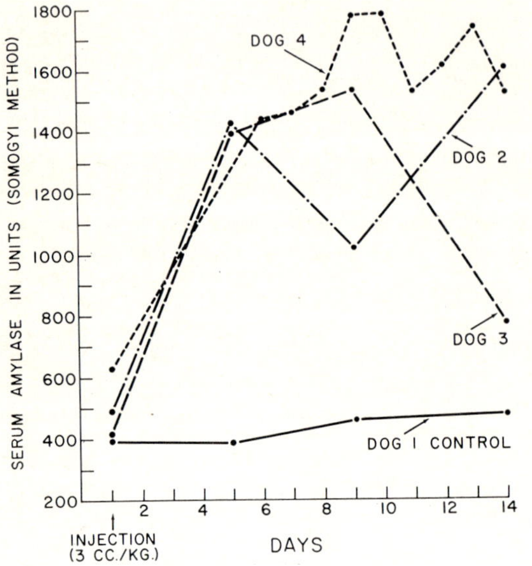


**Fig. 3.** Graph which illustrates elevations in serum amylase values after intravenous injection of rabbit antiserum to canine pancreas into normal dogs.

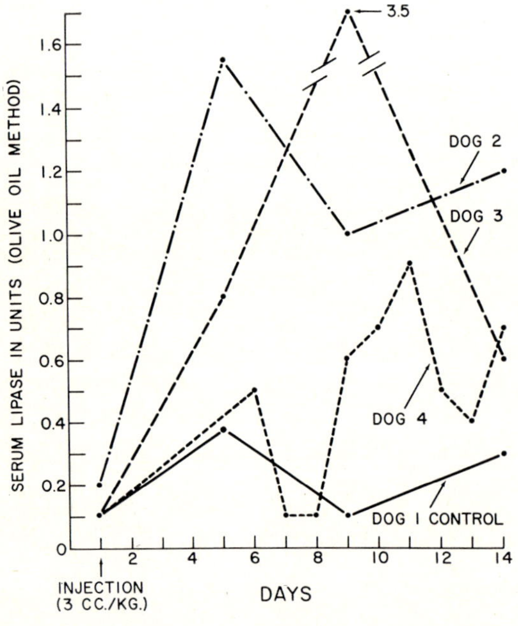


**Fig. 4.** Graph which demonstrates elevations in serum lipase values after intravenous injection of rabbit antiserum to canine pancreas into normal dogs.

factors which react with extracts from homologous pancreatic homogenate. Because of the crude preparation of the pancreatic antigen, plasma proteins and connective tissue were included in small quantities and immunologic reactions between these antigens and the patient's sera cannot be excluded. However, the increased reactivity of the pancreatic extract with the sera from patients with pancreatitis strongly suggests the presence of one or more circulating autoantibodies to human pancreas in these cases. The identification of more than one detectable antigen which reacted with antiserum to human pancreas in the sera of 4 of the patients with pancreatic disease and of 1 of the medical control patients also suggests that more than a single antigen-antibody system is present. In 2 clinical patients, circulating antigens were detected without antibodies being found. The sera from the passively immunized dogs did not contain detectable antigens. It is interesting to postulate from these findings that in the acute phase of the disease the patient disseminates particles of tissue antigen which in turn stimulate the body's immunologic mechanism to produce antibodies. Circulating antigens are apparently rarely found in the chronic phase of the disease when circulating antibodies are abundant.

Waksman[25] points out that antigenic materials which produce experimental autoimmunologic disease are similar in that almost all are, to a certain degree, isolated from the vascular bed. Because of this isolation, they are, in a sense, regarded as alien substances by the immunologic apparatus. Leakage of pancreatic enzymes or precursors into the circulation may thus be analagous to leakage of thyroglobulin from a follicle with subsequent antibody production, cell destruction, and development of Hashimoto's thyroiditis. One might then infer that all nuclear and cytoplasmic constituents, which normally are not accessible to the vascular stream or "antibody-producing cells," are potential antigens to which autoantibodies may be developed.

Thal[22] found circulating precipitating pancreatic antibodies in 32 of 36 patients with chronic pancreatitis and in a large per cent of patients with cystic fibrosis and carcinoma of the pancreas, as well as in occasional patients with lupus erythematosus, ulcerative colitis, and diabetes.

In preliminary studies, immunization of rabbits with specific crystallized pancreatic enzymes dispersed in Freund's adjuvant has not caused production of complementary antiserum. The crystallized pancreatic enzymes in various dilutions did not react with the sera from the human subjects in the present study. This information suggests that the several specific precipitin systems recorded in a few of the clinical cases may represent circulating autoantibodies to one or more cellular constituents other than specific pancreatic enzymes. Thal[22] separated nuclear fractions of human pancreas by differential centrifugation and found that the cytoplasmic fraction alone functioned as an antigen. Human pancreatic juice failed to react with the antiserum, and Thal suggests that the antigen is not derived from the enzymes, but rather from the endoplasmic reticulum of the pancreatic acinar cell. On the other hand, the observation by Robbins and his associates[18] that the sera from patients with lupus erythematosus fix complement with desoxyribose nucleic acid indicates that the antigen in autoimmunologic diseases resides in the cell nucleus.

The importance of distinguishing isoantibodies from true autoantibodies has been emphasized by Mackay.[14] The autoimmunologic status of the demonstable pancreatic antibodies is verified by the recent work of Thal and his associates[23] who found that autologous pancreatic antigen prepared from a specimen removed at operation gave a positive precipitin reaction in a patient with pancreatitis. However, the same author had previously reported the case of another patient with chronic pancreatitis who did not have antibodies reacting with autologous pancreas, although the sera of other patients with pancreatitis did have a positive precipitin reaction against his isologous pancreatic antigen.[24] He also observed that antibodies which were developed in an animal toward its own pancreas reacted with antigens derived from the pancreas of other animals but not with its own pancreas. Mackay and associates[14] found that sera from patients with lupus erythmatosus and macroglobulinemia did not fix complement when tested against antigen prepared from autologous tissues, although strong reactions oc-

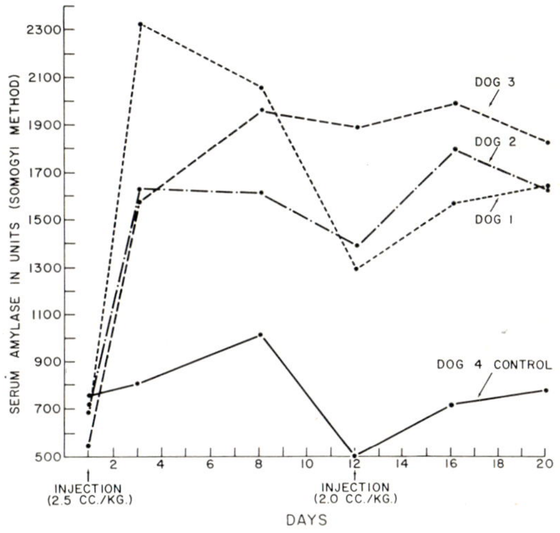


**Fig. 5.** Graph which shows elevations of serum amylase values after repeated injections of rabbit antiserum to canine pancreas into normal dogs.

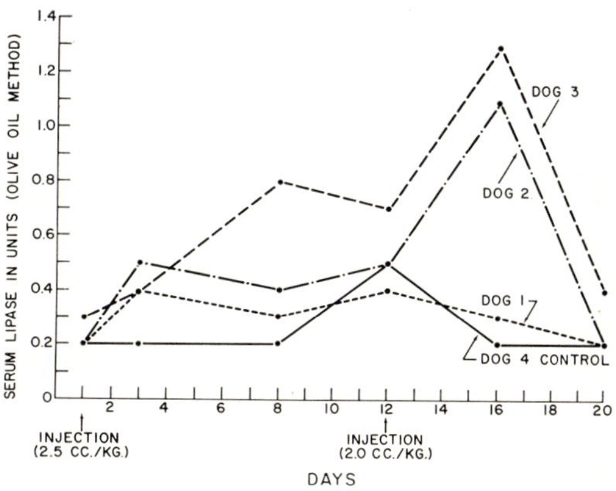


**Fig. 6.** Graph which shows elevations of serum lipase values after repeated injections of rabbit antiserum to canine pancreas into normal dogs.

curred when the same antigens were tested against homologous serum from patients with similar diseases. These findings suggest that only isologous reactions occur when tissue extracts contain substances capable of inhibiting reaction with homologous serum.

The production of specific organic disease by direct sensitization of the normal animal with either homologous or isologous tissue has been reported by several investigators, although these experiments do not definitely implicate circulating autoantibodies as the cause of disease. Rose and Witebsky[21] injected autologous thyroglobulin into the foot pads of rabbits and demonstrated circulating antibodies within 3 weeks. On removal of the remainder of the thyroid gland they found histologic features of typical Hashimoto's goiter. Thal[22, 24] reports histologic pancreatic fibrosis with detectable circulating pancreatic antibodies in dogs after 12 to 18 months of immunization with autologous and homologous pancreatic homogenate.

The important question still unanswered is whether antibodies demonstrated in the autoimmunologic diseases are responsible for the destructive processes, or are merely immunologic by-products of no pathogenetic significance. The critical evaluation of immunologic reactivity, as recorded by ability to produce specific clinical disease by passive transfer of specific antiserum to normal animals, perhaps would be to use antigen, antiserum, and injected animals from the same species. The early work of Masugi[15] demonstrated that clinical and histologic glomerulonephritis could be produced in normal rabbits within 1 week after intravenous injection of duck antiserum to rabbit kidney homogenate. Clinical lesions resembling ulcerative colitis have been produced in dogs by LeVeen and associates[11] by intraperitoneal injection of homologous colon antiserum prepared in rabbits and ducks. In the present study amylasemia and mild lipasemia were produced in dogs by intravenous injections of homologous pancreatic antiserum prepared in rabbits. The failure to demonstrate specific histologic changes in the pancreas of the animals sacrificed 1 month after the antiserum injection despite the development of transient elevations of circulating pancreatic enzyme levels perhaps indicates that an insufficient amount of antiserum was injected or that the animals were sacrificed prematurely. It is interesting to note that the pancreas in 2 of the rabbits immunized against dog pancreas with easily demonstrable antibodies showed no histologic pancreatic disease.

No histologic pancreatic changes were noted by Thal and his associates[23] 3 months after direct immunization with homologous pancreatic homogenate, despite the presence of circulating antibodies. Although Masugi[15] reports histologic kidney changes within 1 month of passive antiserum infusion, several factors are apparent which are not analogous to the present study. His studies indicate that the severity of the disease induced by passive transfer of antiserum varied directly with the ease of detection of antibody in the antiserum and with the amount of antiserum injected into the recipient animals. The kidney is apparently a more labile organ than the pancreas and reflects minor environmental alterations in varied cellular changes much more readily. The histologic appearance of the pancreas in pancreatitis is generally one of fibrosis and scarring with less tendency toward chronic inflammatory and plasma-cell infiltration than is seen in thyroiditis, ulcerative colitis, and glomerulonephritis. The species variance in ability to produce antibodies to heterologous tissue protein is not well understood at the present time. Thus, the antiserum to a heterologous antigen produced by ducks may differ in structure as well as immunologic reactivity from antiserum to the same antigen prepared in rabbits.

The antigen has generally been regarded as a template about which specific antibody-producing cells can manufacture the complementary antibody. More recently Burnet[2-4] has theorized that the information needed to manufacture a given antibody is already inherent in certain mesenchymal cells of the organism. The antigen thus simply selects the cells capable of synthesizing the corresponding antibody and stimulates them to proliferate and to produce more antibody. The capacity to make a given antibody is thus present before antigenic contact. An explanation for immunologic tolerance is provided by the postulation that the immature antibody-producing cell at a certain stage is vulnerable to contact with antigen and that a meeting with the corresponding antigen will destroy or inhibit it before birth.

Although the chemical composition, mode of formation, and pathogenetic significance of the antibodies in autoimmunologic disorders are, in general, poorly understood, their presence, as detected by the precipitin or other immunologic tests, may be of clinical diagnostic value for the present.

## SUMMARY

Autoimmunization has been cited as a possible etiologic factor in the development of unexplained chronic disease in isolated organ systems. The etiology of chronic relapsing pancreatitis in human beings has not been clearly defined, although the recurrent nature of the disease in many instances suggests the possibility of a hypersensitive state.

The clinical results detailed in the present study demonstrate that the sera of 15 of 16 patients with pancreatitis and each of 3 patients with carcinoma of the pancreas contain one or more precipitating antibodies which react with homologous pancreatic homogenate. One or more circulating pancreatic antigens were detected in the sera of approximately half of these patients. Sera from healthy blood donors and patients with various medical diseases rarely showed these reactions.

An attempt was made to create experimental pancreatitis by the injection of rabbit antiserum to canine pancreatic homogenate into healthy dogs. Elevations in serum amylase and lipase levels were detected within 4 days after intravenous infusion of 3 ml. of pancreatic antiserum per kilogram of body weight.

The mechanism underlying the formation of autoantibodies and the pathogenetic significance of the antibodies in autoimmunologic disorders is generally incompletely understood; however, their presence as detected by various immunologic tests may be of diagnostic value at present.

The authors gratefully acknowledge the constructive advice of Drs. Henry E. Weimer and S. H. Lawrence and the technical assistance of Joyce Shiner.

### REFERENCES

1. Broberger, O., and Perlmann, P.: Autoantibodies in human ulcerative colitis, J. Exper. Med. **110:** 657, 1959.
2. Burnet, M.: Auto-immune disease. I. Modern immunological concepts, Brit. M. J. **2:** 645, 1959.
3. Burnet, M.: Auto-immune disease. II. Pathology of the immune response, Brit. M. J. **2:** 720, 1959.
4. Burnet, M.: The clonal selection theory of acquired immunity, Nashville, 1959, Vanderbilt University Press.
5. Ceppellini, R., Polli, E., and Celada, F.: A DNA-reacting factor in serum of a patient with lupus erythematosus diffusus, Proc. Soc. Exper. Biol. & Med. **96:** 572, 1957.
6. Dameshek, W., and Schwartz, S. O.: The presence of hemolysins in acute hemolytic anemia, New England J. Med. **218:** 75, 1938.
7. Gajdusek, D. C.: An "autoimmune" reaction against human tissue antigens in certain acute and chronic diseases. I. Serological investigations, Arch. Int. Med. **101:** 9, 1958.
8. Henry, R. J., and Chiamori, N.: Study of the saccharogenic method for the determination of serum and urine amylase, Clin. Chem. **6:** 434, 1960.
9. Henry, R. J., Sobel, C., and Berkman, S.: On the determination of "pancreatitis lipase" in serum, Clin. Chem. **3:** 77, 1957.
10. Kattus, A., and Weimer, H. E.: Personal communication.
11. LeVeen, H. H., Falk, G., Ostroff, G., and Calem, W. S.: The production of ulcerative colitis by anticolon sera, S. Forum **11:** 3, 1960.
12. Liu, C. T., and McCrory, W. W.: Autoantibodies in human glomerulonephritis and nephrotic syndrome, J. Immunol. **81:** 492, 1958.
13. Mackay, I. R., and Gajdusek, D. C.: An "autoimmune" reaction against human tissue antigens in certain acute and chronic diseases. II. Clinical correlations, Arch. Int. Med. **101:** 30, 1958.
14. Mackay, I. R., Larkin, L., and Burnet,

F. M.: Failure of "autoimmune" antibody to react with antigen prepared from the individual's own tissues, Lancet **273:** 122, 1957.
15. Masugi, M.: Über die experimentelle Glomerulonephritis durch das spezifische Antinierenserum. Ein Beitrag zur Pathogenese der diffusen Glomerulonephritis, Beitr. path. Anat. **92:** 429, 1934.
16. Murray, J. E., Merrill, J. P., and Harrison, J. H.: Kidney transplantation between seven pairs of identical twins, Ann. Surg. **148:** 343, 1958.
17. Ouchterlony, O.: Antigen-antibody reaction in gels. IV. Types of reactions in co-ordinated systems of diffusion, Acta. path. et microbiol. scandinav. **32:** 231, 1953.
18. Robbins, W. C., Holman, H. R., Deicher, H., and Kunkel, H. G.: Complement fixation with cell nuclei and DNA in lupus erythematosus, Proc. Soc. Exper. Biol. & Med. **96:** 575, 1957.
19. Roitt, I. M., Doniach, D., and Campbell, P. N.: The nature of the gamma globulins in lymphadenoid goitre, Biochem. J. **64:** 54P, 1956.
20. Roitt, I. M., Doniach, D., Campbell, P. N., and Hudson, R. V.: Autoantibodies in Hashimoto's disease (lymphadenoid goitre), Lancet **271:** 820, 1956.
21. Rose, N. R., and Witebsky, E.: Studies on organ specificity. V. Changes in the thyroid glands of rabbits following active immunization with rabbit thyroid extracts, J. Immunol. **76:** 417, 1956.
22. Thal, A. P.: The occurrence of pancreatic antibodies and the nature of the pancreatic antigen, S. Forum **11:** 367, 1960.
23. Thal, A. P., Egner, W., and Murray, M. J.: Circulating antibodies in chronic pancreatic disease, S. Forum **10:** 240, 1959.
24. Thal, A. P., Egner, W., and Murray, M. J.: Isoantibody formation in chronic pancreatic disease, Lancet **1:** 1128, 1959.
25. Waksman, B. H.: Experimental allergic encephalomyelitis and the "auto-allergic" diseases, Internat. Arch. Allergy, **14:** 1, 1959.
26. Witebsky, E., and Rose, N. R.: Studies on organ specificity. IV. Production of rabbit thyroid antibodies in the rabbit, J. Immunol. **76:** 408, 1956.

*(For discussion, see page 148.)*

# The role of the parathyroid glands in calcium and magnesium metabolism in acute hemorrhagic pancreatitis

IVAN A. HERNANDEZ, M.D.
SAMUEL R. POWERS, JR., M.D., M.Sc.D.
THOMAS F. FRAWLEY, M.D.
ALBANY, N. Y.
*From the Departments of Surgery and Endocrinology and Metabolism.* *Supported in part by United States Public Health Grant A-2381.*

Acute necrotizing pancreatitis is associated with a significant mortality rate. Death may supervene at the end of a period of profound shock associated with cyanosis, dyspnea, myocardial failure, and acute renal insufficiency. Prompt recognition of the severity of the intravascular and extracellular fluid deficits followed by appropriate correction of the water, colloid, and crystalloid deficit will frequently result in resuscitation of the patient. Unfortunately, these corrective measures may be unsuccessful. While the specific toxic agent responsible for the apparently irreversible vascular collapse remains unidentified, it is frequently associated with depression of the serum calcium concentration and clinical evidence of skeletal muscle irritability. More recently, a fall in serum magnesium levels has also been noted.[3]

A possible relationship between the depressed serum $Ca^{++}$ concentrations and alterations in parathyroid function was suggested by a favorable response to the administration of parathyroid hormone (PTH) by a patient with tetany associated with proved hemorrhagic pancreatitis. Pertinent chemical data from this patient are presented in Fig. 1. Clinically, the administration of PTH was followed by the disappearance of muscle twitching within 6 hours. This response was especially significant since 4 intravenous injections of calcium chloride (1 Gm. each) had failed to alter the clinical or chemical findings. During the next week the patient developed evidence of adrenal insufficiency which was documented by an intravenous ACTH test. The changes in serum $Ca^{++}$ and $PO_4^{\equiv}$, coupled with the response to PTH, suggested the possibility of parathyroid insufficiency as well as the more completely documented adrenal insufficiency.

The correlation of hypocalcemia with a poor prognosis in hemorrhagic pancreatitis prompted an investigation into possible mechanisms which might be concerned with a fall in serum calcium and magnesium concentrations.

Alterations in serum calcium levels may be due to fluctuations in parathyroid function or, conversely, could be the cause of compensatory alterations in parathyroid activity. In order to eliminate any possible effect of changing parathyroid secretion, this study was carried out with parathyroidectomized animals maintained on a constant regimen of replacement therapy with A.T. 10 and constant calcium intake. The effect of acute necrotizing pancreatitis on calcium and magnesium metabolism has been compared in normal and parathyroidectomized animals.

## METHODS

Total parathyroidectomy is difficult to achieve in dogs.[11] A satisfactory technique

Read at the Twenty-second Annual Meeting of the Society of University Surgeons Kansas City, Kan., Feb. 9-11, 1961.

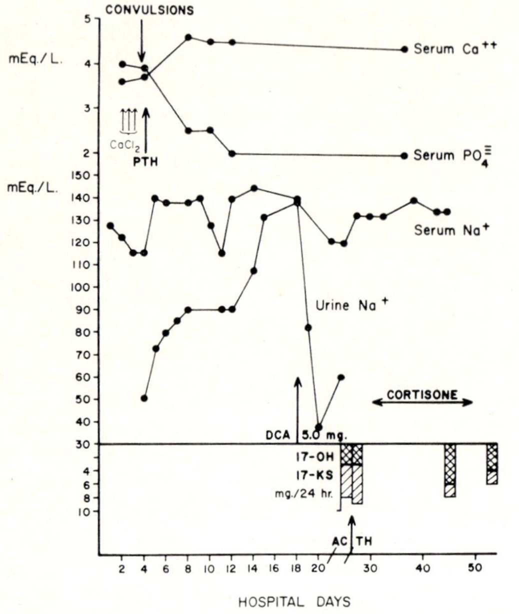


**Fig. 1.** Metabolic studies from a patient with severe hemorrhagic pancreatitis. The presenting signs were peripheral collapse, oliguria, and convulsions.

for total thyroidectomy and bilateral neck dissection has been utilized and the effect of this procedure on serum calcium levels has been followed for periods of up to 9 months in a separate group of animals.

A large midline cervical incision was made from well above the larynx to the manubrium. The sternomastoid and sternohyoid muscles were then mobilized and retracted laterally to expose the carotid sheaths. Both superior thyroid arteries were identified and divided at their origin and then the carotid sheaths were split from this point downward as far as possible into the superior mediastinum. All tissues within the area between the carotids and below the level of the superior thyroid arteries were removed en bloc. The pretracheal fascia and the areolar tissue which surrounds the esophagus were included. The recurrent nerves were stripped clean but left intact. The dissection was then carried as far into the superior mediastinum as possible with removal of all fatty and areolar tissue.

During the immediate postoperative period the animals required PTH and supplemental calcium by oral and parenteral routes. After approximately 1 week a constant program at A.T. 10, thyroid extract, and a fixed calcium diet was instituted. Deprivation of A.T. 10 resulted in a fall in serum calcium levels and the appearance of clinical tetany. When A.T. 10 was discontinued several weeks after parathyroidectomy, the serum calcium level fell, frequently to levels of 3.5 mEq. per liter, but this was not associated with clinical signs of muscular irritability. In 3 animals it was impossible to maintain serum levels in spite of apparently adequate replacement therapy. Completeness of parathyroid removal was checked in each animal subjected to experimental pancreatitis by temporary withdrawal of A.T. 10 and observation of the fall in the serum calcium level. Three animals were followed for 9 months and then the A.T. 10 and high calcium diet were withheld. Serum $Ca^{++}$ levels fell to 3.3, 3.4, and 3.5, but tetany did not develop.

Acute hemorrhagic pancreatitis was produced by the method of Elliott.[4] The duodenum was opened through a small incision just opposite the orifice of the main pancreatic duct and a small catheter was gently in-

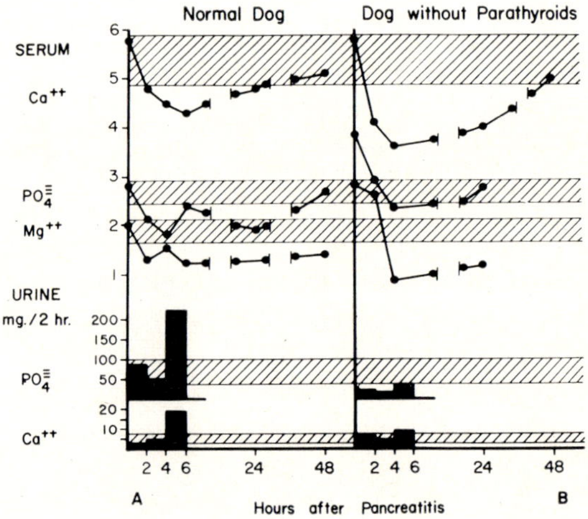


**Fig. 2.** Metabolic studies in a pair of typical experiments. Shaded areas represent the range of values during the control period of all normal dogs in this study. The animal without parathyroid glands was maintained on a constant dose of A.T. 10 throughout the study.

serted for a distance of about 3 cm. Ten milliliters of a 4 per cent solution of sodium taurocholate containing 500,000 U. of crystalline trypsin at a pH of 7.5 was injected under manometric control at a pressure of 10 cm. of water. The catheter was removed without ligation of the duct and the duodenum closed. The quantity and concentration of the injection mixture was worked out by trial and error to produce a moderately severe but nonfatal pancreatitis. After the injection, the pancreas was inspected for evidence of edema and hemorrhage in all animals. All animals subjected to pancreatitis received 1,500 ml. of dextran over an 8-hour period. Blood samples for $Ca^{++}$, $Mg^{++}$, and $PO_4^{\equiv}$ were collected prior to the induction of pancreatitis, then at 2-hour intervals for 6 hours, and also at 24 and 28 hours. Two-hour urine collections were obtained via an indwelling catheter and analyzed for $Ca^{++}$, $PO_4^{\equiv}$, and 17-ketosteroids. $Ca^{++}$, $Mg^{++}$, and $PO_4^{\equiv}$ were determined by standard methods[6-8]; 17-ketosteroids by the method of Callow.[2]

Fourteen dogs with intact parathyroid glands and 14 parathyroidectomized dogs were subjected to pancreatitis. One-half of each group received a single dose of 100 U. PTH 3 hours after development of pancreatitis. Six additional animals with intact parathyroid glands were treated with 12 mEq. of $Mg^{++}$, 1½ and 3 hours after the development of pancreatitis.

## RESULTS

The effect of pancreatitis on $Ca^{++}$, $PO_4^{\equiv}$, and $Mg^{++}$ metabolism in a single pair of experiments is shown in Fig. 2.* The animals with intact parathyroid glands (Group A) showed a fall in serum $Ca^{++}$, $PO_4^{\equiv}$, and $Mg^{++}$ levels. This was associated with a rise in urinary excretion of $PO_4^{\equiv}$ and $Ca^{++}$, indicative of a secondary increase in parathyroid activity. Five of 7 animals in this group demonstrated an increased $PO_4^{\equiv}$ excretion, whereas $Ca^{++}$ excretion was increased in 4. A rise in $Ca^{++}$ excretion did not occur when

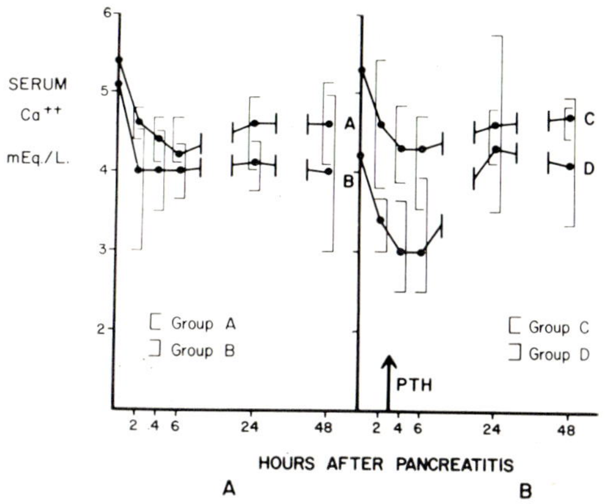


Fig. 3. Serum calcium values for all 4 groups of animals after the development of pancreatitis. Heavy lines represent the averages for each group. Brackets indicate the range of values observed for each group. Groups B and D are parathyroidectomized animals. *B* shows the effect of a single dose of PTH.

the serum $Ca^{++}$ level was below 4.2 mEq. per liter. Fig. 2, *B*, illustrates the chemical changes which occur after pancreatitis in an animal without parathyroid glands (Group B). Serum $Ca^{++}$ and $Mg^{++}$ fall to lower levels than are seen in dogs with intact parathyroid glands and there is no change in urinary $PO_4^{\equiv}$ or $Ca^{++}$ excretion.

Fig. 3 is a summary of the serum $Ca^{++}$ values in all groups of animals. There was a considerable spread of the values within each group so that in addition to the group average, the maximum and minimum concentrations for each period are indicated. Although there is some overlapping between groups, it is apparent that animals without parathyroid glands suffered a more severe and more prolonged fall than was seen in animals with intact parathyroid glands. In addition, the administration of PTH produced a rapid return of serum $Ca^{++}$ values toward the normal range. Only 1 animal in the group without either parathyroid glands or supplemental PTH had a serum $Ca^{++}$ level over 4.0 mEq. per liter at the end of 24 hours, whereas all animals with both parathyroid glands and additional PTH had levels of over 4.2 mEq. per liter. The pres-

*Space limitations preclude the inclusion of the almost 1,000 blood and urine values. These data are available from the Albany Medical College on request.

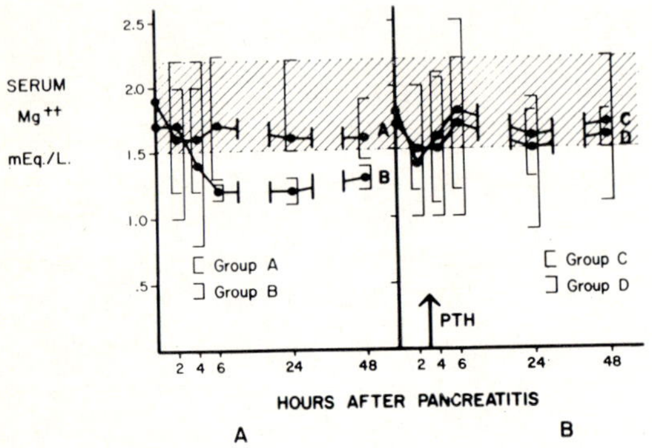


**Fig. 4.** Serum magnesium values after pancreatitis in all groups.

ence of either endogenous or exogenous parathyroid hormone tended to minimize the extent and duration of the hypocalcemia.

Fig. 4 summarizes the changes in serum $Mg^{++}$ levels after the induction of pancreatitis. Intact animals (Group A) suffered a significant decrease in 5 of the 6 experiments in which adequate samples were obtained. The lowest values in this group were 1.2 mEq. per liter. All parathyroidectomized animals without supplemental PTH had serum $Mg^{++}$ levels of less than 1.2 mEq. per liter after the development of pancreatitis. In 1 animal the level fell to 0.8 mEq. per liter. The administration of PTH produced a rise in serum $Mg^{++}$ to the normal range by 24 hours in all animals of Group C and in all but one of Group D. These data suggest that normal or increased amounts of parathyroid hormone will minimize the fall in serum $Mg^{++}$ levels and also that the parenteral administration of PTH will tend to increase the depressed values toward normal. Two additional animals received a constant infusion of $Mg^{28}$ during the induction of pancreatitis. Specimens of fat from the peritoneal cavity showed an eightfold increase in counting rates 3 hours after the introduction of the bile salts—trypsin mixture into the pancreatic duct. Of special interest was the finding of a significant amount of activity in samples of subcutaneous fat from the abdominal wall. Six animals with intact parathyroid glands were treated with 12 mEq. of $Mg^{++}$ by vein at 1½ hours and 3 hours after induction of pancreatitis. No significant change in $Mg^{++}$ occurred but there was an indication that the serum $Ca^{++}$ in this group fell less than that in Group A. The average maximum fall in serum $Ca^{++}$ in the animals treated with $Mg^{++}$ was only 0.8 mEq. per liter as compared with an average fall of 1.4 mEq. per liter in the untreated group.

Serum and urinary $PO_4^{\equiv}$ values were somewhat variable but nevertheless followed certain general patterns. Ten of 15 animals with intact parathyroid glands showed a fall in serum levels and 8 showed a significant increase in urinary excretion. These changes were generally associated with a fall in the serum $Ca^{++}$ level of more than 1 mEq. per liter. Animals without parathyroid glands started with higher $PO_4^{\equiv}$ values in the control period than normal dogs, with the highest values associated with the lowest serum $Ca^{++}$ levels. After the induction of pancreatitis, there was a fall in the serum $PO_4^{\equiv}$ level similar to that seen in animals with intact parathyroid glands, but this was not associated with an increased urinary $PO_4^{\equiv}$ excretion. The reason for this fall in the level of serum $PO_4^{\equiv}$ without an increased urinary loss is not clear.

Excretion of 17-ketosteroids showed no definite pattern in any of the groups. There was no clear-cut evidence of either increased or diminished adrenal cortical function.

## COMMENT

Acute hemorrhagic pancreatitis may result in a significant fall in serum $Ca^{++}$ concentration. The clinical observation of a striking improvement in neuromuscular irritability with a simultaneous rise in serum $Ca^{++}$ levels after the administration of PTH in a patient with pancreatitis suggested the present experimental study. The technique described by Elliott[4] will regularly produce severe necrotizing pancreatitis in the dog and usually results in a significant fall in serum $Ca^{++}$ and $Mg^{++}$ concentrations. The possibility of altered parathyroid function acting either to augment or minimize these changes indicated the desirability of removing the parathyroid glands and maintaining the animals on a fixed replacement regimen. The dosages of A.T. 10 and calcium were sufficient to maintain most of the animals in essentially normal calcium and phosphate balance so that the changes which occurred after pancreatitis developed cannot be ascribed to a deficiency of circulating hormone. If clinical pancreatitis was associated with a hypoparathyroid state, the animals on A.T. 10 maintenance therapy should have been protected instead of suffering a more profound fall in serum $Ca^{++}$ level.

The presence of increased parathyroid activity in normal animals subjected to experimental pancreatitis is indicated by a less profound fall in serum $Ca^{++}$ levels than occurred in the parathyroidectomized group and also by the increased $PO_4^{\equiv}$ excretion. In addition, the administration of exogenous PTH further minimized the chemical alterations after the development of pancreatitis. The mechanism which leads to increased parathyroid activity after a sudden fall in serum $Ca^{++}$ levels is suggested by the studies of Patt and Luckhardt,[9] who perfused parathyroid glands with calcium-free blood and noted the release of a $Ca^{++}$ mobilizing factor. The protective action of circulating PTH on serum $Ca^{++}$ levels is probably due to the ability of PTH to induce bone resorption and hence mobilize bone calcium.[5]

A fall in serum $Mg^{++}$ levels in pancreatitis has been previously reported.[3] The possibility that this is due to precipitation of $Mg^{++}$ in areas of fat necrosis has been substantiated by the studies with $Mg^{28}$ which demonstrated increased quantities of radioactive material, not only in the areas of gross fat necrosis within the peritoneal cavity, but also in subcutaneous fat. It appears that circulating pancreatic enzymes cause lipolysis in central and peripheral fat depots which releases sufficient amounts of free fatty acids to account for the binding of significant quantities of $Mg^{++}$.

The protective action of the parathyroid glands in limiting the fall in serum $Mg^{++}$ concentration, as well as the effect of exogenous PTH in restoring these values to normal, suggests a possible direct action of PTH on magnesium metabolism. This concept is not supported by data from our parathyroidectomized animals prior to the induction of pancreatitis or by the studies of Roberts.[10] Serum magnesium values were essentially identical in all groups with or without replacement therapy. A possible explanation for the rise in serum magnesium level after the injection of PTH comes from the observation that patients with hyperparathyroidism apparently mobilize bone stores of $Mg^{++}$ along with $Ca^{++}$.[1] The action of PTH in producing resorption of bone would liberate $Mg^{++}$ along with $Ca^{++}$ and $PO_4^{\equiv}$ and tend to increase serum levels of all three.[10]

The sequence of metabolic events which occur in hemorrhagic pancreatitis therefore seems to be first a fall in serum $Ca^{++}$ and $Mg^{++}$ levels due to binding of these ions in areas of fat necrosis, both within the peritoneal cavity and in the fat depots. The lowered serum calcium level stimulates the parathyroid glands with increased bone resorption and increased $PO_4^{\equiv}$ excretion. Bone resorption then results in liberation of $Ca^{++}$ and $Mg^{++}$ into the circulation and a rise in serum concentrations.

The clinical significance of hypocalcemia and hypomagnesemia in hemorrhagic pancreatitis or the therapeutic implications of PTH administration was not determined in this study. These studies emphasize that pancreatitis may be accompanied by alterations in serum $Mg^{++}$ level which in turn could account for some of the clinical findings heretofore ascribed to widespread tissue damage or nonspecific toxic materials.

The severity of the pancreatitis and the fluid therapy in this study were deliberately set to insure survival of the animals. Only an occasional animal died and no group of experiments was significantly affected. The response of the animals to PTH was therefore assessed only in terms of biochemical alterations and not in terms of the natural history of the disease. The question of whether the lowered serum $Ca^{++}$ and $Mg^{++}$ levels are merely an indication of the severity of the disease or whether they play a direct role in the fatal outcome remains unanswered. The possibility that the pallor, cyanosis, and peripheral collapse frequently seen in severe pancreatitis might be due at least in part to hypomagnesemia is suggested by the dramatic clinical improvement noted in the patient treated with PTH. Additional clinical studies on the effects of PTH on patients with pancreatitis will have to be carried out to produce a satisfactory answer to this question.

## CONCLUSIONS

1. Experimental pancreatitis results in a significant fall in serum calcium and magnesium concentrations.

2. Lowered serum calcium levels were associated with blood and urinary changes consistent with increased parathyroid activity.

3. Parathyroid hormone of either endogenous or exogenous origin favorably modified the magnitude and duration of the depression of serum calcium and magnesium levels.

4. These experimental studies, supported by metabolic studies in a patient with hemorrhagic pancreatitis, suggest that PTH may have a beneficial effect on the clinical course of patients with depressed serum values of calcium and magnesium in association with acute hemorrhagic pancreatitis.

### REFERENCES

1. Barnes, B. A., Krane, S. M., and Cope, O.: Magnesium studies in relation to hyperparathyroidism, J. Clin. Endocrinol. **17:** 1407, 1957.
2. Callow, R. K.: The chemical estimation of urinary neutral 17-ketosteroids, J. Endocrinol. **5:** 67, 1946-1948.
3. Edmonson, H. A., Berne, C. J., Homann, R. D., Jr., and Wertman, M.: Calcium, potassium, magnesium and amylase disturbances in acute pancreatitis, Am. J. Med. **12:** 34, 1952.
4. Elliott, D. W., Williams, R. D., and Stewart, W. R.: The role of trypsin and of bile salts in the pathogenesis of acute pancreatitis, S. Forum **10:** 533-537, 1958.
5. Engfeldt, B., and Zettergtrom, R.: Biophysical and chemical investigation on bone tissue in experimental hyperparathyroidism, Endocrinology **54:** 506, 1954.
6. Fiske, C. H., and Subbarow, Y.: The colorimetric determination of phosphorus, J. Biol. Chem. **66:** 375-400, 1925.
7. Horner, W. H.: The determination of calcium in biological material, J. Lab. & Clin. Med. **45:** 951-957, 1955.
8. Orange, M., and Rheim, H. C.: Microestimation of magnesium in body fluids, J. Biol. Chem. **189:** 379, 1951.
9. Patt, H. M., and Luckhardt, A. B.: Relationships of a low blood calcium to parathyroid secretion, Endocrinology **31:** 384, 1956.
10. Roberts, B., Murphy, L. M., and Rosenthal, O.: The effect of parathyroid hormone upon serum levels and urinary excretion of magnesium, S. Forum **5:** 509, 1954.
11. Sanderson, P. H., Marshall, F., and Wilson, R. E.: Calcium and phosphorus homeostasis in the parathyroidectomized dog, J. Clin. Invest. **39:** 662, 1960.

## DISCUSSION*

**Dr. William G. Anlyan** (Durham, N. C.). I shall confine my remarks to the paper by Dr. Elliott and his colleagues who have done a fine piece of work. It may be recalled that before this Society in 1957 we presented our arbeit on some of the pathologic and physiologic alterations which result from chronic ductal obstructions with Vinylite injection of the ductal system of the pancreas in dogs. At that time an incidental finding was that 50 per cent of our animals with ductal obstruction followed 6 months or longer had multiple duodenal ulcers. We did not know at that time whether this was purely a pH problem of keeping the alkaline pancreatic juices out of the duodenum or whether there might be a hormonal component responsible for the ulceration. This diligent work by Dr. Elliott and his co-workers would tend to substantiate the latter possibility.

**Dr. Edwin H. Ellison** (Milwaukee, Wis.). The authors are to be congratulated on a beautifully conceived and executed study. I agree with Dr. Elliott that the hyperacidity resulting from exclusion of pancreatic juice from the duodenum either by construction of a fistula or by total pancreatectomy most likely resulted from the impaired digestion of fat. The consistent and marked increase of acid secretions from Heidenhain pouches after obstruction of the pancreatic ducts alone is certainly most significant and suggests not only a gastric secretagogue arising from

*Discussion of papers by Elliott, Taft, Passaro, and Zollinger; Fonkalsrud and Longmire; and Hernandez, Powers, and Frawley.

the pancreatic islets but also raises the question as to whether or not a gastric inhibitor is produced by the acinar cells of the pancreas. Failure to isolate a gastrin-like hormone by Gregory's method from the normal pancreas might be dependent in part upon the presence of this inhibitor substance in the extract. Failure to abolish the hypersecretion by resection of the obstructed pancreas is somewhat disconcerting but also points toward the presence of an inhibitor in normal acini. Similar happenings have also been reported in ulcer patients after removal of a solitary benign ulcerogenic tumor with the vagus nerves and stomach still intact. In these instances hypersecretion subsided gradually which suggested a gradual reduction of the hyperplastic parietal cell mass to normal. With this in mind, I would like to ask Dr. Elliott how long he has observed his animals after resection of the obstructed pancreas.

**Dr. Thomas T. White** (Seattle, Wash.). I certainly have enjoyed listening to these 3 papers, but I will discuss only the first one. First, we have been making chronic pancreatic fistulas for the study of the external secretion of the pancreas for about 6 years. We have made approximately 400 of these, some of which have been maintained for as long as 5 months. To date we have not seen an ulcer in any of these dogs. We have never performed any pouch experiments. Second, no ulcer appeared in 25 totally pancreatectomized dogs used by the department of medicine for glucagon studies. I think that the mechanism for the hypersecretion which Dr. Elliott found in his Heidenhain pouch is illustrated here. Emulsification is needed to produce duodenal inhibition through the enterogastrone mechanism as indicated by Sircus. Both bile and pancreatic juice are needed to produce emulsification. All of these experiments interfere with one or other of the factors which facilitate emulsification.

**Dr. Stanley R. Friesen** (Kansas City, Kan.). I wish to discuss the paper presented by Dr. Elliott. I think it might be appropriate to enlarge a bit on the work that Prof. Gregory of Liverpool is doing. As he reported in the May 14, 1960, issue of *Lancet,* he and his co-workers have been successful in extracting from an ulcerogenic non-insulin-secreting islet-cell pancreatic adenoma a substance which has a high gastrinlike activity and which has no histamine activity. In December, 1960, we had occasion to take care of a patient who had the clinical findings of the Zollinger-Ellison syndrome with marked gastric hypersecretion, an ulcer in the third portion of the duodenum, gastric hyperplasia, duodenal nodularity, and at operation findings of a pancreaticoduodenal islet-cell carcinoma with lymph node and hepatic metastases. I sent tissue from the primary tumor, the lymph node metastases, and the hepatic metastases to Gregory, who found high gastrinlike activity in all 3 of these tissues. No histamine activity was found in these. For control, he is extracting for us tissues from non-islet-cell acinar adenocarcinomas of the pancreas with metastases which show no gastrin activity. We believe this finding of non-histamine, high gastrin activity in the metastases of islet-cell carcinoma is the first such demonstration. This observation strongly supports the humoral theory of the mechanism of the gastric hypersecretion in the Zollinger-Ellison syndrome.

**Dr. Herbert B. Greenlee** (Chicago, Ill.). I would like to discuss Dr. Elliott's paper. We have been doing similar work at the University of Chicago and I have 2 slides which illustrate some of our results. The first demonstrates that after complete and total ligation of the pancreatic ducts, 5 of 6 previously controlled Heidenhain pouch dogs showed a significant rise in the gastric secretory output up to 2½ times that of control levels. We postulated that this effect might be mediated through the gastric antrum. However, the next slide illustrates that a similar increase occurred after pancreatic duct ligation in previously controlled vagotomized and antrectomized dogs. The animals in both series developed hypolipemia which was corrected by feeding raw pancreas, but with no corresponding return of the gastric secretion to control levels.

**Alan P. Thal** (Minneapolis, Minn.). I would like to compliment Drs. Fonkalsrud and Longmire on their very well-presented paper. Our studies on circulating pancreatic antibodies in the human being entirely confirm their finding that the majority of patients with chronic pancreatic disease show circulating antibodies demonstrable both by the Ouchterlony gel-diffusion technique and the Boyden tanned red-cell hemagglutination technique.

The first slide compares an interaction between the gamma globulin of a patient with chronic pancreatitis and antigens derived from the pancreas of various species. It will be seen that this reaction is entirely species specific.

In the second slide, antigens were prepared from the tail of the pancreas and spleen of a patient undergoing caudal pancreatectomy for pancreatitis. The patient's gamma globulin in the central well reacts only with pancreas extract which shows organ specificity.

At the moment, we are studying children with cystic fibrosis and their near relatives. Forty of 42 such children with proved cystic fibrosis have circulating antibodies, whereas only 5 of 108 normal siblings were positive. In addition, 22 of 28 mothers of children with cystic fibrosis showed pancreatic antibodies.

Finally, in long-term experiments, when chronic pancreatitis has been induced in an isolated segment of the uncinate process of the canine pancreas, we have found quite marked chronic pancreatitis in the main pancreas after a period of 12 to 18 months. Analysis of such experiments is hampered by the occurrence of spontaneous chronic pancreatitis in dogs.

**James T. Grace** (Buffalo, N. Y.). I would like to comment briefly on the agar gel diffusion technique. Dr. Richard Metzgar and I have been concerned for some time with the reactivity of various normal and presumably immune human sera with extracts of different types of human tissue, normal and malignant. We were disturbed by the frequency with which lines appeared in the agar plates with all combinations of sera and tissue extracts when antigen-antibody reactions could not be demonstrated by other in vitro serologic tests.

By use of immunoelectrophoresis, we found that the reactive serum components had the mobility of albumin and the reactive tissue extract components migrated in the $alpha_2$ globulin region. Since hemoglobin was present in all of our tissue extracts, and since this also migrates in the $alpha_2$ globulin region, we reacted crystalline albumin with crystalline hemoglobin in agar plates and observed lines similar to the ones which occurred with sera and tissue extracts.

I mention these observations not to point out the binding capacity of albumin for hemoglobin components (this is well known), but rather to point out the problems involved in interpretation of agar gel diffusion reactions when whole serum and hemoglobin-containing tissue extracts are used. We advise caution in ascribing an immunologic basis to such reactions unless this can be substantiated by other serologic methods.

**Dr. Dan W. Elliott** (closing). I certainly appreciate the generous remarks of Drs. Anlyan, Ellison, White, Friesen, and Greenlee. Dr. Ellison asked how long we have watched animals after resection of an atrophic pancreas to see whether or not their hypersecretion would slowly subside. We have with us in our laboratory animals in which this resection was performed last September, about 6 months ago. Their hypersecretion remains unchanged. Since Dr. Friesen mentioned Gregory's analysis of an ulcerogenic tumor, I want to add that this work is also going forward in our laboratory at Columbus. We have used Dr. Gregory's method and have been able to duplicate his findings. We have found a gastrin-like substance in the hepatic metastases of an ulcerogenic tumor which, by electron microscopy, contained secretory granules typical of alpha cells. I appreciate Dr. Greenlee's discussion of this paper since he has obtained findings which are very similar to our own, but previously were unknown to us.

**Dr. Eric W. Fonkalsrud** (closing). I wish to thank the discussers for their very kind and constructive comments on this controversial subject. The early studies by Dr. Thal and his associates, which related pancreatitis to autoimmunologic phenomena, were of considerable help to us in establishing the techniques for the present study. This composite slide shows an immunoelectrophoretic preparation in which the central trough is filled with goat antihuman serum. The well on one side of the trough contains normal human serum and the well on the opposite side is filled with the serum from a patient with pancreatitis. A specific stain for the beta lipoprotein fraction of the serum was used and here we see an abnormal migration of this fraction in the serum from the patient with pancreatitis as compared to its normal location in the control serum. We have seen this altered migration pattern for beta lipoprotein in 2 other patients with pancreatitis and this suggests that perhaps the pancreatic antigen, or a least one of these antigens, might reside in this fraction of the serum. With regard to other methods of immunologic testing, we have used the complement fixation test on the serum of 4 patients with pancreatitis and recorded a positive reaction in 1 patient with a titer of 1 to 8.

# The relative importance of the vagus nerve, antrum, and acid-secreting mucosa in the prevention of experimental peptic ulceration

R. C. HARRISON, M.D.
H. T. G. WILLIAMS, M.B.
W. PISESKY, M.D.
S. HUSAIN, M.D.
O. H. SILBERMANN, M.D.
G. J. FRANCIS, M.D.
J. W. IRVINE, M.D.
EDMONTON, ALBERTA
*From the Department of Surgery and Surgical-Medical Research Institute, University of Alberta*

The continuing controversy about the choice of operation for duodenal ulcer and debate regarding the role of the antrum in ulcer control led us to analyze the relative significance of the various factors which are known to reduce acid secretion. The evidence is very strong that duodenal ulcer is an acid-engendered disease; the acid, of course, is produced by the parietal cells. They are stimulated by 2 major mechanisms, vagal and antral. The vagi stimulate the parietal cells directly, and also stimulate the antrum to produce gastrin. Gastrin is produced in response to antral distention and the presence of food, as well as by vagal stimulation. All three of these responses are greatly modified by the pH existing in the antrum at the time. An autoregulatory control of acid by the antrum and duodenum, dependent on pH, undoubtedly exists, but whether the regulation is accomplished by control of gastrin production alone or by the production of an inhibitor substance as well is not yet clarified.[4] It is well established that the antrum left in an alkaline environment is definitely ulcerogenic, but it is far from clear whether the antrum retained in an acid environment favors or retards the development of peptic ulcer. It is also uncertain how the antral effect is modified by vagal denervation. Besides the vagal and antral stimulation of the acid-secreting parietal cells, there is a minor effect by humoral agents from the intestine and there is a role, as yet unclarified, played by the adrenal glands, pancreas, and other endocrine glands.

As surgeons, we approach the control of duodenal ulcer through the control of acid secretion. This we can do by vagally denervating the acid-secreting parietal cells, vagally denervating the antrum which is left in situ, excising the antrum, or resecting a varying percentage of the acid-secreting portion of the stomach. What is the relative importance of each of these factors in ulcer control? They cannot be studied individually in the human being, and they cannot be studied in experimental animals by pouch methods which only reflect the humoral phases of secretion. We must assess these factors in animals by the reduction in ulcer incidence which results. This approach has been used by a number of authors with the Mann-Williamson dog.[1-3, 6, 7, 9] The accumulated experience of these investigators suggests that vagotomy of the whole

Supported by Grants from the National Research Council of Canada and the City of Edmonton Civic Employees.

Read at the Twenty-second Annual Meeting of the Society of University Surgeons, Kansas City, Kan., Feb. 9-11, 1961.

**Table I.** *The procedures employed*

| *Procedure No.* | *Procedure* | *Antrum* | *Parietal-cell mass** | *No. of dogs* | *No. of ulcers* |
|---|---|---|---|---|---|
| 1 | Pylorectomy | Preserved, vagally innervated | Intact, vagally innervated | 5 | 5 |
| 2 | Pylorectomy and vagotomy | Preserved, vagally denervated | Intact, vagally denervated | 5 | 4 |
| 3 | Vagal denervation of antrum and pylorus | Preserved, vagally denervated | Intact, vagally innervated | 4 | 3 |
| 4 | Antrectomy | Resected | Intact, vagally innervated | 5 | 2 |
| 5 | Antrectomy and vagotomy | Resected | Intact, vagally denervated | 5 | 2 |
| 6 | Hemigastrectomy | Resected | 25% resected, remainder vagally innervated | 5 | 2 |
| 7 | Hemigastrectomy and vagotomy | Resected | 25% resected, remainder vagally denervated | 5 | 1 |
| 8 | Billroth I | Resected | 50% resected, remainder vagally innervated | 5 | 3 |
| 9 | Billroth I and vagotomy | Resected | 50% resected, remainder vagally denervated | 5 | 1 |
| 10 | Segmental | Preserved, vagally denervated | 50% resected, remainder vagally innervated | 5 | 1 |
| 11 | Segmental and vagotomy | Preserved, vagally denervated | 50% resected, remainder vagally denervated | 5 | 2 |
| 12 | Tubular | Preserved, vagally innervated | 50% resected, remainder vagally innervated | 5 | 5 |
| 13 | Tubular and vagotomy (same series as No. 11) | Preserved, vagally denervated | 50% resected, remainder vagally denervated | 5 | 2 |
| 14 | Radical Billroth I | Resected | 75% resected, remainder vagally innervated | 6 | 1 |
| 15 | Radical Billroth I and vagotomy | Resected | 75% resected, remainder vagally denervated | 8 | 1 |
| 16 | Radical segmental | Preserved, vagally denervated | 75% resected, remainder vagally innervated | 7 | 4 |
| 17 | Radical segmental and vagotomy | Preserved, vagally denervated | 75% resected, remainder vagally denervated | 7 | 1 |
| 18 | Radical tubular | Preserved, vagally innervated | 75% resected, remainder vagally innervated | 3 | 2 |
| 19 | Radical tubular and vagotomy (same series as No. 17) | Preserved, vagally denervated | 75% resected, remainder vagally denervated | 7 | 1 |

*The acid-secreting portion of the stomach.

stomach has reduced the incidence of experimental ulcers in the Mann-Williamson preparation, that antrectomy also has been effective, and that vagotomy and antrectomy combined have been even more effective. They were unable, however, to determine whether vagotomy exerted a beneficial effect through denervation of the antrum or through denervation of the acid-secreting mucosa, and were unable to evaluate the effect of resection of increasing amounts of acid-secreting mucosa. The severe nutritional problems inherent in the Mann-Williamson preparation and the fact that it increases acid secretion may have affected their conclusions.

## METHODS

We have previously described[8] an experimental method of ulcer production in the dog which has proved to be very satisfactory for this study (Fig. 1). A 20 cm. length of terminal ileum with its mesentery intact was interposed after division of the first portion of the duodenum. Without the addition of exogenous drugs, 80 per cent of these animals developed deep callous peptic ulcers in the ileal segment. Of particular importance was the fact that their nutrition remained satisfactory and the area proximal to the duodenum could be utilized for methods of ulcer control.

By performing the surgical procedures commonly employed for duodenal ulcer, plus others particularly designed for investigation of the role of the vagus, antrum, and parietal-cell mass, we were able to separate these 3 factors and assess them individually (Fig. 2). In Table I are listed the procedures which were employed, the status of the antrum, the status of the acid-secreting mucosa (parietal-cell mass), and the number of dogs used in each instance. Pylorectomy was performed instead of pyloroplasty because there was insufficient room for pyloroplasty between the pylorus and the short segment of duodenum proximal to the duodenoileal suture line. Vagal denervation of the intact antrum was carried out by division and resuture of the antral-body junction, and clearance of the lesser curvature of the stomach.[5] Vagotomy, when employed, was transabdominal. Tubular gastrectomy and vagotomy results in the same preparation as segmental gastrectomy and vagotomy, so the 1 series of dogs was used to assess both procedures. Each procedure was tested in from 3 to 8 dogs, a total of 90 animals. Generally the ileal insert and the procedure being tested were performed in 1 stage, and if the animals did not die of hemorrhage or perforation they were sacrificed at 3 months and the incidence of true ulcers noted. Only 1 procedure was evaluated in each animal.

## RESULTS

As previously recorded, the ileal insertion procedure itself results in an ulcer incidence of 80 per cent.[8] While the incidence of ulceration associated with each of these procedures is interesting, the number of animals in each series is small and no significant conclusions can be drawn on a comparative basis. On the other hand, when the physiologic variables previously mentioned are compared, the number of animals is significant and the comparisons are probably valid.

There are 3 possible ways to deal with the antrum, (1) retain it as a vagally innervated antrum, (2) retain it as a vagally denervated antrum, or (3) excise it. Table II is a comparison of the ulcerogenic effect between procedures in which the antrum is retained and identical procedures in which it is excised. A significant reduction in ulcer incidence results from antral exci-

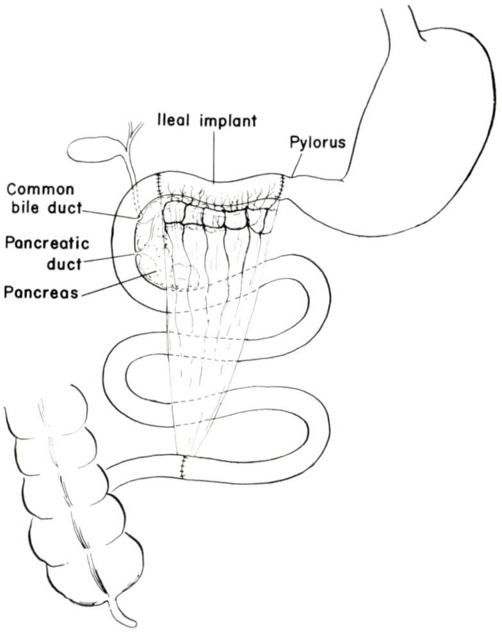


**Fig. 1.** The experimental procedure (from S. Forum 9: 455, 1959).

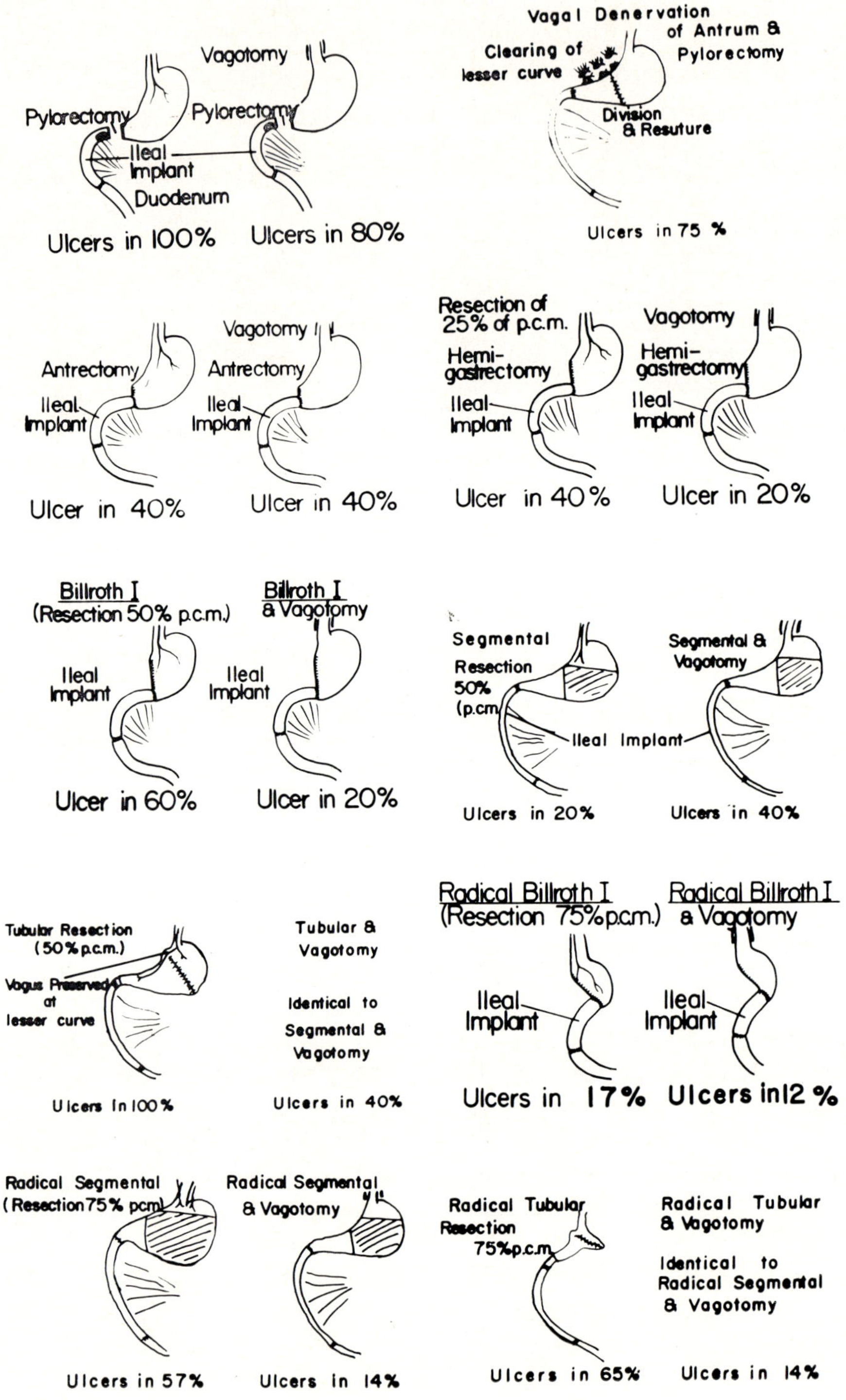


Fig. 2. Illustration of the procedures listed in Table I. Because of the small number of animals in each group, a comparison between procedures is not justified.

sion, but it will be noted that in some instances the preserved antrum is vagally innervated, while in others it is vagally denervated. If the antrum is retained, is its effect modified by vagal innervation? Table III is a comparison of the ulcerogenic effect in 3 series of animals (A, B, and C), in each of which the only variable is a change in the status of the antrum. These 3 series are combined to give more significance to the study, and the percentage of peptic ulceration under these three circumstances noted. Although the antrum is in contact with acid-secreting mucosa in all these procedures, there is a marked reduction in ulcer incidence when the antrum is vagally de-

**Table II.** *Effect of antrectomy in 2 comparable groups*

| *Procedure* | *No. of dogs* | *No. of ulcers* | *Plus antrectomy* | *No. of dogs* | *No. of ulcers* |
|---|---|---|---|---|---|
| Pylorectomy (No. 1) | 5 | 5 | Pylorectomy and antrectomy (No. 4) | 5 | 2 |
| Vagal denervation of antrum and pylorus (No. 2) | 4 | 3 | Pylorectomy and antrectomy (No. 4) | 5 | 2 |
| Pylorectomy and vagotomy (No. 2) | 5 | 4 | Pylorectomy, antrectomy, and vagotomy (No. 5) | 5 | 2 |
| Segmental (No. 10) | 5 | 1 | Billroth I (No. 8) | 5 | 3 |
| Segmental and vagotomy (No. 11) | 5 | 2 | Billroth I and vagotomy (No. 9) | 5 | 1 |
| Tubular (No. 12) | 5 | 5 | Billroth I (No. 8) | 5 | 3 |
| Tubular and vagotomy (No. 13) | 5 | 2 | Billroth I and vagotomy (No. 9) | 5 | 1 |
| Radical segmental (No. 16) | 7 | 4 | Radical Billroth I (No. 14) | 6 | 1 |
| Radical segmental and vagotomy (No. 17) | 7 | 1 | Radical Billroth I and vagotomy (No. 15) | 8 | 1 |
| Radical tubular (No. 18) | 3 | 2 | Radical Billroth I (No. 14) | 6 | 1 |
| Totals | 51 | 29 | | 55 | 17 |
| Per cent ulcer | 57 | | | 31 | |

**Table III.** *Incidence of ulcer when antrum was vagally innervated, vagally denervated, and resected*

| *Group* | *Antrum preserved, vagally innervated* | *No. of dogs* | *No. of ulcers* | *Antrum preserved, vagally denervated* | *No. of dogs* | *No. of ulcers* | *Antrum excised* | *No. of dogs* | *No. of ulcers* |
|---|---|---|---|---|---|---|---|---|---|
| A | Pylorectomy (Procedure No. 1) | 5 | 5 | Vagal denervation of antrum and pylorus (Procedure No. 3) | 4 | 3 | Antrectomy (Procedure No. 4) | 5 | 2 |
| B | Tubular (Procedure No. 12) | 5 | 5 | Segmental (Procedure No. 10) | 5 | 1 | Billroth I (Procedure No. 8) | 5 | 3 |
| C | Radical tubular (Procedure No. 18) | 3 | 2 | Radical segmental (Procedure No. 16) | 7 | 4 | Radical Billroth I (Procedure No. 14) | 6 | 1 |
| | Totals | 13 | 12 | | 16 | 8 | | 16 | 6 |
| | Per cent ulcer | 92 | | | 50 | | | 38 | |

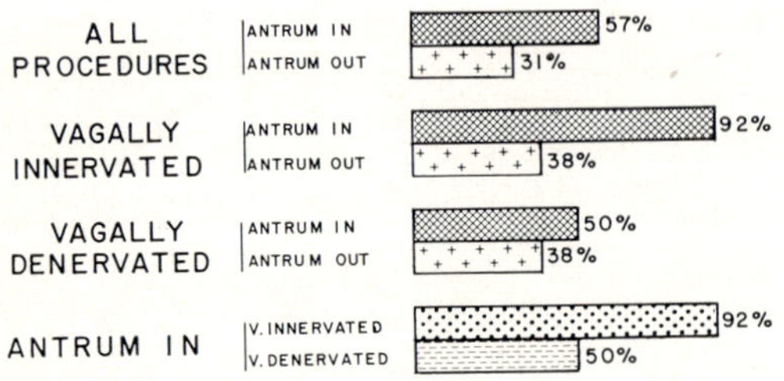


**Fig. 3.** The effect of the antrum on the development of experimental ulcer.

nervated and a further reduction if it is excised. In Fig. 3 these results are expressed as a bar graph.

When one pairs a series of procedures against an identical series with the addition of vagotomy, it is not surprising that the incidence of ulceration is almost halved by the addition of vagotomy (Table IV). There are 2 obvious mechanisms whereby vagotomy could reduce acid secretion and hence the incidence of ulcer. In this study we can evaluate the relative importance of

**Table IV.** *Effect of vagotomy in 2 comparable groups*

| *Procedure* | *No. of dogs* | *No. of ulcers* | *Plus vagotomy* | *No. of dogs* | *No. of ulcers* |
|---|---|---|---|---|---|
| Pylorectomy (No. 1) | 5 | 5 | Pylorectomy and vagotomy (No. 2) | 5 | 4 |
| Antrectomy (No. 4) | 5 | 2 | Antrectomy and vagotomy (No. 5) | 5 | 2 |
| Hemigastrectomy (No. 6) | 5 | 2 | Hemigastrectomy and vagotomy (No. 7) | 5 | 1 |
| Billroth I (No. 8) | 5 | 3 | Billroth I and vagotomy (No. 9) | 5 | 1 |
| Segmental (No. 10) | 5 | 1 | Segmental and vagotomy (No. 11) | 5 | 2 |
| Tubular (No. 12) | 5 | 5 | Tubular and vagotomy (No. 13) | 5 | 2 |
| Radical Billroth I (No. 14) | 6 | 1 | Radical Billroth I and vagotomy (No. 15) | 8 | 1 |
| Radical segmental (No. 16) | 7 | 4 | Radical segmental and vagotomy (No. 17) | 7 | 1 |
| Radical tubular (No. 18) | 3 | 2 | Radical tubular and vagotomy (No. 19) | 7 | 1 |
| Totals | 46 | 25 | | 52 | 15 |
| Per cent ulcer | 54 | | | 29 | |

**Table V.** *Effect of vagotomy on parietal-cell mass (antrum previously denervated)*

| *Antrum vagally denervated, P.C.M.* vagally innervated* | *No. of dogs* | *No. of ulcers* | *Plus denervation of P.C.M.** | *No. of dogs* | *No. of ulcers* |
|---|---|---|---|---|---|
| Vagal denervation of antrum and pylorectomy (No. 3) | 4 | 3 | Pylorectomy and vagotomy (No. 2) | 5 | 4 |
| Segmental (No. 10) | 5 | 1 | Segmental and vagotomy (No. 11) | 5 | 2 |
| Radical segmental (No. 16) | 7 | 4 | Radical segmental and vagotomy (No. 17) | 7 | 1 |
| Totals | 16 | 8 | | 17 | 7 |
| Per cent ulcer | 50 | | | 41 | |

*Parietal-cell mass.

**Table VI.** *Effect of vagotomy on parietal-cell mass (antrum previously excised)*

| *Antrum excised, P.C.M.* innervated* | *No. of dogs* | *No. of ulcers* | *Plus denervation of P.C.M.** | *No. of dogs* | *No. of ulcers* |
|---|---|---|---|---|---|
| Antrectomy (No. 4) | 5 | 2 | Antrectomy and vagotomy (No. 5) | 5 | 2 |
| Hemigastrectomy (No. 6) | 5 | 2 | Hemigastrectomy and vagotomy (No. 7) | 5 | 1 |
| Billroth I (No. 8) | 5 | 3 | Billroth I and vagotomy (No. 9) | 5 | 1 |
| Radical Billroth I (No. 14) | 6 | 1 | Radical Billroth I and vagotomy (No. 15) | 8 | 1 |
| Totals | 21 | 8 | | 23 | 5 |
| Per cent ulcer | 38 | | | 21 | |

*Parietal-cell mass.

denervation of the antrum and denervation of the acid-secreting parietal-cell mass. An analysis of the effect of vagotomy on the acid-secreting mucosa alone can be studied by studying 2 comparable groups, those in which the antrum has been previously denervated by the primary procedure (Table V) and those in which the antrum has been previously excised (Table VI). An analysis of these 2 groups together (Table VII) shows that vagotomy of the parietal-cell mass only reduces the incidence of ulceration slightly, whereas from Table II we have seen that vagotomy of the antrum has a much more marked effect. The effect of vagotomy on the incidence of ulceration is expressed diagrammatically in Fig. 4.

There are 2 series in which the only variable is the percentage of parietal-cell mass excised. They enable us to assess the effect of this factor on the incidence of ulceration (Table VIII). No decrease in ulcer incidence occurs until the extent of excision exceeds 50 per cent, so that if we depend on excision of the acid-secreting mucosa alone for ulcer control, the excision must be extensive. In 5 animals all of the acid-secreting mucosa was excised by the method described by Williams.[11] It is interesting that no ulcers developed. This group is not considered in detail because it does not lend itself to a comparison with those with the other procedures, although it is useful in illustrating the effect of excision of the acid-secreting mucosa (Fig. 5).

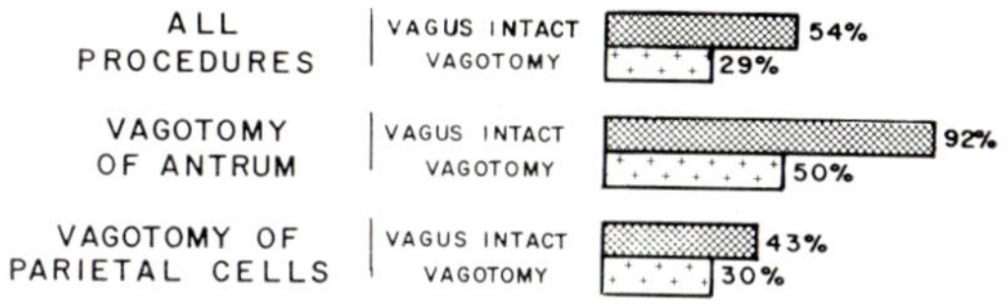


**Fig. 4.** The effect of the vagus nerve on the development of experimental ulcer.

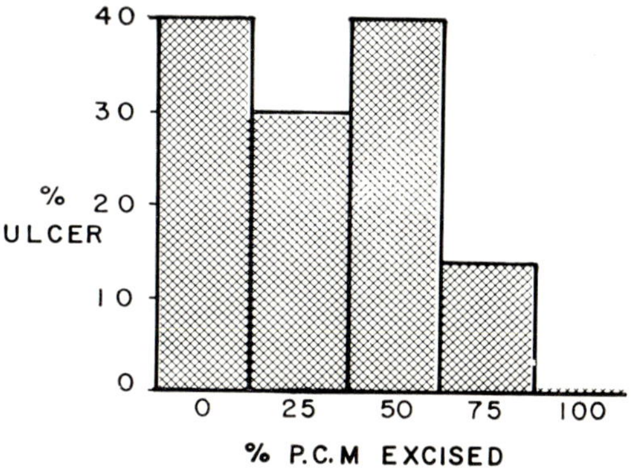


**Fig. 5.** The effect of excision of successive quarters of the parietal-cell mass on the development of experimental ulcer.

**Table VII.** *Effect of vagotomy on parietal-cell mass (combined data)*

| | *Innervated parietal-cell mass* | | *Denervated parietal-cell mass* | |
|---|---|---|---|---|
| | *No. of dogs* | *No. of ulcers* | *No. of dogs* | *No. of ulcers* |
| Totals | 37 | 16 | 40 | 12 |
| Per cent ulcer | 43 | | 30 | |

**Table VIII.** *Effect of parietal-cell excision on subsequent ulcer development*

| Group | No. P.C.M.* excision | No. of dogs | No. of ulcers | 25% P.C.M. excision | No. of dogs | No. of ulcers |
|---|---|---|---|---|---|---|
| A | Antrectomy (No. 4) | 5 | 2 | Hemigastrectomy (No. 6) | 5 | 2 |
| B | Antrectomy and vagotomy (No. 5) | 5 | 2 | Hemigastrectomy and vagotomy (No. 7) | 5 | 1 |
| | Totals | 10 | 4 | | 10 | 3 |
| | Per cent ulcer | 40 | | | 30 | |

*Parietal cell mass.

## COMMENT

Because of our previous work on the autoregulatory role of the antrum these results were surprising. We rather expected that the beneficial autoregulatory role of the antrum exceeded its ulcerogenic capacity, and that its presence in an acid environment would tend to protect against ulceration. We also thought that it would be more effective in this regard if it were vagally innervated. We doubted that vagal stimulation of the antrum and subsequent gastrin production by this mechanism was very significant, for it has been extremely difficult to demonstrate its presence at all by physiologic studies.[10] Nevertheless, these studies on ulcer suggest that the antrum's ulcerogenic effect exceeds its autoregulatory effect, and that this is particularly true if the antrum is vagally innervated. Thus, if the antrum is retained it should be vagally denervated or, better yet, excised. In this paper we are only considering the problem of duodenal ulcer from the point of view of ulcer recurrence, and there are situations such as the difficult duodenum in which preservation of the antrum may be desirable to avoid death. Besides death and ulcer recurrence in duodenal ulcer operations, one must of course consider the important problem of postoperative morbidity.

We were not surprised to find a significant reduction in ulcer incidence by vagotomy, but we were surprised that vagotomy of the antrum is much more significant than vagotomy of the parietal-cell mass.

One might have anticipated a linear reduction in ulceration as increasing amounts of acid-secreting mucosa were excised, but if the results from this small series of animals are valid, such is not the case. They suggest that the addition of a limited excision to antrectomy will not significantly reduce the incidence of ulceration, except that it helps to ensure complete excision of the antrum. It appears that the parietal-cell mass is a target gland being acted upon by several stimuli, and in such a situation elsewhere in the body one does not achieve a significant reduction in effect unless a subtotal resection of the target organ is performed.

From a practical point of view, we, as surgeons, can still elect to approach the problem of ulcer control by vagotomy, excision of the antrum, or excision of the acid-secreting mucosa. What do the presently employed procedures for duodenal ulcer accomplish, and what is the explanation for their effectiveness? If these procedures on dogs truly reflect the situation in clinical duodenal ulcer, our conclusions appear justified.

The Billroth procedures accomplish antrectomy and resection of 25 to 55 per cent of the acid-secreting portion of the stomach. Antrectomy is very effective, but unless the resection takes 75 per cent or more of the whole stomach the excision of the parietal-cell mass is not nearly as effective as the antrectomy. The addition of vagotomy of the residual gastric pouch after resection cannot be expected to accomplish much in reducing the incidence of ulcer. The smaller

| *50% P.C.M. excision* | *No. of Dogs* | *No. of ulcers* | *75% P.C.M. excision* | *No. of dogs* | *No. of ulcers* |
|---|---|---|---|---|---|
| Billroth I (No. 8) | 5 | 3 | Radical Billroth I (No. 14) | 6 | 1 |
| Billroth I and vagotomy (No. 9) | 5 | 1 | Radical Billroth I and vagotomy (No. 15) | 8 | 1 |
| | 10 | 4 | | 14 | 2 |
| | 40 | | | 14 | |

the residual pouch, the less effective it will be. The combination of antrectomy and vagotomy owes most of its effect to the former aspect of the procedure. Segmental resection owes much of its success to vagal denervation of the antrum. Dr. Wangensteen's 70 per cent resection of the acid-secreting mucosa has successfully prevented the development of recurrent ulcer. A contraction of this may prove inadequate. Tubular resection probably failed because the antrum was vagally innervated. Vagotomy with drainage succeeds in the majority of patients because of the effectiveness of vagal denervation of the antrum and, to a lesser extent, because of vagal denervation of the acid-secreting mucosa. In this discussion of choice of surgical procedures for duodenal ulcer, we have considered only the problem of recurrent ulcer. Many other factors enter into the decision, but it is useful to know the relative effectiveness of each surgical maneuver in terms of prevention of ulcer recurrence.

## SUMMARY

In a series of 90 dogs the relative importance of vagotomy, antrectomy, and resection of the acid-secreting body of the stomach in preventing peptic ulceration was investigated. This is a study on an experimental ulcer in a dog, but in the past the correlation between man and the dog has been significant in the field of peptic ulcer.

Although the autoregulatory role of the antrum in acid control is a physiologic fact, its ulcerogenic qualities exceed its beneficial potential. Thus, if it is excised the incidence of peptic ulcer is almost halved. If retained, its ulcerogenic properties are much reduced by vagal denervation.

Vagal denervation of the intact stomach also reduces the incidence of ulceration by almost one-half. When one considers its 2 possible pathways, vagotomy of the acid-secreting mucosa is not nearly as effective as vagal denervation of the antrum.

Resection of the acid-secreting mucosa is of course effective in preventing ulceration, but it must exceed 50 per cent before the incidence of ulcer is significantly reduced.

### REFERENCES

1. Beaver, M. G., and Mann, F. C.: The production of peptic ulcer after section of the gastric nerve, Ann. Surg. **94:** 1116, 1931.
2. Enerson, D. N., Woodward, E. R., Tovee, E. B., Neal, W. B., Sibley, J. A., and Dragstedt, L. R.: Failure of vagotomy to prevent the formation of Mann-Williamson ulcers in dogs, Arch. Surg. **60:** 223, 1950.
3. Harkins, H. N., and Hooker, D. H.: Vagotomy for peptic ulcer; experimental and clinical studies, SURGERY **22:** 239, 1947.
4. Harrison, R. C.: The present status of the gastric antrum—a collective review, Canad. J. Surg. **2:** 295, 1959.
5. McCrea, E. D'A.: The abdominal distribution of the vagus, J. Anat. **59:** 18, 1924.
6. Oliver, J. V.: Effect of vagotomy on development of the Mann-Williamson ulcer in the dog, Arch. Surg. **55:** 180, 1947.
7. Saltzstein, H. C., Sandweiss, D. J., Hammer, J. M., Hill, E. J., and Vandenberg, H. J.: Effect of vagotomy on Mann-Williamson ulcers in dogs, Arch. Surg. **55:** 130, 1947.
8. Silbermann, O. H., Williams, H. T. G.,

Pisesky, W., and Harrison, R. C.: Experimental production of peptic ulceration, a new method, S. Forum **9:** 455, 1959.

9. Storer, E. H., Woodward, E. R., and Dragstedt, L. R.: The effect of vagotomy and antrum resection on the Mann-Williamson ulcer, SURGERY **27:** 526, 1950.
10. Thein, M. P., and Schofield, B.: Release of gastrin from the pyloric antrum following vagal stimulation by sham feeding in dogs, J. Physiol. **148:** 291, 1959.
11. Williams, H. T. G., Pisesky, W., and MacKenzie, W. C.: Total excision of acid secreting gastric mucosa in the dog, S. Forum **9:** 451, 1959.

## DISCUSSION

**Dr. Sam E. Stephenson, Jr.** (Nashville, Tenn.). I want to say how much I enjoyed this presentation of some exhausting work. Anyone working in this area knows the many problems involved. I must say first that we completely agree and over the last 14 years vagotomy and antrectomy has been our procedure of choice for duodenal ulcer. The slide shows untilization of only the ulcer recurrence rate as a method of acceptability. Over the last 14 years we have built up a series of 832 patients. This shows the breakdown of the 804 patients whom we have been able to follow. In this group there have been 5 recurrent ulcers. Of these recurrences, one is a possible incomplete vagotomy. The lady bled massively and because of her shocklike picture, time was not taken to explore the hiatus. A higher resection was performed. Three other patients have a proved incomplete vagotomy. There has been 1 case of a malignant Zollinger-Ellison tumor. This gives an over-all incidence of 0.6 per cent. It is interesting that all of our recurrent ulcers have occurred within the first 24 months after the operation.

**Dr. Lloyd M. Nyhus** (Seattle, Wash.). I, too, agree that we have seen an extremely large group of experiments here today. My only comment is that perhaps each category should be enlarged. For a number of years, we have heard about antral acid inhibition, and therefore we have thought of the antrum in a protective rather than a destructive role. Dr. Harrison and his colleagues have presented studies which seem to incriminate the antrum as a foe. It is important that we understand the basic role of the antrum. The local effect of distention and of secretogogues, which we call the local antral phase, is well known. The most fascinating and most recent area of development has been the release of gastrin by vagal stimulation, called the vagal antral phase. This slide shows the concept of using insulin hypoglycemia to stimulate the vagus nerve and cause a specific release of acid from a Heidenhain pouch. In this experiment, with a denervated pouch, the output of acid relates to the release of gastrin by vagal stimulation. When the vagus nerve has been severed there is marked decrease in the acid output due to vagal stimulation. On the basis of these and other experiments, we have concluded that gastrin release by vagal stimulation represents a significant portion of the total release of gastrin in the spectrum of antral stimulatory mechanisms. Finally, the experience presented here by Dr. Harrison gives additional evidence that the ulcer recurrence rate in patients of less than one-half of 1 per cent reported after approximately 4,000 combined operations, that is, vagotomy plus antrectomy, will remain at this astoundingly low level.

**Dr. R. Cameron Harrison** (closing). I would like to thank Drs. Stephenson and Nyhus for their discussion. With respect to the number of animals, I hope no one will draw any conclusions from the incidence of ulceration noted after each procedure. One cannot draw conclusions from 5 to 8 animals, but the number of animals compared with respect to the vagus, antrum, and parietal-cell mass does provide evidence of the ulcerogenic role.

Earlier this afternoon there was discussion regarding the role of hypersecretion in experimental peptic ulcer. We investigated this in 4 animals using pouch secretion as an index, and were unable to demonstrate any increase in acid secretion after the ileal insert procedure.

It is indeed surprising that the vagal-antral mechanism is so important, as it took physiologists and surgeon-physiologists a very long time to demonstrate that this mechanism even existed.

# The effective period of preventive antibiotic action in experimental incisions and dermal lesions

JOHN F. BURKE, M.D.
BOSTON, MASS.
*From the Department of Surgery, Harvard Medical School, and the Surgical Services, Massachusetts General Hospital*

It has become obvious over the past few years that current antibiotic substances do not control all infections caused by the staphylococcus. Thus, the importance of preventing infection rather than dealing with an already established lesion remains critical. Since antibiotics, under a large variety of circumstances, are known to prevent bacterial growth, it is logical to attempt to use them to prevent such bacterial complications as pneumonia or incisional infections. That they have proved ineffective after a widespread trial in the clinic is clear[1, 2, 5-8, 12-14]; however, the reasons for this failure in terms of the biology of tissue defense remain obscure. Before complete abandonment of the idea of antibiotics as aids in the prevention of bacterial growth in tissue, it would be well to attempt to answer one question—is there any time during the period of development of a primary bacterial lesion during which systemically administered antibiotics are effective in preventing or inhibiting the development of the lesion?

To answer this question it is necessary first to define the period of development of a primary bacterial lesion and, second, to compare the effects of antibiotics at various stages during the development of the experimental lesion. The period of development can be defined as the interval between the arrival of bacterial cells in tissue (primary lodgment) and the creation of a fully developed lesion produced by bacteria and their metabolic products. (Secondary lesions would then include any spread from the original mature focus.) For the experimental primary staphylococcal lesion it has usually been assumed that the period of development covers approximately 24 hours. In this time the lesion reaches maximum size as judged by the perimeters of vision and touch.

In order to determine the time during the development of a primary staphylococcal lesion when antibiotics are effective, as well as the extent of this effectiveness, special experiments were constructed. Lesions and incisions contaminated with staphylococci in a standardized manner[10] were created in the skin of guinea pigs. Antibiotics were given intravenously to separate animals according to graded intervals, some before the introduction of staphylococci and others at stages during the development of the lesions. The lesions or incisions created in the animals treated with antibiotics were compared with the lesions or incisions in control animals not treated, and the effects of the antibiotics were noted. The ability of antibiotics to influence lesions in various stages of development was determined by comparing lesions treated at these various stages with each other and with control lesions not treated. Comparison was made when both test and control lesions were 24 hours old.

## MATERIAL AND METHODS

**Antibiotics.** The antibiotics used were penicillin G potassium, chloramphenicol, erythromycin, and Achromycin. With the

Supported by Grant E-2392 from the National Institutes of Health, United States Public Health Service.

Read at the Twenty-second Annual Meeting of the Society of University Surgeons, Kansas City, Kan., Feb. 9-11, 1961.

exception of chloramphenicol, the antibiotics were made up in an aqueous solution from the powdered form on the day of use. The antibiotics were all given intravenously and, unless indicated otherwise, were given in 1 injection. Penicillin was given in doses ranging between 20,000 and 100,000 U. The usual dose was 20,000 U. Chloramphenicol, erythromycin, and Achromycin were given in doses ranging from 1 to 5 mg. per 100 Gm. The usual dose was 1 mg. per 100 Gm.

**Bacteria.** Strains of *Staphylococcus aureus* were used. Most of the experiments were carried out with strain CN 491 of the Wellcome collection, but the effect of each antibiotic was also determined on lesions created by freshly isolated pathogenic staphylococci. In any experiment the bacteria were sensitive to the antibiotic used as judged by the antibiotic disc method.

**Guinea pigs.** Albino guinea pigs which weighed 250 to 400 grams were used. The skin was prepared by clipping and depilation with Nair.

**Dermal lesions.** Staphylococci from 18-hour nutrient broth cultures were spun down and washed 3 times in isotonic saline solution, after which they were resuspended in a volume of saline solution which equaled the volume of nutrient broth. One-tenth of a milliliter of this suspension was injected intracutaneously into the depilated guinea pig. This method gave circular indurated lesions with a diameter[10] directly related to the dose of viable bacteria. Antibiotic-treated lesions were always compared with nontreated lesions made with the same suspension of bacteria. The skin of the trunk was used in an area posterior to the scapula, anterior to the knee, and dorsal to a line 3 cm. on either side of the ventral midline. The effect of antibiotics 1 hour before and up to 6 hours after the introduction of staphylococci was tested in 4 to 8 animals and usually in duplicate in each animal. The diameters recorded are the means of from 8 to 16 lesions. When injected in this manner, the staphylococcal suspensions caused easily reproducible lesions which consisted of 7 to 10 mm. of induration with a central 2 to 3 mm. of necrosis when measured in 24 hours.

**Experimental incisional infections.** Incisions measuring 2 cm. in length were made with a scalpel. The incisions were made in the same area as that used for dermal lesions. The incisions were carried in depth through the panniculus carnosus and subcutaneous tissue to the deep fascia. These incisions were retracted widely and 0.1 ml. of saline solution or washed and suspended staphylococci, prepared as for the dermal lesion, was used to flood the space provided. Retraction was continued to allow the bacterial suspension to settle in the wound for 3 minutes. The wound was then closed with Michel clips to approximate the skin. Excess bacterial suspension was carefully removed from the skin after closure of the wound. No attempt was made to evacuate the wound before closure.

**Evaluation of antibiotic effect.** Diameters were measured in lesions 24 to 30 hours old and the extent of induration was recorded. In the case of the experimental incisions the diameter of induration was measured when the incisions were between 24 and 30 hours old. In both cases, in addition to the visual measurement, the animals were sacrificed, and the skin containing the lesion

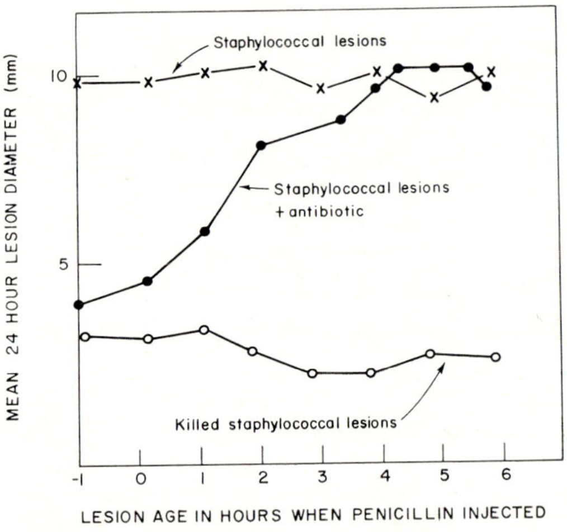


**Fig. 1.** Decreasing effect of penicillin on lesion diameter as lesion age on penicillin injection increases.

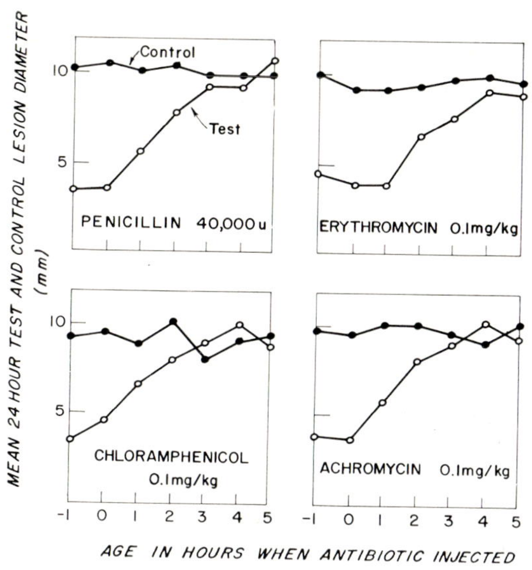


**Fig. 2.** Decreasing effect of 4 antibiotics on lesion size as lesion age on antibiotic injection increases.

or incision was fixed and a histologic section cut transversely across its center. The various antibiotics were given intravenously at hourly intervals from 3 hours before to 6 hours after the injection of staphylococci or the creation of skin incision. Each animal was given a single injection of antibiotics at a time designed to test antibiotic effect on lesions of a certain age. In all experiments the controls were animals in which an exactly similar procedure had been followed, with the exception that antibiotics were not given. In addition, part of the staphylococcal suspension was autoclaved and 0.1 ml. of suspension of killed bacteria was injected in order to determine the lesion size created by bacterial protein.

## EXPERIMENTAL RESULTS

**Dermal lesions.** Compared with control lesions, developing lesions treated with an effective antibacterial substance showed a definite, short period when they were susceptible to antibiotics. This susceptibility was maximum when the antibiotic was in the tissue when the bacteria arrived. Fig. 1 shows the decreasing effect of penicillin (20,000 U.) given intravenously on the further development of staphylococcal lesions as the age of the lesion on injection of penicillin increased from −1 to 6 hours. The antibiotic effect may be judged by the decrease in size of the treated lesion as compared with the control lesion made in animals not given antibiotics. Fig. 1 shows that if penicillin was given 1 hour before staphylococci were injected (−1 hour lesion), the resultant lesion was hardly bigger than that produced by killed bacteria, although the expected lesion would be 10 mm. in diameter. If the antibiotic was given at the same time the bacteria were injected (0 hour lesion), the suppression of the 24 hour lesion was slightly less marked. As the time interval between the injection of bacteria and the administration of penicillin increased, the antibiotic effect decreased. When staphylococci were injected 3 hours before antibiotics were given, the resultant lesion was hardly smaller than the control. Penicillin injected longer than 3 hours after staphylococci had been introduced had no effect on ultimate lesion size. Penicillin in quantities of up to 100,000 U. in single and divided doses has been given to animals with lesions 4 to 16 hours old without any observable effect on the 24 hour lesion size.

The effect of intravenous chloramphenicol, erythromycin, and Achromycin on 24 hour lesion size is plotted in Fig. 2. Again the decreasing susceptibility with increasing lesion age on injection of antibiotics is clearly shown and is the same as that found with penicillin. As with penicillin, massive initial or intermittent therapy with any of the antibiotics produced no observable effect on lesion size after the lesions were more than 3 hours old.

Fig. 3 shows a sequence of photomicrographs of 24 hour dermal infections which illustrate our findings. The control lesion made with 0.1 ml. of sterile saline solution (Fig. 3, *A*) showed almost no changes from normal skin. The lesion made by injection of 0.1 ml. of staphylococcal suspension after the injection of 20,000 U. of penicillin (Fig. 3, *B*) showed slight edema and white-cell infiltration. The lesion made by the injection of 0.1 ml. of the same bacterial suspension, but with penicillin (20,000 U.) not given until the bacteria had been in the tissue 3 hours (Fig. 3, *C*), showed edema, extensive necrosis, and white-cell infiltration with considerable infiltration below the panniculus carnosus.

In these experiments strains of staphylococci sensitive to the antibiotic used were chosen. The effect of antibiotics ineffective against strains of staphylococci in vitro is less predictable. In general, however, antibiotics ineffective in vitro are ineffective in vivo.

**Experimental incisions.** The irregularity in the area of induration and necrosis of experimental incisions was considerably greater than in standard lesions. This made the plotting of induration diameter impractical. There was no measurable induration in incisions not contaminated with staphylococci. The incisions contaminated with staphylococci in animals not given antibiotics contained irregulas areas of induration 11 to 21 mm. wide when measured at right angles to the center of the incision in 24 hours. Necrosis was usually restricted to the wound edge, but was also occasionally seen in 2 to 3 mm. patches in the area of induration well away from the skin edge. The indurated areas had a purple-red discoloration and showed considerable edema.

The titration of the susceptibility of contaminated incisions to systemic antibiotics was run as for the dermal lesions. Incisions were made and contaminated –1 to 5 hours before the intravenous injection of antibiotic.

Incisions made and contaminated 3 hours before the intravenous injection of penicillin, chloramphenicol, erythromycin, or Achromycin in the doses used in treating the dermal lesions resulted in lesions indistinguishable from the control contaminated incisions not treated with antibiotics. The incisions made and contaminated 1 to 2 hours before injection of antibiotics also resulted in lesions which fell in the range of the control contaminated incisions. If, however, the antibiotics were given before the incisions were made, their gross appearance at 24 hours could not be distinguished from the control incisions not contaminated by staphylococci.

Fig. 4 shows a sequence of photomicrographs of 24 hour incisions which illustrate our findings. All incisions were contaminated with the same staphylococcal suspension. The control incision contaminated with saline solution (Fig. 4, *A*) showed very little reaction and almost no white-cell infiltration. In the control incision with staphylococcal contamination, when the animal did not receive penicillin at any time (Fig. 4, *B*), there was great thickening and edema of all layers involved. The inflammatory reaction extended down to and included the abdominal wall muscles and the entire center of the lesion was necrotic. Extensive polymorphonuclear infiltration and multiple areas of necrosis in the dermis and panniculus carnosus were seen. The incision made and contaminated 15 minutes after the intravenous injection of 20,000 U. of penicillin (Fig. 4, *C*) showed a small number of polymorphonuclear cells localized to the area of incision with a small collection of polymorphonuclear cells deep in the dermis. The lesion was not thickened or edematous and the tissue deep to the panniculus carnosus was normal. The incision made and contaminated 3 hours before penicillin was given (Fig. 4, *D*) was remarkably similar to the lesion which developed in the animal in which penicillin was never given (Fig. 4, *B*).

As in the case of dermal lesions, the bacteria in the contaminated incision were maximally susceptible to antibiotics when the antibiotics were in the tissue before the bacteria were introduced. The period of susceptibility appears shorter and more difficult to measure because of the irregularity of the mature lesions, but the major antibiotic effect is over in approximately 1 hour.

## COMMENT

Although the physical events necessary to produce a visual and palpable mature primary lesion require 24 hours, there is evidence[9-11] that the biochemical interac-

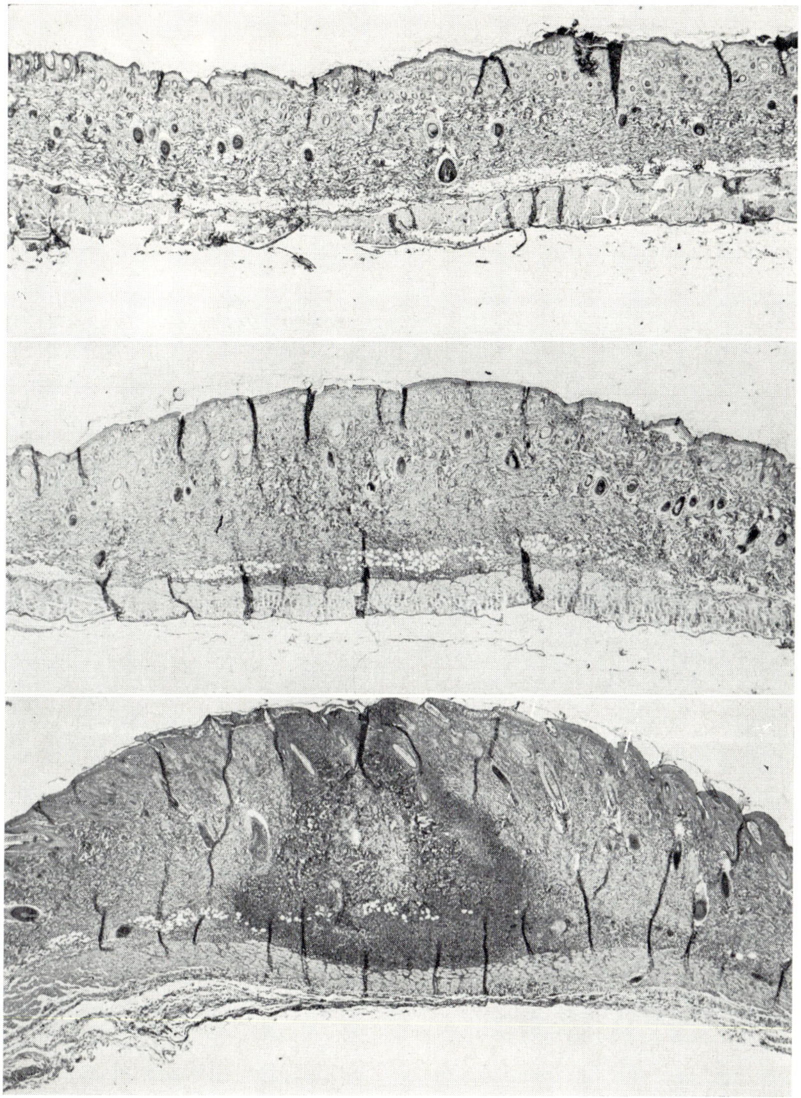

A

B

C

**Fig. 3.** Histologic specimens of control and staphylococcal lesions which show decreasing effect of penicillin as lesion age increases. *A,* Control lesion made with 0.1 ml. saline solution. *B,* Penicillin (20,000 U.) followed by 0.1 ml. live staphylococcal suspension. *C,* Live staphylococcal suspension, 0.1 ml., followed in 3 hours by 40,000 U. penicillin. (×39; reduced 1/3.)

tions between tissue and bacteria which control the size of this lesion take place in a much shorter time. These decisive steps, however, appear to have little direct effect on the internal structure of the area involved. The extensive physical rearrangements, such as induration and necrosis, classically looked upon as the direct action of bacteria on tissue appear (when the total period of primary lesion development is examined) to be only a slowly evolving, indirect result of bacterial action.

If this is true, a developing primary bacterial lesion could be modified during the early short period of decisive biochemical action, but not during the period of slowly evolving induration and necrosis. There is considerable evidence to support this view. Miles and associates[10, 11] have shown that if an animal is deprived of certain portions

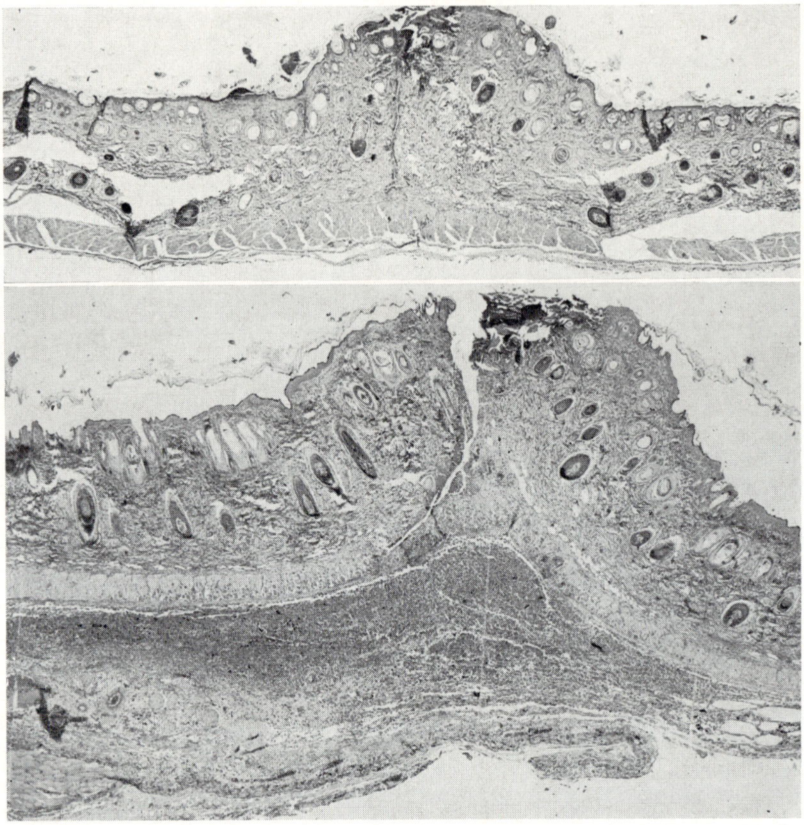

**Fig. 4.** Histologic appearance of control and contaminated incisions. Decreasing effect of penicillin is seen as age of contamination increases. *A,* Control incision contaminated with saline solution. *B,* Experimental incision contaminated with 0.1 ml. staphylococcal suspension. No penicillin was given. *C,* Peni-

of his defenses against bacteria during the first few hours after bacterial invasion, there will be enhancement of the bacterial lesion over that predicted. Equally important, these experiments show that the elimination of the defense mechanisms after this "decisive period" produces no effect on the 24 hour lesion size. Also, vascular events, such as changes in capillary permeability and endothelial stickiness, are restricted to these initial few hours.[3] This evidence is all consistent with the theory that the decisive steps which determine the size of the mature primary bacterial lesion take place very shortly after the bacteria reach the tissue.

In our experiments the effective period of antibiotic action was also restricted to the initial few hours after the arrival of bacteria in tissue. The period of development during which the lesions were found susceptible to antibiotics coincided with that found by Miles and colleagues.[10] Of particular interest is the fact that the period of susceptibility is short and the time of maximum antibiotic effect is soon after the time the bacteria arrive in the tissues. Under these circumstances there does not appear to be a "golden period"[4] when tissue is "infection free" after contamination.

This effective period of preventive antibiotic action is short and the exact time of primary lodgment for the nonpostoperative infection so obscure that the use of antibiotics to prevent primary lesions appears impossible. However, incisions containing bacteria are usually seeded when the wound is open during operation. Thus, the time of primary lodgment is easily predicted. The

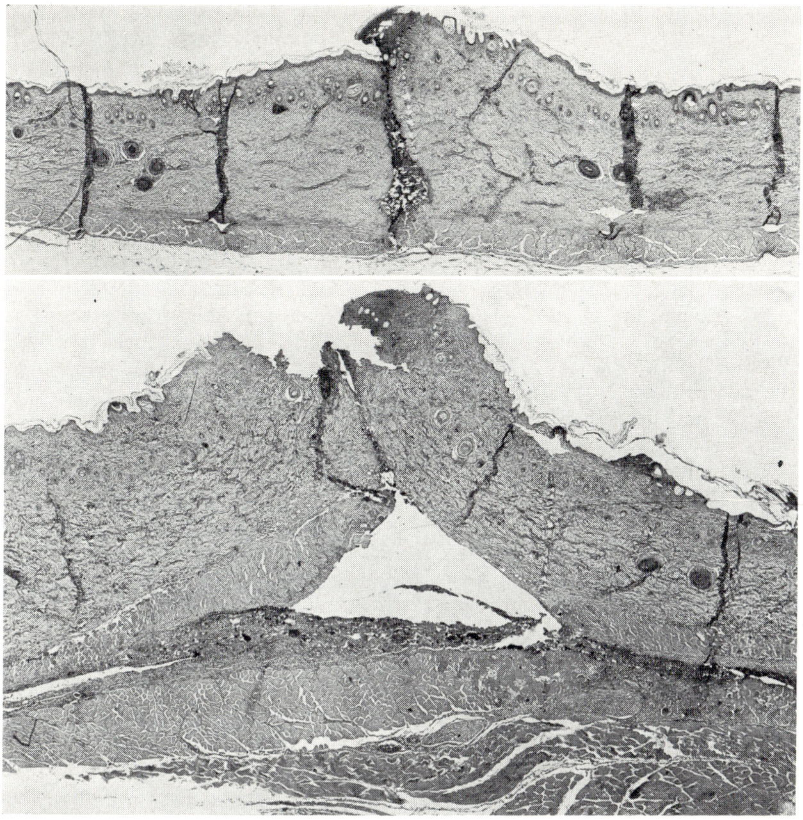

*C*

*D*

cillin (20,000 U.) followed by incision contaminated with 0.1 ml. staphylococcal suspension. *D,* Incision contaminated with 0.1 ml. staphylococcal suspension, followed in 3 hours by 20,000 U. of penicillin. (×39; reduced ⅓.)

fact that the time of the earliest opportunity for incisional contamination can be exactly determined arouses speculation about the absolute failure of the so-called "prophylactic antibiotics." Frequently "prophylactic antibiotics" are started after operation.[14] In these cases the first antibiotic given is at a time at which experimental evidence concerning staphylococcal infection shows clearly that the antibiotic has no effect. This is not to say that antibiotics given before incisions are made will reduce the rate of incisional infections, for the problem is infinitely more complex than the experimental system outlined. Host resistance, foreign material, hematoma, tissue trauma, and so forth, are surely factors in postoperative incisional suppuration. However, if a situation arises in which it appears necessary to give an antibiotic as an aid in preventing bacteria from creating a primary lesion, the evidence indicates it should be given early, so that it is in the tissue when the bacteria arrive.

## SUMMARY

There is a definite short period when the developing staphylococcal dermal or incisional infection may be suppressed by antibiotics. This effective period begins the moment bacteria gain access to the tissue and is over in 3 hours. Systemic antibiotics have no effect on primary staphylococcal infections if the bacteria creating the infection have been in the tissue longer than 3 hours before the antibiotics are given. Antibiotics cause maximum suppression of infection if given before bacteria gain access to tissue.

The author wishes to thank Robert H. Witt for valued technical assistance.

## REFERENCES

1. Altemeier, W. A., Culbertson, W. R., and Vetto, M.: Prophylactic antibiotic therapy, A. M. A. Arch. Surg. **71:** 2, 1955.
2. Appleton, D. M., and Waisbren, B. A.: The prophylactic use of chloramphenicol in transurethral resections of the prostate gland, J. Urol. **75:** 304, 1956.
3. Burke, J. F., and Miles, A. A.: The sequence of vascular events in early infective inflammation, J. Path. & Bact. **76:** 1, 1958.
4. Cole, W. H., and Elman, R.: Textbook of general surgery, New York, 1948, Appleton-Century-Crofts, Inc., ed. 5, p. 1090.
5. Garrod, L. P.: Present position of the chemotherapy of bacterial infections, Brit. M. J. **2:** 756, 1955.
6. Howe, C. W.: Prophylactic antibiotic therapy with special reference to gynecologic surgery. *In* Meigs, J. V., and Sturgis, S. H., editors: Progress in gynecology, New York, 1957, Grune & Stratton, vol. 3, p. 735.
7. Linder, F.: Chirurgische staphylokokkeninfekte und antibiotica, Arch. f. klin. Chir. **287:** 74, 1957.
8. McKittrick, L. S., and Wheelock, F. C., Jr.: The routine use of antibiotics in elective abdominal surgery, Surg. Gynec. & Obst. **99:** 376, 1954.
9. Miles, A. A.: Nonspecific defense reactions in bacterial infections, Ann. New York Acad. Sc. **66:** 356, 1956.
10. Miles, A. A., Miles, Ellen M., and Burke, J.: The value and duration of defence reactions of the skin to the primary lodgement of bacteria, Brit. J. Exper. Path. **38:** 79, 1957.
11. Miles, A. A., and Niven, Janet S. F.: The enhancement of infection during shock produced by bacterial toxins and other agents, Brit. J. Exper. Path. **31:** 73, 1950.
12. Pulaski, E. J.: Discriminate antibiotic prophylaxis in elective surgery, Surg. Gynec. & Obst. **108:** 385, 1959.
13. Sanchez-Ubeda, R., Fernand, E., and Rousselot, L. M.: Complication rate in general surgical cases. The value of penicillin and streptomycin as postoperative prophylaxis—a study of 511 cases, New England J. Med. **259:** 1045, 1958.
14. Tachdjian, M. O., and Compere, E. L.: Postoperative wound infection in orthopedic surgery. Evaluation of prophylactic antibiotics, J. Internat. Coll. Surgeons **28:** 797, 1957.

*(For discussion, see page 184.)*

# Studies of surgically induced pyelonephritis

JOHN H. DAVIS, M.D.
JAMES A. COIL, B.A.
CLEVELAND, OHIO
*From the Department of Surgery, Western Reserve University, and the University Hospitals of Cleveland*

Pyelonephritis continues to hold the interest of the investigator and the clinician. It represents one of the most common infectious diseases, second only to respiratory tract infection. It is found in 10 to 30 per cent of patients who come to autopsy, is frequently asymptomatic during life, is relatively easy to diagnose with quantitative bacteriologic studies, and is frequently preventable or curable in the acute stage with the appropriate antibiotic, yet many of the aspects of pathogenesis are unexplained.

Most commonly, the disease is caused by the gram-negative bacteria, especially *E. coli,* but the "era of antibiotics" has seen an increase in *A. aerogenes, P. vulgaris,* and *Ps. aeruginosa* as the causative organism.

The mechanism whereby the bacteria gain entrance to the kidney is the subject of speculation. One possible source is organisms in the bloodstream secondary to infection elsewhere in the body. Another possibility is that bacteria ascend from an infected lower urinary tract, either by way of the ureter or the periureteral lymphatics. Direct extension from the neighboring colon is also possible. Finally, the infectious process may involve more than one of these routes in some cases.

Many experimental methods of producing pyelonephritis have been devised, but most of them involve some insult to the renal parenchyma. Partial or complete ligation of a ureter with its attendant hydronephrosis permits the development of pyelonephritis after the intravenous injection of bacteria.[3, 8, 14] Direct injection of bacteria into the renal parenchyma[6] or massage of the parenchyma followed by the intravenous administration of bacteria[2] will produce pyelonephritis. Finally, the intravenous administration of bacteria in large concentration will produce the disease with some degree of reproducibility in certain animals.[5, 7]

The development of a simple, reproducible method of producing this disease in the rat was published by Vivaldi[13] in 1959. The studies presented here are based on a modification of this method.

## METHOD

Male Sprague-Dawley rats which weighed 200 to 250 grams were used throughout these studies unless otherwise indicated.

The bacterial infection was created by the introduction of bacteria into the urinary bladder with sterile technique. The animals were shaved over the abdomen and cleansed with Amphyl. A low midline incision was then made and the bladder permitted to fill the wound. With the bladder held with sterile forceps, a 26 gauge sterile needle was inserted into the bladder and an aliquot of urine withdrawn for culture. Through the same needle, the bacteria were introduced in appropriate concentration in a volume that did not exceed 0.2 ml. A sterile sponge was then held over the bladder for a moment to prevent leakage, after which the

Supported in part by a grant from The Diabetes Fund of Greater Cleveland.

Read at the Twenty-second Annual Meeting of the Society of University Surgeons, Kansas City, Kan., Feb. 9-11, 1961.

**Table I.** *Results of variation of the dose of bacteria instilled into the rat bladder*

| *No. of bacteria injected* | *No. of rats* | *No. of kidneys infected* | *% infected* | *Positive urine culture (%)* | *Time of sacrifice (days)* |
|---|---|---|---|---|---|
| $1 \times 10^8$ | 63 | 112/126 | 87 | 93 | 5 |
| Male, surgically induced | 42 | 77/84 | 91 | — | — |
| Female, catheter induced | 21 | 35/42 | 83 | — | — |
| $1 \times 10^5$ | 21 | 22/42 | 52 | 76 | 5 |
| $1 \times 10^3$ | 23 | 12/46 | 26 | 38 | 5 |

bladder was returned to the abdomen and the incision closed with silk sutures. The animals were returned to their cages and permitted food* and water ad libitum.

The animals were sacrificed at the appropriate time and an autopsy performed with sterile technique. The incision was made from xiphoid to pubis and the bladder grasped with a sterile forceps. An aliquot of urine was taken for plating. The kidney pedicles were clamped and each kidney removed, weighed, and sectioned in the midline with aseptic technique used throughout. One-half of the kidney was placed in formalin for histologic study and the remaining half was ground in a sterile mortar in nutrient broth. The appropriate dilutions were made and plated for bacterial colony counting.

A strain of *P. vulgaris,* grown from a human infection and maintained in our laboratory stock cultures, was used in all of the studies. All cultures were 18 hour cultures grown in nutrient broth. The bacterial concentration was estimated in a Coleman Jr. spectrophotometer at 660 $\mu$ prior to injection and the number of viable bacteria actually injected was determined by the back plating technique.

The technique of diverting the ureteral flow on one side was accomplished at the time of bacterial injection. While the abdomen was open, the left ureter was dissected free of surrounding structures and divided with a sharp knife. The posterior peritoneum was incised and a small pouch developed. The proximal end of the ureter was inserted into this pouch and the distal end was ligated. This provided an adequate "bladder" for the duration of the experiments.

*Purina laboratory chow.

## RESULTS

In Table I the results of variation of the dose of bacteria injected into the bladder are presented. The resulting infection is a linear function of the dosage. When the bacteria were given by catheter in the female rat, rather than into the open bladder, the results were not quite as consistent.

The results of keeping the injected dose of bacteria constant ($1 \times 10^8$) but varying the time of sacrifice are seen in Table II. Ninety per cent of the kidneys were infected at 24 hours after the injection and this level was maintained for at least 6 weeks. Some animals began to die from the infection within 5 days of the onset, but the mortality rate was relatively low, about 5 per cent. The mortality rate rose with time, however, and in the 4 to 6 week groups the rate may

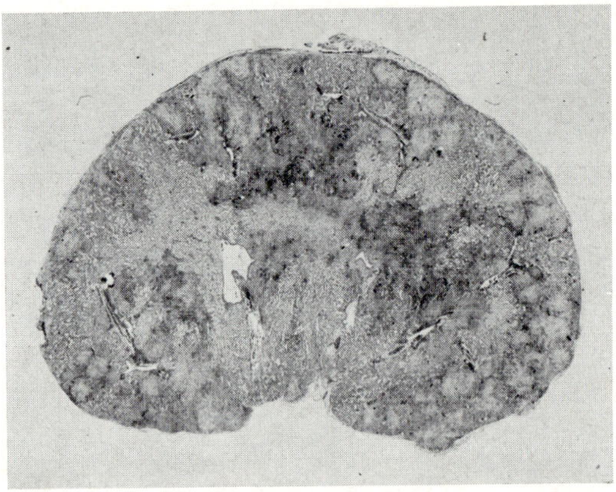

**Fig. 1.** Coronal section of a kidney 5 days after bladder was inoculated with $1 \times 10^8$ *P. vulgaris.* Note the numerous abscesses with marked alteration of architecture. (×7; reduced ⅕.)

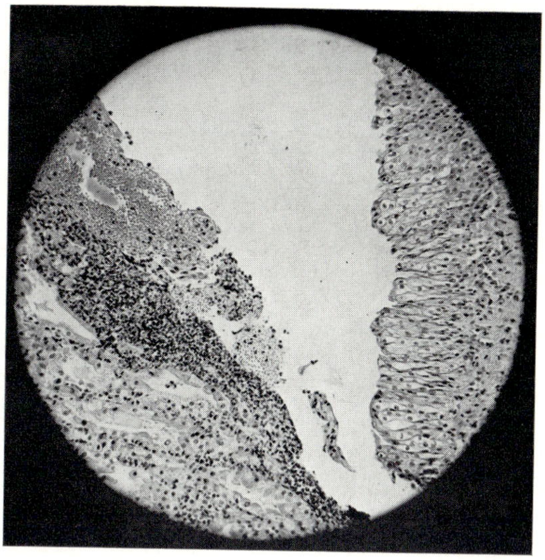

**Fig. 2.** Photomicrograph of renal pelvis. Note normal pelvic mucosa on right and mucosal ulceration on left with extensive inflammatory exudate. The earliest histologic changes appear to be in the pelvis. (×75; reduced 5/11.)

be as high as 50 per cent. The figures given indicate only animals that survived to be sacrificed.

When the bladder was opened at the end of 5 days, many fine granules were seen in the bladder and were typical of the "sand" seen in the human bladder. In animals which survived longer than 2 weeks, frank bladder calculi were very common. These stones were easily palpated through the abdominal wall and account for some of the deaths on the basis of urinary tract obstruction. The calculi removed from the bladder of one of the rats weighed 0.7 Gm.

Chemical analysis of the stones shows them to be calcium-phosphate complexes intermixed with bacteria. The bacterial concentration within the stone proved to be in the range of $10^8$ bacteria.

The pathologic changes in the kidney are demonstrated in Figs. 1 through 4. The lesion appeared to be typical of an ascending type of pyelonephritis. The lesion in the kidney was frequently wedge-shaped, beginning in the renal pelvis and extending out toward the cortex. Cortical abscesses were frequent, but there was always medullary disease associated with it. Occasionally there was pus in the pelvis and tubules without evidence of cortical disease. It must be stated that serial sections throughout the entire kidney were not made so that cortical infection may have been present. In general, cortical infection was easily predicted from the gross specimen because of the presence of numerous abscesses on the surface of the kidney.

The high incidence of infection plus the pathologic picture of an ascending type of pyelonephritis suggested additional experiments to test this hypothesis. A group of 18 rats was infected in the usual manner, except that at the time of infection the left ureter was isolated and divided in approximately the midportion. The distal end was ligated. The upper end was buried in a retroperitoneal pouch which served as a substitute bladder for the duration of the experiment. The problem was to divide the ascending pathway without permitting hydronephrosis to develop. Previous studies in this laboratory, in which partial ureteral ligation was carried out in the rabbit followed by the intravenous injection of bacteria, produced infection only in animals

**Table II.** *Results of kidney infection at varying times after bladder inoculation*

| *No. of rats* | *Time period* | *Positive urine culture* | *No. of kidneys infected* | *Remarks* |
|---|---|---|---|---|
| 10 | 24 hr. | 10/10 | 18/20 | None |
| 6 | 3 days | 4/6 | 10/12 | None |
| 63 | 5 days | 59/63 | 112/126 | Sand in bladder |
| 5 | 9 days | 4/5 | 8/10 | Sand in bladder |
| 2 | 12 days | 2/2 | 3/4 | Sand in bladder |
| 11 | 2 wk. | 10/11 | 17/22 | Sand in bladder |
| 5 | 4 wk. | 5/5 | 10/10 | 0.7 Gm. stones in 1 bladder |
| 7 | 6 wk. | 7/7 | 13/14 | Stones (multiple), scarred kidneys, hypertension |

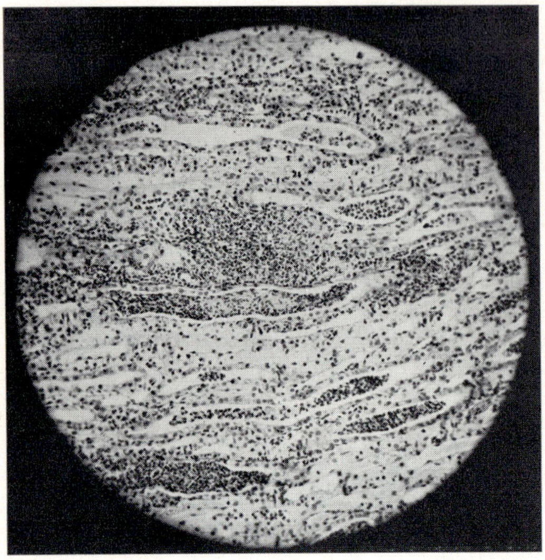

**Fig. 3.** Microscopic section of the renal medulla. Note the many pus-filled tubules as well as the inflammatory exudate in the interstitial space surrounding the tubules. (×150; reduced 5/11.)

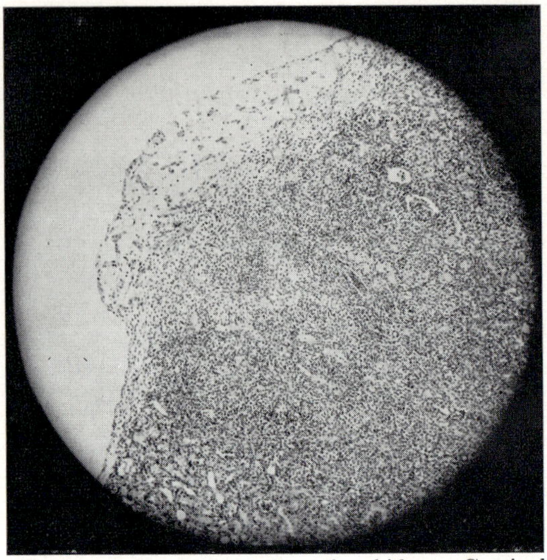

**Fig. 4.** Microscopic section of a kidney. Cortical abscess protrudes above the surface of the kidney. There is almost complete destruction of normal architecture in the area. Animal was sacrificed at 5 days. (×150; reduced 5/11.)

that had developed hydronephrosis. We also tried ureterosigmoidostomy and ureterocutaneous anastomosis in the rat, but technical difficulties prevented satisfactory results. The retroperitoneal pouch worked very well, however, and hydronephrosis was not a problem. The animal would undoubtedly have complications from this pouch if it were followed for a longer period of time. This group of 18 animals was sacrificed on the fifth day and the right kidney was infected in 14 of the 18 animals, but the left kidney was infected in 2 of the 18 animals. In no instance was the left kidney infected while the right was not.

The effects of 3 different antibiotics were tested to determine the role of prophylactic therapy after instrumentation. The antibiotics used were streptomycin, chloramphenicol, and Gantrisin. The strain of Proteus used in these studies was sensitive to all 3 agents.

Four groups were studied with the first 2 antibiotics; (1) drug started 24 hours before the infecting challenge was given, (2) drug started at the same time as the challenge, (3) drug started 24 hours after the challenge, and (4) drug started 72 hours after the challenge. The results are summarized in Table III. Since it appeared to be important to start the antibiotic within 24 hours of the time of challenge, the studies with Gantrisin did not include the time variable. The Gantrisin studies were used to study different dosage levels of the antimicrobial agent.

We have been studying the role of the adrenal steroids in experimental infection and 4 additional groups of animals were used to evaluate hydrocortisone in this preparation. The 4 groups had the drug administered at the same time intervals as the animals treated with streptomycin and chloramphenicol. There appeared to be no effect from the administration of adrenal steroids, at least in the dose used in this experiment.

In several groups of animals peripheral organ (lung, liver, and spleen) studies were made to determine the presence of viable bacteria. Viable bacteria at levels of $10^2$ to $10^4$ organisms per gram of tissue were found in 30 to 50 per cent of the animals. Since the bacterial challenge was given into the bladder, we must assume that these organisms entered the blood stream from the bladder or the subsequently infected kidney.

An additional group of 25 animals was challenged by the same number of bacteria ($10^8$) injected into a tail vein rather than the bladder. Peripheral organ counts were carried out at 5 days in the same manner as when the bacteria were injected into the bladder. The results were similar in that viable bacteria were found in 30 to 50 per cent of the organs tested. Thus, it seems that once the bacteria gain access to the blood stream they are retained in the reticuloendothelial system in viable form.

A final group of 3 rats was challenged with *P. vulgaris* via the bladder and sacrificed at 4 hours. The results were most interesting in that 1 of the animals already had $10^4$ bacteria in the kidney. The entrance of bacteria into the kidney may be assumed to occur within a very short period of time after the challenge.

## COMMENT

The rate of kidney infection after the introduction of *P. vulgaris* into the urinary bladder by surgical means is a linear function of the administered dose. Infection, as judged by the presence of large numbers of viable bacteria in the kidney, starts about 4 hours after injection and reaches a level of 90 per cent by the twenty-fourth hour. The development of the histologic lesion in the kidney requires more time and it has been shown that the classic picture of acute pyelonephritis requires approximately 5 days.

The method whereby the bacteria reach the kidney is not proved beyond doubt, but there is good reason to believe that the infection is of an ascending type. First of all, the pathologic picture is that of an ascending lesion with the initial stage being a pyelitis. The infection subsequently spreads up the tubules and eventually involves the cortex. This sequence of events fits the pathologic description of ascending pyelonephritis. Second, the results of early culture of the ureters and kidneys show that bacteria have reached the kidney within 4 hours of the time they were injected. This finding does not eliminate the possibility of hematogenous spread, but it makes it unlikely. Third, the difference in results obtained when the ureter was interrupted on the left side makes ascending infection the most likely possibility. It would have been more satisfactory if there had been no infection in the left kidney in any of the animals, but this was not the case. There are several possible explanations for this result. Perhaps the most likely would be a technical failure in transplantation of the ureter. This is a small structure in the rat and could easily be missed. Against this is the finding at the time of autopsy of a pouch filled with fluid which appeared to be urine.

**Table III.** *Antibiotic treatment*

| *Group* | *Time drug started* | *No. of rats* | *Abscesses* | *Positive urine culture* | *No. of kidneys infected* |
|---|---|---|---|---|---|
| *Streptomycin, 0.5 mg./day S.C.* | | | | | |
| I | 24 hr. preoperatively | 5 | 0 | 1/5 | 1/10 |
| II | At operation | 4 | 0 | 0/5 | 0/8 |
| III | 24 hr. postoperatively | 5 | 1 | 3/5 | 2/10 |
| IV | 72 hr. postoperatively | 4 | 3 | 3/3* | 6/8 |
| *Chloramphenicol, 5 mg./day I.M.* | | | | | |
| I | 24 hr. preoperatively | 5 | 0 | 3/4* | 4/10 |
| II | At operation | 5 | 0 | 4/4* | 3/10 |
| III | 24 hr. postoperatively | 5 | 0 | 4/5 | 3/10 |
| IV | 72 hr. postoperatively | 4 | 1 | 4/4 | 7/8 |
| *Gantrisin, 1%, in food* | | | | | |
| I | At operation | 10 | 0 | 6/10 | 12/20 |
| *Gantrisin, 2%, in food* | | | | | |
| II | At operation | 6 | 0 | 0 | 0/12 |

*Urine sample lost.
Urine pH was checked on all animals and it remained acid throughout the experiment.

It has been suggested that ascending urinary tract infection occurs through the periureteral lymphatics rather than through the lumen of the ureter.[11] If this is the case, it is possible that with our surgical technique not all of the lymphatics were divided at the time the ureter was divided and thus permitted the ascension of bacteria. We cannot completely eliminate this possibility.

The most likely explanation for 11 per cent involvement of the sectioned side is hematogenous spread of bacteria. I believe we can postulate that after the introduction of bacteria into the bladder an ascending infection occurs, either through the lumen of the ureter or through the periureteral lymphatics to the kidney. Once the bacteria have become established in the kidney they gain access to the blood stream either through the renal vein or into the cisterna chyli via the lymphatic channels. Rattner[12] has demonstrated the passage of bacteria, probably through pyelotubular or pyelointerstitial lymphatics, from the kidney to the lymphatic system. Magoun[10] inoculated the renal pelvis with bacteria and recovered the organism from the vena cava and spleen in 1 animal. In our own studies we have frequently cultured the lungs, liver, and spleen at the time of sacrifice and have found viable organisms in 30 to 50 per cent of the animals. The organisms were plated quantitatively and ranged from $10^2$ to $10^5$ organisms per gram of tissue. These studies demonstrate that the organism being used enters the blood stream at some time during the natural history of the disease. That the bacteremia does not occur from the bladder is suggested by the experiments in which we sectioned the ureter. If the entrance of the bacteria into the kidney were initially hematogenous, both kidneys ought to be involved to a similar degree. Since this was not true in our experiments or in the experiments of Vivaldi,[13] we believe the hypothesis that ascension occurs on the intact side with subsequent bacteremia and secondary involvement of the sectioned side. This hypothesis would only be pertinent in cases in which lower urinary tract infection was the primary disease.

The possibility that pyelonephritis may be a much more frequent sequela of lower urinary tract infection than is generally supposed has been studied by Kass[9] and by Beeson.[1] There is not much argument that acute pyelonephritis may develop from a chronic bladder infection, especially in patients with an indwelling catheter. There has been more controversy over the possibility that pyelonephritis may follow the introduction of a single inoculum of bacteria, such as occurs with instrumentation of the lower urinary tract. Since we can caution against needless catheterization and overzealous instrumentation of the lower urinary tract, but cannot eliminate the need for it in many situations, prevention of infection becomes a problem. As was seen in Table III, complete protection against the development of experimental pyelonephritis was possible when the appropriate antimicrobial drug was administered within 24 hours of the introduction of the bacteria.

The results of a clinical trial of a long-acting sulfonamide in 448 pregnant women who underwent the trauma of childbirth and its attendant catheterization would support this idea. There was a significant reduction in the number of patients who developed bacteriuria after catheterization in the treated group as compared to the control group.[4] Kass[9] was able to completely prevent the pyelonephritis of pregnancy by the prophylactic administration of the appropriate antibiotic during the pregnancy. These studies strongly suggest that this is an area in which prophylactic chemotherapy is not only desirable but mandatory if we are to prevent some of the serious complications that occur.

## SUMMARY AND CONCLUSIONS

1. Surgically induced pyelonephritis is easily produced in the rat by the injection of *P. vulgaris* into the exposed urinary bladder. This results in bilateral pyelonephritis in over 90 per cent of the animals and, if undisturbed, will proceed to chronic

infection with stone formation, abscessed kidneys, and possibly hypertension.

2. This pyelonephritis appears to be an ascending infection secondary to inflammation of the bladder.

3. The bacteria reach the kidney very soon after the bladder inoculation. Preliminary studies show viable bacteria in the kidney within 4 hours of inoculation.

4. The hypothesis is presented that once the kidney becomes infected the bacteria gain entrance to the blood stream and can infect the opposite kidney in which the ureter has been divided to prevent ascension of the bacteria.

5. The experimental infection can be prevented by the administration of the appropriate antimicrobial drug within 24 hours of the time the bladder is inoculated.

6. The suggestion is made that this technique may simulate the events after instrumentation of the lower urinary tract in human beings. If these data are confirmed, the use of prophylactic antibiotics at the time of such instrumentation may be an important factor in decreasing the incidence of postoperative pyelonephritis.

## REFERENCES

1. Beeson, P. B.: Factors in the pathogenesis of pyelonephritis, Yale J. Biol. & Med. **28:** 81, 1955.
2. Braude, A. E., Shapiro, A. P., and Siemienski, J.: Hematogenous pyelonephritis in rats. I. Its pathogenesis when produced by a simple new method, J. Clin. Invest. **34:** 1489, 1955.
3. Davis, J. H.: Unpublished data.
4. Davis, J. H., Rosenblum, J. M., Quilligan, E. J., and Persky, L.: An evaluation of post-catheterization prophylactic chemotherapy, J. Urol. **82:** 613, 1959.
5. DeNavasquez, S.: Experimental pyelonephritis in the rabbit produced by staphylococcal infection, J. Path. & Bact. **62:** 429, 1950.
6. Freedman, L. R., and Beeson, P. B.: Experimental pyelonephritis. IV. Observations on infections resulting from direct inoculation of bacteria in different zones of the kidney, Yale J. Biol. & Med. **30:** 406, 1958.
7. Gorill, R. H.: The establishment of staphylococcal abscesses in the mouse kidney, Brit. J. Exper. Path. **39:** 203, 1958.
8. Guze, L. B., and Beeson, P. B.: Experimental pyelonephritis. I. Effect of ureteral ligation on the course of bacterial infection in the kidney of the rat, J. Exper. Med. **104:** 803, 1956.
9. Kass, E. H.: Bacteriuria and pyelonephritis of pregnancy, A. M. A. Arch. Int. Med. **105:** 194, 1960.
10. Magoun, J. A. H.: Absorption from the urinary tract, J. Urol. **10:** 67, 1923.
11. Murphy, J. J., Shoenberg, H. W., Rattner, W. H., and Scott, R.: The role of the lymphatic system in pyelonephritis, S. Forum **10:** 880, 1960.
12. Rattner, W. H., Myint, M. D., and Murphy, J. J.: The route of transfer of bacteria from the renal pelvis to the circulating blood, Surgery **43:** 298, 1958.
13. Vivaldi, E., et al.: Ascending infection as a mechanism in the pathogenesis of experimental non-obstructive pyelonephritis, Proc. Soc. Exper. Biol. & Med. **102:** 242, 1959.
14. Weyrach, H. M., Rosenberg, M. L., Amar, A. D., and Redor, M.: Effects of antibiotics and vaccination on experimental pyelonephritis, J. Urol. **78:** 532, 1957.

*(For discussion, see page 184.)*

# Management of pulmonary complications of surgical operations (primarily atelectasis) with pancreatic dornase inhalations

EUGENE E. CLIFFTON, M.D.
CARLO E. GROSSI, M.D.
ERNEST R. ESAKOF, M.D.
NEW YORK, N. Y.
*From the Division of Experimental Surgery and Thoracic Surgery, Memorial Hospital for Cancer and Allied Diseases, Sloan-Kettering Cancer Center, and Cornell University Medical College*

Atelectasis and bronchopneumonia are still common and serious postoperative complications. Patients with chronic bronchopulmonary disease, pulmonary fibrosis, and emphysema, heavy smokers, and obese short-necked individuals are most likely to have these complications. These patients develop a diminished respiratory exchange due to thick secretions with resultant atelectasis after anesthesia and surgical procedures. Bronchopneumonia or pneumonitis with antibiotic-resistant organisms follows frequently. Measures such as bronchoscopy and endotracheal suction are traumatic and often ineffective. Expectorants at best are very slow in action. Aerosol therapy with nonspecific detergents may be of value in keeping the tracheobronchial tree clean and moist[2, 12] but have no effect in removing exudate already inspissated. Enzymes such as trypsin,[15, 16, 20, 21] chymotrypsin, and streptokinase-streptodornase (Varidase) have been reported to be effective,[13, 14] but serious reactions including irritation and allergic manifestations are common.[6-9, 17] Human fibrinolysin is effective only in the presence of aspirated blood.

Pancreatic desoxyribonuclease (dornase)[1, 11] has been very effective in liquefying thick secretions and crusts adherent to the tracheobronchial mucosa. It has been without toxic reaction in a large number of patients treated for chronic bronchopulmonary diseases, including bronchiectasis, lung abscess, and tracheitis sicca and in postoperative and post-traumatic atelectasis and pneumonitis.[3-5, 10, 18, 19]

Our experience with pancreatic dornase in over 400 patients will be summarized in this report. The results with the use of this agent as a preoperative measure in patients with purulent bronchiectasis and abscesses, as well as many individuals with emphysema, pulmonary fibrosis, and chronic bronchopulmonary disease, have been particularly satisfactory.

After anesthesia and operation these patients develop thick, tenacious secretions. Because of restriction of respiratory excursion due to wound pain, they fail to cough adequately and atelectasis with or without pneumonitis results from the stasis of secretions.

A careful preoperative evaluation is important and the following preoperative regimen should be instituted in patients with chronic bronchitis, emphysema, and purulent bronchopulmonary disease: (1) pancreatic dornase should be administered for at least 1 day prior to the operation, (2) postural drainage after inhalations of pancreatic dornase may be helpful and is certainly indicated in patients with large amounts of secretions, (3) secretions should be collected and measured for 24-hour periods and culture

Read at the Twenty-second Annual Meeting of the Society of University Surgeons, Kansas City, Kan., Feb. 9-11, 1961.

and sensitivity studies obtained, (4) bronchodilators should be administered in the presence of wheezing or a history of asthma, and (5) instruction for deep breathing and coughing should be given before operation to be instituted as soon as possible after the operation.

## MATERIAL AND METHODS

Pancreatic desoxyribonuclease (dornase*) is a lyophilized powder of bovine origin, (100,000 U. per vial). Routinely 100,000 U. are dissolved in 2 ml. of buffer solution supplied in a separate vial. For certain conditions such as tracheitis sicca the volume may be increased to 4 to 5 ml. The solution must be used immediately because the enzyme, when in solution, loses activity rapidly even if refrigerated. It should not be mixed with other materials.

To be effective the enzyme must come in contact with the involved mucosa. This is accomplished only by delivering a concentrated solution or mist by aerosol with oxygen or a De Vilbiss pump at a flow rate of 5 to 7 L. per minute. The balloon present on some nebulizers should be clamped off and the patient urged to inhale deeply at all times. A hand nebulizer is not adequate in patients who breathe shallowly and have difficulty in inhaling. The Bird or Bennet intermittent positive-pressure apparatus is recommended. The 2 ml. of enzyme solution should be inhaled in 15 to 20 minutes. With a tracheostomy, the enzyme dissolved in 4 to 5 ml. of solution is delivered by means of a small, multiperforated polyethylene catheter inserted for some distance into the trachea. It may also be sprayed directly into the tracheostomy from a syringe with an adapter if first mixed with air. The patient is urged to inhale deeply as the material is instilled.

## RESULTS

**General results.** Pancreatic dornase has been used in several institutions under our direction in over 500 cases. No significant toxic, allergic, or irritative reaction to dornase has been seen in any of these cases. In many patients there is a temporary increase, sometimes marked, in the amount of sputum or secretions raised after the institution of dornase therapy. This may last for several hours or even for a day or more. It is probably due to dissolution of the thick secretions and freeing of material behind a bronchial plug. It always decreases to normal with improvement in the pathologic process.

In the usual patient who had been unable to cough up the thick, tenacious, high-viscosity mucus, within an hour or two the sputum usually becomes thin, is no longer tenacious, and can be coughed up easily. This is particularly noticeable in the weak and aged individual. We have found that endotracheal aspirations can be abandoned even in patients who needed it very frequently before dornase administration. The patient breathes more easily and the secondary effects of obstruction quickly improve. Clinical evidence of atelectasis or bronchopneumonia will clear in a few hours to a day or two and clearing will usually be obvious on roentgenogram by the second or third day, if not sooner. A good result is recorded only in a patient who shows complete return in less than 3 days to the condition which prevailed before the complication occurred. In many cases there is marked improvement within 24 hours. Treatment can be stopped 24 hours after a good result has been obtained.

Pancreatic dornase has been used in over 500 patients without any toxic or allergic reaction. In 3 patients irritation of the pharynx or trachea was found to be due to radiation therapy to the area. In 2 patients nausea was associated with radiation therapy and continued after dornase therapy had been discontinued. We ourselves have directly managed or observed the results in 406 of the 500 patients (Table I).

**Thoracic surgery.** There were 92 patients with serious postoperative atelectasis and pulmonary complications after thoracic procedures (Table II). Of these, 83 had complete relief of the atelectasis or other pul-

*Merck Sharp & Dohme, West Point, Pa.

**Table I.** *Indications for use of pancreatic dornase aerosol*

| *Indication* | *No.* |
|---|---|
| Postoperative atelectasis | 164 |
| Tracheitis sicca and atelectasis | 119 |
| Chronic pulmonary diseases | 59 |
| Preoperative use | 64 |
| Total | 406 |

**Table II.** *Pancreatic dornase for atelectasis after thoracic operations*

| | *No.* | *Days before improvement* | *Results* | |
|---|---|---|---|---|
| | | | *Good* | *No change* |
| *After thoracotomy* | | | | |
| Major atelectasis | 28 | 1 | 24 | 4 |
| Segmental atelectasis | 34 | 1 | 31 | 3 |
| *After pulmonary Resection* | | | | |
| Major atelectasis | 16 | 1 | 14 | 2 |
| Segmental atelectasis | 14 | 2 | 14 | 0 |
| Totals | 92 | 5 | 83 | 9 |

**Table III.** *Pancreatic dornase for atelectasis after head and neck, breast, and abdominal operations*

| | *No.* | *Days before improvement* | *Results* | |
|---|---|---|---|---|
| | | | *Good* | *No change* |
| After head and neck operation | 7 | 1 | 7 | — |
| After breast operation | 5 | 2 | 5 | — |
| After abdominal operation | 60 | 2 | 54 | 6 |
| Totals | 72 | 5 | 66 | 6 |

monary complications within 48 hours and only 9 were unchanged. Thirty patients had undergone pulmonary resections. These patients all were critically ill with fever, tachycardia, dyspnea, and cyanosis. The usual means of control had failed to reverse the process. In all of these patients improvement was noted within a few hours after the first inhalation of dornase, and 28 of the 30 had marked clinical improvement. The 2 in whom the atelectasis failed to clear had tumor obstruction as shown by subsequent bronchoscopy and postmortem examination. None of these patients developed a bronchopleural fistula despite the recent bronchial closure. Sixty-two individuals had undergone exploratory thoracotomy or such procedures as esophagectomy, mediastinal tumor excision, or the chest-wall operation for carcinoma of the breast. Fifty-five of these had an excellent response to dornase therapy. In the entire group treatment was instituted on the second to eighth postoperative day and improvement was noted within the first few hours in most patients.

**Case 1.** H. H., a 58-year-old man, had a resection of middle and lower lobe for squamous carcinoma of the lung. He was readmitted on June 19, 1960, for treatment of a recurrent carcinoma of the lung thought to be present in the right upper lobe. At operation on June 21, 1960, a second primary carcinoma of the trachea 2 cm. above the anterior edge of the right bronchus was found. A large segment of trachea and the upper lobe were removed and primary closure of the tracheal defect carried out. Postoperatively partial atelectasis of the left upper lobe was shown by physical signs and roentgenogram. There was rapid pulse, dyspnea and cyanosis. This persisted in spite of nasotracheal suction and the administration of Alevaire, antibiotics, and expectorants. The patient was given dornase aerosol, 100,000 U., on June 23, 1960, and within 12 hours he began to cough up moderate amounts of thick yellow sputum. There was rapid clearing of the dyspnea and cyanosis and physical examination showed clearing of the atelectasis. On June 25 the roentgenogram showed no atelectasis. There was no bronchopleural or tracheal fistula postoperatively and the chest tubes were removed on the fifth postoperative day. Convalescence was uneventful.

**Case 2.** E. S., a 50-year-old woman, was admitted because of a tumor in the left breast. On Jan. 13, 1959, a left radical mastectomy with chest-wall resection was carried out for carcinoma. By the fourth postoperative day the patient had become dyspneic, cyanotic, and very restless and atelectasis of the left lower lobe was present (Fig. 1). Temperature was 101.4° F. and pulse 120. Alevaire and tracheal aspirations had been unsuccessful in alleviating the atelectasis. At 2:30 P.M. on January 14 dornase was given, and this was repeated in 4 hours. Within 6 hours of the first inhalation the patient began to cough up blood-tinged sputum and became less apprehensive and more alert. Her color was much improved and after this there was steady clinical clearing of the atelectasis. She became afebrile in 48 hours. The chest roentgenogram of January 21 showed clearing of the atelectasis (Fig. 2).

**General surgical procedures.** There were 72 patients treated with dornase for lobar or segmental atelectasis and/or pneumonitis after head and neck, breast, abdominal, or pelvic operations (Table III). It was noted especially in patients with severe incisional pain and splinting of the chest. Over 90 per cent of these patients responded by relief of the pulmonary complication in from a few hours to 2 days. The secretions became very thin and could be raised without difficulty, and there was no need for endotracheal suction.

**Case 3.** M. L., a 63-year-old white man, had an infiltrating carcinoma of the bladder and underwent a radical total cystectomy, pelvic lymph-node dissection, and construction of an ileal bladder on July 19, 1960. On the second postoperative day he developed marked dyspnea and tachycardia, and a fever to 103° F. He was not able to cough up any secretions and endotracheal suction was being carried out at frequent intervals without relief. Oxygen with Alevaire was administered. He remained slightly cyanotic and febrile, with a pulse rate of 120. There was marked diminution of breath sounds in the right base with an elevation of the right side of the diaphragm, and there were fine râles at the left base. Chest roentgenogram on July 22 showed atelectasis of the right lower lobe and a segmental atelectasis on the left (Fig. 3). Dornase aerosol administration was begun on July 22 and within 12 hours the pulse was 100, respirations were normal, the oxygen tent could be discontinued, and the patient began to bring up thick mucous plugs on coughing. Within 48 hours there was clinical evidence of complete resolution of the atelectasis with return of temperature to normal. A repeat chest roentgenogram on July 25 showed clearing of the atelectasis (Fig. 4). This was confirmed by roentgenogram on August 3.

**Tracheitis sicca and atelectasis.** One hundred and nineteen patients with severe tracheitis sicca were treated with pancreatic dornase (Table IV). These were divided into 3 groups, tracheostomy patients, recently laryngectomized patients, and patients who had been operated upon more than 2 months before. The results have been dramatic in patients with an obstructed airway due to thick crusts and tenacious secretions. In over 90 per cent of the patients the crusts have

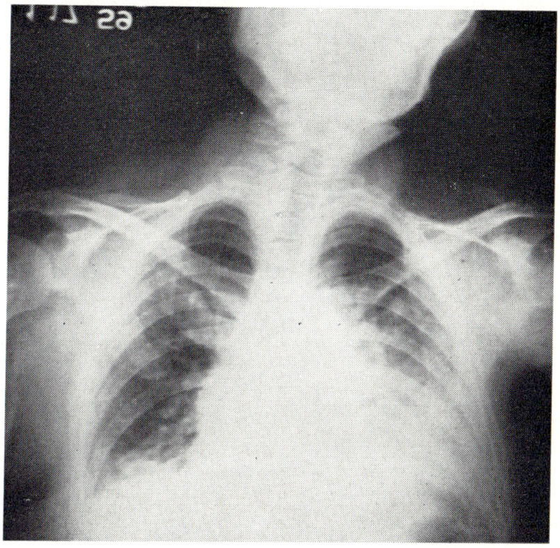

**Fig. 1.** Case 2. Chest roentgenogram taken on Jan. 17, 1959, 4 days after left radical mastectomy and chest-wall resection. Dornase therapy was started the next day.

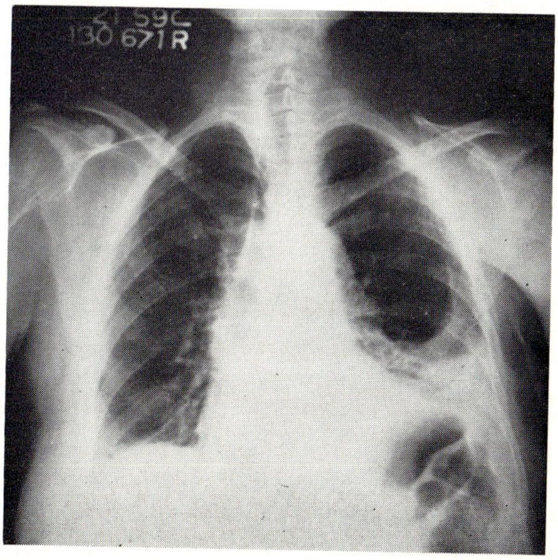

**Fig. 2.** Case 2. Chest roentgenogram taken on Jan. 21, 1959, 3 days after start of dornase therapy, shows the resolution of the atelectasis.

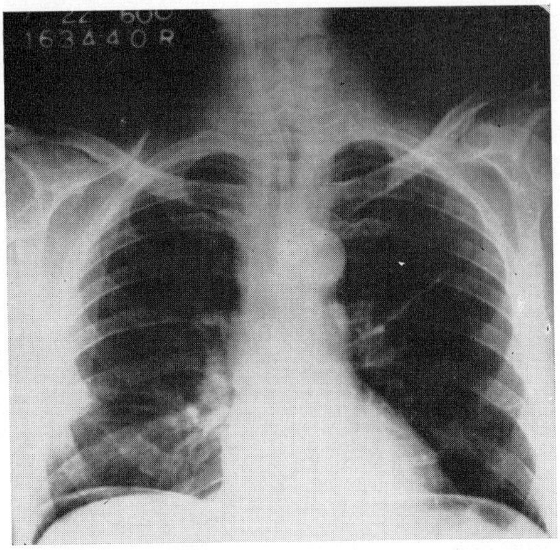

**Fig. 3.** Case 3. Chest roentgenogram taken on July 22, prior to beginning of dornase therapy.

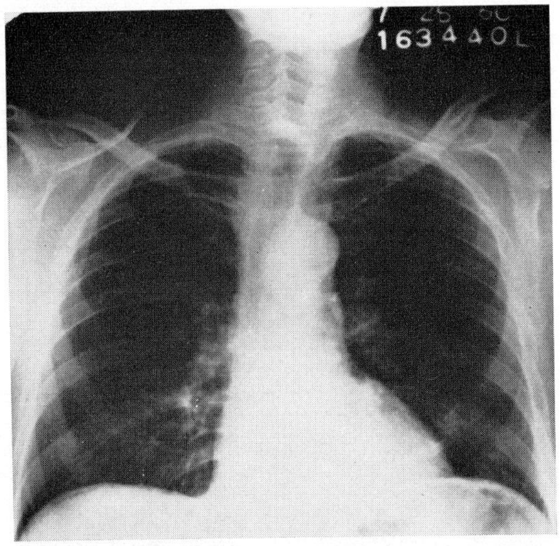

**Fig. 4.** Case 3. Rapid clearing of the atelectasis was seen clinically in 2 days. Follow-up roentgenogram taken on July 25, 1960, shows good aeration of the right lower lobe.

been loosened and the secretions thinned so that the patient could cough them up without difficulty. Partial relief of the obstruction to the airway was usually noted in 30 minutes and a complete return to normal was apparent within 24 hours. Three days of treatment was usually sufficient in these patients. Several patients with recurrence of tracheitis sicca over a period of years have responded well to more than 1 course of enzyme therapy.

One patient developed a serious complication which should be mentioned. The trachea was almost completely obstructed prior to treatment and the obstruction could not be removed mechanically. After the first instillation of dornase he began to breathe more easily and took a deep inspiration with development of an atelectasis. Bronchoscopy was necessary to remove a large plug impacted in the bronchus.

**Chronic bronchopulmonary diseases.** A wide variety of chronic bronchopulmonary diseases have been treated, among them chronic lung abscess, bronchiectasis, asthma, and chronic bronchitis (Table V). In these patients pancreatic dornase should be used only to overcome complications such as atelectasis or pneumonitis, or to prepare the patients for operation, bronchoscopy, bronchography, or other procedures. It has been particularly useful in asthmatic patients with bronchial plugs and in patients with staphylococcal pneumonia after influenza. It is not particularly useful as a method of treatment for the chronic disease itself. Although improvement during the course of therapy is usual, it quickly regresses when the inhalations are discontinued. Six of the 7 patients with chronic lung abscesses showed a marked change with increased drainage of thin pus and more rapid resolution than expected. Apparently, mucopurulent exudate which blocked the bronchial connection was lysed. The one patient who did not respond was later shown to have a tumor which blocked the bronchus.

**Preoperative treatment.** The fourth case report illustrates the successful use of dornase preoperatively in patients with chronic bronchopulmonary disease.

**Case 4.** E. S., a 37-year-old white woman, was admitted on Oct. 16, 1960, with a 2-month history of cough and fever. Three weeks prior to admission she had experienced hemoptysis. At that time a chest roentgenogram taken in another hospital showed an abscess and surrounding pneumonitis in the right lower lobe and calcified lymph nodes

**Table IV.** *Pancreatic dornase in tracheitis sicca*

| | No. | Days before improvement | Results | |
|---|---|---|---|---|
| | | | Good | No change |
| After tracheostomy | 41 | 1 | 37 | 4 |
| After laryngectomy up to 8 weeks postoperatively | 63 | 2 | 63 | — |
| After laryngectomy over 2 months postoperatively | 15 | 2 | 15 | — |
| Totals | 119 | 5 | 115 | 4 |

in the right hilum. Hemoptysis and high fever continued throughout this hospitalization and after admission to Memorial Hospital. At bronchoscopy on October 20 considerable blood was noted coming from the right middle lobe orifice. Three days after bronchoscopy the patient again had a severe hemoptysis accompanied by marked dyspnea, tachycardia, and increased fever and chills. Findings at physical examination were typical of atelectasis of the right middle and lower lobe. On October 25, the chest roentgenogram showed increased infiltration around the abscess and atelectasis of the right lower and middle lobes (Fig. 5). The patient remained toxic with a rapid pulse, cyanosis, and high fever and an emergency operation was planned. During this entire 4-week period she had been treated very actively with antibiotics. After consultation, dornase therapy was started on October 26 (100,000 U. three times a day). In a few hours the patient began to bring up moderate amounts of purulent material and old blood. The chest became clear on auscultation without wheeze, râles, or rub in the area of the right middle and lower lobes and the temperature began to fall in 48 hours. In 72 hours the temperature reached and stayed normal for the first time in 4 weeks. Repeat chest roentgenogram (Fig. 6) on October 31 showed a resolution of the atelectasis and pneumonitis of the right lower lobe with decrease in size of the abscess cavities. The patient was considered ready for operation. Because of the possibility of tuberculosis, at this point an antituberculous drug was instituted. On November 3 a right lower and middle lobectomy was carried out. Pathologic study showed fibrocaseous tuberculosis with multiple abscess formation. The postoperative course was uneventful, the antituberculous regime was continued and the woman was discharged to her home on the eleventh postoperative day.

**Prebronchoscopy.** We have used dornase prior to bronchoscopy in a series of cases to facilitate collection of sputum and secretions for Papanicolaou smears. Preliminary data indicate that the yield of positive diagnoses has been increased by this measure. There has been no indication of sensitivity of the bronchial mucosa to dornase by this direct observation.

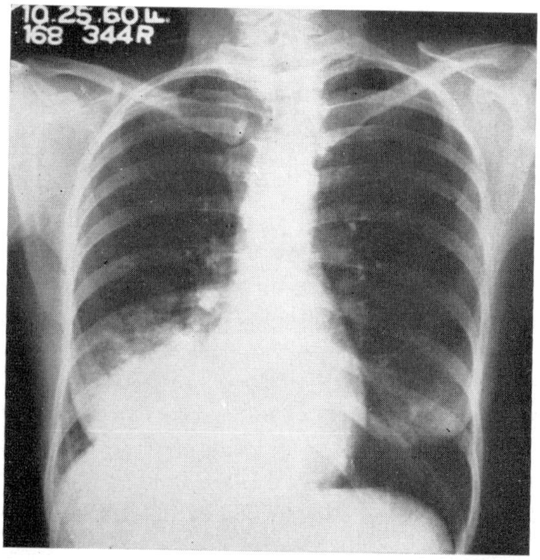


**Fig. 5.** Case 4. Chest roentgenogram taken on Oct. 25, 1960, prior to start of dornase therapy.

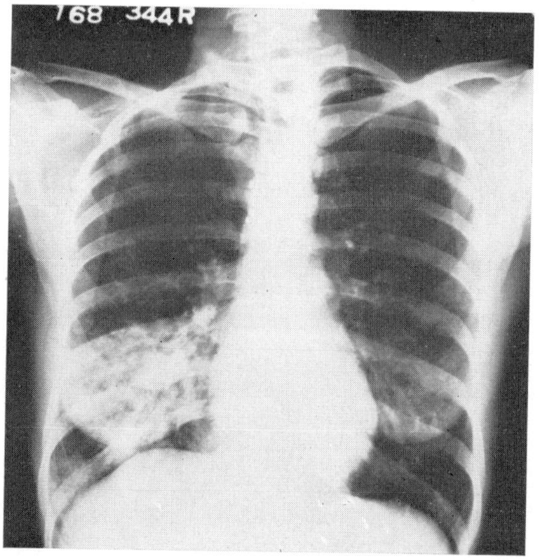


**Fig. 6.** Case 4. Roentgenogram taken on Oct. 31, 1960, after 5 days of dornase aerosol therapy.

**Table V.** *Pancreatic dornase in chronic bronchopulmonary diseases*

| *Diagnosis* | *No.* | *Days of therapy* | *Results* | |
|---|---|---|---|---|
| | | | *Good* | *No change* |
| Lung abscess | 7 | 5 | 6 | 1 |
| Bronchiectasis | 9 | 5 | 9 | — |
| Asthma | 2 | 3 | — | 2 |
| Chronic bronchitis with thick secretions | 41 | 6 | 37 | 4 |
| Totals | 59 | 20 | 52 | 7 |

## COMMENT

With the development of enzymes for clinical use, new concepts of therapy are necessary. Instead of using medications which will affect the enzymatic activity of the tissues or cells secondarily, we can add the enzyme or its inhibitor directly and obtain a much more rapid and dramatic effect. Frequently the enzymatic process which has been activated will continue once the reaction has been triggered by addition of the enzyme from outside. Unusual care must be directed to the use of these agents. The enzyme must be delivered to its site of action. In the present instance the dornase must have contact with the lining of the tracheobronchial tree. It must be delivered in a fine mist to the depths of the bronchi. Enzymes, particularly dornase, lose activity rapidly. In solution it loses much of its activity within 30 minutes, so that it must be used as rapidly as possible. Enzymes are susceptible to inactivation by many chemicals and should not be used with other agents unless they are known to have no inhibiting effect on the enzyme. Enzymes have a specific pH and temperature range for maximal activity, and for clinical use enzymes which can be effective in the physiologic range must be used or they must be adequately buffered in the body to maintain activity.

Dornase is effective without causing tissue irritation when used with the diluent furnished.

Once the secretions are liquefied the decrease in viscosity allows easier expectoration and eliminates the need of repeated endotracheal aspirations which are not only traumatic but also can trigger a reflex bronchospasm with dyspnea and retention of secretions and may introduce infection. In the majority of acutely ill patients with major atelectasis, the use of this enzyme will bring about a rapid mobilization of the tracheobronchial secretions with improvement in the clinical picture and the resolution of the atelectasis.

In thoracic procedures the enzyme has been particularly useful and it has not interfered with the healing of the bronchial stump. Indeed, one might expect that it would be helpful by removing purulent exudate from the area. Dornase aerosol has improved the results of pulmonary resection in marginal-risk patients. In many instances a patient acutely ill with atelectasis in spite of the usual measures showed evidence of resolution of the process within 12 hours of dornase administration. Similar results were obtained in cases of pulmonary complications after abdominal operations.

The preoperative use of this liquefying agent has aided in preparation for operation of patients with chronic bronchitis, bronchiectasis, and diminished respiratory reserve. Particularly in patients with pulmonary lesions in whom lung abscess or bronchiectasis is a major factor, the use of the dornase aerosol has brought about a maximum improvement prior to resectional operation. It has been effective even when postural drainage and bronchoscopy have failed to bring about satisfactory preparation of the patient for thoracotomy. The fact that no reactions have been encountered and that the liquefaction of the secretions is brought about in a short period of hours makes its use easy and desirable. In patients in whom tracheostomy is anticipated the enzyme loosens any crusts or thick secretions and reduces the need for traumatic suction postoperatively.

In patients with tracheitis sicca the local instillation of this material has proved to be very effective. No other treatment has been satisfactory for this serious complication of laryngeal and head and neck operations. Once thick crusts form in the tracheobronchial tree, repeated suctioning results only in local trauma, more bleeding, and greater crust formation. Dornase administered by local instillation has allowed the patient to cough up thick crusts within 30 minutes and the effect is prolonged. After a course of treatment the patient may remain without difficulties for months.

Use of dornase aerosol is indicated also in patients with chronic bronchopulmonary diseases when thick secretions or bronchial plugs are a major problem.

## SUMMARY

1. Over 400 patients with atelectasis or other serious pulmonary complications of operations were given pancreatic dornase aerosol without significant toxic allergic or other undesirable reactions.

2. Rapid clearing of the atelectasis or other pulmonary complications occurred in over 90 per cent of the patients. Improvement occurred in a few hours and complete resolution was noted usually after 1 to 2 days of treatment.

3. Preoperative use of this enzyme in patients with chronic bronchopulmonary disease is advocated.

### REFERENCES

1. Armstrong, J. B., and White, J. C.: Liquefaction of viscous purulent exudates by desoxyribonuclease, Lancet **2:** 739, 1950.
2. Christie, H. E., Meakins, J. F., and Aronovitch, M.: Aerosol therapy in the treatment of postoperative pulmonary atelectasis, Canad. M. A. J. **61:** 388, 1949.
3. Cliffton, E. E.: Pancreatic dornase aerosol in pulmonary endotracheal disease, Dis. Chest **30:** 373, 1956.
4. Cliffton, E. E., and Grossi, C. E.: Pancreatic desoxyribonuclease (dornase) aerosol in treatment of bronchopulmonary complications and tracheitis sicca, Cancer. In press.
5. Cliffton, E. E., and Grossi, C. E.: Pancreatic dornase aerosol in postoperative atelectasis, Am. J. Surg. **100:** 447, 1960.
6. Craven, J. F.: Treatment of obstructive atelectasis by aerosol administration of proteolytic enzymes, J. Pediat. **42:** 228, 1953.
7. Farber, S. M., Gorman, R. D., Wood, D. A., Grimes, O. F., and Pharr, S. L.: Enzymatic débridement; particular reference to trypsin and desoxyribonuclease in the control of cough and sputum associated with tuberculosis, J. Thoracic Surg. **27:** 45, 1954.
8. Farber, S. M., Pharr, S. L., Wood, D. A., and Frost, J. K.: Enzymatic therapy in diseases of the chest, Lab. Invest. **4:** 362, 1955.
9. Limber, C. G., Reiser, H. G., Roettig, L. C., and Curtis, O. M.: Enzymatic lysis of respiratory secretions by aerosol trypsin, J. A. M. A. **149:** 816, 1952.
10. Lynch, B., Cliffton, E. E., and Lewis, J.: Tracheitis sicca. Successful enzymatic treatment with pancreatic desoxyribonuclease (dornase), New England J. Med. **256:** 495, 1957.
11. McCarty, M.: Purification and properties of desoxyribonuclease isolated from beef pancreas, J. Gen. Physiol. **29:** 123, 1946.
12. Miller, J. B., Brown, L. J., Goldfarb, P. M., Leight, M., McVey, L., Phillips, S. C., Sellers, D. F., and Zeiman, H.: Alevaire inhalations for eliminating secretions in asthma, sinusitis, bronchitis and bronchiectasis of adults, Ann. Allergy **12:** 611, 1954.
13. Miller, J. M., Surmonte, J. A., and Long, P. H.: Intrabronchial use of streptokinase-streptodornase in treatment of slowly resolving pneumonia, Dis. Chest. **23:** 149, 1953.
14. Muenster, J. J., Flance, I. J., and Sweeney, B.: Treatment of unresolved pneumonia with streptokinase-streptodornase, Am. J. Med. **12:** 376, 1952.
15. Peck, M. E., and Levin, S.: Atelectasis: physiopathology and treatment, special reference to its occurrence in bulbar poliomyelitis and to a suggested therapeutic aid by the intrabronchial administration of trypsin, J. Thoracic Surg. **24:** 619, 1952.
16. Prince, H. E., Etter, R. L., and Jackson, R. H.: Aerosol trypsin therapy in the treatment of asthma, Ann. Allergy **12:** 25, 1954.
17. Roettig, L. C., Reiser, H. G., Habeeb, W., and Mark, L.: The use of trypsin in chest disease, Dis. Chest **21:** 245, 1952.
18. Segal, M. S., and Goldstein, H.: Pancreatic dornase aerosols in bronchopulmonary diseases, Ann. New York Acad. Sc. **68:** 138, 1957.
19. Solomon, A., Herschfus, J. A., and Segal, M. S.: Aerosols of pancreatic dornase in bronchopulmonary disease, Ann. Allergy **12:** 71, 1954.
20. Steigman, A. J., and Scott, C. H.: Trypsin in poliomyelitis patients with tracheotomy, J. A. M. A. **150:** 1403, 1952.
21. Unger, L., and Unger, A. H.: Trypsin inhalations in respiratory conditions with thick sputum, J. A. M. A. **152:** 1109, 1953.

## DISCUSSION*

**Dr. William A. Altemeier** (Cincinnati, Ohio). All three of these papers have been very interesting. I would like to confine my remarks, however, to the paper by Drs. Burke and McDermott because of mutual interests. I think this paper has been particularly well conceived and executed and that the results are both significant and important. Similar experiments have been conducted at the University of Cincinnati by two of my residents, Drs. Alexander and McGloin. They have shown a similar high degree of prophylactic effectiveness of aqueous penicillin given to guinea pigs, provided that the injection of penicillin was started before challenge by the hemolytic *Staphylococcus aureus* or at the time of challenge. If the injection of penicillin was delayed for 4, 8, or 12 hours after challenge by bacteria, there was no significant prophylactic effect. There is evidence, however, to suggest that the period in which penicillin may have any prophylactic effect may not be fixed to 3 or 4 hours. In previous similar experiments performed by Drs. MacMillan and Culbertson in my laboratory with *Clostridium welchii,* it was found that a significant degree of protection could be obtained for as long as 12 hours after a challenge with these organisms, provided that the bacterial suspensions injected were free of toxin. Under such circumstances, a 40 per cent survival was obtained when the injections of penicillin were delayed 8 to 12 hours after challenge and the dose increased fiftyfold. We intend to repeat the experiments with the *Staphylococcus aureus* and use a saline suspension of washed cells free of toxin to make sure that the effects we are seeing in the first 3 hours are not due to a significant degree to the coexistent toxin and the suspension.

**Dr. Frank Spencer** (Baltimore, Md.). I was impressed that Dr. Burke has found that only a few hours in difference in the starting of antibiotic therapy made a significant difference in the rate of infection. Similar observations, however, were reported by Dr. H. W. Scott about a year ago in studies of contaminated grafts in the abdominal aorta.

We have been interested in the reasons for the ineffectiveness of postoperative antibiotics in the reduction of wound infections. Two speculations have been (1) that the organism might be encapsulated in a wound hematoma and thus is inaccessible to circulating antibiotics given after operation or (2) that penicillin in customary dosages might be ineffective, whereas massive doses of penicillin would be effective. A similar approach has been found effective in the treatment of bacterial endocarditis. On the basis of these considerations, we are performing a study of the routine use of antibiotics in patients who undergo clean abdominal operations on a random sampling basis. At the beginning of anesthesia the patients are given 1 Gm. of chloromycetin by intravenous injection and also 500,000 U. of penicillin. Subsequently, each hour for the subsequent 24 hours 500,000 U. of penicillin is given and at 8-hour intervals 1 Gm. of chloromycetin. At the end of 24 hours a total of 3 Gm. of chloromycetin and 12,000,000 U. of penicillin have been given. All antibiotics are stopped at this time.

Only initial results are available at this time, as less than 200 patients have been studied. It is of interest, however, that the infection rate in the group which received the massive doses of antibiotics is about one-half of that occurring in the group not given antibiotics.

**Dr. Paul V. Harper** (Chicago, Ill.). Dr. John Sommer in Dr. Vermeulen's laboratory at the University of Chicago has been pursuing for several years this question of experimental pyelonephritis in the rat, and he also found that when infection was introduced into the bladder through the suprapubic route the obstructed kidney occasionally became infected. However, while infection was introduced into the animal's bladder through a small polyethylene urethral catheter, the obstruction of the ureter apparently gave complete protection to the kidney on that side so that it was unnecessary to postulate the seeding of the obstructed kidney via the hematogenous route from the other kidney. Dr. Sommer also injected through the urethral catheter into these animals' bladders indigo carmine at physiologic volumes and pressures. The direct observations of the ureters showed that there was reflux of the dye up into the kidney in the great majority of the animals. This accounts adequately, I think, for the existence in the rat of ascending infection. This reflux of urine up the ureters has not been demonstrated in the human being, so it appears that this beautiful and unequivocal evidence for ascending infection in the rat cannot be construed in any way to demonstrate the existence of a similar phenomenon in man.

**Dr. Willard E. Goodwin** (Los Angeles, Calif.). These remarks are confined to the paper on experimental pyelonephritis and in a way echo what Dr. Harper has just said. This is a very nice study, and I agree completely—*for rats.* However, none of this audience should go home believing that the same thing is true of human beings. If it were, instrumentation of the urinary tract of a human patient would be impossible. In human beings this situation can occur under conditions of chronic vesical-neck obstruction with vesicoureteral reflux.

*Discussion of papers by Burke; Davis and Coil; and Cliffton, Grossi, and Esakof.

The poor little rat, however, has no protection against reflux. I invite you to consider a simple experiment. Fill the rat's bladder with indigo carmine which is visible with the naked eye. It will run upward into both kidneys as you watch. If you squeeze the bladder a little bit, you can see it run into the renal veins. Ultimately it will turn the whole rat blue. This probably explains Dr. Harper's animals which got infections after ureteral ligation. The spread was from the bladder to the other kidney, thence to the blood stream, and to the kidney with the ligated ureter.

We have performed the experiment of overfilling the bladder with indigo carmine and India ink in rats, rabbits, dogs, cats, and human subjects. The rabbit and the rat both show vesicoureteral reflux. Dogs, cats, and human beings, unless they have some obstructive lesion, do not exhibit this phenomenon. There seems to be a species difference. The rat is probably not the best animal in which to study pyelonephritis in relation to bladder infections. It may be that this simple species difference is one of the things that has lead to some of the current erroneous conclusions about pyelonephritis and the catheter.

It is very interesting, indeed, to know what happens to rats, but let us not necessarily apply this information to the human being. The poor rat can't help itself.

**Dr. Ed Howes** (Hartford, Conn.). I want to comment on the magic 6 hours after wounding. Fredrich, one of the forgotten men in surgery, professor of surgery at Leipzig at the end of the nineteenth century, first called attention to this 6 hours in a scientific investigation. This work was carried out shortly after bacteria were discovered, cultured, and stained. He wondered why all wounds did not become infected. When he crushed tissue or put in dirt with bacteria, all wounds became infected. But if he removed the crushed tissue or dirt within the first 6 hours, few wounds became infected. With later removal, more and more became infected until, after 12 hours, all again were infected. This experiment is the scientific basis for débridement (Arch. klin. Chir. 57: 288, 1898).

Débridement was first practiced in World War I when its application was immediately confused with primary closure of the wounds. The experience was enough, however, to show that it would be successful if carried out within 6 hours. Policard and Desplas showed that bacteria begin to multiply in the wound after this period.

In World War II, when the sulfa drugs and penicillin were introduced, this period was lengthened slightly to 8 hours.

Previously I showed that if susceptible bacteria were put into a crushed wound, nearly 100 per cent prevention of infection could be obtained if the antibiotic was introduced within the first 4 hours. After 6 hours, more and more wounds became infected, although the bacteria were still susceptible to the antibiotic. The only other change that could be found was that the bacteria were now inside leukocytes where the antibiotic could not reach them (Ann. Surg. 124: 268, 1946).

It is interesting to hear that the 6 hours still exist.

**Dr. John F. Burke** (closing). I agree with Dr. Howes absolutely. What we have shown you today is a limited case, a specific example, and cannot be carried over directly into complex situations such as surgical wounds. I think the most important point is that the lesions shown reached their maximum at 24 hours, but could not be altered after 3 hours. These were primary lesions without secondary spread. This does not only pertain to alteration by antibiotics. Other experiments have shown that host factors which tend to limit the size of a primary lesion must be blocked in this first 3 hours in order to produce a lesion bigger than predicted. It appears that the biochemical exchange between host and invading bacteria is over in a short period close to exact time of invasion—in our experimental lesions and wound infections, 3 hours. If you would alter this lesion, you have to do it during this period.

**Dr. John H. Davis** (closing). I would like to make just 2 comments. Dr. Harper mentioned injecting the urinary bladder with bacteria through a catheter rather than through a surgical incision. We have used this technique but have given it up because in some instances a mixed infection resulted. The problems are great enough with only one bacterial strain and so we have limited ourselves to the surgical technique.

In answer to Dr. Goodwin, I certainly agree that the results in the rat do not necessarily apply to man. There is, however, some evidence by high-speed cineroentgenography that vesicoureteral reflux occurs in normal human beings. I thank the discussers for their comments.

# Prolonged survival of a renal homograft in a dog treated with 6-mercaptopurine

J. C. PIERCE, M.D.
R. L. VARCO, M.D.
ROBERT A. GOOD, M.D.
MINNEAPOLIS, MINN.

In 1958 Schwartz and associates[13] reported a marked suppression of antibody formation to bovine serum albumin in rabbits when 6-mercaptopurine was given simultaneously with the antigen. In the following 2 years, Meeker[10] and Schwartz[12] and their colleagues demonstrated a significant prolongation of the survival of skin homografts in rabbits by treatment with 6-mercaptopurine. These experiments led us to study the effect of this antimetabolite on the survival of organ homotransplants in another species. The kidney was chosen because its rejection pattern in the dog has been well studied,[5] it has a sharp rejection end point, and standard methods for evaluating its functional survival were available.[14]

## METHODS

Mongrel dogs immunized for distemper and rabies which weighed from 10 to 26 kilograms were anesthetized intravenously with pentobarbital, 30 mg. per kilogram, and the skin was treated with pHisoHex and tincture of Zephiran. With sterile technique, the right kidney was excised through a subcostal incision and implanted into the left side of the recipient's neck by anastomosis of the renal vessels to the external jugular vein and common carotid artery end-to-end with No. 6-0 silk. Total ischemia time ranged from 16 to 50 minutes. The ureter was cut to 10 cm. in length and was brought out to the surface for a skin ureterostomy.[8] (In the first few experiments, a plastic cannula was tied into the ureter but because this was followed by stenosis in 2 to 3 weeks, it was abandoned.) During the operation 1,000 ml. of normal saline solution was given intravenously to promote diuresis. In the later experiments atropine, 0.6 mg., was given intravenously 30 minutes prior to the pentobarbital, and tracheal suction was performed at the conclusion of the operation. Transplants were performed reciprocally in 34 dogs and unilaterally in 17. 6-Mercaptopurine,* 3 to 6 mg. per kilogram, was given intravenously before the implantation of the transplant into the recipient. It was found to be essential that the parenteral form of the drug be freshly prepared on the day when given because it rapidly lost its potency in solution. In 3 experiments the drug was started the day prior to transplantation, but this appeared to have no particularly beneficial effect. For 8 to 12 days after operation the drug was given daily by mouth in gelatin capsules. After this it was given every second day and dosage was adjusted for changes in the weight of the dog. A different regimen was followed in dogs which received 4 to 5 mg. per kilogram daily. This dose was continued until the white blood cell count fell. At that time the dose was reduced.

Achromycin, 250 mg., was given intravenously at the beginning of the operation and procaine penicillin, 400,000 to 900,000 U., was given intramuscularly daily thereafter. In the earlier experiments the dogs were

Supported by grants from the United States Public Health Service and the Minnesota Heart Association.

Read at the Twenty-second Annual Meeting of the Society of University Surgeons, Kansas City, Kan., Feb. 9-11, 1961.

*Supplied as Purinethol through the courtesy of Dr. D. S. Searle, Burroughs, Wellcome and Co.

also given streptomycin, 1.0 to 2.0 Gm., intramuscularly daily, but this was discontinued because of respiratory depression. Bacitracin ointment was applied to the ureterostomy site at operation. Each dog received 0.6 ml. of multivitamins* daily and canned meat 2 to 7 times per week, in addition to dog biscuit ad libitum. Finally, the dogs were exercised daily, usually by running them up and down stairs.

Continuing function of a homograft was determined by profuse wetting of the coat of the dogs below the ureterostomy each day. This has proved a reliable index except for occasional false-negative results. At weekly intervals 50+ ml. of urine was collected from the ureterostomy for urinalysis.

## RESULTS

A total of 51 dogs treated with 6-mercaptopurine received renal homografts. Of these, there were 11 technical failures in that the homografts functioned for 3 days or less. In 2 dogs the drug was discontinued after 2 and 4 days and function ceased at 7 and 8 days, respectively. The results in the remaining 38 dogs are presented in Table I. Fifteen of the transplants functioned for 15 or more days, 4 of these functioned for over 30 days, and 1, No. 398, functioned and is continuing to function for over 400 days. The mortality rate increased sharply to 80 per cent in animals treated with 6-mercaptopurine at the 5 mg. per kilogram level. Most of the dogs that died had bronchopneumonia. A few developed a toxic syndrome characterized by anorexia, diarrhea, rapid weight loss, leukopenia, and jaundice.

**Hematologic studies.** In most dogs the hematocrits were maintained at a constant level. The anemia which developed in some dogs responded to an increase in meat ration. The erythrocyte sedimentation rate uncorrected for hematocrit showed an inconstant rise to the range 25 to 50 mm. per hour during the time of active homograft rejection. In dog No. 398 the erythrocyte sedimentation rate rose initially to 55, but after the first 2 months it remained in the range 0 to 15 until excision of the recipient's second kidney. The white blood cell count generally fell below 8,000 per cubic millimeter in 1 to 2 weeks. There was marked variation, however. Dog No. 2937 maintained a white blood cell count of over 10,000 for 4 weeks while on 5 mg. per kilogram per day of 6-mercaptopurine. In dog No. 398 the white blood cell count fell initially to 7,000 to 8,000 for about 2 months, after which it was 9,000 to 14,000. In the differential leukocyte count, the lymphocyte fraction was usually depressed to the range 1 to 12 per cent. In dog No. 398, after being depressed for the first 3 months, the lymphocyte fraction ranged from 18 to 37 per cent.

**Urine studies.** The specific gravity ranged from 1.000 to 1.032. In dog No. 398 the urine did not become concentrated until 1 month after implantation.

Results of tests for urine protein were usually negative until 1 to 2 weeks prior to rejection, when they became positive. In dog No. 398 it was intermittently negative and positive.

**Weight of host dogs.** The weights of the dogs usually decreased for 1 to 2 weeks

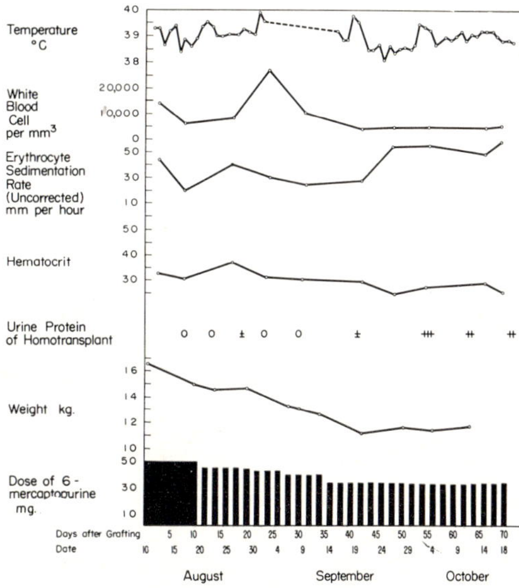


**Fig. 1.** Clinical course of renal homograft recipient No. 1750 treated with 6-mercaptopurine.

*Abdec drops, Parke, Davis & Company.

and then were maintained at 20 to 30 per cent below operative weight; dog No. 398 decreased in weight from 12.2 to 10.0 kilograms in 10 days and then over the succeeding 5 months increased to 15.0 kilograms.

Studies in dog No. 1750, in which the transplant functioned for 70 days before death, are presented in Fig. 1.

**Bromsulphalein excretion.** Table II summarizes the results of Bromsulphalein excretion in 9 dogs after a test dose of 5 mg. per kilogram. There was no impairment of function after as long as 89 days with 6-mercaptopurine, 3 mg. per kilogram, given every second day.

**Clearance studies and blood urea nitrogen.** Serial para-aminohippuric acid (P.A.H.) and creatinine clearances[14] were performed on the homotransplant in dog No. 398 (Table III). Each value represents the mean of 3 successive collection periods

**Table I.** *Survival of renal homografts and mortality rate related to initial dosage level of 6-mercaptopurine*

| *Initial dosage level of 6-mercaptopurine (mg./Kg.)* | *Duration of function (days)* | *Median days functioned* | *Total No. of homografts* | *No. of dogs dying during treatment* | *Mortality rate (%)* |
|---|---|---|---|---|---|
| 1.0 | 5, 7 | 6 | 2 | 0 | 0 |
| 3.0 | 4, 4, 4, 6, 7, 7 | | | | |
| | 7, 8, 9, 9, 11, 11, 11* | | | | |
| | 12, 12,* 13, 14, 14 | | | | |
| | 15, 16, 17, 17,* 18 | | | | |
| | 18,* 21,* 31,* 70* | | | | |
| | 270+ | 12 | 28 | 7 | 25 |
| 4.0 | 17, 17,* 22 | 17 | 3 | 1 | 33 |
| 5.0 | 10,* 12,* 14,* 20, 31* | 14 | 5 | 4 | 80 |
| | | | 38 | 12 | 32 |

*Died with functioning renal homograft.

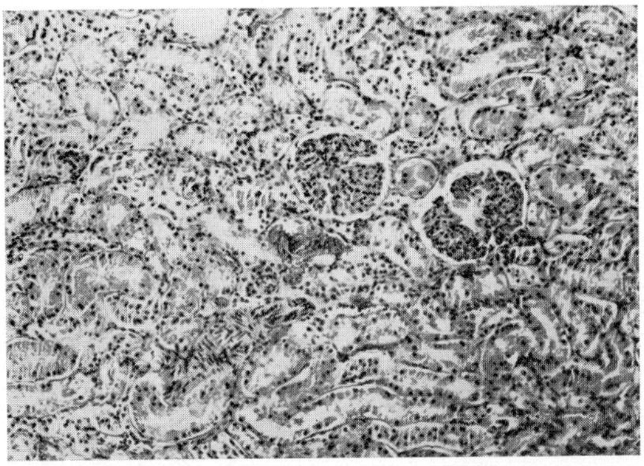

**Fig. 2.** 6-Mercaptopurine-treated kidney homotransplant, which functioned until the death of the host dog (No. 3897), on the seventeenth day postoperatively. Note the absence of lymphocytic and plasmacytic infiltration. (Hematoxylin and eosin; ×80.)

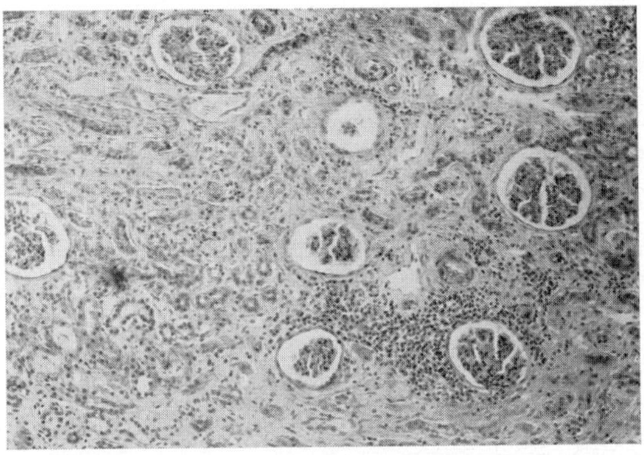

**Fig. 3.** 6-Mercaptopurine-treated kidney homotransplant, which functioned until death of the host dog (No. 1750), on the seventieth day postoperatively. Note the moderate amount of lymphocytic and plasmacytic infiltration, the marked tubular atrophy, and the thickening of Bowman's capsule. (Hematoxylin and eosin; ×80.)

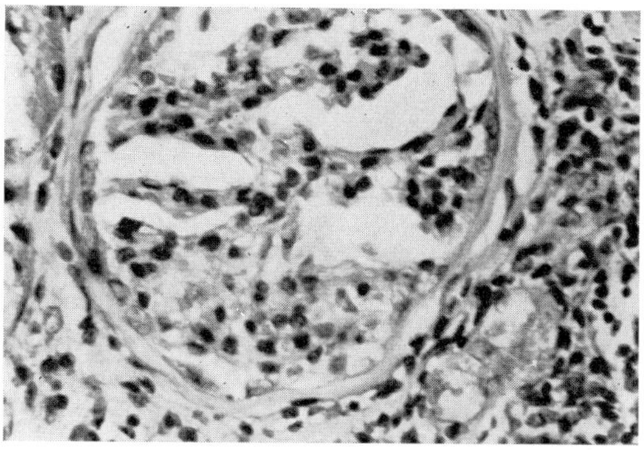

**Fig. 4.** Glomerulus from kidney homotransplant of 6-mercaptopurine-treated dog No. 398 which shows cresent formation, thickening of Bowman's capsule, and periglomerular infiltration of plasma cells. (Hematoxylin and eosin; ×330.)

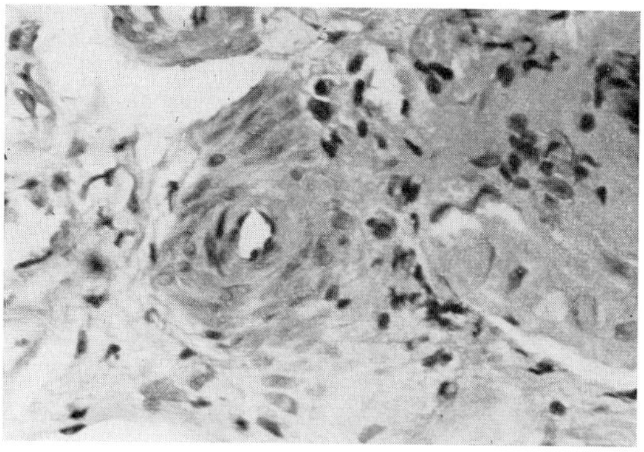

**Fig. 5.** Artery from kidney homotransplant of 6-mercaptopurine-treated dog No. 398 13 days after the last dose of the drug. (Hematoxylin and eosin; ×330.)

of at least 15 minutes each, corrected for the weight of the dog. Simultaneous studies were performed on the recipient's own kidneys on 3 occasions. The means for the P.A.H. and creatinine clearances of the recipient lie within 1 standard deviation of the values cited by Smith.[14] The mean values for the P.A.H. and creatinine clearances of the homografted kidney during the first 163 days after transplantation were 53 and 65 per cent of normal, respectively, with allowance for the fact that normal is based on 2 kidneys. After excision of the recipient's own kidneys, these clearances increased to 80 per cent of normal for P.A.H. and 110 per cent for creatinine, which suggested hypertrophy of the transplant. Blood urea nitrogen in this same dog showed a maximal rise to 32 mg. per cent after removal of the recipient's second kidney (Table IV). When 6-mercaptopurine was stopped the maximum value during the next 19 days was 26.2 mg. per cent.

**Pathology.**

*Kidney homotransplants.* Gross examination of the kidney transplants which were still functioning when the host dog died showed an absence of swelling and hemorrhage, and a minimal gain in weight (Table V). Microscopic examination showed no round-cell infiltration in one-half of these cases and minimal to moderate round-cell infiltration in the remainder (Figs. 2 and 3). In the 4 kidneys which functioned for more than 30 days there was tubular atrophy with interstitial fibrosis and thickening of the basement membrane of the capillary tufts and Bowman's capsule in many of the glomeruli (Fig. 4). A few of the arterioles showed hypertrophy of the muscularis and intimal proliferation (Fig. 5). Two of the transplants showed acute pyelonephritis. Biopsies of the kidney of dog No. 398 at 255 days when 6-mercaptopurine treatment was stopped and 13 days later both showed moderate numbers of round cells consisting principally of plasma cells as demonstrated by methyl green-pyronine stain (Figs. 6 and 7). The glomeruli, tubules, and arterioles showed

**Table II.** *Effect of 6-mercaptopurine* on Bromsulphalein excretion in dogs*

| *Dog. No.* | *BSP (mg. %)* | *Days on 6-mercaptopurine* |
|---|---|---|
| 398 | 3.0 | 89 |
| 1748 | 0.3 | 27 |
| 26 | 1.3 | 21 |
| 1750 | 0.6 | 14 |
| 1275 | 1.7 | 12 |
| 1260 | 3.7 | 13 |
| 1150 | 0.5 | 15 |
| 1262 | 1.5 | 13 |
| 1082 | 4.8 | 19 |
| Means | 1.9 | 24.8 |

*Three milligrams per kilogram daily for 9 to 10 days, then every other day.

the lesions noted in other transplants which functioned for over 30 days. Host kidneys in the above animals were normal except for acute tubular degeneration consistent with postmortem change and 1 kidney which showed minimal glomerulonephritis. Therefore, the lesions which occurred in the transplanted kidneys were not the result of 6-mercaptopurine treatment.

Transplants which stopped functioning before the death of the host showed typical gross and microscopic lesions of homograft rejection (Fig. 8). Grossly the kidneys were tensely swollen with hemorrhage at the corticomedullary junction and had increased in weight to up to 3 times their weight at transplantation. Microscopically there was dense cellular infiltration of lymphocytes, plasma cells, and some macrophages.

The spleens from treated host animals in which the kidneys were functioning at the time of death were decreased in weight in comparison to spleens from treated hosts in which transplants were re-

**Table III.** *Clearance studies on renal homograft and the recipient's kidneys in dog No. 398*

| Date | Day after grafting | Clearances (ml./min./Kg.*) Homograft P.A.H. | Homograft Creatinine | Recipient's kidneys P.A.H. | Recipient's kidneys Creatinine |
|---|---|---|---|---|---|
| June 10, 1960 | 32 | 3.9 | 1.8 | — | — |
| July 19, 1960 | 71 | 3.7 | 1.4 | — | — |
| Aug. 23, 1960 | 105 | 3.9 | 1.4 | 11.3 | 4.2 |
| Sept. 22, 1960 | 135 | 2.8 | .98 | 8.9 | 3.2 |
| Oct. 20, 1960 | 163 | 2.4 | 1.2 | 11.2 | 5.6 |
| | Mean values | 3.2 | 1.4 | 10.5 | 4.3 |
| Nov. 16, 1960 | 190 | Left nephrectomy | | — | — |
| Dec. 7, 1960 | 211 | Right nephrectomy | | — | — |
| Dec. 27, 1960 | 231 | 5.4 | 2.3 | — | — |
| Jan. 15, 1961 | 251 | 5.4 | 2.4 | — | — |
| | Normal values for a 2-kidney dog[14] | | | 13.5 ± 3.26 | 4.3 ± 1.01 |

*Homograft corrected to weight of donor dog (16.9 kilograms) and recipient's kidneys corrected to median weight of recipient dog (13.0 kilograms).

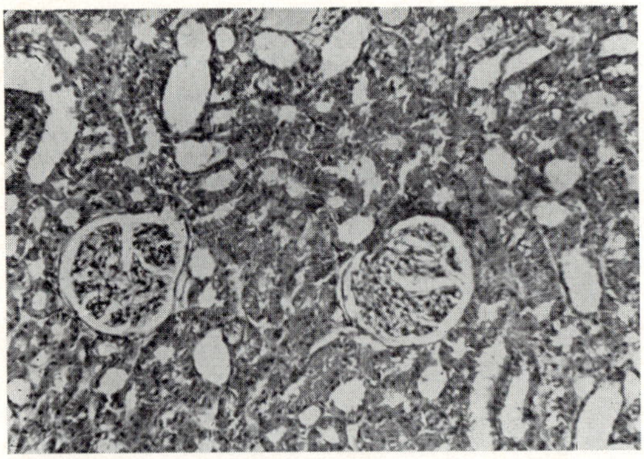

**Fig. 6.** The kidney homotransplant from dog No. 398 13 days after 6-mercaptopurine treatment had been withdrawn. (Hematoxylin and eosin; ×80.)

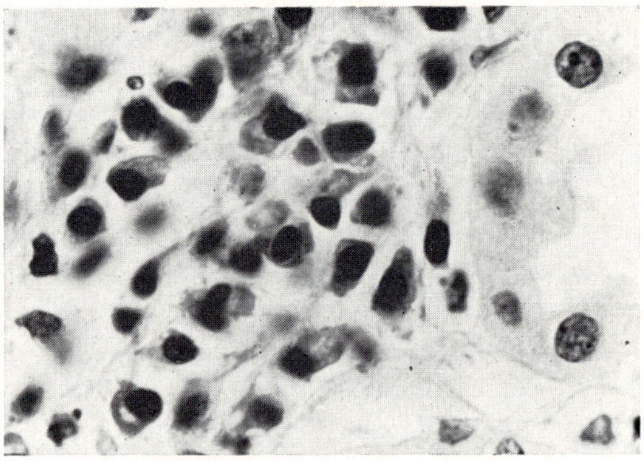

**Fig. 7.** Plasma-cell infiltrate in the cortex of dog No. 398's kidney homotransplant on the last day of 6-mercaptopurine treatment (255 days after transplantation). (Methyl green-pyronine; ×830.)

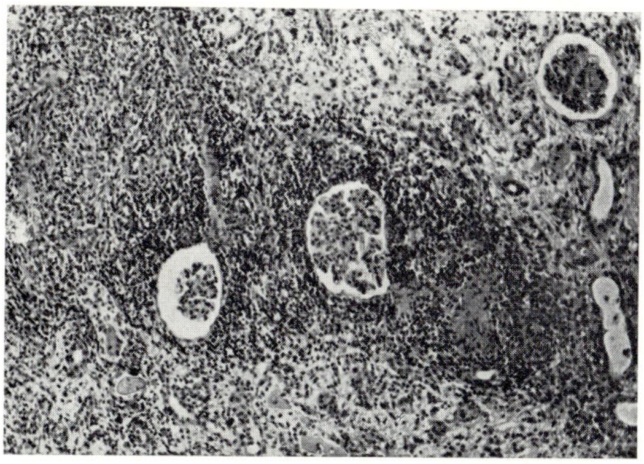

**Fig. 8.** Homotransplanted kidney from 6-mercaptopurine-treated dog No. 2048 which shows the lymphocytic and plasmacytic infiltration characteristic of the homograft reaction which was found in treated kidneys that stopped functioning. (Hematoxylin and eosin; ×80.)

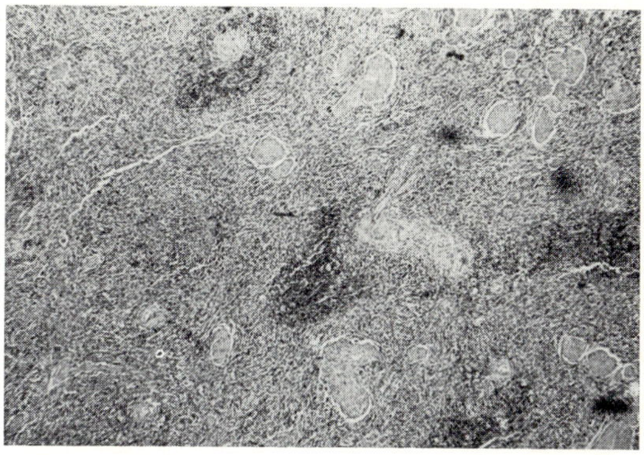

**Fig. 9.** Spleen from tolerant dog No. 2691 after 13 days of 6-mercaptopurine treatment at 5 mg. per kilogram. Note the loss of all lymph follicles except for small, irregular collections of lymphocytes. (Hematoxylin and eosin; ×30.)

**Table IV.** *Results of blood urea nitrogen determinations on kidney homograft recipient No. 398*

| *Date* | *Day after grafting* | *BUN (mg. %)* |
|---|---|---|
| Oct. 14, 1960 | 158 | 5.0 |
| Oct. 21, 1960 | 165 | 16.2 |
| Nov. 16, 1960 | 191 | 13.0 (excision of recipient's left kidney) |
| Nov. 21, 1960 | 196 | 17.5 |
| Nov. 23, 1960 | 198 | 12.0 |
| Nov. 25, 1960 | 200 | 17.0 |
| Dec. 7, 1960 | 212 | 14.0 (excision of recipient's right kidney) |
| Dec. 9, 1960 | 214 | 28.0 |
| Dec. 12, 1960 | 217 | 31.7 |
| Dec. 16, 1960 | 221 | 22.0 |
| Dec. 19, 1960 | 224 | 25.5 |
| Dec. 22, 1960 | 227 | 28.0 |
| Jan. 6, 1961 | 242 | 27.0 |
| Jan. 19, 1961 | 255 | Kidney, spleen, and lymph node biopsies, last dose of 6-mercaptopurine |
| Jan. 20, 1961 | 256 | 17.0 |
| Jan. 21, 1961 | 257 | 21.5 |
| Jan. 23, 1961 | 259 | 17.0 |
| Jan. 24, 1961 | 260 | 25.0 |
| Jan. 26, 1961 | 262 | 20.0 |
| Jan. 28, 1961 | 264 | 26.2 |
| Jan. 30, 1961 | 266 | 24.0 |
| Feb. 3, 1961 | 270 | 17.5 |
| Feb. 7, 1961 | 274 | 21.0 |

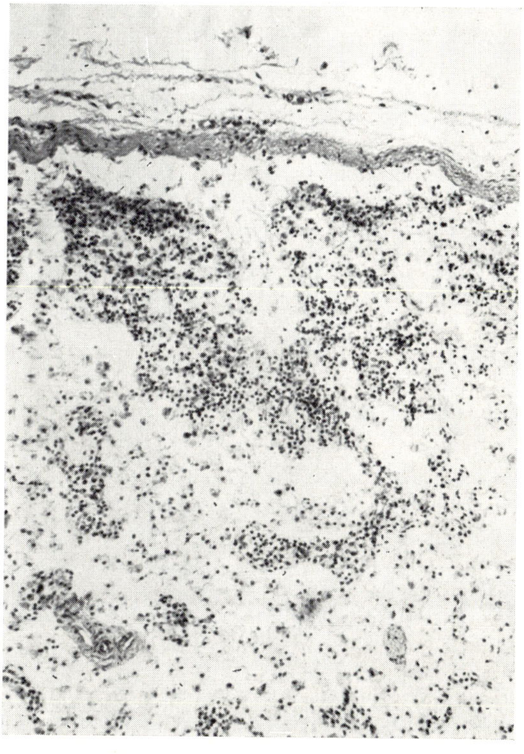

**Fig. 10.** Mesenteric lymph node from 6-mercaptopurine-treated dog No. 1750 at 70 days. Note loss of lymph follicles and thinning of the cortex and medullary cords. (Hematoxylin and eosin; ×125.)

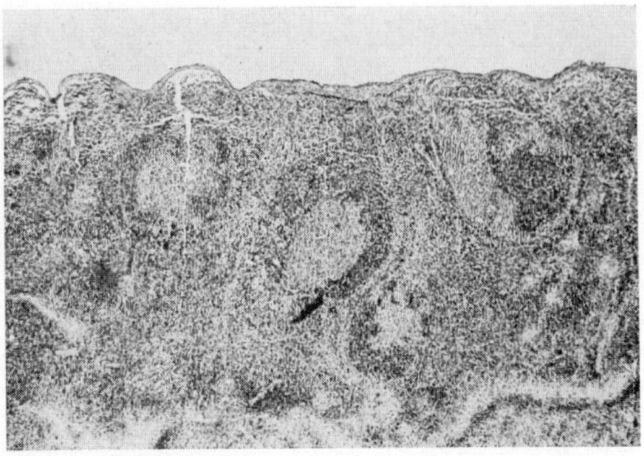

**Fig. 11.** Mesenteric lymph node from 6-mercaptopurine-treated dog No. 398 after 255 days of treatment. Note the thick cortex containing active lymph follicles with well-developed mantle zones. (Hematoxylin and eosin; ×30.)

jected. The means and standard deviations (corrected for the weight of the animal) were 1.6 ± 0.5 and 3.8 ± 1.4 Gm. per kilogram, respectively. The microscopic findings paralleled the gross. Spleens from "tolerant hosts" showed loss of most lymph follicles and absence of mitotic figures. Lymphocytes and plasma cells were more affected than reticulum cells (Fig. 9). Spleens from "intolerant" hosts showed preservation of many lymph follicles, although they were generally decreased in size and the mantle zone was absent. Mitotic figures were present in the germinal centers. Thus, the success of 6-mercaptopurine in suppressing the homograft reaction correlates well with the suppression of lymphocyte production in the spleen.

Mesenteric lymph nodes from "tolerant" hosts, although not decreased in size grossly, showed thinning of the cortex, loss of primary follicles, and decrease in the medullary cords (Fig. 10).

Dog. No. 398, in contrast with other tolerant hosts, showed primary follicles in a mesenteric lymph node and secondary follicles containing many mitotic figures in the spleen (Figs. 11 and 12).

## COMMENT

Calne[2] reported the survival of 2 renal homotransplants in nephrectomized dogs treated with 6-mercaptopurine for 21 and

**Table V.** *Pathology of renal homografts treated with 6-mercaptopurine*

| | *Dog No.* | *Initial dosage level of 6-mercaptopurine (mg./Kg.)* | *Days of function* | *Weight gain (Gm.)* | *Cellular infiltration in cortex* |
|---|---|---|---|---|---|
| Functioned until death of host | 49 | 3 | 11 | – | 0 |
| | 316 | 3 | 12 | – | 0 |
| | 2691 | 5 | 12 | – | 0 |
| | 2933 | 5 | 14 | 1.3 | 0 |
| | 2528 | 3 | 17 | 3.5 | + |
| | 3897 | 4 | 17 | 1.0 | 0 |
| | 1916 | 3 | 18 | – | + |
| | 1638 | 3 | 21 | 4.5 | 0 |
| | 26 | 3 | 31 | – | + |
| | 2937 | 5 | 31 | 0.9 | +++ |
| | 1750 | 3 | 70 | – | ++ |
| | 398* | 3 | 255+ | – | +++ |
| Stopped functioning before death of host | 2593 | 3 | 7 | 46 | ++++ |
| | 1840 | 3 | 11 | 42 | ++++ |
| | 1150 | 3 | 14 | 68 | +++ |
| | 1262 | 3 | 16 | 93 | ++++ |
| | 2122 | 3 | 17 | 118 | ++++ |
| | 2975 | 5 | 20 | 88 | ++++ |
| | 2815 | 4 | 22 | 80 | ++++ |

*Kidney is still functioning.
+ = a few scattered cells.
++ = small foci of cells.
+++ = large foci of cells.
++++ = confluent cellular infiltration.

A B
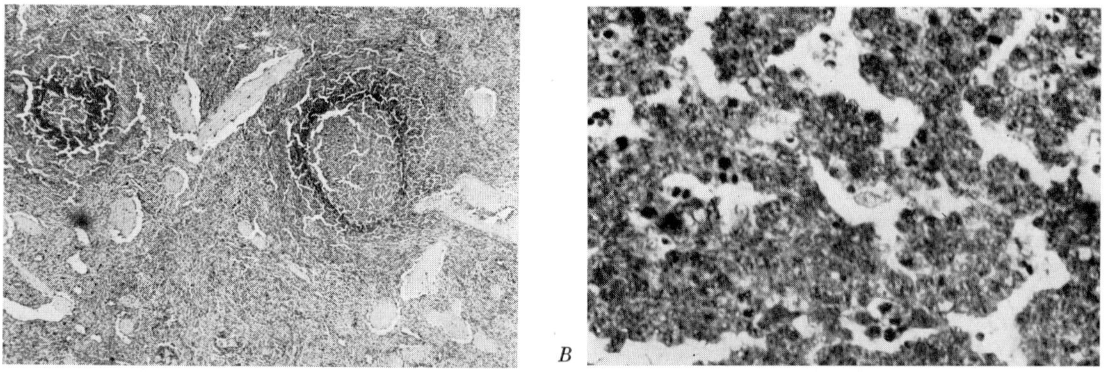

**Fig. 12.** *A*, Spleen from 6-mercaptopurine treated dog No. 398 after 255 days of treatment shows active lymph follicles with prominent mantle zones (×30). *B*, The germinal centers contain many cells undergoing mitosis (×330). (Hematoxylin and eosin.)

47 days when the dogs died of pneumonia. Blood urea levels at time of death were 40 mg. per cent. No homograft reaction was found in either transplant by microscopy.

Zukoski and colleagues[15] obtained functional survival of renal homografts in nephrectomized dogs for 25, 27, and 34 days. They also reported complete suppression of gross and microscopic evidences of the homograft reaction in 4 dogs 14 to 15 days after transplantation. Biopsies which showed only a mild reaction were obtained in 9 other treated dogs. Treatment at 5 mg. per kilogram for 14 days completely eliminated the lymph follicles in the spleen and lymph nodes. These 2 studies together with the data presented here show that 6-mercaptopurine can block the homograft reaction to kidneys in dogs, at least temporarily.

At the biochemical level 6-mercaptopurine is first converted to 6-mercaptopurine ribonucleotide by the action of a 5′-phosphate pyrophosphorylase enzyme and α-5-phosphoribosyl-pyrophosphate.[3] Evidence for the necessity of this step is that tumor cells and strains of bacteria which are resistant to 6-mercaptopurine lack this enzyme.[4, 9] The 6-mercaptopurine ribonucleotide then competatively inhibits the conversion of inosine ribonucleotide to adrenine ribonucleotide.[7, 11] It does not, however, inhibit the incorporation of adenine or adenine nucleotide into nucleic acids. One report suggested that 6-mercaptopurine might itself be incorporated into desoxyribonucleic acid and ribonucleic acid.[6] A later study, however, has failed to support this.[1]

At the cellular level, histologic studies have shown that in instances in which 6-mercaptopurine has prolonged renal homograft survival there is absence or a definite depression of lymphocytic infiltration into the graft. The mechanism by which these cells damage kidneys is not clear, but the presence of glomerular and arteriolar lesions in kidney homografts which survive for more than 30 days suggests that these structures may be involved in addition to the tubules as sites for the action of the lymphocytes. In addition, production of lymphocytes in the spleen and lymph nodes is dramatically de-

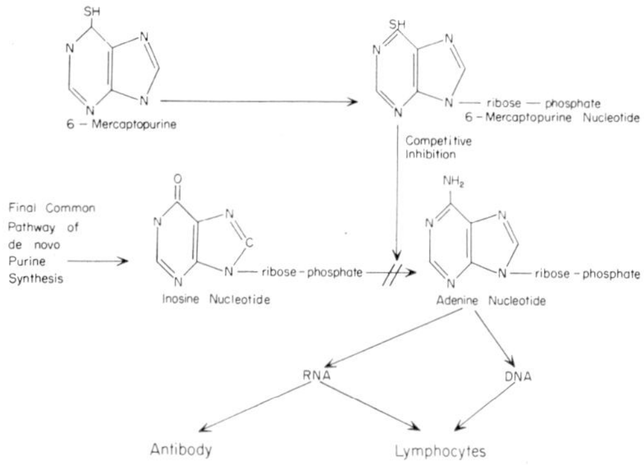


**Fig. 13.** Site of action of 6-mercaptopurine in blocking the homograft rejection mechanism.

pressed in most instances when the reaction in the graft has been prevented. Cells which are produced may be ineffectual in damaging the graft because of blockade of their production of antibody secondary to reduction of ribonucleic acid synthesis by 6-mercaptopurine. These relationships are summarized in Fig. 13.

## SUMMARY

1. In 51 dogs treated with 6-mercaptopurine, 15 renal homografts survived for 15 days or more. One of these is still functioning after 400 days.

2. The homograft reaction can be prevented temporarily by 6-mercaptopurine in some dogs, as confirmed by both gross and microscopic criteria.

3. Four renal homografts which functioned for more than 30 days showed glomerular and arteriolar lesions in addition to tubular lesions and round-cell infiltration.

4. The mechanism of action of 6-mercaptopurine is discussed.

The authors wish to express their appreciation for the helpful advice of Dr. S. J. Zak and the technical assistance of Mr. A. LeDoux, Miss D. Melcher, Mr. J. Maney, and Mrs. R. Weiner.

### REFERENCES

1. Brockman, R. W.: Mechanism of resistance to 6-mercaptopurine: metabolism of hypoxanthine and 6-mercaptopurine by sensitive and resistant neoplasms, Cancer Res. **20:** 643, 1960.
2. Calne, R. Y.: The rejection of renal homografts inhibition in dogs by 6-mercaptopurine, Lancet **1:** 417, 1960.
3. Carter, C. E.: Reaction of 6-mercaptopurine with inosine- and with guanosine-5′-phosphate pyrophosphorylase purified from *E. coli,* Biochem. Pharmacol. **2:** 105, 1959.
4. Davidson, J. D.: Studies on the mechanism of action of 6-mercaptopurine in sensitive and resistant L1210 leukemia in vitro, Cancer Res. **20:** 225, 1960.
5. Dempster, W. J.: Kidney homotransplantation, Brit. J. Surg. **40:** 447, 1953.
6. Elion, G. B., Bieber, S., and Hitchings, G. H.: The fate of 6-mercaptopurine in mice, Ann. New York Acad. Sc. **60:** 297, 1954.
7. Hakala, M. T., and Nichol, C. A.: Studies on the mode of action of 6-mercaptopurine and its ribonucleoside on mammalian cells in culture, J. Biol. Chem. **234:** 3224, 1959.
8. Lapchinsky, A. G.: Recent results of experimental transplantation of preserved limbs and kidneys and possible use of this technique in clinical practice, Ann. New York Acad. Sc. **87:** 539, 1960.
9. Lieberman, I., and Ove, P.: Enzyme studies with mutant mammalian cells, J. Biol. Chem. **235:** 1765, 1960.
10. Meeker, W., Condie, R., Weiner, D., Varco, R., and Good, R.: Prolongation of skin homograft survival in rabbits by 6-mercaptopurine, Proc. Soc. Exper. Biol. & Med. **102:** 459, 1959.
11. Salser, J. S., Hutchison, D. J., and Balis, M. E.: Studies on the mechanism of action of 6-mercaptopurine in cell-free preparations, J. Biol. Chem. **235:** 429, 1960.
12. Schwartz, R., Dameshek, W., and Donovan, J.: The effect of 6-mercaptopurine on homograft reactions, J. Clin. Invest. **39:** 952, 1960.
13. Schwartz, R., Stock, J., and Dameshek, W.: Effect of 6-mercaptopurine on antibody production, Proc. Soc. Exper. Biol. & Med. **99:** 164, 1958.
14. Smith, H.: Principles of renal physiology, New York, 1956, Oxford University Press, p. 32.
15. Zukoski, C. F., Lee, H. M., and Hume, D. M.: The prolongation of functional survival of canine renal homografts by 6-mercaptopurine, S. Forum **11:** 470, 1960.

## DISCUSSION

**C. F. Zukoski** (Richmond, Va.). In our studies on the effect of 6-mercaptopurine on functional survival of renal homotransplants, bilateral nephrectomies were performed in the dogs at the time of the transplantation. As controls for these studies, bilaterally nephrectomized dogs with no renal homograft lived an average of 7.5 days. Ten dogs with bilateral nephrectomy and a renal homograft without 6-mercaptopurine therapy lived an average of 15 days. In the dogs given 6-mercaptopurine therapy, 3 of 18 lived for 32, 42, and 66 days with normal blood urea nitrogen. We have not noticed the glomerular lesions which Dr. Pierce mentioned.

**Dr. Willard E. Goodwin** (Los Angeles, Calif.). Drs. Pierce and Varco are to be complimented on an interesting and timely piece of work. It is from efforts such as this that we may someday learn to deal with the homograft rejection reaction.

We continue to be extremely interested in the problem of renal homotransplantation. Dr. Matt Mims, one of our residents, had a canine homotransplanted kidney which lived for 114 days after transplantation and was normal at the time of the death of the animal. The significant thing about this experiment, we think, was that the recipient had received chyle lymphocytes from the donor in large amounts before, during, and after the transplantation. We do not know why this allowed the unrelated homotransplanted kidney to live longer than the expected time, but we believe that in some way it affected the rejection reaction.

I also want to mention briefly a recent homotransplantation experience in a patient. A 22-year-old girl was the recipient of her mother's kidney in September, 1960. Before transplantation, an attempt was made to reduce the circulating lymphocytes by the administration of nitrogen mustard followed by Cytoxan, which was later followed by renal homotransplantation. The initial result was satisfactory. However, after about a month, she began to reject her mother's kidney as expected. This rejection was halted by massive doses of corticosteroids (specifically, prednisone, 200 mg. a day). She died 20 weeks and 3 days after the transplantation of pneumonia and overwhelming sepsis which could not be controlled during the administration of the massive doses of adrenal steroids.

You will note that she did not survive as long as Dr. David Hume's untreated patient, who lived 5½ months with a homotransplanted kidney from an unrelated donor. The significant things that we think we learned from this adventure in human renal homotransplantation were that (1) renal decapsulation at the time of the original operation was helpful, (2) the lymphocytes could be depressed with nitrogen mustard and this may have had some effect, and (3) massive doses of adrenal corticosteroids are capable of postponing rejection for weeks and even months. Although similar experiments have been tried in animals with smaller doses of cortisone, the prolongation of the rejection period was very slight. Before this experience, we did not realize that it was possible to block the rejection in this way.

Since genetic and immunologic factors governing the rejection reaction seem at present to be unmodifiable in the human being, it seems to us that a possible future solution may follow the sort of excellent work and approach we have heard this morning from Drs. Pierce and Varco. In addition to suppression of the rejection reaction by various poisonous drugs, it may be hoped that rejection can be delayed by the use of steroids until a possible adaptation may take place.

**Dr. J. C. Pierce** (closing). I would like to thank Drs. Zukowski and Goodwin for their remarks and to report the latest studies on dog No. 398. 6-Mercaptopurine treatment was stopped 3 weeks ago, at which time the transplant had functioned for 255 days. A biopsy 2 weeks later showed no appreciable increase in cellular infiltration of the transplant. Two and one half weeks after withdrawal of 6-mercaptopurine, 197 ml. of urine was collected which showed a trace of protein. The blood urea nitrogen was 21 mg. per cent. It is too early yet to know whether the kidney is slowly rejecting or whether tolerance has been induced.

# Perfusion and replacement of the canine liver

PAUL J. KESTENS, M.D.
WILLIAM V. McDERMOTT, JR., M.D.
BOSTON, MASS.
*From the Department of Surgery, Harvard Medical School, and the Surgical Services, Massachusetts General Hospital*

With the advent of satisfactory pump-oxygenator systems for use in extracorporeal circulation, satisfactory metabolic studies in isolated and perfused organs and systems should prove feasible. Our initial studies in the isolated and perfused canine liver have been reported.[2] Maintenance of a normal liver by perfusion techniques has proved particularly troublesome in the dog because of the frequency, in fact almost the inevitability, of the "outflow block" phenomenon. This problem has driven many investigators to utilize other species which may not be as available or as satisfactory in size. The history of efforts at perfusion of the mammalian liver has been reviewed and the results evaluated in terms of flow, oxygen consumption, and so forth.[3]

In the course of more than 100 attempts at perfusion of canine livers, it has been possible to overcome the "outflow block" phenomenon and to maintain a normally functioning organ for as long as 8 hours.

Because of the potentialities of utilization of this type of technique for tumor perfusion in man, the hepatectomized host dog has been maintained during the perfusion and replacement of the liver attempted in 16 of the experiments.

Selected studies from the last 36 perfusions will be reported in detail.

Supported by United States Public Health Grant No. A-362 (C 8) and by the Medical Foundation of Boston.

Read at the Twenty-second Annual Meeting of the Society of University Surgeons, Kansas City, Kan., Feb. 9-11, 1961.

## METHODS

In the last 36 isolated liver perfusions, a standardized technique has been used in which both hepatic artery and portal vein have been perfused with blood under physiologic conditions of pressure and oxygen saturation. The outflow was collected by gravity in a graduated reservoir (I), pumped to a second reservoir (II), and filtered. From there, the circuit was divided, with a portion going directly to the portal reservoir (III) and a portion going to the disc oxygenator. The oxygenated blood was again divided with a portion going to reservoir III to provide a mixture of venous and oxygenated blood for the portal inflow and the remainder passing to the second pump to provide fully oxygenated blood for the arterial inflow. The exact details of the equipment, operative procedure, and method of isolation and perfusion are described minutely in a previous report[3] and need not be repeated here. A schematic representation of the circuit is shown in Fig. 1. The circuit is similar to that used with the previously described standardized technique but has the addition of a splanchnic bypass from the splenic vein to the left jugular vein as well as from the infrahepatic vena cava to the right jugular vein. These bypasses are essential to the maintenance of the hepatectomized host if replant is to be attempted. All experiments were carried out in the special operating room of the vascular laboratories, where the temperature of the entire room could be controlled and studies carried out at either normothermic or hypothermic levels.

Flow rates were measured directly or by means of calibrated pumps, and pressures were read from manometers at appropriate points in the circuit.

Plasma pH levels were determined immediately in the operating room on a Beckman pH meter. Other biochemical determinations (total carbon dioxide, oxygen saturation, glucose, lactate, parameters of liver function, and so forth) were carried out by standard techniques.

## RESULTS

In the last 36 isolated perfusions carried out by the standardized technique described, there were 2 failures due to technical errors. In the remaining 34 experiments, flow rates were highly satisfactory once circulation was well established. In 16 of the perfusions which were carried on for 4 hours or more, and in which no experiments were introduced which might alter flow or pressure significantly, reasonably normal indices were maintained. In Fig. 2, the average flows, pressures, pH, carbon dioxide tension, and carbon dioxide levels are recorded with the range of measurement recorded during the 16 isolated perfusions. The average outflow from the liver has been over 400 ml. per minute (about 1.2 ml. per minute per gram of liver tissue in these animals). The flow rates were considerably higher than any pub-

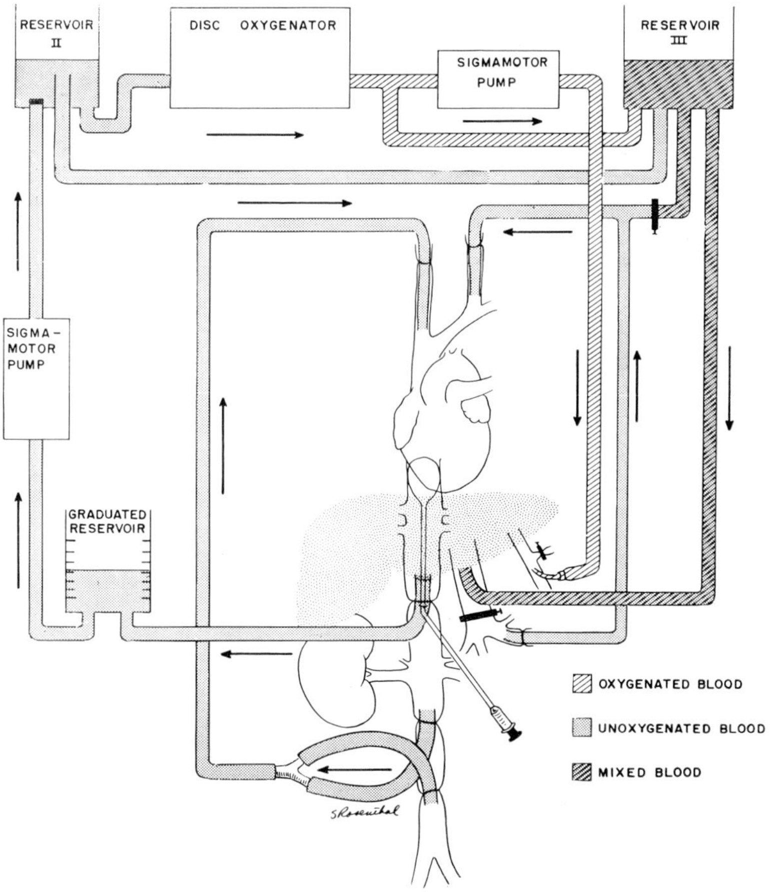


**Fig. 1.** A diagrammatic representation of the system used for total isolation, perfusion, and replacement of the canine liver.

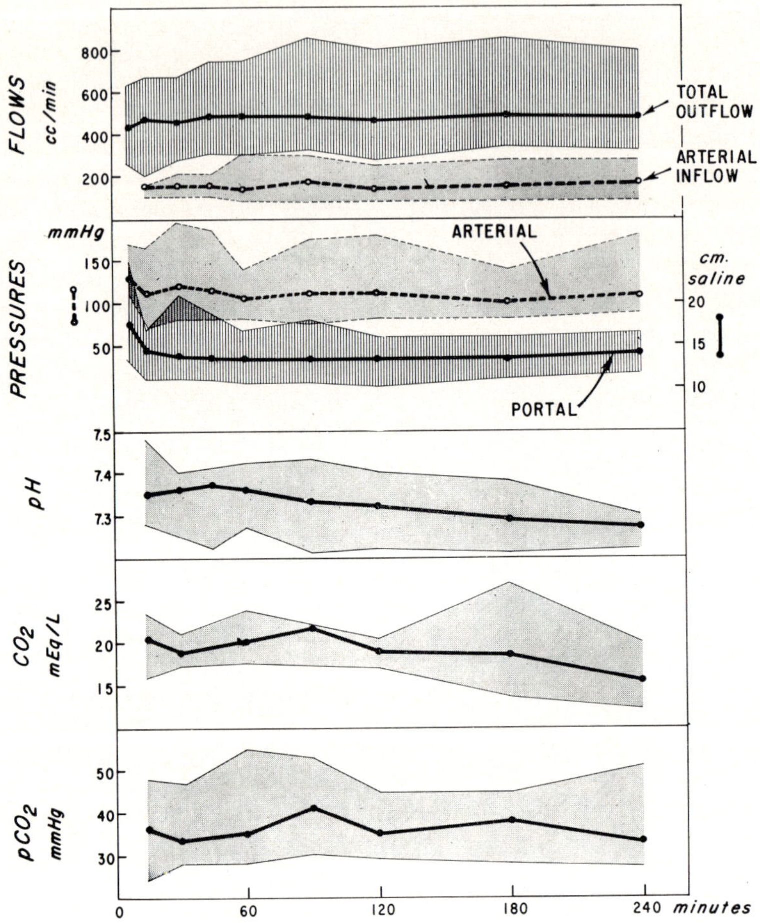


**Fig. 2.** Selected indices in 16 liver perfusions.

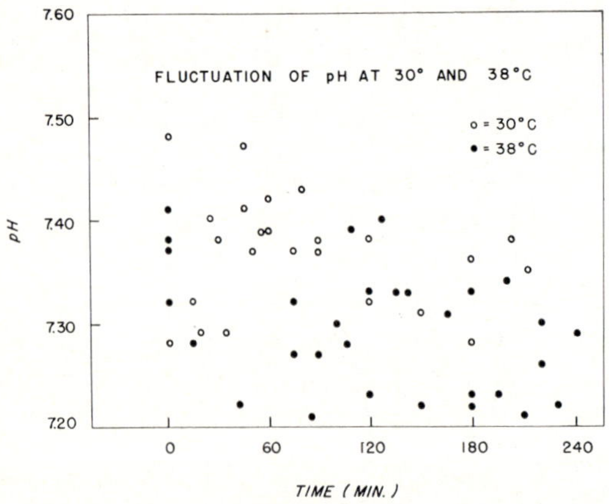


**Fig. 3.** Changes in pH which occur during perfusion under normothermic and hypothermic conditions.

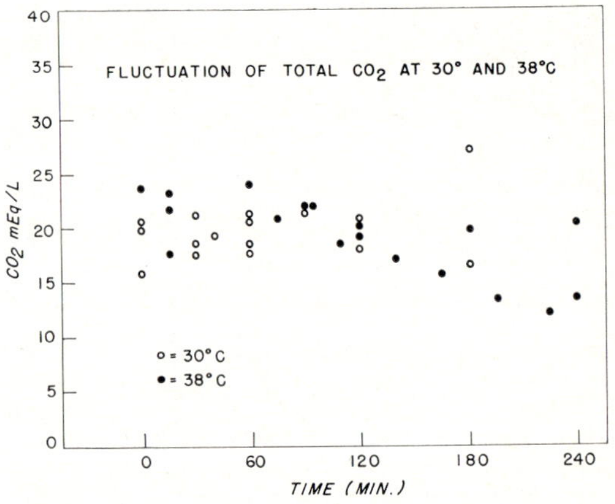


**Fig. 4.** Changes in total carbon dioxide which occur during perfusion under normothermic and hypothermic conditions.

lished data on any species which has come to our attention and fall within the range reported in studies on the intact dog by Blalock and Mason.[1]

The pH levels always showed a tendency to fall but were maintained within normal range by the addition of bicarbonate every 30 minutes; the amount added varied according to the change in pH, but the average was 8 mEq. per hour. It is not surprising that the induction of hypothermia (30° C.) by alteration of the temperature of the room prevented the fall in pH which invariably occurred at normothermic levels unless bicarbonate was added at regular intervals. These data are shown in a scattergram (Fig. 3).

The carbon dioxide and the carbon dioxide tension values were also well maintained with only a very slight fall during a 4-hour perfusion period. Unless bicarbonate is added, however, the carbon dioxide content tends to fall during a perfusion and over the period of 4 hours, a change of 6 to 10 mEq. per liter may be observed. At hypothermic levels (30° C.), however, no appreciable change occurs (Fig. 4).

Liver function was well maintained as indicated by bile excretion of 8 ml. per hour with over 90 per cent of bilirubin in the conjugated form, excellent clearance of added ammonia, and bromsulphthalein retention of 6 per cent or less in 45 minutes. Transaminase levels in general were not elevated, although on a few occasions, particularly toward the end of a long perfusion, there was a tendency for the level to rise.

Oxygen consumption averaged better than 15 ml. per minute (0.04 ml. per minute per gram of liver) under normothermic conditions, which testifies to the excellent metabolic rate maintained during the perfusion.

**The "outflow block" phenomenon.** A number of factors appeared to induce an "outflow block" in our early perfusions and the picture of a dark, congested liver with increasing resistance and decreasing flow occurred with discouraging frequency. Eventually this barrier to successful perfusion studies disappeared when a standard-

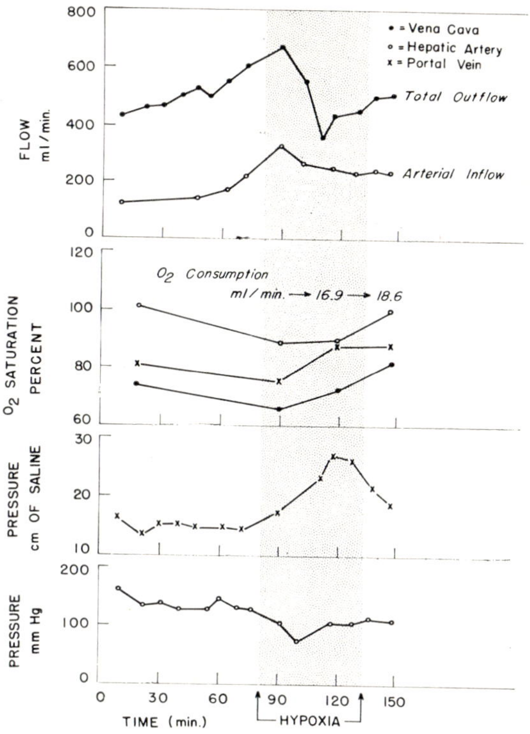


**Fig. 5.** Effect of anoxia on flow and pressure in the perfused liver.

ized and technically satisfactory method was established in which pH, oxygenation, carbon dioxide, and carbon dioxide tension levels were maintained in the normal range. In our experience, satisfactory perfusions and the maintenance of a metabolically normal liver could not be maintained by perfusion through the portal vein alone, even when fully oxygenated blood was used. Hypoxia, induced by lowering the oxygen saturation of hepatic arterial blood, caused a rapid fall in total outflow, a rise in portal pressure and in portal bed resistance, and the typical picture of a blue, congested liver. There was no significant change in arterial pressure, flow, or resistance (Fig. 5). The effects of a low carbon dioxide tension, induced by use of 100 per cent oxygen in the oxygenator, were quite different, however. Under these circumstances the outflow also decreased but the portal pressure and flow remained constant. There was less congestion but the arterial inflow decreased and the

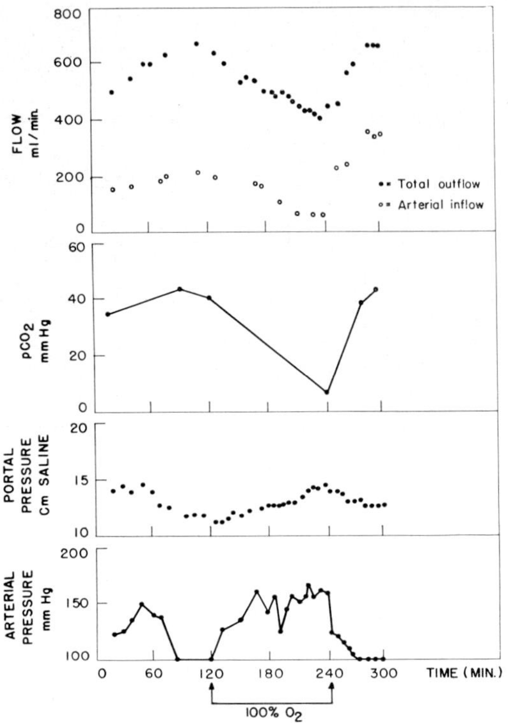


**Fig. 6.** Effect of low carbon dioxide tension on flow and pressure in the perfused liver.

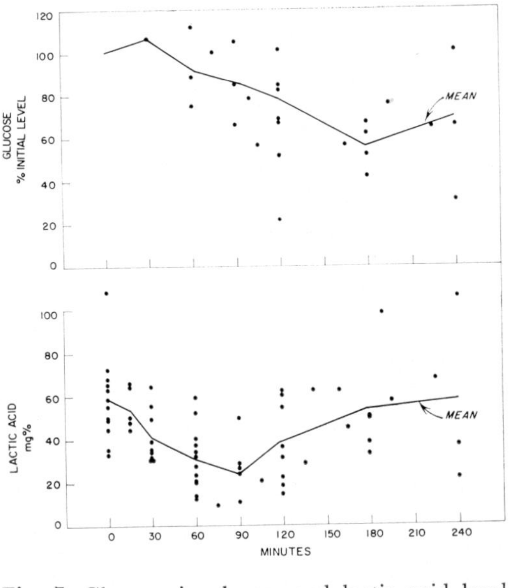


**Fig. 7.** Changes in glucose and lactic acid levels during perfusion of the liver.

arterial pressure and resistance rose (Fig. 6). Eventually this sequence of events resulted in progressive liver anoxia and an increasing resistance in the portal bed also, but even after a period of 2 hours, restoration of normal flow could be achieved if the carbon dioxide tension was restored to normal.

**Carbohydrate metabolism.** Frequent measurements of blood glucose and lactic acid levels were made during a number of the satisfactory perfusions. The results are shown in Fig. 7. Because infusions of glucose were given during operation and before the actual isolation of the liver, the initial levels were quite variable; therefore changes have been shown as per cent of the initial level in order to maintain uniformity in the presentation of the data. It is of particular interest that glucose levels fell steadily during the first 3 hours of perfusion and even after that showed only a slight tendency to rise. This indicates that the liver was utilizing glucose at a rapid rate and these observations are confirmed by liver biopsy before and after perfusion (Fig. 8). These histologic sections and special staining with periodic acid oxidation, followed by Schiff's reagent with a saliva control, showed that a tremendous accumulation of glycogen in the hepatic cells had occurred. A metabolically unsatisfactory liver perfusion results in the release of glucose rather than the synthesis of glycogen. This has been characteristic in previous reports in which this aspect of the metabolism of the perfused liver has been discussed. To our knowledge, this is the first perfusion preparation in which glycogenesis has been accomplished.

Lactic acid levels in the perfusate also fell during the initial phases, although levels in stored blood from the donor measured at the same time rose steadily. After about 1½ hours, however, lactic acid levels, in distinction to glucose levels, began a slow, steady rise which necessitated maintenance of a normal pH with added bicarbonate as previously mentioned. This pattern occurred at hypothermic levels (Figs. 9 and 10) even though oxygen utilization was considerably depressed.

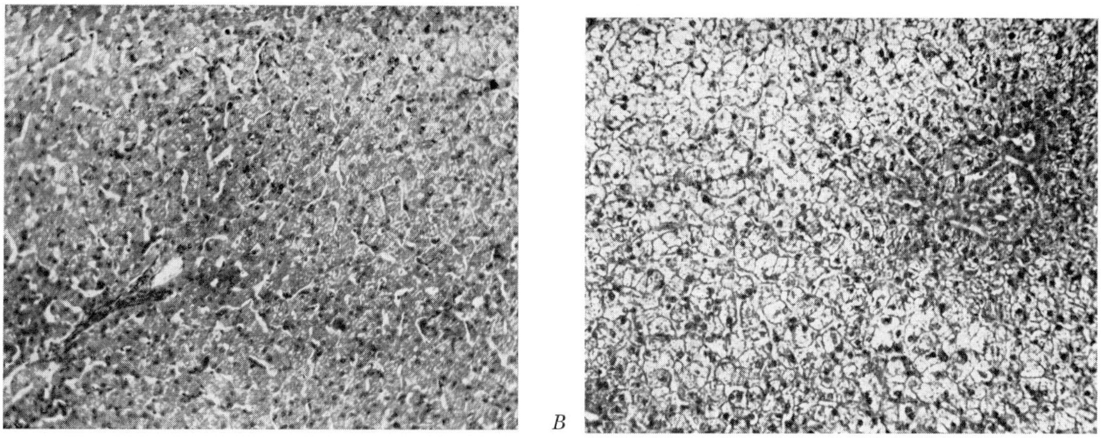

A B

**Fig. 8.** Microscopic sections of the liver which show the tremendous increase in glycogen during perfusion. *A,* Before perfusion. *B,* After perfusion.

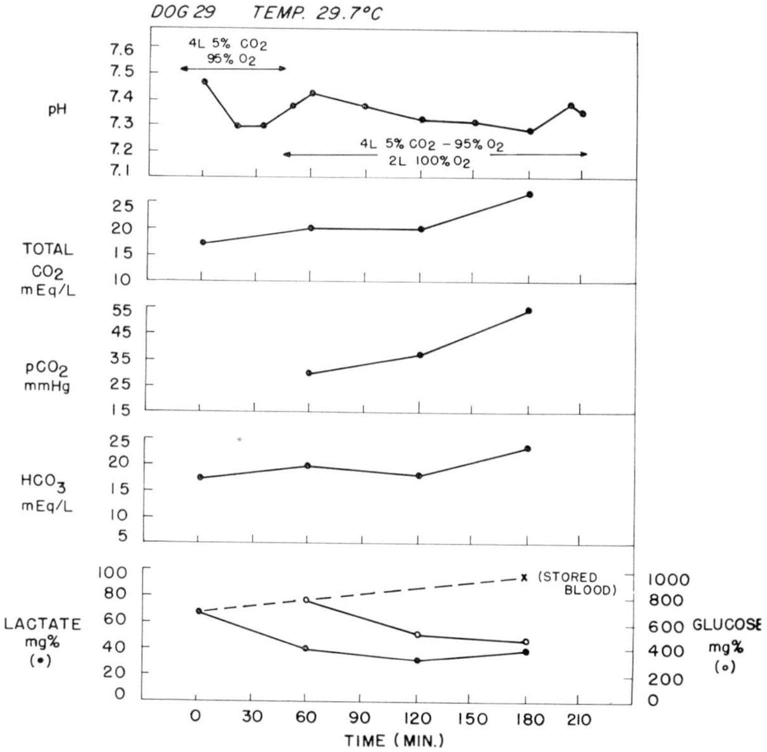


**Fig. 9.** Changes in glucose and lactic acid levels during perfusion and changes in lactic acid levels of stored blood under hypothermic conditions.

It is difficult to draw any conclusions from a single experiment but the effects of glucagon and insulin were tested in 1 perfusion after preliminary studies on flow and carbon dioxide tension changes had been investigated. When normal flow was re-established, successive injections of glucagon and insulin were given in the hepatic arterial inflow (Fig. 11). This appeared to result in a rise in glucose level after injection of

**Table I.** *Liver function after replacement of the perfused canine livers*

| Dog | Duration of perfusion | Ammonia ($\gamma$ %) | | BSP retention (%) | | Serum glutamic oxaloacetic transaminase (U.) | |
|---|---|---|---|---|---|---|---|
| | | 2 weeks | 3-10 months | 2 weeks | 3-10 months | 2 weeks | 3-10 months |
| $P_1$ | 75 | 107 | — | 22 | — | — | — |
| $P_3$ | 150 | 107 | 72 | 8 | 1 | 25 | 20 |
| $P_{14}$ | 60 | | 87 | 1 | 1 | 25 | 50 |
| $P_{25}$ | 90 | 95 | 85 | 7 | 4 | 330 | — |
| $P_{27}$ | 180 | | — | 7 | — | 338 | — |

glucagon and a fall after insulin injection. The second dose of insulin, however, had no apparent effect. During this whole phase of the experiment there was an unexpected decrease in lactic acid levels even though pH levels were falling with the re-institution of the carbon dioxide–oxygen mixture in the oxygenator.

**Replantation of the perfused liver.** In 16 of the experiments, the hepatectomized animal was supported during the period of isolation and perfusion of the liver, and then the liver was restored to its normal location. This added to the complexities of the apparatus, required additional shunts to prevent splanchnic pooling (Fig. 1), and presented additional metabolic and coagulation problems in the donor animals. There were 8 deaths in the immediate postoperative period, 4 of which were due to technical problems and 2 to a persistent and refractory clotting defect. There were 3 late deaths, 1 of which was due to hemorrhagic pancreatitis. The other 2 dogs showed no recognizable cause of death. Thus, there were 5 long-term survivors available for study and observations. The results of liver function tests are given in Table I. Except for elevations in the glutamic–oxaloacetic transaminase in the early postoperative period, the replanted liver maintained satisfactory function and the dogs appeared healthy and well nourished. All 5 long-term survivals were sacrificed at intervals ranging from 3 to 10 months and microscopic sections showed normal liver cells and architecture. There were no thrombotic occlusions in any of the re-established vascular pathways.

## COMMENT

These studies as reported can be divided into 3 major phases, (1) the technical and metabolic aspects inherent in the establishment of a satisfactory perfusion system which would permit maintenance of the normally functioning liver totally isolated from the animal, (2) preliminary metabolic studies designed to make use of this experimental tool to clarify various problems in liver physiology, and (3) technical problems associated with replantation of the isolated liver after a period of perfusion.

The major problem which has been encountered over the years by investigators who attempted to establish an isolated liver for perfusion purposes was the frequent occurrence of an "outflow block" which prevented a satisfactory perfusion and resulted in a liver unsatisfactory for metabolic studies. The phenomenon of the "outflow block" is most prominent in the dog and has led other investigators to seek other species for perfusion experiments. It may well be that the sphincter mechanisms described in the hepatic veins of the dog contribute to this problem, but by the time a standardized system of creating a satisfactory perfusion system in the canine liver had been established, it became apparent that there is no single mysterious factor which was the cause of this block. Failure of proper oxygenation

| *Albumin/globulin (Gm. %)* | | *Bilirubin (mg. %)* | | *Alkaline phosphatase (Bodansky units)* | | *Thymol turbidity (U.)* | |
|---|---|---|---|---|---|---|---|
| *2 weeks* | *3-10 months* | *2 weeks* | *3-10 months* | *2 weeks* | *3-10 months* | *2 weeks* | *3-10 months* |
| — | — | — | — | — | — | — | — |
| — | 4.6/1.7 | — | 0.2 | 12.4 | 3.6 | — | 1.5 |
| 3.3/1.8 | 4.4/1.7 | 0.2 | 0.4 | 2.2 | 5.6 | — | — |
| 3.6/1.6 | 3.3/2.3 | 0.2 | 0.4 | 16.2 | 3.3 | 0.3 | — |
| — | 4.3/1.8 | — | — | 21.0 | — | — | — |

is probably the most important factor. Even a very transient period of anoxia of the liver will result in an "outflow block" in the intrahepatic portal bed and the liver will become swollen, blue, and congested. Once this occurs it is frequently irreversible, although on occasions, by careful adjustment of the inflow circuits, it has been possible to re-establish a good flow and to decompress gradually the congested intrahepatic vascular bed. If a rapid and smooth transfer can be accomplished from the normal inflow to the liver to the perfusion circuit, success can be expected in a large percentage of cases and an outflow of 400 ml. per minute can be expected and maintained for many hours.

These studies have demonstrated some of the factors which affect the flow through the liver. A period of hypoxia of 30 to 60 minutes' duration results in a steady fall in the total outflow from the perfused liver and a rise in the portal pressure. The arterial inflow and pressure remain constant during this metabolic alteration. These changes are reversible when oxygen is again introduced. If total anoxia occurs, however, or if prolonged hypoxia (greater than 90 minutes) is carried out, the liver will become increasingly blue and congested and gradually an irreversible stage of "outflow block" is reached which renders further attempts at restoration of normal flow impossible.

Induction of low carbon dioxide tension in the perfusion circuit by eliminating carbon dioxide from the oxygenator has a different effect. Again the total outflow decreases as the carbon dioxide tension falls, but under these circumstances the portal pressure and flow remain constant and the deficit in total flow is attributable almost entirely to the decrease in arterial inflow. Concomitant with the decrease in arterial inflow, the pressure rises in the arterial circuit which indicates that a block has been established in the arteriolar intrahepatic vascular bed.

While undoubtedly almost any metabolic abnormality will affect the perfused liver and induce alterations in pressure and flow in the various components of the complex intrahepatic vascular bed, the alterations induced by hypoxia and by low carbon dioxide tension appear to be the most consistently reproducible. As might be expected, however, for a satisfactory perfusion, it is essential to maintain a normal pH as well as satisfactory oxygenation and carbon dioxide tension.

Since the major portion of our efforts over the past 2 years has been directed toward the establishment of a satisfactory perfusion of the canine liver and study of the metabolic factors which may alter pressure and flow in the various circuits, specific metabolic studies directed toward liver function under these circumstances have been preliminary in nature. The most interesting observations to date have been concerned with carbohydrate metabolism. It has been extremely interesting and encouraging that, as described in the results of the experiments, this isolated and perfused liver utilizes glucose in the formation of glycogen at a highly satisfactory rate. During perfusions of up to 3 hours there has been a steady fall in the initial glucose level. In the past, isolated and perfused livers have almost invariably shown a production of glucose from stored glycogen and attempts to establish a positive delta across the perfused liver bed have been unsuccessful. Apparently this is a very sensitive index of liver function and the formation of glycogen requires a liver which functions at very nearly normal levels. After roughly 3 hours of perfusion, it has been quite common to see the glucose level rise again, which suggests that after this period of time and despite continued satisfactory outflow, liver function begins to fail to some extent and the previously synthesized glycogen begins to release glucose back into the circuit. Concomitant studies with lactic acid have shown that during the initial phases of perfusion lactic acid levels will fall steadily which indicates metabolism by the liver of the lactic acid which is formed by glycolysis in the red blood cells. After about 1½ hours of perfusion, however, the lactic acid levels begin to rise steadily during the remaining period of the perfusion. The exact reasons for this remain to be clarified. It is possible that the metabolism of glucose and lactic acid by the isolated liver is competitive. Some preliminary studies suggest that lactic acid may be cleared more rapidly and over a longer period of time in a circuit of relative hypoglycemia.

Preliminary studies of the effect of glucagon and insulin on this isolated liver are presented mainly to demonstrate some of the areas which can be studied effectively with this preparation. These initial studies and others in progress suggest that there is a very definite effect of insulin on the iso-

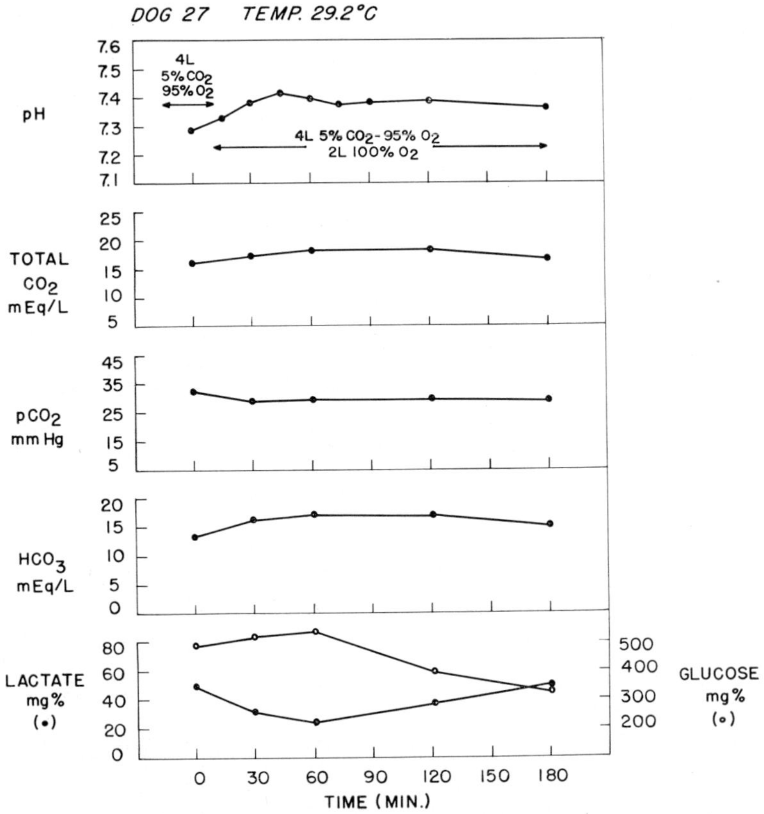


**Fig. 10.** Changes in glucose and lactic acid levels during perfusion under hypothermic conditions.

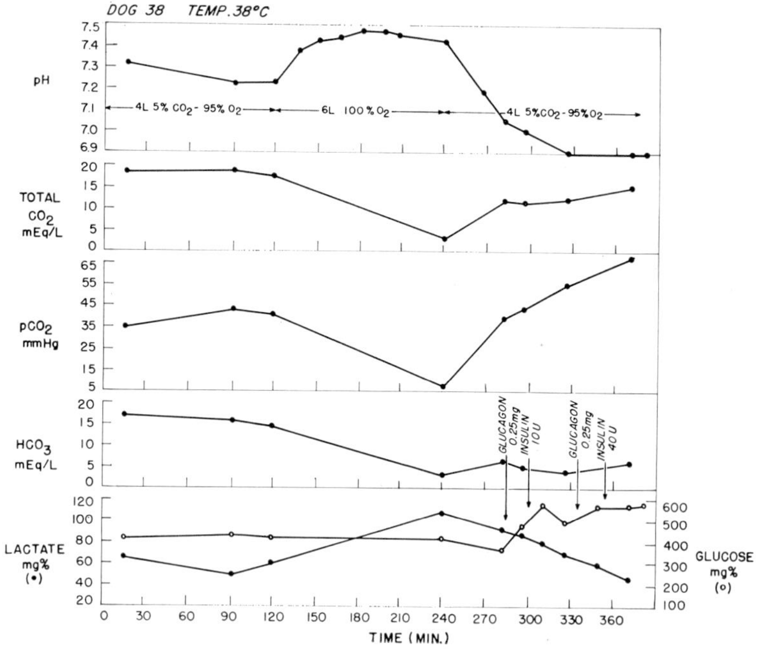


**Fig. 11.** Effect of glucagon and insulin on blood glucose and lactic acid levels during perfusion.

lated liver, a point which has been controversial for many years.

The observations made on replacement of the isolated and perfused liver relate in many ways to the excellent studies on homotransplantation of the canine liver carried out by Moore and his associates.[4] These confirm the technical feasibility of transplantation of the liver once the immunologic block associated with homotransplantation has been solved. These replacement studies were also carried out with a view toward studying the feasibility, dosage levels, and types of perfusion circuits which could be utilized in man for the treatment of isolated malignant disease of the liver, either primary or metastatic. The technical and metabolic problems of maintaining an isolated and perfused liver simultaneously with the maintenance of a hepatectomized donor, followed by restoration of the normal vascular circuits, are obvious. The success rate in these experiments was not high, but certainly demonstrated the complete feasibility of achieving success in an increasing percentage of cases.

## SUMMARY AND CONCLUSIONS

1. A technique of isolation and prolonged perfusion of the canine liver in which both inflow tracts are utilized has been described. The establishment of normal flow and pressure and the maintenance of normal pH, oxygen consumption, and carbon dioxide tension during the perfusion, as well as the support of normal liver function during the procedure, have been described.

2. Preliminary studies of carbohydrate metabolism in the isolated and perfused liver have been reported. Demonstration of the feasibility of maintaining glycogenesis in this preparation is stressed.

3. The feasibility of restoring the isolated liver to the hepatectomized donor animal after a period of a prolonged perfusion is described.

### REFERENCES

1. Blalock, A., and Mason, M. F.: Observations on the blood flow and gaseous metabolism of the liver of unanesthetized dogs, Am. J. Physiol. **117:** 328-334, 1936.
2. Kestens, P. J., Austen, W. G., and McDermott, W. V., Jr.: Biochemical and physiological

studies on the viable extracorporeal liver, S. Forum **10:** 225-229, 1960.

3. Kestens, P. J., Farrelley, J., and McDermott, W. V., Jr.: A technique of isolation and perfusion of the canine liver, J. Surg. Res. **1:** 58, 1961.
4. Moore, F. D., Wheeler, H. B., Demissianos, H. V., Smith, U., Balankura, O., Abel, K., Greenberg, J. B., and Dammin, G. J.: Experimental whole-organ transplantation of the liver and of the spleen, Ann. Surg. **152:** 374-387, 1960.

## DISCUSSION

**Dr. Ben Eiseman** (Denver, Colo.). During the past 2 years our studies have centered about pump-oxygenator perfusion of the pig liver completely isolated and removed from the donor animal. I wish to make 6 very brief comments. (1) We, too, have been plagued by the temporary outflow block that occurs near the onset of perfusion and which is of uncertain etiology. As experience has increased, it has become less of a problem. Our impression is that avoidance of liver hypoxia by perfusion of the hepatic artery via a long limb from the oxygenator prior to cutting off portal venous flow is of most benefit in the prevention of such hepatic venous blockade. (2) We utilize physiologic pressures but higher flow rates which are in the neighborhood of 1 ml. per gram of liver per minute. (3) We maintain physiologic temperatures at all times since one cannot be certain that complex enzyme activity will return to normal immediately upon rewarming from hypothermic levels. (4) The pH is kept near 7.4 by suitable alteration of the oxygen-carbon dioxide ratio in the oxygenator. (5) Our findings concerning glucose utilization are similar to Dr. McDermott's. The glucose is utilized, glycogen broken down, and a relatively high level of glucose more or less maintain by some inner glucostat. (6) Finally, we have found that the perfused liver converts ammonia to urea at a fantastic rate. We have perfused a human liver from a fresh cadaver and believe that such a technique offers promise for the future treatment of patients with severe liver failure.

**Dr. Lloyd M. Nyhus** (Seattle, Wash.). You have heard of experiments with the dog and the pig. I would like to pursue the subject of the calf. With the apparatus we have been using, which is quite similar to that which Dr. Eiseman described, complete isolation is established. For physiologic studies, we also have believed that we should maintain body temperature as much as possible and we have taken great care to do so. You may remember that in our report at this meeting last year, we first experimented with the dog but were disenchanted by the marked edema, as Dr. McDermott has mentioned. We therefore began experiments with the calf. This slide shows a calf liver with minimal edema in the holding container after several hours of perfusion. We have been extremely careful to keep tubing and other parts of our apparatus sterile since we believed that the defects in our study of 18- or 24-hour perfusions might have been due to bacterial contamination. In the next slide, you will note that between 6 and 8 hours, the amount of accumulation remained about the same. As time progressed, there was a rather significant amount of change, but much less than we had previously seen with the dog liver. We believe that we have perfected our technique quite nicely in the calf and are eager to apply what we have learned in the calf to the dog.

**Dr. Oscar Creech, Jr.** (New Orleans, La.). I want to ask Dr. McDermott if he has observed any changes in hepatic outflow with changes in temperature; that is, any differences with low temperatures and with high.

**Dr. William V. McDermott, Jr.** (closing). I was extremely interested in the comments of Drs. Eiseman and Nyhus on their very intriguing work. There is a typographic error in the program. The average flow was 390 ml. per minute with a range of about 250 to 800. The flow usually increased once established as oxygenation improved and our average flow now runs around 600 ml. per minute after the first hour of perfusion. I envy Dr. Nyhus' opportunity to switch to the calf from the dog. The supply of calves in New England is limited and we were restricted to use of the dog. I would be interested in knowing, if Dr. Nyhus goes back again to the dog, if he can overcome the outflow block problem. I am sure that it is possible, although it is much more difficult than in the calf. In answer to Dr. Creech's comments, if the temperature is brought to hypothermic levels, there is much less difficulty with outflow block. However, the metabolic conditions are altered a great deal, as you might imagine. Oxygen consumption drops and we were interested in maintaining normal temperatures if possible because the ultimate objective of this preparation was to study metabolic parameters under normal conditions.

# Blood coagulation factors in liver disease

WILLIAM T. WEAVER
WILLIAM G. ANLYAN
R. W. POSTLETHWAIT
With technical assistance of E. K. Spada
DURHAM, N. C.
*From the Department of Surgery, Duke University Medical Center, and the Durham Veterans Administration Hospital.*

The coagulation of blood is obviously of primary concern to the surgeon but the intricate steps of the complicated system of multiple reactions between various proteins which result in coagulation is not part of his everyday working information, nor should it be. Some knowledge of coagulation is necessary, however, in the surgical management of patients with diseases of the liver and biliary system. These patients present certain problems involving blood coagulation because the liver is involved in the synthesis of most of the reactants involved in the clotting process. The usual estimation of prothrombin time by the Quick one-stage method provides useful information, but in some situations has serious shortcomings. The reaction is not specific. A patient can have a nearly normal prothrombin time and still have hemorrhagic tendencies clinically. This is important in the management of patients who are being given anticoagulant drugs as well as those with liver damage.

Owren[5] discovered that prothrombin, previously regarded as a single coagulation factor, was in reality 3 substances of similar structure, prothrombin, proaccelerin (factor V), and proconvertin (factor VII). Suitable laboratory methods for the determination of these individual substances have been developed. Quick verified the complex nature of "prothrombin" and separated it into 2 fractions. One he called "labile factor" because it disappeared on storage with oxalated plasma. The other, which was not sensitive to storage, was called "stable factor."[5] Additional evidence indicated that labile factor and factor V were the same and Owren[5] stated, "it must be assumed that the labile factor of Quick is identical with pro-accelerin." Semantically, a cumbersome group of synonyms has developed. Factor V is also called "labile factor," "proaccelerin," "plasma Ac globulin," and "plasma prothrombin conversion factor," whereas factor VII is also known as "stable factor" and "proconvertin." We prefer to use the terms "factor V" and "factor VII" (Fig. 1).

Specific prothrombin determinations may also be of interest in these patients. The validity and specificity of this procedure is based on the fact that the only variable is the concentration of prothrombin, since factors V and VII, as well as fibrinogen, are provided in optimal amounts before the determination is made.[11]

## PURPOSE

The purpose of this study was to evaluate the changes in various coagulation factors (prothrombin by the Quick one-stage method, factor V, factor VII, and specific prothrombin) in 116 patients who had clinical

Supported by United States Public Health Service Grant No. H-2616 (C4) and Duke University Center for Aging Grants M-2109 and H-3583.

Read at the Twenty-second Annual Meeting of the Society of University Surgeons, Kansas City, Kan., Feb. 9-11, 1961.

Factor V (labile proaccelerin)
Antihaemophilic globulin (AHG)
Platelet factor III
Christmas factor (PTC-factor IX)
Factor VII (stable proconvertin)
Stuart (factor X)
Plasma thromboplastin antecedent (PTA)

↓

Thromboplastin

↓

Prothrombin ⟶ Thrombin
Thrombin + Fibrinogen ⟶ Fibrin

**Fig. 1.** Simplified blood coagulation mechanism.

evidence of liver disease. In all patients laboratory determinations were also made of total protein, albumin-globulin ratio, bilirubin, alkaline phosphatase, cholesterol, Bromsulphalein retention, and thymol flocculation and turbidity.

A variety of conditions are associated with hypoprothrombinemia, including obstructive jaundice, biliary fistula, sprue, celiac disease, intestinal fistula, gastrocolic fistula, intestinal polyposis, intestinal obstruction, postoperative gastric retention, ulcerative colitis, sterilization of the bowel preoperatively, congestive heart failure, thyrotoxicosis, myxedema, anemia, and severe acute infections.[5, 10] The difficulties of determining the exact status of liver function are well known, but a group of patients with liver damage should provide a means of comparison of the factors which may be deficient in the hypoprothrombinemic state. A study of these incompletely understood blood factors in the full range of patients with liver disease, therefore, might produce information of 3 types, (1) whether or not liver damage existed, (2) the extent of the liver damage, and (3) clues to aid in differential diagnosis. The response to parenteral administration of vitamin $K_1$ to these patients might also be of interest.

## METHODS

The patients were divided into 5 groups according to the nature of the pathologic lesion. Group I consisted of 61 patients with cirrhosis of the liver, many of whom were being evaluated as candidates for a surgical portasystemic shunt (Fig. 2). Group II was composed of 20 patients with biliary obstruction. Two patients had pancreatic carcinoma and the remainder had choledocholithiasis as the obstructing lesion. Group III was made up of 7 patients with hepatocellular damage secondary to toxins or infection. Two of them were suspected of having arsenic intoxication, 1 had sarcoid, and the remaining 4 had hepatitis. Group IV consisted of 8 patients in whom carcinoma of the liver, either primary or secondary, was the major hepatic disease. Group V was composed of 20 patients in whom no definite liver disease was demonstrated, although the clinical courses were compatible with mild hepatitis (Fig. 3).

After the base line coagulation and liver function studies had been obtained, vitamin $K_1$ emulsion (50 mg. of Mephyton) was administered intravenously and the coagulation studies repeated after 6 and 24 hours. It has been shown that coagulation factors respond more promptly to the natural oil-soluble vitamin K compounds than to synthetic water-soluble preparations.[10] Mephyton is a 1 per cent lecithin solution of natural vitamin $K_1$.

Coagulation factors were determined by the Quick[7] one-stage prothrombin time test, Owren's[4] method for specific prothrombin determination, Wolf's[12] modification of Stefanini's method for estimation of factor V, and F. Koller's[2] procedure for factor VII determination.

**Experimental groups.** Two groups of dogs were studied. Group I consisted of 10 dogs with experimental carbon tetrachloride–induced cirrhosis in the laboratory of Dr. Bernard Fisher at the University of Pittsburgh. Blood samples for the coagulation studies were obtained before and after the intravenous administration of vitamin $K_1$ emulsion, 50 mg. Group II was made up of 10 mongrel dogs in which the common bile duct was ligated under intravenous Nembutal anesthesia. Serum bilirubin, transaminase, phosphatase, and the coagulation factors were checked twice a week for an average period of 2 weeks.

## RESULTS

**Evaluation of individual coagulation factors.** Quick one-stage prothrombin test (Q. O. S.) is the standard laboratory method for the "routine prothrombin determination." Of the 116 patients, 28 (24.1 per cent) had abnormal values. Patients in all groups were considered to have an abnormal value if the result was 70 per cent of normal or lower. This test was second only to that for factor VII in the degree of sensitivity to liver damage.

Specific prothrombin determination, based primarily on the concentration of prothrombin, was not as sensitive as the standard Quick one-stage method for determination of prothrombin, since only 22 (19 per cent) of the 116 patients showed abnormal levels.

Factor V appeared to be the least sensitive of all and only 14 (12 per cent) of the 116 patients had an abnormal deficiency. All but 2 of these were patients with cirrhosis, the exceptions being 1 from the obstructive jaundice group and 1 from miscellaneous groups.

Factor VII was the most sensitive of all factors studied; 38 (32.8 per cent) of the 116 patients showed an abnormality of this factor. It was especially sensitive in the patients in the group with cirrhosis; 26 (42.5 per cent) of the 61 patients with cirrhosis had abnormal levels. To a lesser degree this was true in patients with obstructive jaundice, since 25 per cent had subnormal levels. This is shown graphically in Figs. 4 and 5. All patients in each of these groups were placed in order of ascending factor VII levels and the other factors for the individual patients were plotted against the factor VII line. This shows that factor VII levels were consistently lower than those of the other factors. In the cirrhotic group, only patients with an albumin level of less than 3 Gm. per cent and/or a Bromsulphalein retention of greater than 10 per cent were selected and in the biliary obstruction group only patients with a bilirubin of greater than 1 mg. per cent are represented on the illustrations. Table I shows the percentage of

**Table I.** *Percentage of patients with abnormal findings*

| | *Quick test (%)* | *Factor VII (%)* | *Specific pro-thrombin (%)* | *Factor V (%)* |
|---|---|---|---|---|
| Over-all series | 24.1 | 32.8 | 19.0 | 12.0 |
| Cirrhosis | 27.8 | 42.5 | 18.0 | 19.7 |
| Obstruction | 25.0 | 25.0 | 15.0 | 5.0 |
| Hepatocellular disease | 14.3 | 28.6 | 28.6 | 0 |
| Carcinoma | 12.5 | 25.0 | 37.5 | 0 |
| Miscellaneous | 20.0 | 15.0 | 15.0 | 5.0 |

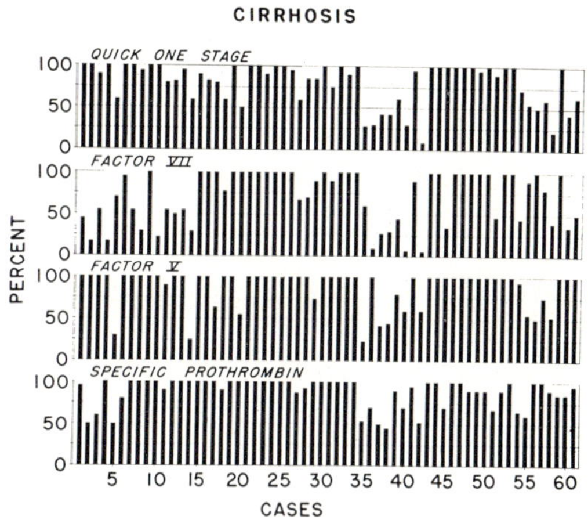


**Fig. 2.** Coagulation factors of patients with cirrhosis.

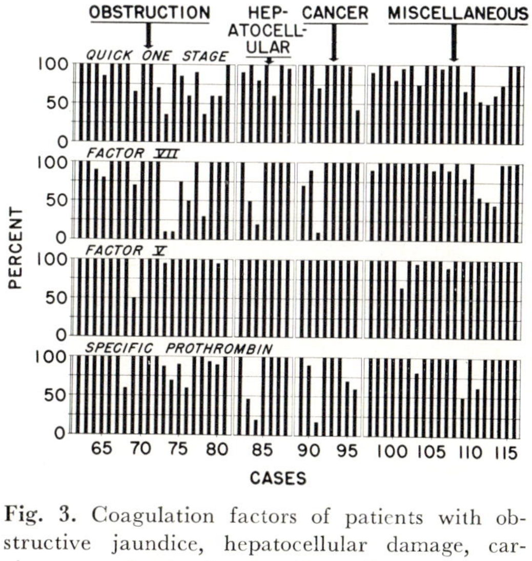


**Fig. 3.** Coagulation factors of patients with obstructive jaundice, hepatocellular damage, carcinoma, and miscellaneous liver disease.

patients with abnormal findings in each group.

**Results of vitamin $K_1$ stimulation.** All patients who had obstructive jaundice and low coagulation factors responded to vitamin $K_1$ emulsion by increasing the titer of the individual deficient factors. None of the patients in this group showed any progressive decline in blood factors after being given vitamin $K_1$. Patients with cirrhosis fell into 2 groups according to the effect of vitamin $K_1$. Nine patients had an increase in coagulation factors, whereas 5 patients showed a progressive decline of these factors in spite of vitamin $K_1$ stimulation. In the latter group, the degree of hepatic damage apparently had progressed to a degree that the liver was unable to synthesize the deficient factors (Fig. 6).

In the experimental studies of the 10 dogs with carbon tetrachloride—induced cirrhosis, 2 had depressed factors in the abnormal range and were refractory to vitamin $K_1$ stimulation. The rest of the dogs did not achieve liver damage of a degree sufficient to elicit a decline in coagulation factors. Most values remained at 100 per cent. Five of the 10 dogs which had ligation and division of the common bile duct developed a coagulation factor deficit and all responded in a positive manner to vitamin $K_1$.

## COMMENT

For the normal synthesis of prothrombin several conditions are necessary, a sufficient supply of vitamin $K_1$ (extrinsic from the diet and intrinsic via intestinal bacteria), the presence of bile salts in the intestine for the absorption of vitamin $K_1$, and enough healthy liver cells to produce sufficient enzymatic activity to synthesize prothrombin. The relationship of vitamin $K_1$ to the formation of prothrombin is not clear. Apparently it does not enter into the construction of the molecule of prothrombin, but is essential to its synthesis.[10] The same is probably true for factor VII. Factor V, which is also manufactured by the liver, is less dependent on vitamin $K_1$ and, in fact, may be completely independent of a vitamin $K_1$ influence.[9]

From the pathophysiologic standpoint, low values of coagulation factors are basically due to 2 factors, the inability to absorb vitamin $K_1$ because of the unavailability of bile salts (biliary obstruction) and decreased hepatic function (cirrhosis, hepatitis, and so forth). If this is true, patients and dogs with biliary obstruction should respond to parenterally given vitamin $K_1$ by forming new coagulation factors and should show a rise in titer in prothrombin, factor V, and factor VII. Patients and animals with damaged livers would not show this response. This was borne out in both animal and patient studies, and factor VII was unusually sensitive in this regard.

A reliable method for the estimation of hepatocellular function would be of great value in differential diagnosis as well as providing information relative to operability

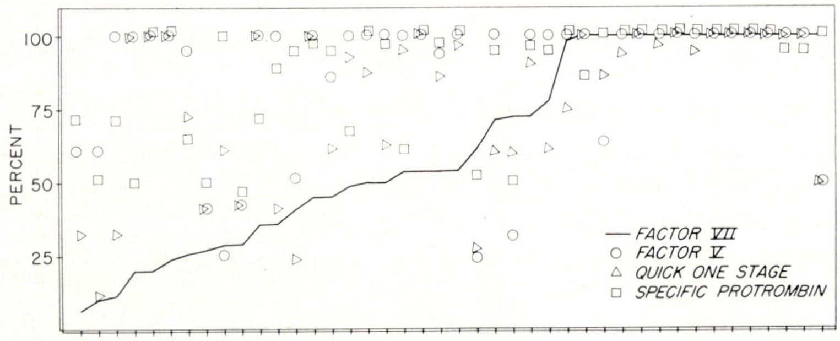


**Fig. 4.** Patients with cirrhosis arranged in ascending order of factor VII values.

of patients with liver disease. Sjostrom[9] has shown that patients of this type are more sensitive to Warfarin than normal control patients and has postulated the use of this test in patient evaluation. However, this would mean partial anticoagulation in a patient prior to operation. Esophageal varices would be a contraindication for this test. Since the majority of these surgical patients are given vitamin $K_1$ preoperatively for therapeutic reasons, the concomitant measurement of the coagulation factors previously described adds information of diagnostic importance.

The response to vitamin $K_1$ infusion appears to be of greater usefulness in the differentiation between hepatocellular damage and biliary obstruction when the blood coagulation factors are studied individually instead of by the one-stage Quick prothrombin determination.

## CONCLUSIONS

An effort has been made to bring information on blood coagulation which has been developed largely in the laboratory into the field of clinical surgery. Interest in the relationship between liver disease and blood coagulation is not new.[6] Through newer laboratory methods, however, refinements in our knowledge can be made. In a series of 116 patients with clinical evidence of liver disease, determinations of various coagulation factors (Quick one-stage prothrombin, specific prothrombin, factor V, and factor VII tests) were performed as well as a battery of liver function tests. The results indicate that of the newer factors studied, factor VII is unusually sensitive to liver damage and provides more information in this regard than the standard or "routine" prothrombin test by the Quick one-stage method. This is especially evident in patients with cirrhosis. Factor V and specific prothrombin tests are probably not as sensitive as the Quick one-stage prothrombin test; however, they might provide additional information in the evaluation of the individual patient.[8] The response to intravenously administered vitamin $K_1$ emulsion in the differentiation between hepatocellular damage and biliary obstruction is clearer when the individual factors are determined than when only the Quick one-stage prothrombin test is used.

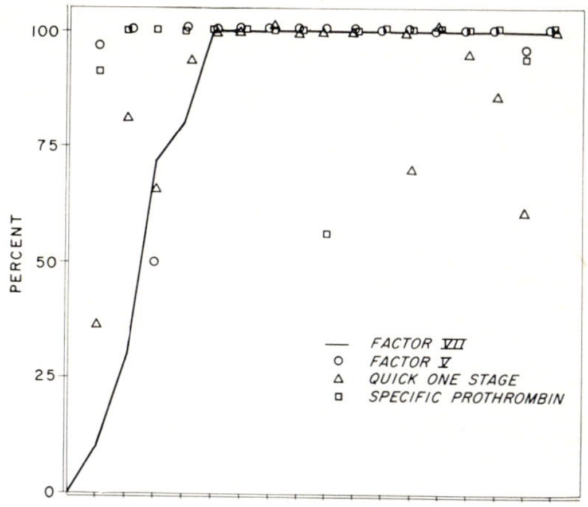


**Fig. 5.** Patients with obstructive jaundice arranged in ascending order of factor VII values.

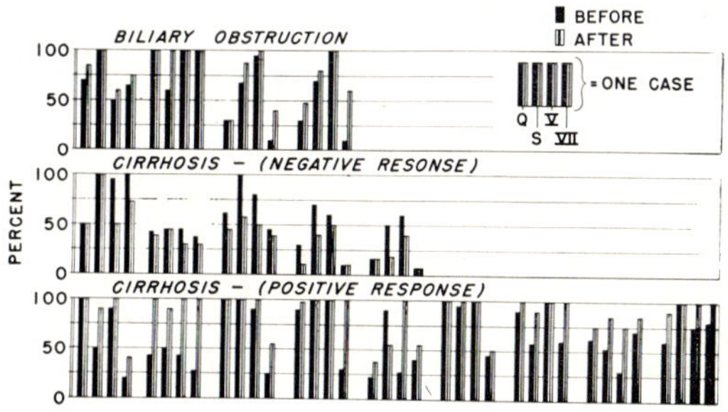


**Fig. 6.** Response of blood factors to vitamin $K_1$ in patients.

## REFERENCES

1. Gamble, J. R., Dennis, E. W., Coon, W. W., Hodgson, P., Willis, P. W. III, and MaCris, J. A.: Clinical comparison of vitamin K and water-soluble vitamin K in combating hypoprothrombinemia, A. M. A. Arch. Int. Med. **95:** 52, 1955.
2. Koller, F., Loeliger, A., and Duckert, F.: Experiments on a new clotting factor (factor VII), Acta haemat. **6:** 1, 1951.
3. Matsuoka, M., Satake, Kiyoto, and Fukazawa, Masara: Fibrinogen level in hepatic diseases with special reference to fibrinogen levels in liver cancer, liver cirrhosis and other cancerous diseases, Acta Hepat. Jap. **1:** 61, 1960.

4. Owren, P. A.: Blood clotting and allied problems, Tr. Josiah Macy Jr. Foundation, 1952, p. 98.
5. Owren, P. A.: Prothrombin and accessory factors, Am. J. Med. **14:** 201, 1955.
6. Petrein, G.: Untersuchungen über die Blutgerinnung bie icterus nebst einigen Worten über die sog cholamischen Blutungen, Acta chir. scandinav. **58:** 488, 1925.
7. Quick, A. J.: Tr. first conf. of blood clotting and allied problems, Josiah Macy Jr. Foundation, 1948, p. 170.
8. Rieben, W.: The construction and clinical significance of the coagulohepatogram, J. Clin. Path. **5:** 257, 1952.
9. Sjostrom, B.: The activity of prothrombin and proconvertin plasma in diseases of the biliary tract. A clinical study, Acta chir. scandinav. **113:** 1, 1957.
10. Stefanini, M., and Dameshek, W.: The hemorrhagic disorders, New York, 1955, Grune & Stratton, Inc.
11. Tocantins, L. M.: The coagulation of blood, New York, 1955, Grune & Stratton, Inc., p. 94.
12. Wolf, P.: A modification of routine laboratory use of Stefanini's method of estimating factor V in human oxalated plasma, J. Clin. Path. **6:** 34, 1953.

## DISCUSSION

**Dr. Grossi** (New York, N. Y.). I want to compliment the authors on a very interesting paper. In the past year, Dr. Rousselot, Dr. Moreno, and I, at St. Vincent's Hospital of the City of New York, have been studying coagulation defects in 80 patients with cirrhosis. Although defects in prothrombin were found by the Quick method, the greatest defect was found in factor VII and spontaneous fibrinolytic activity. In 30 patients studied during portacaval shunts, administration of vitamin $K_1$ did not affect factor VII, while Quick time and factor V did respond. In our series, 40 per cent of cirrhotic patients had spontaneous euglobulin fibrinolytic activity and 17 per cent had whole-clot lysis. An inhibitor of fibrinolysin, $\epsilon$-aminocaproic acid, has been used in these patients. When 2 Gm. of $\epsilon$-aminocaproic acid was given intravenously, there was inhibition of euglobulin fibrinolytic activity and whole-clot lysis for 4 to 6 hours. These coagulation defects are not considered significant in the production of the abrupt bleeding from varices in which powerful hemodynamic forces are the responsible factors.

**Dr. William G. Anlyan** (closing). I thank Dr. Grossi for his comments. Most of our patients with cirrhosis were also being evaluated for portasystemic shunts.

# Evidence for histamine as the agent responsible for gastric hypersecretion after portacaval shunt

WILLIAM SILEN, M.D.*
BEN EISEMAN, M.D.**
DENVER, COLO.
*From the Department of Surgery, University of Colorado Medical Center, and Denver Veterans Administration Hospital*

It is now a well-established fact that gastric hypersecretion develops after portacaval shunt in dogs.[4, 7, 11, 16, 23] Although many of the characteristics of such hypersecretion have been defined and several plausible etiologic factors already eliminated,[3, 4, 6, 14, 23] the true mechanism responsible for this phenomenon remains unclear. The possible role of histamine as the final common stimulator of the parietal cells of the stomach[5] suggested the evaluation of its importance in the causation of gastric hypersecretion after portacaval shunts.

Various investigators have reported a variety of findings consistent with the hypothesis that histamine is released into the portal circulation by feeding and that hepatic bypass of histamine-containing portal blood may be responsible for hypersecretion after portacaval shunts. In 1953, Anrep and associates,[1] utilizing a bioassay method for determination of histamine, noted that portal venous blood uniformly contained greater quantities of this substance than did hepatic venous or peripheral arterial blood. The observation by Updike and colleagues[24] and Irvine and Code[12] that the levels of free histamine in the urine of normal dogs were markedly elevated after a protein meal, but not after a meal of bread and milk, was strikingly reminiscent of our own finding that the gastric hypersecretion after portacaval shunt was most marked after protein ingestion.[23] Schayer and Ivy[21] found that after administration of $C^{14}$-labeled histidine and an antihistaminase (aminoguanidine) to rats, much greater quantities of $C^{14}$-labeled histamine were found in the urine after feeding than in the starved animal. The same investigators later observed that after the subcutaneous injection of $C^{14}$-labeled histidine, the ingestion of food caused a 35 and 52 per cent decrease, respectively, in the amount of $C^{14}$-labeled histamine of the small intestine and stomach when compared with the findings in fasting animals.[22] Schayer and Ivy concluded from these experiments that histamine definitely was released from the stomach and small intestine by feeding.

In 1955, Livingston and Code[17] reported that injection of histamine via the portal vein reduced the amount recovered in the urine. Silen and Eiseman[23] showed that secretion from canine Heidenhain pouches was much greater when histamine was given systemically than when it was given as an intraportal infusion at the same rate and concentration. The suggestion was made that the liver could inactivate the gastric secretory properties of histamine and that the hepatic bypass of histamine-containing portal blood might be the mechanism responsible for gastric hypersecretion after portacaval shunts. Irvine and his group[13] made similar observations and reached the same con-

Supported by United States Public Health Service Grant A-2934 (now A-4889).

Read at the Twenty-second Annual Meeting of the Society of University Surgeons, Kansas City, Kan., Feb. 9-11, 1961.

*Present address: University of California Medical Center, San Francisco, Calif.

**Present address: University of Kentucky Medical Center, Lexington, Ky.

clusions. The findings of Lebedinskaja[16] and Gerez and Weiss[11] that the pepsin content of the gastric juice falls while the volume and acidity increase after portacaval shunt are consistent with this hypothesis, since exogenously-administered histamine causes similar changes in gastric secretion.

The development of more sensitive techniques for the estimation of the extremely small quantities of histamine in plasma has made it possible to investigate the importance of this substance as a physiologic stimulant of gastric secretion.

## METHODS

**Studies in normal dogs.** The response of peripheral arterial plasma histamine levels to the ingestion of a standard protein meal has been studied 25 times in 18 normal dogs. The test meal consisted of 2 cans of a commercial dog food (Pard), which contains 11.0 per cent protein and 4.5 per cent fat. The meal was consumed over a 5- to 10-minute period. Samples of blood for plasma histamine analysis were obtained from the femoral artery before and 90, 180, and 360 minutes after completion of the test meal. Arterial rather than venous blood was utilized because it represents blood similar to that presented to the stomach via its arterial circulation, and because it is probable that most histamine is lost during a single circuit through the tissues.[5]

**Studies in dogs with portacaval transposition.** Eight normal dogs utilized in the previous study and an additional 4 dogs were subjected to portacaval transposition as described by Child and associates.[2] After a suitable recovery period, the response of the peripheral arterial plasma histamine levels to the test meal of Pard was studied 23 times in the manner described. Heidenhain pouches were prepared in 6 of the 12 dogs, and in these animals pouch secretions were collected at 30-minute intervals after ingestion of the test meal during the performance of the histamine tests. The volume of each 30-minute specimen was measured and the free acid determined by titration with 0.1 N sodium hydroxide solution.

**Comparison of the plasma histamine content of portal venous versus hepatic venous or femoral arterial blood.** These studies were carried out to determine whether portal venous blood plasma contained consistently greater quantities of histamine than either hepatic venous or femoral arterial blood. In 9 unanesthetized dogs, the plasma histamine content of portal venous and either hepatic venous or femoral arterial blood was determined before and at 90-minute intervals after the protein test meal. The tests extended over a 6-hour period. A total of 15 experiments were performed with either indwelling polyethylene catheters or London cannulae for simultaneous sampling of portal and hepatic venous blood. In 9 experiments, the plasma histamine content of portal blood was compared with that of hepatic venous blood, whereas in 6 experiments femoral arterial blood was obtained for comparison with portal blood.

**Determination of the histamine content of the plasma.** The method of Lowry and co-workers[18] was used for all determinations of the histamine content of the plasma. This method, as outlined by the authors, consists of 5 main steps, (1) extraction of the histamine from the plasma with trichloracetic acid, (2) concentration of histamine and separation from many other amines by adsorption on Decalso, (3) formation of the colored derivative of histamine with dinitrofluorobenzene (DNFB), (4) further concentration and separation of this derivative from DNFB derivatives of remaining amines by extraction into methyl-n-hexylketone, followed by extraction into hydrochloric acid, and (5) measurement of the color in microcuvettes at 360 m$\mu$.

Recovery of known amounts of histamine is remarkably constant at 75 to 80 per cent in our work as reported by Lowry and his group. Because of the constancy of the recovery, measurement of changes in histamine is valid. Standards were carried through the entire process with each set of tests, thus correcting for the incomplete recovery. Duplicate determinations were made on each sample of plasma with a 7 per cent variation. The mean value of duplicate determinations is reported in each instance. It is to be stressed that the dangers of positive error from the release of leukocytic histamine are great, since histamine is 2,000 times as concentrated in the leukocytes as in the plasma. All samples of blood were drawn extremely carefully into cold siliconized syringes and the plasma was separated quickly in a refrigerated centrifuge. Hemolysis was used as an indication of excessive trauma to the cellular elements of the blood. Lowry and associates have shown that this method is quite specific for histamine in that only 1.7 μg. per liter of apparent histamine in the plasma is not destroyed by histaminase. The accuracy of the method of histamine determination was further tested at intervals by (1) ascertaining the proportionality of spectrophotometer readings and varying known amounts of histamine and (2) by the addition of known amounts of histamine to samples either before or after adsorption on the Decalso.

## RESULTS

**Studies in normal dogs.** The histamine content of the plasma rose in each of the 25 tests after the test meal. The peak usually occurred 180 minutes after the meal but on a few occasions took place at 90 minutes. The mean fasting level of plasma histamine in the femoral artery blood was 14.5 ± 0.99 μg. per liter. The mean peak level of plasma histamine after ingestion of the test meal was 23.9 ± 2.6 μg. per liter (Fig. 1). The difference between these two values is highly significant ($p = < 0.01$). This constitutes a 65 per cent mean rise in arterial plasma histamine level after feeding of the test meal.

**Studies in dogs with portacaval transposition.** In each of the 23 tests in these 12 dogs, a rise in arterial plasma histamine level was demonstrated. The peak occurred 180 minutes after the test meal in almost every instance. The mean fasting level and the mean peak level of plasma histamine after the test meal were 11.3 ± 0.79 and 33.6 ± 7.7 μg. per liter, respectively (Fig. 1). The difference between these two values is highly significant ($p = < 0.01$) and represents a mean rise of 197 per cent. The difference between the rises in plasma histamine levels above fasting values after feeding in the normal and in the dogs with transposition is suggestive but not statistically significant ($p = 0.1$). It is interesting to note that the fasting values of plasma histamine in dogs with portacaval transposition were slightly lower than those in normal dogs.

In the 8 dogs which underwent tests both before and after portacaval transposition there was no statistical difference between fasting levels of plasma histamine before and after the shunt. The peak values of plasma histamine after ingestion of the test meal were considerably greater after portacaval transposition in 5 of the 8 dogs (Fig. 2) and were approximately the same in 3 dogs. Whether or not more frequent sampling of blood would have detected differences in the latter 3 dogs remains conjectural. This was not carried out because of the large volumes of blood necessary for these determinations.

In the 6 animals in which secretion from a Heidenhain pouch was determined simultaneously with histamine determinations after the test meal, the pouch secretions usually reached a peak slightly before the peak value in plasma histamine levels was noted (Fig. 3). Because the pouch secretion achieved after such a test meal represents

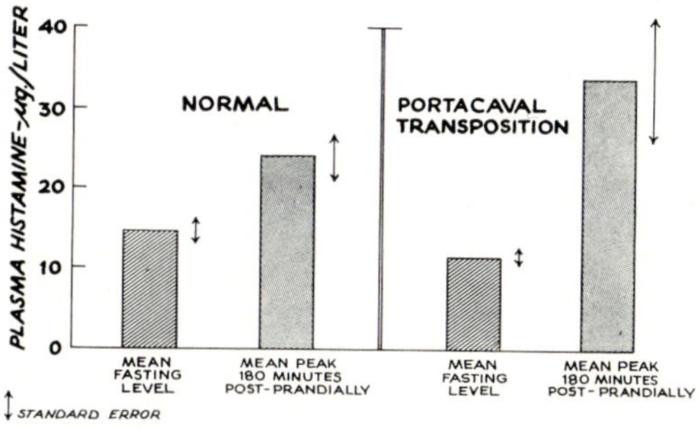


**Fig. 1.** Mean fasting and mean peak postprandial peripheral arterial plasma histamine levels in normal dogs (25 tests) and in dogs with portacaval transposition (23 tests).

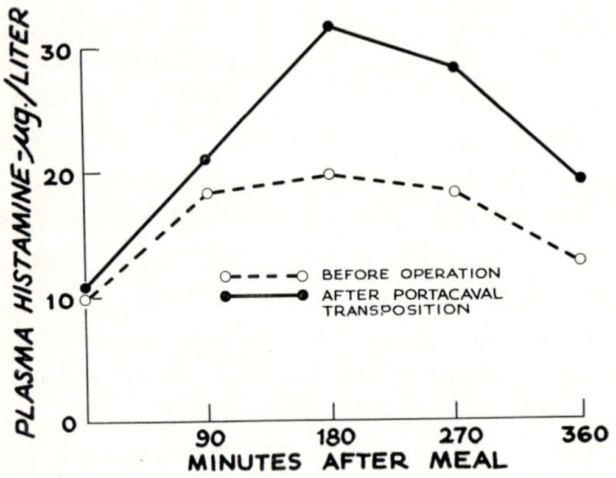


**Fig. 2.** Representative response of peripheral arterial plasma histamine level to protein test meal in the same animal before and after portacaval transposition. Five of the 8 dogs studied in this manner had similar responses, whereas no differences between pre- and postshunt tests were noted in the remaining 3 animals.

the sum of a variety of stimuli, it is difficult to correlate the rises in plasma histamine levels with the changes in pouch secretion. The early peak in secretion may well represent antral phase secretion. The later high rate of secretion of gastric juice still present when the histamine levels of the plasma are highest may represent intestinal phase secretion, especially since previous observations by us and many others[3, 14, 23] point to accentuation of the intestinal phase as most important in the hypersecretion after portacaval shunt.

**Comparison of the plasma histamine content of portal venous versus hepatic venous or femoral arterial blood plasma.** The histamine content of portal venous blood plasma rose to much higher levels than that of hepatic venous or femoral artery blood in every instance after the test meal (Fig. 4). The mean fasting level of portal plasma histamine was 11.9 ± 1.5 μg per liter and the mean peak level after the meal was 31.6 ± 7.0 μg. per liter. The corresponding values for the hepatic vein or femoral artery samples were 12.0 ± 1.3 and 16.0 ± 1.8 μg. per liter, respectively. The difference between the rises in plasma histamine levels of portal venous versus hepatic venous or femoral arterial blood after the test meal was statistically significant ($p = < 0.03$ and $> 0.02$). The fasting levels of plasma histamine found in the portal blood did not differ significantly from those in the hepatic vein or femoral artery blood. The peak levels of histamine invariably were reached at 180 minutes after the meal in all specimens. Responses were similar whether hepatic venous or femoral arterial blood was compared with portal blood.

## COMMENT

Our data show that in both normal dogs and in dogs with portacaval transposition, a highly significant rise in arterial plasma histamine level occurs after a protein test meal. Although the mean rise in histamine level after feeding in the dogs with portacaval transposition was 197 per cent as opposed to only a 65 per cent rise in the normal dogs, these differences are only suggestive and are of borderline statistical significance. The greater rise in the arterial plasma histamine level evoked by the test meal after shunt in the majority of the dogs studied both before and after portacaval transposition lends greater importance to the observed differences, however. The most significant data which corroborate the thesis that histamine is released into portal blood after feeding are those which show the striking differences between the histamine

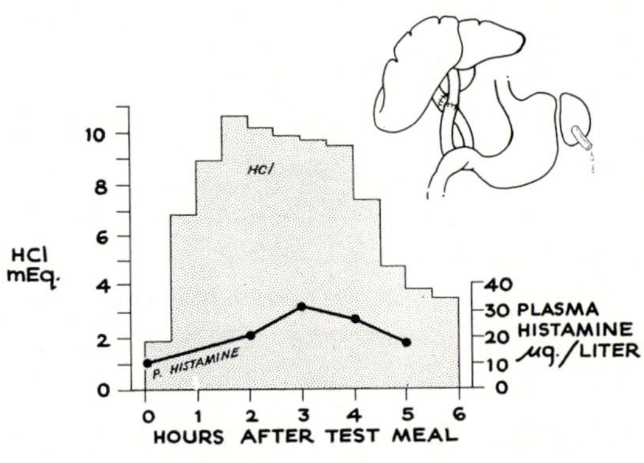


**Fig. 3.** Comparison of response of Heidenhain pouch secretion and peripheral arterial plasma histamine level to test meal after portacaval transposition.

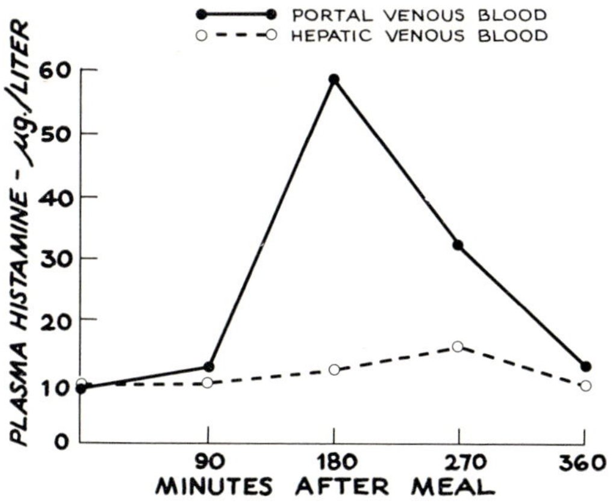


**Fig. 4.** Representative response of plasma histamine level in portal and hepatic venous blood to test meal in a normal dog.

content of the portal and hepatic venous or femoral arterial blood. Thus, in the presence of a portacaval shunt, large amounts of histamine-containing portal blood are shunted into the systemic circulation and are delivered to the stomach without being exposed to inactivation by the liver during the first circuit. The previous demonstration that the liver largely inactivates the gastric secretory activity of histamine[23] strengthens the validity of this hypothesis. Our finding that the peak values of the histamine content of the plasma occur 3 hours after ingestion of the test meal is consistent with the contention that the gastric hypersecretion after portacaval shunt is an accentuation of the intestinal phase of gastric secretion.[3, 6, 14, 23]

It is not very surprising that the fasting levels of plasma histamine do not differ significantly in the normal dogs or dogs with transposition, despite the fact that previous studies showed that the fasting pouch secretion rises after portacaval shunting.[23] The amounts of histamine released into the portal circulation may be so small during fasting that they are undetectable by present methods. Such minute quantities could provide sufficient potentiation of vagal and antral stimuli to account for the rises in fasting secretion as well as the slightly increased gastric secretory response to carbohydrate and fat after portacaval transposition.[23] This explanation is supported by the studies of Öbrink,[20] who showed that there is probably no threshold value for the effect of histamine on gastric secretion and that the slightest amount of histamine given intravenously by continuous injection will initiate secretion.

The studies reported demonstrate clearly that histamine is released into portal blood after protein ingestion in dogs. However, a considerable volume of conflicting evidence appears in the literature as to the presence or absence of histamine in the blood during periods of gastric secretion. Koskowski's[15] report in 1933 alone contends that smooth-muscle reacting substances are increased in the blood during digestion in both man and dogs. These experiments have been criticized as being poorly controlled, and the possibility has been suggested that smooth-muscle reacting substances other than histamine may have caused the observed changes.[5] On the other hand, MacIntosh[19] was unable to demonstrate a rise in the histamine content of whole arterial blood after feeding. One milligram of histamine, estimated by MacIntosh as producing a peak rate of gastric secretion equivalent to that which occurs after a meat meal, caused only doubtful rises in blood histamine levels. Emmelin and associates[8] and Emmelin and Kahlson[9] and others showed that no rise in histamine content of the arterial blood plasma could be observed while gastric secretion was elicited by the intravenous administration of histamine. When large doses of histamine exceeding the amount necessary for maximal gastric secretion are given, rises in histamine content in the plasma are detected and are related in a linear fashion to the dosage of this agent.[8, 20]

Several factors may be responsible for these paradoxical findings. It is important to recognize that the bioassay method of histamine determination utilized in all of the cited studies is scarcely sensitive enough to detect accurately the very small amounts of histamine in plasma. Bioassay also has the inherent drawback of requiring the extracts used to be free of all substances which can stimulate or inhibit the contraction of the smooth muscle. In addition, the studies by MacIntosh[19] with this method of histamine determination were performed on whole blood and changes in the histamine content of the plasma might easily have been masked by the relatively large amount of histamine in the leukocytes. Furthermore, it is highly probable that histamine is metabolized extremely rapidly and is greatly diluted in the blood after its release. These factors also contribute to the difficulty in its detection. We believe that these considerations tend to negate the fact that MacIntosh[19] was unable to find changes in whole-blood histamine after feeding and that the other investigators cited[8, 9, 10] could not detect changes in plasma histamine when histamine was administered intravenously in dose ranges sufficient to stimulate gastric secretion submaximally.

Although our experiments and those of Irvine and associates[13] suggest that the histamine in portal blood may arise from exogenous sources, such as ingested protein, the exact origin of the histamine is not known. The importance of endogenous sources of histamine and the factors controlling its release into the portal blood remain to be determined.

## SUMMARY

1. A statistically highly significant rise in the plasma histamine content of peripheral arterial blood occurs after protein ingestion in both normal dogs and in dogs with portacaval transposition, with a somewhat greater rise in the latter group.

2. Plasma histamine levels of portal blood rise to consistently higher values than do those of hepatic venous or femoral arterial blood in normal dogs after protein ingestion.

3. Hepatic bypass of histamine-containing portal blood may well be the cause for gastric hypersecretion after portacaval shunt, especially that which occurs after protein ingestion.

## REFERENCES

1. Anrep, G. B., Barsoum, G. S., and Talaat, M.: Release of histamine by the liver, J. Physiol. **120:** 419, 1953.
2. Child, C. G., III, Barr, D., Holswade, G. R., and Harrison, C. S.: Liver regeneration following portacaval transposition in dogs, Ann. Surg. **138:** 600, 1953.
3. Clarke, J. S., McKissock, P. K., and Cruze, K. Studies on the site of origin of the agent causing hypersecretion in dogs with portacaval shunt, SURGERY **46:** 48, 1959.
4. Clarke, J. S., Ozeran, R. S., Hart, J. C., Cruze, K., and Crevling, V.: Peptic ulcer following portacaval shunt, Ann. Surg. **148:** 551, 1958.
5. Code, C. F.: Histamine and gastric secretion, Ciba Clin. Sympos., Boston, 1956, Little, Brown & Company, p. 189.
6. Cornish, P. G., Silen, W., Eiseman, B., and Woods, L. P.: Further studies on the mechanism of gastric hypersecretion after portacaval shunts, S. Forum **11:** 351, 1960.
7. Dubuque, T. J., Jr., Mulligan, L. V., and Neville, E. C.: Gastric secretion and peptic ulceration in the dog with portal obstruction and portacaval anastomosis, S. Forum **8:** 208, 1958.
8. Emmelin, N.: On the presence of histamine in plasma in a physiologically active form, Acta physiol. scandinav., vol. 11, suppl. 34, 1945.
9. Emmelin, N., and Kahlson, G. S.: Histamine as a physiological excitant of acid gastric secretion, Act physiol. scandinav. **8: 289,** 1944.
10. Emmelin, N., Kahlson, G., and Wicksell, F.: Histamine in plasma and method of its estimation, Acta physiol. scandinav. **2:** 123, 1941.
11. Gerez, L., and Weiss, A.: Über die magensaftsekretion bei eckscher fistel, Ztschr. ges. exper. Med. **100:** 281, 1937.
12. Irvine, W. T., and Code, C. F.: Gastric secretion and free histamine in urine, Am. J. Physiol. **195:** 202, 1958.
13. Irvine, W. T., Duthie, H. L., Ritchie, H. D., and Waton, N. G.: The liver's role in histamine absorption from the alimentary tract, Lancet **1:** 1064, 1959.
14. Kohatsu, S., Gwaltney, J. A., Nagano, K., and Dragstedt, L. R.: Mechanism of gastric hypersecretion following portacaval transposition, Am. J. Physiol. **196:** 841, 1959.
15. Koskowski, W.: Les propiétés dynamiques du sang au cours de la digestion et leurs changements dans différentes conditions expérimentales, J. physiol. et path. gén. **31:** 697, 1933.
16. Lebedinskaja, S. I.: Über die magensekretion bei eckschen fistelhunden, Ztschr. ges. exper. Med. **88:** 264, 1933.
17. Livingston, R. H., and Code, C. F.: Role of

the liver in the conjugation of histamine in intact animals, Am. J. Physiol. **181:** 428, 1955.

18. Lowry, O. H., Graham, H. T., Harris, F. B., Priebat, M. K., Marks, A. R., and Bregman, R. U.: The chemical measurement of histamine in blood plasma and cells, J. Pharm. & Exper. Therap. **112:** 116, 1954.
19. MacIntosh, F. C.: Histamine as a normal stimulant of gastric secretion, Quart. J. Exper. Physiol. **28:** 87, 1938.
20. Öbrink, K. J.: Studies on the kinetics of the parietal secretion of the stomach, Acta physiol. scandinav. vol. 15, suppl. 51, 1948.
21. Schayer, R. W., and Ivy, A. C.: Evidence that histamine is a gastric secretory hormone in the rat, Am. J. Physiol. **189:** 369, 1957.
22. Schayer, R. W., and Ivy, A. C.: Release of $C^{14}$-histamine from stomach and intestine on feeding, Am. J. Physiol. **193:** 400, 1958.
23. Silen, W., and Eiseman, B.: The nature and cause of gastric hypersecretion after portacaval shunts, SURGERY **46:** 38, 1959.
24. Updike, E. H., II, Code, C. F., and Hallenbeck, G. A.: Excretion of free histamine in urine during gastric secretion stimulated by humoral mechanisms, Am. J. Physiol. **195:** 197, 1958.

*(For discussion, see page 237.)*

# Experimental ascites. II. The effects of portacaval shunts on ascites produced with an internal vena cava cannula

MARSHALL J. ORLOFF, M.D.*
GILBERT B. SNYDER, M.D.
DENVER, COLO.

*From the Department of Surgery, University of Colorado School of Medicine*

Considerable recent evidence indicates that hepatic venous outflow obstruction plays a major role in the pathogenesis of ascites associated with liver disease. The anatomic studies of corrosion casts of human livers by Madden and associates[5] and the investigation of volume changes in the hepatic vascular bed by Welch and associates[13] have demonstrated that in cirrhosis with ascites there is a striking diminution in the size of the hepatic venous outflow tract. Also, histologic studies by Madden and associates clearly showed obstruction of the hepatic veins within the liver in patients with ascites.

Recognition of the importance of "outflow block" in cirrhotic ascites has led to attempts to decompress the liver by a number of different surgical techniques. In general these have consisted of operations aimed at reducing the inflow of blood to the liver, such as the end-to-side portacaval shunt and ligation of the hepatic artery and its branches and, more recently, procedures directed at reducing the inflow to and improving the outflow from the liver, such as the portacaval H graft of Theron and Allen,[11] the side-to-side portacaval shunt employed by Welch and associates,[13] and the double portacaval shunt of McDermott.[6] The rationale of the latter operations is based on evidence that retrograde flow of blood may occur in the valveless portal vein which therefore is capable of functioning as an outflow tract when there is obstruction within the liver.[2, 4, 7, 12]

In a separate communication,[8] a method is described for the production of massive ascites in dogs by insertion of a polyvinyl cannula into the inferior vena cava at the level of entrance of the hepatic veins. This technique, originated by Kling and Allen,[3] results in gradual selective occlusion of the hepatic veins without production of an elevation of pressure in the inferior vena cava. The development of such a method has made it possible to investigate the effects of portal-systemic shunting procedures on ascites resulting from hepatic venous outflow obstruction. The present investigation was undertaken to experimentally establish a basis for the clinical use of these procedures.

## METHODS

**Operation.** The method used to produce ascites is described in detail in a separate communication from this laboratory.[8] Briefly, it consisted of insertion of a polyvinyl cannula* into the abdominal inferior vena cava and positioning of it at the level of entrance of the hepatic veins where it was anchored

Supported in part by United States Public Health Service Grant No. A-3048.

Read at the Twenty-second Annual Meeting of the Society of University Surgeons, Kansas City, Kan., Feb. 9-11, 1961.

*Markle Scholar in Medical Science. Present address: Department of Surgery, University of California School of Medicine, and Harbor General Hospital, Los Angeles, Calif.

*Natvar "400" tubing made by Natvar Corporation, Woodbridge, N. J., and supplied by Electrical Specialty Co., Denver, Colo.

to the vessel wall (Fig. 1). The cannula measured 3 to 3.5 inches in length, 0.025 inch in wall thickness, and varied in outer diameter from 0.375 to 0.438 inch. The tubes were siliconized on the internal surface but the external surface was not altered. All operations were performed with sterile technique through a right thoracoabdominal incision under intravenous pentobarbital sodium anesthesia. Heparin in a dose of 1 to 1.5 mg. per kilogram of body weight was administered intravenously prior to insertion of the cannula. The dogs received 5 per cent dextrose in water intravenously in a dose of 30 to 50 ml. per kilogram of body weight during the operation, and postoperatively were offered food and water ad libitum. All animals were given procaine penicillin intramuscularly in a daily dose of 600,000 U. on the day of operation and for 3 days postoperatively.

Ninety healthy adult male and female mongrel dogs varying in weight from 19 to 28 kilograms were used as subjects and were divided into 3 groups (Fig. 2). Group I consisted of 47 control animals which were subjected to insertion of the internal vena cava cannula alone. These dogs are described in detail in a separate report.[8] Group II was made up of 33 animals in which insertion of the cannula was combined with a side-to-side portacaval shunt (Fig. 3). The shunt was created immediately after insertion of the prosthesis. The opening in the abdominal inferior vena cava through which the prosthesis was introduced was used for the anastomosis, which measured 3 to 3.5 cm. in length. An elipse of vessel wall was removed from both the vena cava and portal vein in order to insure a wide connection and 2 continuous sutures of No. 5-0 vascular silk were employed to perform the anastomosis. Group III consisted of 10 dogs in which insertion of the cannula was combined with an end-to-side portacaval shunt (Fig. 3). As in Group II, the shunt was performed after insertion of the cannula. An elipse of vena cava wall was excised, and the end of the portal vein was beveled in order to create a large anastomosis which was accomplished with 2 continuous sutures of No. 5-0 vascular silk. The portal vein was ligated on the splanchnic side of the bifurcation.

In 3 animals in Group II, the side-to-side shunt was taken down several months after its construction. This was performed through a long transverse subcostal incision on the right side. The anastomosis was simply divided between vascular clamps and the separated vessels were individually reconstructed with continuous No. 5-0 vascular silk sutures.

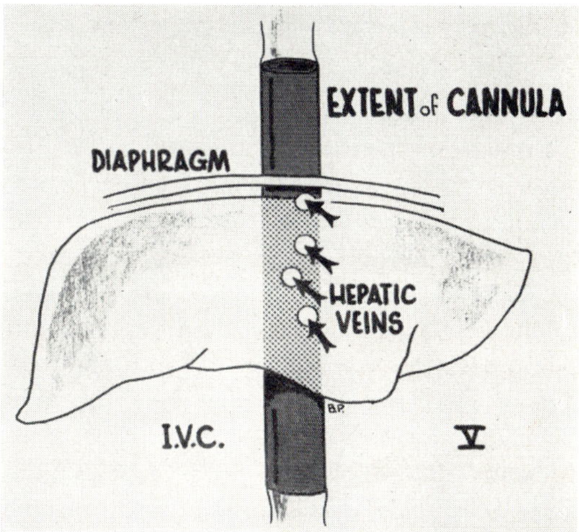


**Fig. 1.** Polyvinyl cannula in place in the inferior vena cava opposite the orifices of the hepatic veins. The reactive polyvinyl chloride produces gradual occlusion of the hepatic veins with resultant hepatic venous outflow obstruction and ascites.

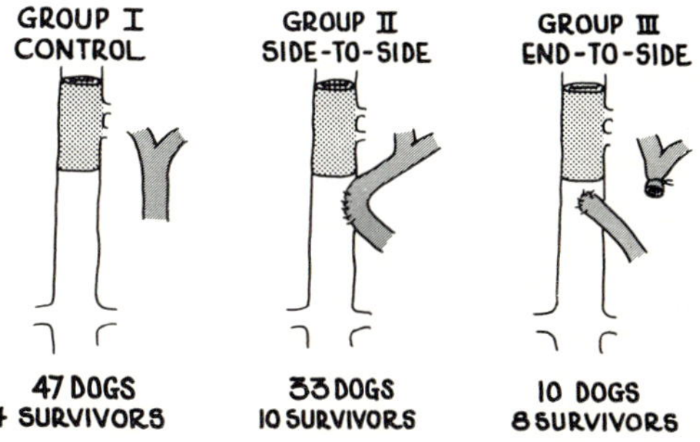


**Fig. 2.** The 3 groups of dogs involved in this study. Thirty-two of the 90 animals were long-term survivors.

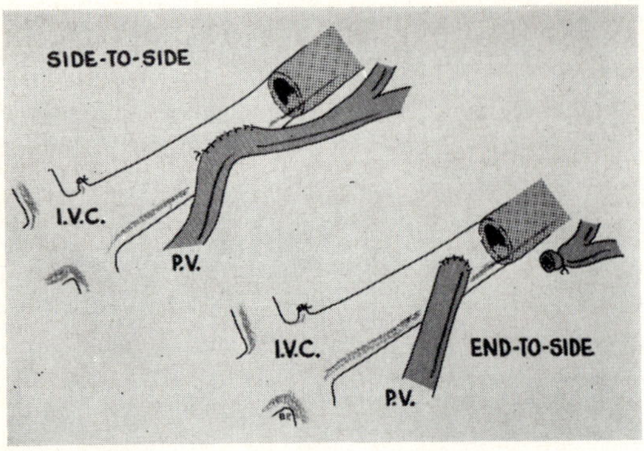


**Fig. 3.** The types of portacaval shunts which were studied. In Group II, insertion of the vena cava cannula was combined with a side-to-side portacaval shunt and in Group III insertion of the cannula was combined with an end-to-side portacaval shunt.

**Pressures.** Pressures in the abdominal inferior vena cava and portal vein were determined by needle puncture at the start of the operation and again after insertion of the cannula and completion of the shunt. A spinal manometer filled with a heparin and saline solution was employed and the base line of reference was the level of the vein in which the pressure was being measured. Pressure determinations were repeated in several animals in Groups I and II some months after operation.

**Angiograms.** Angiography of the inferior vena cava was performed 3 weeks to 10 months postoperatively in most animals which survived for more than 2 weeks. This was accomplished under light intravenous pentobarbital anesthesia with 70 per cent Urokon in a dose of 25 ml. which was injected rapidly through a vena cava catheter positioned just superior to the orifices of the renal veins. Eight roentgenograms were obtained serially at 1-second intervals.

**Paracentesis.** All animals were subjected to abdominal paracentesis when ascites was first apparent clinically, and intermittently thereafter. Paracentesis was performed with a large trocar under local anesthesia from a position underneath a special table which contained an opening through which the dog's abdomen protruded.

**Autopsies.** All animals which did not die were eventually sacrificed. The viscera were studied grossly, with particular attention given to the liver, portal vein, and vena cava. Patency of the cannulae and of the portacaval shunts was carefully ascertained. The liver was examined microscopically.

## RESULTS

### Mortality rate.

*Long-term survival.* Fourteen of 47 control animals (30 per cent), 10 of 33 dogs with side-to-side protacaval shunts (30 per cent), and 8 of 10 dogs with end-to-side portacaval shunts (80 per cent) were considered long-term survivors in that they were alive for a sufficient length of time to have developed ascites if it were going to occur.

*Early death.* Fifty-eight animals died within 2 weeks of operation. The majority of these (71 per cent) died within 48 hours postoperatively from what was believed to be acute hepatic congestion resulting from a tight-fitting cannula which produced sudden occlusion of the hepatic veins. Eight dogs died from incidental complications such as pneumonia and wound infections, 1 dog was lost, and the cause of death could not be determined in the remaining 8 animals.

**Pressures.** Table I shows the changes in pressure in the inferior vena cava and portal vein which occurred after insertion of the cannula and completion of the shunt. In all but 1 of the 47 control dogs in Group I there was a fall in vena cava pressure, presumably due to obstruction to the entrance into the vena cava of hepatic venous blood. At the same time, there was a rise in portal venous pressure in 38 of the 47 control animals (81 per cent), believed to have resulted from hepatic venous outflow obstruction with back pressure on the portal system.

In Group II, 28 of the 33 animals (85 per cent) with side-to-side shunts had an increase in vena cava pressure, presumably as a consequence of shunting of splanchnic blood into the vena cava and perhaps, in addition, due to the passage of hepatic blood by retrograde portal flow into the systemic circulation. Four animals showed no change in vena cava pressure and in 1 there was a slight fall. Thirty of the 33 dogs (91 per cent) experienced a fall in portal venous pressure due to decompression of the splanchnic bed into the lower pressure vena cava.

All 10 animals with end-to-side shunts in Group III had a rise in vena cava pressure due to shunting of the relatively high-pressure portal system into the low-pressure caval system. After insertion of the cannula and ligation of the portal vein, but prior to performance of the shunt, portal pressure on the splanchnic side of the ligature was increased in all animals. Of greater interest, portal pressure on the hepatic side of the ligature after insertion of the cannula was increased in 70 per cent of the dogs (mean of 2.5 cm. saline) and in the remaining 30 per cent decreased only slightly (mean of 2 cm. saline). In no instance did the portal pressure on the hepatic side of the occlusion fall markedly as might be expected in a vessel without branches or retrograde flow.

In 4 control dogs and 5 animals with side-to-side shunts, determinations of pressures by direct needle puncture were repeated 1 to 9 months after operation (Table II and Fig. 4). Two animals in each group had patent cannulae while the remaining 5 dogs had occluded cannulae. The portal venous pressure increased markedly to hypertensive levels in all control animals as a result of progressive outflow block, while the vena cava pressure did not change significantly in the dogs with patent prostheses and increased only slightly in those with blocked cannulae. The failure to develop a marked increase in vena cava pressure after occlusion of the cannula was probably due to the development of a profuse collateral circulation. In the animals with side-to-side shunts, the portal pressures did not change significantly in those with patent cannulae. In those with thrombosis of the cannulae, increased portal pressures were found but the levels remained within the normal range and did not reach the hypertensive levels observed in the controls. The pressures in the vena cava in dogs with shunts showed a similar pattern, with only small changes occurring in those with patent cannulae. In the dogs with occluded cannulae, the vena cava pressures increased, but the increments were not as great as are seen, for example, after band constriction of the thoracic inferior vena cava.

In 3 animals with side-to-side shunts, all of which had thrombosis of the cannulae, the anastomosis was taken down 3 to 7½ months after the initial operation (Table

**Table I.** *Pressures in abdominal inferior vena cava and portal vein immediately before and after insertion of cannula and performance of portacaval shunt*

| | No. of dogs | *Inferior vena cava pressure (mean, cm. saline)* Initial | Final* | Change | % animals | *Portal vein pressure (mean, cm. saline)* Initial | Final* | Change | % animals |
|---|---|---|---|---|---|---|---|---|---|
| Group I, control | 47 | 7.5 | 3.8 | −3.7 | Fall, 98, no change, 2, rise, 0 | 11.5 | 13.5 | +2.0 | Rise, 81, no change, 15, fall, 4 |
| Group II, side-to-side | 33 | 6.6 | 7.9 | +1.3 | Rise, 85, no change, 12, fall, 3 | 11.1 | 7.5 | −3.6 | Fall, 91, no change, 6, rise, 3 |
| Group III, end-to-side | 10 | 6.2 | 7.7 | +1.5 | Rise, 100 | 11.7 | Occluded splanchnic,† 13.7 | +2.0 | Rise, 100 |
| | | | | | | | Occluded hepatic† 14.1 | +2.4 | Rise, 70, fall, 30 |

*Final pressure determined at end of operation just prior to wound closure.
†Occluded splanchnic and occluded hepatic indicate the side of the occluding ligature on which the portal pressure was determined before the shunt was constructed.

**Table II.** *Pressure measurements in the abdominal inferior vena cava and portal vein in 9 dogs in Groups I and II repeated 1 to 9 months after insertion of the cannula and performance of the shunt*

| | Dog No. | Cannula patency | Interval between measurements (mo.) | Pressures (cm. saline): Inferior vena cava: Initial* | Repeat | Change | Portal vein: Initial* | Repeat | Change |
|---|---|---|---|---|---|---|---|---|---|
| Group I, control | 59-423 | Patent | 1 | 3.5 | 3.0 | −0.5 | 14.5 | 26.5 | +12.0 |
| | 60-22 | Patent | 4½ | 2.5 | 3.0 | +0.5 | 13.5 | 23.4 | + 9.9 |
| | 60-43 | Occluded | 4½ | 4.0 | 8.0 | +4.0 | 15.3 | 27.0 | +11.7 |
| | 60-176 | Occluded | 2½ | 8.0 | 10.0 | +2.0 | 15.5 | 25.6 | +10.1 |
| Group II, side-to-side | 59-542 | Patent | 7 | 5.5 | 7.5 | +2.0 | 5.5 | 7.5 | + 2.0 |
| | 60-271 | Patent | 9 | 4.4 | 6.8 | +2.4 | 6.8 | 7.4 | + 0.6 |
| | 59-331 | Occluded | 5 | 9.0 | 18.0 | +9.0 | 8.0 | 16.0 | + 8.0 |
| | 59-459 | Occluded | 3 | 10.4 | 17.0 | +6.6 | 8.0 | 16.6 | + 8.6 |
| | 59-501 | Occluded | 7½ | 6.8 | 12.2 | +5.4 | 4.2 | 12.2 | + 8.0 |

*Initial pressure refers to pressure at end of initial operation measured after insertion of cannula and in Group II after completion of shunt.

**Table III.** *Pressures in the abdominal inferior vena cava and portal vein in 3 ascites-free dogs with side-to-side shunts obtained before and immediately after the shunts were taken down*

| Dog No. | Cannula patency | Interval to takedown (mo.) | Pressures (cm. saline): Inferior vena cava: Control | After shunt | Before take-down | After take-down | Portal vein: Control | After shunt | Before take-down | After take-down | Ascites (L.): Before take-down | After take-down |
|---|---|---|---|---|---|---|---|---|---|---|---|---|
| 59-331 | Occluded | 5 | 9.0 | 9.0 | 18.0 | 14.0 | 10.4 | 8.0 | 16.0 | 25.0 | 0 | 2.7 |
| 59-459 | Occluded | 3 | 9.0 | 10.4 | 17.0 | 14.0 | 12.0 | 8.0 | 16.6 | 20.0 | 0 | 1.6 |
| 59-501 | Occluded | 7½ | 6.4 | 6.8 | 12.2 | 10.8 | 10.6 | 4.2 | 12.2 | 18.5 | 0 | 3.8 |

III and Fig. 5). After obliteration of the shunt there was an increase in portal pressure and a fall in vena cava pressure, indicating that the shunt had been functioning to decompress the liver and splanchnic bed.

**Ascites.** Twelve of 14 surviving control dogs developed massive persistent ascites, first detected clinically between 9 and 44 days postoperatively and varying in amount from 1.5 to 11.5 L. The failure of 2 animals to develop ascites was due, as shown by autopsies, to low insertion of the cannula which allowed the large superior hepatic vein to escape fibrotic occlusion.

Nine of 10 long-term survivors with side-to-side portacaval shunts remained free of ascites during observation periods of 2 to 9 months. One animal which died 12 weeks postoperatively was found to have 500 ml. of ascitic fluid at autopsy although repeated paracenteses during life, including an abdominal tap 1 week before death, had failed to indicate the presence of ascites. This dog died, presumably as a result of acute gastric dilatation, 36 hours after angiography performed under general anesthesia.

In 3 animals with side-to-side shunts which were free of ascites, the anastomosis was taken down 2, 5, and 7¼ months, respectively, after the initial operation. The cannulae in all 3 animals had been shown by angiography to be blocked. At the second operation the shunts were found to be patent, the livers to be normal, and the peritoneal cavities to be free of fluid. After operation all 3 dogs promptly developed ascites and died in 4, 12, and 24 days, respectively (Table III). At autopsy, the liver in each dog was greatly enlarged and congested, and the abdominal cavity contained straw-colored ascitic fluid varying in amount from 1,600 to 3,800 ml.

All 8 surviving dogs with end-to-side portacaval shunts developed persistent massive ascites and subsequently died from the resultant inanition. The ascites was detected clinically from 15 to 36 days postoperatively and varied in amount from 2.2 to 8.7 L.

**Angiograms.** Inferior vena cava angiography was attempted in 28 of the 32 long-term survivors, 3 weeks to 10 months postoperatively. In 7 control animals, 9 dogs with side-to-side shunts, and 8 dogs with end-to-side shunts the procedure was satisfactory in that the vena cava was clearly visualized. The cannulae were found to be patent in 3 of 7 controls (43 per cent), 3 of 9 dogs with side-to-side shunts (33 per cent), and in 4 of 8 dogs with end-to-side shunts (50 per cent) (Figs. 6 through 8). In the remaining animals, 58 per cent of the total, the prosthesis was blocked and numerous large collateral vessels were seen carrying the dye from the vena cava to the heart (Figs. 9 through 11).

**Autopsies.** Postmortem examinations were performed in all but one of the long-term survivors, a dog from Group II. In 1 additional control animal the cannula was lost during the autopsy and the question of patency cannot be answered. Six control animals died from inanition associated with ascites 21 to 60 days postoperatively and the remaining 8 were sacrificed 5 weeks to 10½ months after operation. Three animals with side-to-side shunts died 12 weeks to 4 months after operation from incidental causes (pneumonia, aspiration during angiography, and acute gastric dilatation after angiography), 3 died with ascites after the shunts were taken down, and 4 were sacrificed 6 to 9 months after operation. All 8 animals with end-to-side shunts died in 1½ to 3½ months of operation from inanition associated with massive ascites.

In all of the animals, the cannula was

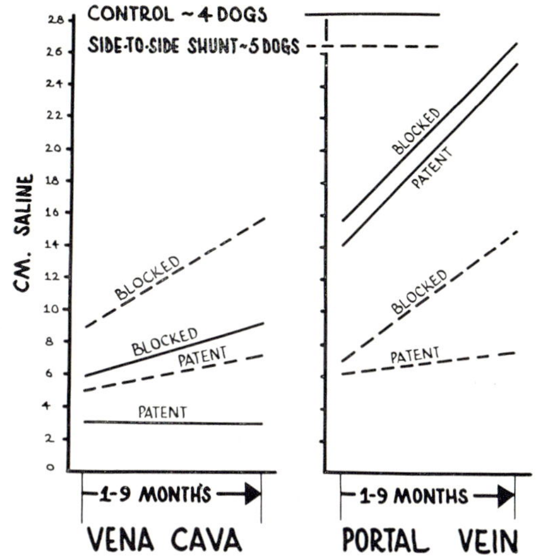


**Fig. 4.** Graph which shows pressures in the inferior vena cava and portal vein at the initial operation and again 1 to 9 months postoperatively in 4 control dogs *(solid line)* and 5 dogs with side-to-side shunts *(dash line)*. Mean pressures of each group are plotted.

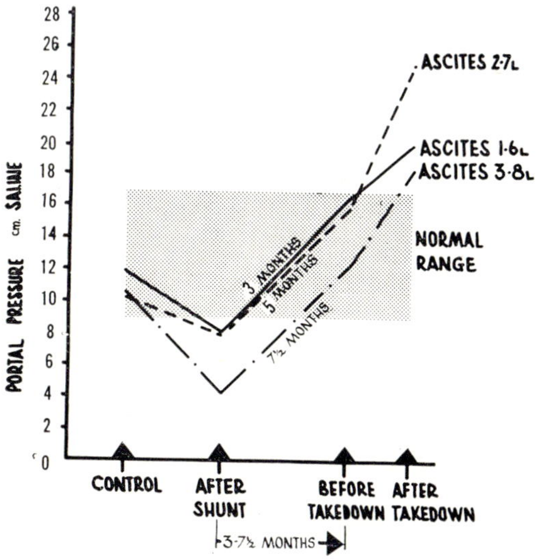


**Fig. 5.** Portal pressures in 3 dogs with side-to-side shunts which were taken down 3 to 7½ months postoperatively. Note the immediate rise in portal pressure after takedown of the shunt and the development of ascites.

**Table IV.** *Comparison of control dogs, dogs with side-to-side shunts, and dogs with end-to-side shunts with regard to ascites and patency of cannulae and shunts*

| | *No. of dogs* | *No. ascitic* | *Clinical onset of ascites (days)* | *Volume of ascites (L.)* | *Angiogram patency of cannula (%)* | *Autopsy patency* | |
|---|---|---|---|---|---|---|---|
| | | | | | | *Cannula (%)* | *Shunt (%)* |
| Group I, control | 14 | 12 | 9-44 | 1.5-11.5 | 43 | 46 | — |
| Group II, side-to-side | 10 | 1 | 0 | 0.5 | 33 | 56 | 100 |
| Group III, end-to-side | 8 | 8 | 15-36 | 2.2- 8.7 | 50 | 50 | 100 |

surrounded by a smooth, shiny neointima which completely occluded the orifices of the hepatic veins. It is believed that this fibrous material deposited on the endothelium of the vena cava resulted from reaction to the polyvinyl prosthesis.

In 6 of 13 control dogs (46 per cent), 5 of 9 animals with side-to-side shunts (56 per cent), and 4 of 8 animals with end-to-side shunts (50 per cent), the cannula was patent, an over-all incidence of 50 per cent. In 1 animal there was a discrepancy between the angiogram and the postmortem findings. The autopsy showed patency of the cannula 1 month after the angiogram had shown occlusion. In the remaining dogs, the prosthesis contained an organized thrombus in association with which there were numerous large collateral veins attached to the vena cava below the level of occlusion. All of the shunts were widely patent. In all control animals, in all animals with end-to-side shunts, and in the 3 dogs in which the side-to-side shunts had been divided, the liver was greatly enlarged, hard, and congested and microscopic studies showed intense hepatic congestion. In addition, with the exception of the 2 control animals mentioned previously, massive ascites was present at death. In contrast, the liver was normal in dogs with intact side-to-side shunts, including the only animal in this group with ascites (500 ml.) alluded to previously.

## COMMENT

The insertion of a polyvinyl cannula in the inferior vena cava opposite the hepatic vein orifices produced progressive hepatic venous outflow obstruction, marked hepatic congestion with enlargement of the liver, portal hypertension, and persistent massive ascites. With the exception of 2 dogs in which the cannula had been positioned incorrectly, all long-term survivors had complete occlusion of all hepatic veins. The experimental preparation used in this investigation, therefore, may be regarded as one with an outflow block of high grade.

The side-to-side portacaval shunt was found to be very effective in preventing the sequelae of hepatic venous outflow obstruction. None of the 10 animals in this group developed hepatomegaly or congestion of the liver. In the dogs in which determinations of portal pressure were repeated several months after operation, there was no significant change in those with patent cannulae, and in those with obstructed cannulae the elevations of portal pressure did not reach the hypertensive levels observed in the controls. Nine of 10 dogs remained free of ascites and the 1 dog in which 500 ml. of ascitic fluid was found at autopsy appeared to have developed ascites as a terminal phenomenon in association with acute gastric dilatation. The latter condition may or may not have been related. Taking down the portacaval shunt in 3 dogs which had been free of ascites resulted in a significant rise in portal pressure and the prompt appearance of ascites and hepatomegaly.

It has been proposed that the side-to-side portacaval shunt owes its effectiveness to its ability to provide both splanchnic and hepatic decompression. If this proposal is to be proved valid, evidence that the portal vein may function as an outflow tract in which retrograde flow of blood may occur is of crucial importance. Such evidence has been provided in the human being by the perfusion experiments of Herrick in 1907[2] and more recently by the studies in cirrhotic patients of Longmire and associates,[4] Warren and Muller,[12] and Mulder and Murray.[7] The results of the present investigation regarding pressure determinations on the hepatic side of the occluded portal vein after insertion of the cannula lend support to the studies in human subjects. In 70 per cent of the animals there was a rise in portal pressure on the hepatic side and in the remaining dogs there was only a slight fall. Because the portal vein was free of branches on the hepatic side of the occlusion, the elevation of pressure could only have resulted from retrograde flow of blood.

Since the vena cava cannula remained patent in only 56 per cent of the animals with side-to-side shunts, an obvious question concerns the failure of the dogs with thrombosis of the cannula to develop ascites as occurs, for example, in animals with constriction of the thoracic inferior vena cava. This question cannot be answered with certainty, but clues to the answer may be found in the results of pressure determinations and in the angiograms. In animals with cannula thrombosis in the control group, vena cava pressures increased only slightly after occlusion and in the group with side-to-side shunts, the vena cava pressures, while higher than in the controls, did not reach the levels usually found in dogs with bands constricting the thoracic inferior vena cava. Also, the livers in the latter group did not become congested and the portal pressures did not reach hypertensive levels. All of these findings indicate that the shunt continued to function in the face of a blocked

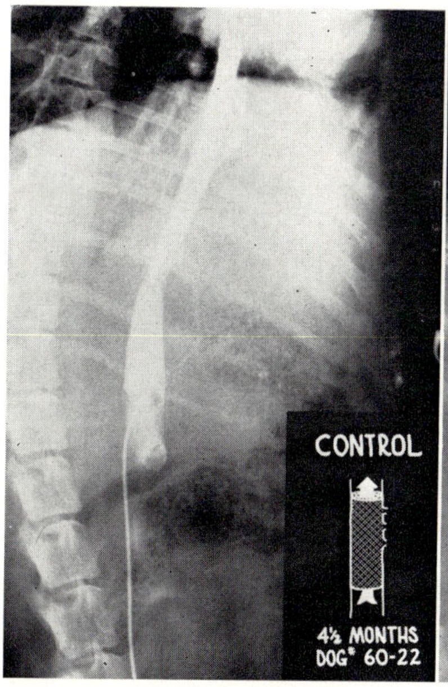


6

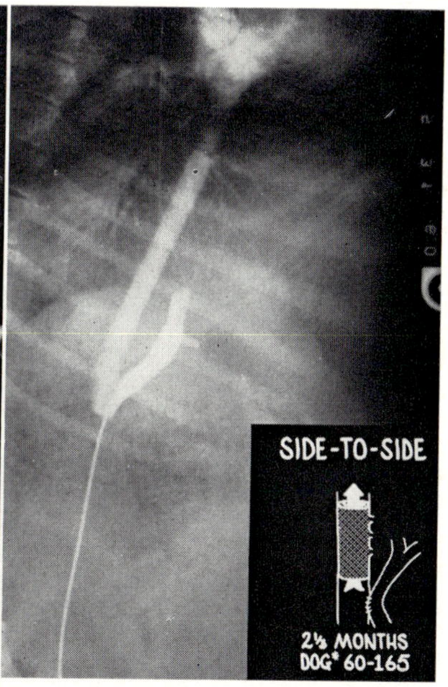


7

**Fig. 6.** Vena cava angiogram from a control dog performed 4½ months postoperatively shows a patent cannula. The animal had 4 L. of ascitic fluid.

**Fig. 7.** Vena cava angiogram from a dog with a side-to-side shunt performed 2½ months postoperatively shows a patent cannula. The catheter was threaded into the hepatic limb of the portal vein where the dye was injected and produced a striking demonstration of retrograde portal flow. The animal was free of ascites.

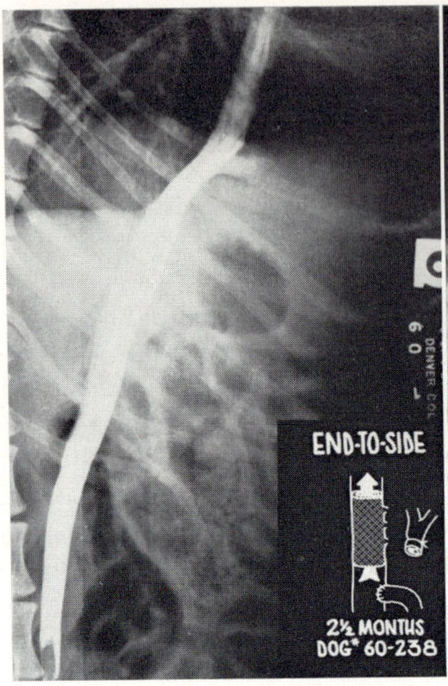


8

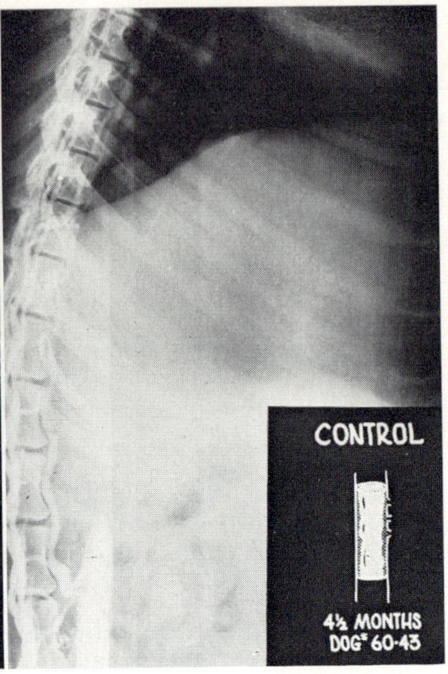


9

**Fig. 8.** Vena cava angiogram from a dog with an end-to-side portacaval shunt performed 2½ months postoperatively shows a patent cannula. The shunt was not visualized since the flow of splanchnic blood was in the direction of the vena cava. The animal had 5 L. of ascitic fluid.

**Fig. 9.** Vena cava angiogram from a control dog shows a blocked cannula and large collateral vertebral and spinal veins by-passing the block and carrying dye to the heart.

cannula, a contention which is supported by the prompt development of ascites in 3 animals when the anastomosis was taken down. All animals with an obstructed cannula were shown by angiography to have developed a profuse collateral circulation bypassing the obstruction. Particularly prominent were the vertebral and spinal veins which connected with the azygos and hemiazygos veins emptying into the superior vena cava (Figs. 9 through 11). It is proposed, therefore, that the gradual development of thrombosis in association with the enlargement of collateral vessels may explain the continued effectiveness of the portacaval shunt in providing hepatic and splanchnic decompression.

The end-to-side portacaval shunt was uniformly ineffective in preventing congestion of the liver and ascites. All of the animals in this group developed hepatomegaly and massive ascites. While the end-to-side shunt is known to reduce the flow of blood to the liver, splanchnic decompression alone was not capable of counteracting the effects of the high-grade outflow block produced by the internal vena cava cannula. Operations such as the end-to-side portacaval shunt and ligation of the hepatic artery which are aimed at reducing the flow of blood to the liver have been recommended as treatment for cirrhotic ascites and some evidence indicates that they may be effective.[1, 10] However, many surgeons have abandoned the "inflow reducing" procedures because of failure to obtain consistent success with their use in ascites.[6, 9] The results of this investigation provide support for the use of combined hepatic and splanchnic decompression as the preferable approach to the treatment of ascites resulting from hepatic venous outflow obstruction, when a surgical procedure is believed indicated.

## SUMMARY AND CONCLUSIONS

The effects of portacaval shunts on ascites produced with an internal vena cava cannula were evaluated in 90 dogs. Forty-seven animals were subjected to insertion of the vena cava cannula alone, 33 animals had insertion of the cannula combined with a side-to-side portacaval shunt, and in 10 animals insertion of the cannula was combined with an end-to-side portacaval shunt. Thirty-two animals survived the operation for long periods. The majority of animals which failed to survive died shortly after operation as a result of acute hepatic venous occlusion produced by a tight-fitting cannula.

Insertion of the cannula alone resulted in an immediate rise in portal pressure and a fall in vena cava pressure in most of the control dogs, while in the animals with shunts this pressure pattern was reversed. In the dogs with end-to-side shunts, portal pressure on the hepatic side of the ligated portal vein increased in 70 per cent, which indicated the occurrence of retrograde blood flow. Redetermination of pressures in 9 animals after an interval of several months showed little change in the dogs with side-to-side shunts which had patent cannulae, while the controls developed portal hypertension. In dogs with side-to-side shunts and occluded cannulae, the portal pressure increased but not to hypertensive levels which indicated that the shunts continued to function in the face of thrombosis of the cannula. The development of extensive collateral channels was believed responsible for the continued effectiveness of these shunts.

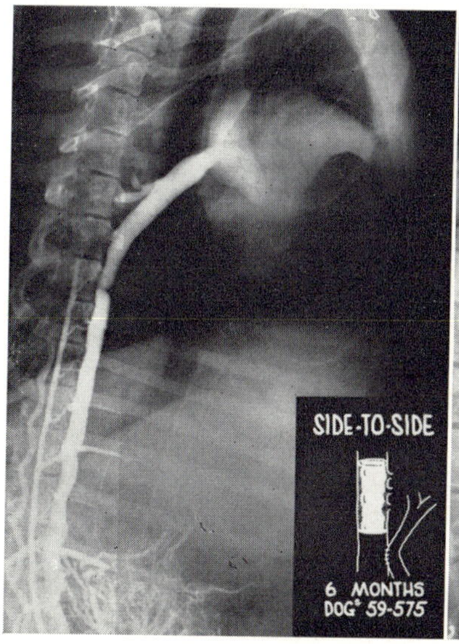


10

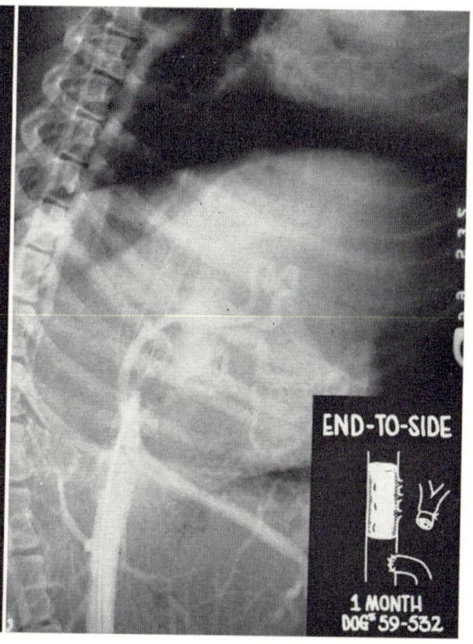


11

**Fig. 10.** Vena cava angiogram from a dog with a side-to-side shunt and a blocked cannula shows profuse collateral circulation emptying into the azygos and hemiazygos veins and thence into the superior vena cava. An outline of the blocked cannula can be seen medial to the dye-filled collaterals.

**Fig. 11.** Vena cava angiogram from a dog with an end-to-side shunt and a blocked cannula shows abundant collateral vessels as well as a dye-filled portal vein entering the vena cava. An outline of the occluded cannula can be seen.

Vena cava angiography and autopsies showed patency of the shunts in 100 per cent of the dogs and patency of the cannulae in 50 per cent. The dogs with thrombosis of the cannulae were found to have developed a profuse collateral circulation bypassing the obstruction in the vena cava.

Twelve of 14 surviving control dogs developed hepatomegaly and massive persistent ascites varying from 1.5 to 11.5 L. Two control dogs did not develop ascites because of low insertion of the cannula with resultant failure to occlude all of the hepatic veins. All 8 surviving dogs with end-to-side shunts developed hepatomegaly and massive ascites. In contrast, 9 of 10 long-term survivors with side-to-side shunts remained free of ascites for periods of up to 9 months, and none of these dogs had hepatomegaly. Takedown of the side-to-side anastomosis of 3 ascites-free animals was followed by the prompt appearance of portal hypertension, hepatomegaly, and ascites.

The side-to-side portacaval shunt proved to be a very effective means of preventing experimental ascites associated with hepatic venous outflow obstruction, while the end-to-side shunt was without effect. The results of this investigation, therefore, provide support for the clinical use of combined hepatic and splanchnic decompression in the treatment of ascites associated with liver disease and outflow block.

## REFERENCES

1. Barker, H. G., and Reemtsma, K.: The portacaval shunt operation in patients with cirrhosis and ascites, SURGERY **48:** 142, 1960.
2. Herrick, F. C.: An experimental study into the cause of the increased portal pressure in portal cirrhosis, J. Exper. Med. **9:** 93, 1907.
3. Kling, S., and Allen, P. B. R.: The effects of gradual complete occlusion of the hepatic veins, S. Forum **9:** 550, 1959.
4. Longmire, W. P., Jr., Mulder, D. G., Mahoney, P. S., and Mellinkoff, S. W.: Side-to-side portacaval anastomosis for portal hypertension, Ann. Surg. **147:** 881, 1958.
5. Madden, J. L., Lore, J. M., Jr., Gerold, F. P., and Ravid, J. M.: The pathogenesis of ascites and a consideration of its treatment, Surg. Gynec. & Obst. **99:** 385, 1954.
6. McDermott, W. V., Jr.: The double portacaval shunt in the treatment of cirrhotic ascites, Surg. Gynec. & Obst. **110:** 457, 1960.
7. Mulder, D. G., and Murray, J. F.: An evaluation of the side-to-side portacaval shunt, S. Forum **11:** 278, 1960.
8. Orloff, M. J., and Snyder, G. B.: Experimental ascites. I. Production of ascites by gradual occlusion of the hepatic veins with an internal vena cava cannula, SURGERY. In press.
9. Ravdin, I. S.: The complexity of liver disease—surgical steps toward solution, Ann. Roy. Coll. Surgeons **20:** 71, 1957.
10. Rienhoff, W. F., Jr., and Woods, A. C., Jr.: Ligation of hepatic and splenic arteries in treatment of cirrhosis with ascites, J. A. M. A. **152:** 687, 1953.
11. Theron, P., and Allen, J. C.: Ascites: clinical and experimental study, Acta med. scandinav. **152:** 145, 1955.
12. Warren, W. D., and Muller, W. H., Jr.: A clarification of some hemodynamic changes in cirrhosis and their surgical significance, Ann. Surg. **150:** 413, 1959.
13. Welch, C. S., Welch, H. F., and Carter, J. H.: The treatment of ascites by side-to-side portacaval shunt, Ann. Surg. **150:** 428, 1959.

*(For discussion, see page 237.)*

# Sodium excretion after intrasplenic and systemic injections of sodium chloride in normal dogs and after portacaval shunt

EARL F. WOLFMAN, JR., M.D.
G. D. ZUIDEMA, M.D.
R. M. ONEAL, M.D.
J. TURCOTTE, M.D.
R. KOWALCZYK, PH.D.
CHARLES G. CHILD, III, M.D.
ANN ARBOR, MICH.
*From the Department of Surgery, The University of Michigan Medical School*

Many patients with cirrhosis of the liver and ascites have a predilection for maintaining a positive sodium balance while excreting greater-than-normal quantities of aldosterone in the urine. This relationship between sodium retention and increased aldosterone excretion can frequently be reversed by portal decompression, and a successful shunt is often followed by relief of the ascites. Why a portacaval shunt induces sodium excretion is not clear. Postshunt natriuresis has been presumed to be due to a decreased secretion of aldosterone by the adrenal cortex. Recently, however, Mittelmann and his associates[6] have shown that after a portacaval shunt some patients with ascites and cirrhosis excrete sodium freely while the urinary aldosterone excretion may even increase. This apparent paradox of an increased urinary excretion of both sodium and aldosterone after portal decompression has not been adequately explained. It seems, then, that secondary hyperaldosteronism is not solely responsible for sodium retention and ascites in some cases of advanced cirrhosis of the liver. Furthermore, a decreased urinary excretion of aldosterone is not a necessary accompaniment of the natriuresis that may occur after portacaval shunt.

This study was undertaken to explore mechanisms whereby a portacaval shunt might influence sodium excretion. Since orally ingested fluids and electrolytes enter the portal circulation and traverse the liver before entering the systemic circulation, it was postulated that intrahepatic compensatory mechanisms might exist to regulate the caprices of oral intake. As early as 1921 Lamson and Roca[5] observed that the rate of disappearance of intravenously injected isotonic salt solutions was decreased 4 times or more when the liver was excluded from the circulation. We reasoned that if the liver was integrated into the control of sodium and water metabolism this mechanism might be modified by a portacaval shunt. Our experiments, therefore, were designed to detect differences in body management of sodium and water when these are injected in isotonic concentrations into the portal and systemic venous circuits in both normal dogs and dogs with end-to-side portacaval shunts.

## METHODS

For ready accessibility, the spleens of 12 adult female dogs weighing between 12 and 18 kilograms were explanted subcutaneously into the left lateral abdominal wall (Fig. 1).

Supported by United States Public Health Service Grants H-4260 and B-2290, and Contract No. DA-49-007-MD-1016, Department of the Army.

Read at the Twenty-second Annual Meeting of the Society of University Surgeons, Kansas City, Kan., Feb. 9-11, 1961.

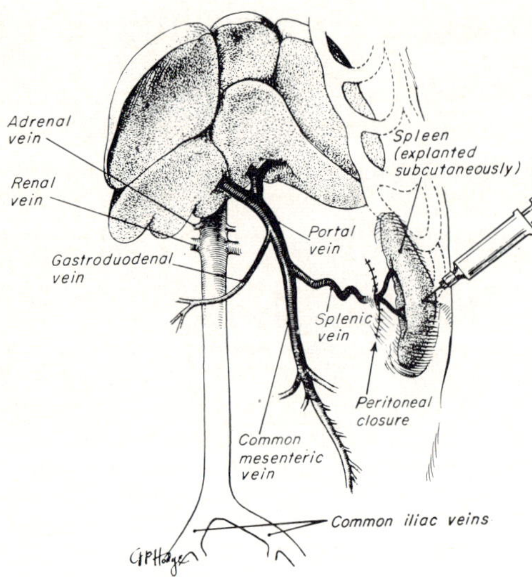


**Fig. 1.** Normal dogs. The spleen has been operatively explanted into a subcutaneous position in the left lateral abdominal wall.

In 6 of these dogs, normal in all respects save for the splenic explantation, patterns of sodium and water excretion were studied. All dogs received standard kennel rations throughout the entire period of study. Two weeks after explantation of the spleen they were lightly anesthetized intravenously with thiopental (25 mg. per kilogram), and positioned supine on an operating table in reverse Trendelenburg position with the head elevated 30 degrees. A blood specimen was obtained for creatinine studies and the urinary bladder catheterized with a No. 20 Fr. Robinson catheter. A 30-minute urine specimen was collected prior to the saline infusion. Next, a splenic puncture was made with a 20 gauge needle attached to a syringe. When venous blood was encountered, the syringe was removed and 500 ml. of 0.9 per cent saline solution administered in a 30-minute interval. Bladder urine was collected at 30-minute intervals, beginning with the splenic infusion and continuing for 5 hours. A postinfusion blood specimen was also obtained for creatinine studies. All urine specimens were placed in ice immediately, and later, after measurement of the volume, were analyzed for osmolality and sodium content. Pre- and postinfusion creatinine clearances were calculated. Postoperatively the animals received Gantrisin, 1.0 Gm. twice daily, to prevent urinary tract infections that otherwise occurred. One week later the procedure was repeated, except that 500 ml. of 0.9 per cent saline solution was injected into the systemic venous circuit through the femoral vein.

In the remaining 6 dogs end-to-side portacaval shunts were fashioned (Fig. 2). Infusions of isotonic saline solution were made into the spleens and femoral veins of these animals which were identical to those made in the normal dogs. At the conclusion of the final infusion, the patency of the shunt was confirmed by splenoportography.

## RESULTS

The mean 5-hour sodium excretions of the normal animals after the infusion of 500 ml. of 0.9 per cent saline solution through the spleen was 16.1 mEq. of sodium. In dogs with end-to-side portacaval shunts only 4.1 mEq. of sodium was excreted (Table I). On statistical analysis of the results, the normal animals were found to

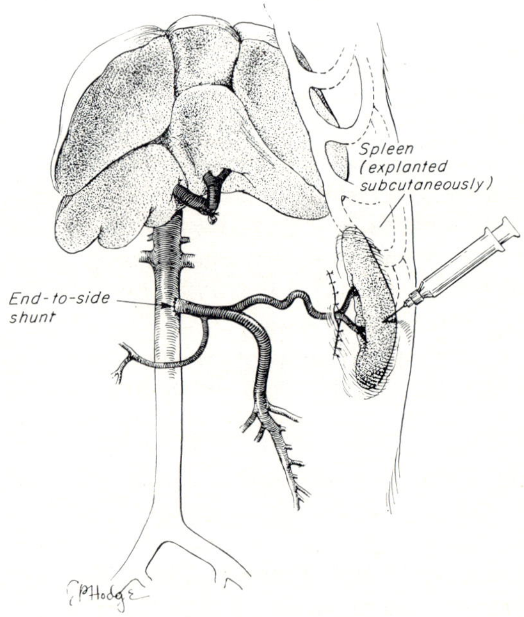


**Fig. 2.** Dogs with shunts. The spleen has been explanted subcutaneously and an end-to-side portacaval shunt performed.

**Table I.** *Mean 5-hour urinary sodium excretions after infusion of 500 ml. of 0.9 per cent saline into spleens and femoral veins of normal dogs and those with end-to-side portacaval shunts*

| | *Spleen (mEq. Na)* | *Femoral vein (mEq. Na)* |
|---|---|---|
| Normal dogs | 16.1 | 28.1 |
| Dogs with portacaval shunts | 4.1 | 10.1 |

have excreted a mean of 16.1± $\sigma$ 4.97 mEq. of sodium in 5 hours. The median 5-hour sodium excretion of this group was 14.95 mEq. and the average deviation from the median ± 3.52 mEq. of sodium. Animals with shunts excreted a mean of 4.1± $\sigma$ 2.65 mEq. of sodium in 5 hours. The median 5-hour sodium excretion of these dogs was 4.4 mEq. and the average deviation from the median ± 1.95. Further analysis with the t-distribution test as described by Snedecor[12] gives a t value of 4.76. This result indicates that the differences observed between the sodium excretions of these 2 groups of animals could be a chance observation in less than 1 in 1,000 instances.

When 0.9 per cent saline solution was injected into the femoral veins in the normal dogs and those with shunts the mean 5-hour sodium excretions were 28.1 and 10.1 mEq. of sodium, respectively. In each group more sodium was excreted after femoral vein infusions than after splenic infusions. Perhaps this is due to the more rapid access of the infused solutions to the systemic circuit when they are administered directly into the femoral vein rather than into the spleen.

Table II is a summary of the mean sodium and urine volume excretions in both groups of dogs before and after the infusion of 500 ml. of 0.9 per cent saline solution into the speens and femoral veins. During the 5-hour period of this study, the normal dogs compensated for the isotonic increase in extracellular fluid volume, caused by either the portal or systemic infusion of normal saline solution, by increasing both the urinary concentration of sodium and the volume of urine. Animals with shunts, in response to the same infusions, exhibited a similar increase in the concentration of sodium excreted, but failed to show any significant increase in volume of urine. The animals with portacaval anastomoses demonstrated no appreciable tendency to retain more sodium under normal circumstances than did the normal dogs. This fact is supported by preinfusion excretions of 0.50 and 0.58 mEq. of sodium in 30 minutes in the normals as compared to 0.25 and 0.53 mEq. of sodium in 30 minutes in the shunted dogs.

One dog in this study which originally served as a normal animal later underwent an end-to-side portacaval shunt and the saline infusions were repeated. Table III shows the difference in response of this animal when the shunt was present.

## COMMENT

This study demonstrates that dogs with end-to-side portacaval shunts retain sodium in significantly greater amounts than those without shunts when isotonic sodium chloride is given either through the portal or systemic venous circuits. Normal animals respond to this isotonic increase in the volume of the extracellular fluid by increasing the concentration of sodium in the urine and the volume of urine. The urinary volumes increased more than the sodium concentration. Dogs with portacaval shunts responded to similar infusions by failing to increase significantly the volume of urine excreted but increasing the concentration of urinary sodium.

The sodium retention observed in the animals with shunts after isotonic saline administration deserves further elucidation. Infusions in these animals, whether into the spleen or femoral vein, immediately enter the systemic venous system and are, therefore, similar in this respect to the femoral vein infusions in normal dogs (Fig. 2). Yet the response of the shunted animals differs from that of the controls in that significant sodium and water retention occurs. Even though dogs are known to have very labile glomerular filtration rates, pre- and post-

**Table II.** *Mean sodium and urine volume excretions before and after infusion of 500 ml. of 0.9 per cent saline into spleens and femoral veins of normal dogs and those with end-to-side portacaval shunts*

| | *Normal dogs* | | *Dogs with end-to-side portacaval shunts* | |
|---|---|---|---|---|
| | *Spleen* | *Femoral vein* | *Spleen* | *Femoral vein* |
| Mean 30-min. excretion of Na prior to infusion (mEq. Na/ml. urine) | 0.14 | 0.16 | 0.06 | 0.08 |
| Mean 5-hr. excretion of Na after infusion (mEq. Na/ml. urine) | 0.20 | 0.24 | 0.08 | 0.16 |
| Mean 30-min. excretion of Na prior to infusion (mEq. Na/30 min.) | 0.50 | 0.58 | 0.25 | 0.53 |
| Mean 30-min. excretion of Na after infusion (mEq. Na/30 min.) | 1.62 | 2.81 | 0.43 | 1.01 |
| Mean 30-min. excretion of urine prior to infusion (ml. urine/min.) | 0.12 | 0.12 | 0.14 | 0.22 |
| Mean 5-hr. excretion of urine after infusion (ml. urine/min.) | 0.27 | 0.39 | 0.18 | 0.21 |
| Mean 30-min. excretion of urine prior to infusion (ml. urine/30 min.) | 3.6 | 3.6 | 4.2 | 6.6 |
| Mean 30-min. excretion of urine after infusion (ml. urine/30 min.) | 8.1 | 11.7 | 5.4 | 6.3 |

infusion creatinine clearance tests were performed. The results were found to vary greatly in the same dog and no correlation was present between the glomerular filtration rates determined and the presence or absence of a portacaval shunt. Since all of the dogs in this study were given identical infusions under similar circumstances, it is unlikely that the observed differences in sodium and water excretion between the 2 groups were due to changes in the glomerular filtration rates.

The outstanding difference between the 2 groups of animals studied is the impaired hepatic function that results from the decreased hepatic blood flow in animals with end-to-side portacaval shunts. Heer and associates[3] found hepatic blood flow reduced approximately 49 per cent when an end-to-side portacaval shunt was performed in otherwise normal dogs. Associated with this reduced hepatic blood flow was a significant impairment of hepatic function as measured by serum albumin concentration, decreased tolerance to dietary protein, increased blood ammonia levels, and increased Bromsulphalein retention. Thus, it may be postulated that the failure of the animals with shunts to compensate for an acute isotonic expansion of the extracellular fluid volume is related to hepatic dysfunction which occurs as a direct result of the Eck fistula. Conceivably, the normal liver contains receptors that respond to extracellular fluid volume changes in the portal venous system.

Although there was significant sodium retention in the dogs with shunts during the 5-hour period of study, these animals showed little tendency to retain sodium under other circumstances. For example both groups of dogs were given identical kennel rations, and under these circumstances the mean 30-minute excretion of sodium prior to infusion was 0.50 and 0.58 mEq. of sodium for the normal animals, and 0.25 and 0.53 mEq. of sodium for those with shunts. This indicates that despite a significant retention of sodium and water by the dogs with shunts in response to an acute isotonic expansion of the volume of the extracellular fluid, these animals ultimately could compensate for these expansions. Perhaps this delayed excretion of sodium and water is accomplished by volume receptors located in other areas or it may be due to the same mechanisms present within the normal liver now responding to a relative increase in hepatic arterial inflow associated with an expanded extracellular fluid volume.

The regulation of extracellular fluid volume and tonicity have been discussed for more than a decade. Such discussions have been concerned with specific locations and modes of action of osmoreceptors and volume receptors.[1, 2, 4, 8-11, 15, 18, 19] Even though the specific location of such receptors, as well as their afferent and efferent pathways, remains unknown, their clinical significance is emphasized when one encounters certain patients with profound disturbances in the tonicity or volume of the extracellular fluid. In regard to volume receptors, not only their location, but also the mechanisms by which they act, remain obscure. At the present time, 2 physiologic processes appear to be involved. Strauss[13] has summarized evidence which indicates that the supraoptico-hypophyseal system is responsive to critical changes in the extracellular fluid volume. Also, since extracellular volume is dependent upon its total solute, of which sodium and potassium are the most important elements, aldosterone secretion appears to be part of this regulatory process. Heretofore, little attention has been given to the liver and its possible role in the regulation of the volume of extracellular fluid.

Welch and colleagues[16] have stated that the sine qua non of ascites formation associated with cirrhosis is an hepatic blood outflow block, probably postsinusoidal in location. They relate the formation of ascites under such circumstances entirely to mechanical factors associated with increased vascular hydrostatic pressure relationships in

**Table III.** *Response of 1 dog (No. 60-119) to infusion of 500 ml. of 0.9 per cent saline into spleen and femoral vein both as a control and with an end-to-side portacaval shunt*

| | *Spleen* (*mEq. Na*) | *Femoral vein* (*mEq. Na*) |
|---|---|---|
| Normal | 14.9 | 28.3 |
| Portacaval shunt | 0.7 | 3.7 |

the congested liver. However, our data indicate a predilection for sodium retention in a functionally impaired liver alone, in the absence of a mechanical postsinusoidal block. Certainly, if receptor mechanisms are normally present within the liver, the superimposition of cirrhosis and a state of hepatic congestion could cause varying degrees of interference with their action. Therefore, portal decompression might well be effective in controlling ascites by permitting the receptors to again respond to volume changes now heralded by the hepatic arterial inflow, even though the total hepatic blood flow remains reduced.

Dogs with portacaval shunts, although increasing the concentration of sodium excreted, showed virtually no increase in the volume of urine in response to the infusions. This observed dissociation of sodium and water excretion is at variance with the mechanisms described by Wolff and associates[17] as compensatory for increases in extracellular fluid volume in liver disease. They suggest that an increase in the volume of extracellular fluid leads to decreased secretion of aldosterone resulting in decreased renal tubular reabsorption of sodium, a decrease in total-body sodium, and a decreased extracellular fluid tonicity. This results in a decrease in water intake and posterior pituitary antidiuretic activity, thus producing a decreased tubular reabsorption of water and decreased total-body fluids. They also postulated that in some patients with hepatic disease, defective intrahepatic breakdown of aldosterone leads to an increase of circulating aldosterone and secondary activation of the antidiuretic mechanism. Such a theory can be questioned for several reasons. First intravenously administered aldosterone has a duration of action of 8 hours or more.[7, 14] It is unlikely that during the 5-hour period of this study the increased excretion of sodium in normal dogs could be entirely due to a decrease in aldosterone secretion combined with an excessively rapid metabolic degradation of any circulating aldosterone. Furthermore, a similar increase in the concentration of sodium excreted was found in the dogs with shunts, yet the total amount of sodium excreted was significantly less. Second, our data demonstrate a tendency of animals with shunts and secondarily impaired hepatic function to retain water in excess of sodium. Welch and associates have also observed this phenomenon in ascitic patients. Third, Mittlemann and his group[6] attempted to relate the disappearance of ascites and the increased sodium excretion that is often seen after portacaval shunt to decreased aldosterone excretion postoperatively. All 6 patients studied by them demonstrated marked sodium retention and increased urinary excretion of aldosterone in association with ascites preoperatively. In 4 of the 6 patients the inverse relationship between the urinary excretions of aldosterone and sodium was found postoperatively. The 2 other patients, both of whom did not regain ascites, showed an increased excretion of aldosterone and sodium postoperatively. These data indicate that even though the aldosterone excretion remained high, the increased excretion of sodium in these 2 cases was associated with an increased excretion of water postoperatively.

## SUMMARY

Experimental evidence is presented that demonstrates significant sodium and water retention in dogs with end-to-side portacaval shunts in response to isotonic saline infusions into the portal and systemic venous circuits. These data suggest that there are mechanisms located within the liver that aid in the regulation of the extracellular fluid volume, and these are closely integrated with the antidiuretic mechanism of the posterior pituitary gland as well as the adrenal cortex.

### REFERENCES

1. Drury, D. R., Henry, J. P., and Goodman, J.: The effects of continuous pressure breathing on kidney function, J. Clin. Invest. **26:** 945, 1947.
2. Grage, T. B., Winter, J., and Zimmermann, B.: Studies of extracellular volume in the regulation of antidiuretic hormone, S. Forum **11:** 129, 1960.
3. Heer, F. W., Silvius, D. E., and Harper, H. A.: The relation between hepatic blood flow and function in normal dogs and dogs with cirrhosis after portacaval shunt or transposition, S. Forum **11:** 282, 1960.
4. Henry, J. P., and Pearce, W. J.: The possible role of cardiac atrial stretch receptors in the induction of changes in urine flow, J. Physiol. **131:** 572, 1956.
5. Lamson, P. D., and Roca, J.: The liver as a blood concentrating organ, J. Pharmacol. & Exper. Therap. **17:** 481, 1921.
6. Mittelmann, A., Gore, D. O., and Barker, H. G.: The effect of portacaval shunting on urinary aldosterone excretion, S. Forum **10:** 291, 1959.
7. Muller, A. F., Mach, E., and Naegeli, H.: Comparison of the effect of aldosterone and Cortexone (desoxycorticosterone) on electrolyte excretion in man, Acta endocrinol. **20:** 113, 1955.
8. Peters, J. P.: The role of sodium in the production of edema, New England J. Med. **239:** 353, 1948.
9. Peters, J. P., Welt, L. G., Sims, E. A. H., Orloff, J., and Needham, J.: A salt wasting syndrome associated with cerebral disease, Tr. A. Am. Physicians **63:** 57, 1950.
10. Sieker, H. O., Gauer, O. P., and Henry, J. P.: The effect of continuous negative pressure breathing on water and electrolyte excretion by the human kidney, J. Clin. Invest. **33:** 572, 1954.
11. Sims, E. A., Welt, L. G., Orloff, J., and Needham, J. W.: Asymptomatic hyponatremia in pulmonary tuberculosis, J. Clin. Invest. **29:** 1545, 1950.
12. Snedecor, G. W.: Statistical methods, Ames, 1956, The Iowa State College Press, pp. 85-101.
13. Strauss, M. B.: Body water in man, Boston, 1957, Little, Brown & Company.
14. Thorn, G. W., Sheppard, R. H., Morse, W. I., Reddy, W. J., Beigelman, P. M., and Renold, A. E.: Comparative action of aldosterone and 9-alpha-fluorohydrocortisone in man, Ann. New York Acad. Sc. **61:** 609, 1955.
15. Verney, E. B.: Antidiuretic hormone and factors which determine its release, Proc. Roy. Soc., London, s. B. **135:** 25, 1947.
16. Welch, C. S., Welch, H. F., and Carter, J. H.: The treatment of ascites by side to side portacaval shunt, Ann. Surg. **150:** 428, 1959.
17. Wolff, H. P., Koczorek, Kh. R., and Buchborn, E.: Aldosterone and antidiuretic hormone (Adiuretin) in liver disease, Acta endocrinol. **27:** 45, 1958.

18. Wolfman, E. F., Jr., Coon, W. W., and Kahn, E. A.: The recognition and management of severe hypertonicity of the extracellular fluid associated with cerebral lesions, SURGERY **47:** 410, 1960.
19. Wolfman, E. F., Jr., Coon, W. W., Reifel, E., Iob, V., and McMath, M.: Severe hypertonicity of the extracellular fluid associated with cerebral lesions, SURGERY **47:** 929, 1960.

## DISCUSSION*

**Dr. James S. Clarke** (Los Angeles, Calif.). I would like to discuss the first of these 3 excellent papers. Drs. Silen and Eiseman have presented further evidence supporting the hypothesis that histamine is an agent which originates in the gut and may be shunted around the liver, thus causing gastric hypersecretion. However, there are several observations which suggest that this may not be the whole story. One is their finding that the fasting levels of histamine do not seem to be different in dogs with shunts and in dogs without shunts. This may be simply a limitation of the technique. Second is their own finding, as well as that of Dr. Gregory of Liverpool, that the response of the hypersecretion which occurs after shunt to inhibitory pharmacologic agents, such as atropine, is not the same as the response of histamine-induced secretion. Third, Castaneda and his colleagues from Minneapolis have shown that acid secretion caused by stimulation of an isolated antral pouch, which is presumably due to gastrin, is increased in dogs which have a portacaval shunt.

Finally, I would like to suggest that this general hypothesis might account for the findings of increased gastric secretion after pancreatic duct ligation which were presented by Dr. Elliott yesterday. Dr. Dragstedt showed that dogs which have the pancreatic exocrine secretions diverted from the intestinal tract develop weight loss, hypolipemia, and fatty livers. Weight loss at least was seen in some of Dr. Elliott's dogs. In interpreting the effect on gastric secretion of pancreatic operations, all of which involve diversion of pancreatic juice from the gut, one might look at the liver and ask whether it is fatty, whether its content of histaminase is normal, and whether postprandial plasma histamine curves remain unchanged when hypersecretion appears.

**Dr. William V. McDermott, Jr.** (Boston, Mass.). These were 3 very stimulating papers and I want to comment very briefly on each of them. With regard to the paper by Drs. Silen and Eiseman, the increased gastric secretory activity after a shunt is certainly well recognized and well established by now. This report presents evidence to implicate, in part at least, histamines bypassing the liver as being one of the factors involved. Clinically this increased gastric secretory activity is reflected by an increase in the incidence of peptic ulceration after shunt. We have recently reviewed the 237 elective portal systemic shunts constructed up to 1958 at the Massachusetts General Hospital and have found that there is an over-all incidence of 15 per cent of peptic ulceration. In several cases hemorrhage has been a serious and occasionally lethal complication. The paper given by Drs. Orloff and Snyder has been of particular interest to us because of our efforts to reverse cirrhotic ascites. We have believed that part of the pathogenesis of the rather complicated metabolic problem of cirrhotic ascites in man has been hemodynamic and has been related not only to congestion in the splanchnic bed, but also in the intrahepatic vascular bed, in other words, a partial outflow block. Methods of inducing experimental ascites are not entirely applicable to man because man does not present the pure Budd-Chiari syndrome and in no instance of cirrhotic ascites have we found the hepatic pressure to rise after occlusion of portal veins. But nonetheless, it does remain high and the intrahepatic portal bed does remain congested, which suggests that an outflow block or postsinusoidal block is at least a part of the mechanism which produces ascites. In attempting to correct this, we have applied combined splanchnic and hepatic decompression by use of the double shunt which is similar in concept to the use of the side-to-side shunt by Dr. Welch and his associates and others.

In reviewing the over-all results of shunt operations in 40 patients who had intractable ascites at the time of construction of the shunt, the results have been very good if the double or side-to-side portacaval shunt has been used. In 17 cases there have been 2 deaths, but 14 of the 15 survivors have had rapid, complete, and permanent dissipation of the ascites. The end-to-side portacaval shunt has been less satisfactory, but has in many instances ultimately resulted in the dissipation of ascites. The appearance of sodium in the urine is rather delayed as compared to the rapid appearance of sodium after the construction of a side-to-side or double shunt and the ascites will frequently persist for weeks or even months. On 2 occasions, patients with only minimal ascites have, in the postoperative phase after construction of end-to-side shunt, developed severe intractable ascites which persisted for some months after the operation. A splenorenal shunt, of course, is basically a small side-to-side shunt and the results have more or less fallen in between the results of the other 2 types. In regard to the paper presented by Dr. Wolfman and his associates, I

*Discussion of papers by Silen and Eiseman; Orloff and Snyder; and Wolfman, Zuidema, Oneal, Turcotte, Kowalczyk, and Child.

wonder if these metabolic effects could be related to failure of clearance of aldosterone by the partially damaged liver.

**Dr. Harold G. Barker** (New York, N. Y.). I enjoyed these 3 papers very much and wish to compliment the essayists. I want to comment briefly on Dr. Orloff's paper. He has shown very nicely that dogs with side-to-side shunts avoid the ascites that normally follows hepatic vein obstruction, whereas dogs with end-to-side shunts get the ascites in spite of the shunt. This implies that a side-to-side shunt would relieve the ascites in patients with Budd-Chiari syndrome and we have had the opportunity to try this with good success. It is important, however, that we not construe the results of this study as an argument in favor of side-to-side shunting in patients with ascites from cirrhosis of the liver. Some of you will remember that we presented before this society last year the results of our study on the use of end-to-side shunts in cirrhotic ascites. We have found no reason to date to lose faith in this operation. I wonder if Dr. Orloff would comment on the wide variability in survival rates between the 3 groups of dogs from 80 per cent for those with end-to-side shunts down to 25 per cent for the controls.

**Dr. W. Dean Warren** (Charlottesville, Va.). I would also like to comment on the very nice paper of Drs. Orloff and Snyder. Although we do not believe that the intrahepatic pressure is the most important factor in the development of ascites in patients, it certainly is one of the 2 or 3 physiologic derangements which leads to ascites. Because of this, we believe the side-to-side portacaval shunt is most certainly indicated in cirrhosis with ascites because of the markedly diminished outflow resistance which is brought about by this operation. With this procedure, there can occur a marked fall in sinusoidal pressure with little change in the arterial perfusion of the sinusoidal bed. In a number of patients there has been a documented increase in flow to the liver although the sinusoidal pressure has been greatly reduced. Because of this beneficial effect in the hemodynamic status of the liver, we feel that the side-to-side portacaval shunt is the operative procedure to be utilized in such patients.

**Dr. William Silen** (San Francisco, Calif.). I would like to thank Drs. Clarke and McDermott for discussing this paper. With reference to the lack of difference between the fasting levels of plasma histamine in the shunt and nonshunt normal dogs, I think it is important to recognize that one can give histamine exogenously in quantities sufficient to produce gastric secretion and yet may not be able to measure this amount of histamine in the blood with present methods. Thus, minute increments in plasma histamine may be physiologically active in causing increased gastric secretion in the fasting dog with a shunt but may not be detectable by any presently known means. Second, with regard to our inhibition studies, it is true that atropine inhibits the gastric hypersecretion after portacaval shunt, whereas it does not inhibit secretion induced by exogenously administered histamine. The reasons for this discrepancy are not clear, but some authors have indicated that endogenous and exogenous histamine may react quite differently. We are now conducting human studies and our results are certainly in the direction of those which we found in the animals. In conclusion I would like to say that everyone has always wondered whether or not histamine plays a physiologic role in gastric secretion and I think these studies certainly indicate that it does.

**Dr. Marshall J. Orloff** (closing). I wish to thank Drs. Barker, McDermott, and Warren for their comments. As you know, all three of these men have made important and pioneer contributions to our knowledge of portal hypertension and ascites. Dr. Barker asked for an account of the marked differences in mortality rates between the group with side-to-side shunts and the group with end-to-side shunts. It is difficult, with the internal vena cava cannula technique, to control precisely the amount of hepatic venous outflow obstruction produced by the cannula and, as we indicated, the major cause of early death in all of the groups was acute hepatic vein occlusion from a tight-fitting cannula. However, as time went on and we developed more experience, our ability to estimate the amount of occlusion improved. The end-to-side shunt group was our most recent one and our only explanation for the improved survival rate in this group is that we had greater experience with the procedure. We do not believe that the lower mortality rate can be interpreted as having resulted from some beneficial effect of the end-to-side shunt.

It is very true that the results of these experiments in dogs may not have direct application to man, as do so few experiments in animals. However, there is not too much question that an important factor in the pathogenesis of ascites associated with liver disease is hepatic venous outflow block. I believe that there has been sufficient substantiation of the existence of this phenomenon in man to give us confidence that it is at least partly responsible for ascites. In this sense, and perhaps only in this sense, our experiment is comparable to what is found in human beings. We would find it difficult to completely ignore the striking beneficial effect of side-to-side portacaval shunt on the sequelae of outflow block in the dog or the lack of benefit from end-to-side shunt, alhtough we agree that one should be cautious in applying these findings to man, particularly since cirrhosis is a very complex disease.

**Dr. Earl F. Wolfman, Jr.** (closing). I would like to thank the discussers for their comments and stress the point that our use of the end-to-side portacaval shunt in this experimental protocol was designed to obtain information regarding the underlying physiologic disturbances in the liver. It is not to be construed as an endorsement of any one particular type of shunt in the surgical management of portal hypertension. In regard to Dr. McDermott's question as to whether or not the sodium retention observed could be due to increased circulating levels of aldosterone resulting from a failure of liver conjugation, I doubt this. We found that shunted animals responded to isotonic saline infusions by excreting a relatively normal concentration of sodium in the urine. The basic defect was the failure to excrete an increased urinary volume. This observation was not previously unknown, although we were unaware of it at the time we undertook this study. Lamson and Roca in 1921 demonstrated that when isotonic saline was infused into animals with hepatic arterial occlusion and Eck fistulas, the rate of disappearance of the infused solutions was reduced fourfold as compared to that in normal animals. It is happenstance that some 40 years later we confirmed this aspect of their work. In summary, I think it is fairly important to keep an open mind and to recognize that cirrhosis and the ascites associated with it probably has more than one cause. Certainly mechanical hydrostatic pressure relationships are important, but we must consider these in relationship to basic underlying physiologic processes. If these can be determined and clarified, perhaps we can then select the proper operation for a given patient.

# Experimental studies of factors which influence hepatic metastases. VIII. Effect of anticoagulants

BERNARD FISHER, M.D.
EDWIN R. FISHER, M.D.*
PITTSBURGH, PA.
*From the Department of Surgery, Laboratory of Surgical Research and Pathology, University of Pittsburgh*

Renewed interest has recently become focused upon the manner in which circulating tumor-cell emboli are arrested in the vascular system and ultimately become overt metastases. After histologic studies in man and animal, numerous investigators[3, 14, 21-26] have reported in detail upon the sequence of events which occurs in this phenomenon. Of particular distinction in this regard is the work of Wood[26] in which the fate of blood-borne cancer cells was followed in the living animal by means of serial microcinematography. From these reports, and from our own observations, it seems that almost immediately after the lodgment of tumor cells and prior to the onset of further events in their conversion to metastases, such cells become enmeshed in intravascular thrombi. Wood concluded from his experiments that the failure of embolic tumor cells to establish metastases might well be "related to their inability to attach securely to the endothelium and evoke the formation of a surrounding thrombus."

The necessity of such a clot for development of metastases, while not proved, is also suggested by the few reports in which anticoagulants were reputed to retard tumor growth and reduce the number of metastases. Wood and associates mentioned that heparin and dicumarol reduced the incidence of lung tumors in Swiss mice injected with cells of the Lewis bladder carcinoma 150 and in C57BL/6 mice inoculated with Lewis sarcoma 241 tumor-cell suspensions.[28] Similarly, Cliffton and Grossi[6] noted a marked reduction in the incidence of metastases when human plasmin (fibrinolysin) was administered to rabbits inoculated intravenously with V2 carcinoma or Brown-Pearce carcinoma-cell suspensions. More recently[13] they found a reduction in pulmonary metastases when rats which received human plasmin were intravenously injected with Walker 256 carcinoma cells. Jolles and Greening[15] implanted fragments of sarcoma S37 into Balb/C mice and found that if they injected heparin at the site of the transplant they could reduce the number of "takes."

In order to obtain more detailed information concerning the use of anticoagulants in metastasis inhibition, during the past 8 months we resorted to an evaluation of the effect of heparin and human plasmin upon the development of experimentally induced hepatic metastases.

## MATERIALS AND METHODS

Adult female Sprague-Dawley rats,* which weighed 175 to 200 grams, were used to evaluate the effect of heparin and plasmin upon induced hepatic metastases. They were housed in individual cages and permitted water and laboratory chow† ad libitum.

Supported by the Mary J. Baers Memorial Grant for Cancer Research from the American Cancer Society.

Read at the Twenty-second Annual Meeting of the Society of University Surgeons, Kansas City, Kan., Feb. 9-11, 1961.

*Senior Research Fellow, United States Public Health Service.

*Holtzman Farms, Madison, Wis.
†Purina.

The tumor utilized in this study, the Walker carcinoma,[8] has been propagated in our laboratory since January, 1957. The technique used to prepare tumor-cell suspensions, as well as the method of intraportal injection of tumor cells used with rats receiving 2,000 and 5,000 U. of plasmin and their controls, has already been described in detail.[9] Animals in this study were lightly anesthetized with ether, subjected to celiotomy, and injected intraportally via a large mesenteric vein with 0.5 ml. of saline-plasma solution containing 5,000 tumor cells. It was not feasible to inject tumor cells in this manner into animals that were heparinized prior to or shortly after their inoculation. The mortality rate from hemorrhage consequent to laparotomy and venous puncture was prohibitive. After the use of numerous variations of technique, the experiment was conducted with a minimum of deaths by insertion of short lengths of polyethylene tubing (PE 50, outer diameter 0.038 inch) via a tributary into the portal vein 4 days prior to the onset of heparinization and tumor-cell injection. The tubes were anchored in place by a silk ligature and tunneled subcutaneously to emerge from the back of each animal's neck. Tumor cells (5,000 in 0.5 ml. of saline-plasma solution) were injected via the tubes into both the animals given heparin and their controls. These rats were lightly anesthetized with ether during the inoculation. A similar technique was employed with the group which received 1,000 U. of plasmin and their controls.

From preliminary experiments it was found that by the subcutaneous injection of 700 U.S.P. units (7 mg.) of heparin* per 100 Gm. of body weight at 9:00 A.M. and 9:00 P.M., the clotting time of animals, as determined by the capillary tube method, could be maintained continuously over 30 minutes. All animals which received heparin were maintained on this regimen for 2, 4, or 7 days.

Plasmin solutions were prepared immediately before use. This was done by dissolv-

*Liquaemin sodium, Organon Inc.

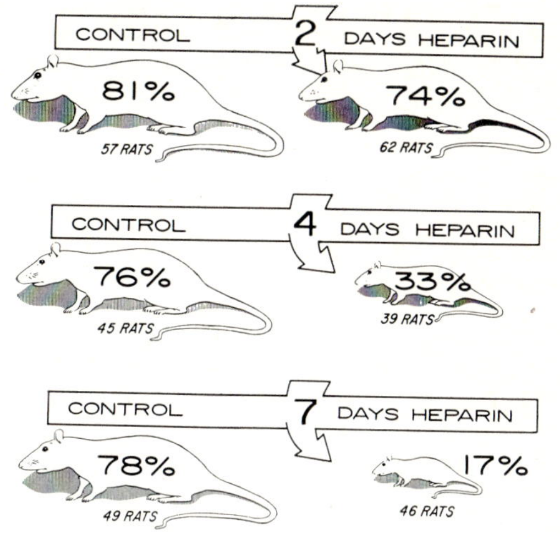


**Fig. 1.** Animals heparinized at time of tumor-cell injection and maintained on heparin for 2, 4, and 7 days.

ing 50,000 U.* in an appropriate volume of 5 per cent dextrose in water so that 1 ml. contained either 1,000, 2,000, or 5,000 U. All injections of fibrinolysin were via a femoral vein which had been exposed by a short incision in the groin. With a 27 gauge needle, the solution (1 ml.) was injected under direct vision so that there was no question as to the route of administration. Three to 5 minutes were taken to infuse each dose of fibrinolysin.

The fibrinolytic activity of plasma was determined by the euglobulin fibrinolytic method described by Cliffton and Cannamela.[5] By this procedure the time required to lyse a standard clot in a test tube was measured. It was also determined by the plate method of Astrup[1] whereby the lysis of a preformed clot was observed in a semiquantitative fashion.

## RESULTS

**Effect of heparin** (Figs. 1 and 2). The injection of heparin 4 hours prior to the intraportal inoculation of 5,000 Walker carcinoma cells and the maintenance of heparinization for subsequent 48 hours resulted in no significant alteration in the incidence

*Thrombolysin, Merck Sharp & Dohme. Courtesy of Dr. N. H. Schimmel.

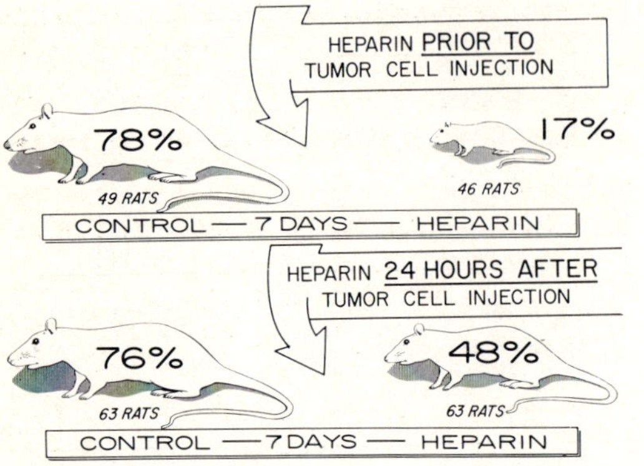


**Fig. 2.** Comparison of effect of heparinization maintained for 7 days when started prior to tumor-cell injection and 24 hours after tumor-cell injection.

of hepatic metastasis. When examined 14 days after tumor-cell injection, 81 per cent of 57 unheparinized control rats exhibited tumor and 74 per cent of the 62 rats which had received heparin demonstrated metastases.

If heparinization was continued for 4 days instead of 2, a significant difference in the incidence of metastases occurred between the control and treated groups. Whereas 34 of 45 (76 per cent) of the former had liver metastases, only 13 of 39 (33 per cent) of the latter showed such tumor growth.

Heparin administration for 7 days resulted in a striking reduction in the number of animals with tumor. With such a regimen only 8 of 46 (17 per cent) had liver neoplasm in contrast to 38 of 49 (78 per cent) rats in the control group. It was also evident that the liver tumors which did grow in the animals treated with heparin were smaller and fewer in number than those in the control animals. The animals without tumor in both the control and treated groups were resutured and permitted to survive for another week, at which time they were reexamined. Six of the 11 animals with liver tumor at 2 weeks demonstrated metastases, while only 4 of the 38 in the heparinized group grew tumor during the additional week.

In 63 rats heparin administration was begun 24 hours after the injection of tumor cells and was continued for 7 days. Some decrease in the incidence of metastases occurred, but this was not as pronounced as when heparinization was instituted prior to tumor-cell injection. Thirty (48 per cent) of such heparinized rats had liver metastases, while 76 per cent of 63 control animals exhibited neoplasms.

In acute experiments heparinized and nonheparinized rats were injected via the portal vein with 400,000 tumor cells. Almost simultaneously a 1 ml. sample of blood was aspirated from a hepatic vein between the liver and diaphragm. When smears were examined for tumor cells, there was no apparent difference between the number of such cells in the blood of heparinized animals and the number in the blood of the unheparinized animals.

**Effect of plasmin (fibrinolysin).** The greater the dosage of plasmin employed the more pronounced and prolonged was the fibrinolytic activity of the euglobulin fraction of plasma as observed by the time for lysis of a standard clot in a test tube (Table I) or by the lysis of a preformed clot on a

**Table I.** *Fibrinolytic activity of the euglobulin fraction of plasma after injection of 1,000, 2,000, and 5,000 U. of plasmin*

| *Units of plasmin injected* | *Standard clot lysis time (Time after injection of plasmin)* | | | | |
|---|---|---|---|---|---|
| | *15 min.* | *30 min.* | *1 hr.* | *2 hr.* | *24 hr.* |
| 0 (control) | > 24 hr. | – | – | – | – |
| 1,000 | 1 hr., 14 min. | 3 hr., 2 min. | 11 hr., 21 min. | > 24 hr. | > 24 hr. |
| 2,000 | 34 min. | 2 hr., 7 min. | 9 hr., 54 min. | 9 hr., 5 min. | > 24 hr. |
| 5,000 | 27 min. | 52 min. | 1 hr., 58 min. | 18 hr. | > 24 hr. |

Each value is the average of 3 rats.

plate (Fig. 3). Variation occurred from animal to animal, and was most pronounced in all dosages 1 and 2 hours after plasmin injection.

To evaluate the effect of the plasmin upon the development of metastases, experiments were performed with injections of 1,000, 2,000, or 5,000 U. either just prior to tumor-cell injection or 2, 4, and 8 hours after (Fig. 4). When 1,000 U. of plasmin was injected 15 minutes prior to inoculation of tumor cells, 28 of 63 rats (44 per cent) demonstrated tumor after 2 weeks, whereas 36 of 58 control animals (62 per cent) had liver metastases. Of the 32 animals receiving 2,000 U. prior to tumor-cell injection, only 4, or 13 per cent, had metastases, whereas 40 per cent of controls were found to have tumor. If 2,000 U. of plasmin was injected 2, 4, or 8 hours after tumor-cell inoculation, less of an inhibition resulted. Twenty-seven, 28, and 30 per cent of such animals demonstrated metastases.

The use of 5,000 U. of plasmin was no more effective than the use of smaller amounts. While 40 per cent of control rats developed metastases, 21 per cent of those injected prior to tumor-cell inoculation were tumor positive after 14 days. This dosage used 2 and 4 hours after injection of tumor cells was without effect.

Similarly, this amount of plasmin was not effective in abolishing the stimulative effect which liver trauma exerts upon the development of hepatic metastases (Fig. 5). Eight of 18 (44 per cent) control animals injected with tumor cells had liver tumor 14 days later. In 19 the liver was massaged just after cell injection and 69 per cent were positive. Nineteen others were similarly handled, except that they received 5,000 U. of plasmin prior to tumor-cell injection and liver manipulation. Of these, 13, or 68 per cent, also grew tumor.

As in heparinized rats, blood was aspirated from the hepatic vein simultaneouly with the injection of tumor cells into plasmin-treated animals and their controls. No difference in number of cells was apparent in the 2 groups.

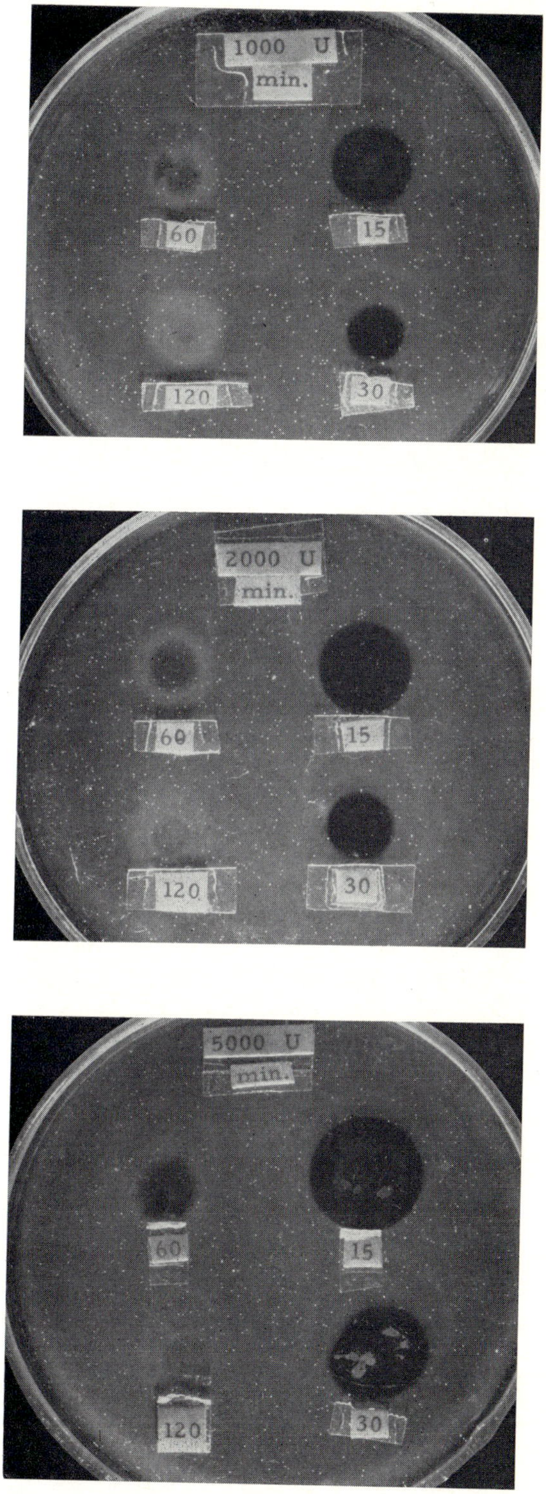


**Fig. 3.** Example of fibrinolytic activity of the euglobulin fraction of plasma 15, 30, 60, and 120 minutes after administration of 1,000, 2,000, and 5,000 U. of human plasmin.

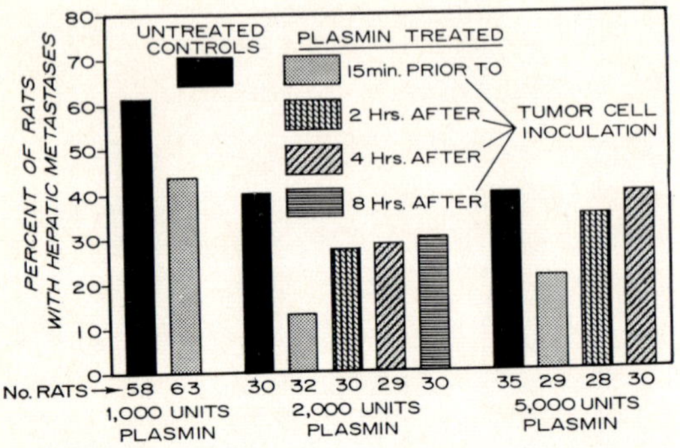


**Fig. 4.** Effect upon metastases of 1,000, 2,000, and 5,000 U. of human plasmin administered 15 minutes before and 2, 4, and 8 hours after tumor-cell injection.

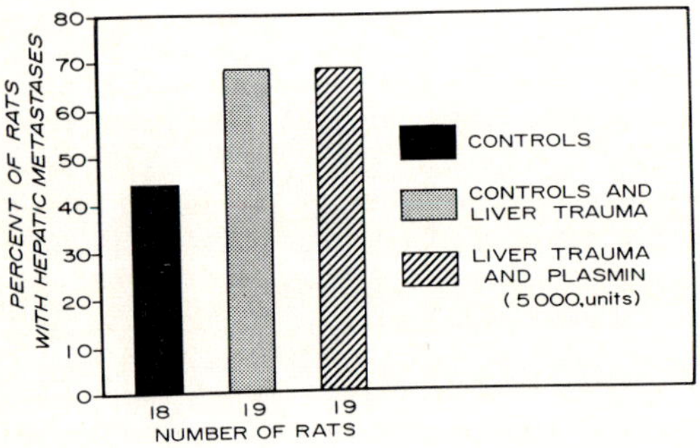


**Fig. 5.** Effect of human plasmin given prior to tumor-cell injection and liver manipulation.

## COMMENT

Willis[25] has suggested that the most critical time insofar as the fate of embolic tumor cells is concerned is the period between their lodgment and their attainment of an extravascular position. While the evidence is meager, it is convincing that extravascular invasion of tumor cells may occur within a matter of hours after their introduction into the circulation. Warren and Gates[24] found tumor-cell growth beyond pulmonary capillaries by 3 hours and established perivascular growth by 12 hours. Wood,[26] using a rabbit ear chamber for in vivo study of metastasis formation by V2 carcinoma, observed such invasion as early as 3 hours and, rarely, after as long as 48 hours. Recently Kinsey and associates[16] inoculated the Cloudman S91 melanoma into DBA mice and 36 hours later observed "suspected" extravascular tumor cells. By 48 hours there was no question of their extravascular location.

These data are significant in the consideration of chemotherapy as an adjuvant to cancer operations. It is presumed that the greatest effectiveness of chemotherapeutic agents so used is upon circulating tumor cells or, at least, upon those still confined to the vascular system. Indeed, experimental evidence suggests that this is so, for when McDonald and associates[19] administered nitrogen mustard of triethylene thiophosphoramide (thio-TEPA) shortly after the intraportal inoculation of Walker tumor cells, marked suppression of metastases resulted. If, however, the drugs were administered 48 hours after injection of tumor cells, no such effect occurred. A subsequent report by these investigators[20] indicated that drug administration after as short a time as 6 hours was ineffectual. Similarly, Kramer and his group[17] noted a decrease in effectiveness of thio-TEPA in reducing pulmonary metastases in mice when administered more than 6 hours after inoculation with sarcoma 37 and after 48 hours when Cloudman S91 melanoma was used. Thus, there seems to be a relationship between the effectiveness of a chemotherapeutic agent and the time of extravascular invasion of tumor cells.[16]

Our observation that both heparin and plasmin given hours after injection of tumor cells were less effective than when they were administered prior to inoculation suggests that anticoagulants hinder the attainment of an extravascular position by tumor cells, possibly through interference with the initial sticking of cancer cells to the vascular endothelium and/or the formation of intravascular thrombi. By use of these agents to prolong the residence of tumor cells within blood vessels, perhaps the effectiveness of chemotherapeutic agents as adjuvants to surgical procedures may be promoted. This possibility is currently being investigated.

The finding that protracted anticoagulation with heparin (4 to 7 days) in contrast to shorter therapy was necessary to produce striking inhibition of metastatic development suggests that tumor cells, though not enmeshed in thrombi, may remain entrapped and viable in their intravascular position in the liver for at least several days and are capable of developing into metastases when heparin is discontinued.

After prolonged heparinization and presumably inhibition of thrombus formation, the reduction in metastases may be due to (1) loss of viability of the tumor cells, (2) a delay in tumor growth under such conditions, (3) achievement of a dormant state by the tumor cells, (4) a dislodgment of tumor cells and their transport away from the liver, or (5) heparin itself exerting a cancerocidal effect. No specific evidence in absolute support of any of these possibilities is forthcoming from this study, but that some of them are unlikely is suggested. It was previously reported by us[11] that if animals were subjected to laparotomy and liver manipulation 14 days after intraportal tumor-cell injection and re-examined 1 week later, a striking number which had had no metastases at first examination had them at 21 days in contrast to the control rats which were not operated upon. This phenomenon was not observed in the group of animals heparinized for 7 days, which suggests that tumor cells were no longer viable or no longer resident in the liver. Multiple re-explorations to stimulate the growth of dormant tumor cells, such as we have previously performed,[10] were not carried out.

The possibility that heparin itself was exerting a direct effect upon tumor cells was considered. There is some evidence that heparin may act as a mitotic inhibitor both in vitro[12, 29] and in vivo.[2, 18] Balazs and Holmgren,[2] using an intraperitoneal inoculation of solid Ehrlich carcinoma, reported a slight increase in survival time of animals when heparin treatment was begun after transfer of tumor. More recently, Lippman[18] demonstrated a decrease of mitotic index in Ehrlich ascites tumor cells after a single, but not repeated, injection of heparin. She found no effect on the survival time of treated animals. Animals were injected by us intraportally and subcutaneously with tumor-cell suspensions prepared in a heparin-saline solution. Growth of tumor was not prevented or delayed. Rats inoculated subcutaneously with tumor and systemically heparinized for 7 days likewise seemed to grow tumor as proficiently as the untreated rats.

Apparently the effect of heparin was not achieved by its interference with the lodgment of tumor cells in the liver, for metastases did occur after withdrawal of heparin when it had been administered for 48 hours. Also, it was found that after tumor-cell inoculation no greater number of such cells traversed the liver and were to be found in the hepatic vein blood of heparinized rats than was seen in controls.

Our results with human plasmin substantiate the findings of Grossi and colleagues[13] that this fibrinolytic agent may reduce the incidence of metastases. We, however, were unable to elicit the dramatic effect which they obtained, in spite of the use of much larger amounts of plasmin in some instances. This may be due in part to the fact that their Walker tumor was carried in the ascitic form, while ours was a solid tumor. Moreover, our results pertained to the effect upon hepatic metastases, while theirs were concerned with such growth in the lung. It is reasonable to suggest that a difference exists in the "soil" of the lung and the liver insofar as support of tumor growth is concerned.

Why a single dose of plasmin, with its brief fibrinolytic activity when administered prior to tumor-cell inoculation, should be effective in inhibiting growth of metastases in contrast to the necessity for prolonged heparinization is not clear. The variation in fibrinolytic response from animal to animal, the in vitro measurement of fibrinolytic activity by use of the euglobulin fraction of plasma with antiplasmin removed as an index of in vivo action, the presence of a high antiplasmin titre in rat blood, and the complexities and incomplete knowledge of the fibrinolytic system[4, 7] all make speculation as to mode of action under the conditions of our experiments unwarranted.

As with heparin, and as reported by Grossi and colleagues[13] for plasmin, no direct effect of human fibrinolysin upon the viability of tumor cells could be elicited. It was of interest that plasmin failed to interfere with the augmentory effect of trauma upon metastatic incidence and that it was without effect when given several hours after the injection of tumor cells. This suggests that extravascular migration of such cells may occur with rapidity.


## SUMMARY

During the course of investigation of factors which influenced the development of experimentally induced hepatic metastases, tumor-cell thrombi in intrahepatic portal vein radicles were frequently noted. Since studies by others suggest the importance of such thrombi in the conversion of tumor emboli to metastases, it was deemed worthwhile to evaluate the effect of heparin and human plasmin (fibrinolysin) upon the "take" and growth of hepatic metastases.

When 5,000 Walker carcinoma tumor cells were injected intraportally into heparinized rats and heparinization was continued for the subsequent 48 hours, no significant alteration in the incidence of hepatic metastases resulted. Fourteen days after tumor inoculation, 81 per cent of control animals and 74 per cent of heparin-treated rats demonstrated hepatic tumor. If, however, heparinization was maintained for 4 and 7 days, 33 per cent of the former and only 17 per cent of the latter had metastases. When heparin administration was begun 24 hours after tumor-cell injection and was continued for 7 days, the effect achieved was not as striking. Hepatic tumor was observed in 48 per cent of such rats.

The administration of human plasmin prior to tumor-cell inoculation inhibited the formation of hepatic metastases. When 2,000 U. was administered, 13 per cent of the animals demonstrated tumor in comparison to 40 per cent in the untreated control animals. Injection of fibrinolysin 2, 4, or 8 hours after injection of tumor was ineffectual.

Consideration is given to the mechanism of action of these agents. It is suggested that they hinder the attainment of an extravascular position by tumor cells. Since there seems to be a relationship between the effectiveness of a chemotherapeutic agent and this extravascular migration, the possibility is considered that anticoagulants may prolong the residence of tumor cells within blood vessels and thus improve the effectiveness of chemotherapeutic agents as adjuvants to surgical procedures.


## REFERENCES


1. Astrup, T., and Mullertz, S.: The fibrin plate method for estimating fibrinolytic activity, Arch. Biochem. & Biophys. **40:** 346, 1952.
2. Balazs, H., and Holmgren, H.: Effect of sulfomucopolysaccharides on growth of tumor tissue, Proc. Soc. Exper. Biol. & Med. **72:** 142, 1949.
3. Baserga, R., and Saffiotti, U.: Experimental studies on histogenesis of blood-borne metastases, A. M. A. Arch. Path. **59:** 26, 1955.
4. Brinkhous, K. M., and Roberts, H. R.: Thrombolysis and thrombolytic agents a brief review, J. A. M. A. **175:** 96, 1961.
5. Cliffton, E. E., and Cannamela, D.: Fibrinolytic and proteolytic activity of a human plasminogen prepared from fraction III of human plasma, J. Appl. Physiol. **6:** 42, 1953.
6. Cliffton, E. E., and Grossi, C. E.: Effect of human plasmin on the toxic effects and growth of blood-borne metastasis of the Brown-Pearce carcinoma and the V2 carcinoma of rabbit, Cancer **9:** 1147, 1956.
7. Cohen, S. I., and Warren, R.: Fibrinolysis, New England J. Med. **264:** 79, 128, 1961.
8. Fisher, E. R., and Fisher, B.: Electron microscopic, histologic and histochemical features of the Walker carcinoma, Cancer Res. **21:** 527, 1961.
9. Fisher, E. R., and Fisher, B.: Experimental studies of factors influencing hepatic metastases. I. The effect of number of tumor cells injected and time of growth, Cancer **12:** 926, 1959.
10. Fisher, B., and Fisher, E. R.: Experimental evidence in support of the dormant tumor cell, Science **130:** 918, 1959.
11. Fisher, B., and Fisher, E. R.: Experimental studies of factors influencing hepatic metastases. III. Effect of surgical trauma with

special reference to liver injury, Ann. Surg. **150:** 731, 1959.
12. Goerner, A.: The influence of anticlotting agents on transplantation and growth of tumor tissue, J. Lab. & Clin. Med. **16:** 369, 1931.
13. Grossi, C. E., Agostino, D., and Cliffton, E. E.: The effect of human fibrinolysin on pulmonary metastases of Walker 256 carcinosarcoma, Cancer Res. **20:** 605, 1960.
14. Iwasaki, T.: Histological and experimental observations on the destruction of tumour cells in the blood vessels, J. Path. & Bact. **20:** 85, 1915-1916.
15. Jolles, B., and Greening, S. G.: Effect of heparin upon tumour growth, Acta Unio Internat. cancr., Louvain **16:** 682, 1960.
16. Kinsey, D. L., Price, E. B., Jr., and Smith, R. R.: Effectiveness of chemotherapy in relation to extravascular invasion by embolic tumor cells, Cancer **13:** 733, 1960.
17. Kramer, W. M., Eck, R. V., and Smith, R. R.: Prevention of experimental lung metastases with triethylene thiophosphoramide (thio TEPA), Surg. Gynec. & Obst. **106:** 427, 1958.
18. Lippman, M.: The growth-inhibitory action of heparin on the Ehrlich ascites tumor in mice, Cancer Res. **17:** 11, 1957.
19. McDonald, G. O., Livingstone, C., Boyles, C. F., and Cole, W. H.: The prophylactic treatment of malignant disease with nitrogen mustard and triethylene thiophosphoramide (thio TEPA), Ann. Surg. **145:** 624, 1957.
20. Morales, F., Bell, M., McDonald, G. O., and Cole, W. H.: The prophylactic treatment of cancer at the time of operation, Ann. Surg. **146:** 588, 1957.
21. Saphir, O.: The fate of carcinoma emboli in the lung, Am. J. Path. **23:** 245, 1947.
22. Schmidt, M. B.: Die verbreitungswege der karcinome und die beziehung generalisierter sarkome zu den leukämischen neubildungen, Gustav Fischer Verlag (Jena), 1903.
23. Walther, H. E.: Krebsmetastasen, Benno Schwabe and Co. (Basel), 1948.
24. Warren, S., and Gates, O.: The fate of intravenously injected tumor cells, Am. J. Cancer **27:** 485, 1936.
25. Willis, R. A.: Spread of tumours in the human body, St. Louis, 1952, The C. V. Mosby Company, ed. 2.
26. Wood, S., Jr.: Pathogenesis of metastasis formation observed in vivo in the rabbit ear chamber, A. M. A. Arch. Path. **66:** 550, 1958.
27. Wood, J. S., Jr., Holyoke, E. D., and Yardley, J. H.: An experimental study of the influence of adrenal steroids, growth hormone, and anticoagulants on pulmonary metastasis formation in mice, Proc. Res. **2:** 157, 1956.
28. Wood, J. S., Jr., Yardley, J. H., and Holyoke, E. D.: The relationship between intravascular coagulation and the formation of pulmonary metastases in mice injected intravenously with tumor suspension, Proc. Am. A. Cancer Res. **2:** 260, 1957.
29. Zahl, P. A.: The action of bacterial toxine on tumors. VIII. Factors in their use for cancer therapy, J. Nat. Cancer Inst. **11:** 279, 1950.

## DISCUSSION

**Dr. Eugene E. Cliffton** (New York, N. Y.). This is an excellent piece of work and one that is of tremendous importance to us, the surgeons. We have all operated on patients with carcinoma only to lose the patient shortly thereafter to metastases. At present there is a tremendous interest in tumor cells in the blood, and we are finding more and more instances in which there are cells in the circulating blood even in patients who survive for a long time. The important factor is how these cells produce metastases and how they can be controlled. We have studied the effect of anticoagulants on production of pulmonary metastases. In our original work with VX-2 carcinoma, a thromboplastic tumor, we were able to decrease the number of pulmonary metastases and with the Brown-Pearce carcinoma the rate of liver metastases was decreased.

With the Walker 256 carcinosarcoma in rats, we were able to decrease the transplantability of tumor by subcutaneous injection of blood in weanling rats with fibrinolysin and heparin. This effect lasted for only 2 hours, the duration of effectiveness of a single injection. Using a cecal tumor by implantation of Walker 256 cells, we were able to determine the effect of manipulation of a resectable tumor. With manipulation, there was a sharp peak of cells to 6,000 per ml. in the blood stream. In 5 minutes this returned to normal. With an unresectable tumor, cells are present in the circulation at all times, but manipulation results in a sharp increase in the number, again for only a few minutes. If fibrinolysin or heparin is given prior to manipulation the peak is much smaller but prolonged in the resectable lesion, which indicates that the cells remain in circulation. With the unresectable lesions the peak is hardly noticeable. The number of "takes" with subcutaneous inoculation of blood is also much less.

# Regional perfusion of the pelvis: consideration of the "leakage" problem

WALTER LAWRENCE, JR., M.D.
PAUL KUEHN, M.D.
SHYUNIGHI MORI, M.D.
J. W. POPPELL, M.D.
BAYARD CLARKSON, M.D.
NEW YORK, N. Y.
*From the Departments of Surgery and Chemotherapy, and the Division of Experimental Surgery and Physiology, the Memorial Sloan-Kettering Cancer Center*

The unique approach of regional perfusion for cancer chemotherapy introduced by Creech[4] is based on the assumption that a therapeutically significant drug concentration may be maintained in the desired area while systemic dosage is kept within safe limits. The efficiency of isolation of the anatomic area to be perfused is of paramount importance in the achievement of this aim. The purpose of this presentation is to examine the phenomenon of "leakage" during regional perfusion in the pelvis, an anatomic area that not only offers problems in vascular isolation but also will present many therapeutic opportunities if this general treatment method proves worthwhile.

A number of methods have been employed for the estimation of mixing between the perfusion and systemic circuits. Most of these employ an intravascular indicator, such as T-1824,[5] RISA,[10, 12] or $Cr^{51}$-tagged red blood cells,[1] and the concentration of this substance is measured in intermittent blood samples or by external counting from some portion of the nonperfused areas.[10] Limb perfusion has proved to be well-isolated in such studies, primarily because of the ease of efficient tourniquet application. Perfusion of other anatomic areas, where tourniquet control of collateral blood vessels is not feasible, has in general been associated with an unusual degree of cross circulation or "leakage."[1] Pelvic perfusion has been a prime example of such a "high leakage" system because of the absence of a cephalad tourniquet.

The use of an indicator as described to estimate cross circulation between 2 vascular circuits initially seemed quite straightforward. We have become increasingly aware, however, that the data obtained from such studies were extremely difficult to evaluate from the standpoint of regional administration of chemotherapeutic agents. Without attempting to assess the clinical effectiveness of this regional treatment method, we would like to present some of our observations on "leakage" during clinical and experimental pelvic perfusion with the extracorporeal pump-oxygenator.

## METHODS

**Surgical procedures.** The data on conventional regional pelvic perfusion in man were obtained from 7 patients subjected to pelvic perfusion by a technique similar to that originally described by Creech[4] and Austen and his associates.[1] The aorta and vena cava were mobilized at laparotomy and the larger collateral vessels controlled by ligature. The arterial and venous catheters were inserted

Read at the Twenty-second Annual Meeting of the Society of University Surgeons, Kansas City, Kan., Feb. 9-11, 1961.

retrograde from the groin into the femoral artery and saphenous vein. After occlusion of the aorta and vena cava, leg tourniquets were inflated and circulation of the pelvis carried out by means of an oxygenator (97.5 per cent oxygen and 2.5 per cent carbon dioxide) and 2 Sigmamotor pumps. After our initial trials with a disposable bubble oxygenator (Abbott), we then employed a small modification of the Kay-Cross rotating disc oxygenator. Hyperthermia (40° to 41° C.) in the perfusion circuit was also utilized.

Pelvic perfusions were performed on a series of 25 dogs by a similar technique. The arterial and venous catheters in animals were inserted into the lumbar aorta and vena cava, distal to the sites of occlusion, and leg tourniquets were omitted from this canine perfusion system. In most of the experimental perfusions and in 3 of the clinical perfusions, additional control of collateral flow was attempted by means of a paraspinal lumbar rubber tourniquet placed behind the ureters, colon, and great vessels and passed around the posterior muscle mass. The perfusion rates employed in all of these pelvic perfusions were adjusted so that pressure in the arterial line of the perfusion circuit was always lower than systemic blood pressure.

A subsequent modification of the procedure just described has been carried out in 6 additional clinical pelvic perfusions and 10 additional pelvic perfusions in the dog. With this method the aorta and vena cava are occluded by means of balloon-tipped catheters inserted through the groins, as described by Watkins and co-workers,[11] and collateral flow is controlled by a specially constructed, broad pneumatic tourniquet that encloses the abdomen. This technique is described in detail elsewhere,[8] but pertinent illustrative data from these studies are also included in this study.

**Laboratory procedures.** The intravascular indicators used in these studies were RISA or the subject's red blood cells tagged with $Cr^{51}$.[9] For comparative studies $Na^{24}$ and $K^{42}$ were also used to study the mechanics of mixing of nonmetabolized substances with extravascular distribution. Radioactivity of 1 ml. samples of heparinized whole blood ($Cr^{51}$, $K^{42}$) or plasma (RISA, $Na^{24}$) were determined in duplicate with a well scintillation counter. When 2 isotopes were utilized simultaneously, the radioactivity in respect to the individual isotopes was calculated from 2 separate determinations spaced 1 day apart. The differences in "half-life" of the isotopes concerned were then used to determine the proportion of each isotope in the samples.

$$\text{Formula I: } cpm_o x = \frac{cpm_t - fy\,(cpm_o)}{fx - fy}$$

$$\text{Formula II: } cpm_o y = cpm_o - cpm_o x$$

Where:
- x = Isotope of longer half-life.
- y = Isotope of shorter half-life.
- $cpm_o$ = Original (Day 1) total net counts per minute.
- $cpm_t$ = Day 2 total net counts per minute.
- fx = Decay factor for isotope x.*
- fy = Decay factor for isotope y.*

*To determine fx and fy:

$$fx = \frac{cpm_t \text{ (x standard)}}{cpm_o \text{ (x standard)}}$$

$$fy = \frac{cpm_t \text{ (y standard)}}{cpm_o \text{ (y standard)}}$$

The concentration of Methotrexate in plasma samples was determined microbiologically by a modification of the technique described by Burchenal and colleagues.[2] The plasma concentration of 5-fluorouracil (FU) and 5-fluoro-2-deoxyuridine (FUDR) was determined either spectrophotometrically or by microbiologic assay employing *Streptococcus faecalis* (SFO) in a modified assay media as developed by Flynn,[6] or by both methods simultaneously. FU and FUDR were separated electrophoretically prior to microbiologic assay when indicated.

**Procedures for study of loss from perfusion circuit.** In most of these studies of leakage the isotope ($Na^{24}$, $K^{42}$, RISA, or $Cr^{51}$-tagged red blood cells) was mixed thoroughly with the fresh heparinized blood prior to its use for priming the oxygenator. In studies in which an intravascular indicator was introduced into the systemic circuit, it was given intravenously at the onset of the actual perfusion. Drug administration was carried out through the arterial line of the

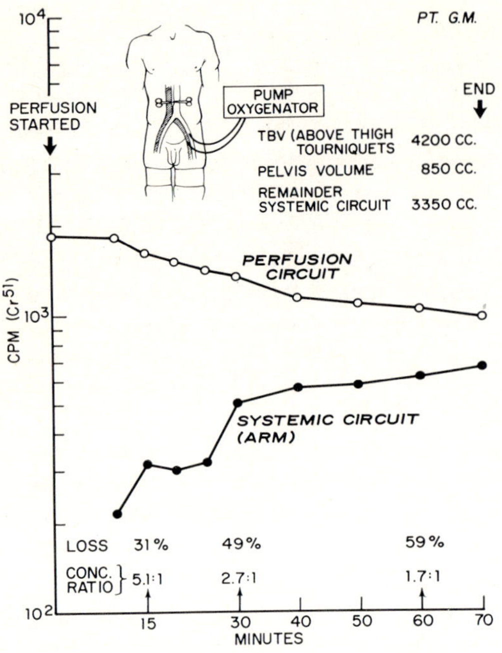


**Fig. 1.** Data obtained during typical clinical pelvic perfusion by standard technique (see inset). $Cr^{51}$-tagged red blood cells in perfusion circuit and serial blood samples taken from systemic circuit (arm) and perfusion circuit. Leakage is expressed both as per cent loss and concentration ratio.

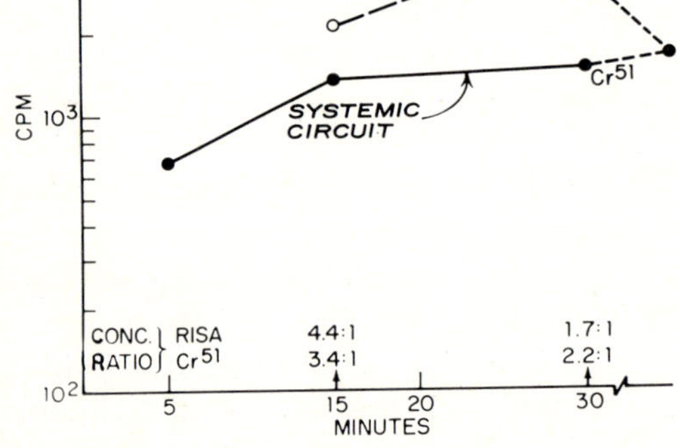


**Fig. 2.** Simultaneous measurement of leakage into and out of the perfusion circuit during a clinical pelvic perfusion similar to that in Fig. 1.

extracorporeal system after adequate function of the artificial circulation had been established (usually within 5 minutes of onset of the actual perfusion procedure). In our early studies the arterial line of the oxygenator system was used for obtaining samples of the perfusion circuit, but in all subsequent studies the venous line has been employed as a source of perfusion circuit measurements. Peripheral or systemic circuit measurements were carried out on samples obtained from a Lindeman needle in an antecubital vein in patients undergoing perfusion and from carotid artery catheters in the dog.

## OBSERVATIONS

During the course of our study of pelvic perfusion we have been concerned with the therapeutic implications of leakage as it is usually measured. From our modest experience with this form of regional perfusion, an attempt will be made to discuss (1) means of expressing the degree of cross circulation, (2) possible significance of such measurements in regard to localization of chemotherapeutic agents, and (3) efforts to improve anatomic isolation of this strategic area.

**Means of expressing leakage.** The graph in Fig. 1 is an example of the type of mixing curve that is obtained during a typical clinical pelvic perfusion ($Cr^{51}$-tagged red blood cells were placed in the perfusion circuit.) A relatively simple means of describing the changes that occur is to compare the concentrations of $Cr^{51}$-tagged red blood cells in the 2 circuits by "concentration ratios." However, since we are interested in the percentage loss of the chemotherapeutic agent placed in the perfusion circuit, it is tempting to calculate the percentage loss of $Cr^{51}$-tagged red blood cells from the perfusion circuit. Such a calculation should be quite simple since the concentration of the indicator in the systemic circuit as well as the total quantity of indicator originally placed in the perfusion circuit are known.

The formula that can be utilized for accumulated per cent leakage of $Cr^{51}$-tagged red blood cells at time t is:

$$\% \text{ leakage } Cr^{51}\text{-tagged R.B.C.} = \frac{\text{c.p.m./c.c. R.B.C. (time t)} \times \text{volume systemic circuit RCM}}{\text{total c.p.m. } (Cr^{51}) \text{ injected into perfusion circuit}} \times 100$$

The missing quantity for this calculation is the volume of the systemic circuit outside of the actual area of perfusion. This can be estimated as suggested by Austen[1] but this introduces a rather inaccurate quantity into the calculation.

If it is assumed that the net loss of blood from the perfusion circuit is equal to the net quantity of blood passing from the systemic to the perfusion circuit, the relative volumes of the systemic and perfusion circuits can be calculated from the curves shown in Fig. 1. For example, data on $Cr^{51}$ concentrations in the 2 circuits at 15 and 60 minutes could be introduced into 2 simultaneous equations with the systemic and perfusion circuit volumes as the 2 "unknowns." These equations can then be solved for the volume relationship between the circuits. In this instance, the perfusion circuit (including the oxygenator) was found to be equal to 0.51 times the systemic circuit. The total blood volume (above thigh tourniquets) was determined preoperatively and found to be 4,200 ml. By these calculations the systemic circuit volume was found to be 3,350 ml. The per cent of the original isotope lost from the perfusion circuit at time t could then be calculated. In this patient, 49 per cent of the total isotope had been lost from the perfusion circuit by 30 minutes, and by the end of the perfusion the loss was 59 per cent. This approaches almost complete mixing of the 2 circulations as can be seen in Fig. 1.

These calculated values for per cent loss from the perfusion circuit in this patient, as well as the concentration ratios (perfusion-systemic), are similar to those found in most clinical pelvic perfusions although there is some degree of variability. Of 7 pelvic perfusions in which similar studies were made, the median values for concentration ratios were 4:1 (3.2 to 5.2:1) in 15 minutes, 2.2:1 (1.7 to 2.7:1) at 30 minutes, and 1.5:1 (1.1 to 1.8:1) at 60 minutes. All of these data describe the loss of intravascular isotope from the perfusion circuit into the active systemic circuit.

The transfer rate of isotope from the systemic circuit into the perfusion circuit usually occurs at a similar rate in such poorly isolated systems. Fig. 2 demonstrates this by showing the data from a clinical pelvic perfusion in which another intravascular isotope (RISA) was added to the systemic circuit and measurements of both $Cr^{51}$-tagged red blood cells and RISA in the 2 circuits carried out simultaneously. When regional isolation of an anatomic area is markedly improved so that few collateral channels are available for transfer, other factors may lead to marked disproportion in flow rates in and out of the perfusion circuit. Fig. 3 is a good example of this phenomenon in a perfusion in which the isotope (RISA) was introduced into the systemic circuit. This pelvic perfusion system shows no dilution of systemic blood by the perfusion blood at any time, despite increasing radioactivity in the perfusion circuit. This indicates a steady flow of blood into the perfusion circuit with little or no loss, a situation which obviously cannot persist for long periods.

The calculation outlined for determination of the percentage loss from the perfusion circuit depends on knowledge of the systemic blood volume outside the perfusion circuit. This calculated volume is based on equations which assume that (1) transfer out of and into the perfusion circuit occurs at a relatively constant rate, and (2) the volumes of the individual circuits remain constant throughout the perfusion procedure because of equal transfer into and out of the perfusion circuit. However, it has become quite clear from subsequent studies that neither of these 2 assumptions is uniformly valid. Data from systemic circuit samples in the 10- to 30-minute period in Fig. 1 demonstrates this variability in rate of transfer into the systemic circuit, and we have noted more striking

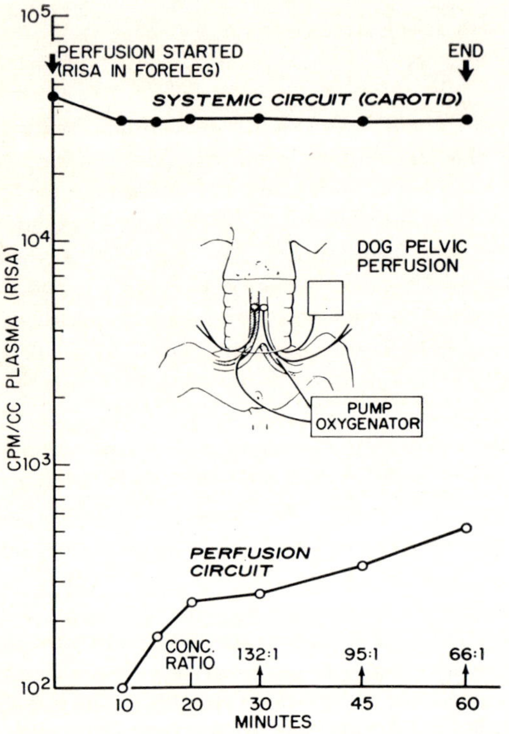


**Fig. 3.** Data obtained during experimental pelvic perfusion utilizing an abdominal pneumatic tourniquet to control losses through collateral vessels. Indicator (RISA) placed in systemic circuit and data demonstrate small loss into perfusion circuit but no transfer from perfusion circuit into systemic circuit.

changes in rate of transfer in other studies. In addition, the virtual volume of the perfusion circuit can actually vary in the pelvis itself by vasomotor changes in the vessels, and the volume of reservoir frequently cannot be maintained at a steady level during perfusion. This is particularly true of the better isolated perfusion systems as disproportionate transfer rates are more likely to occur.

In addition to requiring 2 assumptions that are frequently false, this calculation of per cent loss has the error produced by reentry of indicator after its initial escape from the perfusion circuit. There may also be differing rates of equilibration of the various indicators within the individual circuits. For all these reasons, most of the comparative data to be presented on other drugs or indicators will be expressed as ratios of the concentrations of these substances in the 2 circuits. This means of expression requires less "compounding" of the actual data obtained and, for anatomically similar systems, such concentration ratios appear to be a valid means of demonstrating differences. This simple means of describing the data does not give a quantitative estimate of the amount of isotopic material lost from the regional circuit, but consideration of subsequent data with substances of larger volumes of distribution demonstrates that accurate quantitation of loss of intravascular isotope, even if possible, would not even give an approximation of the drug dosage to the systemic or nonperfused circuit.

**What do leakage measurements mean?** The volume of distribution of the different chemotherapeutic agents, the relative concentrations in or outside the cells, the rates of metabolism, and the renal excretion of the agents will all lead to errors in estimation of drug loss solely on the basis of the systemic concentration measurements. For these reasons, we attempted a study to compare the leakage of purely intravascular isotopes (RISA and $Cr^{51}$-tagged red blood cells) with nonmetabolizable radioactively tagged ions of larger distribution patterns. $Na^{24}$, which diffuses into the extracellular space, seemed an ideal indicator for such a study.

Data from a pelvic perfusion in the dog in Fig. 4 in which both $Na^{24}$ and $Cr^{51}$ red blood cells were added to the perfusion circuit demonstrate a greater concentration gradient from the perfusion to the systemic circuit for the extracellular isotope ($Na^{24}$) than for the intravascular isotope ($Cr^{51}$-tagged red blood cells). In 3 dogs the transfers of $Cr^{51}$-tagged red blood cells and $Na^{24}$ were studied simultaneously and in 2 additional dogs these comparisons were made between RISA and $Na^{24}$ (Figs. 5 and 6). In each instance, the concentration ratios between the 2 circuits were consistently greater for $Na^{24}$ than for the intravascular isotope. Since the volume of distribution of $Na^{24}$ in the systemic circuit is essentially 4 times that of the plasma, it still seemed possible that the total loss of isotope might be greater for $Na^{24}$ than for $Cr^{51}$-tagged red blood cells or RISA. The comparison of total loss for the 2 isotopes used simultaneously in the same experiment was therefore expressed as a ratio by the formula:

$$\frac{\text{Loss } Cr^{51} \text{ R.B.C.}}{\text{Loss } Na^{24}} = \frac{\dfrac{Cr^{51} \text{ c.p.m./c.c. R.B.C.}}{\text{Total } Cr^{51} \text{ dose}}}{\dfrac{Na^{24} \text{ c.p.m./c.c. plasma} \times 4}{\text{Total } Na^{24} \text{ dose}}} \times \frac{\text{Hct*}}{\text{1-Hct}}$$

*With simultaneous study of RISA and $Na^{24}$ the same formula can be used except for omission of the factor $\frac{\text{Hct}}{\text{1-Hct}}$.

The actual volume of the systemic circuit does not need to be calculated for this comparison as described in the previous calculations, since this type of ratio only expresses the total loss of $Cr^{51}$-tagged red blood cells in relation to the total loss of $Na^{24}$. Despite the difference in volume of distribution of the 2 isotopes, the total loss of RISA or $Cr^{51}$-tagged red blood cells was always greater than the total loss of $Na^{24}$, and this difference increased with time (Table I).

When the radioactive isotope of potassium ($K^{42}$) was studied simultaneously with $Cr^{51}$-tagged red blood cells, it was found that the concentration gradient between the 2 circuits was even greater for $K^{42}$ than it was for $Cr^{51}$ (Fig. 7). Undoubtedly, complete equilibration of the $K^{42}$ did not occur within the perfusion circuit during this time, but the ratio of concentrations in the 2 circuits was, nonetheless, strikingly different.

In view of the data which demonstrated greater concentration gradients and smaller losses between the circuits with isotopes of larger volumes of distribution than the vascular tree, it seemed wise to study the ratio of concentrations of chemotherapeutic agents between the circuits. It can be seen in Table II that the ratios of concentrations of drug between the 2 circuits were considerably greater than were found with either $Na^{24}$, RISA, or $Cr^{51}$-tagged red blood cells. This is also shown graphically in Figs. 5 and 6. In these studies, the role of urinary excretion of the agent from the systemic circuit was eliminated by clamping both ureters during the experimental perfusion. In these experiments, Methotrexate demonstrated concentration ratios between the 2 circuits almost identical to the concentration ratios obtained with $Na^{24}$ (Fig. 5 and Table II). This is not surprising in view of the data presented by Freeman[7] which demonstrated the volume of distribution for Methotrexate to be approximately that of the extracellular space. Almost total recovery in the urine of an intravenous dose also suggests minimal metabolism of the drug by the tissues. The fluorinated pyrimidines (FU and FUDR) showed much greater concentration ratios between the circuits than was noted with $Na^{24}$ (Figs. 4 and 6 and Table II). This can probably be explained by published data which demonstrate distribution of FU in the total body water[3] after intravenous injection. All of these studies with radioactive indicators or drugs seemed to demonstrate that the volume of distribution of the substance concerned played a major role in its quantitative rate of loss from the perfusion circuit.

The role of the volume of distribution of a chemotherapeutic agent or radioactive

**Table I.** *Experimental pelvic perfusion (dogs): comparison of total loss from perfusion circuit of 2 isotopes with intravascular (RISA or $Cr^{51}$-tagged red blood cells) and extracellular ($Na^{24}$) volumes of distribution*

| Dog No. | Isotopes studied simultaneously | Total loss of RISA or $Cr^{51}$-tagged R.B.C. / Total loss of $Na^{24}$: 20-30 min. | 60 min. |
|---|---|---|---|
| 700 | $Na^{24}$, $Cr^{51}$ | 2.75 | 3.03 |
| 833 | $Na^{24}$, $Cr^{51}$ | 1.56 | 1.65 |
| 398 | $Na^{24}$, $Cr^{51}$ | 1.41 | — |
| 384 | $Na^{24}$, RISA | 1.59 | 1.97 |
| 315 | $Na^{24}$, RISA | 1.34 | 1.47 |

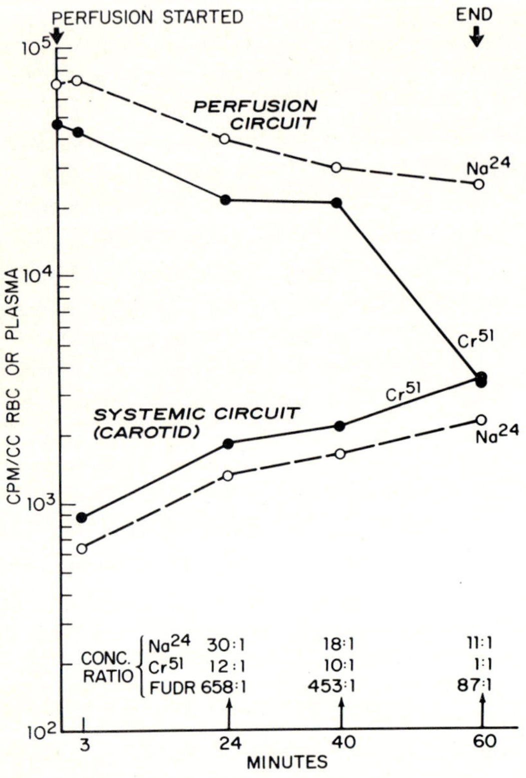


**Fig. 4.** Comparison of concentrations in perfusion and systemic circuits of $Cr^{51}$-tagged red blood cells, $Na^{24}$, and FUDR during experimental pelvic perfusion (dog).

isotope being studied in the postperfusion "flush" procedure was also of interest. For purposes of comparison of the efficiency of the indicator-free "flush," the residual concentration of the substance in question was expressed as a per cent of the "preflush" concentration (Table III). In each of 3 experiments on dogs, the effectiveness of the "flush" with 1 L. of dextran was greater for the intravascular isotope than it was for the extracellular isotope. The ability of this procedure to clear the fluorinated pyrimidines from the perfusion circuit was definitely less than the ability to clear the circuit of $Na^{24}$. The data obtained for Methotrexate in this regard were actually quite similar to those obtained with $Na^{24}$. Data from the same procedure in 4 patients subjected to pelvic perfusion (Table IV) also show a greater residual drug concentration and less efficient clearing of the perfusion circuit than was noted with the intravascular isotope. While the total loss of these agents during the perfusion is less than expected from the usual studies of intravascular isotopes, the proportion of the original dose that remains in the local area after perfusion and the clearing procedure is completed is apparently much greater than would be expected from data with RISA or $Cr^{51}$.

**Efforts to improve regional isolation of the pelvis.** After initial experience with the standard procedure for pelvic perfusion, we became very dissatisfied with the degree of regional isolation that was achieved. In an attempt to improve this in our pelvic perfusions in dogs, we utilized a transverse laparotomy incision and applied a rubber tube tourniquet to the entire paraspinal muscle group. This tourniquet was placed behind the ureters, colon, aorta, and vena cava at the level of the major vessel occlusion. As can be seen in Fig. 8, this did improve the degree of vascular isolation to some extent. There was great variability in the leakage measurements, however, despite uniformly vigorous attempts to ligate all visible collaterals and apply the tourniquet as firmly as possible. Fig. 9 demonstrates the wide range of concentration ratios obtained in 20 dogs subjected to pelvic perfusion in this manner. The median values for concentration ratios between the perfusion and systemic circuits were 14 to 1 in 15 minutes, 6.8 to 1 in 30 minutes, and 5.4 to 1 in 60 minutes. Despite the variability in degree of isolation achieved by this technique, we then applied a rubber tube tourniquet in a similar fashion to 3 patients during pelvic perfusion. Placement of the tourniquet in man was less satisfactory because of elevation of the tourniquet by the projecting bodies of the lumbar vertebrae. This technical problem seemed to be overcome by placement of multiple laparotomy pads in each lumbar gutter to achieve a more cylindrical mass for the tourniquet, but all 3 patients had mixing curves at the time of perfusion that were almost identical to those obtained with the standard procedure. This, then, was no

**Table II.** *Experimental pelvic perfusion (dogs): comparison of concentration ratios (perfusion/systemic) of isotopes and drugs studied simultaneously*

| Dog No. | Indicator and drug | Concentration ratio | | | |
|---|---|---|---|---|---|
| | | 15-20 min. | 30 min. | 40 min. | 60 min. |
| 315 | $Na^{24}$ | — | 27.3:1 | — | 11.0:1 |
| | RISA | — | 9.3:1 | — | 4.7:1 |
| | 5-FU | — | 95:1 | — | 104:1 |
| F102 | $Cr^{51}$-tagged R.B.C. | 20:1 | 5.7:1 | 4.5:1 | — |
| | FUDR | 432:1 | 57:1 | 53:1 | — |
| F103 | $Cr^{51}$-tagged R.B.C. | 7.5:1 | — | 6.1:1 | 5.5:1 |
| | FUDR | 192:1 | — | 198:1 | 186:1 |
| 700 | $Na^{24}$ | 29.9:1 | — | 18.3:1 | 10.8:1 |
| | $Cr^{51}$-tagged R.B.C. | 11.9:1 | — | 9.7:1 | 1:1 |
| | FUDR | 658:1 | — | 453:1 | 86.7:1 |
| 312 | $Na^{24}$ | — | 14.1:1 | — | 11.0:1 |
| | RISA | — | 7.6:1 | — | 5.5:1 |
| | Methotrexate | — | 15.3:1 | — | 11.8:1 |

**Table III.** *Experimental pelvic perfusion (dogs): effectiveness of terminal "flush" of perfusion circuit (1,000 ml. dextran)*

| Dog No. | Indicator and drug | Concentration in venous line of perfusion circuit | | Residual (as % of concentration) |
|---|---|---|---|---|
| | | Before flush | After flush | |
| 700 | $Na^{24}$ | $5.27 \times 10^3$ c.p.m./ml. | $7.92 \times 10^2$ c.p.m./ml. | 15 |
| | $Cr^{51}$ | $8.24 \times 10^3$ c.p.m./ml. | $9.11 \times 10^2$ c.p.m./ml. | 11 |
| | FUDR | 520 γ/ml. | 200 γ/ml. | 38 |
| E315 | $Na^{24}$ | $2.02 \times 10^4$ c.p.m./ml. | $4.03 \times 10^3$ c.p.m./ml. | 20 |
| | RISA | $1.62 \times 10^4$ c.p.m./ml. | $3.91 \times 10^2$ c.p.m./ml. | 2 |
| | 5-FU | 447 γ/ml. | 218 γ/ml. | 49 |
| E312 | $Na^{24}$ | $1.58 \times 10^4$ c.p.m./ml. | $5.82 \times 10^3$ c.p.m./ml. | 37 |
| | RISA | $2.34 \times 10^4$ c.p.m./ml. | $2.78 \times 10^3$ c.p.m./ml. | 12 |
| | Methotrexate | 20 γ/ml. | 7.6 γ/ml. | 38 |

**Table IV.** *Effectiveness of terminal "flush" of pelvic perfusion circuit in patients (1,500 ml. "drug-free" blood)*

| Patient | Indicator and drug | Plasma concentration (venous line perfusion circuit) | | Residual (as % of plasma concentration) |
|---|---|---|---|---|
| | | Before flush | After flush | |
| L. C. | RISA | $1.08 \times 10^5$ c.p.m./ml. | $3.76 \times 10^3$ c.p.m./ml. | 3.5 |
| | Methotrexate | 112 γ/ml. | 10 γ/ml. | 8.9 |
| M. S. | RISA | $3.77 \times 10^4$ c.p.m./ml. | $8.05 \times 10^2$ c.p.m./ml. | 2.1 |
| | Methotrexate | 260 γ/ml. | 18 γ/ml. | 7.0 |
| V. T. | RISA | $1.16 \times 10^4$ c.p.m./ml. | $2.0 \times 10^3$ c.p.m./ml. | 17.2 |
| | FUDR | 2675 γ/ml. | 860 γ/ml. | 32 |
| M. G. | RISA | $1.53 \times 10^4$ c.p.m./ml. | $2.40 \times 10^3$ c.p.m./ml. | 16 |
| | FUDR | 1975 γ/ml. | 680 γ/ml. | 34 |

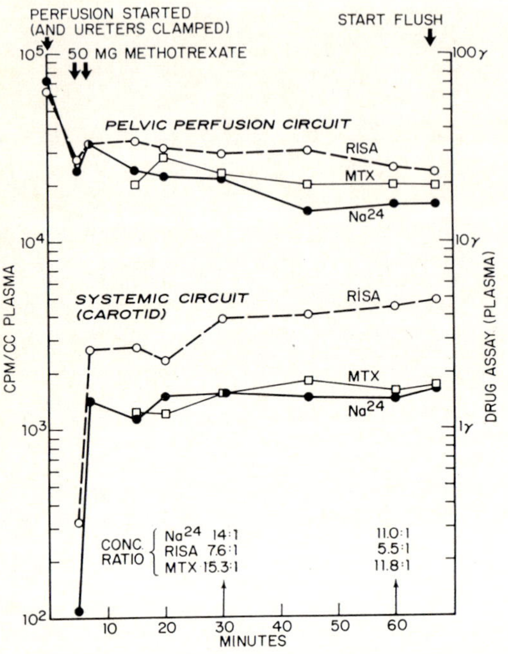


**Fig. 5.** Comparison of concentrations in perfusion and systemic circuits of RISA, $Na^{24}$, and Methotrexate during experimental pelvic perfusion (dog). Note similarity of concentration gradients of $Na^{24}$ and Methotrexate.

improvement on the clinical procedure as originally outlined.

In view of the fact that a major problem in regional isolation of the pelvis seemed to be the absence of an efficient cephalad tourniquet, a large pneumatic tourniquet was then applied to the entire abdomen of the dog and perfusion carried out after lumbar aortic and vena caval occlusion had been produced by balloon-tipped catheters. This method did improve the vascular isolation during regional perfusion as shown in Fig. 3. After a number of preliminary trials in the laboratory, this general isolation method has been applied to pelvic perfusion in 6 patients (Fig. 10). Anatomic isolation was virtually complete in 5 of these 6 patients; in 1 patient the reason for poor isolation was a technical error in placement of catheters. The limiting factor in this procedure has been the evidence of ischemia in the liver from prolonged intraperitoneal pressure, but it is hoped this problem may be solved by the use of hypothermia. Our preliminary experiences with this technique will be de-

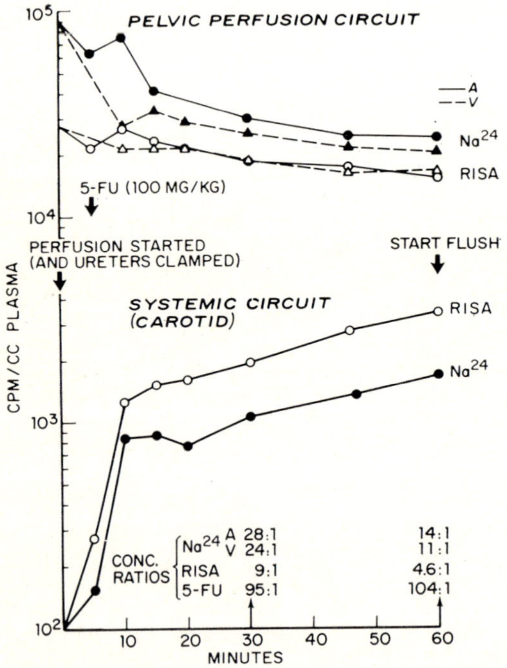


**Fig. 6.** Comparison of concentrations in perfusion and systemic circuits of RISA, $Na^{24}$, and 5-fluorouracil during pelvic perfusion in dog.

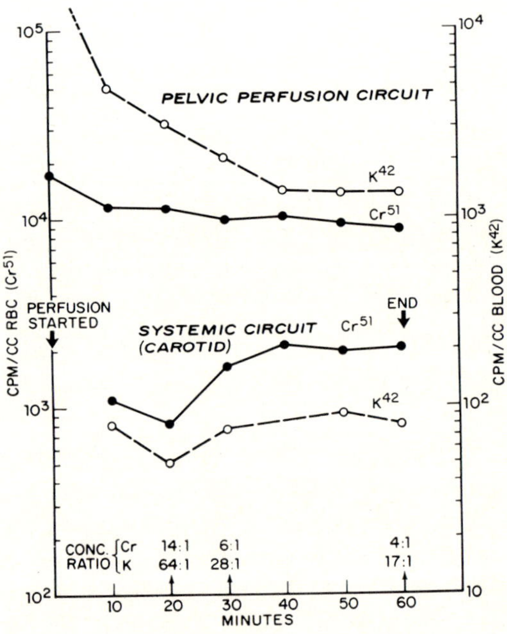


**Fig. 7.** Comparison of concentrations in perfusion and systemic circuits of $Cr^{51}$-tagged red blood cells and $K^{42}$ during pelvic perfusion in dog.

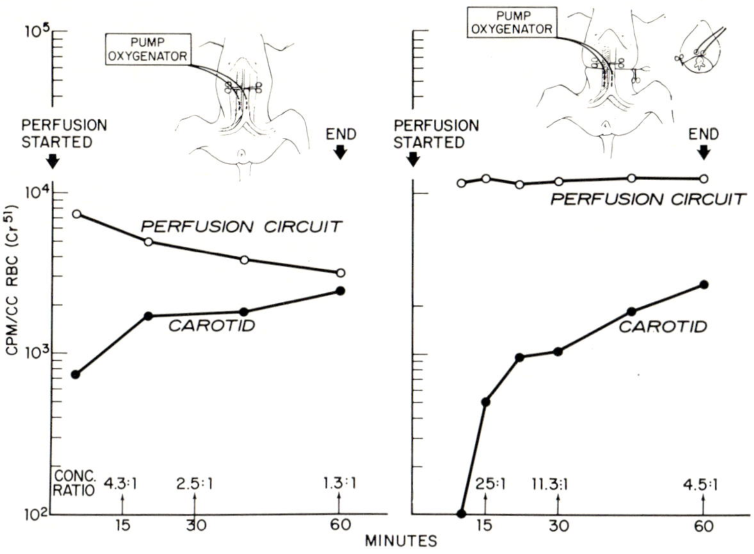


**Fig. 8.** A study of efficiency of isolation of experimental pelvic perfusion with $Cr^{51}$. Graph on left demonstrates typical data obtained with simple occlusion of lumbar aorta and vena cava with perfusion distally. Graph on right demonstrates improvement in isolation produced by addition of paraspinal rubber tourniquet (see inset).

scribed in more detail elsewhere,[8] but the idea is presented here as a possible solution to the problem of isolation of collateral vessels in pelvic perfusion.

## COMMENT

These studies have given us a different concept of partially isolated systems of regional perfusion. Although there is an interstitial fluid interface between the perfusion circuit and the remainder of the body, the transfer rates of nonvascular isotopes that were observed indicate that the transfers do occur entirely or almost entirely through vascular channels. Probably only the portion of the isotope or chemotherapeutic agent that is in the plasma carries on a significant degree of mixing with the tissues to be protected. The volume of distribution of the agent in the perfusion, as well as its rate of incorporation in the cells or in the metabolism of the tissues perfused, appears then to be of much greater import in determining expected drug loss than is estimation of vascular leakage (Fig. 11). In pelvic per-

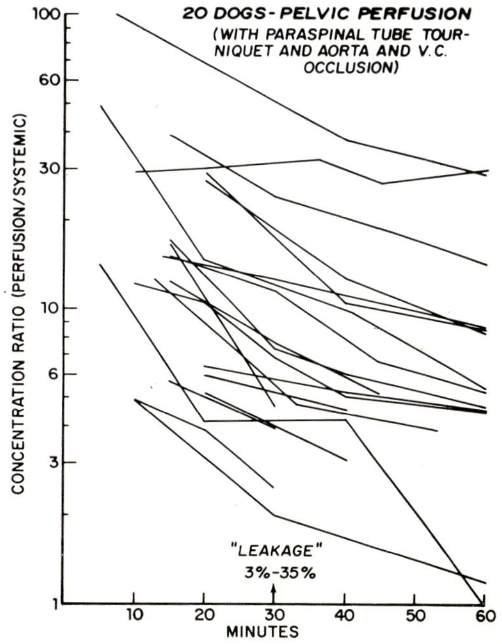


**Fig. 9.** Marked variability in efficiency of isolation achieved during experimental pelvic perfusion with a uniform technique. Data from 20 perfusions compared by means of concentration ratios between perfusion and systemic circuits.

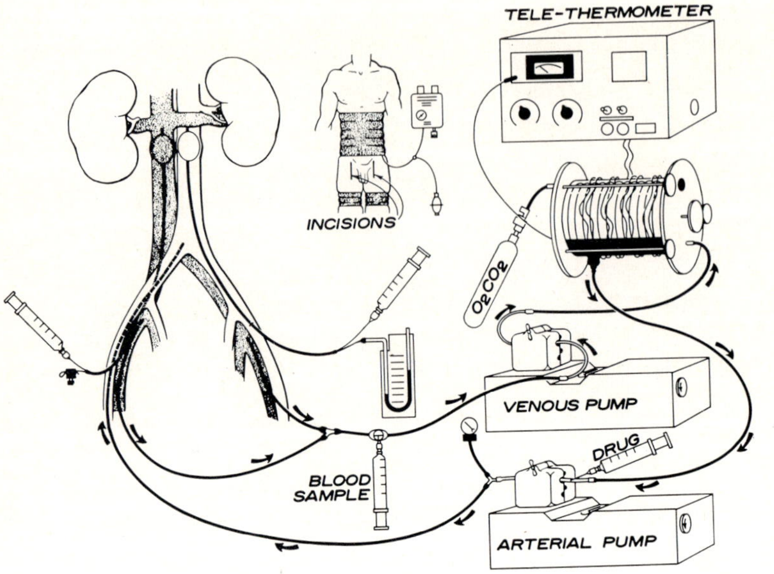


**Fig. 10.** Diagram of clinical pelvic perfusion method utilizing abdominal pneumatic tourniquet.

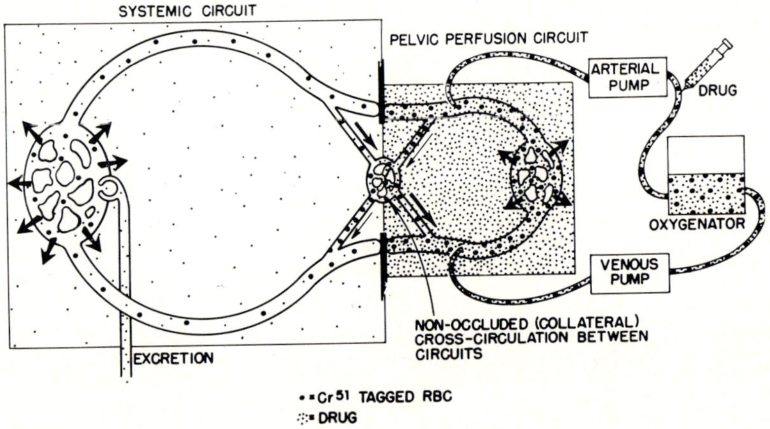


**Fig. 11.** Diagrammatic concept of factors which affect concentrations of intravascular indicator ($Cr^{51}$-tagged red blood cells or RISA) and a chemotherapeutic agent in perfusion systemic circuits when isolation is incomplete.

fusion, a rapidly fixed or metabolized agent such as nitrogen mustard may be the preferable agent, but antimetabolites might be more effectively used in high leakage systems than intravascular isotope studies would lead us to believe, in view of their extravascular distribution. The inefficiency of clearing of the circuit of these agents at the end of the perfusion may even be a more limiting factor with this technique than losses which occur during the perfusion itself. What appears to be a rapidly mixing system still has many possible advantages from the standpoint of regional chemotherapy. Efforts to improve isolation similar to those presented should be continued, however, in view of the great therapeutic opportunity in this unique anatomic area.

## SUMMARY

Data on losses (or leakage) during clinical and experimental pelvic perfusion have been presented. An effort has been made in these studies to determine the relationship between the findings with various isotopes and the behavior of chemotherapeutic agents in these systems. It was found that the volume of distribution of the substance concerned was a primary factor affecting leakage. In view of the significantly smaller losses of isotopes and agents that had extravascular distribution, intravascular samples ($Cr^{51}$ or RISA) did not accurately reflect the transfer of specific chemotherapeutic agents. These studies also demonstrated less efficient clearing of drugs from the perfusion circuit by the "terminal flush" than could be accomplished with the intravascular isotopes. The therapeutic implications of these studies, as well as procedures employed to improve anatomic isolation, have been discussed.

We appreciate the help and encouragement of our colleagues R. J. Booher, R. Brasfield, D. Karnofsky, C. J. McPeak, H. T. Randall, and P. Vanamee. We are also indebted to W. Brown, M. Hood, E. Masle, and A. M. O'Connor for technical assistance.

### REFERENCES

1. Austen, W. A., Monaco, A. P., Richardson, G. S., Baker, W. H., Shaw, R. S., and Raker, J. W.: Treatment of malignant pelvic tumors by extracorporeal perfusion with chemotherapeutic agents, New England J. Med. **261:** 1037, 1959.
2. Burchenal, J. H., Waring, G. B., Ellison, R. R., and Reilly, H. C.: A simple method for determination of levels of amethopterin in blood and urine, Proc. Soc. Exper. Biol. & Med. **78:** 603, 1951.
3. Chauduri, N. K., Montag, B. J., and Heidelberger, C.: Studies on fluorinated pyrimidines: III. The metabolism of 5-fluorouracil-2 $C^{14}$ and 5-fluoro-orotic-2 $C^{14}$ acid in vivo, Cancer Res. **18:** 318, 1958.
4. Creech, O., Jr., Krementz, E. T., Ryan, R. F., and Winblad, J. N.: Chemotherapy of cancer; regional perfusion utilizing extracorporeal circuit, Ann. Surg. **148:** 616-632, 1958.
5. Edelman, S., Greenspan, E. N., and Baronofsky, I. D.: Recent advances in medicine and surgery; isolation-perfusion in cancer chemotherapy, New York J. Med. **60:** 2877, 1960.
6. Flynn, L. M., Williams, V. B., O'Dell, B. L., and Hogan, A. G.: Medium for assay of vitamins with lactic acid bacteria, Anal. Chem. **23:** 180, 1951.
7. Freeman, M. V.: The fluorometric measurement of the absorption, distribution and excretion of single doses of 4-amino-10 methyl pteroylglutamic acid (amethopterin) in man, J. Pharmacol. & Exper. Therap. **122:** 154, 1956.
8. Lawrence, W., Jr., Kuehn, P., Masle, E. T., and Miller, D. G.: An abdominal tourniquet for regional chemotherapy, J. Surg. Res. In press.
9. Read, R. C.: Studies of red cell volume and turnover using radiochromium—description of a new "closed" method of red cell volume measurement, New England J. Med. **250:** 1021, 1954.
10. Stehlin, J. S., Clark, R. L., White, E. C., Smith, J. L., Griffin, A. C., Veese, R. H., and Healey, J. E.: Regional chemotherapy for cancer; experience with 116 perfusions, Ann. Surg. **151:** 605, 1960.
11. Watkins, E., Jr., Hering, A. C., Luna, R., and Adams, H. D.: The use of intravascular balloon catheters for isolation of the pelvic vascular bed during pump-oxygenator perfusion of cancer chemotherapeutic agents, Surg. Gynec. & Obst. **111:** 464-468, 1960.
12. Woodhall, B., Hall, K., Mahaley, S., and Jackson, J.: Chemotherapy of brain cancer: experimental and clinical studies in localized hypothermic cerebral perfusion, Ann. Surg. **150:** 640, 1959.

*(For discussion, see page 271.)*

# Abdominal perfusion for cancer chemotherapy with hypothermia and hyperthermia

WILLIAM W. SHINGLETON, M.D.
ROY T. PARKER, M.D.
STEPHEN MAHALEY, M.D.
DURHAM, N. C.
*From the Departments of Surgery and Obstetrics and Gynecology, Duke University Medical Center*

Techniques for perfusion of certain body areas, including the pelvis, were first described by Creech and his associates[2] in 1958. A technique for abdominal and liver perfusion was first described by Shingleton[10] in 1959. An integral part of the procedure for abdominal and liver perfusion was the use of general body hypothermia (31° to 32° C.) outside of the perfused area to protect bone marrow, combined with hyperthermia (38° to 39° C.) of tissues within the perfused area to enhance drug action. Since isolated pelvic perfusion has been found by Stehlin[13] to be associated with a relatively large "circulatory leak," hypothermia and hyperthermia, as used in abdominal perfusion, have been made a part of the technique in pelvic perfusion. This report concerns a further description of the use of temperature differential in localized body areas as an adjunct to abdominal and pelvic perfusion for cancer chemotherapy.

## METHOD

The circulatory isolation of the abdominal visceral area during perfusion consisted of cannulation of the abdominal aorta and inferior vena cava via femoral vessels and clamping of the aorta and vena cava just above the diaphragm through a right thoracotomy.[9] Tourniquets were applied to the upper thighs.

The perfusion unit consisted of a dual channel, independently variable torque conversion Sigmamotor pump, a Travenol bubble oxygenator into which blood and 100 per cent oxygen were pumped, a Harrison-Brown heat exchanger, a bubble trap, and 4 blood filters that were included in the circuit to remove fibrin clots. A rotameter (flowmeter) was used to record perfusion flow, and systemic arterial and perfusion arterial pressures were measured by Statham strain gauges connected to an Offner recorder.

After induction of general anesthesia, general body hypothermia to 31° to 32° C. was produced by use of a Therm-O-Rite blanket. Tourniquets on the upper thighs were inflated. The extracorporeal circulation unit was primed with 1,500 ml. of heparinized donor blood. This blood was heated to 41° to 42° C. by circulation through the heat exchanger. After occlusion of the aorta, vena cava, and azygos vein, the blood in the extracorporeal unit was perfused through the abdominal area for a period of 20 to 30 minutes. One of the alkylating agents was introduced either in divided doses at 5-minute intervals into the inflow catheter of the perfusion circuit or mixed in the blood in the circulation unit. The drugs used were either A-139, 1.0 to 3.0 mg. per kilogram, Cytoxan, 40 mg. per kilogram, L-phenylalanine mustard, 2 mg. per kilogram, or

Supported in part by Research Grant No. CY-4860, National Cancer Institute, Department of Health, Education and Welfare.

Read at the Twenty-second Annual Meeting of the Society of University Surgeons, Kansas City, Kan., Feb. 9-11, 1961.

nitrogen mustard, 0.75 mg. per kilogram.* After conclusion of the perfusion, 1,000 ml. of blood were then "flushed" through the perfused area. Occlusion of the aorta and vena cava was released, catheters were removed from the femoral vessels, and these vessels repaired.

For pelvic perfusion, the abdominal aorta and vena cava were clamped just above the bifurcation. The femoral artery and vein were cannulated. Tourniquets were placed around the upper thighs. All other aspects of the procedure were the same as with abdominal perfusion.

## RESULTS

Twenty-five patients with advanced abdominal or pelvic malignancies have undergone perfusion. The data on patients who have had abdominal perfusion are shown in Table I. The data on patients who have had pelvic perfusion are shown in Table II.

Figs. 1 and 2 depict the differences in tissue temperature used within the perfused segment and outside of the perfused area during abdominal and pelvic perfusions.

There was no immediate operative death. Death has not occurred because of bone marrow depression. One patient who had pelvic perfusion with A-139, 3 mg. per kilogram of body weight, for advanced carcinoma of the cervix, developed partial bilateral sciatic nerve paralysis that has persisted for 2 months after the procedure. In retrospect, this was thought to be due to an excessive dosage of A-139 for pelvic perfusion under these conditions. A majority of the patients had advanced disease at the time of perfusion. Death after perfusion has been due to further spread of the disease. Reduction in tumor size has been observed in some patients. Most of the patients have had rather pronounced relief from pain after the procedure. A sufficient number of patients with similar tumor types and extent of disease is not yet available for evaluation of the effect of the procedure on survival time.

*A-139 is 2, 5-diethylenimino-3, 6-bis (2 methoxyethoxy)-1, 4-benzoquinone; Cytoxon is N, N-bis (β-chloroethyl)-N′, O-propylene phosphoric acid ester diamide monohydrate; L-phenylalanine mustard is 3-[p-(Bis {2′-chlorethyl} amino) phenyl] - L-alanine; and nitrogen mustard is methyl - bis (β-chloroethyl) amine.

## COMMENT

The evidence for the protective effect of hypothermia on bone marrow exposed to alkylating agents comes from 4 sources, (1) theoretical considerations, (2) animal survival experiments, (3) radioisotope studies, and (4) clinical results.

**Theoretical considerations.** A theoretical basis for the protection may be derived from the temperature coefficient of the alkylating process itself. For example, with nitrogen mustard, Bergel[1] has observed a temperature coefficient of 2 for each 10-degree change. Schmahl[8] and Woodhall[14] have found that the lethal effects of alkylating agents on experimental animal tumors are significantly increased with increases in incubation temperature. It was on this basis that Woodhall[14] introduced the technique of heating the perfused blood during perfusion of the head and neck region. Increase in blood viscosity, which occurs with hypothermia,[4] may alter the volume and pattern of blood flow through cooled tissues and result in less contact of alkylating agent with sensitive bone marrow.

**Animal survival experiments.** Shingleton[11] reported a significant protection against bone marrow depression and death from lethal doses of nitrogen mustard when dogs were cooled to 31° to 32° C. prior to administration of the drug. The mortality rate was 9 per cent in a group of 11 dogs under hypothermia, as compared to 90 per cent in a control group of 11 dogs at normal body temperature. Histologic studies of bone marrow from these animals showed a specific protective effect of hypothermia, possibly related to alterations of blood flow which occurred with cooling.

**Radioisotope studies.** Using $P^{32}$-labeled thio-TEPA, Rochlin[7] has shown a decrease in drug uptake in tissue of the hind leg of a dog during hypothermia (80° F.) and an increased uptake during hyperthermia (101° F.). We recently have used $C^{14}$ ethyl–labeled nitrogen mustard during abdominal perfusion in dogs.[12] In these experiments, to be reported in detail later, 15 μc of $C^{14}$ ethyl-labeled nitrogen mustard was introduced into the perfusion circuit. It was found that the leak into areas outside the perfused segment was significantly diminished when the nonperfused tissues were cooled to 31° to 32° C. It has been suggested that this effect possibly is related to an increase in blood viscosity that occurs with tissue cooling. Furthermore, it was found that "circulatory leak," as measured with the $I^{131}$-labeled albumin technique, and "drug leak," as measured by $C^{14}$-labeled nitrogen mustard, are significantly different when these substances are introduced simultaneously into the perfusion circuit of an animal undergoing abdominal perfusion. In this study, the circulatory leak was estimated to be 35 per cent and the drug leak was estimated to be 15 per cent during 20 minutes of perfusion. The extent of drug leak will depend to a great extent upon the speed of reactivity of the specific drug used in perfusion. The leak with nitrogen mustard, a highly reactive compound, would be much less than with longer acting agents such as Cytoxan. Analysis of intestinal and liver tissue samples for radioactivity showed a decrease in uptake of the labeled nitrogen mustard when these tissues were cooled to 31° to 32° C., and an increase when the tissues were warmed to 39° C.

**Clinical results.** The results of abdominal and pelvic perfusion, combined with differential temperature control of restricted body areas, indicate that this procedure permits the introduction of dosages of alkylating agents 3 to 4 times greater than safe systemic therapy and into a volume estimated to be less than 50 per cent of the total blood volume. These calculations suggest a blood concentration of drug 6 to 8 times greater than can be achieved by systemic adminis-

**Table I.** *Abdominal perfusion*

| *Patient* | *Age* | *Sex* | *Weight (Kg.)* | *Diagnosis* | *Perfusion drug* | *Follow-up* | *Lowest WBC* | *Post-operative day* |
|---|---|---|---|---|---|---|---|---|
| D. A. | 28 | F | 44.8 | Carcinoma of colon | Cytoxan, 40 mg./Kg. | Died, 4 mo. | 3,100 | 7 |
| E. B. | 26 | F | 38.3 | Carcinoma of cervix | A-139, 1.5 mg./Kg. | Died, 2 mo. | 7,850 | 11 |
| L. C. | 48 | F | 44.3 | Carcinoma of cervix | A-139, 1.5 mg./Kg. | Died, 4 mo. | 7,400 | 6 |
| W. C. | 35 | M | 53.7 | Malignant melanoma | L-phenylalanine mustard, 2 mg./Kg. | Living, 3 mo. | 1,075 | 13 |
| A. H. | 26 | M | 66.6 | Hodgkin's disease | Nitrogen mustard, 0.75 mg./Kg. | Died, 1 mo. | 700 | 6 |
| J. J. | 42 | F | 67.3 | Carcinoma of ovary | Cytoxan, 40 mg./Kg. | Died, 3 mo. | 437 | 8 |
| F. P. | 41 | F | 33.2 | Carcinoma of ovary | A-139, 1.5 mg./Kg. | Died, 1 mo. | 3,100 | 2 |
| E. R. | 21 | F | 56.3 | Retroperitoneal adenocarcinoma | A-139, 2 mg./Kg. | Living, 1 mo. | 2,600 | 10 |
| W. R. | 34 | M | 61 | Leiomyosarcoma | A-139, 1.5 mg./Kg. | Living, 14 mo. | 3,500 | 4 |
| J. S. | 66 | M | 53.7 | Carcinoma of pancreas | Cytoxan, 40 mg./Kg. | Died, 3 mo. | 900 | 9 |
| D. S. | 33 | M | 67.1 | Carcinoma of rectum | Cytoxan, 40 mg./Kg. | Living, 12 mo. | 1,820 | 11 |
| J. Sm. | 54 | M | 81.2 | Carcinoma of pancreas | A-139, 3 mg./Kg. | Died, 1 mo. | 320 | 10 |
| V. S. | 49 | F | 46.5 | Carcinoma of pancreas | A-139, 2 mg./Kg. | Died, 3 mo. | 5,425 | 5 |
| B. S. | 60 | M | 61.5 | Carcinoma of pancreas | Cytoxan, 40 mg./Kg. | Died, 4 mo. | 2,150 | 13 |

**Table II.** *Pelvic perfusion*

| *Patient* | *Age* | *Sex* | *Weight (Kg.)* | *Diagnosis* | *Perfusion drug* | *Follow-up* | *Lowest WBC* | *Post-operative day* |
|---|---|---|---|---|---|---|---|---|
| G. B. | 56 | F | 73 | Carcinoma of ovary | A-139, 2 mg./Kg. | Living, 8 mo. | 4,100 | 4 |
| A. D. | 55 | F | 73.2 | Carcinoma of cervix | Cytoxan, 40 mg./Kg. | Died, 2 mo. | 113 | 7 |
| T. E. | 40 | F | 60 | Carcinoma of ovary | A-139, 1.5 mg./Kg. | Died, 3 mo. | 5,400 | 20 |
| M. G. | 54 | F | 51 | Carcinoma of cervix | A-139, 3 mg./Kg. | Died, 5 mo. | 8,250 | 7 |
| V. M. | 54 | F | 54 | Carcinoma of cervix | Cytoxan, 40 mg./Kg. | Living, 14 mo. | 1,480 | 11 |
| Z. M. | 39 | F | 97 | Carcinoma of ovary | Cytoxan, 40 mg./Kg. | Living, 17 mo. | 5,320 | 5 |
| L. L. | 31 | F | 56.6 | Carcinoma of cervix | A-139, 3 mg./Kg. | Living, 3 mo. | 2,700 | 16 |
| L. R. | 47 | F | 70.4 | Carcinoma of cervix | Cytoxan, 40 mg./Kg. | Died, 4 mo. | 350 | 8 |
| F. S. | 39 | F | 48.4 | Carcinoma of cervix | A-139, 1 mg./Kg. | Died, 5 mo. | 4,850 | 4 |
| R. S. | 41 | F | 43.2 | Carcinoma of rectum | A-139, 2 mg./Kg. | Living, 2 mo. | 4,200 | 7 |
| L. W. | 56 | M | 55.2 | Carcinoma of buttocks | Cytoxan, 40 mg./Kg. | Died, 3 mo. | 15,775 | 1 |

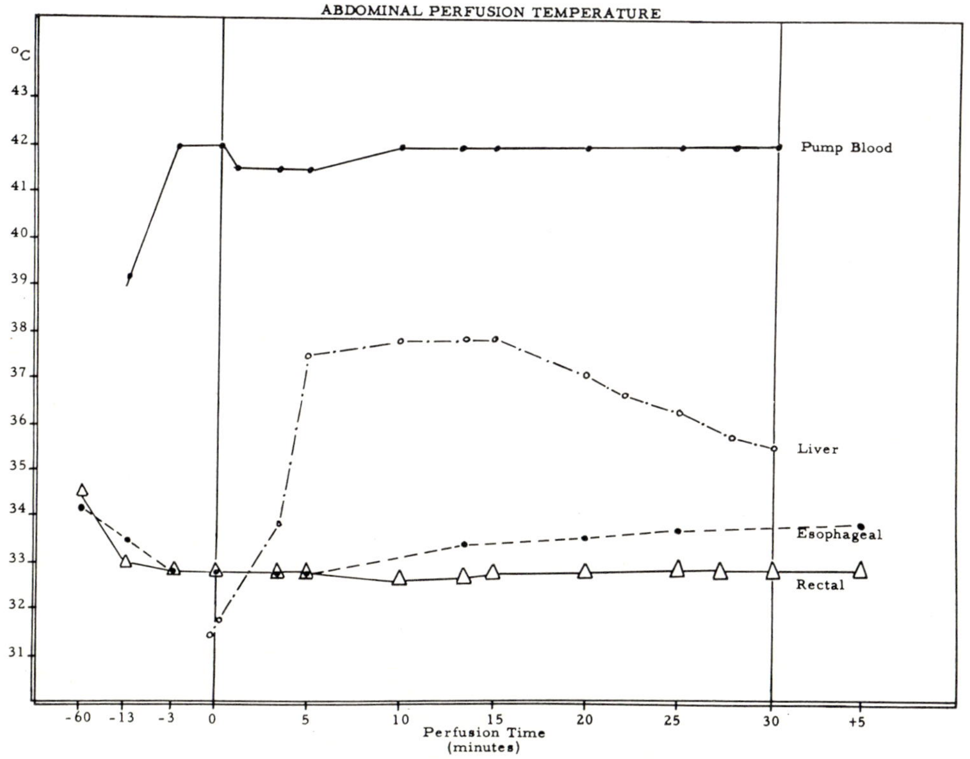


**Fig. 1.** Graph shows data obtained during abdominal perfusion under general body hypothermia. The perfused blood was introduced at a temperature of 41° C. Note the rise in liver temperature which occurred, with no appreciable change in the rectal and esophageal temperature.

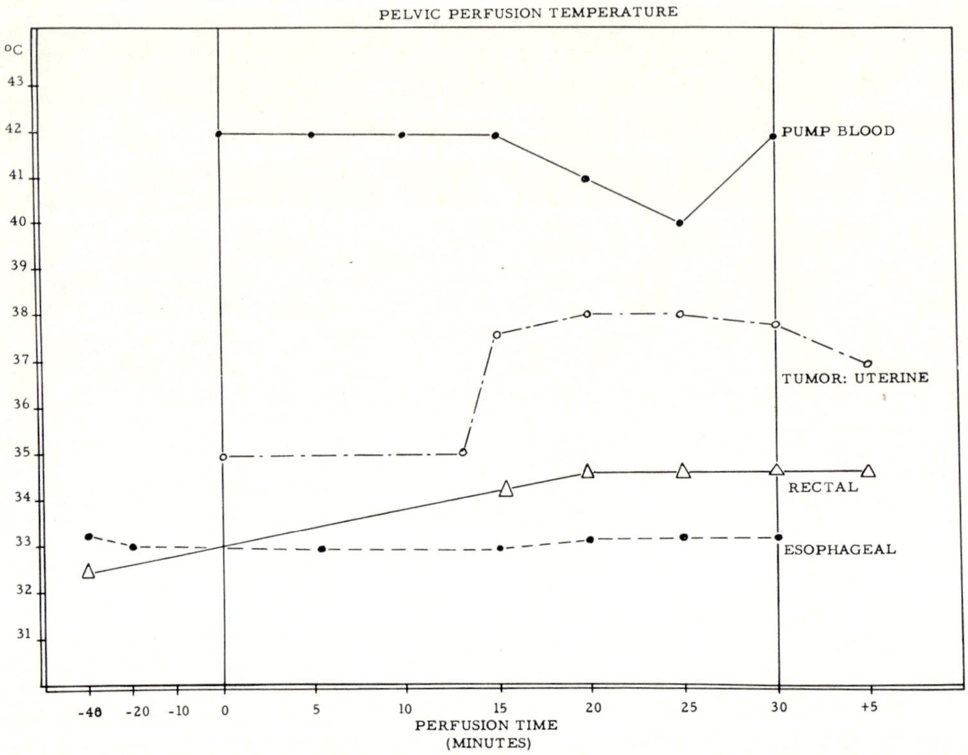


**Fig. 2.** Graph shows data obtained during pelvic perfusion under general body hypothermia. The perfused blood was introduced at a temperature of 41° C. Note the rise in uterine temperature which occurred, with no appreciable change in the rectal and esophageal temperature.

tration. No electrolyte disturbance and no serious damage to the function of the gastrointestinal tract, liver, or kidney have been found in patients after the procedure.[9] A low flow rate (200 to 300 ml. per minute) has been used. It is suggested that by utilization of hypothermia outside of the perfused area the necessity for an involved and difficult anatomic dissection for circulatory isolation during abdominal perfusion, as recently suggested by Hitchcock,[5] or during pelvic perfusion, as suggested by Stehlin,[13] is avoided. The necessity for bone marrow transfusion, as suggested by Jessiman,[6] during pelvic perfusion is also avoided. Additional studies are needed to define more accurately optimum flow rate, tissue oxygen tension and temperature, and specific uptake of drug in tumor tissue as compared to normal tissue. The feasibility of heating tumor-bearing areas of the body to even higher temperatures than reported here has been suggested by Gilchrist[3] in order to further enhance tumorcidal effects of the agents administered. It was found that by electromagnetic heating the temperature in the liver of a dog can be raised to 45° C. for 30 minutes without apparent damage to the organ.

## SUMMARY

Regional perfusion of the abdominal visceral and/or pelvic areas with an alkylating agent has been carried out in 25 patients with abdominal malignancies. General body hypothermia for bone marrow protection outside of the perfused area, with rapid rewarming of tissues within the perfused area to enhance drug action, has been used with perfusion in all patients. No operative death has occurred. Nine patients in the group developed a significant leukopenia after the procedure; however, no fatality can be directly attributed to bone marrow failure. The only major complication has been a bilateral partial sciatic paralysis in 1 patient perfused for Stage IV cervical cancer in whom a high dose of drug was used. Relief of pain has occurred in a majority of patients after perfusion. Nine of 25 patients are alive from 2 to 14 months after perfusion. The average survival time after perfusion in the 16 dead patients was 3 months. All patients died from progression of malignant disease.

The authors wish to express their appreciation to Mrs. Jacqueline Lancaster, Mrs. Jane Mahaley, and Mrs. Lucie Krueger for their technical assistance in these studies.

**REFERENCES**

1. Bergel, F.: Quoted by Henderson, I., in discussion of Shingleton, W., and Parker, R.: Abdominal perfusion with hypothermia and hyperthermia, Cancer Chemotherapy Report, No. 10, p. 37, 1960.
2. Creech, O., Krementz, E. T., Ryan, R. F., and Winblad, J. N.: Chemotherapy of cancer: regional perfusion utilizing an extracorporeal circuit, Ann. Surg. **148:** 616, 1958.
3. Gilchrist, R. K.: Potential treatment of cancer by electromagnetic heating, Surg. Gynec., & Obst. **110:** 499, 1960.
4. Gollan, F.: Discussion of paper by Shingleton, W., and Parker, R.: Abdominal perfusion with hypothermia and hyperthermia, Cancer Chemotherapy Report, No. 10, p. 37, 1960.
5. Hitchcock, C., Bascom, J., Strobel, C., Mueller, G., and Shepard, R.: Selective intra-arterial perfusion of total abdominal viscera for carcinoma, Surg. Gynec. & Obst. **111:** 484, 1960.
6. Jessiman, A.: Pelvic perfusion technique, Cancer Chemotherapy Report, No. 10, p. 5, 1960.
7. Rochlin, D.: Discussion of paper by Shingleton, W., and Parker, R.: Abdominal perfusion with hypothermia and hyperthermia, Cancer Chemotherapy Report, No. 10, p. 37, 1960.
8. Schmahl, D., and Druckrey, H.: Beitrage zum Wirkungsmechanismus von N-oxyd-lost, Naturwiss. **9:** 199, 1956.
9. Shingleton, W. W., Parker, R., and Mahaley, S.: Abdominal perfusion for cancer chemotherapy, Ann. Surg. **152:** 583, 1960.
10. Shingleton, W. W., Reeves, J. W., Keppel, R. A., Mahaley, S., and Taylor, H. M.: Studies on abdominal organ perfusion for cancer chemotherapy, Ann. Surg. **151:** 741, 1960.
11. Shingleton, W. W., and Smith, A. G.: Hypothermia against lethal dose of mechlorethamine, A. M. A. Arch. Surg. **82:** 400, 1961.
12. Shingleton, W. W.: Unpublished data.
13. Stehlin, J. S., Clark, R., White, E., Smith, J., Griffin, A., Jesse, R., and Healey, J.: Regional chemotherapy for cancer: Experiences with perfusions, Ann. Surg. **151:** 605, 1960.
14. Woodhall, B., Pickrell, K., Georgiade, N., Mahaley, M. S., and Dukes, H.: Effect of hyperthermia upon cancer chemotherapy; Application to external cancers of head and face structures, Ann. Surg. **151:** 750, 1960.

*(For discussion, see page 271.)*

# The effect of increased oxygen tension on the tumoricidal effect of nitrogen mustard

EDWARD T. KREMENTZ, M.D.
LYNN KNUDSON
NEW ORLEANS, LA.
*From the Department of Surgery, Tulane University School of Medicine*

Cancer chemotherapy by regional perfusion with use of a pump-oxygenator has produced encouraging results when conventional chemotherapy has been of little benefit.[2, 10, 11, 19, 22, 23, 25] Current interest in regional perfusion has focused attention on the role of oxygenation of the perfusate.[2, 18, 23] In the beginning, the duration of perfusion was short, isolation incomplete, and no attempt was made to control the temperatures of the perfusate. Thus, little injury to normal tissues would have resulted even if unoxygenated blood were used. At present, however, perfusion is carried out under hyperthermic conditions, with more complete isolation, for longer periods, and with highly reactive agents. These conditions probably necessitate the use of an oxygenated perfusate to minimize tissue damage.

Another factor to be considered is the effect of increased tissue oxygen tension on the action of alkylating agents. Thomlinson and Gray[5, 6, 13, 14] in Great Britain have shown that the effect of irradiation on normal tissue and on several tumor-host systems is potentiated by an increase in the tissue oxygen tension. Churchill-Davidson,[5, 6] at St. Thomas's Hospital, utilizing a pressure chamber in which patients can be kept at 3 atmospheres of oxygen during treatment, gives convincing clinical evidence of improved response to irradiation.[5, 6] In this country, confirmatory experimental work has been reported by Hollcroft,[15] who used a transplantable lymphosarcoma, and by Beck and Reick,[4] who used sarcoma 180.

Alexander and Stacey[1] have demonstrated that the biologic changes produced by alkylating agents and ionizing irradiation are due to damage of desoxyribonucleic acid (DNA) molecules. The only difference is that the alkylating agent must diffuse into the cell and some of the DNA molecules are more accessible than others to its action.

Clark[7, 8] has shown that the oxygen tension in tissues may be increased to 600 mm. Hg during whole body perfusion with a bubble oxygenator, depending upon the volume of tissue perfused, the temperature and flow rate of the perfusate, and the degree of oxygen saturation. It had been demonstrated in our laboratory that the tissue oxygen tension in the hind limb of the dog is increased to 450 per cent of normal with the bubble oxygenator currently used and that toxicity of 5-fluorouracil increases about 20 per cent with addition of oxygen to the perfusate.[20]

The effect of increased oxygen tension on the action of alkylating agents in human beings has been difficult to assess. Consequently, it was thought that experiments with standard transplantable tumors in mice might indicate whether or not there is any potentiation of the cancericidal action of

Supported in part by United States Public Health Service Grant CY-3782, The Greater New Orleans Cancer Association, Inc., The Anna Fuller Fund for Medical Research, and The Frost Foundation.

Read at the Twenty-second Annual Meeting of the Society of University Surgeons, Kansas City, Kan., Feb. 9-11, 1961.

alkylating agents under conditions of increased tissue oxygen tension.

## EXPERIMENT OBSERVATIONS

The oxygen pressure chamber utilized for these experiments consisted of a 20-quart commercially available pressure cooker in which a multidirectional oxygen jet was inserted in the center of the floor. Oxygen introduced under pressure through this jet was circulated throughout the chamber, and was released through the escape valve during the experiments. The valve allowed a maximum pressure of 20 pounds per square inch, confirmed by the gauge on the oxygen tank. The passage of oxygen through the chamber allowed for free circulation of gases and removal of accumulated carbon dioxide.

**Experiment 1.** This study consisted of the inoculation of CFW mice with approximately 5 million Ehrlich ascites tumor cells in 0.1 ml. of normal saline solution obtained from pooled ascitic fluid from 5 donor mice. The animals were identified, separated into groups of 4, and distributed to provide for cage control. On the second day after the injection of tumor cells, mice from 2 groups were placed in an oxygen chamber with pressure of 20 pounds per square inch for 15 minutes. The animals from the remaining 2 groups were left in their cages. Immediately after exposure to oxygen, 1 group of mice in the pressure chamber and 1 group remaining in the cages were given 1 mg. per kilogram of body weight of nitrogen mustard in 0.2 ml. of normal saline solution intraperitoneally. After the administration of the drug, the 2 original groups were again subjected to oxygen pressure of 20 pounds per square inch for 30 minutes. All mice were then returned to their cages. On the seventh day after treatment, the mice were sacrificed and a quantitative determination of the number of tumor cells present in the abdominal cavity was made by Baillif's[3] modification of the method of Klein.[17] Seventy-seven groups of 4 mice each were available for study. However, a number of other groups had to be discarded in their entirety when 1 or more of the mice died.

Table I shows the results in 77 groups of mice in the study. The table gives the average cell counts and the range of cell counts within each group. These data have been graphically summarized in Fig. 1. There is no significant difference between the untreated mice and those subjected to high oxygen pressure. The difference between the groups treated with mustard and those which received no drug was highly significant. In addition, the average number of tumor cells in the group treated with nitrogen mustard and oxygen under pressure is significantly lower than the average number in those treated with nitrogen mustard alone. This difference would be observed by chance less than once in 1,000 times under the given assumptions.

**Experiment 2.** One hundred Swiss mice were divided into 4 groups of 25 each, identified, and distributed to provide for cage controls. The mice were injected with 5 million ascites tumor cells intraperitoneally and, 2 days later, were treated in the same fashion as described in Experiment 1. The mice were returned to their cages and kept under observation until the day of death, which was recorded. All surviving animals were autopsied on the thirtieth day after treatment. This experiment was repeated 4 times so that each group contained approximately 400 mice. Twelve animals which died on the day of treatment were not included in the study.

**Table I.** *Effect of increased oxygen tension and nitrogen mustard on Ehrlich ascites tumor (77 experiments in CFW mice)*

| *Cell counts (millions)* | *$HN_2$ and $O_2$** | *$HN_2$* | *$O_2$* | *Air* |
|---|---|---|---|---|
| Range | 0-959 | 7-729 | 2-911 | 3-850 |
| Mean | 84.6 | 117.6 | 380.2 | 375.9 |

*One milligram per kilogram of body weight of nitrogen mustard and 100 per cent oxygen under 20 pounds pressure per square inch for 30 minutes.

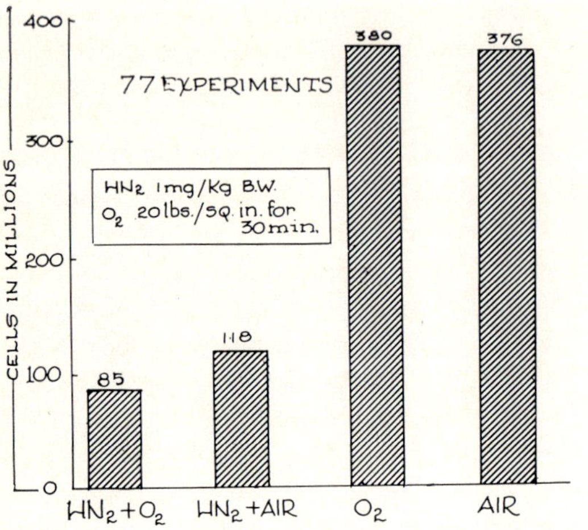


**Fig. 1.** Effect of increased oxygen tension and nitrogen mustard on tumor cell count in mice with Ehrlich ascites tumor.

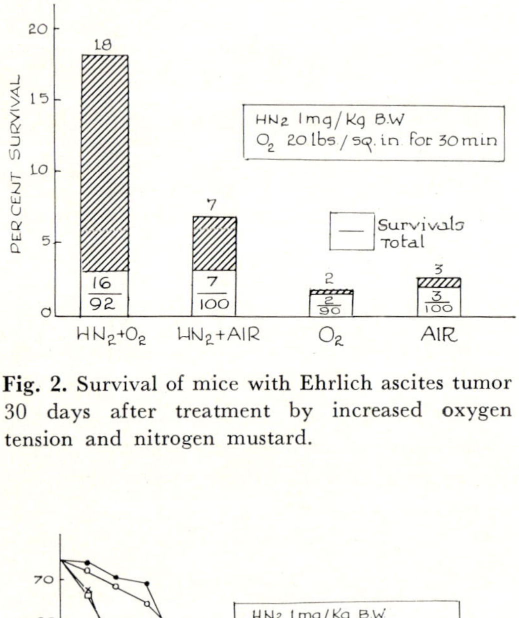


**Fig. 2.** Survival of mice with Ehrlich ascites tumor 30 days after treatment by increased oxygen tension and nitrogen mustard.

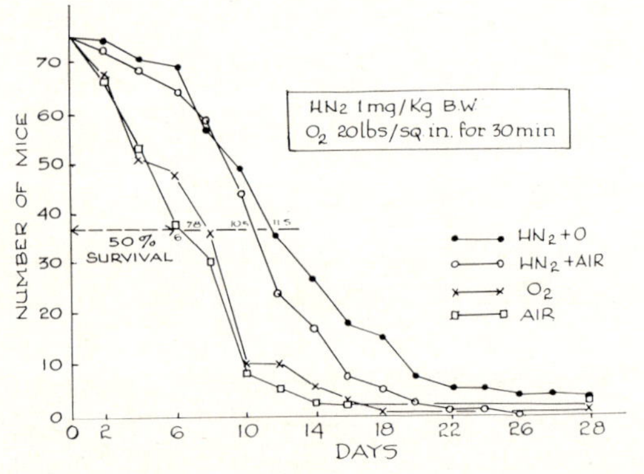


**Fig. 3.** Survival of mice with sarcoma-37 treated by increased oxygen tension and nitrogen mustard.

Results of this experiment are seen in Table II and more graphically in Fig. 2. Table II shows the survivors with Ehrlich ascites tumor on the thirtieth day treated under the conditions indicated. Eighteen per cent of the group treated with nitrogen mustard and oxygen under pressure survived to the thirtieth day and 7 per cent survived when treated with nitrogen mustard alone. Two per cent of the group treated with oxygen survived as compared to 3 per cent in the control group. The difference between the number of survivors in the group treated with nitrogen mustard and oxygen and the number in the group treated with nitrogen mustard and air is statistically significant at the 1 per cent level with the chi square test.

**Experiment 3.** One hundred Swiss mice were divided into 4 groups. The animals were identified, distributed to provide for cage controls, and inoculated with the ascitic form of Sarcoma 37 which is a transplantable carcinosarcoma.[24] The mice received approximately 800,000 to 1 million cells in 0.1 ml. of normal saline solution obtained from pooled ascitic fluid from 5 donor mice. Two days after the inoculation of the tumor cells, the mice were treated in a fashion identical to that described in Experiment 3. The day of death was recorded and on the thirtieth day after treatment the remaining animals were sacrificed. This experiment was repeated 3 times so that a total of 75 mice in each group were evaluated.

The results of this experiment, depicted in Fig. 3, show the survival curves for the mice with Sarcoma 37 treated with nitrogen mustard and oxygen. Examination of these curves shows that, at 30 days, there were 2 surviving mice in the group treated with drug and oxygen (1 with tumor), 1 in the oxygen-treated group, and 2 in the air-treated group (none with tumor). The 50 per cent survival times for the 4 groups were 11.5 days (drug and oxygen), 10.5 (drug and air), 7.8 (oxygen), and 6.0 (air). Furthermore while all points on the nitrogen mustard and oxygen curve, with 1 exception, show better survival than the drug and air curve, these

2 curves are not separated by statistically significant differences as is seen from a Mann-Whitney test. While the data seem to suggest that the action of nitrogen mustard is potentiated by increased oxygen tension with Sarcoma 37, larger numbers of mice or a second treatment introduced at day 6 may produce an increased separation of the curves. In any event, the data are suggestive enough to warrant further investigation.

**Experiment 4.** This experiment was conducted in the same manner as the second experiment with the exception that 2 studies with 5 groups of 10 mice each were performed. The additional group consisted of mice that had been made polycythemic by intraperitoneal transfusions of pooled, washed red blood cells. This technique has been described previously.[18] The recipient mice were given 0.5 ml. of a red blood cell suspension for 3 successive days, were inoculated with tumor on the day after the transfusions, and treated 2 days later. Hematocrits obtained at the time of treatment ranged from 62 to 78 per cent; the hematocrits of the control mice ranged from 50 to 55 per cent. Days of death were recorded and surviving mice were sacrificed at the twenty-eighth day after treatment.

Table III shows the number of mice which survived at the end of the experiment and the number of mice with tumor. Thirty per cent of the mice with elevated hematocrits treated with nitrogen mustard and oxygen under pressure survived 28 days, 10 per cent of the mice treated with nitrogen mustard and oxygen under pressure survived, and none of the remaining groups contained surviving animals. It should be noted that the 50 per cent survival times showed reversal of the 28-day observations. The group treated with drug and air had the greatest number of survivors, followed by the group treated by drug and oxygen, then the group given drug and oxygen with polycythemia. It is of interest to note that a control group of another experiment, consisting of polycythemic mice with ascites, had no prolongation of life. The number of animals in these groups is too small to warrant a statistical analysis and the experiment is a preliminary one.

## DISCUSSION

Experiments 1 and 2 indicate that the therapeutic effect of nitrogen mustard is potentiated by increased oxygen tension. Had the exposure of the mice to increased oxygen tension alone produced any therapeutic effect, it would be necessary to determine whether the effect was potentiative, additive, or synergistic.[12, 21] As no therapeutic effect from the increased oxygen tension was observed, the increase in survival or reduction in number of tumor cells from the combined treatment indicate potentiation of the therapeutic effect of the alkylating agent. Experiment 3 was performed with Sarcoma 37 to determine whether or not the results could be duplicated with another tumor-host system. While suggestive information was obtained, additional study is needed.

One problem has been to find a tumor-host drug system that, with appropriate dose

**Table II.** *Effect of increased oxygen tension and nitrogen mustard on 30-day survival of mice with Ehrlich ascites tumor*

| *Experiments* | *$HN_2$ and $O_2$* | *$HN_2$* | *$O_2$* | *Air* |
|---|---|---|---|---|
| 1. Survivors/treated | 6/25 | 0/25 | 2/25 | 2/25 |
| 2. Survivors/treated | 1/23 | 1/25 | 0/25 | 0/25 |
| 3. Survivors/treated | 5/21 | 3/25 | 0/21 | 1/25 |
| 4. Survivors/treated | 4/23 | 3/25 | 0/25 | 0/25 |
| Total survivors/treated | 16/92 | 7/100 | 2/96 | 3/100 |
| Survivors/with tumor | 13 | 7 | 2 | 2 |
| Survivors (%) | 18 | 7 | 2 | 3 |

**Table III.** *Effect of polycythemia, increased oxygen tension, and nitrogen mustard on survival of mice with Ehrlich ascites tumor*

| *Experiments* | *$HN_2$ and $O_2$ (Polycythemia*)* | *$HN_2$ and $O_2$* | *$HN_2$* | *$O_2$* | *Air* |
|---|---|---|---|---|---|
| 1. Survivors/treated | 2/10 | 0/10 | 0/10 | 0/10 | 0/10 |
| 2. Survivors/treated | 4/10 | 2/10 | 0/10 | 0/10 | 0/10 |
| Total survivors†/treated | 6/20 | 2/20 | 0/20 | 0/20 | 0/20 |
| Survivors (%) | 30 | 10 | 0 | 0 | 0 |

*Hematocrit approximately 70 per cent at treatment.

†Survivors sacrificed at twenty-eighth day. All contained tumor.

of drug, will show the effect of increased oxygen tension on tumoricidal action of the alkylating agents. Another experiment, not reported here, involved the treatment of mice with sarcoma 180 with 3 mg. per kilogram of body weight of TSPA.[18] In a few experiments, the sarcoma 180 treated with TSPA and increased oxygen tension showed better regression than in the other groups but no consistent conclusions could be obtained and this study was abandoned. In addition to those with alkylating agents, similar studies should be carried out with the antimetabolites and the antibiotic group of tumoricidal drugs as well as with different tumors and animals.

One fact that warrants discussion concerns the mechanism by which increased oxygen tension is obtained. It is generally considered that a patient breathing pure oxygen will completely saturate the available hemoglobin and that the resultant oxygen tension will approximate 140 mm. Hg.[16] Increasing the available hemoglobin by producing a polycythemic individual may cause further increase in the oxygen tension but any great increase will necessitate the use of the bubble oxygenator or a high pressure chamber. This increase in oxygen tension results from oxygen being dissolved in or supersaturating the plasma, and tissue oxygen tension responds almost immediately to this increase.[9]

It is our belief that potentiation, while of importance, is only one of a number of factors which contribute to improved results after perfusion. These factors include intra-arterial administration of drug (high dosage), protection of the host against the toxic effects of the alkylating agents, and regulation of perfusion pressure.[10, 19]

The explanation that Churchill-Davidson has presented for the use of the high-pressure chamber with radiation is pertinent.[6] He believes that tumor cells are protected by the low oxygen concentration about them and this protection can be abolished by increasing the partial pressure of oxygen respired. The low oxygen concentration in the tumor is mainly due to the distance of the solid masses of tumor cells from their capillaries. It has been determined by theoretical calculation that these cells fall into zones of diminished radiosensitivity. In addition, evidence has been presented which indicates slowing or stagnation of blood in the tumor capillaries from congestion, necrosis, thrombosis, edema, and infection associated with the tumor. These factors, which tend to lower the tumor oxygen tension, would be overcome by the use of the high-pressure chamber.

Similarly, the pump-oxygenator would increase the oxygen tension as well as adequately providing for perfusion of tumor tissue.

## CONCLUSION

The cancericidal effect of nitrogen mustard on an Ehrlich ascites tumor in mice is potentiated by increased tissue oxygen tension.

The authors wish to express their appreciation to Phillip Good, Instructor in Biostatistics, Tulane University School of Medicine, for the preparation of the statistical analyses used in this paper.

## REFERENCES

1. Alexander, P., and Stacey, K. A.: Comparison of the changes produced by ionizing radiations and by the alkylating agents: evidence for a similar mechanism at the molecular level, Ann. New York Acad. Sc. **68:** 1225, 1958.
2. Austen, W. G., Monaco, A. P., Richardson, G. S., Baker, W. H., Shaw, R. S., and Raker, J. W.: Treatment of malignant pelvic tumors by extracorporeal perfusion with chemotherapeutic agents, New England J. Med. **261:** 1037, 1959.
3. Baillif, R. N.: Graduated loading of the reticuloendothelium and growth rate of the Ehrlich mouse ascites tumor, Cancer Res. **16:** 479, 1956.
4. Beck, L. V., and Reick, Virginia: Variation of oxygen supply on the susceptibility of tumor tissue to the Growth inhibiting effects of x-radiation, Proc. Am. A. Cancer Res. **2:** 279, 1958.
5. Churchill-Davidson, I., Sanger, C., and Thomlinson, R. H.: High pressure oxygen and radiotherapy, Lancet **1:** 1091, 1955.
6. Churchill-Davidson, I., Sanger, C., and Thomlinson, R. H.: Oxygenation in radiotherapy. II. Clinical application, Brit. J. Radiol. **30:** 406, 1957.
7. Clark, L. C., Jr., Helmsworth, J. A., Kaplan, S., Sherman, R. T., Taylor, Z.: Polarographic measurement of oxygen tension in whole blood and tissues during total bypass of the heart, S. Forum **4:** 93, 1953.
8. Clark, L. C., Kaplan, S., Matthews, E. C., Edwards, F. K., and Helmsworth, J. A.: Monitor and control of blood oxygen tension and pH during total body perfusion, J. Thoracic Surg. **36:** 488, 1958.
9. Clowes, G. H. A., Jr.: Extracorporeal maintenance of circulation and respiration, Physiol. Rev. **40:** 827, 1960.
10. Creech, Oscar Jr.: General considerations in cancer chemotherapy Cancer Chemotherapy Report, No. 10, p. 1, 1960.
11. Creech, Oscar, Jr., Krementz, E. T., Ryan, R. F., and Winblad, J. N.: Regional perfusion utilizing an extracorporeal circuit, Ann. Surg. **148:** 616, 1958.
12. Gaddum, J. H.: Pharmacology, London, 1948, Oxford University Press.
13. Gray, L. H.: Oxygenation in radiotherapy. I. Radiobiological considerations, Brit. J. Radiol. **30:** 403, 1957.
14. Gray, L. H., Conger, A. D., Ebert, M., Hornsey, S., and Scott, O. A. C.: The concentration of oxygen dissolved in tissues at the time of irradiation as a factor in radiotherapy, Brit. J. Radiol. **26:** 638, 1953.
15. Hollcroft, J. W., Lorenz, E., and Matthews, M.: Factors mediating the effect of x-irradiation on regression of a transplanted lymphosarcoma, J. Nat. Cancer Inst. **12:** 751, 1952.
16. Ito, I., Kolff, W. J., and Effler, D. B.: Prevention of overoxygenation during treatment with a heart-lung machine in cardiac operations, Cleveland Clin. Quart. **25:** 9, 1958.
17. Klein, G.: Use of Ehrlich's ascites tumor of mice for quantitative studies on the growth and biochemistry of neoplastic cells, Cancer **3:** 1052, 1950.
18. Krementz, E. T., Harlin, R., and Knudson, L.: The enhancement of chemotherapy by increased tissue oxygen tension; Cancer Chemotherapy Report **10:** 125, 1960.
19. Krementz, E. T., Creech, O., Jr., Ryan, R. F., and Wickstrom, J.: Treatment of malignant tumors of the extremities by perfusion with chemotherapeutic agents, J. Bone & Joint Surg. **41-A:** 6, 1959.
20. Ryan, R. F., Winblad, J. N., Hottinger, G. C., and Creech, O., Jr.: Effects of various perfusates in isolated vascular beds using an extracorporeal circuit, S. Forum **9:** 195, 1958.
21. Salter, W. T.: A textbook of pharmacology, Philadelphia, 1952, W. B. Saunders Company.
22. Shingleton, W. W., Reeues, J. W., Jr., Keppel, R. H., Mahaley, M. S., Jr., and Taylor, H. M.: Studies on abdominal organ perfusion for cancer chemotherapy, Ann. Surg. **151:** 5, 1960.
23. Stehlin, J. S., Jr., Clark, R. L., Jr., White, E. C., Smith, J. L., Jr., Griffen, A. C., Jesse, R. H., Jr., and Healey, J. E., Jr.: Regional chemotherapy for cancer, Ann. Surg. **151:** 4, 1960.
24. Steward, H. L., Snell, K. C., Dunham, L. J., and Schlyen, S. M.: Transplantable and transmissible tumors of animals, Sec. 12, Fasc. 40, Armed Forces Institute of Pathology. Washington, D. C., 1956.
25. Woodhall, B., Hall, K., Mahaley, S., Jr., and Jackson, J.: Chemotherapy of brain cancer; experimental and clinical studies in localized hypothermic cerebral perfusion, Ann. Surg. **150:** 4, 1959.

## DISCUSSION*

**Dr. W. Glenn Young, Jr.** (Durham N. C.). In discussing the papers by Drs. Shingleton and Lawrence, I would like to mention a technique that we have been using for the treatment of

*Discussion of papers by Lawrence, Kuehn, Mori, Poppell, and Clarkson; Shingleton, Parker, and Mahaley; and Krementz and Knudson.

carcinoma of the lung and other intrathoracic neoplasms, in which differential pelvic perfusion hypothermia is utilized. With an extracorporeal pump-oxygenator and heat exchanger system, dogs were perfused via the femoral artery with the outflow catheter in the inferior vena cava. It was possible to obtain a significant temperature gradient between the upper and lower halves of the body. In the animal shown in the slide, the esophageal temperature was maintained in the region of 35° C., with the temperature in the pelvis and rectum below 25° C. When the maximal temperature gradient was reached, nitrogen mustard (1.5 mg. per kilogram) was administered into the jugular vein. The next slide shows the sternal bone marrow 1 week later. It was very hypocellular and myeloid elements were absent. On the other hand, the pelvic bone marrow was well preserved with almost normal cellularity. This finding has been confirmed in clinical studies. Using a relatively high flow rate, one also obtains some degree of isolation between the upper and lower circulatory systems. When radioactive iodinated serum albumin was injected into the jugular vein during the perfusion, the concentration remained quite high in the superior vena cava as opposed to the concentration in the inferior vena cava.

**Dr. J. Bradley Aust** (Minneapolis, Minn.). The 3 preceding papers are representative of some of the best work going on in the field of isolated perfusion. The factors of leakage, flow rate, temperature, and oxygenation are all of importance and are being investigated. Leakage from the isolated circuit, as measured by tagged albumin or chromium, is of significance only to the extent that it parallels the actual leakage of the agent used. With use of agents as rapidly fixed as nitrogen mustard, even the large leakages obtained in pelvic perfusion do not cause great difficulty with bone marrow depression. In over 50 perfusions with nitrogen mustard we have never seen a bone marrow depression in any of our patients. On the other hand, agents which have prolonged activity, such as phenylalanine mustard, require minimal leakage and washout techniques to prevent systemic toxicity. Another important factor in any discussion of leakage is the flow rate used and the differential pressure in the isolated region as contrasted to the systemic circulation. If the pressure in the systemic circuit is higher, blood tends to flow into the region perfused in preference to leaking out. The effect of temperature in control of isolated perfusion has interested us and we have studied the active life of nitrogen mustard in various solutions at different temperatures. As blood is heated the nitrogen mustard has a shorter and shorter active life span. We have been concerned that nitrogen mustard put into heated blood would be inactivated before it reached the tumor. With an isolated dog limb as a model and by measuring the amount of nitrogen mustard entering and leaving the limb, one can by difference calculate the amount of nitrogen mustard taken up by the limb. Under these circumstances, if oxygen tension is lowered in the perfused circuit, there is a greater uptake of nitrogen mustard. Does this mean we should not oxygenate our blood? I cannot answer that question. The crucial information is how much agent is getting to the tumor and how much the tumor is taking up. Today Dr. Krementz has pointed out that in all probability the nitrogen mustard uptake of cancer is greater under high oxygen tension and so we are caught in the horns of a dilemma. If we use high oxygen in the circuit we know that the total uptake of the region is not as good; however, we have no information regarding the differential uptake by the tumor which is the crucial knowledge needed.

**Dr. Walter Lawrence, Jr.** (closing). I want to thank Drs. Aust and Young for their comments, and I could not agree more with what Dr. Aust has said about "leakage." I think that the point we were trying to make with some of our data was that the indicator leak has nothing to do with any specific drug and each drug is different in its leakage behavior. Actually, in regard to nitrogen mustard, it really becomes unreasonable to measure leaks. We were particularly interested in using antimetabolites in perfusion, and particularly pelvic perfusion, because we have been so discouraged by our nitrogen mustard results clinically. This is what led to these studies. In regard to Dr. Young's comment about iliac marrow protection for high-dose chemotherapy of the thorax, we have tried a slightly different approach to this. By using the same pneumatic abdominal tourniquet and aortic occlusion with balloon catheter above the celiac axis, we have found differential marrow changes similar to those he showed on his slide. I would like to ask Dr. Shingleton one question because we have tried his total abdominal perfusion as well, on only 1 patient, with balloon catheters to occlude the vena cava and the aorta above the liver instead of thoracotomy. We were somewhat concerned and confused by the persistence of the low rectal temperatures during the perfusion. We wondered whether we were really getting adequate perfusion in some of the areas we were trying to treat. When we did this with hyperthermia in our perfusion circuit we still maintained a low rectal temperature just as he has shown.

**Dr. W. W. Shingleton** (closing). I would like to thank Drs. Young, Lawrence, Aust, and Krementz for their comments.

In regard to Dr. Lawrence's question concerning the rectal temperature during abdominal perfusion, I would like to report that we have found that the use of a rectal thermometer is a very inaccurate way to measure changes in tissue temperature during hypothermic—hyperthermic perfusion. A thermister placed in the liver or other abdominal viscera will give a more accurate measurement of changes in tissue temperature. In regard to Dr. Krementz's comment about the "extensive surgery" involved in the technique described, I would like to reply that the only surgical procedure involved is a right thoracotomy (patient's diagnosis previously established by laparotomy) and cannulation of the femoral vessels. Since hypothermia is relied upon to protect against leak, extensive dissection to isolate collateral circulation is avoided.

**Dr. Edward T. Krementz** (closing). I would like to mention one thing about the abdominal perfusion that Dr. Shingleton reported. We have treated 1 patient by this method and are inclined to think that this is a little too much surgical manipulation for patients with advanced malignant disease. If, however, the end results prove to be satisfactory, we will change our minds.

The problem of nerve damage after perfusion with alkylating agents should be mentioned and I want to caution the audience about this danger. We have had 10 or more patients who have experienced nerve damage. This has occurred with seventh, eighth, or ninth cranial nerves or the brachial plexus after administration of high doses of nitrogen mustard in relatively confined areas and is a complication to avoid if you are planning to use perfusion chemotherapy.

In regard to Dr. Aust's remarks, we are aware of his work concerning the better utilization of nitrogen mustard after increased concentrations of carbon dioxide. We have started experiments with the high pressure chamber to check this observation using 95 per cent oxygen and 5 per cent carbon dioxide. Mice cannot tolerate any more carbon dioxide under pressure than this and they die with the use of 10 per cent carbon dioxide. We have no other data available as yet about this problem.

# Techniques of obtaining and preparing suspensions of spleen and bone marrow for the treatment of supralethally irradiated dogs

JERROLD K. LONGERBEAM, M.D.*
RICHARD C. LILLEHEI, M.D., Ph.D.**
EDMUND YUNIS, M.D.
SADEK HILAL, M.D.
MINNEAPOLIS, MINN.
*From the Departments of Surgery, Radiology, and Laboratory Medicine, University of Minnesota Medical School*

The protective effects of various bone marrow and spleen preparations against total-body irradiation in small animals have been well demonstrated.[3, 7, 13] The use of these same tissue preparations in larger animals and in man has met with less success, and more frequently than not investigators have reported the failure of spleen or bone marrow autografts to protect dogs against supralethal or even lethal total-body irradiation.[1, 21] Yet Alpen and Baum[2] have reported that infusions of autologous bone marrow will protect lethally irradiated dogs. Moreover, Mannick and his group[15] have reported the recovery of supralethally irradiated dogs given autologous bone marrow. Thomas and co-workers[23] have shown that bone marrow homografts between sibling dogs may be successful if doses of total-body irradiation of 1,500 r are used prior to the infusion of several billion cells. Recently we have reported that suspensions of autologous spleen will also protect lethally and supralethally irradiated dogs.[12] Interestingly enough, whole-organ autologous transplants of the spleen or spleen shielding have not protected the dog as have the cell suspensions, which indicates that homogenization of the spleen releases or makes available certain substances and/or cells which are not available from the intact splenic autograft or from the shielded spleen.

Supported by United States Public Service Grant A-3361.
Read at the Twenty-second Annual Meeting of the Society of University Surgeons, Kansas City, Kan., Feb. 9-11, 1961.
*Giannini Fellow.
**Markle Scholar.

During the course of these experiments, and in similar experiments with autologous bone marrow, techniques have been developed for obtaining and preparing suspensions of spleen or bone marrow which have resulted in larger yields of viable cells than previously have been reported. It is our belief that failure to obtain cells in large numbers or to handle the cells properly after they have been obtained is the chief reason for the conflicting reports of their efficacy in protecting the dog against lethal total-body irradiation. This belief is strengthened by the data of Urso and Congdon[25] who have shown that the survival rate in small animals after lethal total-body irradiation is proportional to the number of viable cells infused.

The methods presently used for obtaining and preparing splenic and bone marrow suspensions in this laboratory along with the results of experiments in which such preparations have been used to protect dogs against lethal and supralethal total-body irradiation form the basis of this report.

## MATERIALS AND METHODS

Adult mongrel dogs of both sexes weighing from 10 to 25 kilograms have been used throughout this study. The sole method of selection has been to use dogs in apparent good health in which white blood cell counts were under 15,000 and hematocrits were 40 per cent or above. The dogs were not immunized against canine distemper or hepatitis and were not isolated before or after irradiation from new stock dogs which continually come into the kennels.

The irradiation was delivered with a 250 KVP, 30 Ma. unit. The filter was 0.5 mm.[3]; half-value layer, 1.5 mm.[3]; focal skin distance, 120 cm.; and field size, 80 cm. in diameter. The radiation was given at the rates of 4.45, 10, or 22.6 r per minute, one-half of the total being given through each of 2 lateral parts. Doses used are stated as "minimum tissue doses" and were calculated at the midsagittal plane of the dog, which is to say that no tissue received less than the stated dose and some may have received up to 178 per cent of the stated dose.

Peripheral blood and bone marrow specimens were obtained prior to irradiation for hematocrits, nucleated cell counts, and differential counts. The animals were studied during the postirradiation course with daily hematocrits, white blood cell counts and platelet and reticulocyte counts. Periodic bone marrow studies were also performed. All animals were followed carefully until death or until complete hematologic and clinical recovery. All dogs that died were autopsied and the survivors were sacrificed at periods varying from 1 to 12 months, except for a small representative group which will be followed indefinitely. All irradiated animals received daily intramuscular injections of penicillin, 400,000 U., streptomycin, 0.5 Gm., and neomycin, 0.25 Gm., until white blood cell counts increased above 4,000 and the animals were clinically well. Parenteral fluids and/or gavage feedings of milk, cream, or meat were also given when indicated.

**Preparation of splenic suspension.** Dogs which had been fasted for 18 hours were anesthetized with pentobarbital sodium and their abdomens opened aseptically. The gastrosplenic ligament was divided, leaving the spleen pedicled on the splenic artery and vein. To empty the spleen of blood before removal, 0.25 mg. of epinephrine in 5 ml. of saline solution was injected intravenously. Then when the spleen had tightly contracted, the splenic vessels were divided and it was removed. Immediately after this, the splenic artery was cannulated and the spleen perfused at 4° C. with 200 to 300 ml. of Tis-U-Sol* which contained 0.1 mg. heparin, 100 U. of penicillin, and 100 μg streptomycin per milliliter. The pH of the Tis-U-Sol was adjusted to 7.2 by the addition of a concentrated solution of sodium bicarbonate. This initial perfusion cooled the spleen rapidly, removed any residual sinusoidal blood, and prevented clotting during subsequent manipulation of the splenic cells. The splenic vein was then clamped and the spleen allowed to distend by the additional infusion of 500 to 1,500 ml. of Tis-U-Sol at 4° C. This step greatly facilitated the subsequent separation of splenic cells from the stroma. The spleen was then sliced into strips approximately 2 mm. in thickness, and the strips transferred individually to a 30 mesh stainless steel screen disc, which had a pore diameter of 570 μ.[9] The splenic pulp was forced through the screen by gentle pressure of the gloved finger, and was then transferred to a plastic beaker containing one of the suspending solutions. The stroma of the spleen was discarded.

This pulp containing the splenic cells was then further broken up by passage through a series of stainless steel screens with 40, 60, and 100 mesh per inch and a pore diameter of 380, 150, and 130 μ, respectively. Nylon or siliconized stainless steel syringes with interchangeable stainless steel screen discs were used for this procedure.[27] The final cell suspension was diluted to a total volume of at least 250 ml. with suspending solution.

Fig. 1 shows the equipment necessary for the preparation of this homogenate. The resulting suspension contained very few small clumps of cells and could be given intravenously without filtration provided that it was given at a rate of 100 ml. per

*Baxter Laboratories.

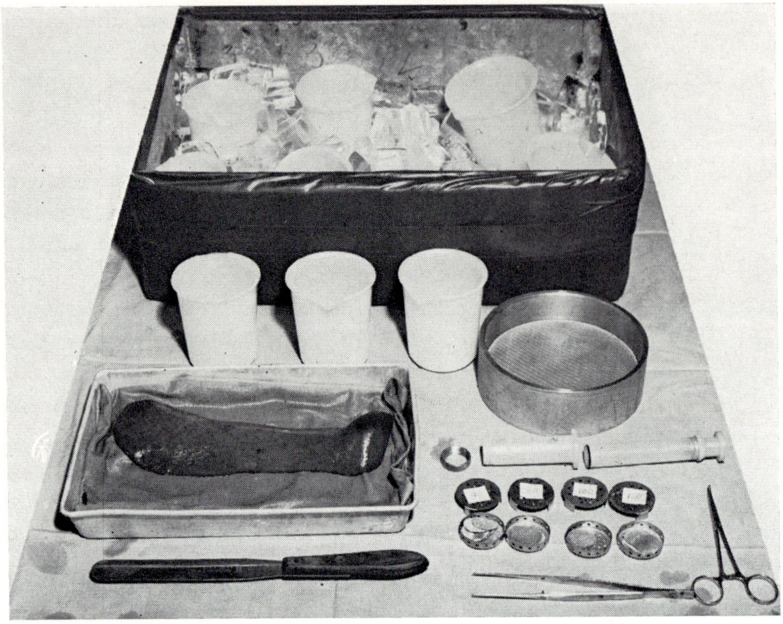

**Fig. 1.** Equipment necessary for preparation of splenic suspension.

hour or less. Two of 45 dogs died in an acute state during the infusion of this suspension but in each case they had been given 250 ml. of suspension containing more than 10 and 21 billion cells, respectively, in less than 30 minutes. The remaining dogs showed no ill effects from these splenic infusions.

By these techniques yields of 2 to 35 billion cells were obtained in 45 animals, with an average yield of 10.1 billion cells and a viability of 60 to 70 per cent, as determined by the trypan blue dye exclusion technique. Supravital staining techniques to determine cell viability in cell suspension has only recently been worked out and is still being modified.[18, 22] Some of these techniques are completely unreliable. The trypan blue technique, modified by one of us (S. H.) to give a method which we believe produces reliable and reproducible results, is reported here in greater detail.

**Trypan blue dye exclusion technique for testing cell viability.** A routine nucleated cell count was performed on an aliquot portion of the cell suspension with a standard white blood cell—diluting pipette, a hemacytometer, and 2 per cent acetic acid as the diluent. With cell count as a guide, the aliquot sample was diluted with the suspending solution to give a cell concentration of approximately 20,000 nucleated cells per mm.[3] The resulting sample was diluted 1.1 with a 1 per cent solution of trypan blue in GKN solution or normal saline solution and allowed to stand for 10 minutes at room temperature. A nucleated cell count was repeated on this final dilution with the white blood cell pipette and the hemacytometer, but TC 199 or the original suspending solution was substituted for the 2 per cent acetic acid. This left a background of intact red cells, but they did not interfere with the counting. If the red cells are lysed there is always a possibility of damage to the nucleated cells, which results in an inordinately low viability count.

The total number of nucleated cells was obtained by multiplying the number of cells counted in the 4 large corner squares by all of the diluting factors, times 1,000 to convert to cell per milliliter,[3] and finally times the total number of milliliters of the splenic or bone marrow suspension.

At the same time, a differential viability count was performed in the hemacytometer under high power, counting approximately 200 cells. Living cells were characterized by their ability to exclude dye and therefore remained unstained. Cells exhibiting nuclear or cytoplasmic staining, or those with stained vacuoles, or those with distorted cell membranes were considered to be dead.

**Final preparation and administration of the splenic homogenate.** During the various manipulations of the splenic cells, all containers were kept in an ice bath to insure maximum viability of the cells. After the final passage through the finest mesh screen, the suspension was transferred to Fenwal plastic bags and stored in the refrigerator until used. At the time of reinfusion, the cell suspension was also cooled by placing the Fenwal bag in an ice bath.

Suspensions of splenic cells have also been prepared by the use of tissue presses, homogenizers of the Potter type, and by controlled enzymatic digestion of the spleen with trypsin, but all these methods have been discarded in favor of the present technique because they were either time-consuming and/or gave poor yields of viable cells.

While the splenic suspension was being prepared, the abdominal incision of the dog was closed and the dog transported to the therapy room, where the prescribed dose of total body irradiation was given. The suspension of autologous spleen cells was given to the dog intravenously immediately upon completion of the irradiation.

**Preparation of bone marrow suspensions.** Necropsy and biopsy studies in a group of 7 dogs showed that the highest concentrations of myeloid and erythroid elements (the richest marrow) were in the bones which are listed in Table I, in decreasing order of bone marrow concentration. However, when accessibility and volume are considered in addition to the richness of the bone marrow, the humeri, femurs, iliac crests, and ischia are the best sites for aspiration (Fig. 2). Observations on excised and sagittally sectioned bones showed that the humoral marrow cavity can be entered longitudinally via the relatively thin cortex of the anatomic neck and greater tuberosity. The proximal one-half of the humoral marrow cavity can also be entered transversely with a needle inserted through the thin cortex of the anterior lateral crest which extends inferiorly from the greater tuberosity (Fig. 3). Both of these routes were used by us for complete aspiration of the humerus.

The femoral marrow cavity can be entered longitudinally via a recess formed by the junction of the neck and trochanter of the femur. The femoral cortex of the posterior lateral surface of the trochanter is also relatively thin and permits a transverse approach to the upper one-third of the femoral marrow cavity. Both of these approaches were used for complete aspiration of the femur (Fig. 3).

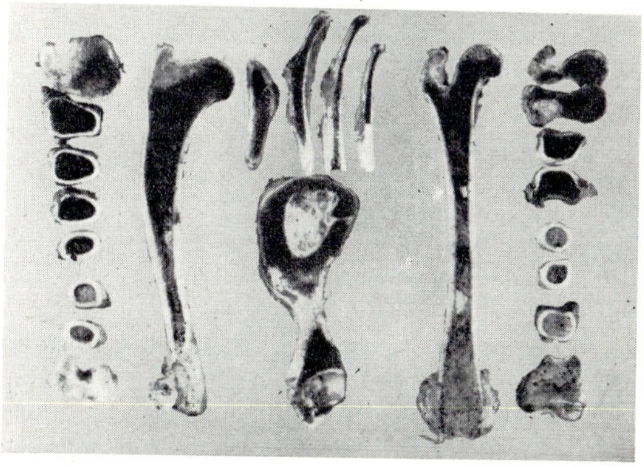

**Fig. 2.** Sagittal and cross sections of humerus, ileum, ischium, and femur in the dog show the areas of "rich" bone marrow.

**Table I.** *Bone marrow hematocrits from various bones which show nucleated cell content*

| *Bone* | *No. of bones* | *Myeloid and erythroid elements (%)* |
|---|---|---|
| Sternum | 9 | 7.7 |
| Humerus | 9 | 7.0 |
| Rib | 6 | 6.8 |
| Femur | 9 | 5.5 |
| Iliac crest | 9 | 4.7 |
| Ischium | 3 | 3.9 |
| Tibia | 2 | 1.0 |

The iliac marrow cavity can be entered at various sites along the posterior margin of the crest, and finally the ischial marrow cavity is entered through the tuberosity.

A Bierman needle, 16 gauge, was used to enter the humeri and femurs transversely and to aspirate the iliac crest. Longitudinal aspirations from the shafts of the humeri, femurs, and also from the ischia were performed with 16 gauge, 4½ inch spinal needles. Most of the red marrow in the humerus is in the upper one-half and in the femur the red marrow is in the upper one-third. Therefore, needles longer than 4½ inches are unnecessary in the dog. During aspiration the needles were rotated and the plane of aspiration changed frequently in order to aspirate the entire marrow cavity.

This simple percutaneous multipuncture technique yields as many as 20 billion cells (exclusive of nucleated peripheral blood cells) from a single dog. Moreover, yields of 8 to 12 billion cells are not uncommon. The total number of cells obtained in a typical dog from each of the bones mentioned is listed in Table II. The last column shows the total number of viable bone marrow cells obtained after corrections had been made for nucleated peripheral blood cells and per cent viability. Both humeri have

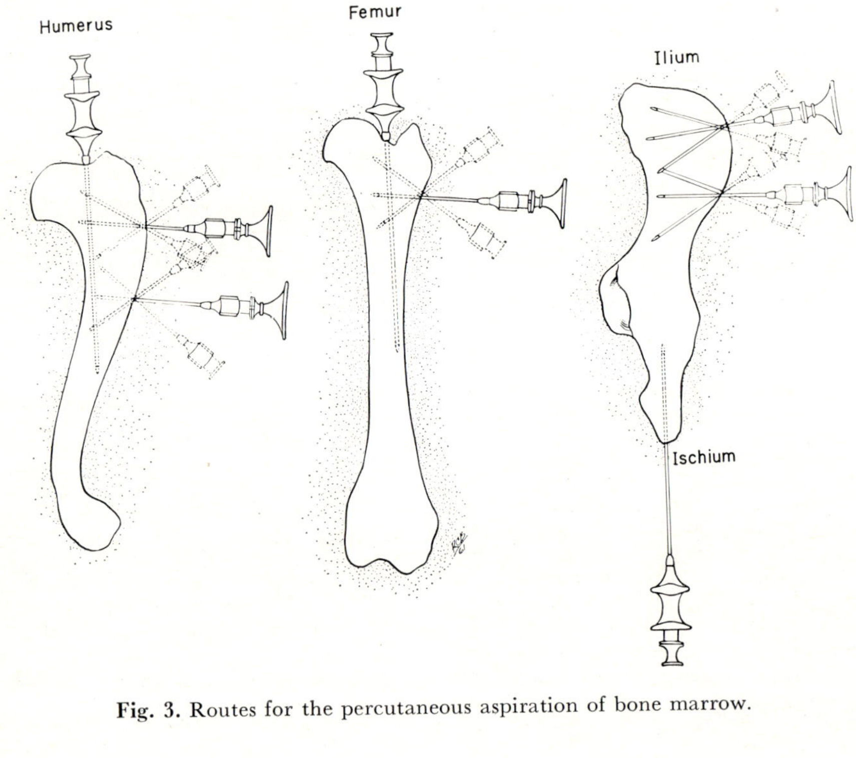


**Fig. 3.** Routes for the percutaneous aspiration of bone marrow.

**Table II.** *Sources of bone marrow*

| *Bone* | *Volume removed/ml.* | *Total cells (×10⁹)* | *W.B.C.* (×10⁹)* | *B.M.C. (×10⁹)* | *% viable* | *No. viable B.M.C. (×10⁹)* |
|---|---|---|---|---|---|---|
| Right humerus | 64 | 33.1 | 0.64 | 2.67 | 68 | 1.83 |
| Left humerus | 270 | 6.97 | 3.21 | 3.76 | 66 | 2.50 |
| Femur | 33 | 1.38 | 0.33 | 1.05 | 67 | 0.71 |
| Iliac crest | 18 | 0.70 | 0.18 | 0.52 | 54 | 0.28 |
| Ischium | 12 | 0.36 | 0.12 | 0.24 | 53 | 0.13 |

*Amount of marrow obtained from various bones by percutaneous aspirational techniques.

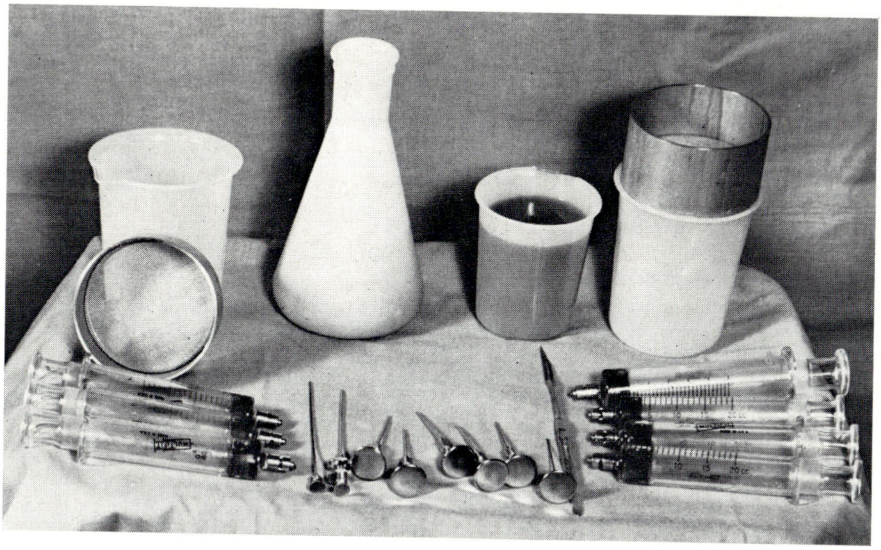

**Fig. 4.** Equipment for obtaining and preparing bone marrow suspensions.

been aspirated to show that removal of 4 times the volume from a single bone does not necessarily increase the yield of bone marrow cells by the factor of 4. The optimum volume to be removed depends both upon the bone being aspirated and the size of the dog. In general, we have found that aspirating 50 to 150 ml. from the humerus, 25 to 75 ml. from the femur, and 10 to 15 ml. from the iliac crest and ischium gives optimal yields of marrow.

**Procedure for use of bone marrow autografts.** The dog to be irradiated was anesthetized with pentobarbital sodium. The sites for bone marrow aspiration were shaved and washed with pHisoHex and benzalkonium chloride. Heparin, 0.75 mg. per kilogram, was given intravenously to facilitate aspiration and to prevent clotting of the bone marrow in the syringe prior to adequate mixing with the suspending solution. Siliconized 30 ml. syringes containing 2 to 5 ml. of the same suspending solution used for the spleen cells were used to aspirate each 5 to 10 ml. of bone marrow. The marrow was collected in sterile plastic Erlenmeyer flasks packed in ice. At the conclusion of the aspiration, the marrow was filtered through a 60 mesh stainless steel screen with a pore diameter of 150 $\mu$. This removed particles of bone and many fat globules. The marrow was not centrifuged, but was transferred directly to plastic Fenwal bags and stored in the refrigerator until the time of infusion. The equipment used for obtaining and preparing bone marrow suspension is shown in Fig. 4.

After removal of the marrow, the dog was irradiated and immediately the autologous marrow was returned to the dog intravenously at a rapid rate (200 to 300 ml. per hour).

All objects with wettable surfaces such as syringes, needles, and screens that came in contact with spleen or bone marrow cells were washed in a mild detergent, rinsed 8 times in tap water, then 8 times in distilled water, air dried, and resiliconized prior to reuse.[17]

**Suspending solutions, pH, and anticoagulants.** It is not enough merely to obtain large numbers of bone marrow or spleen cells to protect animals from the lethal effects of total body irradiation. Equally important are the solution in which the cells are stored, the pH of the solution, temperature of storage, and the anticoagulant used.

Any of the balanced salt solutions used in tissue culture which have an osmolarity of 280 to 300 milliosmoles per liter and a

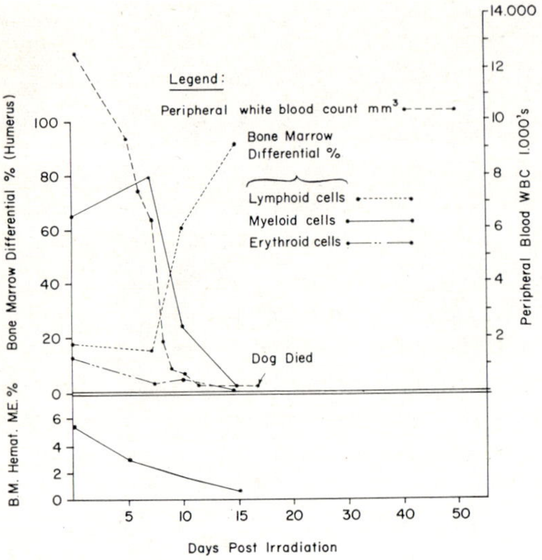


**Fig. 5.** Changes in bone marow and peripheral blood in the lethally irradiated and untreated dog.

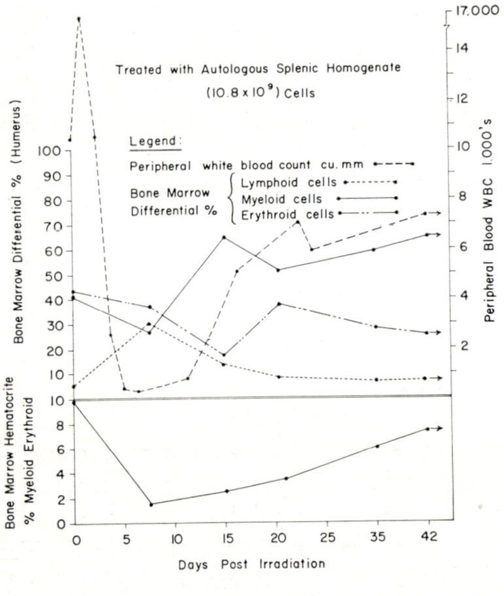


**Fig. 6.** Change in bone marrow and peripheral blood in the lethally irradiated and treated dog.

pH adjusted to 7.2 to 7.4 are satisfactory for cell suspension.[24] The solutions used in this study have included Tis-U-Sol, TC 199,* and a solution developed in this laboratory.[8] Penicillin and streptomycin were added to each of these solutions to give a concentration of 100 U. per milliliter of penicillin and 100 $\mu$g per milliliter of streptomycin.

Either heparin or ethylenediamine tetracetate (EDTA) has been used to prevent coagulation in these suspensions. The concentration of heparin used in solution for suspension of spleen cells has been 0.05 mg. per milliliter and for suspension of bone marrow cells 0.1 mg. per milliliter of heparin has been used. More recently EDTA has been used as the anticoagulant for suspension of both bone marrow and spleen cells. A neutral isotonic solution of EDTA was prepared by dissolving 2.25 Gm. of the disodium salt and 1.50 Gm. of the tetrasodium salt in 100 ml. of distilled water. The resulting 3.75 per cent solution of EDTA had a pH of approximately 7.2 and an osmolarity of 288 milliosmoles per liter. This solution of EDTA was added to the suspending solution in a sufficient quantity to bring the final concentration of EDTA to 1.5 mg. per milliliter (that is, 4 ml. of 3.75 per cent EDTA solution to 100 ml. of suspension solution).

## ASPECTS OF ACUTE IRRADIATION ILLNESS IN THE DOG

**Clinical course in untreated dogs.** Control dogs which received 300 to 600 r total body irradiation usually showed the first effects of irradiation by the second or third postirradiation day. Appetites declined and these animals drank only water or perhaps milk, but eschewed all solid food. By the fourth or fifth day, the dogs appeared tired and listless, and forced feeding was frequently necessary either by placing meat in the posterior pharynx or giving milk or cream by stomach tube. In the 300 to 600 r dosage range, only a few dogs spontaneously vomited and this was limited to the fourth to seventh days. When necessary dogs were maintained on parenteral fluids during this period. Diarrhea was not a problem in the 300 to 600 r range.

**Clinical course in treated dogs.** Dogs given 500 to 900 r total body irradiation and treated successfully with splenic or bone marrow suspensions usually had a marked

*Difco Laboratories.

amelioration of clinical symptoms, especially at the lower levels of irradiation. The severity of symptoms, in general, paralleled the amount of irradiation given, but there was an inverse relationship between the severity of symptoms and the total number of viable cells infused, so that a dog receiving 900 r and a very large number of cells might have a mild clinical course, while a dog given 600 r and receiving a small number of cells might have a severe clinical course.

At 900 r and over, symptoms were more severe even in the treated animals. Vomiting was frequent during the first week, and a watery, bloody diarrhea occasionally appeared about the fifth day. Three dogs in the treated group developed a severe diarrhea and died of an acute necrotizing hemorrhage enteritis.

**Hematologic aspects of irradiation illness in the dog.** In lethally irradiated control dogs (300 to 600 r) the white blood cell count had moderately increased on the first postirradiation day, but by the third day the count had begun a steady decline. In control animals, the nadir of the white blood cell count (usually less than 200 cells per cubic millimeter) was reached in 6 to 8 days and death usually followed in 24 hours. In lethally irradiated animals that recovered as a result of treatment with bone marrow or splenic suspensions, the white blood cell count rarely fell below 300 cell per cubic millimeter. The nadir, which was also reached in 6 to 8 days, was followed by a progressive and rapid increase in the white blood cell count, which correlated with an improving clinical course. The cellularity of the bone marrow decreased concomitantly with the peripheral white blood cell count. Differential bone marrow counts showed a progressive decrease in erythroid, myeloid, and lymphoid elements, but a much slower decrease (and therefore a relative increase) in lymphoid elements (Fig. 5). By the time of death on the eighth or ninth day, the only cells found in the hypocellular marrow were lymphocytes, plasma cells, and large vagocytic histiocytes.

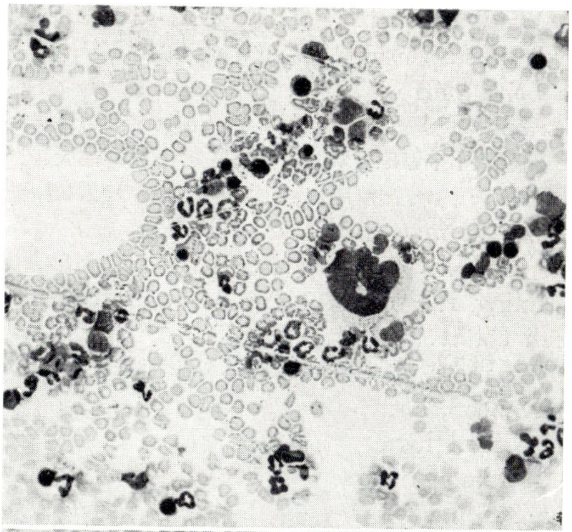

*A*

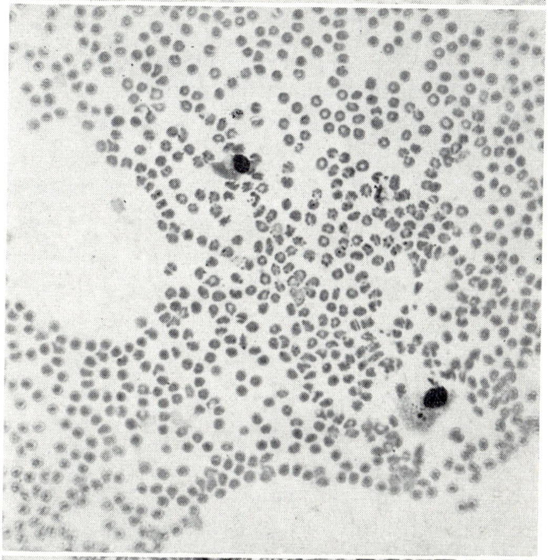

*B*

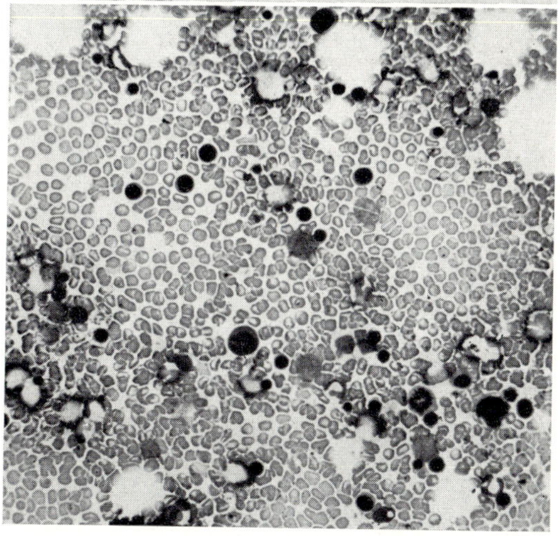

*C*

**Fig. 7.** Bone marrow changes in a lethally irradiated dog treated with autologous bone marrow. *A*, Control bone marrow (×300). *B*, Bone marrow at 7 days (×300). *C*, Marrow at 21 days (×240).

Dogs treated with bone marrow and splenic suspensions, after irradiation, showed a bone marrow picture identical to that described for untreated controls until the eighth or ninth day, at which time myeloid and erythroid series of cells reappeared in the bone marrow. This reappearance of cells in the bone marrow correlated with a beginning rise in the peripheral white blood cell count (Fig. 6). By the fourteenth day, bone marrow regeneration was usually well advanced, and by the twenty-first day often appeared hyperplastic (Fig. 7).

**Pathologic aspects.** Death from acute irradiation illness in the control dogs usually occurred in 8 or 9 days, while the occasional death in dogs unsuccessfully treated with splenic or bone marrow suspension occurred between the ninth and fourteenth days.

In all of these dogs, both treated and untreated, the characteristic finding at autopsy was a fibrinoid hemorrhagic bronchopneumonia. In addition, the bowel wall was usually thin and pale, and scattered petechial mucosal hemorrhages, and minute mucosal ulcerations were present. At radiation doses above 900 r, the petechial hemorrhages in the bowel were more numerous, but in only 3 animals did it appear severe enough to contribute to the cause of death. Epicardial and subendocardial petechial hemorrhages were present in approximately 10 per cent of the animals, and were more numerous at higher irradiation doses, but again they were probably of little clinical significance. The spleen in the control dogs was usually small and weighed less than 25 grams. These spleens, as well as the lymph nodes, showed marked hypocellularity on microscopic examination.

**Late deaths.** A small group of treated animals lived beyond the second week only to die in 3, 4, or 5 weeks. Although hematologic recovery was apparently complete, these animals remained anorexic and gradually lost weight in spite of continued forced feedings until they were emaciated "shells" with hunch backs and ruffled hair. It is interesting that Urso and Congdon[25] have described an identical syndrome in lethally irradiated small animals that have been given just barely enough bone marrow cells to permit prolonged but not permanent survival. In small animals given larger doses of bone marrow, this syndrome did not occur. The dogs which developed this syndrome were also found to have received a borderline number of cells (1.5 to 2 × $10^9$ cells).

## RESULTS

**Effect of temperature and pH.** A pilot study has been performed to determine the effects of temperature and pH upon the viability of cell suspensions stored for short periods of time. In Table III the effects of storage at 5° and 25° C. are shown. There is a slightly more rapid decline in viability at the higher temperature, but in this small study it does not appear to be as important a factor as has been reported.[16] Careful adjustment of the pH is of great importance for maintaining viability, since at a pH of 6.8 or below there is a lower initial as well as a more rapid decline in viability than is evident at a pH of 7.2 to 7.4 (Table IV).

During the developmental stage of the technique for the preparation of splenic suspensions, 16 dogs were treated with splenic suspension prepared from spleens which were neither cooled nor perfused and no attention

**Table III.** *Effects of storage temperature on bone marrow viability*

| *Temperature (C.)* | *No. of specimens* | *Viability (%)* | | |
|---|---|---|---|---|
| | | *Initial* | *2 hr.* | *4 hr.* |
| 5° | 5 | 61.5 | 54.8 | 48.7 |
| 25° | 5 | 60.9 | 53.5 | 41.8 |

**Table IV.** *Effects of diluents and pH on bone marrow viability*

| | *pH* | *No. of specimens* | *Viability (%)* |
|---|---|---|---|
| Tis-U-Sol heparin | 6.3 | 4 | 57 |
| Tis-U-Sol heparin | 6.8 | 2 | 67 |
| 199-EDTA | 6.9 | 2 | 75 |
| Hilal's | 6.6 | 2 | 51 |
| Hilal's | 7.2 | 2 | 81 |

Table V

| Group | No. of dogs | Procedure | Dosage of total body irradiation (r) | No. of survivors | % survival |
|---|---|---|---|---|---|
| 1 | 21 | Controls | 300-600 | 1 | 4.6 |
| 2 | 15 | Autografts of intact spleen | 500 | 1 | 7.3 |
| 3 | 11 | Shielding of spleen | 500 | 3 | 27 |

was given to adjustment of the pH. None of these dogs, all of whom were given 600 r total body irradiation, survived, and they are not included in the present report.

**Results in total body irradiation experiments.** The individual experiments in this part of the study can be classified into 6 groups. The first 3 groups (Table V) have been reported on previously and are briefly summarized.

*Group I.* Of 20 dogs in this control group given 300 to 600 r total-body irradiation, only 1 dog survived and this dog received only 300 r.

*Group II.* In this group of 15 dogs a splenectomy was performed and the abdomen was closed temporarily. The spleen was cooled to 4° C. while the dog was being given 500 r of total-body irradiation. The spleen was immediately replaced after the irradiation as a whole-organ autograft by reanastomosis of the splenic artery and vein.[12] This procedure did not give significant protection against the irradiation, even though the splenic vessel anastomoses were usually patent at autopsy.

*Group III.* In the 11 dogs in Group III the spleen was pedicled around the splenic vessels and shielded in a lead box outside the abdominal cavity while the dog was given 500 r total-body irradiation. In each case the spleen received less than 25 r measured dose. Again, this procedure did not provide significant protection against lethal total body irradiation.

*Group IV.* The 21 dogs in this group were given 500 to 700 r total-body irradiation. The spleen was removed aseptically, and while the dog was being irradiated a suspension was prepared from the entire spleen by the method described. The splenic suspension was given intravenously immediately after irradiation. The clinical course in these dogs, especially in those receiving only 500 r, was distinctly different than in the preceding groups. The dogs remained alert and active in their cages. Anorexia and vomiting did not occur and these dogs continued to take water and milk voluntarily. The white blood cell count began to decline at about the same time as in the first 3 groups, but in the survivors never fell below 300 cells per cubic millimeter, and a rapid return of the white blood cell count to normal usually began about the eighth or ninth postirradiation day. The bone marrow also became very hypocellular. Only a few cells of the lymphoid and plasma cell series were present by the eighth or ninth day. By the fourteenth day regeneration of bone marrow was usually well under way and at the end of 3 weeks, the bone marrow appeared normal or hyperplastic. Typical signs of irradiation illness appeared with increasing doses of irradiation, but these dogs, in general, were not nearly as ill as their counterparts in the control group. Of 10 dogs receiving 500 r, 9 survived and 3 of 6 given 600 r survived, while at 700 r, 2 of 4 survived. When these results are analyzed in terms of the total number of viable cells given, the results are more meaningful (Table VI). In dogs which received less than 3 billion splenic cells, the survival rate was 50 per cent, but in those which received more than 3 billion cells, the survival rate was increased to 79 per cent. Furthermore, dogs receiving the largest number of cells usually had the mildest clinical course.

*Group V.* Twenty-nine dogs were given doses of total-body irradiation varying from 500 to 1,000 r. Each of these dogs was treated with an autologous bone marrow suspension prepared as described. The re-

**Table VI.** *Group 4, autologous spleen cell infusions: survival correlated with lymphoid cell dose*

| *Radiation dose (r)* | *Less than 3.0 × 10⁹ viable cells* | | | *Greater than 3.0 × 10⁹ viable cells* | | |
|---|---|---|---|---|---|---|
| | *No. of dogs* | *No. of survivors* | *% survival* | *No. of dogs* | *No. of survivors* | *% survival* |
| 500 | 2 | 1 | 50 | 8 | 8 | 100 |
| 600 | 4 | 2 | 50 | 3 | 2 | 66 |
| 700 | – | – | – | 4 | 2 | 50 |
| Totals | 6 | 3 | 50 | 15 | 12 | 79 |

**Table VII.** *Group 5, autologous bone marrow infusions: survival correlated with bone marrow dose*

| *Radiation dose (r)* | *Less than 2.0 × 10⁹ viable cells* | | | *Greater than 2.0 × 10⁹ viable cells* | | |
|---|---|---|---|---|---|---|
| | *No. of dogs* | *No. of survivors* | *% survival* | *No. of dogs* | *No. of survivors* | *% survival* |
| 500 | 1 | 0 | 0 | 4 | 4 | 100 |
| 600 | 2 | 0 | 0 | 4 | 3 | 75 |
| 700 | 3 | 1 | 33 | 3 | 3 | 100 |
| 900 | 3 | 0 | 0 | 4 | 4 | 100 |
| 1000 | 3 | 1 | 33 | 2 | 1 | 50 |
| Totals | 12 | 2 | 17 | 17 | 15 | 88 |

sults of this experimental group are shown in Table VII. Seventeen of 29 dogs survived, an over-all survival rate of 59 per cent. If examined in terms of the total number of viable bone marrow cells given, it is evident that dogs which received less than 2 billion cells had a survival rate of 17 per cent, and in dogs which received more than 2 billion cells, the survival rate was increased to 88 per cent. The clinical and hematologic course in the surviving dogs in this group was almost identical to that of the surviving dogs in Group IV. With increasingly higher doses of irradiation, the symptoms of radiation illness were intensified, but in dogs which received the largest number of cells, the symptoms were ameliorated at all irradiation dose levels.

## COMMENT

The experiments reported have all been carried out under ordinary laboratory conditions with adult mongrel dogs in apparent good health which were not isolated from other stock dogs. Although isolation units and a kennel-raised strain of dogs are desirable and no doubt would increase the number of survivors, they are not mandatory and, indeed, such conditions are impossible to attain in most experimental laboratories.

The techniques of preparing bone marrow and splenic suspension described are effective and uncomplicated and require a minimum of equipment. Any of the balanced salt solutions suitable for tissue culture work, to which antibiotics and anticoagulants have been added in the concentrations indicated are satisfactory suspending solutions. Careful adjustment of the pH of the suspending solution to 7.2 and cooling of the suspension to 4° C. during the entire in vitro period will increase viability of the cells.

Investigators have reported that small animals can be protected against lethal total-body irradiation by a variety of splenic and bone marrow preparations, including even cell-free extracts of spleen.[6] There is evidence, however, that even in small animals the greatest protection is afforded by viable cells, and the protection is proportional to the number of cells given.[20, 25] The results reported here seem to be in agreement with the latter statement, since the degree of protection afforded was proportional to the number of viable cells given. Also, dogs which received the largest number of cells had the mildest clinical courses. This would suggest, but not prove, a cellular rather than a humoral factor as the protective agent.

There is some evidence that dividing cells are necessary for protection against total-body irradiation.[4] If true, this would account for the apparently somewhat greater effectiveness of bone marrow cells as compared to spleen cells observed in these experiments, because bone marrow contains a higher percentage of dividing cells. The possibility that a humoral factor is present and is operating to stimulate regrowth of bone marrow and lymphatic cells has not been excluded. This is particularly true with splenic suspensions, in which stained smears have shown many fragmented cells from which humoral factors may well have been released. Further studies are in progress to evaluate this potential humoral factor.

These initial studies with bone marrow and splenic infusions have all been concerned with autologous tissue. It has been our thought that in this type of transplantation, as well as with whole-organ autotransplants, the mastery of principles underlying successful autotransplantation will greatly aid in solving similar problems with homologous transplants of all kinds.

The immediate goal is to be able to protect dogs up to 2,000 r. This goal may be achieved if experiments in progress indicate that the protective effects of spleen and bone marrow suspensions are additive. If dogs can be consistently protected by a combination of spleen and bone marrow at these levels, consideration will be given to using similar techniques to treat disseminated cancer in patients. It is encouraging that the spleen is infrequently involved in disseminated carcinoma.

The eventual goal, which is perhaps somewhat remote even though the work is already in progress, is to use these techniques for the successful grafting of homologous spleen and bone marrow in animals. Thomas[23] has indicated that some of the late deaths in dogs treated with irradiation followed by bone marrow homografts may have been due to the failure of the infused homologous bone marrow to restore lymphoid function and immunologic defenses in the lymph nodes and spleen of the recipient, even though bone marrow in the recipient was completely restored. Perhaps suspensions of both homologous spleen and bone marrow will restore not only the hematopoietic tissues but also the immune mechanisms of lymph nodes and spleen of the recipient. Again, radiation in doses up to 1,500 to 2,000 r and perhaps higher[26] will apparently be necessary to destroy the animal's own immune mechanism if homografts are to be successful. If such a radiation chimera can be produced in the hematopoietic and lymphatic tissues of a recipient dog, then whole-organ homografts, taken from the donor of the spleen and bone marrow cells, can also be transferred successfully to this animal. The technical aspects of transferring whole-organ grafts of such organs as stomach, small intestine, kidneys, liver, and the heart have already been mastered in this as well as in other laboratories.[5, 10, 11, 14, 19]

## SUMMARY

Techniques have been developed to obtain and process splenic and bone marrow cell suspensions which have produced large yields of viable cells, up to 22 billion viable spleen cells and 20 billion viable bone marrow cells. These preparations of autologous spleen and bone marrow cells have protected dogs maintained in standard laboratory conditions and given lethal or supralethal total body irradiation. The degree of protection afforded appears to be approximately proportional to the total number of viable cells given. For a given number of cells, bone marrow cells appear to be slightly more protective than spleen cells, especially at the higher levels of irradiation. This may be due to the higher percentage of dividing cells in the bone marrow. The data presented favor the theory that the protection resulting from the use of these suspensions in lethally irradiated dogs is on a cellular rather than a humoral basis, but humoral factors have not been excluded.

The immediate goal of this study is to afford protection to dogs from up to 2,000 r, perhaps by a combination of bone marrow and splenic infusions, after which consideration will be given to the use of this technique to treat disseminated cancer in patients. The ultimate goal is to produce a radiation chimera in which whole-organ homografts can be carried out.

We acknowledge gratefully the aid of Mrs. Betty Jane Points and Miss Cecelia Mi, laboratory technologists, and Mr. Donald Battles and Miss Marlene George in carrying out these experiments. Neomycin was furnished as Mycifradin by The Upjohn Company.

## REFERENCES


1. Allen, J. G., Emerson, D. M., Landy, I. J., Head, L. R., and Basinger, C. E.: The cause of death from total body irradiation. An analysis of the present status after 15 years of study, Ann. Surg. **146:** 322, 1957.
2. Alpen, E. L., and Baum, S. J.: Modification of x-radiation lethality by autologous marrow infusion in dogs, Blood **13:** 1168, 1958.
3. Congdon, C. C.: Experimental treatment of total body irradiation injury, Blood **12:** 746, 1957.
4. Congdon, C. C., McKinley, T. W., Sutton, H., and Urso, P., Jr.: The effects of transfusion of blood showing extreme leucocytosis on survival of x-irradiated mice, Radiation Res. **4:** 424, 1956.
5. Dempster, W. J.: Kidney homotransplantation, Brit. J. Surg. **40:** 447, 1953.
6. Ellinger, F.: Protection of guinea pigs against death by cell-free spleen extract, Science **126:** 1179-1180, 1957.
7. Fishler, M. C., Cole, J. L., Bond, V. P., and Milne, W. L.: Therapeutic effect of rat bone marrow injection in rats exposed to lethal whole body x-radiation, Am. J. Physiol. **177:** 236-242, 1954.
8. Hilal, S.: Unpublished data.
9. Kaltenbach, J. P.: The preparation and utilization of whole cell suspension obtained from solid mammalian tissues, Exper. Cell Res. **7:** 568, 1954.
10. Lillehei, R. C., Goott, B., and Miller, F. A.: The physiological response of the small bowel of the dog to ischemia including prolonged in vitro preservation of the bowel with successful replacement and survival, Ann. Surg. **150:** 543, 1959.
11. Lillehei, R. C., Longerbeam, J. K., Goott, B., Hilal, S., and Yunis, E.: Horizons in abdominal surgery, Postgrad. Med. **29:** 272, 1961.
12. Lillehei, R. C., Longerbeam, J. K., Hilal, S., and Yunis, E.: Studies on the treatment of acute radiation sickness in dogs with various preparations of spleen, SURGERY **48:** 716-723, 1960.
13. Lorenz, E., and Congdon, C. C.: Modification of lethal irradiation injury in mice by injection of homologous or heterologous bone marrow, J. Nat. Cancer Inst. **14:** 955-961, 1954.
14. Lower, R. R., Stofer, R. C., and Shumway, N. E.: Homovital transplantation of the heart, J. Thoracic Surg. **41:** 196, 1961.
15. Mannick, J. A., Lochte, H. L., Ashley, C. A., Thomas, E. D., and Ferrebee, J. W.: Autografts of bone marrow in dogs after lethal total-body radiation, Blood **15:** 255, 1960.
16. Mannick, J. A., Lochte, H. L., Jr., Thomas, E. D., and Ferrebee, J. W.: In vitro and in vivo assessment of the viability of dog marrow after storage, Blood **15:** 517, 1960.
17. Martin, S. P., and Green, R.: Methods for the study of surviving leucocytes, Meth. M. Res. **7:** 136, 1958.
18. Monroe, D. E., Scala, A. R., and Jewell, M.: Methods of measuring viability of ascites cells. Dye exclusion and respiration as affected by depletion, poisons, and viruses, Cancer Res. **19:** 945, 1959.
19. Moore, F. D., Wheeler, H. B., Demissianos, H. V., Smith, L. L., Balankura, O., Abel, K., Breenber, J. B., and Dammin, G. J.: Experimental whole-organ transplantation of the liver and spleen, Ann. Surg. **152:** 374, 1960.
20. Smith, W. W., Marston, R. Q., and Cornfield, J.: Patterns of hemapoietic recovery in irradiated mice, Blood **14:** 737-747, 1959.
21. Sullivan, R. D., Stecher, G., and Sternberg, S. S.: Value of bone marrow and spleen cell suspensions for survival of lethally irradiated dogs, J. Nat. Cancer Inst. **23:** 367-383, 1959.
22. Tennant, J. R.: Studies on mouse leukemia, M.S. thesis, The Graduate School, University of Minnesota, 7-33, 1957.
23. Thomas, E. D., Ashley, C. A., Lochte, H. L., Jr., Jaretzki, A., III, Sahler, O. D., and Ferrebee, J. W.: Homografts of bone marrow in dogs after lethal total-body radiation, Blood **14:** 720, 1959.
24. Tullis, J. L., editor: Blood cells and plasma proteins: their state in nature, New York, 1953, New York Academic Press, Inc., p. 276.

25. Urso, P., and Congdon, C. C.: The effect of the amount of isologous bone marrow injected on the recovery of hematopoeitic organs, survival and body weight after lethal irradiation injury in mice, Blood **12:** 251-260, 1957.
26. Webb, R. L., Jacob, S. W., Stone, J. H., and Dumphy, J. E.: Resistance of bone marrow to direct radiation, S. Forum **11:** 35-36, 1960.
27. Wilson, R. E.: Technics of human bone marrow procurement by aspiration from living donors, New England J. Med. **261:** 781, 1959.

*(For discussion, see page 297.)*

# Studies in the preservation of bone marrow

VICTOR RICHARDS, M.D.
MAXIM PERSIDSKY
SAN FRANCISCO, CALIF.
*From the Department of Surgery, Presbyterian Medical Center, and the San Francisco Institute of Medical Research*

It has been amply demonstrated that a variety of animals will survive lethal doses of irradiation if given intravenous infusions of living bone marrow or other hematopoietic cells. Similarly, fatal doses of radiomimetic agents, often used in cancer chemotherapy, can be tolerated in animals, provided that viable bone marrow is administered in either isologous or homologous form. Efforts to adapt the implications of these experimental observations to problems in man have recently been made, and the initial observations of McGovern and associates[7] have been extensively reviewed in a recent paper by Mathé[6] on the application of hematopoietic cell grafts to the treatment of leukemias and allied diseases in man. Autologous marrow clearly restores bone marrow with hematopoietic cells, replacing those which have been destroyed by irradiation or chemotherapy. Homologous cells, unfortunately, are rejected through the homograft reaction or, if they remain viable, may initiate secondary homologous immune disease. Surgeons have been interested for years in the problems of homologous tissue transplantation, but more recently have been confronted with the more urgent problem of preservation and transplantation of autologous marrow incident to the extensive use of radiomimetic agents in cancer chemotherapy.

Ferrebee and colleagues[2] have studied the collection, storage, and preparation of viable marrow for a number of years. More recently, Pegg and Kemp[9] have reported on the collection, storage, and administration of autologous human bone marrow. Regardless of whether autologous marrow, fetal marrow, or cadaver marrow has been utilized, investigators have in general preserved the marrow by the slow freezing method of Polge and his co-workers.[13] This method consists basically of the addition of glycerol to the preparation of the marrow in approximately 15 per cent concentration and slow freezing of the marrow at the rate of about 1° C. per minute down to –79° C., then storage at this low temperature.

The mechanism by which glycerol acts against death of cells during freezing and thawing has been most extensively studied on red blood cells by Lovelock.[4] His studies suggested that glycerol protects the red blood cells during freezing by preventing excessive salt concentrations in cells, owing to the growth of extracellular ice crystals. The glycerol, then, may prevent lethal intracellular dehydration incident to the crystallization of ice during the freezing process. Lovelock has suggested that any one of a number of nontoxic nonelectrolytes of low molecular weight might serve the same function. However, his own experiments have

Supported by Office of Naval Research Contract Nonr-3168 (00) and United States Public Health Service Grant C-4881.

Read at the Twenty-second Annual Meeting of the Society of University Surgeons, Feb. 9-11, 1961.

failed to show any compound more effective than glycerol.

The marrow cell is basically different from the red blood cell in that it is a nucleated cell. Its survival during freezing with glycerol might be entirely different, and it appears desirable to study the protecting effects of many substances other than glycerol on the marrow cell. Furthermore, glycerol should be removed from the cells prior to intravenous infusion. This removal of glycerol from the thawed cell suspensions is tedious and inconvenient, and damage to the cell may occur during the thawing process from osmotic lysis.

Clearly, there are several basic problems in the preservation of marrow which require continued study; (1) the search for substances other than glycerol that would be desirable preservatives during the freezing process, (2) methods of assessing the viability of frozen marrow cells, (3) the effects of various storage temperatures, different freezing velocities, and possibly even freeze-drying techniques in the preservation of marrow, and (4) the study of the mechanism of cell death during the freezing and thawing process.

The purpose of this presentation is to relate our experiences in the preservation of marrow with respect to (1) the substances used to preserve marrow during the freezing and thawing process, (2) the effects of different cooling velocities and the time of the initiation of ice formation, and (3) the methods of assessing cell survival by the use of tissue culture techniques followed by phase microscopy of the preserved marrow cell.

## BASIC INSTRUMENTATION FOR STUDIES IN MARROW PRESERVATION

The photomicrography and cinemicrography of the marrow cells during the freezing process was accomplished by use of the instrument originally designed by Rapatz and Luyet[14] and perfected here by Persidsky. This instrument is illustrated in Fig. 1. Basically, it consists of a horizontal micro-

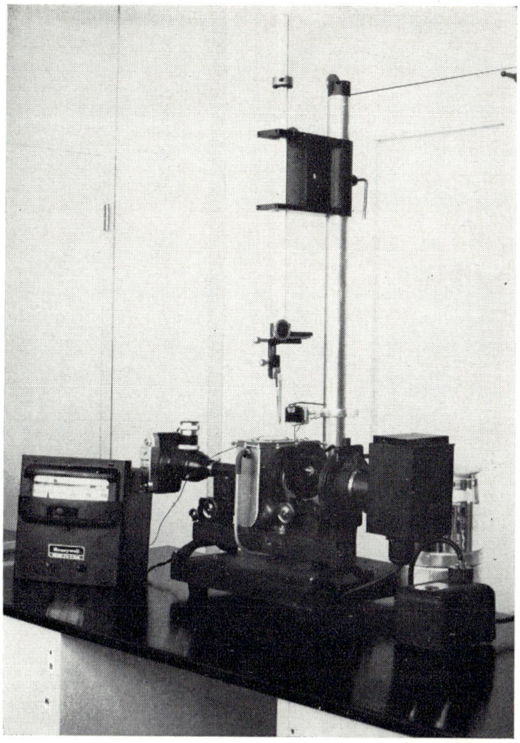

**Fig. 1.** Apparatus used for photomicrography.

scope, the stage of which is replaced by a thermoinsulated chamber containing an alcohol or isopentane bath, depending upon the temperature used. The temperature of the fluid in the bath is lowered by the aspiration of liquid nitrogen through the enclosed space between the chamber, and the thermoinsulation is regulated by the Brown Puls Pyr-O-Vane Controller. This thermoregulator activates the solenoid valve which controls the aspiration of liquid nitrogen through the chamber and thereby holds the temperature at a constant level according to the predetermined setting on the thermoregulator. A specimen holder on a movable vertical carrier immerses the preparation. The specimen is embodied between 2 cover slips sealed with petroleum jelly. The specimen carrier brings the specimen into the bath and carries it into proper position with respect to the microscope objective. The instrument has been so designed that phase microscopy is also possible with this temperature-controlled system.

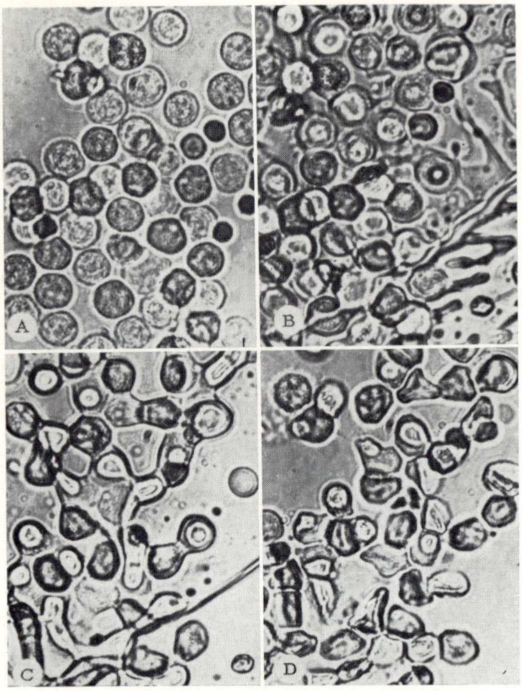


**Fig. 2.** Photomicrographs of freezing marrow *A,* Before ice forms (0° C.), *B,* ice crystals forming (−6° C.), *C,* before thawing of ice (0° C.), and *D,* after thawing (0° C.).

The details of construction and operation of the instrument will be described in a separate paper.[11] Fig. 2 shows photomicrographs of freezing marrow.

## A SIMPLIFIED FREEZING SYSTEM

The Polge method of freezing consists of lowering the temperature of the medium at 1° C. per minute. It involves rather elaborate equipment and does not permit visibility or manipulation of the specimen during the freezing process. As an outgrowth of our new refrigerating system for the microscope stage, we have developed in our laboratory a simple apparatus for permitting controlled cooling rates with freedom to observe and manipulate the specimen during the freezing process. This apparatus consists of a coil of copper tubes immersed in an alcohol bath in a Dewar flask which contains a power stirrer. Liquid nitrogen is aspirated through the copper coil by means of a vacuum line. The rate of flow of the liquid nitrogen is controlled by a needle valve. The temperature of the bath is measured by a thermocouple and recorded by a recording galvanometer. Adjustment of the needle valve permits setting of the cooling rate of the bath at 1° C. per minute (Fig. 3).

The details of this apparatus will be described in a separate publication.[12]

## METHODS OF ASSESSING VIABILITY OF MARROW CELLS AFTER FREEZING

A critical problem in the study of preservation of bone marrow is the determination of the viability of the marrow after freezing in a simple, yet quantitative, manner. We have considered 5 possible methods; (1) tissue culture techniques followed by phase microscopy of the cultured marrow, (2) quantitative injections of isologous marrow into a lethally irradiated inbred strain of mice, (3) interference microscopy of the frozen marrow cell, (4) uptake of tritiated thymidine by preserved marrow contained in Millipore diffusion chambers in isologous and homologous animals, and (5) the leak of fluorescent dyes from the cells during freezing and thawing measured with a Turner fluorometer.

Of these various methods, we shall report on the tissue culture method, followed by phase microscopy. This has proved to be the simplest and most reliable method and permits the assessment of crucial initial factors in the freezing and thawing process. The work reported has been verified by initial experiments on the injection of preserved marrow into lethally irradiated animals. We are beginning the study of marrow by interference microscopy and fluorometry, but have no corroborative data on these methods at the present time.

## THE TISSUE CULTURE TECHNIQUE FOLLOWED BY PHASE MICROSCOPY

A simple tissue culture method has been adapted for the quantitative evaluation of cell viability after different methods of freezing and preservation of marrow. After incubation, living cells adhere to strips of cover glasses placed in horizontal culture bottles containing a mixture of Hank's solution and serum. After 24 hours of incubation, the cover glasses are washed to remove the dead cells and cell viability is estimated by the use of the phase-contrast microscope. The live cells are usually elongated, often have small processes, and appear bright in "negative" phase-contrast illumination. Their cytoplasmic content appears uniform and the nucleus is barely recognizable. Dead cells, on the other hand, show a sharply delineated nucleus, frequently pyknotic, granulated cytoplasm, or else may be very small and compact. Many dead cells appear dark in phase-contrast illumination. The total number of live cells in each of 5 random fields was counted to quantitate the cell viability. Fig. 4 is a photograph of cells after tissue culturing on a cover slip under phase microscopy. The red blood cells, nucleated marrow cells and the live and dead cells can be easily distinguished.

## METHODS OF LOW TEMPERATURE PRESERVATION

All the experiments that will be reported were conducted on rat bone marrow.

**Control.** Bone marrow cells obtained from the femur were suspended in a culture medium consisting of 3 parts of rat serum and 1 part of Hank's solution. This suspension was placed in a 15 c.c. Kimox serum bottle which was horizontally inclined. A narrow strip of a glass cover slip was placed in each bottle. After 24 hours of incubation at 37° C., viable cells were found attached to the glass cover slip. The dead cells which were not attached to the cover slip were removed by washing the cover slip in a 10 per cent dextrose-saline solution. The viable cells in 5 randomly selected microscopic fields were counted under ×40 magnification with phase-contrast microscopy. The viable and the dead cells could be easily counted and a quantitative assay of the effects of various methods of cold temperature preservation could be analyzed.

**The effects of various concentrations of glycerol as a protective agent.** Glycerol was used more or less as the control medium in the light of numerous experiments by

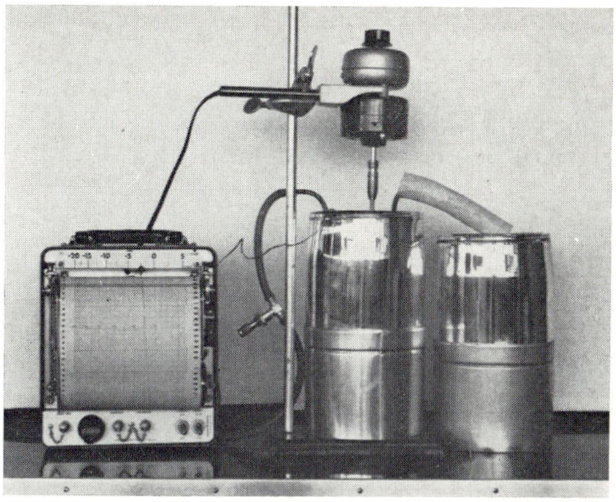

Fig. 3. Simplified cooling apparatus.

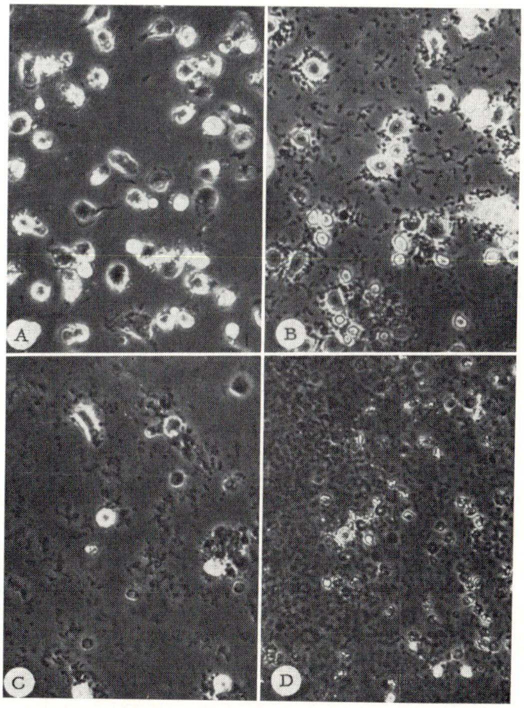


Fig. 4. Phase microscopic studies of cultured marrow cells. *A,* Almost all cells are alive (refractive) with active cellular processes. *B,* Many cells are alive; some are dead. *C,* Most cells are dead; some are alive. *D,* Almost all cells are dead.

many workers. After a short exposure to 15 per cent glycerol at room temperature, in the same culture medium as the control, cells were analyzed under the phase microscope. Many cells began to exhibit a bubble-like expansion in the cell membrane. The membrane finally burst and with loss of continuity of its membrane the cell died. Such cells were dark under the phase-contrast microscope, while the other cells which were intact remained bright and highly refractive. After prolonged exposure of 1 or 2 hours to glycerol in a 20 per cent concentration, the majority of the cells were found to undergo bubble-like transformation and death. In 10 per cent glycerol, however, only a small percentage of cells were affected in this way. The 15 per cent glycerol was intermediate in this respect. After the exposure of cells to the effect of glycerol they were washed and cultured. At the 10 per cent glycerol concentration, 56 per cent of the cells remained alive. At the 15 per cent concentration, only 25 per cent remained alive and at the 20 per cent concentration, only 15 per cent remained alive. In plotting, the results of the cell count in the control group (not exposed to glycerol) have been taken as the 100 per cent figure. It was found that 10 per cent glycerol was the most satisfactory concentration when freezing was employed with tissue culture technique (Fig. 5).

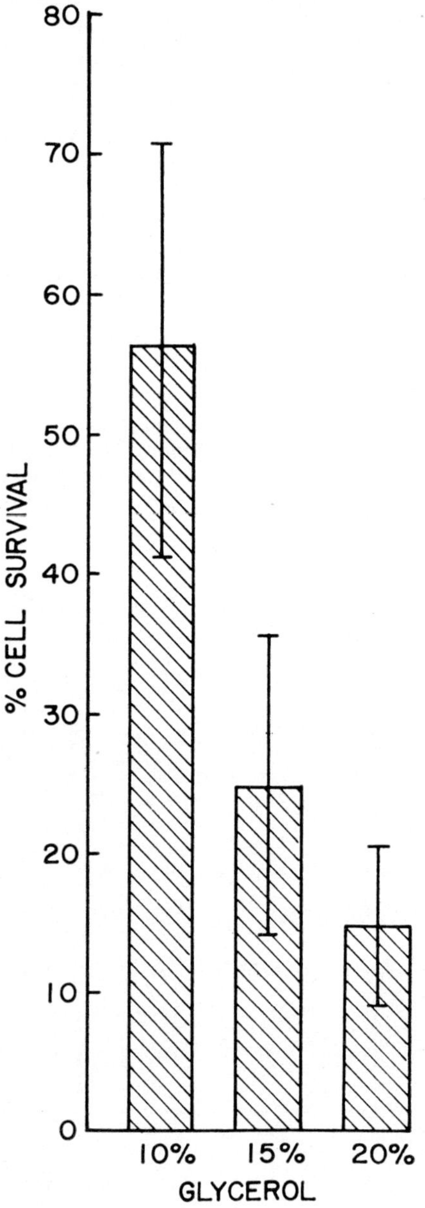


**Fig. 5.** Control effects of glycerol on cultured cells.

**The evaluation of the standard Polge technique of freezing.** The protective effect of various concentrations of glycerol on preserved marrow, with the standard Polge technique of freezing, was evaluated. Concentrations of glycerol ranging 5, 10, 15, to 20 per cent were studied. Several different freezing velocities in the first stage of freezing (down to –25 °C.) were studied, with 1 ml. of cell suspension in 10 ml. test tubes. Lowering of the temperature at 1° per minute down to 25° C. was found better than the faster freezing velocities. The second stage of freezing was always to –79° C. in an alcohol bath. After 10 minutes of exposure to these low temperatures, the material was thawed rapidly in a 38° C. water bath and survival of cells was found to be only 5 to 6 per cent by the tissue culture technique.

The seeding of ice formation was found to be an important variable in cell survival. Spontaneous ice formation takes place at about –20° C., but with the simple freezing methods described, initiation of ice formation could be made to occur at any desired

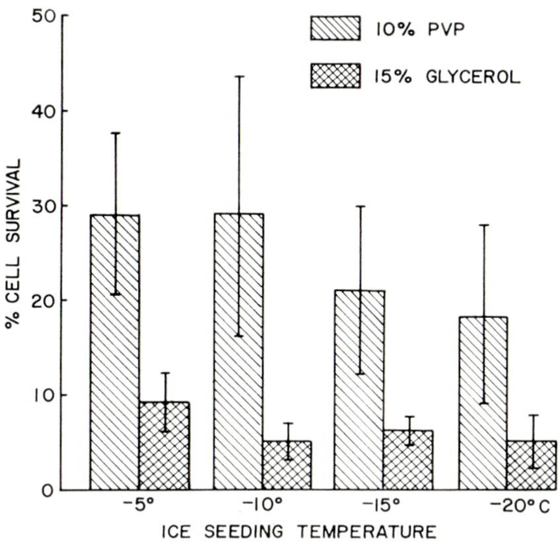


**Fig. 6.** Effects of temperature of ice seeding, glycerol versus PVP.

temperature merely by touching the specimen with a metal rod cooled in liquid nitrogen. Seeding of ice was performed at –5° C. Spontaneous freezing with the temperature lowered at 1° per minute took place between –18 and –25° C. in the medium containing 15 per cent glycerol. The temperature of initiation of ice formation did not have striking effects on the result, but in general the seeding of ice formation at –5° C. gave the best results and averaged about 9 per cent survival. The effect of seeding ice formation at different temperatures with 15 per cent glycerol treatment is illustrated in Fig. 6.

**Comparative study of the protecting effect of other substances in the freezing of cells.** Low molecular weight, nontoxic compounds such as choline chloride and sorbital were studied. The protecting effect of polyvinylpyrrolidone (PVP), however, was studied in greater detail and is reported.

Effects of freezing cells with polyvinylpyrrolidone of 30,000 molecular weight (Plasdone C), 5, 10, 15, or 20 per cent, were examined. Ten per cent was found to be the most satisfactory concentration of polyvinylpyrrolidone in the preservation of marrow by freezing (Fig. 7). The effect of different temperatures of seeding of ice formation under polyvinylpyrrolidone protection was also studied. With the seeding at –5° C., 29 per cent of the cells on the average were found to survive freezing in polyvinylpyrrolidone of 10 per cent concentration.

The addition of 10 per cent polyvinylpyrrolidone to the culturing medium had a very good effect on cell growth. In the control studies without polyvinylpyrrolidone, the number of cells surviving was counted, and this was used at the 100 per cent survival point in the calculation of survival data. The addition of polyvinylpyrrolidone also stabilized the cell suspension and protected it from clumping after freezing and thawing.

The effects of polyvinylpyrrolidone on preservation of marrow are compared with the use of 10 per cent glycerol at various temperatures of ice seeding in Fig. 6.

## COMMENT

We sought to answer 5 basic questions in our studies on the freezing and preservation of marrow. (1) What is the effect of the freezing velocity on the per cent of cell survival? (2) What substances are protective at optimal freezing velocities? (3) At what temperature should ice formation be initiated during the freezing of cells? (4) What is the mechanism of cell death during freezing and thawing? (5) Are there protective

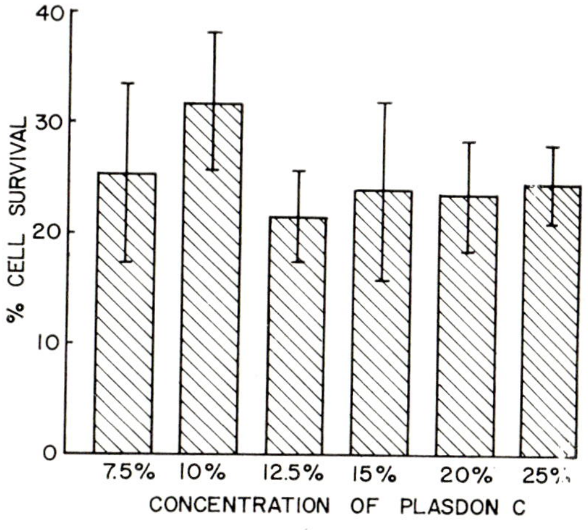


**Fig. 7.** Effects of different concentrations of PVP.

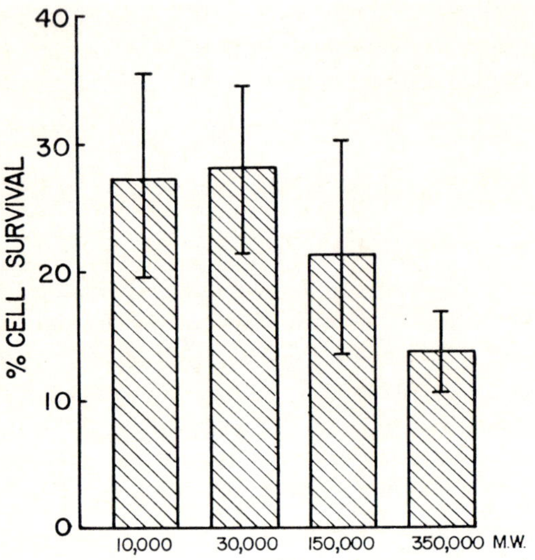


**Fig. 8.** Effects of different molecular weights of PVP.

substances which will permit not only freezing and thawing but also freeze-drying of the marrow cells?

Luyet[5] has studied extensively the mechanism of growth of ice crystals in aqueous solutions and the effect of rapid cooling in hindering crystallization. He has pointed out that the types of ice formations vary with the temperature at which crystallization begins. In the temperature ranges from –3 to –10 degrees, ice crystallizes as hexagonal prisms, stars, or rosettes. Very rapid cooling hinders crystallization and permits the freezing of water in an amorphous, vitreous, or "glasslike" state. According to Luyet, the vitreous or "glasslike" state is just one stage in a complex crystallization process related to cooling velocity and temperature of the frozen water. The details of "particular" or intermediate ice patterns in gels and the periodic phenomena in the freezing of solutions have been studied very carefully by Persidsky and Luyet.[10] The effects of slow and rapid freezing of blood on the pattern of ice formation in blood have been extensively studied by Rapatz and Luyet,[15] and these authors have also analyzed in a detailed fashion the effects of glycerol on the type of ice formation in frozen blood. They have also demonstrated the types of recrystallization that occur on warming and thawing of the frozen blood specimen. Rinfret and Dobbler[16] believe that rapid freezing velocities are so important in the preservation of blood that they have developed a simple, practical procedure for freezing blood in droplet form. The droplets are allowed to impinge on a continuously renewed surface of liquid nitrogen at –196° C. We have tried to evaluate the effects of different freezing velocities in the preservation of marrow and our studies indicate that with marrow cells, slow freezing at the rate of 1° C. per minute, in the manner of Polge, is optimal. We have also demonstrated that the crystallization of water is optimally begun at –5° C. We are undoubtedly producing ice crystals of fairly large size and the fact that optimal survival of cells occurs with this slow freezing velocity is additional evidence that ice crystal formation per se is not necessarily lethal to cells. Assuredly, these crystals are forming primarily in the intercellular spaces and intracellular freezing is not taking place until a much lower temperature is reached.

Lovelock,[4] in his studies of substances protective against freezing injury to red blood cells, has concluded that it is the concentration of salts that is primarily responsible for freezing injury and that the lipoproteins appear to be the most sensitive cell constituents. According to Lovelock's hypothesis, salt which concentrates in solution during freezing acts upon the red blood cells and renders them permeable to cations. The cells then accumulate electrolytes and become susceptible to osmotic lysis when exposed to the lowered osmolarity of the medium after thawing. When freezing is slow and ice crystals are extracellular, flexible animal cells can adapt themselves to their altered shapes without suffering irreparable mechanical injury. Cell death, according to Lovelock, results from the denaturing effect of high salt and solute concentration attending the dehydration that accompanies freezing. Actually, intracellular water would pass through the pores of the cell membrane, if such exists, and freeze in the extracellular spaces, thereby producing the intracellular dehydration and high salt concentration. Some water, of course, is firmly bound within the cell as bound water, and it is postulated that most mammalian cells can tolerate the removal of up to 75 per cent of the water without suffering irreparable change. Lovelock's theory further postulates that the introduction of a material which would be nontoxic to the cell and which could fairly freely diffuse across the cell membrane might prevent excessive intracellular dehydration and thereby prevent cell death during freezing. Glycerol, which was discovered initially in 1949 by Polge, and his group[13] to protect bull spermatozoa from injury by freezing, is such a substance. In theory, however, any nontoxic compound of low molecular weight should prevent freezing and thawing damage. Bender and associates[1] studied the preservation of bone marrow cells in mice and tested experimentally some of the postulates of Lovelock. They demonstrated that polyhydric alcohols of low molecular weight, namely ethylene glycol, glycerol, erythritol, ribitol, mannitol, and sorbitol would preserve enough viable bone marrow cells after freezing to protect lethally irradiated mice on isologous frozen marrow transplantation. They also demonstrated that marrow cells can tolerate a temperature of –196° C. just as well as a temperature of –70° C. Similarly, they showed that cells frozen in solutions of sugars, such as inositol, glucose, and lactose, could also be preserved in a viable fashion after freezing. Another organic compound of low molecular weight, choline chloride, was also effective. Quantitation of cell survival was extremely difficult in their experiments, but the biologic endpoint of preservation of life by transplantation of the frozen isologous marrow cells after lethal total body irradiation seems conclusive. Curiously enough, they tried PVP in 7 per cent concentration and found it completely ineffectual, but they continued to use it in 3.5 per cent suspension in Tyrode solution, since PVP prevents the clumping of marrow cells during the freezing and thawing process. They concluded that the protective compounds must enter the cell to protect against freezing and thawing damage and warned that different species of animals may have different cell permeabilities. To summarize, then, current theories of freezing injury postulate that cell death may occur in 1 or all of 3 fashions: (1) direct pressure from extracellular ice formation (mechanical injury), (2) ice formation within the cell (intracellular freezing probably results in crystals sufficiently large and numerous to break the cell protoplasm and membrane), and (3) excessive concentration of electrolytes within the cells and denaturation of the cell proteins incident to the dehydration accompanying extracellular ice formation and the rehydration on thawing.

Glycerol, which has generally proved to be the most effective agent preserving the viability of cells undergoing freezing and thawing injury, may act by (1) decreasing the crystallization velocity, (2) diluting the hypertonic solutions resulting from the separation of pure ice, (3) facilitating supercooling, or (4) permitting the formation of amorphous or vitreous semicrystals at a small size at low temperatures.

Our results indicate that PVP (Plasdone C), in concentrations of 10 per cent, was considerably superior to 15 per cent glycerol in the preservation of rat bone marrow. Ten per cent PVP also proved to be beneficial for cell growth in the tissue culture method. It prevented the clumping of cells after freezing and the maximal cell surivival occurred when ice formation was induced at about –5° C. The molecules of PVP are obviously far too large to penetrate the cell membrane and its protective action against freezing injury cannot be by the binding of intracellular water incident to the penetration of PVP within the cell. The pharmacologic aspects of PVP, a synthetic polymer of acetylene, ammonia, and formaldehyde, are not completely understood. It is essentially nontoxic and is rapidly excreted through the kidneys, but may be stored in small amounts in the reticuloendothelial system. It has a curious "vehicle" function and can chemically bind certain molecules such as dyes, bilirubin, penicillin, insulin, and various bacterial and viral toxins. It is not metabolized.[3] We have postulated that PVP forms a protective coat around the cell membrane and plugs the "pores" in the cell membrane which are necessary for the transport of water across the cellular membrane. This coating or protecting effect may vary with temperature, but the escape of intracellular water must be prevented early enough in the dehydration process incident to extracellular ice formation that intracellular freezing in all probability does not occur. We are extremely anxious, therefore, in our future work to study the transport of substances in and out of the cell during the freezing process under PVP protection.

One of the tremendous advantages of PVP over glycerol is that it permits not only survival from freezing and thawing injury, but also facilitates drying of living frozen tissue and cells. Glycerol may be a good preservative from the standpoint of prevention of freezing injury, but unfortunately it is nonvolatile and concentrates during drying, leaving the dried product in anhydrous glycerol. The glycerol, of course, is both intra- and extracellular and live mammalian cells cannot be obtained after drying in a glycerolated medium.

Of great interest is the recent demonstration by Merryman[8] on the drying of living mammalian cells. He clearly points out that the preservation of cells by freezing involves not only the injury incident to freezing, but also a second comparable insult relative to thawing, since the processes of freezing and thawing are inseparable in the use of frozen material. An alternate pathway by which cells could return from the frozen state would be drying after freezing. Merryman has demonstrated that reconstitution and viability of living cells after freeze-drying is only possible at the final drying process and reconstitution process requires 40 per cent dextran or PVP. He postulates that drying is a two-step process. The initial process is drying down to about 10 per cent of residual water, which represents the tightly bound water within the cell. Further removal of the water from the cell, without the application of dextran or PVP, irreparably damages it. He postulates also that dextran or PVP in the rehydrating solution provides a protecting "blanket that coats the cell and plugs the hole until the membrane recovers its integrity." The dextran or PVP preserves the integrity of the pore or hole in the cell membrane so that proper rehydration can take place on reconstitution of the cell with water. Merryman's experiments were performed initially with red blood cells and subsequently with bull spermatozoa. Obviously, the demonstration of the preservation of marrow cells under PVP protection during freezing opened to us the possibility of studying freeze-drying of marrow cells. Initial work in this direction has already begun.

## SUMMARY

We have studied the problem of preservation of bone marrow cells by freezing, employing the techniques of microphotography and tissue culturing of frozen marrow with assessment of viability quantitatively under the phase-contrast microscope. Results have been verified by biologic experiments in which frozen isologous marrow was injected into lethally irradiated mice. We have reported on detailed studies with rat bone marrow.

Freezing velocity has been studied. We have found a freezing velocity of 1 degree per second in the temperature range of 0 to –27° C. as most desirable. The temperature at which ice formation is initiated has been studied and the most desirable temperature for initiation of ice formation is –5° C. with the slow freezing process. Different protective substances have been evaluated with respect to 15 per cent glycerol as the control. We have found that PVP with molecular weight 30,000 in 10 per cent concentration gives superior results to 15 per cent glycerol in the preservation of marrow. It is postulated that the mechanism of protection from freezing injury under PVP consists in coating of the cell with PVP, plugging the "pores" in the cell membrane, and preventing intracellular electrolyte concentration, ice formation, and excessive dehydration mechanisms whereby the cell is killed by freezing. PVP possesses the added advantage that it permits freeze-drying, a technique not possible with preservation under glycerol.

### REFERENCES

1. Bender, M. A., Phanthe Tran, and Smith, L. H.: Preservation of viable bone marrow cells by freezing, J. Appl. Physiol. **15:** 520-524, 1960.
2. Ferrebee, J. W., Atkins, L., Lochte, H. L., Jr., McFarland, R. B., Jones, A. R., Dammin, G. J., and Thomas, E. D.: The collection, storage and preparation of viable cadaver marrow for intravenous use, Blood **14:** 140-147, 1959.
3. Gropper, A. L., Raisz, L. G., and Amspacher, W. H.: Collective review—plasma expanders, Internat. Abstr. Surg. **95:** 521-542, 1952.
4. Lovelock, J. E.: Haemolysis of human red blood-cells by freezing and thawing, Biochim. et biophys. acta **10:** 414, 1953.
5. Luyet, B.: On the mechanism of growth of ice crystals in aqueous solutions and on the effect of rapid cooling in hindering crystallization. In Parkes, A. S., and Smith, A. U., editors: Recent advances in freezing and drying, Springfield, Ill., 1960, Charles C Thomas, Publisher.
6. Mathé, G.: Application of hematopoietic cell grafts to the treatment of leukemias and allied diseases—a critical review, Blood **16:** 1073-1088, 1960.
7. McGovern, J. J., Jr., Russell, P. S., Atkins, L., and Webster, E. W.: Treatment of terminal leukemic relapse by total body irradiation and intravenous infusion of stored autologous bone marrow obtained during remission, New England J. Med. **260:** 675-683, 1959.
8. Merryman, H. T.: Drying of living mammalian cells, Ann. New York Acad. Sc. **85:** 729-734, 1960.
9. Pegg, D. E., and Kemp, N. H.: Collection, storage and administration of autologous human bone marrow, Lancet **2:** 1426-1433, 1960.
10. Persidsky, M., and Luyet, B.: Some particular ice patterns observed in the freezing of gelatin gels, Biodynamica **8:** 145-163, 1960.
11. Persidsky, M., and Richards, V.: Unpublished data.
12. Persidsky, M., and Richards, V.: Unpublished data.
13. Polge, C., Smith, A. U., and Parks, A. F.: Revival of spermatozoa after vitrification and dehydration at low temperatures, Nature **164:** 666-668, 1949.
14. Rapatz, G., and Luyet, B.: Apparatus for cinemicrography during rapid freezing, Biodynamica **7:** 346-350, 1957.
15. Rapatz, G., and Luyet, B.: Microscopic observations on the development of the ice phase in the freezing of blood, Biodynamica, **8:** 195-239, 1960.
16. Rinfret, A. P., and Dobbler, G. F.: Observations on the freezing and thawing of blood in droplet form, Biodynamica, **8:** 181-194, 1960.

### DISCUSSION*

**Dr. George L. Jordan, Jr.** (Houston, Texas). We have been interested in bone marrow transplantation and total body irradiation, and during the past 2½ years we have performed experiments similar to those presented today. Some of our results, however, are at variance with the conclusions of Dr. Longerbeam and associates. We have had survivals after 850 r total body irradiation with doses of marrow of less than 2 billion cells. We have not investigated the effect of extremely high doses, however, and it is certainly possible that very high doses may give better protection. Within the past year we have studied autologous spleen transplants and have observed protection at relatively high doses of total body irradiation. In fact, the survival rate at 850 r is 75 per cent, which is better than the survival rate after treatment with autologous marrow in our laboratories. We have not observed a detrimental effect of homologous spleen and bone marrow when given after low doses of total body irradiation. Animals so treated have clinical courses and survival times similar to those of the controls.

In one of Dr. Lillehei's earlier presentations he raised a question concerning the mechanism of protection after autologous spleen administration and suggested the possibility of a protective action upon the animal's own marrow rather than repopulation with splenic cells. We have conducted experiments to determine whether or not acellular extracts of spleen cells will give protection. They do not. We have also administered splenic cells after irradiation of the spleen and these cells have failed to give protection.

**Dr. Mannick** (Richmond, Va.). In Richmond we also have been interested for some time in

*Discussion of papers by Longerbeam, Lillehei, Yunis, and Hilal; and Richards and Persidsky.

the problem of total body irradiation and marrow transplantation and I would like to mention briefly 1 or 2 things which seem to us to make interpretation of results in this field somewhat difficult. The first of these is the problem of the relative biologic effectiveness of the radiation used. Two years ago from the laboratory of Drs. Thomas and Ferrebee in Cooperstown, we reported a series of dogs in which autologous bone marrow permitted survival after total body irradiation in doses ranging from 600 to 1,500 r. Off hand, 1,500 r sounds like a lot more than the 1,000 r that Dr. Longerbeam and Dr. Lillehei gave their dogs. However, the dogs in Cooperstown were irradiated with a double cobalt 60 source. By convention this radiation has a relative biologic effectiveness of 1.0, whereas I believe Drs. Longerbeam and Lillehei used 250 KVP x-ray which would have a relative biologic effectiveness of 1.4. Thus, in actual fact, the 1,000 r at Minnnesota would equal 1,400 r at Cooperstown. This sort of discrepancy may very well account for some of the variation in results reported in the literature.

The second difficulty, I think, is that of deciding when one has actually achieved a marrow autograft. Of course, there is no convenient cell marker which tells one whether or not a peripheral leukocyte has been formed by the graft of autologous marrow, or whether this cell has come from residual hematopoietic tissue left in the host. I think this question is particularly pertinent in view of the fact that Dr. Thomas' group has recently reported survival of dogs after 1,375 r total body irradiation without marrow transplantation of any sort. The treatment in these cases has consisted merely of administration of antibiotics, blood transfusions, and parenteral fluids. In our own laboratory we are now able to keep dogs alive after 700 r of total body x-irradiation without the use of a marrow graft. These facts have forced us to discard our previous ideas of an absolute $L.D._{100}$ radiation dose for dogs, and cast some doubt upon results previously attributed to marrow grafts.

I might say finally that I hope that the 35 billion cells reported in the abstract really were spleen cells and not marrow cells. Otherwise, I am sure that we're going to have to come to Minnesota to get our dogs. The slide shows a few of the bones we have removed from one animal in an attempt to find out how much marrow could be obtained from a mongrel dog. After opening up the bones and curetting out all the marrow, we found we could harvest about 8 billion cells from the entire dog. It is obviously impossible to obtain more marrow cells by inserting a needle into the marrow cavity than by removing all marrow with a curette at autopsy.

**Dr. Jerrold K. Longerbeam** (closing). We appreciate very much the helpful comments of Drs. Jordan and Mannick. Both have made significant contributions to the field of tissue transplantation. The work that Dr. Mannick and his colleagues have done was partially responsible for our undertaking this study. In response to Dr. Jordan's question concerning homografts of bone marrow and spleen, homografts have been performed in a small series of dogs. At radiation doses below 1,000 r, the dogs have appeared more acutely ill and have died, on the average, about a day earlier than controls, but this is not statistically significant. When homografts of bone marrow have been used with radiation doses above 1,000 r, we have achieved prolonged but not permanent survivals. With regard to Dr. Mannick's question, the 35 billion cells were obtained from the spleen, but we have obtained as many as 20 billion bone marrow cells in the dog by aspiration techniques, so it is difficult for me to explain what is wrong with Richmond dogs. I thought only Boston dogs were different from the rest. I would like to emphasize one more point. Since our success in treating total body irradiation with cell infusions has correlated fairly well with the total number of cells given, further investigations into techniques of obtaining and preserving cells appear to be worthwhile.

# Meeting of the Society of University Surgeons, Kansas City, Kan., February 9-11, 1961

RALPH A. DETERLING, JR., M.D.
BOSTON, MASS.

The Twenty-second Annual Meeting of the Society of University Surgeons was held in Kansas City, Kan., Feb. 9-11, 1961, where the Society was the guest of the University of Kansas Medical Center.

On Thursday morning, February 9, members and guests convened in Battenfeld Auditorium of the University of Kansas Medical Center. This day the program was devoted to papers by the host Department of Surgery. Dr. David W. Robinson, presiding, introduced Dr. C. Arden Miller, Dean of the School of Medicine and Director of the Medical Center. After a brief introductory address by Dr. Miller, a word of welcome was added by Dr. Frank Allbritten, Jr., Professor and Chairman of the Department of Surgery. The papers then presented were:

1. Induced hyperthermia in rats. Dale Brett, M.D., and Paul Schloerb, M.D.
2. Cardiac function after elective cardiac arrest. Don R. Miller, M.D., Peter Rasmussen, M.D., and Bernard Klionsky, M.D.
3. Hand contamination as a source of surgical infection. Robert F. Cavitt, M.D.
4. Correlation of serum enzymes with liver disease. Robert T. Manning, M.D.
5. Tubular excretion of organic bases. L. A. Peters, M.D.
6. Transplantation studies on 20-methylcholanthrene-induced leukemia. C. A. Hardin, M.D., and A. A. Werder, Ph.D.
7. Redistribution of blood flow and preferential shunting after Arfonad. James W. Bickley and C. Frederick Kittle, M.D.
8. Histochemical studies in congenital pyloric stenosis. Stanley R. Friesen, M.D.

Dr. Leonard F. Peltier presided over the remainder of the morning session which followed a coffee break.

9. A human hemoglobin with markedly lowered oxygen affinity. Kurt Reissmann, M.D., and William E. Ruth, M.D.
10. Effect of alcohol on hemorrhagic shock. Dean T. Gettler, M.D.
11. Cardiac output during and after various operations. Alfred Heilbrunn, M.D., and Frank F. Allbritten, Jr., M.D.
12. Evaluation of renal function by creatinine clearance test. Perry W. Nadig, M.D.
13. Pharmacologic evidence for a cardiac sphincter mechanism. Evan L. Frederickson, M.D.
14. Prophylactic treatment of fat embolism with lipase. Federico Adler, M.D., and Leonard F. Peltier, M.D.
15. Laminagraphy and stereotaxic surgery. Charles Brackett, M.D.

After an excellent buffet luncheon at the auditorium, the afternoon session proceeded with Dr. Stanley R. Friesen presiding.

16. Physiologic changes with prolonged veno-arterial perfusion. William A. Reed, M.D.
17. The father of American surgery. George F. Sheldon and L. R. C. Agnew, M.D.
18. "Third space" edema formation after small intestinal trauma. David C. Smisson, M.D., and Paul R. Schloerb, M.D.
19. The effect of kidney hyperthermia on renal tolerance to ischemia. Dean Gettler, M. D., Floyd Colip, and Paul R. Schloerb, M.D.

An opportunity was then given the members and guests to visit the remarkable Clendening Library with its fabulous rare book section.

The local program concluded with an interesting look at postgraduate education, a field in which the University of Kansas has rendered distinguished service for many years. Dr. C. Frederick Kittle presided over the symposium, entitled "Continuing Education for the Surgeon." Dr. Mahlon Delp, Chairman of the Department of Medicine, spoke on postgraduate education and its problems, and Dr. Frank Allbritten, Jr., then reported on the experience in surgery at the University of Kansas. Dr. David Ruhe, Director of the Department of Audio-Visual Education, commented on communications, audio-visual aids and continuing education. Dr. Maurice Visscher, Chairman of the Department of Physiology at the University of Minnesota described the role of basic sciences in the postgraduate training of surgeons.

That evening, an enjoyable dinner dance was held in the Grand Ballroom of the Hotel Muehlebach. The Scientific Program presented by the members of the Society on February 10 and 11 is published in this issue of SURGERY.

*Volume 50 Number 2*

# SURGERY

AUGUST, 1961

Clinical surgery

# The use of hypothermia in the closure of atrial septal defects in children

W. T. MUSTARD, M.D.
R. J. BAIRD, M.D.
G. A. TRUSLER, M.D.
TORONTO, CANADA
*From the Department of Surgery, The Hospital for Sick Children*

The beneficial effects which could be expected from the use of hypothermia in cardiac operations were initially appreciated and demonstrated by W. G. Bigelow.[1] The method was utilized by F. J. Lewis in the performance of the first successful "direct-vision" repair of an atrial septal defect in September, 1952.[12] At the present time, 3 different surgical methods are widely used to correct atrial septal defects—the atrial well, cardiac bypass, and general body hypothermia.

The purpose of this article is to review our experience with the method of general hypothermia for the closure of atrial septal defects in children. At the end of June, 1960, 157 patients with atrial septal defects had been operated upon at The Hospital for Sick Children, Toronto; hypothermia had been used in 105 of the operations (Table I). Atrial septal defects associated with total anomalous pulmonary venous drainage or with a separate ventricular septal defect are excluded from this review.

Received for publication Oct. 4, 1960.

## ISOLATED OSTIUM SECUNDUM ATRIAL SEPTAL DEFECT

**Signs and symptoms.** The ages of the 95 children at time of operation varied from 2 to 15 years; the average age was 9 years. Fifty-nine were girls and 36 were boys.

Although the usual complaint was of increased shortness of breath on exercise, over one-third of the children had no symptoms. The physical signs of this defect have been well described elsewhere. Mild congestive failure was present in only 3 children and cyanosis on effort in only one.

All but 2 showed some variant of the incomplete right bundle branch block pattern in the electrocardiogram. The mean axis of the QRS complex lay between +60° and −150° in all and in 75 per cent between +60° and +150°. The frontal vector

**Table I.** *The use of hypothermia in 105 cases of atrial septal defect*

| *Defect* | *No. of patients operated upon* | *No. of cases in which hypothermia used* |
|---|---|---|
| Isolated ostium secundum atrial septal defect | 102 | 95 |
| Ostium secundum atrial septal defect plus partial anomalous pulmonary venous drainage | 10 | 2 |
| Ostium secundum atrial septal defect plus pulmonary stenosis | 6 | 4 |
| Ostium secundum atrial septal defect plus mitrial valve abnormality | 3 | 1 |
| Ostium primum atrial septal defect | 3 | 2 |
| Ostium primum atrial septal defect plus cleft mitral valve | 17 | 0 |
| Ostium primum atrial septal defect plus cleft mitral valve and tricuspid valve | 3 | 1 |
| Common atrioventricular canal | 13 | 0 |
| Totals | 157 | 105 |

was inscribed in a clockwise direction in all cases in which it could be computed.[4]

Preoperative right-heart catheterization was performed in 92 of the 95 patients; in only 3 was the systolic pressure in the pulmonary artery over 50 mm. Hg. At operation, 73 of the defects were located in the central portion of the atrial septum and 2 were found in the superior portion. In 18 the inferior margin extended to the entrance of the inferior vena cava (Fig. 1).

**Method of operation.** As experience was gained, the surgical technique was modified. Only the present technique is described.

The children were anesthetized with thiopental (2.5 per cent) and intubated under succinylcholine relaxation (1 mg. per 3 pounds).[2] They were ventilated with a nitrous oxide–oxygen mixture until spontaneous respiration returned. Halothane was then added and was used as required until the time of inflow occlusion.[2] From then on, usually nitrous oxide only was required. Respiratory control was established as soon as operation was begun and hyperventilation maintained until the chest was closed.

The patients were cooled within a refrigerating blanket and ice bags were added to the axillary and inguinal areas. The skin was not moistened. Both rectal and esophageal temperatures were monitored and the cooling was controlled so that the esophageal temperature did not drop below 29° C. and the rectal temperature below 30° C. The temperature at which the operation was begun varied somewhat with the size of the child, but was usually around 33° to 34° C. At the time of inflow occlusion, the esophageal temperature was 29° to 31° C. and warming had commenced.

The chest was opened with a sternum-splitting incision; neither pleural cavity was entered. The superior and inferior venae cavae were encircled by umbilical tapes which were passed through rubber tubes and used as tourniquets. Two parallel rows of silk sutures were inserted in the lateral wall of the right atrium (Fig. 2, *A*). Traction on the ends of these sutures aided in the application of the Satinsky clamp and was a safety factor in case the clamp should slip once the atriotomy had been made. After the right atrium had been opened within the confines of the clamp, stay sutures of fine silk were inserted. Blind finger exploration of the interior of the right atrium is no longer performed.

The operating table was then rolled to the patient's left, so as to place the atrial septum in a horizontal plane. Before the cavae were occluded, the anesthetist further oxygenated the patient and also injected a small quantity of relaxant in order to prevent diaphragmatic movements while the heart was open. At this stage, 500 ml. of heparinized blood was attached to the intravenous tubing and was used to replace the blood lost during the cardiotomy.[18] As soon as the cavae had been occluded, the entire heart was firmly compressed several times so as to empty it of blood; the Satinsky clamp was then removed. The aorta, pulmonary artery, and pulmonary veins were not occluded; the coronary arteries were not perfused; and a cardioplegic agent was not injected.

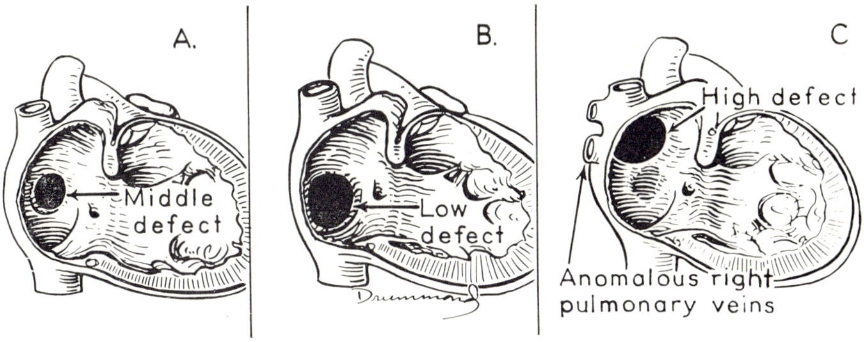


**Fig. 1.** Three varieties of ostium secundum atrial septal defect.

The sucker used to empty the right atrium of blood and to control the slight venous flow which comes from the coronary sinus was fashioned so that it would act as a retractor for the right edge of the incision (Fig. 2, *B*). A similarly shaped hollow retractor was used for the left side of the incision and through it carbon dioxide was passed.[15] Thus the operation proceeded in a dry field, under a blanket of carbon dioxide, and with a minimum of instruments.

The atrial septal defect was visualized, the superior end was picked up, and a waxed No. 2-0 silk suture inserted. Traction on this suture allowed a more accurate definition of the important inferior end of the defect. It is not our practice to excise the eustachian valve of the inferior vena cava, but rather to display its anatomy and then, if the atrial defect extends down to the inferior vena cava, to place the lower suture on the left atrial side of the septum. Care was taken to avoid the region of the coronary sinus lest conduction disturbances occur. The lower stitch was then continued to an over-and-over fashion to the superior end of the defect. The knot which united it to the upper suture was formed but it was not tied until all air and carbon dioxide had been extruded from the left atrium. This was accomplished by the anesthetist by inflation of the lungs while the surgeon held the superior portion of the atrial septal defect open. The knot was then "snugged up" under the protection of the blood. The inferior vena cava was released first in order to double-check its patency. With the long suture and the 2 stay sutures held up, the Satinsky clamp was easily reapplied as the right atrium filled with blood.

The right atriotomy was closed by a continuous running silk suture. The pericardial cavity was drained by a No. 16 Fr. rubber catheter and the anterior mediastinum by a No. 20 Fr. polyethylene catheter. The lower half of the pericardium was closed with silk,

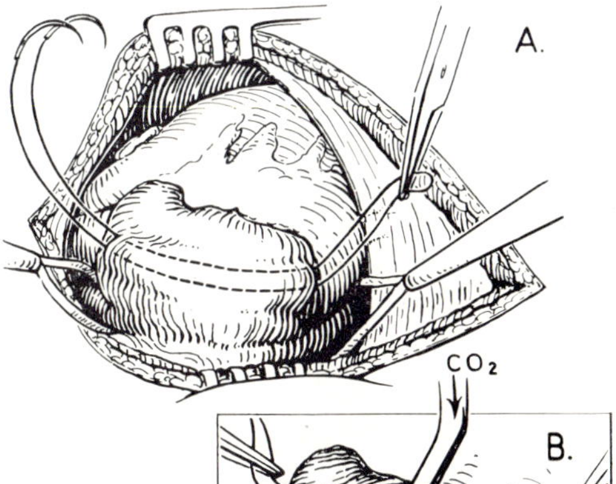


**Fig. 2.** *A*, The insertion of 2 parallel rows of sutures in the lateral wall of the right atrium. *B*, The use of a right-angled sucker and cannula for delivery of carbon dioxide as retractors.

the sternum with wire. Hemostasis was meticulous. Intradermal wire was used for the skin closure.

**Results of operation.** The morbidity resulting from this procedure was low. There have been 4 cases of wound infection of which only one, osteomyelitis of the lower sternum, was a cause for prolonged hospitalization. One patient developed a staphylococcal pericarditis which responded rapidly to treatment. No child in this series required postoperative bronchoscopic suction. Heart block did not occur, although 1 child had atrial flutter for 3 months.

There have been 3 cases of cerebral gas emboli, 1 with air and 2 with carbon dioxide. In 2 of the children the gas was also noted in the coronary arteries and ventricular fibrillation occurred during operation. The children remained unconscious for 1 to 3 days postoperatively. They were all treated by prolonged hypothermia, as described by Williams.[19] All have recovered completely and have no detectable neurological sequelae.

Incomplete closure of the atrial septal defect was suspected clinically in 2 children and proved by postoperative cardiac catheterization. In 1 child, prolonged cardiac massage had been required to overcome ventricular fibrillation and we believe that the recurrence occurred at this time. This recurrence was large enough to demand a second operative procedure. The other recurrence was small (10 per cent rise in atrial oxygen saturation) and further treatment was not recommended.

In the entire series of 95 patients, there was only 1 death from the initial operation. This child died 16 hours after the operation (September, 1957) from cardiac tamponade. The child with the severe recurrence described was operated upon a second time 2 years after the initial procedure; she died on the operating table from an atrial tear which occurred during the thoracotomy. Thus, the hospital mortality rate from this procedure was 2.1 per cent.

The other 92 patients are thought to be entirely cured of the defect. Postoperative cardiac catheterization has been performed on 14 other patients and in none has there been evidence of a persistent left-to-right shunt.

## ATRIAL SEPTAL DEFECT AND PULMONARY STENOSIS

We have operated upon 6 children with a combination of valvular pulmonary stenosis and atrial septal defect of the ostium secundum type. Cardiac bypass was used in 2, hypothermia in 4. The preoperative systolic gradient across the pulmonary valve varied from 52 mm. Hg to 77 mm. Hg. In the first period of inflow occlusion (average of 3 minutes), the pulmonary artery was opened and the pulmonary valve dealt with. With a second period of inflow occlusion (average of 4 minutes), the atrial septal defect was closed. All 6 children have done well. We prefer to use hypothermia in the correction of this lesion, as the coronary flow is then at a minimum and the pulmonary valvotomy is performed in a much drier field.

## ATRIAL SEPTAL DEFECT ASSOCIATED WITH PARTIAL ANOMALOUS PULMONARY VENOUS DRAINAGE

Of the 10 patients operated upon, hypothermia has been used in only 3. In each case in which hypothermia was used, the presence of the anomalous venous drainage was not suspected preoperatively. One child had come to operation without a right-heart catheterization.

In the first case, 2 anomalous right pulmonary veins were present—1 entering the right atrium and 1 entering the superior vena cava. The atrial septal defect was of the high "sinus venosus" type; a left superior vena cava was also present. The defect was corrected by ligation of the right superior vena cava below the azygos vein and above the entrance of the superior pulmonary vein and by then sewing the anterior edge of the atrial septal defect to the lateral wall of the right atrium so that the inferior pulmonary vein and the right superior vena cava were directed into the left atrium. A 5-minute period of inflow occlusion was required.

In the second case, the right superior pulmonary vein entered the upper portion of the right atrium and was associated with a centrally placed atrial septal defect. The defect was enlarged superiorly to give a longer anterior margin which was then sewn to the lateral wall of the right atrium so as to direct the blood from the pulmonary vein into the left atrium. A 7½-minute period of inflow occlusion was required.

In the third case, 3 veins from the right lung entered the right atrium through separate ostea and the atrial septal defect was again centrally placed. After careful assessment of this situation by finger palpation, it was decided to reoperate with the use of cardiac bypass. This anomaly was corrected uneventfully 2 weeks later.

Although neither of the 2 patients in whom the defect was corrected under hypothermia has undergone postoperative catheterization, they have no clinical evidence of a persistent defect and no evidence of superior vena caval obstruction. In spite of the good result obtained in these 2 cases, we believe that all such patients should (if diagnosis is made preoperatively) be operated upon with cardiac bypass. A pulmonary vein entering the superior vena cava will be diagnosed on careful catheterization, but one entering the right atrium may be missed. If so, and it is encountered at operation being performed with the technique of general hypothermia, it can usually be dealt with satisfactorily. We agree with the suggestion of F. J. Lewis that a single vein entering high in the superior vena cava might well be left untouched.[10]

## OSTIUM SECUNDUM ATRIAL SEPTAL DEFECT ASSOCIATED WITH ABNORMAL MITRAL VALVE

We have operated upon only 2 patients with Lutembacher's syndrome (atrial septal defect plus mitral stenosis). Cardiac bypass was used. One other patient, a 9-year-old boy suffering from rheumatic mitral incompetence and an atrial septal defect of secundum type, was operated upon under hypothermia in November, 1957. Only the atrial septal defect was corrected and the child has done well since the operation. With the methods now available to correct abnormal mitral valves, cardiac bypass would of course be used in all such cases.

## THE OSTIUM PRIMUM GROUP

The electrocardiographic criteria required to accurately diagnose the ostium primum atrial septal defect were not crystallized until late in 1958.[8] Prior to that time, 3 members of this group had been operated upon with the hypothermic method.

In October, 1956, a 13-month-old girl with pulmonary hypertension and severe symptoms was operated upon with hypothermia of 29° C. She died during the operation and postmortem examination showed an ostium primum atrial septal defect with associated complete clefts in the aortic leaflet of the mitral valve and the septal leaflet of the tricuspid valve.

In June and October, 1958, 2 boys, age 12 and 13, were brought to operation for ostium secundum defects. There was no preoperative evidence of mitral or tricuspid valvular insufficiency. At operation under hypothermia, the defects were found to be of the ostium primum type and both were repaired by direct suture. Although the mitral and tricuspid valves were only superficially examined at operation there is still no sign that they are incompetent. Both children are asymptomatic and although only one has undergone postoperative catheterization, both the defects appear to be completely closed. On rechecking the electrocardiograms, the axes of the QRS complex were seen to be –70° and –130° and the frontal vectors were inscribed in a counterclockwise direction mainly above the horizontal plane.

All patients with the ostium primum defects who come to operation today are operated upon with the aid of cardiac bypass. In this manner the valves can be carefully examined and repaired, a patch

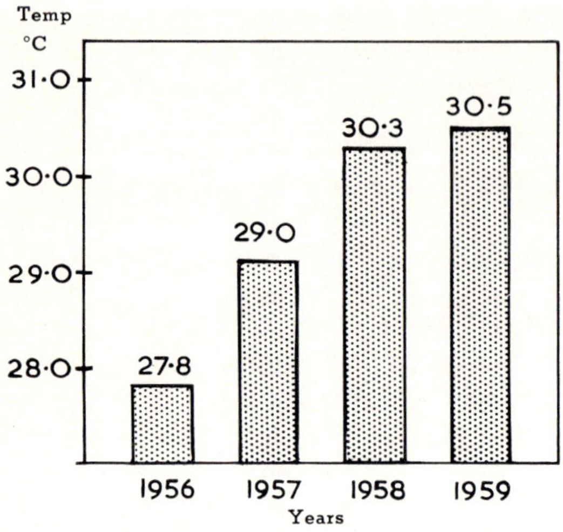


Fig. 3. The change in degree of hypothermia utilized during the closure of atrial septal defects.

may be used in the atrial septal defect if necessary, and the conducting tissue can be carefully guarded.

## DISCUSSION

**The degree of hypothermia.** In the first few cases in which hypothermia was used, there was a tendency to allow the body temperature to drift too low. The ease of producing hypothermia in a child, the practice of wetting the skin during cooling, and the belief that temperatures of 24° to 27° C. were safe, were major factors contributing to this tendency.

Table II and Fig. 3 illustrate the gradual change in the degree of hypothermia employed. Today, instead of a rectal temperature of 27° to 28° C. the lowest temperatures sought are an esophageal temperature of 30° to 31° C. and a rectal temperature of 31° to 32° C. At such temperatures, the oxygen consumption of the body is reduced to almost half that of normal and periods of circulatory occlusion of up to 8 minutes are quite safe.[1]

**Use of cardioplegic agents.** In June, 1957, Lam[9] reported the use of acetylcholine to produce cardiac arrest during intracardiac operations with the aid of cardiac bypass. By the production of cardiac arrest, a still field was obtained and the oxygen requirements were reduced. This technique was used in 14 children operated upon with general hypothermia during the period of May, 1957, to August, 1958. The practice was discontinued after it was seen that the duration of inflow occlusion was lengthened and the incidence of ventricular fibrillation increased (Table III). Neostigmine has not been used.

The incidence of ventricular fibrillation in the last 70 patients operated upon without arrest has been 8 per cent (6 cases). The incidence of ventricular fibrillation described by Swan and associates[17] after the use of neostigmine was 12 times in 100 patients. Evan Bedford and his group[3] have reported an incidence of ventricular fibrillation of 2 out of 40 patients in whom neostigmine was used. In both series, adult patients were included.

**The use of coronary perfusion.** As the heart of each patient in this series has either produced an adequate output immediately after the release of the inflow occlusion (80 cases) or else has responded quickly to cardiac massage and defibrillation (15 cases), we do not believe that coronary perfusion is necessary.[13, 16] The common use of "hypoxic arrest" in cardiac bypass has shown that no true damage is done to the myocardium during such a short period of circulatory arrest. If arrest of longer than 8 minutes is required, then the repeated inflow occlusion technique described by Johnson[7] is more advisable. Our comments in this matter are colored, of course, by the fact that all the patients in our series were children. The myocardium of adults may require more protection.

**Table II.** *The changing level of hypothermia used during the surgical repair of isolated ostium secundum atrial septal defects*

| *Year* | *Average lowest rectal temperature (C.)* | *% patients cooled to under 30° C. (rectal)* |
|---|---|---|
| 1956 | 27.8 | 100 |
| 1957 | 29.2 | 86 |
| 1958 | 30.3 | 38 |
| 1959 | 30.5 | 3 |

**Table III.** *The use of acetylcholine arrest in the repair of ostium secundum atrial septal defects*

| | *No. of cases* | *Ventricular fibrillation* | *Time of inflow occlusion* |
|---|---|---|---|
| No arrest | 81 | 10 (12%) | 4 min. 10 sec. |
| Acetylcholine arrest | 14 | 5 (36%) | 6 min. 20 sec. |

**Occlusion of other vessels.** It is not necessary to occlude the pulmonary veins,[11] as the blood level remains constant in the left atrium and blood does not enter the operative field unless the anesthetist inflates the lungs. Some authors advocate clamping the aorta low enough to occlude the coronary vessels in order to reduce coronary sinus venous return, to avoid coronary air embolism, and to maintain tachycardia.[9, 16] The coronary sinus return in our children has been found to be very limited in amount and easily handled by the sucker. If any air or carbon dioxide is trapped in the left side of the heart, then perhaps it is better to have it enter the coronary rather than the cerebral arteries; in the former location it can be massaged out again.[5] We see no need to occlude the pulmonary artery.[11, 17] It has not been our practice to temporarily occlude the carotid vessels as the circulation is restored; this procedure may be indicated in view of our 3 cases of cerebral air embolism.

**The operative approach.** In January, 1958, the approach was changed from a right thoracotomy with an extension across the sternum, but not into the left pleural cavity, to a sternum-splitting incision. This approach is rapid, there is little bleeding, excellent exposure is obtained, and postoperative pain and pulmonary complications are minimized. Its main disadvantage is cosmetic, for a scar is left at the base of the neck—a scar which has a great tendency to keloid formation. It is our hope that the use of an intradermal wire will improve the appearance of this scar. Wound infection is rare in children and the one patient with sternal osteomyelitis responded rapidly to adequate treatment.

After trying several methods of draining the pericardium and mediastinum after this approach, we have settled on the one described in the section on surgical technique.

**Completeness of closure.** Ten of the first 19 children with isolated ostium secundum defects closed by this technique were catheterized postoperatively. The residual defects demonstrated in 2 patients had both been suspected clinically prior to catheterization. Seven other patients have been catheterized postoperatively and none has shown evidence of an incomplete closure.

**The advantages and disadvantages of the method.** Excellent results have been reported from centers where the "open-well" technique of Gross has been used.[6] McGoon and associates[14] report 51 instances of atrial septal defects closed by this method with no deaths and insignificant morbidity. We have had no experience with such a method, but believe that the ability to see the defect must add some advantages in both ease and completeness of closure.

Cardiac bypass undoubtedly has some advantages. Unforeseen complicating factors such as anomalous veins, abnormal mitral or tricuspid valves, or ostium primum defects can be handled more safely. With the present accuracy of cardiologic diagnosis, however, such cases will rarely be encountered unexpectedly. If they are, most of them can be handled satisfactorily within the time limits imposed by this technique. The fact that some cannot is the main criticism of the hypothermic technique.

The advantage of cardiac bypass must be compared with such disadvantages as the quantity of fresh blood required, the lengthened operating time, the postoperative bleeding problems, and other problems intrinsic to a more complicated technique.

## SUMMARY

The experience of the group at The Hospital for Sick Children, Toronto, in the use of hypothermia for the closure of atrial septal defects is presented. One hundred and five children have been operated upon with this technique up to the end of June, 1960. The modifications of the technique as used in this hospital are described and discussed.

## REFERENCES

1. Bigelow, W. G., Lindsay, W. K., and Greenwood, W. F.: Hypothermia, Ann. Surg. **132:** 849, 1950.
2. Conn, A. W., Allan, D., and Junkin, C. I.: Anaesthesia with hypothermia for closure of atrial septal defects in children, Canad. Anaesth. Soc. J. **6:** 327, 1959.
3. Evan Bedford, D., Holmes Sellors, T., Somerville, W., Belcher, J. R., and Besterman, E. M. M.: Atrial septal defect and its Surgical treatment, Lancet **1:** 1255, 1957.
4. Evans, J., Rowe, R. D., and Keith, J. D.: The clinical diagnosis of atrial septal defect in children, Am. J. Med. **30:** 345, 1961.
5. Geohegan, T., and Lam, C. R.: Cardiac resuscitation following standstill, ventricular fibrillation and coronary embolism, Am. Surgeon **20:** 928, 1954.
6. Gross, R. E., Watkins, E., Pomerany, A. A., and Goldsmith, E. J.: A method for surgical closure of interauricular septal defects, Surg. Gynec. & Obst. **96:** 1, 1953.
7. Johnson, J., and Kirby, C.: Intermittent inflow occlusion for the direct visual repair of atrial septal defects, J. Thoracic Surg. **37:** 314, 1959.
8. Kiely, B., Adams, P., Anderson, R. C., and Lester, R. G.: The ostium primum syndrome, A. M. A. J. Dis. Child. **96:** 381, 1958.
9. Lam, C. A., Gahagan, T., Mota, C., and Green, E.: Induced cardiac arrest (cardioplegia) in open-heart surgical procedures, SURGERY **43:** 7, 1958.
10. Lewis, F. J.: High defects in the atrial septum, J. Thoracic Surg. **36:** 1, 1958.
11. Lewis, F. J., and Niazi, S. A.: A technique employing hypothermia for the repair of atrial septal defects, Surg. Gynec. & Obst. **106:** 751, 1958.
12. Lewis, F. J., and Taufic, M.: Closure of atrial septal defects with the aid of hypothermia, SURGERY **33:** 52, 1953.
13. Mahoney, E. B., Manning, J. D., Deweese, J. A., and Schwartze, S. I.: Clinical results of correction under hypothermia of atrial septal defects and pulmonary valvular stenosis, J. Thoracic Surg. **38:** 292, 1959.
14. McGoon, D. C. M., DuShane, J. W., and Kirklin, V. W.: Surgical treatment of atrial septal defects in children, Pediatrics **24:** 992, 1959.
15. Nichols, H. T., Morse, D. P., and Hirose, T.: Coronary and other air embolization occurring during open-heart surgery, SURGERY **43:** 236, 1958.
16. Riberi, A., Grice, P., Rodriguez, R., Kajikun, H., and Schumacker, H. B.: Prolongation of safe period of inflow occlusion in hypothermic state by coronary and carotid artery perfusion with oxygenated blood, J. Thoracic Surg. **32:** 399, 1956.
17. Swan, H., Kortz, A. B., Davies, D. H., and Blount, S. G.: Atrial septal defect, secundum. An analysis of 100 patients undergoing open surgical repair, J. Thoracic Surg. **37:** 52, 1959.
18. Waddell, W. G., Fairley, H. B., and Bigelow, W. G.: Improved management of clinical hypothermia based upon related biochemical studies, Ann. Surg. **146:** 542, 1957.
19. Williams, G. R., Jr., and Spencer, F. C.: The clinical use of hypothermia following cardiac arrest, Ann. Surg. **148:** 462, 1958.

## ADDENDUM

Since this paper was submitted for publication an additional 45 children have undergone operative closure of atrial secundum defects with no deaths and no recurrences (no recatheterization).

# Lung and heart complications of the treatment of hydrocephalus by ventriculoauriculostomy

J. L. EMERY, M.D.
H. B. HILTON, M.R.C.P.E.
SHEFFIELD, ENGLAND
*From the Department of Pathology, Children's Hospital*

For over half a century[9] the ideal surgical palliative treatment for hydrocephalus has consisted of shunting excess cerebrospinal fluid into the blood stream. There have been progressive technical advances in this field, with use of segments of veins,[18] arteries,[2, 6, 13, 15] rubber tubes,[5, 10] polyethylene tubes,[12] ball valves with tetrafluorethylene tubes,[20] and, more recently, the Spitz-Holter valve with nonwettable tubing which enables excess cerebrospinal fluid to be drained directly into the heart.

A large number of children have now been treated with the Spitz-Holter valve,[4, 16, 17] but the old problem of occlusion of the shunt channel appears in some cases to be replaced by a new series of complications. Two of Anderson's[1] series of 36 children died with pulmonary embolism. Three of Carrington's[4] series of 50 children died with septicemia, and 8 of MacNab's[16] 60 children had clot formation in the superior vena cava and heart.

We have become increasingly aware of a new pattern of pathologic lesions which have developed as a result of the cerebrocardiac shunts and the present paper is an attempt to describe them.

## CASES AND FINDINGS

The material studied came from necropsies on 15 patients with hydrocephalus in which ventriculoauriculostomy with the Spitz-Holter valve had been performed. The children were from a series of over 100 so treated by Mr. R. B. Zachary in the Children's Hospital, Sheffield. In all but 2 of the cases the hydrocephalus was associated with a meningomyelocele and its associated deformities. The other 2 cases appeared to be primary hydrocephalus, probably due to aquiductal deformities. Death occurred between the ages of 18 days and 2 years, 10 months. The valve had been in situ from between 3 days and 2 years, 2 months.

Some details of the cases and the gross necropsy findings are presented in Table I. In the 15 children, 7 only showed necropsy evidence of meningitis, and in 5 of these 7 there was evidence of infection in the lung with emboli. In one of the latter, death occurred 11 days after the insertion of the valve.

The lesions found fall into 2 groups, cardiac and pulmonary. The cardiac lesions included partial or complete occlusion of the veins entering the right auricle, and thrombi of varying size attached to the end of the catheter, auricular wall, or to the tricuspid valve. The lung lesions included massive pulmonary alveolar hemorrhage in a child dying 4 days after insertion of the valve, multiple emboli of great variation in size and number, focal arteritis, and 1 peculiar case of hemosiderosis.

The lesions which were discovered are discussed in the order of their incidence (Table II).

**Emboli in the pulmonary circulation.** Multiple emboli were found in pulmonary vessels in all but 1 child, who died with massive pulmonary hemorrhage 4 days after insertion of the valve. In some cases the emboli were obviously recent and lay with-

Received for publication Oct. 4, 1960.

**Table I.** *Details of the gross necropsy findings of 15 children who died after ventriculoauriculostomy with the Spitz-Holter valve*

| *Age at death* | *Period valve had been in situ* | *Valve tube entering auricle (Spitz-Holter valve)* | *Postmortem findings* | |
|---|---|---|---|---|
| | | | *Heart* | *Lungs* |
| 2 yr., 10 mo. | 2 yr., 2 mo. | Thrombosis of right jugular vein and innominate vein; no thrombus around catheter tip | Ulceration of endocardium of right auricle, 10 by 10 mm., with vegetation | Emboli with vascular occlusions but no gross infarction |
| 18 days | 5 days | End of tube entered tricuspid valve; no thrombi | No gross lesion | Recent emboli; small areas of vasculitis |
| 11 mo. | 7 mo. | Thrombus around catheter tip | Vegetations on tricuspid valve and right auricle wall | Massive pulmonary thrombosis |
| 1 mo. | 6 days | Thrombus around catheter tip | Acute pericarditis, endocarditis, endocardial ulceration | Septic infarcts; massive pulmonary thrombosis |
| 1 yr. | 5 mo. | Thrombosis in superior vena cava and innominate vein; catheter clear | Thrombus on wall of right atrium passing through tricuspid valve | Pulmonary hemosiderosis; small emboli; intimal degeneration |
| 2 mo. | 11 days | Thrombosis in superior vena cava and innominate vein; catheter clear | No gross lesion | Suppurative emboli; pleurisy with effusion |
| 10 mo. | 8 mo. | No thrombi | No gross lesion | Terminal thrombosis |
| 2 mo. | 4 days | No thrombi | No gross lesion | Collapse of lung with massive intra-alveolar hemorrhage |
| 3 mo. | 2 mo. | Small thrombus around catheter | Ulceration of endocardium of right auricle; mural endocarditis, tricuspid valve vegetations | Recent and old organized emboli |
| 1 yr. | 7 mo. | Tip of catheter in inferior vena cava; thrombus only around catheter in superior vena cava | No gross lesion | Mural thrombi in pulmonary arteries; acute focal vasculitis; bronchopneumonia |
| 5 mo. | 5 wk. | Thrombus about tip of catheter | Thrombus attached to tricuspid valve | Suppurative emboli |
| 2 yr., 4 mo. | 2 yr. | Catheter had passed from left jugular vein up innominate vein on right side; old thrombosis of all these veins present | No gross lesion | Multiple nonsuppurative emboli; *Torula histolytica* infection |
| 8 mo. | 4 mo. | Thrombus around tip of catheter | No gross lesion | Suppurative emboli |
| 15½ mo. | 8 mo. | Valve removed just before death; thrombosis of left and right jugular vein and right subclavian vein | No gross lesion | Suppurative emboli |
| 8 mo. | 3 mo. | Valve removed just before death | No gross lesion | Multiple nonsuppurative emboli; bronchopneumonia |

in the lumina of medium-sized arteries (Fig. 1, *A*), but in the majority of instances they completely occupied small arteries and showed varying degrees of organization. Thus it is not certain whether many of the small lesions were emboli or local thrombus formations.

The changes in the surrounding tissues varied considerably. In many instances there appeared to be no edema or cellular infiltration of the vessel walls or surrounding tissues although the emboli were vascularized and being eliminated.

**Occlusion of veins entering the heart.** In every instance the catheter entering the heart was surrounded by a collar of dense, fibrinous material as it lay within the jugular vein. This collar extended varying distances down the catheter into the auricle. In several instances the clot had propagated from the jugular into the innominate and subclavian veins. In 1 case the catheter had passed from one innominate vein to the other and the whole of the superior vena caval system appeared to be completely occluded.

**Thrombosis around the distal end of the catheter.** As mentioned, the catheter was always surrounded by a collar of fibrinous material, but the end of the tube did not appear to be occluded. Attached to the end of the fibrinous collar were variable masses of fibrinous clot and Fig. 2 shows one of these. This was a large mass which entered and obstructed the tricuspid valve and apparently caused clinical tricuspid incompetence.

In 1 case in which a large thrombus of this type was found, the clinicians had observed abnormal heart murmurs over the right side of the thorax and the presence of a thrombus occluding the tricuspid valve was diagnosed before death.

In 2 instances there was no clot attached to the end of the catheter, but massive pulmonary embolism had occurred.

In surveying the cases, we gained the impression that the majority of the large pulmonary emboli came from fibrinous thrombi attached to the end of the catheter.

**Table II.** *Lesions in heart and lungs in 15 children who died after ventriculo-auriculostomy with Spitz-Holter valve*

| *Lesion* | *No. of cases* |
|---|---|
| Multiple small "emboli" in pulmonary circulation | 14 |
| Complete or partial occlusion of veins entering heart | 13 |
| Thrombus around distal end of catheter | 10 |
| Other lesions of pulmonary vessels | |
| Early mycotic aneurysm formation | 7 |
| Periarteritis | 8 |
| Intimal degeneration | 4 |
| Thrombus formation on wall of right atrium with or without extension to tricuspid valve | 6 |
| Ulceration of auricular endocardium due presumably to trauma by catheter | 4 |
| Massive pulmonary embolism | 2 |
| Pulmonary hemosiderosis | 1 |

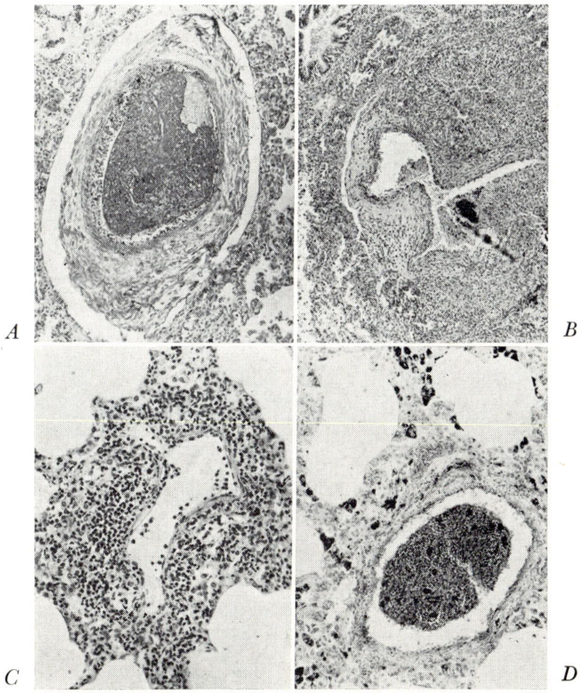


**Fig. 1.** *A,* Cross section of a medium-sized artery in lung which contains a thrombus. *B,* Artery in which part of the wall is necrosed. Black area is a mass of organisms. *C,* Small blood vessel in the lung which shows acute periarteritis. *D,* Lung which shows a blood vessel and alveoli. The section has been stained for iron. Black-stained cells are iron-containing macrophages in the alveoli. Black iron deposition can also be seen deep to the wall of the blood vessels almost in the center of the photograph.

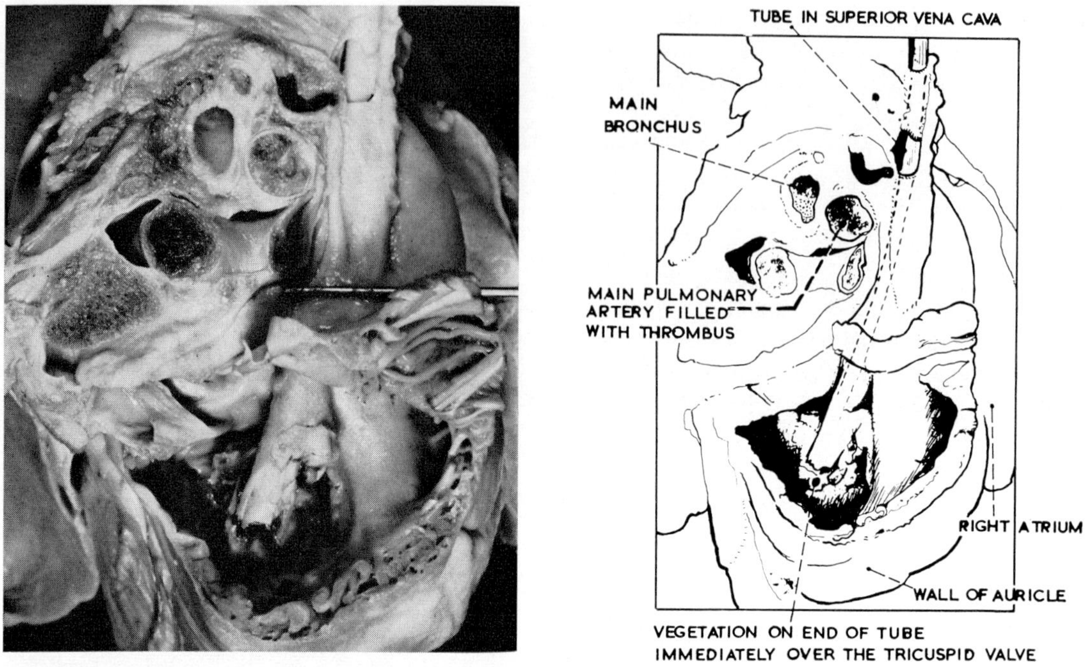


*A*

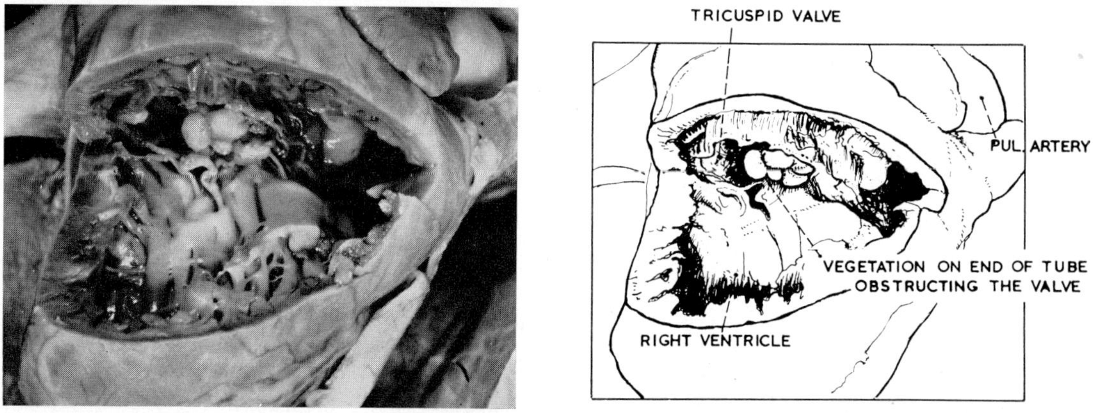


*B*

**Fig. 2.** *A,* The right lung cut across the hilum and the right atrium opened from above. The course of the catheter through the vena cava and entering the auricle can be seen, and a broken mass of thrombus is visible on the end of the catheter. The main pulmonary artery, adjacent to the main bronchus, is completely occluded by thrombus. *B,* The view looking up onto the free edge of the tricuspid valve through a wedge-shaped opening in the right ventricle.

**Other lesions of pulmonary vessels.**

*Mycotic aneurism formation.* In 7 cases intra-arterial thrombi were associated with suppuration, destruction of the arterial wall, and extension into the surrounding tissue. One such lesion is shown in Fig. 1, *B.*

*Periarteritis.* In several cases the first impression on superficial examination of the sections was that the lungs showed multiple areas of bronchopneumonia. Closer inspection showed that the local areas of inflammation were not associated with the bronchioles, but surrounded small blood vessels and in 8 cases multiple foci of periarteritis were found (Fig. 1, *C*). In these cases the vessels did not appear to contain thrombi and in some vessels cut longitudinally the periarteritis appeared to be completely focal and quite independent of any local intimal change.

*Intimal degeneration.* In 4 cases, intimal degeneration in the form of swollen, thickened intimal cells was found. This intimal change was not associated with any inflammatory infiltration. The latter lesions, however, are difficult to interpret in the light of the artefact found at postmortem examination.

**Thrombus formation on the wall of the right atrium.** In 6 cases the wall of the right atrium contained one or more plaques of smooth, yellow vegetation. These areas were not propagated thrombi from the superior vena cava and appeared to have arisen at the site of some trauma to the auricle. In several instances it was difficult to understand how trauma from the catheter could have occurred. In 2 instances the vegetations had progressed on the surface of the tricuspid valve and partially occluded the lumen.

**Local pericarditis.** In 1 instance in which catheter trauma was likely, there was local pericarditis over the area of vegetation.

**Massive pulmonary thrombosis.** In 2 cases the child died suddenly and unexpectedly and the major necropsy finding was complete occlusion of the pulmonary arteries by embolus. These emboli had apparently come from thrombotic masses already described around the end of the catheter in the auricle.

**Pulmonary hemosiderosis.** One child showed a remarkable clinical picture. After the insertion of Spitz-Holter valve and shunt, the child developed progressive anemia which necessitated repeated transfusions. At necropsy the lung was found to be indurated and brown. Microscopy of sections stained for iron showed many iron-laden macrophages within the alveoli and deposits of iron in and around the walls of small arteries (Fig. 1, *D*). The site of periarterial iron deposition corresponded exactly with the areas of periarteritis found in other cases. No inflammatory changes were seen. Sections stained for elastic tissue did not convince us that there was any primary defect in structure of the lung and we were forced to conclude that there was some relationship between the presence of the cerebrocardiac shunt and the hemosiderosis.

## DISCUSSION

The introduction of the Spitz-Holter valve appears to be associated with 2 groups of pathologic lesions in the heart and lungs; first, the local and embolic effects of thrombi on the end of the tube in the cardiac auricle, and second, lesions in the lung that appear to be independent of the presence of thrombi or embolism (that is, periarteritis, intimal degeneration, and possibly hemolysis and hemosiderosis). Since we do not know the constituency of cerebrospinal fluid throughout the history of these patients, we cannot say whether the changes in the pulmonary blood vessels are due to infected cerebrospinal fluid entering the pulmonary circulation or to a reaction of the vessel wall to what may be essentially a foreign cerebrospinal fluid protein.

The thrombotic lesions are more easy to understand and are probably of greater immediate clinical importance, as in 2 of the patients that died, cardiac signs developed with apparent tricuspid incompetence. Surgical interference and the removal of a large thrombus in the auricle appear to be a practical possibility.

The lesions that we have found in the lungs are very like those described in the older literature after endocarditis of the ductus arteriosus.[3, 7, 11] It is very important that pyrexia and periods of crepitations in the lung be treated seriously and not dismissed as being small areas of bronchopneumonia. If a child who has such a tube and shunt entering the auricle develops meningitis or pneumonia, it should be treated medically as acute bacterial endocarditis.

The patients discussed here are dead, but the frequency of small lesions in these cases suggests that similar lesions are probably present in children alive with these shunts. Unusual pulmonary and cardiac symptoms and signs are thus likely to occur in such cases and merit special clinical study.

## SUMMARY

Children who die after ventriculoauriculostomy shunt with the Spitz-Holter valve showed the presence of multiple lesions in the pulmonary circulation.

In addition to emboli and thrombi, there were local arteritis, periarteritis, and mycotic aneurysm formation. One child had pulmonary hemosiderosis.

Large thrombi attached to the end of the auricular catheter had caused tricuspid incompetence.

With any clinical infection, particularly of the meninges and lungs in children treated with such shunts, an associated acute endocarditis should be suspected.

Photographs were taken by Mr. Rickus and the drawings were made by Mr. Foster.

### REFERENCES

1. Anderson, F. M.: Ventriculo-auriculostomy in treatment of hydrocephalus, J. Neurosurg. **16:** 551-557, 1959.
2. Beck, C.: Discussion of Andrews, E. W.: A case of hydrocephalus treated by continuous drainage through a glass tube, Surg. Gynec. & Obst. **10:** 327, 1910.
3. Boldero, H. E. A., and Bedford, D. E.: Infective endocarditis in congenital heart disease, involving the pulmonary artery, Lancet **2:** 747-749, 1924.
4. Carrington, K. W.: Ventriculo-venous shunts using the Holter valve as a treatment of hydrocephalus, J. Michigan M. Soc. **58:** 373-383, 1959.
5. Cushing, H.: Studies in intracranial physiology and surgery. The third circulation. The hypophysis. The gliomas, London, 1926, Oxford University Press, chap. 12, p. 146.
6. Enderlen, L.: Zur Behandlung des Hydrocephalus, Beitr. klin. Chir. **76:** 889-890, 1911.
7. Fischer, R., and Schur, M.: Mykotische Endokarditis und Endarteritis der Arteria pulmonalis bei offenem Ductus Botalli, Klin. Wchnschr. **11:** 114-116, 1932.
8. Fleming, H. A., and Seal, R. M. A.: Staphylococcal infection following cardiac surgery, Thorax **10:** 327, 1955.
9. Gartner: Cited by Kausch.[14]
10. Haynes, I. S.: Congenital internal hydrocephalus. Its treatment by drainage of the cisterna magna into the cranial sinuses, Ann. Surg. **57:** 449-484, 1913.
11. Horder, T. J.: Infective endocarditis, with an analysis of 150 cases and with special reference to the chronic form of the disease, Quart. J. Med. **2:** 289, 1908.
12. Ingraham, F. D., Matson, D. D., Alexander, E., Jr., and Woods, R. P.: Studies in the treatment of experimental hydrocephalus, J. Neuropath. & Exper. Neurol. **7:** 123-143, 1948.
13. Kanavel, A. D.: Discussion of Andrews, E. W.: A case of hydrocephalus treated by continuous drainage through a glass tube, Surg. Gynec. & Obst. **10:** 327, 1910.
14. Kausch, W.: Die Behandlung des Hydrocephalus der kelinen Kinder, Arch. klin. Chir. **87:** 709-796, 1908.
15. McClure, R. D.: Hydrocephalus treated by drainage into a vein of the neck, Johns Hopkins Hosp. Bull. **20:** 110-113, 1909.
16. MacNab, G. H.: The Spitz Holter valve, J. Neurol. Neurosurg. & Psychiat. **22:** 82, 1959.
17. Nulsen, F. E., and Spitz, E. B.: Treatment of hydrocephalus by direct shunt from ventricle to jugular vein, S. Forum **2:** 299-408, 1952.
18. Payr, E.: Drainage der Hirnventrikel mittelst frei transplantirter Blutgefasse; Bemerkungen über Hydrocephalus, Arch. klin. Chir. **87:** 801-885, 1908.
19. Pudenz, R. H.: Experimental and clinical observations on the shunting of cerebrospinal fluid into the circulatory system. *In* Clinical Neurosurgery, Baltimore, 1958, Williams & Wilkins Company, vol. 5, chap. 6, pp. 98-114.
20. Pudenz, R. H., Russel, F. E., Hurd, A. H., and Shelden, C. H.: Ventriculo-auriculostomy: a technique for shunting cerebrospinal fluid into the right auricle; preliminary report, J. Neurosurg. **14:** 171-179, 1957.

# Measurement of arterial flow in the lower extremities with radioisotopes

JOHN E. APPLEN, M.D.
GEORGE S. LERMAN, M.D.*
PAUL E. WALKER, M.D.
STATEN ISLAND, N. Y.
*From the United States Public Health Service Hospital*

Radioisotopes have previously been used in attempts to determine the rate of blood flow in extremities. Their use was provoked by general dissatisfaction with the older methods of oscillometry, plethysmography, and colorimetry.

Radioactive sodium and $I^{131}$-labeled serum albumin have been the agents chiefly employed. Scintillation counters have proved most satisfactory as detection devices. Two general methods have been used; first, determination of the build-up of activity in a region after intravenous injection,[2, 5] and second, measurement of the rate of removal of a labeled diffusable local injection into the tissue.[4] Scintillation counters placed regionally are then used to determine the rate of build-up, or "wash-out," of the substances.

In practical application these methods have heretofore had 4 inherent deficiencies. First, in measuring build-up after intravenous injection the prolonged time needed to achieve intravascular mixing has led to sources of error. The slow mixing of the isotope reflects in late "contamination" of the curve which causes significant errors. Second, recently arterial injections of substances have been tried in order to diminish the mixing time.[1] Technical difficulties with this method, such as control of the speed of injection and geometric distortion produced by the injection, might impose a problem. In addition, if build-up curves were attempted over the lower leg after injection into the femoral artery, any pathologic process proximal to the point of injection might be missed. We have eliminated slow mixing as a source of error more simply by using a tourniquet technique. Third, dosage has also been a problem inasmuch as there are significant variations in the tissue–vascular space ratio in human beings, depending on obesity, muscle mass, and so forth. Fourth, the "wash-out" methods in which $Na^{24}$ is chiefly employed have the disadvantage of being influenced too greatly by local conditions such as edema, spasm, and actual tissue distortion from the injection.[3]

The shortcomings of the methods mentioned with their apparent inaccuracies and procedural complexity have relegated them to the research laboratory. There has been a need for a relatively simple, accurate, and objective method of evaluating patients with claudication-like symptoms. We have developed a method which satisfies these prerequisites. The method has been effectively used as a screening device and as an adjunct to arteriography.

The first portion of our study was conducted on laboratory animals. The object was to produce controlled arterial insufficiency and determine the relative efficiency of the radioisotope build-up method in reflecting the degree of arterial insufficiency.

## STUDIES IN DOGS

**Method and materials.** Twenty-seven dogs were studied in the laboratory under pentobarbital anesthesia. After heparinization, the

Received for publication Sept. 29, 1960.

*Present address: Veterans Administration Hospital, St. Louis, Mo.

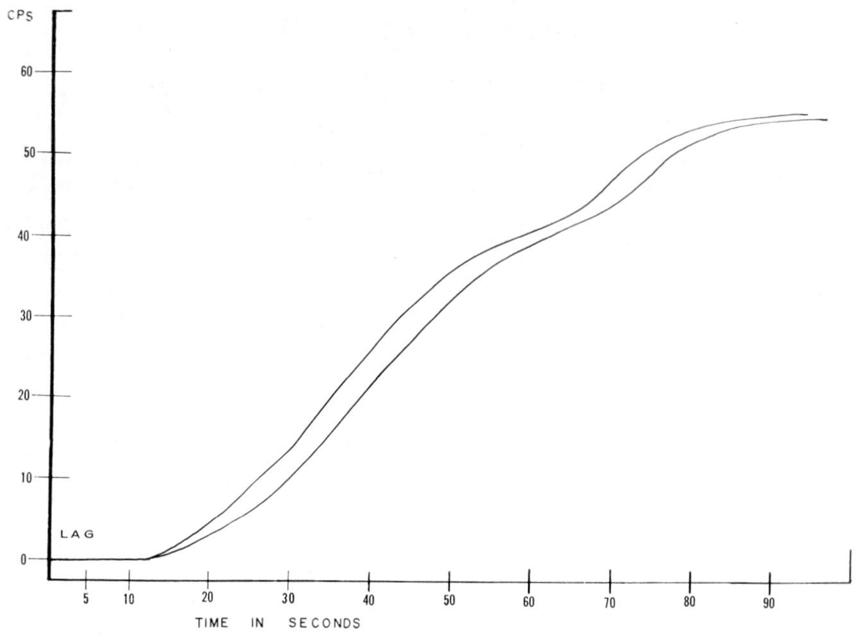


**Fig. 1.** This graph represents the uniformity of isotope response in 2 dogs of equal weight given equal dosages of $I^{131}$.

right femoral artery was cannulated to divert the blood through a recording flowmeter* and return it to the femoral artery at the level of the bifurcation of the profunda femoris. Readings on the flowmeter were interpreted in milliliters per minute. When the rate of flow had stabilized, albumin $I^{131}$ was rapidly injected through a catheter placed high in the brachial vein. A probe scintillation counter† placed against the popliteal area of the right leg below the cannulated femoral artery then recorded the rate of build-up of radioactivity as arterial blood flowed into the leg.

**Results.** The curves obtained in normal dogs were found to have a striking geometric uniformity and displayed 4 different features (Fig. 1): (1) an initial lag period of 10 seconds, (2) a sharp primary rise reaching a plateau at 30 seconds, (3) a secondary upward slope, and (4) an end point achieved after 90 seconds which did not fluctuate.

The slope of the curve and the magnitude of the end point were directly proportional to the dosage of $I^{131}$ per pound weight. Fig. 1 illustrates the identical response in 2 dogs of similar weight given equal dosages of the tracer.

We next attempted to produce arterial occlusion in the dog comparable to the syndrome seen in arteriosclerosis obliterans. After interruption of the generous collateral flow to the right leg, the iliac artery was partially occluded. The resultant degree of diminished blood flow in the leg was then measured with the mechanical flowmeter. After stabilization, the tracer was injected into the brachial vein in standard dosages. The degree of reduction in flow afforded by partial ligation of the iliac artery was reflected in the radioisotope build-up curve. Fig. 2 depicts the response in 4 animals which received 0.3 $\mu c$ of $I^{131}$ per pound. The upper curve is that of a normal dog. The 3 succeeding lower curves represent the graded slower response in animals with 75 per cent, 50 per cent, and 25 per cent of normal flow. It will be noted that the lag period and time to maximum response are progressively prolonged with increased oc-

*Rotameter and recording unit No. 45, Clifford Wilson, Indianapolis, Ind.

†NRD Radimax scintillation counter, NRD Instrument Company, St. Louis, Mo.

clusion and the slopes of the curves are lowered accordingly.

## STUDIES IN HUMAN SUBJECTS

**Materials and methods.** We next attempted to apply this method to human beings. Sixty patients, both normal and abnormal, have been tested. Abnormal patients were those with arteriographically proved occlusive disease. Except for the omission of the mechanical flowmeter and substitution of direct needle puncture in an antecubital vein for the brachial vein cut-down, the procedure was the same initially as that used in the animal studies. Two-tenths of a microcurie per pound was found to be a safe, workable dose of the tracer material.

After injection of the tracer into the vein the response curves achieved over the lower leg were found to be similar to those found in dogs. The lag period was more prolonged, however, and it was noted that some of the patients with proved arterial occlusion had build-up curves not unlike those seen in the lower range in normal patients. This apparently was due to slower mixing of the tracer material which had been introduced by direct venipuncture to simplify the technique.

This error was obviated by application of an arterial tourniquet to the thigh of the leg being studied immediately prior to the injection and for a period of 2 minutes thereafter. A tourniquet pressure of 450 mm. was maintained during this period. There were no untoward effects from the tourniquet, even in patients with postoperative grafts. The use of the tourniquet allowed the isotope to be homogenously distributed everywhere except in the leg in which flow was being measured. Upon rapid release of the tourniquet, the tagged blood was suddenly allowed to flow into the leg and the geometry of the arterial bolus was reflected in counts per second by the recorder attached to the scintillation counter. Fig. 3 shows that the response in normal human subjects is extremely predictable.

**Results.** In 20 normal subjects tested by this method the lag time was found to vary only 2 seconds. The range was from 2.0 to 4.0 seconds. In 10 consecutively studied patients with proved occlusive disease the lag period varied from 10 seconds to infinity

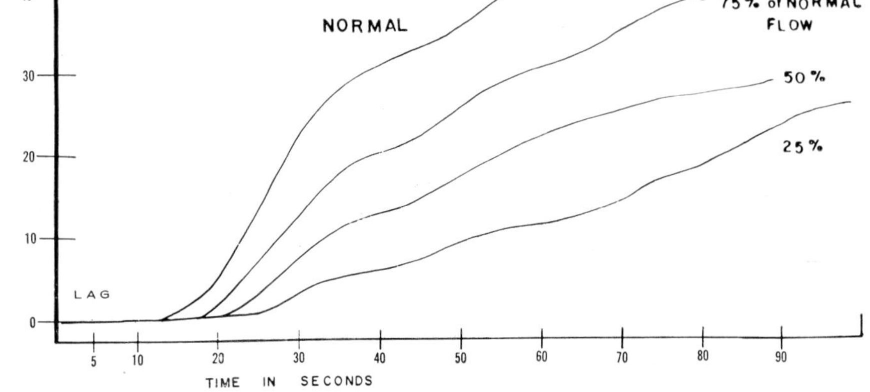


**Fig. 2.** Curves representing isotope response in a normal animal contrasted to the responses achieved in dogs with progressive occlusion of the femoral artery.

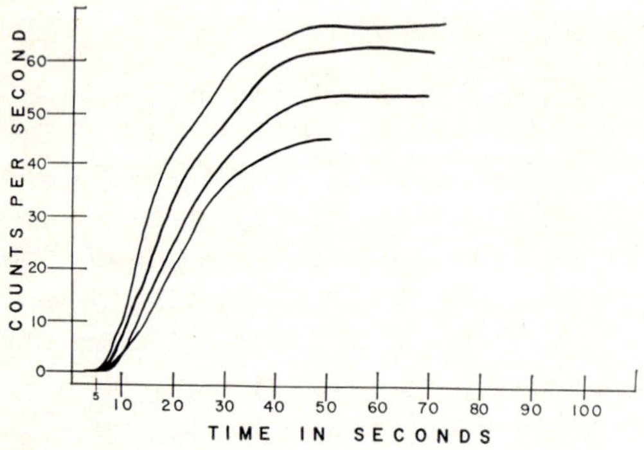


**Fig. 3.** Isotope response pattern in normal human subjects. Note the relatively short lag time. The time needed to reach maximum concentrations ranges from 30 to 40 seconds.

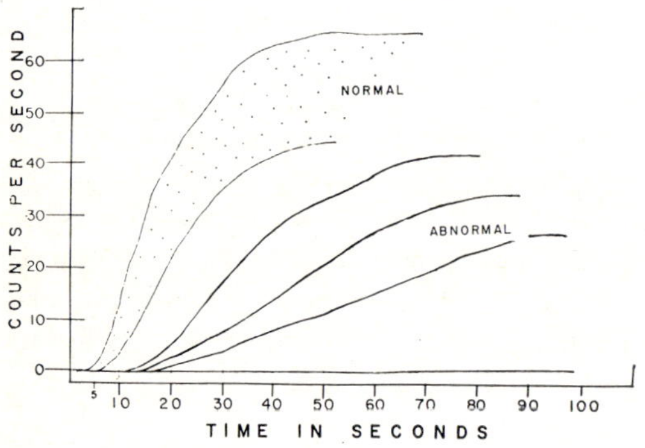


**Fig. 4.** Illustration of the range of isotope response in normal subjects as contrasted to patients with proved arterial occlusive disease. Note the increasing lag time and delay of maximum response with disease.

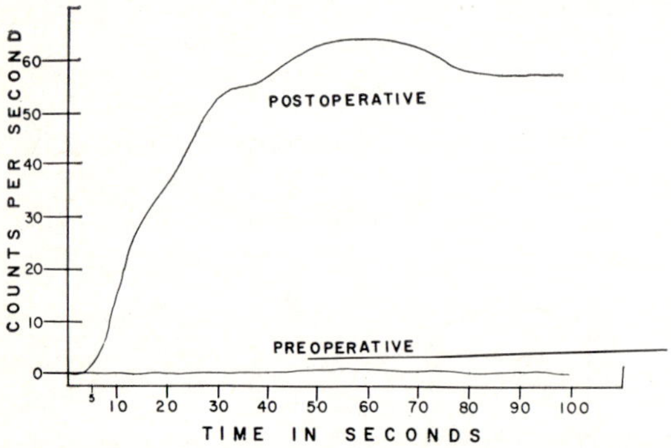


**Fig. 5.** Pre- and postoperative results in a patient with occlusion of a femoral graft. The graft was replaced surgically and the build-up curve improved dramatically.

(Fig. 4). This characteristic tends to separate clearly the normal from the abnormal group.

Normal patients were found to have a steeper slope.

The end point was achieved in from 30 to 50 seconds in normal subjects. The time to end point in the abnormal group varied from 65 to 120 seconds.

It is significant that the rapidity of response in abnormal subjects was grossly proportional to the degree of obstruction evidenced clinically. For example, the uppermost curve in the abnormal group was that of a patient who had occlusion of the superficial femoral artery with sufficient collateral circulation to give him a palpable popliteal pulse. The lowermost curve was that of a postoperative femoral graft patient who, 1 year after operation, entered the hospital with acute occlusion of the graft and developed a white, pulseless limb. At the time of operation there was complete ischemia of the leg, as suggested by the lack of any response to the isotope test.

Fig. 5 depicts the pre- and postoperative response of the latter patient, who underwent a successful regrafting procedure and had return of the pedal pulses.

## DISCUSSION

With the procedure described, a vascular space exists distal to the tourniquet which is free of radioactive material. This space has volume, $V_t$.

After the release of the tourniquet this volume (V) can be divided into 2 subvolumes, $V_1$ and $V_2$. $V_1$ equals that part of the original volume ($V_t$) that is filled with radioactive material. $V_2$ equals that part of the original volume (V) that is devoid of radioactive material. Thus, $V_1 + V_2 = V_t$ (equation 1). The blood containing radioactive material proceeds down the femoral artery and its branches until it reaches the arterioles. During this flow toward the arterioles no mixing need be postulated.

The release of blood from the arterioles into the capillary beds and subsequent collecting venules then occurs. The collecting venules will now contain blood with radioactive material and also nontagged blood. Thus, the collecting venules will represent the radioactivity of the blood arriving at the arterioles mixing with the blood free of radioactivity. This mixing occurs because of the arteriolar sphincters which may retard emptying of some of the arterioles. It is at this collecting region that mixing occurs.

This assumed mechanism can be expressed as equation 2,

$$\frac{dV_2}{dt} = \frac{(F \times A)}{(Vt)} \times V_2 = {}^{-}kV_2$$

where $k = \frac{F \times A}{V_t}$, F equals an equivalent flow in milliliters per area times time, A equals an equivalent area, and $V_t$ equals total vascular volume of the limb. F and A are equivalent values and constants since the actual flow and cross sectional area change from point to point over the vascular tree.

The negative sign implies a continuing decrease in $V_2$ from time zero (the release of the tourniquet).

Integrating equation 2,

$$V_2 = V_2^{o}e^{-kt},$$

where $V_2^{o} = V_2$ at t = O, but at t = O, $V_2 = V_t$. Thus, equation 3 is

$$V_2 = V_t e^{\frac{-FA}{V_t}t}$$

But from equation 1 ($V_t = V_1 + V_2$), substituting equation 3,

$$V_t = V_1 + V_t e^{\frac{-FA}{V_t}t} \text{ or } V_1 = V_t\ (1 - e^{-kt})$$

The radioactivity is proportional to $V_1$

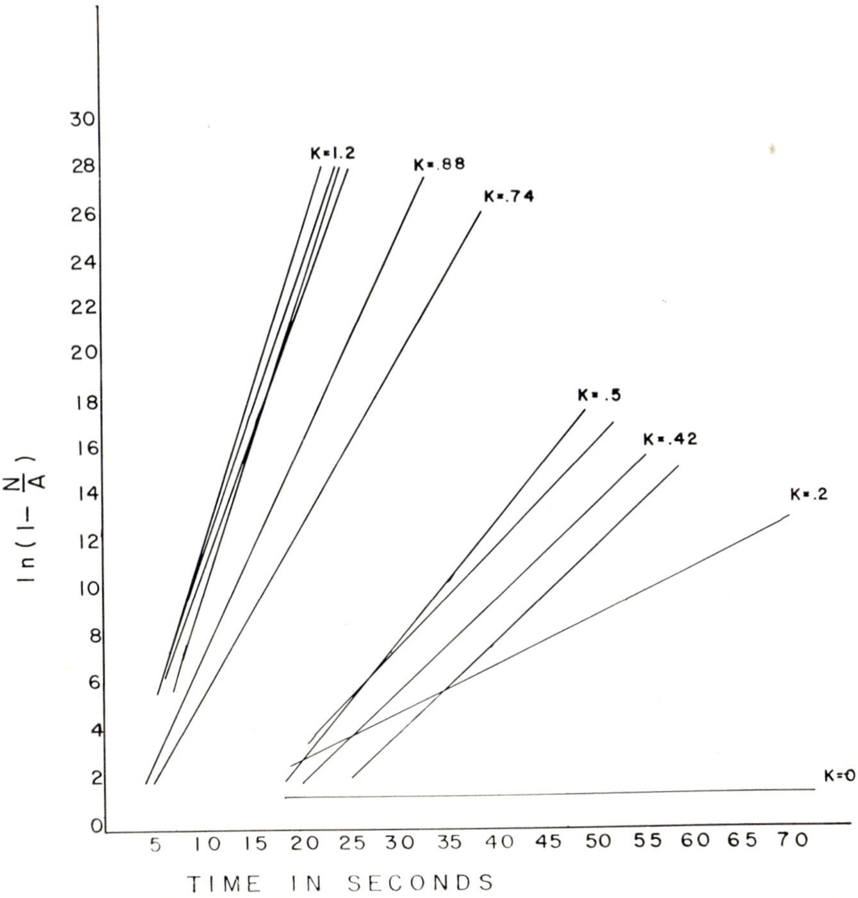


**Fig. 6.** Graph shows how k relates to the slope of the curves achieved by plotting ln $(1-\frac{N}{A})$ versus time. The slope, or k, decreases with disease. k values below 16 indicate arterial occlusive disease.

Table I

| Age | Signs and symptoms | $k \times 10^2$ | Relaxation time T (sec.) | Lag time (sec.) |
|---|---|---|---|---|
| 27 | Control | 7.4 | 13.5 | 3.0 |
| 39 | Control | 6.4 | 15.6 | 4.0 |
| 46 | Control | 8.0 | 12.5 | 3.5 |
| 51 | Control | 7.0 | 14.3 | 3.0 |
| 54 | Control | 7.0 | 12.2 | 2.0 |
| 56 | Control | 12.2 | 8.2 | 2.0 |
| 56 | Control | 11.5 | 8.7 | 2.0 |
| 60 | Control | 10.0 | 10.0 | 2.0 |
| 39 | Iliac block | 3.0 | 33.3 | 7.5 |
| 49 | Femoral block | 4.0 | 25.0 | 11.5 |
| 55 | Femoral block | 5.0 | 20 | 7.5 |
| 57 | Femoral block | 5.1 | 19.5 | 10.5 |
| 60 | Femoral occlusion | 4.0 | 25.0 | 7 |
| 61 | Femoral occlusion | 4.3 | 22.8 | 7.5 |
| 64 | Midfemoral block | 4.1 | 24.4 | 15 |
| 65 | Femoral block | 4.0 | 25.0 | 6 |
| 54 | Complete graft occlusion | 0 | 00 | (No response) |

and after a sufficient time has elapsed $V_1$ equals $V_t$. Thus, in equation 4,

$$N = A\left(1 - e^{-\frac{FA}{V_t}t}\right)$$

where N equals radioactive counts at a time t and A equals maximum of radioactive counts achieved after complete filling.

Plotting N versus t, we get curves of the same shape as our experimentally derived response curves, which verifies our assumption as to the mechanics of flow, at least to the first order approximation.

The constant $k - \frac{FA}{V_t}$, as previously mentioned, thus depends on flow, crossectional area, and the vascular volume $V_t$. The flow is dependent on a number of variables, the most important being tube diameter, blood pressure, elasticity of the arterial and arteriolar system, viscosity of the blood, and the pulsatile character of the blood flow. Of these parameters, tube diameter is the primary determination of F, since the resistance to flow varies inversely with the fourth power of the tube radius. It seems, therefore, that the value of the parameter $\frac{FA}{V_t} = k$ should correlate well with the presence and degree of narrowing and obstruction resulting from arterial occlusive disease.

$\frac{FA}{V_t}$ has the dimension of reciprocal seconds and is the reciprocal of the relaxation time T $\left(T = \frac{V_t}{FA}\right)$.

T represents the relaxation time of the filling process which is the time necessary for the radioactive material to wash in to 1/e of the total volume $V_t$.

Plotting $\ln\left(1 - \frac{N}{A}\right.$ versus time in seconds), a series of straight lines results, the slope of which is the disease constant $k = \frac{FA}{V_t}$. For convenience we have plotted log base 10 and T represents the time needed to fill 1/10 of the volume $V_t$ with radioactive material.

These curves exhibit 3 features, at first a lag time, then a straight-line portion, and at the end an upward deviation from the straight line.

Table I summarizes the experimental results. The plots on patients with known arterial disease gave very good straight lines after an initial lag period. On controls, the best straight line through a set of points was chosen. It is possible that the more rigid arterial walls of the experimental patients gave rise to less nonlinear flow effects than the elastic arterial walls of the control group.

## SUMMARY

A method in which radioactive iodinated serum albumin is utilized for the evaluation of the rate of blood flow in extremities has been presented. The reliability of the method was tested in the laboratory on animals and substantiated by mathematical analysis. The efficiency of the method is undeniable and it is safe. The dosage of the tracer used is less than that used for a thyroid uptake test.

Use of the mathematical expression of the curve allows the examiner to plot the results in such a manner that previous annoying sources of error are automatically corrected and a numerical index of flow is achieved. Use of a numerical expression permits ready recognition of diminished flow in a simple standard manner and provides a base line that can be re-evaluated during the course of therapy.

## REFERENCES

1. Dobson, E. L., and Warner, G. F.: Clearance rates following intra-arterial injections in the study of peripheral vascular beds, *in* Bruner, H. D., editor: Methods in medical research, Chicago, 1960, The Year Book Publishers, Inc., vol. 8, pp. 242-248.
2. Halligan, E. J., Gibbs, J. C., Grieco, R. U., and McKeown, J. D.: An evaluation of peripheral arteriosclerotic insufficiency utilizing radioactive iodinated human serum albumin, Surg. Gynec. & Obst. **102:** 511-516, 1956.
3. Hyman, C.: Peripheral blood flow measurements: tissue clearance, *in* Bruner, H. D., editor: Methods in medical research, Chicago, 1960, The Year Book Publishers, Inc., vol. 8, pp. 242-248.
4. Kety, S. S.: Quantitative measurement of regional circulation by the clearance of radioactive sodium, Am. J. M. Sc. **215:** 353, 1952.
5. Smith, B. C., and Quimby, E. H.: Use of radioactive sodium in studies of circulation in patients with peripheral vascular disease, Surg. Gynec. & Obst. **79:** 142-147, 1944.

# Venous occlusion of the terminal ileum: an experimental study

BENJAMIN B. JACKSON, M.D.
LOUISVILLE, KY.
*From the University of Louisville School of Medicine**

The basic unit of the intestinal organ, the cell, should have prime consideration as pathologic processes impinge upon its normal function. The goal of this experimental study was to relate the alterations in the gross appearance of the dying intestinal cell to its oxygen tension and pH. In an effort to compile data on the oxygen tension and hydrogen ion concentration in the cellular environs, we studied a strangulated segment of terminal ileum viewed through a plastic abdominal window. It was hoped that a less artificial environment for study of venous occlusion might be obtained with the use of the abdominal window.

This paper represents a study of venous occlusion in an apparently closed loop of terminal ileum in 10 dogs in which abdominal windows had been placed.

## EXPERIMENTAL METHOD

**Plastic window insertion.** The technique for inserting a plastic window in the anterior abdominal wall of the dog has been previously described.[6] Two weeks were allowed before strangulation experiments were performed. Fourteen dogs had Plexiglas windows implanted in the abdominal wall, but 4 were excluded because of adhesions and infection. A screw tap was placed at one end of the plastic window so that studies could be carried out without removing the window (Figs. 1 and 2).

Received for publication Dec. 21, 1960.

*Work begun at the laboratories of surgical research at Harvard Medical School and completed at the University of Louisville School of Medicine.

**Strangulation obstruction technique.** With the animal under light Nembutal anesthesia (10 mg. per kilogram), a segment of ileum 30 cm. in length approximately 30 cm. from the ileocecal valve was chosen as the site of obstruction. The veins draining this segment were ligated. This portion of the terminal ileum was manipulated into a circular loop and a linen ligature was loosely applied so as not to prevent arterial inflow. The closed loop was returned to the peritoneal cavity via the screw opening in the Plexiglas window.

**Methods of measuring oxygen tension.** The apparatus was adapted from the tensiometer designed by Davies and Brink[3] and utilized by Montgomery and Horowitz[7-9] (Fig. 3). It consisted of a platinum electrode in a fixed low voltage. The resultant current was proportional to the oxygen tension in the cellular environment and could be read as deflections on a galvanometer.

Fluctuations in the oxygen tension attributable to temperature and precipitation of proteins on the electrode were minimized by utilization of a constant voltage of lv. and by reading the galvanometer 10 seconds after the application of the electrode to the bowel wall. A 60-second interval was allowed between readings and an average of 3 readings was recorded at any given time. The electrode pierced the gut wall for about 2 mm. at an angle of 60 degrees. Calibration of the electrode was obtained by determination of oxygen tension in nonviable bowel in saline solution of known oxygen tension. Corrections were made for temperature.

In order to demonstrate that the oxygen tension measured was in the tissue, readings were taken from normal bowel and 60 minutes after arterial occlusion. If the arterial supply was restored and the animal was permitted to breathe 100 per cent oxygen, the segment improved remarkably in color in 30 seconds. However, the oxygen tension remained at a low level for approximately 120 seconds and then increased rapidly. This was construed as some evidence that the oxygen tension in the cells or interstitial fluid was being measured rather than the oxygen tension in the small peripheral vessels.

**Method of measuring pH.** A modification of the technique employed by Claff and Swenson[1] was used. A microglass electrode

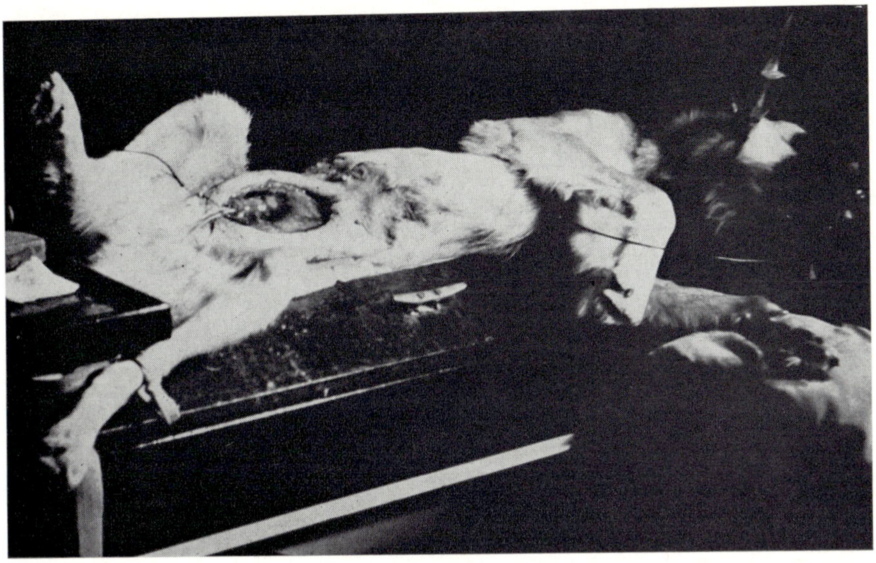

**Fig. 1.** Animal with Plexiglas abdominal window undergoing strangulation experiment under continuous light Nembutal anesthesia.

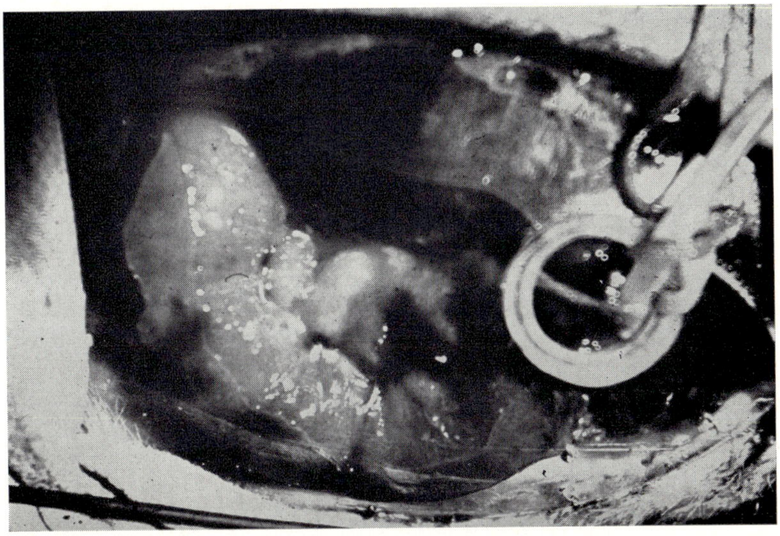

**Fig. 2.** Close-up view of abdominal window. Note the strangulated segment.

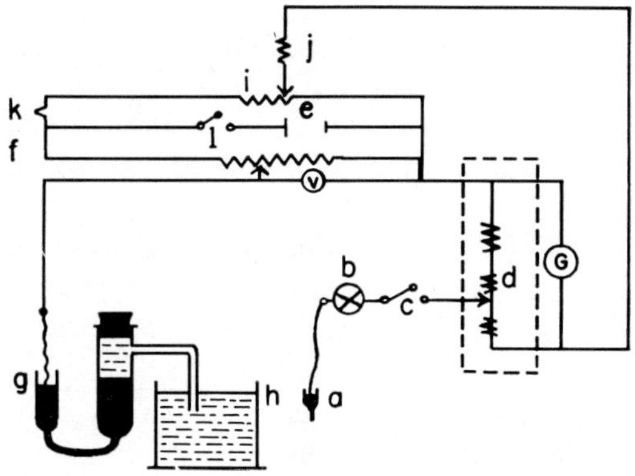


**Fig. 3.** Diagram of the circuit of the oxygen tensiometer. *a,* Electrode tip (cathode); *b,* selector switch; *c,* electrode switch; *d,* Aryton shunt resistance to 65,000 ohms; *e,* dry cell (1.5 v.); *f,* variable resistance; *g,* calomel half cell (anode); *h,* 0.85 per cent sodium chloride in beaker; *i,* variable resistance (500 ohms); *j,* fixed resistance (2 million ohms); *k,* fixed resistance (40,000 ohms); and *l,* main switch. *G,* Rubicon galvanometer, and *V,* voltmeter. The circuit is completed after the insertion of the animal's tongue in the beaker of saline solution and the electrode in the bowel wall.

which required as little as 0.05 ml. of fluid was used for determination of the hydrogen ion cencentration (Fig. 4).

The microtube was inserted beneath the serosa for about 2 mm. at an angle of 60 degrees and allowed to fill by capillary attraction. The subsequent measurement of the electromotive force coincided with the technique of Claff and Swenson. Using a standard acetate reference buffer solution with a tolerance error ± 0.02, we recorded reproducible results within the tolerance of the buffer solution.

## EXPERIMENTAL DATA

**Gross appearance of bowel and mesentery.**

*Normal bowel.* The mesentery was approximately 2 mm. thick, smooth, glistening, and pale pink. Mesenteric vessels coursed through it, producing vascular arcades. The bowel diameter was approximately 1.2 cm. and the bowel wall was 3 to 4 mm. in thickness. The serosal surface had a bluish pink hue. The antimesenteric border was irregular from peristaltic indentations. At least 4 types of movement could be discerned; pendular, constrictive, rotary, and long undulating waves. The degree of activity appeared to have a direct relationship to the height of the pulsations of the mesenteric arteries.

*Thirty minutes after venous occlusion.* The mesentery had doubled in thickness and appeared hemorrhagic with mottled areas of cyanosis. Arterial pulsations could be observed easily. The serosa was smooth, glistening, and moist. The diameter of the bowel was 1.75 cm. Constrictive and pendular types of peristalsis were present. The color of the bowel was red to pink with mottled areas of congestion. There were numerous transverse indentations which extended to the antimesenteric border of the bowel. Dilated mural vessels lay prominently in these grooves. The bowel looked as if it has been converted into thousands of tiny sphincters approximately 2 mm. apart.

*One hour after venous occlusion.* The mesenteric vessels lay in deep furrows at 2 to 6 cm. intervals. The mesentery looked like ballooned triangles with the bases nearest the gut wall. There was little change in the general appearance of the bowel wall except for mottled congestion.

*Two hours after venous occlusion.* The mesentery appeared to be overriding the intestine and dissecting the serosa from the longitudinal muscle layer. The mesentery was 1.5 cm. thick and looked spongy, wet, and granular. The diameter of the intestine was 2.25 cm. Infinitesimal trauma to the intestinal wall which produced spasm caused occlusion of the bowel lumen. Small spastic areas appeared as pasty, bluish-white depressions. Some of the capillaries had ruptured and gave the gut a flea-bitten appearance. The intestinal wall had increased to 0.55 cm. in thickness. Arterial pulsations could be seen. The most pronounced change remained in the mesentery.

*Three to 5 hours after venous occlusion.* The mesentery had shortened and produced a peristalsis-like effect. Dissection of the serosa continued. More fibrin had accumulated on the surface of the gut and mesentery. Not infrequently a capillary bed with all its arborizations could be made out with small knobs which represented rupture of the limbs of the capillary tree. The antimesenteric border was irregular and looked cyanotic. The diameter of the gut was 2.4 cm. The arterial pulsations were no longer visible.

*Five to 8 hours after venous occlusion.* The mesentery had increased to 2.2 cm. in thickness. The mesenteric triangles were adherent from the deposition of fibrin. It seemed that there was little transudation of fluid into the peritoneal cavity, but that the fluid was sequestered in the layers of the bowel wall. The diameter of the bowel had increased to 2.6 cm. There were numerous cyanotic areas that contained hematomas of dark black blood. The mural veins had formed straight, dilated lines accentuated by dark blood. Pendular peristalsis was present.

*Eight to 12 hours after venous occlusion.* The mesentery was 2.4 cm. in thickness and was very granular. Dissection of the serosa had ceased due to the disproportionate increase in the gut wall. The bowel had a reddish-blue tinge. The hematomas were numerous and were becoming confluent. In areas along the antimesenteric border, some of the hematomas had ruptured and left large drops of black, incoagulable fluid on the serosal surface. Thromboses were prominent in the vasa recta and the arcuate vessels. Merely touching the serosa would cause it to break. The bowel wall had thickened to 0.85 cm. Temperature had declined from 38° to 27° C. No peristalsis was evident.

*Twelve to 15 hours after venous occlusion.* The condition of the mesentery was unchanged. The bowel had a bluish-black color with a granular feel. The antimesenteric border was bathed in a black, incoagulable fluid from the herniated hematomas. The line of demarcation between the strangulated loop and the bowel above and below was quite striking. Cyanosis was most pronounced as transverse streaks leading into the mesenteric furrows. The mesentery was 2.5 cm. thick. The diameter of the intestine was 2.8 cm. and the gut wall was 1.4 cm. in thickness. The entire loop had a diffusely black color. The gut wall was smooth and motionless at this stage.

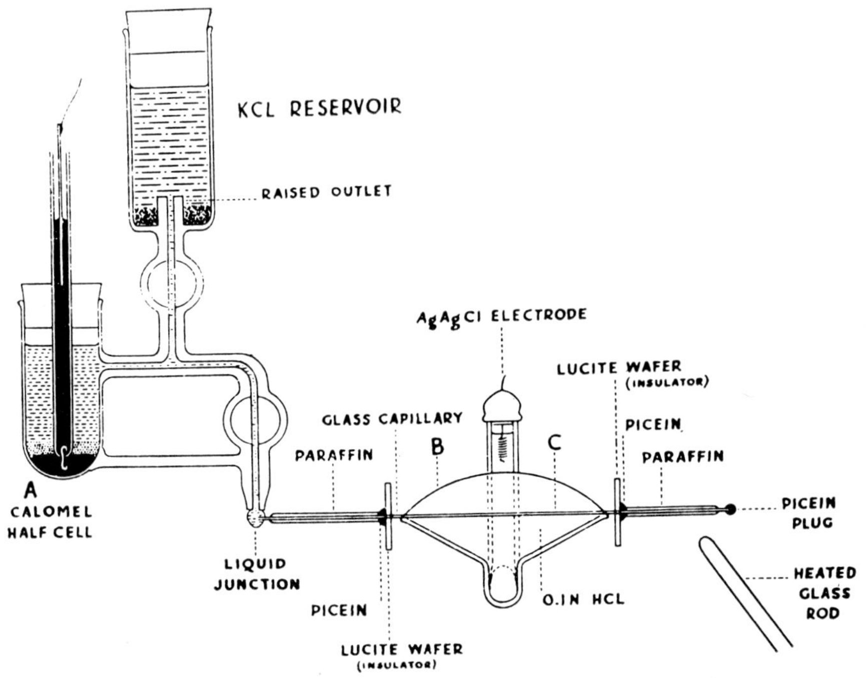


Fig. 4. Diagram of pH meter.

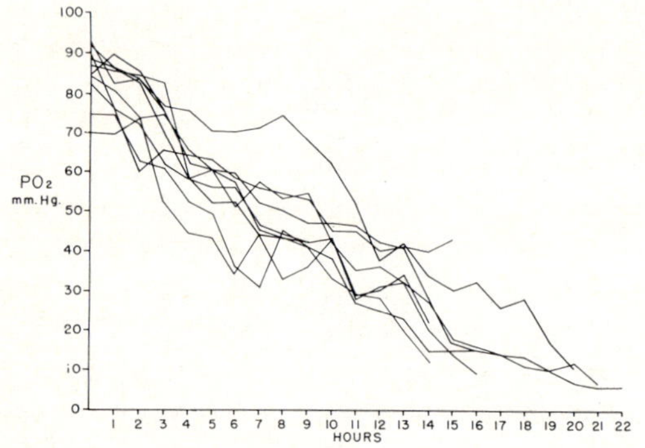


**Fig. 5.** Alterations in oxygen tension in 10 dogs with venous occlusion of 1 foot of terminal ileum.

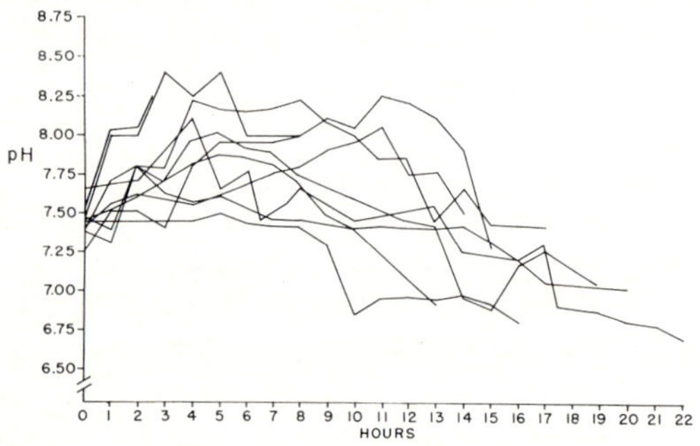


**Fig. 6.** Changes in pH recorded in 10 dogs after venous occlusion of 1 foot of terminal ileum.

*Fifteen to 20 hours after venous occlusion.* No visible changes in the bowel could be recorded from this point.

**Peritoneal fluid.** During the experiment 35 to 160 ml. of transudate was collected. The weight of the bowel at the time of death had increased an average of 301 per cent. Initially the fluid was clear, serous, and odorless. Between 6 and 12 hours the fluid had become incoagulable and had the odor of decaying blood. After the fourteenth hour the fluid had become thick and dark red to black in color. With the window technique it was impossible to calculate fluid loss from peritoneal absorption or dilution.

## DISCUSSION

In this series of experiments the greatest decrease in oxygen tension was between 2 and 12 hours (Fig. 5). The measurement of oxygen tension in the cells declined as time after occlusion increased but the cells appeared to utilize oxygen for 18 to 20 hours. It may be that further oxygen utilization represented bacterial metabolism rather than consumption by the intestinal cells. However, the fact that the oxygen tension in the dying tissue was not equal to the oxygen tension of the air would indicate that some type of cellular activity persisted. In spite of continuing cellular respiration, numerous thromboses in the mural vessels and vasa recta made it impossible to restore normal oxygen consumption after 18 to 20 hours. Even if thromboses were not present, the edema and hemorrhage into the bowel wall, no doubt, would preclude adequate oxygenation.

Rising intercellular pressure as evinced by the gradual increase in size and weight of the bowel wall probably also contributed to the reduction in the diffusion gradient of oxygen to the cells. Intercellular pressure must be equal to the arterial inflow pressure at the end of 14 to 16 hours of obstruction, for there was no detectable increase in the weight of the bowel and mesentery after that time interval. Additional studies will be required to relate intercellular pressure to oxygen tension and pH.

There was an alkaline pH in the period of greatest oxygen decline (Fig. 6). As bowel ischemia increased, cellular autolysis began. Oxygen deprivation and changing pH may alter the structure of the cell membrane and make it more permeable. With a postulated increase in cell membrane permeability, there could be an ingress of alkaline salts from the blood into the interior of the cell.[5, 10] This mechanism may account for the paradoxical alkalinity which occurred between the second and fourteenth hours after venous occlusion. The cellular environment is in reality acidic, but this is masked by the collection of alkaline fluids.

The physical appearance of the bowel after 12 to 14 hours of venous occlusion in a closed loop had a fairly accurate biochemical correlation. After 12 hours, there was no motility of the diffusely black and edematous bowel. There were herniated hematomas on the antimesenteric border. The serosa broke upon gentle touch, the temperature had declined 9° C., and the bowel wall had become sausage-shaped and approximately twice its original thickness. There was much variation, but it appears that the point of irreversible necrosis is reached when the serosa will break upon touch, the bowel wall has increased to twice its thickness when compared with the normal bowel below the strangulation, and the temperature has decreased 8 to 10° C. After a 12- to 14-hour period of venous strangulation, there was a critical decline in oxygen tension and evidence of rising hydrogen ion concentration.

The average length of survival of the 10 dogs after venous ligation in an apparently closed loop of a 1-foot segment of terminal ileum was 13.4 hours.

It is not to be inferred that these observations are necessarily basic. Rather, they tend to confirm and amplify the conclusions of previous investigators.

## SUMMARY AND CONCLUSIONS

1. An attempt was made in 10 dogs to correlate oxygen tension and pH changes with gross appearance in a hypoxic segment of terminal ileum.

2. The greatest decline in oxygen tension occurred in a 10-hour period between 2 to 12 hours after venous occlusion.

3. Acidic pH was recorded after 14 hours of venous obstruction but it is believed that an ingress of alkaline body fluids masked the true degree of cellular autolysis in the early hours of venous occlusion.

4. The point of irreversible necrosis in this series of experiments occurred after 14 hours of venous ligation and was grossly reflected in rupture of the serosa, increase in the bowel wall to twice its original thickness, and temperature decline from 38° to 27° C. The gross changes in hemorrhagic infarction closely paralleled declining oxygen tension and pH.

## REFERENCES

1. Claff, C. L., and Swenson, O.: Micro-glass electrode technique for determination of hydrogen ion activity of blood and biological fluids, J. Biol. Chem. **152:** 519-522, 1944.
2. Consolazio, C. F., Johnson, R. E., and Marsh, E.: Metabolic methods, St. Louis, 1951, The C. V. Mosby Company.
3. Davies, P. W., and Brink, F.: Micro electrodes for measuring oxygen in animal tissue, Rev. Scient. Instruments **13:** 524-535, 1942.
4. Dole, M.: The glass electrode, London, 1941, John Wiley & Sons, Inc.
5. Goldstein, L.: A study of the mechanism of activation of the cell and nuclear membranes in the chaetopterus egg, Biol. Bull. **105:** 87-102, 1953.
6. Jackson, B. B.: Observation on intraperitoneal adhesions, Surgery **44:** 507, 1958.
7. Montgomery, H., Sinsser, H. F., and Horowitz, O.: Oxygen tension of tissue by the polariographic method, Circulation **2:** 845-849, 1950.
8. Montgomery, H., and Horowitz, O.: Oxygen tension in tissue by the polariographic method, J. Clin. Invest. **29:** 1120-1130, 1950.
9. Montgomery, H., and Horowitz, O.: Oxygen tension by the polariographic method, J. Clin. Invest. **27:** 550, 1948.
10. Roselthal, S. M., and Tabor, H.: Electrolytes and chemotherapy in experimental burns and traumatic shock and hemorrhage, Arch. Surg. **51:** 244-252, 1945.

# Renal tubular necrosis: its relation to norepinephrine administration

W. CHUNG, M.D.
V. ŠIMA, M.D.
KARLOVY VARY, CZECHOSLOVAKIA
*Departments of Pathology and Surgery, County General Hospital (OUNZ)*

Nephropathies characterized by tubular lesions have been ascribed to a number of etiologic factors—burns, blackwater fever, transfusions with incompatible blood, sulfonamide intoxication, toxemias of pregnancy, uteroplacental damage, mercury poisoning, severe trauma, and shock.[4] Recently Boughton and Sommers[1] have described patients who at autopsy were found to have massive necrosis of the renal tubules and attributed the lesion to a combination of shock and administration of levarterenol, a vasopressor amine. Moyer and associates,[7] however, have reported that in the normotensive subject norepinephrine causes reduction of renal blood flow because of vasoconstriction, but in the hypotensive subject it markedly improves function. In view of the widespread usage of vasopressor agents in combating surgical shock, the question of possible renal complications is of more than mere academic interest. The present communication is a preliminary report of 11 instances in which renal lesions identical to those described by Boughton and Sommers were found at autopsy. The possible pathogenetic mechanism is discussed with regard to the alleged effects of vasopressor amines in normotensive and hypotensive states.

## MATERIAL AND RESULTS

The patients studied represented a variety of surgical conditions (Table I). With the exception of those in Cases 1 and 5, all underwent either emergency exploratory operation of the abdomen or an elective procedure. Norepinephrine* administration in 5 per cent glucose infusions was instituted in the postoperative period immediately upon recognition of a state of peripheral circulatory collapse. The time interval between diagnosis of circulatory collapse and norepinephrine administration did not exceed a maximum of 1 hour. The dosage rate was varied in each case so as to restore and maintain normal blood pressure. In the majority of cases the patients died suddenly not long after termination of norepinephrine administration.

Necropsy was performed, on the average, within 8 hours after death. Nonprotein nitrogen was determined on blood obtained at autopsy.

Grossly, the kidneys were in no way remarkable. Microscopically, the renal lesion was quite distinctive and fairly uniform in all the patients. The intact glomeruli and the loops of Henle in the cortex stood out in marked contrast against a background of deeply eosinophilic, structureless tubules (Figs. 1 and 2).

The glomeruli were swollen and usually occupied the entire Bowman's space. Cellularity was not increased (Fig. 3). Along the rim between the swollen glomeruli and the capsule occasional desquamated epithelial cells and scanty amounts of proteinous ma-

Received for publication Oct. 3, 1960.

*Levarterenol hydrotartarate (Spofa).

terial were found. This was often but not invariably the case. The epithelium of Henle's loop appeared to be slightly swollen, but aside from this no abnormality could be seen either in nuclear or cytoplasmic structure. Very rarely small amounts of proteinous material were seen in their lumina.

Both the proximal and distal segments of the convoluted tubules were necrotic and showed complete dissolution of nuclei. The cytoplasm was coarsely granular and projected into the tubular lumina, either partially or completely occluding them. The interstitial spaces around the tubules were somewhat edematous, but free of inflammatory cells. The basal membrane was undamaged. In a few instances it was not discernible in the most severely damaged areas.

The medulla presented no pathologic changes. Casts were often found but were considered nonspecific and incidental.

In patients who underwent bile tract operations the liver was always examined in order to exclude possible hepatorenal syndromes, the pathogenesis of which is still obscure and not properly a part of the present study.

Appraisal of the severity of the tubular necrosis with regard to the total dose or the dosage rate of norepinephrine administration did not show any particular relationship. Neither did the nonprotein nitrogen bear any relationship to the amount of norepinephrine.

## DISCUSSION

There are 2 generally accepted causes of tubular necrosis. One is toxins, either bacterial or chemical, and does not concern

**Table I.** *Patients with renal tubular necrosis who received norepinephrine*

| *Case No.* | *Age* | *Sex* | *Diagnosis* | *Operation* | *Total dose (mg.)* | *Duration (hr.)* | *μg/hr.* | *Non-protein nitrogen** |
|---|---|---|---|---|---|---|---|---|
| 1 | 63 | F | Pyosalpinx with generalized peritonitis† | None | 6 | 48 | 125 | 73 |
| 2 | 31 | F | Sigmoid cancer | Sigmoidectomy | 20 | 10 | 2,000 | 146 |
| 3 | 51 | M | Internal abdominal injuries | Laparotomy, suture of ruptured intestinal loops | 15 | 8 | 1,880 | 216 |
| 4 | 38 | M | Pelvic fracture | Laparotomy | 40 | 72 | 550 | 200 |
| 5 | 24 | M | Ruptured appendix with generalized peritonitis† | None | 10 | 9 | 1,100 | 185 |
| 6 | 47 | F | Choledocholithiasis | Choledocholithotomy | 6 | 2 | 3,000 | 200 |
| 7 | 47 | F | Bronchiectasis | Lobectomy | 14 | 4 | 3,500 | 160 |
| 8 | 65 | F | Choledocholithiasis | Choledocholithotomy, cholecystectomy | 32 | 18 | 1,777 | 155 |
| 9 | 61 | M | Hemorrhagic pancreatitis | Laparotomy | 40 | 27 | 1,481 | 174 |
| 10 | 51 | F | Ruptured appendix with generalized peritonitis | Appendectomy | 22 | 18 | 1,222 | 180 |
| 11 | 68 | M | Carcinoma ventriculi | Gastrectomy | 24 | 14 | 1,714 | 163 |

*Postmortem.

†Clinically undiagnosed.

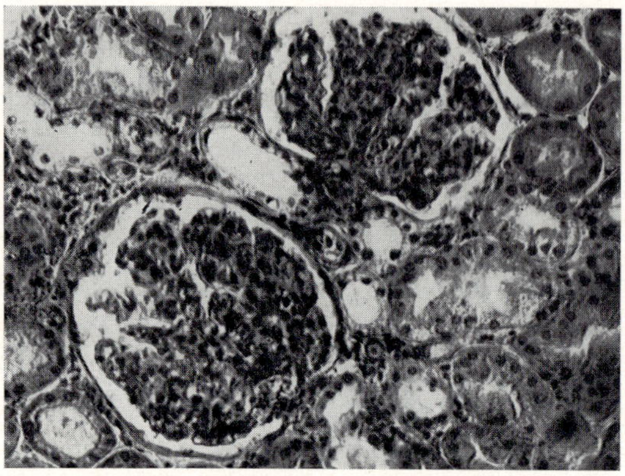

**Fig. 1.** Normal kidney. (Hematoxylin and eosin; ×170.)

us in this discussion. The other is ischemia. In spite of the number of excellent studies[5, 8] on tubular necrosis, it is still far from clear how ischemia acts in producing a selective necrosis of the convoluted tubules. The glomeruli, the loops of Henle, and the collecting ducts are known to be notably resistant to ischemia.

It is perhaps appropriate at this point to recall briefly the vasculature of the kidney. The renal artery, upon entry into the kidney, gives rise to the arcuate branch which courses between the cortex and the medulla. The interlobular artery passes off from the arcuate and traverses the cortex, sending the short vasa afferentia to the glomeruli. Beyond the glomeruli the vasa efferentia divides into 2 channels, one going to the peritubular network and the other (rectae) to the medulla (presumably in close association with the ascending and descending loops of Henle). The important point is that blood supplying the convoluted tubules and the medulla is, for all practical purposes, postglomerular in origin. The paraglomerular contribution is negligible, if at all operative. If ischemia intervenes, it is curious, then, why one segment, the proximal and distal tubule, should be injured while the other, Henle's loop and the collecting duct, remains intact.

Two problems arise, first, to explain how ischemia in general causes selective tubular necrosis, and, second, to explain how norepinephrine acts in producing the same type of lesion.

With regard to the first question, the usual explanation advanced is that the tubular epithelium represents a highly differentiated structure and hence is more vulnerable to ischemic injury than other segments of the nephron.[11] This concept was perhaps tenable at one time when the collecting ducts were considered merely inert conduits without functional significance. Today it is clear that, on the contrary, the ducts are highly specialized structures. In the countercurrent multiplier system proposed by Wirz,[13] it is precisely in the ducts that the glomerular filtrate is concentrated for final disposal, a process which requires an eminently high degree of differentiation.

A more plausible explanation for the genesis of tubular necrosis is to found in the new theory of plasma skimming in the renal vessels. It was originally proposed by Pappenheimer and Kinter[2, 3, 9] to provide a better account of certain fundamental facts peculiar to renal physiology, that is, constancy of renal blood flow, glomerular filtration, and arteriovenous oxygen difference over a wide range of arterial pressure.

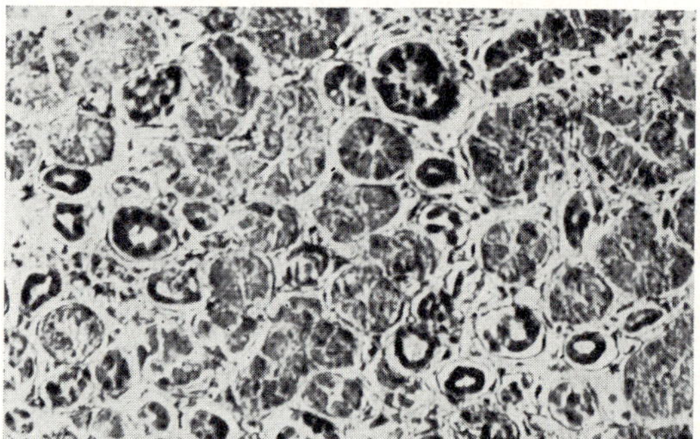

**Fig. 2.** Complete necrosis of the proximal and distal segments of the convoluted tubules with dissolution of structure and swelling of cytoplasmic remains. The dark structures interspersed among the necrotic tubules are the intact loops of Henle. The interstitial tissue shows moderate edema. (Hematoxylin and eosin; ×170.)

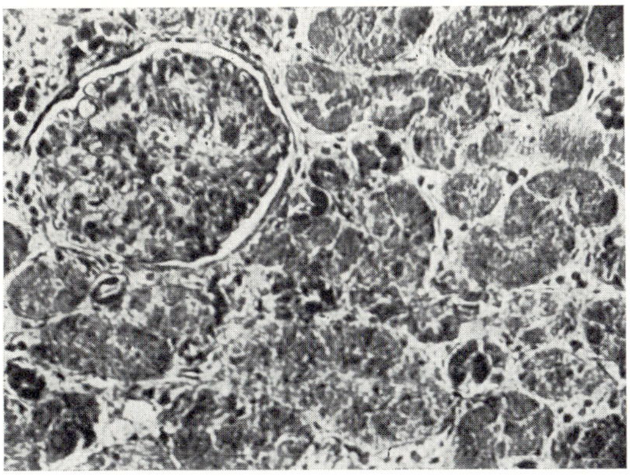

**Fig. 3.** Granular eosinophilic masses of necrotic tubular epithelium surrounding a swollen but otherwise intact glomerulus. Compare with Fig. 1. (Hematoxylin and eosin; ×170.)

The fundamental physical basis for this theory is a high velocity axial flow of red blood cells combined with branching networks which drain off plasma from the periphery of the flow stream. The degree of separation is dependent on the corpuscular content and the kinetic energy. With normal corpuscular content there is with each increment in arterial pressure a greater separation of blood into 2 streams. The net effect is increased vascular resistance due to increased viscosity, since the latter increases as a function of the third power of the red blood cell concentration. Such a mechanism would maintain renal blood flow and glomerular filtration at relatively constant rates regardless of wide arterial pressure fluctuations. In addition, shunting of the cell-poor moiety into the peritubular capillary system would imply a lower oxygen uptake from the blood stream and thus a low arteriovenous oxygen difference.

The critical assumption in the theory is a peculiar geometry of the renal vessels at 2 points. It is assumed that the afferent arterioles and the arteriole to the peritubular network branch off from their respective vessels at right angles so as to drain off the plasma much more effectively as the blood stream is separated.

Let us consider now how cell separation can produce selective ischemia of the tubules and necrosis. At a renal arterial pressure of 140 mm. Hg and a normal hematocrit of 0.45, the intrarenal hematocrit is 0.20. (The intrarenal hematocrit is one of the important points which demonstrate a redistribution of red blood cells and plasma in the kidney tissue.) Let us assume that for each 100 ml. of blood flowing through the kidney, 8 ml. of cells and 48 ml. of plasma pass through the tubules. This gives an intrarenal hematocrit of 0.14, which is fairly close to the value experimentally determined by Pappenheimer and Kinter and which indicates that most of the intrarenal hematocrit is contributed by the peritubular blood. The 8 ml. of erythrocytes bathing the tubules provides 3.5 ml. of oxygen. The rectae, on the other hand, contain 37 ml. of erythrocytes capable of delivering 16.1 ml. of oxygen to Henle's loop and the collecting ducts. Consequently, there is, under physiologic conditions, an uneven supply of oxygen to the nephron.

Let us now assume that there is a 60 per cent reduction in renal blood flow, due either to blood loss or internal redistribution of total blood, with roughly normal corpuscular content. Further, let us assume that shock is still in its reversible phase and that the renal arterial pressure is reduced to about 96 mm. Hg. This would mean that such a reduction in kinetic energy, with normal corpuscular content, would, as a first approximation, produce an intrarenal hematocrit of 0.28, or a reduction in cell separation by a factor of 1.4. The cell separation would still be of such a magnitude as to make the effect of decreased oxygen supply always much more severely felt in the convoluted tubules than in the loops of Henle and the collecting ducts.

It is probably the peculiar anatomic arrangement and the functional mechanism of cell separation which make the tubular epithelium more susceptible to ischemic damage than other parts of the nephron. The kidneys hence possess an intrinsic mechanism which, although admirably effective under a variety of conditions, can in certain circumstances be to their own detriment.

**Table II.** *Tubular sodium loss in hypotensive patients after norepinephrine administration (calculated from data of Moyer[7])*

| Patient | | Glomerular filtration rate (inulin) | Plasma Na (mEq./L.) | Filtered Na load* (mEq./L.) | Excreted Na (mEq./min.) | % excreted Na lost through tubules* |
|---|---|---|---|---|---|---|
| W. H. | C | 3 | 130 | 0.39 | 8 | 95 |
| | $V_1$ | 114 | 128 | 14.5 | 20 | 27 |
| | $V_2$ | 92 | 128 | 11.8 | 19 | 38 |
| | $B_1$ | 67 | 133 | 8.9 | 25 | 64 |
| | $B_2$ | 155 | 134 | 20.7 | 451 | 95 |
| M. C. | C | 10 | 135 | 1.4 | 39 | 96 |
| | $V_1$ | 60 | 127 | 7.6 | 179 | 96 |
| | $V_2$ | 78 | 127 | 9.9 | 192 | 95 |
| | $B_1$ | 82 | 123 | 10.0 | 188 | 94 |
| L. M. | C | — | 135 | — | 0 | — |
| | $V_1$ | 5 | 135 | 0.7 | 61 | 99 |
| | $V_2$ | 16 | 131 | 2.1 | 152 | 98 |
| | $B_1$ | 23 | 125 | 2.8 | 663 | 99 |
| | $B_2$ | 119 | 123 | 14.6 | 108 | 87 |
| T. H. | C | 128 | 136 | 17.5 | 124 | 85 |
| | $V_1$ | 137 | 135 | 18.5 | 114 | 84 |
| | $V_2$ | 140 | 135 | 18.9 | 129 | 85 |
| | $B_1$ | 184 | 136 | 25.0 | 276 | 91 |

*Calculated.

C, Control during shock.

$V_1$, Partial restoration of blood pressure with a vaso-pressor agent.

$V_2$, Complete restoration of blood pressure with a vasso-pressor agent.

$B_1$, Immediately after transfusion of blood.

$B_2$, Follow-up study.

It is believed that the illustration given provides a fairly good account of the genesis of tubular ischemia and necrosis. This is not to be construed that in its present form the theory does not raise a number of problems which still remain to be investigated. It does, however, offer a unifying concept, the predictions of which are amenable to experimental verification.

With regard to the effect of norepinephrine, it has been reported by Moyer and colleagues[7] that in the hypotensive state there is an improvement in renal function and blood flow. They suggest that the improvement is due to the ambivalent behavior of norepinephrine which causes differential vasoconstriction between the kidney and the remainder of the general circulatory bed. A re-evaluation of their data shows that their conclusions are completely untenable. First, analysis of the relationship between sodium excretion and urine flow shows an abnormally exaggerated osmotic diuresis, indicating impairment of tubular function. Furthermore, all of the filtered sodium was lost in the urine with no tubular reabsorption. Indeed, practically all of the urinary sodium was derived from nonfiltered sources, that is, tubular sources (Table II). This in itself is clear evidence of tubular dysfunction, if not frank necrosis. Consequently, it cannot be accepted as proved that norepinephrine has a beneficial effect on renal function as Moyer claims. In fact, the evidence is to the contrary.

Norepinephrine reduces renal blood flow by vasoconstriction.[10] Assuming that cell separation is in operation, the net effect would be the same as described previously, that is, deprivation of oxygen to the convoluted tubules first and foremost. If this vasoconstriction takes place under circumstances of a pre-existing reduction in renal blood flow such as in hypotension, the ischemic effect would be additive. Boughton and Sommers[1] originally implicated the combination of shock and norepinephrine as the cause of tubular necrosis in their patients.

But they were unable to explain the pathogenetic mechanism.

Additional evidence that vasopressor amines can produce tubular necrosis comes from experimental studies with serotonin (5-hydroxytryptamine). This substance, which is allied to norepinephrine in its vasoconstrictive properties, has been shown to be capable of producing renal necrosis and both tubular and massive cortical necrosis.[6, 12]

We have been impressed by the fact that a number of patients receiving equal or greater doses of norepinephrine than in the present series failed to show any morphologic signs of tubular necrosis. It appears that this may be due to either extreme hypotension or extreme vasoconstriction (physiologic or pharmacologic). These are the 2 conditions under which cell separation no longer operates in the renal vessels. In extreme hypotension (below a critical level) the kinetic energy available is insufficient to divide the blood into 2 streams. Similarly, extreme vasoconstriction reduces the velocity of blood flow to such a degree that axial streaming no longer obtains. In either case the normal unequal oxygen distribution would be nullified in order to compensate for a decrease in over-all oxygen supply. In effect, this would represent a check mechanism for extreme variations detrimental to renal function.

The importance of possible deleterious effects of norepinephrine administration lies perhaps not so much in the production of frank tubular necrosis as in the development of various degrees of tubular dysfunction. The latter is probably much more common than is suspected and, unless the clinician bears it in mind, can easily go unnoticed. This does not mean that it is of no significance. In the postoperative period, when the proper functioning of the body's homeostatic mechanisms is of the utmost importance, any unbalancing of homeostasis such as in tubular dysfunction with consequent loss of base conservation, to mention but one aspect, would prolong recovery and impair wound healing.

## SUMMARY

A preliminary report of studies now in progress is presented on the effect of norepinephrine on the kidneys. It describes the postmortem finding of massive necrosis of the convoluted tubules with sparing of the glomeruli, the loops of Henle, and the collecting ducts. The lesion is attributed to the administration of norepinephrine. The pathogenesis of the lesion is discussed and is based on considerations of the theory of cell separation in the renal vessels.

### REFERENCES

1. Boughton, A. J., and Sommers, S. C.: Renal changes in shock treated with levarterenol (Levophed), Am. J. Clin. Path. **28:** 29, 1957.
2. Kinter, W. B., and Pappenheimer, J. R.: Renal extraction of PAH and diodrast-$I^{131}$ as a function of arterial red cell concentration, Am. J. Physiol. **185:** 391, 1956.
3. Kinter, W. B., and Pappenheimer, J. R.: Role of red blood corpuscles in regulation of renal blood flow and glomerular filtration rate, Am. J. Physiol. **185:** 399, 1956.
4. Kolff, W. J.: Acute renal failure: causes and treatment, M. Clin. North America **39:** 1041, 1955.
5. Lucké, B.: Lower nephron nephrosis, Mil. Surgeon **99:** 371, 1946.
6. MacDonald, R. A.: Pathogenesis of lesions induced by serotonin, Am. J. Path. **35:** 297, 1959.
7. Moyer, J. H., Morris, G., and Beazley, H. L.: Renal hemodynamic response to vasopressor agents in the treatment of shock, Circulation **12:** 96, 1955.
8. Oliver, J., MacDowell, M., and Tracey, A.: The pathogenesis of acute renal failure associated with traumatic and toxic injury: renal ischemia, nephrotoxic damage, and the ischemic episode, J. Clin. Invest. **30:** 1307, 1951.
9. Pappenheimer, J. R., and Kinter, W. B.: Hematocrit ratio of blood within the mammalian kidney and its significance for renal hemodynamics, Am. J. Physiol. **185:** 377, 1956.
10. Pullman, T. N., and McClure, W. W.: The response of the renal circulation to constant-speed infusions of l-norepinephrine, Circulation **9:** 600, 1954.
11. Sheehan, H. L., and Moore, H. C.: Renal cortical necrosis and the kidney of concealed accidental hemorrhage, in Page, I. H., and Corcoran, A. C., editors: American lecture

series, Springfield, Ill., 1952, Charles C Thomas, Publisher, No. 167.

12. Waugh, D., and Pearl, M. J.: Serotonin-induced acute nephrosis and renal cortical necrosis in rats, Am. J. Path. **36:** 431, 1960.

13. Wirz, H., Hargitay, B., and Kuhn, W.: Lokalisation des Konzentrierungsprozesses in der Niere durch direkte Kyroskopie, Helvet. physiol. et pharmacol. acta **9:** 196, 1951.

# Mannitolization. I. The prevention and therapy of oliguria associated with cross-clamping of the abdominal aorta

KEVIN G. BARRY MAJOR, MC, USA
ARTHUR COHEN, LIEUTENANT COLONEL, MC, USA
PRESTON LeBLANC, B.S.
WASHINGTON, D. C.
*From the Department of Metabolism, Division of Medicine, Walter Reed Army Institute of Research, and the Department of Surgery, Walter Reed General Hospital*

Cross-clamping of the abdominal aorta (CCAA) is necessary during abdominal aneurysmectomy. Many satisfactory operative procedures are complicated by oliguria, acute renal failure, and death. Powers[10] reported a 30 per cent incidence of oliguria and 4 fatal cases of acute renal failure which occurred after CCAA in a 12-month interval at Albany Hospital. Twenty per cent of the deaths associated with elective aneurysmectomy at the Mayo Clinic[12] are due to acute renal failure. Recovery from acute renal failure which complicates cross-clamping of the abdominal aorta is a rarity.

The lengthening life span and technical surgical advances increase yearly the number of elderly, poor-risk patients acceptable for aneurysmectomy and requiring CCAA. Therefore, the development of a safe method which protects against CCAA oliguria and acute renal failure is urgent and important. The only previously reported method requires the use of ganglionic blocking agents to maintain the systolic blood pressure at 70 to 80 mm. Hg during the operation.[10] The maintenance of hypotension in these elderly patients might increase the risk of cerebrovascular accidents and myocardial infarctions. Therefore, a more innocuous therapy is needed.

Studies at Walter Reed Army Medical Center in which dogs were utilized have shown that an abrupt decrease in renal blood flow, glomerular filtration rate, and urinary flow occurs when CCAA is performed.[6] One of the authors (A. C.) has found a similar abrupt fall in urinary flow in man when the aortic clamp is applied during aneurysmectomy.[8] Mannitol has been utilized by the Walter Reed Army Medical Center group to protect against epinephrine-induced fatal renal failure in dogs.[7] Water loading alone was unsuccessful.

The authors have successfully used intravenous mannitolization for the prevention and therapy of CCAA oliguria in human beings. It is the authors' judgment that the urgent need for safe protection against acute renal failure complicating aneurysmectomy warrants publication of a preliminary report. It is hoped that many centers will give this innocuous therapy prompt clinical trial.

## METHODS

Mannitol is a 6-carbon hexahydric alcohol. It is distributed in the extracellular fluids and freely filtered at the glomerulus. It is not reabsorbed from the renal tubules. It is inert and nontoxic.[5] Theoretically, as a result of the noted properties, and in our experience, mannitol is the most effective and least toxic renal osmotic solute available.

Mannitolization was used by one of the authors (K. G. B.) for therapy in refractory

Received for publication Oct. 10, 1960.

cardiac and cirrhotic fluid retention unresponsive to the usual spectrum of diuretic regimens. The excellent results led to its use in cases of acute left and right heart failure. The diuresis was prompt and massive with parallel clinical improvement within 2 hours of initiation of mannitolization.[1] Mannitolization was then tried in 1 patient with acute cerebral edema after an open-heart operation. Again, prompt diuresis was obtained. Many of the patients studied were in precarious cardiopulmonary condition because of combinations of myocardial, valvular, and coronary heart disease. In over 50 trials, no evidence of circulatory overload or other deleterious effect was found.

The initial use of intravenous mannitolization in CCAA occurred when Patient 1 manifested oliguria after aneurysmectomy. A 50 ml. ampule of 25 per cent mannitol was heated to dissolve all crystals and aspirated into a preheated syringe. It was administered at approximately body temperature directly intravenously over a 3-minute period. The same procedure was followed in Patient 2. Since the therapy was effective in these oliguric patients, it was decided to try mannitolization prophylactically to prevent oliguria during CCAA. This was successfully accomplished in Patients 3 and 4.

An infusion of 5 per cent mannitol in water was initiated in Patient 3 after intubation, bladder catheterization, and urinary collection during a control period. An infusion rate of 10 ml. per minute was used until vigorous diuresis was established and then infusion flow rate was adjusted to maintain urinary flow rate every 10 minutes. During the period of CCAA a 20 per cent infusion at a maintenance flow rate was used. Para-amino-hippurate clearance was used to measure effective renal plasma flow; glomerular filtration was measured by insulin and endogenous creatinine clearance studies. The results are described in Case 3. The treatment of Patient 4 was performed as an emergency when our supply of mannitol was limited. Therefore, a smaller amount of mannitol was administered and administration was interrupted for 82 minutes. The experience with these 2 cases, especially the finding that effective renal plasma flow and glomerular filtration rate decreased abruptly when the aorta was clamped despite continuing diuresis (Case 1) prompts us to propose the following protocol:

1. oral water load, 20 ml. per kilogram, 0500 hours, day of operation
2. 0 to 10 minute control urine collection after intubation and urinary bladder catheterization
3. 10 minutes to approximately 45 minutes prior to clamp application, 5 per cent mannitol at 15 ml. per minute until urine flow stable for 10 minutes; then adjustment of infusion rate to equal urinary flow rate
4. 45 minutes prior to clamping, 20 per cent mannitol infusion rate adjusted to equal urinary flow rate
5. clamp application to abdominal closure; 5 per cent mannitol infusion adjusted to equal urinary flow

N.B. Infusion of 20 per cent mannitol for at least 30 minutes prior to cross-clamping takes priority over all other steps.

## CASE REPORTS

**Clinical study in postclamping oliguria.**

*Case 1.* A 73-year-old white woman underwent aortic cross-clamping for resection of aneurysm on April 15, 1960. The aorta was cross-clamped above the right renal artery for 13 minutes. Fig. 1 demonstrates the occurrence of oliguria with urinary output averaging 14 ml. per hour and urinary specific gravity dropping from 1.020 to 1.013 during the 30 hours prior to the intravenous administration of mannitol. After the administration of 12.5 Gm. of mannitol over a 5-minute period, urinary output increased dramatically to 125 ml. the third hour after administration. The rate of intravenous fluid administration was not increased until after diuresis had been established. Also, the urinary specific gravity had followed the course usually seen in early renal failure and the blood urea nitrogen had risen from a preoperative value of 13 mg. per 100 ml. to 25 mg. per 100 ml. The failure of the urinary specific gravity to rise after mannitol had been given suggests that the patient was not dehydrated at the time of administration, since it has been our experience in other studies that the dehydrated patient will have urinary specific gravities of approximately 1.035 after mannitol infusion.

*Case 2.* A 67-year-old white man underwent sigmoidal resection for carcinoma on April 20, 1960. At the time of operation an aortic aneurysm was discovered and removed. Cross-clamping of the aorta below the renal arteries was necessary. During the first 10 postoperative hours, the hourly urinary output averaged 6.5 ml. with a specific gravity of 1.016 as illustrated in Fig. 2. After administration of 12.5 Gm. of mannitol intravenously over a 5-minute period, the output increased dramatically to 20 ml. within 1 hour and 50 ml. per hour by 3 hours. In contrast to Case 1, the urinary specific gravity rose to 1.024, which is more commensurate with normal hydration. Again, the rate of fluid administration was not increased until diuresis had been established.

*Comment.* These cases represent 2 instances in which a medical regimen for acute renal failure was considered. The patient in Case 1 was over 72 hours postoperative and showed the usual milestones of acute renal failure as measured in terms of adequate hydration, stable blood pressure, specific gravity of 1.013, and rising blood urea nitrogen associated with oliguria. The failure to increase urinary specific gravity after mannitol administration was also suggestive of normal or overhydration. It should be recalled that the therapy once recommended for early post-traumatic oliguria included rapid administration of dextrose and water. Subsequently, it was thought that any beneficial effect was simply in the restoration of circulating blood volume or rehydration. Recently, the use of osmotic diuretics for hemoglobinuria in burn patients has been recommended.[4, 11] The possibility that mannitol, via its osmotic diuretic and probable homeostatic effects on the kidneys, may be therapeutic in early severe oliguria must be investigated.

Mannitolization abolished consideration of an acute renal failure regimen in these cases and reassured the authors concerning the patient's renal status in management. The delivery of urine in large amounts to the specimen bottle is the most important consequence of mannitolization in these cases of oliguria.

**Clinical studies in the prevention of oliguria after aortic cross-clamping.**

*Case 3.* A 63-year-old white man without previous history of cardiovascular renal disease and normal results of studies relative to these systems was noted to have an abdominal aneurysm on physical examination prior to radiation therapy of a nasopharyngeal malignancy. An elective aneurysmectomy in which a bifurcation graft was utilized was performed May 17, 1960. The changes of urinary flow associated with the operative procedure and mannitolization are illustrated in Fig. 3. Mannitol was used as a 5 per cent solution except during the period of cross-clamping of the aorta. During this 58-minute interval, 20 per cent mannitol was infused. A urinary flow rate of over 6 ml. per minute was obtained prior to clamping. Urinary flow continued to rise over 7 ml. per minute during occlusion of the aorta. Vital signs remained stable and the patient excreted over 3,000 ml. of urine during the 24-hour period subsequent to operation. Postoperatively, the blood urea nitrogen, serum electrolytes, and urinalysis remained unremarkable. Urinary specific gravity varied from 1.010 to 1.028.

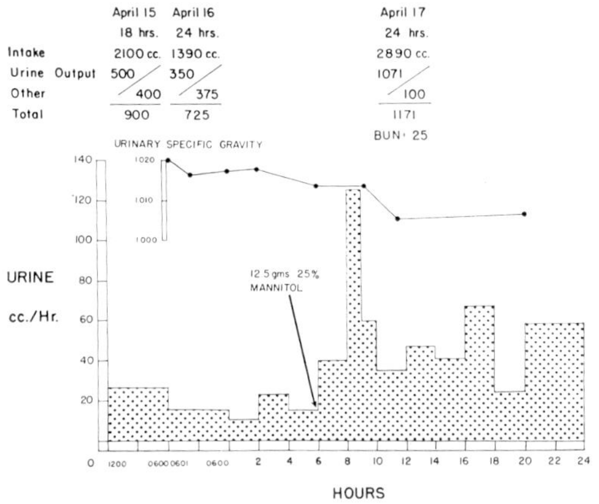


**Fig. 1.** Study of Case 1 was initiated at 1200 hours, April 15, upon admission to recovery ward after operation. Contiguous time intervals are plotted along the abscissa. The time scale is expanded on April 17 to emphasize the prompt diuresis after mannitolization. Arrow indicates initiation of a 3-minute mannitol infusion. Note drop in specific gravity from April 15 to 17. The further decrease during mannitol diuresis may indicate overhydration or intrinsic renal dysfunction.

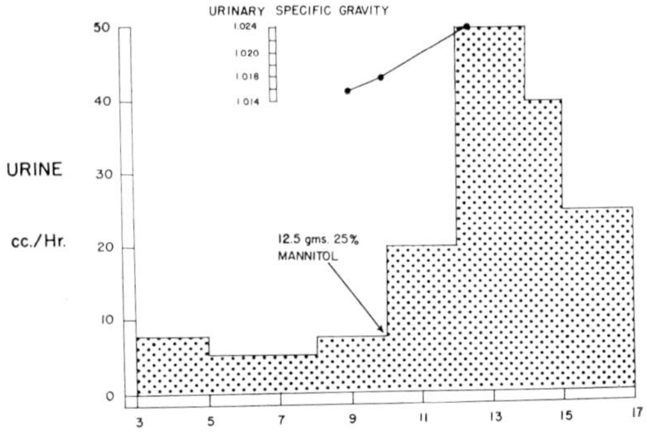


**Fig. 2.** Study of Case 2 was initiated 3 hours after operation. Note prompt diuresis after mannitolization. Arrow indicates time at which 3-minute mannitol infusion was started. Urinary specific gravity rose slightly during diuresis, possibly indicating normal hydration.

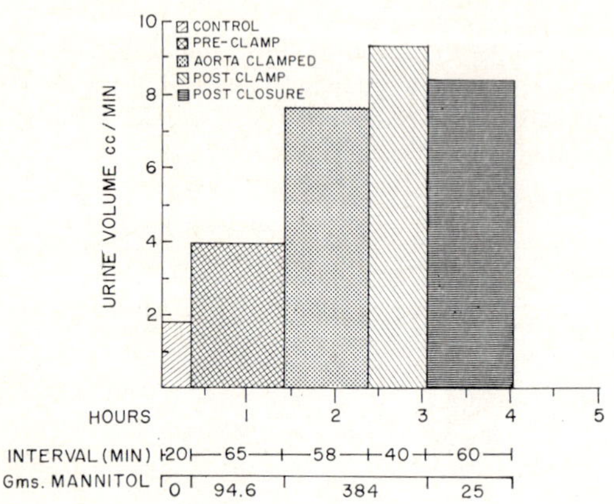


**Fig. 3.** Study of Case 3 was initiated after intubation and bladder catheterization. Time scale is contiguous. Control urine was collected prior to operation and postclosure specimens upon its completion. Below abscissa, concordant with time scale, are plotted time interval for each phase of the study and quantity of mannitol infused per interval. Five per cent mannitol was infused except during CCAA, when a 20 per cent solution was used. Note acceleration of urine flow which persisted through interval of aortic clamping.

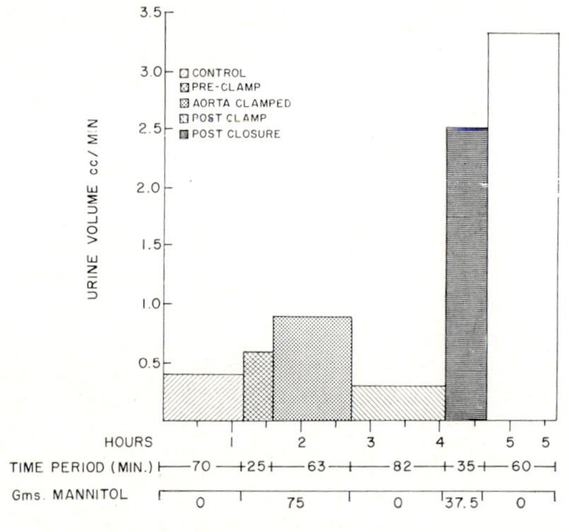


**Fig. 4.** Study of Case 4 was initiated after intubation and urinary bladder catheterization. The time scale is contiguous. Control urine was collected prior to operation and postclosure urine upon its completion. Below the abscissa concordant with the time scale are plotted the time interval for each phase of the study and the quantity of mannitol infused per interval. Mannitolization with a 15 per cent solution in water established an adequate urine flow during CCAA. Note the abrupt decrease of urine flow during the interruption of mannitol infusion and its dramatic increase upon resumption of the infusion.

*Case 4.* A 66-year-old white woman was admitted June 2, 1960, because of severe abdominal pain during the preceding 48 hours. A pulsatile abdominal mass was found and the diagnosis of abdominal aortic aneurysm with impending rupture was made. Pertinent history included hypertension of 20 years' duration, episodes of cerebral vascular encephalopathy in 1945 and 1955, anterior wall myocardial infarction followed by chronic congestive heart failure in 1956, and diabetes mellitus which had required hypoglycemic therapy since February, 1960. Physical examination showed a blood pressure of 180/100 and confirmed the impression of abdominal aneurysm. The blood urea nitrogen was 22, and albuminuria and pyuria were present. Emergency laparotomy showed an aortic aneurysm beginning just below the renal arteries and extending to the aortic bifurcation. A bifurcation graft was required. Fig. 4 illustrates the variation in urinary flow correlated with the surgical procedure and mannitolization. The control period followed intubation and bladder catheterization. The mannitol supply was limited, so 75 Gm. was administered as a 500 ml. infusion over an 88-minute period. The urine flow is not comparable to that in Case 3, probably because of the limited amount of mannitol and rate of infusion utilized. However, an adequate urinary flow was obtained and sustained throughout the 63-minute period of aortic cross-clamping. The diuresis obtained with mannitolization was highlighted by the fall in urinary flow to 0.3 ml. per minute during the 82-minute interval when the patient received no mannitol and the increase to 2.5 per minute promptly upon the reinstitution of a 15 per cent mannitol infusion as shown in period 5. During the 24 hours subsequent to operation, the urinary volume totaled 1,280 ml. Six days postoperatively the blood urea nitrogen was 23 mg. per cent and a random urinary specific gravity determination on an aglycosuric specimen was 1.020.

*Comment.* The use of prophylactic mannitolization in these 2 patients illustrates 2 important features. First, mannitol as used in these patients caused no observable toxicity. The patient in Case 4 had severe chronic cardiovascular disease with congestive heart failure and diabetes, but showed no evidence of overloading of the circulatory system during or after mannitolization. Second, mannitol produced a diuresis throughout aortic cross-clamping which cannot be obtained by simple water loading and which would be hazardous to attempt with other osmotic agents such as sodium chloride or hypertonic glucose.[3]

## DISCUSSION

Oliguria and acute renal failure associated with cross-clamping of the aorta in human beings is a dread and usually fatal complication. Vigorous programs in basic and clinical research into the mechanisms and prevention of acute renal failure are being actively pursued in many centers.[3, 6, 10, 12] When one of the authors (K. G. B.) found mannitol, a 6-carbon hexitol, effective and safe for use in diuretic therapy for refractory fluid retention, acute left ventricular failure, and cerebral edema, study of mannitolization in patients subjected to CCAA during aneurysmectomy was undertaken.[1]

Experimental studies have shown a marked decrease in renal blood flow, glomerular filtration rate, and urine flow associated with aortic cross-clamping below the renal arteries in animals.[6, 10] The performance of parallel studies in patients is not ideal or precise. However, studies at the Walter Reed Army Medical Center have shown a marked decrease in urine flow during and after aortic cross-clamping in the human being.[8] Patient 3 showed an increasing diuresis during cross-clamping despite abrupt decrease in renal plasma flow (CPAH) and glomerular filtration rate ($C_I$, $C_{cr}$). It is believed that mannitol prevented the expected associated decrease in urine flow.

Mannitol is freely filtered at the glomerulus and is not reabsorbed. The high osmotic activity of mannitol is thus concentrated throughout the tubular lumina. Increased renal fluid volume without significant change in general circulatory hemodynamics may occur. It has been shown by Bounous[3] and others that hypertonic glucose causes an increase in renal blood flow accompanied by an increase in cardiac output and circulating blood volume. Bounous believes that the changes in renal blood flow are related more to blood sugar levels than to change in cardiac output or blood volume. Mannitol has approximately the same particle size as glucose, but is limited to the extracellular space, is not reabsorbed from the renal tubules, and is not metabolized. Therefore, given in equivalent amounts, its renal osmotic effect should be more marked and of longer duration. We believe that this is the case. Therefore, mannitol held in the tubular lumen may cause an increase in fluid volume localized to the tubular lumen discouraging tubular collapse. There may be a local increase of nutrients necessary for renal tissue metabolism which protects the kidney during subsequent decreased renal blood flow caused by aortic cross-clamping. The protective effect of mannitol against experimental epinephrine renal shutdown[7] may operate through a similar mechanism.

Since a high concentration of mannitol in the tubular fluid is needed prior to clamping, it is recommended that 20 per cent mannitol be infused for 30 minutes prior to CCAA.

Experimental studies to elucidate the mechanism of mannitol protection against the renal effects of CCAA are planned.

## SUMMARY

Cross-clamping of the abdominal aorta (CCAA) is regularly accompanied by oliguria. Acute renal failure is a serious and frequently fatal complication of CCAA.

This preliminary report is prompted by the dramatic effectiveness of intravenous mannitolization in overcoming oliguria after CCAA in 2 patients and in preventing oliguria during CCAA in 2 patients.

It is proposed that this safe and apparently successful technique for the prevention of CCAA oliguria be given clinical trial in other hospitals.

The authors gratefully acknowledge Dr. Richard T. Smith, Director, Medical Services, Merck Sharp & Dohme, for supplying the mannitol.

### REFERENCES

1. Barry, K. G., Cohen, A., Knochel, J. P., Whelan, T. J., Jr., Beisel, W. R., Vargas, C. A., and LeBlanc, P. C., Jr.: Mannitol infusion. II. Prevention of acute functional renal failure during resection of aneurysm of abdominal aorta, New England J. Med. **264:** 967, 1961.
2. Barry, K. G., and Berman, A. R.: Mannitol infusion. III. Acute effect of intravenous infusion of mannitol on blood and plasma volumes, New England J. Med. **264:** 1085, 1961.
3. Bounous, G., and Shumacker, H. B., Jr.: Influence of blood sugar levels upon renal blood flow, Ann. Surg. **151:** 441, 1960.
4. Dudley, H. A., Batchelor, A. D., and Suther-

land, A. B.: The management of haemoglobinuria in extensive burns, Brit. J. Plastic Surg. **9:** 275, 1957.

5. Ellis, F. W., and Drentz, J. C., Jr.: Sugar alcohols: metabolism and toxicity studies with mannitol and sorbitol in men and animals, J. Biol. Chem. **141:** 147, 1941.
6. Gagnon, J. A., Bolt, D. A., Clarke, R. W., and Geever, E. F.: The effects of lower aortic occlusion on renal function in the dog, SURGERY **47:** 240, 1960.
7. Hatcher, C. R., Jr., Gagnon, J. A., and Clarke, R. W.: The effects of hydration on epinephrine induced renal shutdown in dogs, S. Forum **9:** 106, 1959.
8. Herndon, E. G., Jr., and Cohen, A.: Unpublished data.
9. Last, J. H., McDonald, G. O., Jones, R. A., and Bond, E. E.: Rates of equilibration of inulin and mannitol between plasma and interstitial water in edematous states, J. Lab. & Clin. Med. **39:** 62, 1952.
10. Powers, S. R., Boba, A., and Stein, A.: The mechanism and prevention of distal tubular necrosis following aneurysmectomy, SURGERY **42:** 156, 1957.
11. Schilling, J. A., Ginn, H. E., Richardson, W. R., and Dunlap, H. E.: A new approach to the therapy of the severely burned patient, Ann. Surg. **150:** 756, 1959.
12. Sheranian, L. O., Edwards, J. E., and Kirklin, J. W.: Late results in 110 patients with abdominal aortic aneurysm treated by resectional placement of aortic homograft, Surg. Gynec. & Obst. **109:** 309, 1959.
13. Smith, H. W.: The kidney, New York, 1951, Oxford University Press, pp. 768-780.
14. Smith, W. W., Finklestein, N., and Smith, H. W.: Renal excretion of hexitols and their derivatives and endogenous creatinine-like chromogen in dog and man, J. Biol. Chem. **135:** 231, 1940.

# Postoperative endocarditis due to Candida: clinical observations and the experimental production of the lesion

THEODORE COOPER, M.D., PH.D.
ANDREW G. MORROW, M.D.
WILLIAM C. ROBERTS, M.D.
LLOYD G. HERMAN, PH.D.
BETHESDA, MD.
*From the Clinic of Surgery, National Heart Institute, The Department of Pathologic Anatomy and the Sanitary Engineering Branch, The National Institutes of Health*

Postoperative endocarditis is an infrequent but dreaded complication of operations for the correction of congenital or acquired heart disease.[2, 3] The rarity of the disease is somewhat surprising since all intracardiac procedures result in some damage to the endocardium and foreign bodies in the form of sutures or prosthetic materials are usually inserted. Although a certain number of microorganisms are probably introduced into the circulation in the course of every cardiac operation, the size of this inoculum can be minimized by vigilant asepsis and the defense mechanisms of the patient will ordinarily prevent the development of infection. Also, in many clinics, antibiotics are routinely administered during the early postoperative period, although the role of such prophylaxis in preventing postoperative endocarditis has not been established.

The most lethal form of postoperative endocarditis is that in which the responsible organism is a fungus.[7] Only 2 patients who developed postoperative fungal endocarditis have been described in the surgical literature[4, 6] and in each the disease was recognized only at autopsy. Three patients in this clinic have developed mycotic endocarditis after operations for rheumatic heart disease. Although the infections were recognized and treatment was undertaken, each patient died.

Received for publication Oct. 3, 1960.

This experience prompted an investigation of methods for the production of fungal endocarditis in experimental animals and of the factors which influence the development of the disease. In the present report, the results of these studies are presented as well as brief clinical descriptions of the patients in whom endocarditis occurred.

## CASE REPORTS

**Case 1.** G. V., a 45-year-old man, had acute rheumatic fever at the age of 25 and symptoms of dyspnea and easy fatigability had been noted for several years before his admission. The clinical findings indicated the presence of mitral stenosis. This diagnosis was confirmed at cardiac catheterization when he was found to have a mean left atrial pressure of 22 mm. Hg and an end diastolic gradient of 15 mm. Hg across the mitral valve. In April, 1958, a closed mitral commissurotomy was performed. The valve leaflets were mobile and a satisfactory valve opening was accomplished by digital fracture of the commissures. The patient tolerated the operation well and the postoperative course was uneventful except for the development of atrial fibrillation which could not be converted with quinidine. He was given 1.0 Gm. of streptomycin and 1.2 million units of penicillin daily for 8 days postoperatively and penicillin orally for an additional week. The patient was discharged from the hospital 20 days after operation. Two weeks later he developed fever, sweating, and weakness which persisted in spite of treatment by his physician. When readmitted 9 weeks after operation he was found to have low grade fever and enlargement of the spleen. An apical systolic murmur, not present at the time of his discharge, was audible. Blood cultures revealed a heavy growth of *Candida parakrusei.* In spite of intensive treatment with amphotericin B, the patient died 5 weeks after the presence of the infection had been proved. At autopsy active endocarditis which involved the mitral valve and left atrium was evident and *Candida* was cultured from the vegetations present. Microscopic sections of a vegetation on the anterior mitral leaflet demonstrated the presence of abundant moniliform organisms. Infarcts in the spleen, kidney, liver, lung, and hilar lymph nodes all contained the organism.

**Case 2.** M. S., a 39-year-old housewife, had had chorea at the age of 9 and an attack of acute rheumatic fever at the age of 29. Since the age of 34 she had experienced increasing cardiac disability. On clinical examination she was in evident cardiac failure and the murmurs of mitral stenosis and regurgitation were audible. At left-heart catheterization the mean left atrial pressure was 34 mm. Hg, an end diastolic gradient of 11 mm. Hg was recorded across the mitral valve, and the contour of the left atrial pressure pulse indicated gross mitral regurgitation. In November, 1958, an open surgical repair of the mitral valve was undertaken. During complete cardiopulmonary bypass, for a period of 1 hour, a posterior annuloplasty was performed and the anterior commissure opened. After operation the patient's course was smooth but her convalescence was slow. She was given 1.0 Gm. of streptomycin daily for 5 days, 1.2 million units of penicillin daily for 14 days and penicillin orally for an addi- oxygenator at the end of the perfusion grew only tional 16 days. A culture of blood taken from the a Flavobacterium which was thought to be a laboratory contaminant. The patient was discharged 4 weeks after operation. Three and one-half months after operation the patient was readmitted because of progressive cardiac failure and fever. *Candida guilliermondi* was grown from the blood in pure culture. Therapy with amphotericin B was initiated, but the patient died 2 weeks after treatment was begun. At autopsy 2 vegetations were present on the mitral valve and one on the right coronary cusp of the aortic valve. Cultures and microscopic sections of these vegetations showed them to be *Candida guilliermondi.* Embolic abscesses were found in the spleen, kidney, brain, and spinal cord.

**Case 3.** H. D., a 48-year-old dentist, presented with a history of rheumatic fever and the physical findings of aortic stenosis. Left-heart catheterization showed an elevated left atrial pressure, a left ventricular pressure of 250/40 mm. Hg, a brachial artery pressure of 130/70 mm. Hg, and a cardiac output of 6.4 L. per minute. The peak systolic gradient of 120 mm. Hg across the aortic valve indicated severe stenosis. Aortic valvulotomy under direct vision was performed in June, 1959. During the course of the operation cardiopulmonary bypass was employed for 25 minutes. All 3 commissures of a densely calcified valve were opened and a gratifying fall in the pressure gradient was apparent in the operative pressure records. Cultures of blood taken from the heart-lung machine after the operation grew *Candida guilliermondi.* Postoperatively the patient's course was apparently uncomplicated. He was given 1.0 Gm. of streptomycin daily for 5 days and 1.2 million units of penicillin daily for 13 days. He was discharged 16 days after operation. About 2 weeks later the patient experienced spiking fever which persisted in spite of antibiotics given by his physician. He was readmitted 6 weeks after operation. At this time numerous blood cultures showed *Staphylococcus aureus* and *Candida guilliermondi.* Antibiotic therapy was initiated promptly and the antifungal agent, amphotericin B, was also employed. Subsequent blood cultures became negative for *Staphylococcus aureus* but continued to show growth of the Candida. Since maximal doses of amphotericin were ineffective, another antifungal agent, designated RO-2, was employed separately and in conjunction with amphotericin and antibiotic agents. The progress of the infection was essentially unaltered, however, and the patient died 4 months after treatment was begun. Three vegetations, the largest of which was 2.5 cm. in diameter, were found on the aortic valve at autopsy (Fig. 1, *A* and *B*). *Candida guilliermondi* was cultured from the blood and the organisms were visible in microscopic sections (Fig. 1, *C* and *D*). Infected infarcts were found in the spleen and brain.

A more complete description of the clinical courses of these patients and the details of their therapy will be reported elsewhere.[1]

## EXPERIMENTAL METHODS

In 14 mongrel dogs which weighed 11 to 24 kilograms, aortic regurgitation was created by the technique previously described by Roshe and Morrow.[8] After induction of anesthesia with thiopental sodium and endotracheal intubation, the right thorax was entered through the fourth intercostal space. During inflow occlusion, the ascending aorta was opened and a disc of tissue 3.9 mm. in diameter was excised from the base of the right coronary aortic leaflet. Circulation was restored and the aortotomy was closed. Four to 6 weeks after operation 12 of the animals were utilized for fungal inoculation and the 2 remaining ones served as uninoculated controls.

Initial studies in normal dogs were carried out to determine the magnitude of inoculum which would maintain a blood level of organisms for several minutes. After the intravenous injection of 32 million cells of *Candida guilliermondi* into normal dogs, it could be grown from blood sampled 5 to 10 minutes later. Consequently, all inoculations into the experimental animals consisted of 32 million or more organisms. Saline suspensions of cultures grown from the blood of patient H. D. were used as the source of *Candida guilliermondi.*

Three controls dogs which had not been operated on and 12 with aortic regurgitation were inoculated. The controls and 3 of those with aortic regurgitation were given no drugs. Of the remaining 9 dogs with aortic lesions, 5 were given 800,000 U. of penicillin and 0.5 Gm. of streptomycin intramuscularly on each of 8 days and 4 received 100 mg. of tetracycline intramuscularly daily for this period. In all animals venous blood cultures were drawn at weekly or biweekly intervals for a period of 3 months. At death, autopsy was performed immediately, and cultures of heart blood, of vegetations if present, and of apparently involved organs were obtained. Tissue was then placed in formalin and prepared for microscopic study.

## RESULTS

The results of the study are summarized in Table I.

**Inoculated controls with normal aortic valve.** Negative blood cultures were obtained

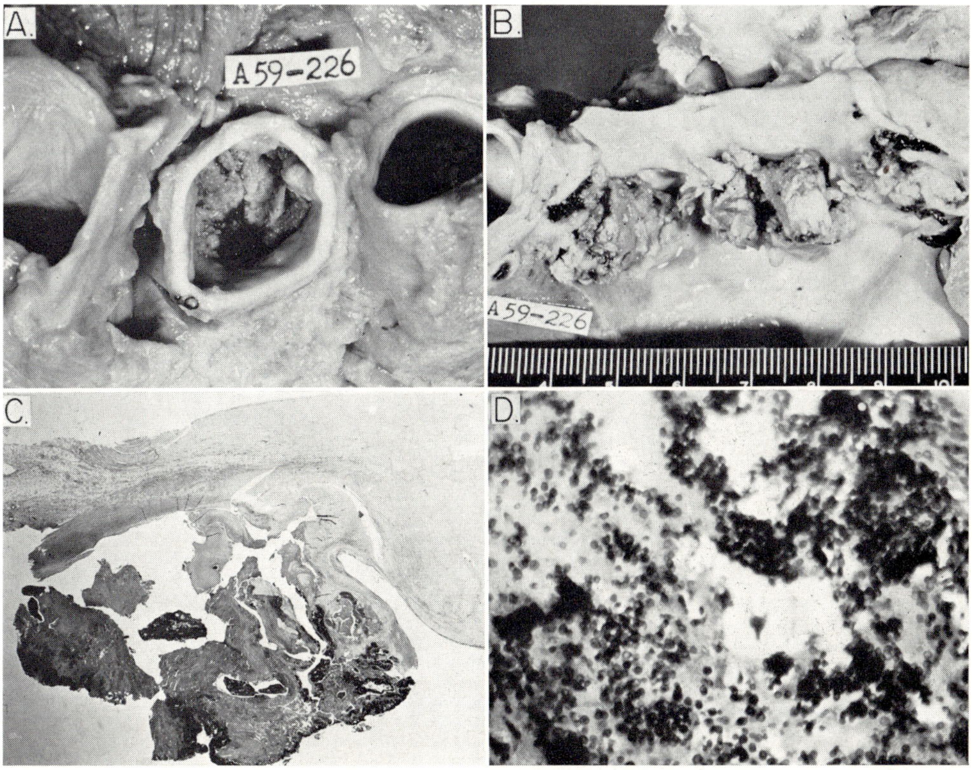


**Fig. 1.** Gross and microscopic photographs of the heart of patient H. D. *A,* The aortic valve as seen from above. Large fungating vegetations nearly occlude the valve orifice. *B,* The left ventricular outflow tract, aortic valve, and aorta have been opened. Vegetations nearly fill each aortic sinus of Valsalva. *C,* Microscopic section through one of the vegetations (PAS; ×10). The darker areas are colonies of Candida. The ventricular surface of the aortic cusp is free of vegetation. *D,* High power view of one of the colonies of Candida shown in C. (PAS; ×495). Only spore forms are present and hyphae are absent.

**Table I.** *Results of intravenous inoculation of Candida guilliermondi in dogs*

| Group | No. of dogs | During life: Positive blood cultures | During life: Signs of illness | At autopsy: Positive blood or tissue culture | At autopsy: Valvular vegetations |
|---|---|---|---|---|---|
| Inoculated controls, normal aortic valve | 3 | None | None | None | None |
| Inoculation, aortic regurgitation, no antibiotics | 3 | None | None | None | None |
| Inoculation, aortic regurgitation, penicillin and streptomycin | 5 | 4 | 2 | 3 | 3 |
| Inoculation, aortic regurgitation, tetracycline | 4 | 1 | 1 | 1 | 1 |
| Aortic regurgitation, no inoculation, no antibiotics | 2 | None | None | None | None |

in all animals over the entire period of observation. The dogs gained weight, were active, and showed no signs of being ill. At postmortem examination none had evidence of endocarditis or other diseases attributable to the inoculation of the organisms.

**Inoculation, aortic regurgitation, and no antibiotics.** These 3 animals showed no positive blood cultures over 7 test periods. They gained weight and showed no evidence of being ill. At sacrifice no evidence of active endocarditis was present. The right coronary leaflets were scarred and thickened. The holes in them were rimmed by fibrous tissue. In one animal the perforation in the valve was healed. The viscera were free of signs of emboli.

**Inoculation, aortic regurgitation, and administration of penicillin and streptomycin.** Four of these 5 animals evidenced at least 1 positive blood culture during 6 sampling periods. Two showed repeatedly positive cultures. One dog died 6 days after inoculation, apparently in heart failure. At postmortem examination pleural fluid was present and the heart was dilated. A small (6 mm.) vegetation was present around the regurgitant orifice in the right coronary cusp. The spleen contained septic emboli. Cultures of heart blood and of the spleen were positive for *Candida guilliermondi.* A second animal died 1 month after inoculation in severe heart failure with passive congestion. An ulcerative vegetation 1 cm. in diameter was present on the aortic valve. Infarcts were grossly evident in the spleen. Cultures of the vegetation on the right coronary cusp yielded *Candida guilliermondi* and a gram-negative bacterium. A third animal at sacrifice demonstrated a 2.4 cm. vegetation on the right coronary cusp which extended through the ventricular septum into the right ventricle, probably through a tract inadvertently made by the punch during operation (Fig. 2, *A* and *B*). There were infarcts in the kidneys and spleen. Cultures of the vegetation were positive for *Candida guilliermondi* and moniliform organisms were seen on microscopic section of the valve (Fig. 2, *C* and *D*). In the remaining animals the hearts were normal except for the regurgitant lesions in the aortic leaflets.

**Inoculation, aortic regurgitation, and tetracycline administration.** One of 4 animals showed a positive culture during the observation period. This animal did not gain weight but otherwise did not appear ill. At sacrifice a vegetation 0.5 cm. in diameter was present on the right coronary cusp. Culture of the vegetation was positive for *Candida guilliermondi* although no organisms were seen on microscopic section of the valve. In the remaining animals the hearts were normal except for the regurgitant lesions in the aortic leaflets.

**Aortic regurgitation, no inoculation, and no antibiotics given.** The hearts of these 2 animals showed no evidence of endocarditis.

The regurgitant orifices were patent and minimally scarred.

## DISCUSSION

The experimental study described demonstrates that fungal endocarditis can be produced in the dog when a site for its localization is provided by damage to an aortic leaflet. Although the number of experimental animals in the study was not large the results imply that antibiotic administration after inoculation with *Candida guilliermondi* facilitated the development of the lesion. This finding was not a surprising one, since it is commonly observed that long-term antibiotic therapy increases susceptibility to fungal infection in other areas of the body.[9] The selection of penicillin, streptomycin, and tetracycline in the investigation was based solely on the fact that postoperative patients commonly receive these drugs. The dosage employed was arbitrary. It is possible that other antibiotics or dosage schedules might alter or enhance the experimental occurrence of the lesion.

All 3 patients whose cases are reported had been treated prophylactically with penicillin and streptomycin and again one must speculate as to the role of these agents in the development of the infections. It has recently been advocated that antibiotics not be given routinely after cardiovascular oper-

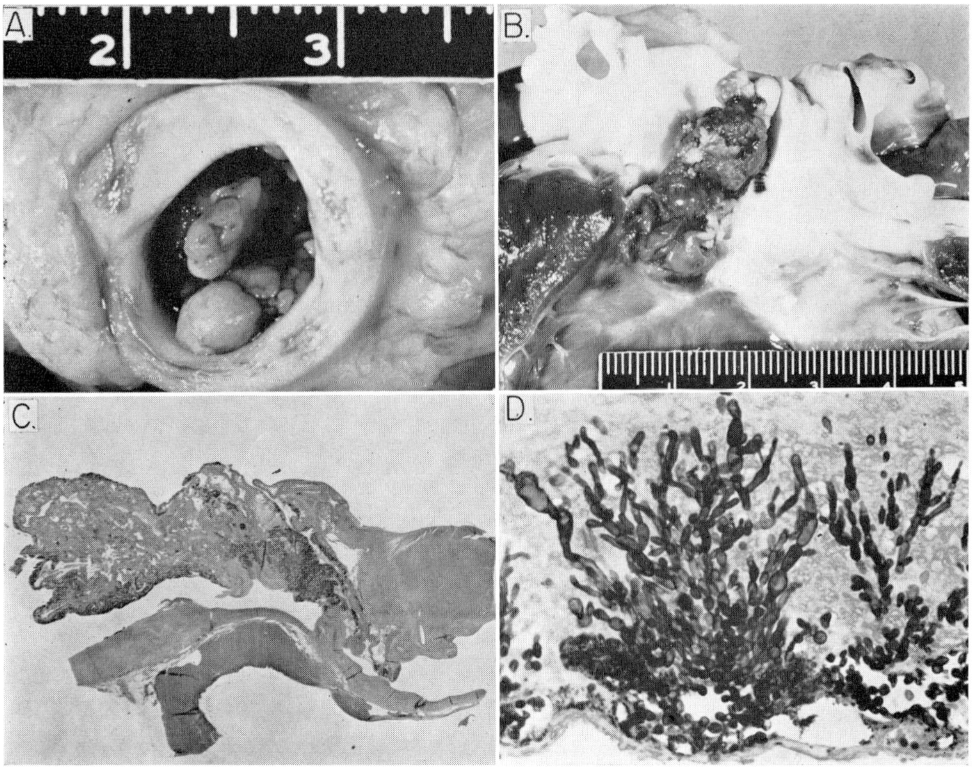


**Fig. 2.** Gross and microscopic photographs of the heart of a dog in which mycotic endocarditis was experimentally produced. *A,* The aortic valve as seen from above. A large vegetation obstructs the valve orifice. *B,* View taken after the left ventricle, aortic valve, and aorta were opened. The vegetation arises in the right coronary aortic cusp, which had previously ben perforated, and protrudes into the ascending aorta. *C,* Microscopic section through the vegetation demonstrated in *B.* (Hematoxylin and eosin; ×4). The darker areas are colonies of Candida. *D,* High power photomicrograph of Candida organisms (Methenamine silver; ×515). The hyphae forms are predominant here as contrasted to the spore forms shown in Fig. 1.

ations,[5] but until wider experience has validated this suggestion it is unlikely that the practice will be widely embraced. Prevention of endocarditis, therefore, depends upon minimizing the opportunity for inoculation, particularly at operation. In one of the 3 patients described, *Candida guilliermondi* was obtained from culture of the pump-oxygenator blood at the termination of operation and suggested a source of contamination in the operating room. An extensive bacteriologic survey, however, yielded no positive cultures for Candida from any furnishings, supplies, equipment, or instruments. Each patient had had cardiac catheterization shortly before operation and it was thought that the organism might have been introduced at this time and that the infections were already established at the time of operation. The organism was never found during a detailed survey in the catheterization laboratory, however, and the source of the organisms remains obscure.

Recognition of fungal endocarditis before death in these patients was possible because of awareness of its occurrence and of the practice of routinely inoculating blood cultures into media suitable for the growth of fungi as well as bacteria. Although success in treating Candida endocarditis has not been reported, early recognition of the disease will certainly permit a study of its natural history and provide opportunity for the trial of more effective agents as they become available.

## SUMMARY

Three patients are described in whom endocarditis due to a "nonpathogenic" Candida occurred after operations for acquired heart disease. In each the disease was recognized in life but therapeutic measures were in vain. This experience suggested an experimental study in which fungal endocarditis was produced in dogs rendered vulnerable to infection by the previous production of aortic regurgitation. Endocarditis due to Candida only occurred in animals which were given antibiotics after inoculation with the organism, which suggests a relationship between the use of these agents and the occurrence of the disease. This method for the experimental production of fungal endocarditis may provide a useful preparation for studies of new chemotherapeutic agents developed for the treatment of this presently universally fatal infection.

### REFERENCES

1. Andriole, V. T., Kravetz, H. M., Roberts, W. C., and Utz, J. P.: Candida endocarditis: clinical and pathological observations. In press.
2. Heins, H. L., Jr., and Linde, L. M.: Bacterial endocarditis after surgery for congenital heart disease, Circulation **20:** 712, 1959.
3. Hoffman, F. G., Zimmerman, S. L., Bradley, E. A., and Lapidus, B.: Bacterial endocarditis after surgery for acquired heart disease: report of two cases and review of the literature, New England J. Med. **260:** 152, 1959.
4. Hyun, B. H., Dawson, E. A., and Pence, R. E.: Bacterial and mycotic endocarditis following cardiac surgery, J. Thoracic Surg. **35:** 298, 1958.
5. Kittle, C. F., and Reed, W. A.: Antibiotics and extracorporeal circulation, J. Thoracic Surg. **41:** 34, 1961.
6. Koelle, W. A., and Pastor, B. H.: *Candida albicans* endocarditis after aortic valvulotomy, New England J. Med. **255:** 997, 1956.
7. Merchant, R. K., Louria, D. B., Geisler, P. H., Edgcomb, J. H., and Utz, J. P.: Fungal endocarditis: review of the literature and report of three cases, Ann. Int. Med. **48:** 242, 1958.
8. Roshe, J., and Morrow, A. G.: Experimental production of graded aortic insufficiency, Surg. Gynec. & Obst. **101:** 305, 1955.
9. Zimmerman, L. E.: Candida and Aspergillus endocarditis, with comments on the role of antibiotics in dissemination of fungus disease, Arch. Path. **50:** 591, 1950.

# Surgical management of mycotic aneurysms

DONALD C. NABSETH, M.D.
RALPH A. DETERLING, JR., M.D.
BOSTON, MASS., AND NEW YORK, N. Y.
*From the Department of Surgery, Tufts University School of Medicine, Columbia University College of Physicians and Surgeons, and the Surgical Service of the Presbyterian Hospital*

An aneurysm which results from infection in the wall of an artery is currently regarded as a "mycotic aneurysm." Osler[18] is credited with originating the term. In 1885 he described a 30-year-old man with malignant endocarditis who, at autopsy, was found to have 4 separate aneurysms of the aortic arch which were caused by "mycotic endarteritis." Although syphilitic aneurysms arise from the action of micro-organisms on the arterial wall, they are commonly differentiated from the mycotic variety. Review of the literature shows rather loose usage of the term "mycotic" in reference to lesions of blood vessels. In general, all aneurysms which result from the presence of bacteria or fungi are accepted as belonging in the mycotic group. The object of this paper is to report our experience with 5 cases of this rare type of aneurysm and to stress the important features of surgical management.

## CASE REPORTS

**Case 1.** E. B., a 31-year-old woman, was admitted to the hospital in June, 1948, with the chief complaint of low-back pain of 5 months' duration. There was no history of any previous illness. On physical examination a tender pulsatile mass was found in the region of the umbilicus. A systolic bruit was present. At operation a fusiform aneurysm of the abdominal aorta was found surrounded by dense inflammatory tissue. Biopsy of tissue surrounding the aneurysm showed acute inflammation. Proximal aortic constriction was instituted with the use of a rubber band wrapped in polyethylene film. A bilateral lumbar sympathectomy was performed. There was complete relief of back pain. When last seen in May, 1959, the patient was free of symptoms.

**Case 2.** S. K., a 25-year-old man, was admitted to the hospital with the diagnosis of subacute bacterial endocarditis. There was a history of rheumatic fever between the ages of 10 and 14 years. He appeared as a thin, pale, chronically ill patient. The temperature was 38.3° C. and pulse 100. Two fresh petechiae were seen in the left fundus. Blood cultures showed *Streptococcus viridans.* Two weeks after admission the patient developed a painful pulsatile mass in the lateral aspect of the right thigh. Operation showed a saccular mycotic aneurysm involving the descending branch of the lateral circumflex artery. The aneurysm was excised. At a follow-up visit 1½ years later, the patient was found to be well.

**Case 3.** L. E., a 12-year-old Chinese girl, was admitted to the hospital on Jan. 7, 1953, with the diagnosis of subacute bacterial endocarditis. She had acute rheumatic fever 4 years previously. Mitral insufficiency, mitral stenosis, and aortic stenosis were present. While being treated with bed rest and antibiotics, the patient experienced the gradual onset of periumbilical pain 2 weeks after admission. One week later a tender pulsatile mass was felt above the level of the umbilicus. At operation an aneurysm of the superior mesenteric artery was found. This was surrounded by dense inflammatory tissue. No further operative procedure was attempted because of aneurysmal involvement of all primary branches of the artery and the critical condition of the patient. Immediately after the operation, the patient was completely free of abdominal pain. The abdominal mass became firm, decreased in size, and was non-

Received for publication Oct. 10, 1960. Resubmitted Jan. 3, 1961.

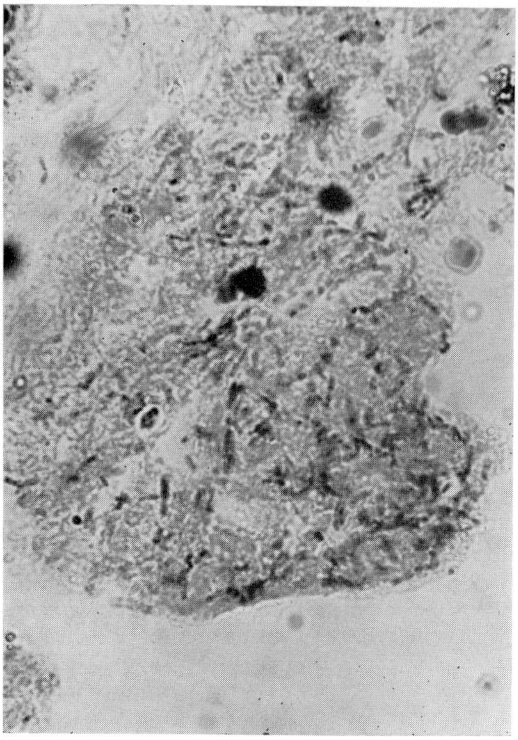

**Fig. 1.** Microscopic section of blood clot contained in mycotic aneurysm in Case 4. Gram-negative rod-shaped bacteria were identified as *Salmonella choleraesuis*.

pulsatile. Two years later the abdominal mass had completely disappeared and the patient was free of symptoms.

**Case 4.** E. Y., an 80-year-old man, was admitted to the hospital on Aug. 2, 1956, with a tender pulsating mass in the left thigh which had been present for 2 days. Physical examination showed a large (10 cm. diameter) pulsatile mass in the medial aspect of the midportion of the left thigh. The overlying skin appeared red and tense. Because of rapid expansion of the mass an emergency operation was required on the second hospital day. A large false aneurysm was found arising from the distal aspect of the superficial artery. This was excised and the resulting arterial defect was bridged with an arterial homograft. Disruption of the homograft occurred 5 days later. A culture of the aneurysm revealed *Salmonella choleraesuis* (Fig. 1). The homograft was removed and the artery was ligated. Two months later a second arterial perforation occurred at the site of previous ligature. *Salmonella choleraesuis* was again cultured from the artery. The wound healed. Four months later low thigh amputation was necessary for progressive ischemia of the left foot.

**Case 5.** C. M., a 30-year-old housewife, was admitted to the hospital on March 17, 1959, because of pain and swelling in the right popliteal area of 2½ months' duration. A heart murmur had been discovered 2 years prior to admission. There was no history of rheumatic fever. Physical examination showed a Grade II systolic murmur in aortic and mitral areas. Temperature was 38° C. There was a tender pulsatile mass (6 by 5 cm.) in the right popliteal space (Fig. 2). During 2 weeks of observation, the aneurysm gradually enlarged. Thorough study failed to show the etiology of the aneurysm. Nine negative blood cultures were obtained and the fever continued unchanged. A right lumbar sympathectomy was performed. Four days later the popliteal aneurysm was excised (Fig. 3). The resulting arterial defect was bridged by a plastic arterial prosthesis (woven Teflon). Culture of the aneurysm showed streptococcus. The patient was given large doses of penicillin and streptomycin and the fever gradually returned to normal. When seen 2 years later she was asymptomatic. The graft continues to function well.

## DISCUSSION

A patient with a mycotic aneurysm usually presents a dual problem in therapy; namely, the antibiotic treatment of bacterial endocarditis or septicemia, and the surgical treatment of aneurysm. Prior to the availability of antibiotic drugs, surgical procedures for mycotic aneurysms associated with bacterial endocarditis tended to complicate the course or precipitate the termination of an almost invariably fatal disease. Today the antibiotic drugs have led to a situation in which the surgeon is called to treat an aneurysm in the presence of manageable endocarditis or septicemia.

Spontaneous cure of mycotic aneurysms has rarely occurred.[16, 18] Case 3 is a striking example of the spontaneous disappearance of an aneurysm which may occasionally occur. In this instance, a 12-year-old girl with subacute bacterial endocarditis developed an aneurysm of the superior mesenteric artery. Surgical exploration and biopsy confirmed the presence and nature of the aneurysm. Because of the unfavorable location of the aneurysm, the marked local inflammatory reaction, and the critical condition of the patient, a further surgical procedure was not attempted. Postoperatively, the patient was remarkably free of the pain and the aneurysm was felt to be smaller and firmer. Presumably thrombosis occurred. When last seen 2 years later this patient had no evidence of aneurysm.

In addition to being usually associated with a blood stream infection, mycotic aneurysms differ from the syphilitic and arteriosclerotic varieties in several important respects. Occurring commonly in young people, the infected aneurysm is usually found in an otherwise normal arterial tree which has an excellent capacity for the development of collateral circulation and responds well to sympathetic denervation. Second, the rapidly developing type of mycotic aneurysm which may proceed to rupture within a few days, as in Case 4, demands an urgency of surgical treatment not usually necessary in other types of aneurysms. Third, special surgical considerations regarding the technical handling of the aneurysm and adjacent arteries are prompted by the fact that the operation is necessarily performed in an infected field.

A variety of surgical procedures have been used in the treatment of mycotic aneurysms (Table I). Proximal (Hunterian) ligation or proximal and distal ligation with or without excision proved to be the most acceptable methods before the antibiotic era. In view of the septic nature of the condition and the failure of antibiotic therapy to consistently eliminate infection from the aneurysm, we believe that excision of the sac is a primary objective. When the aneurysm is located in a noncritical artery, that is, one in which ligation does not appreciably alter function or viability of the part it supplies, it is usually well treated by simple ligation and excision. This is illustrated by Case 2. Even when located in more critical sites, such as the superior mesenteric, common iliac, and femoral arteries, good results have been obtained after extirpation of the aneurysm with proximal and distal ligation of the artery.[1, 4, 9, 19] Success in these instances was attributed to development of collateral arterial channels secondary to gradual vascular occlusion associated with the aneurysm.

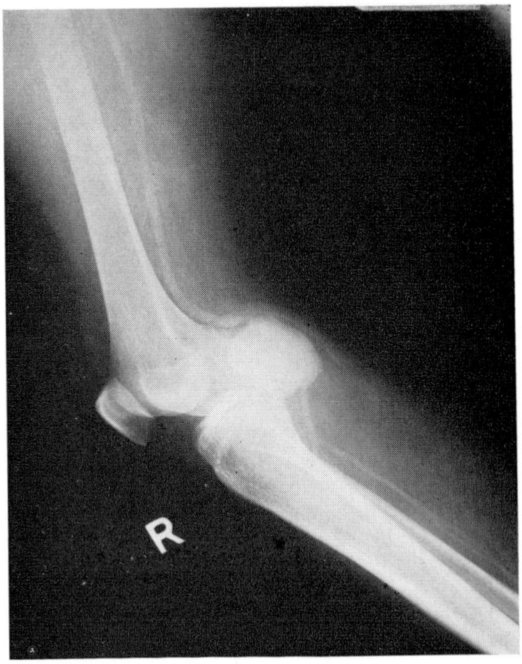


**Fig. 2.** Arteriogram shows the aneurysm of the popliteal artery described in Case 5.

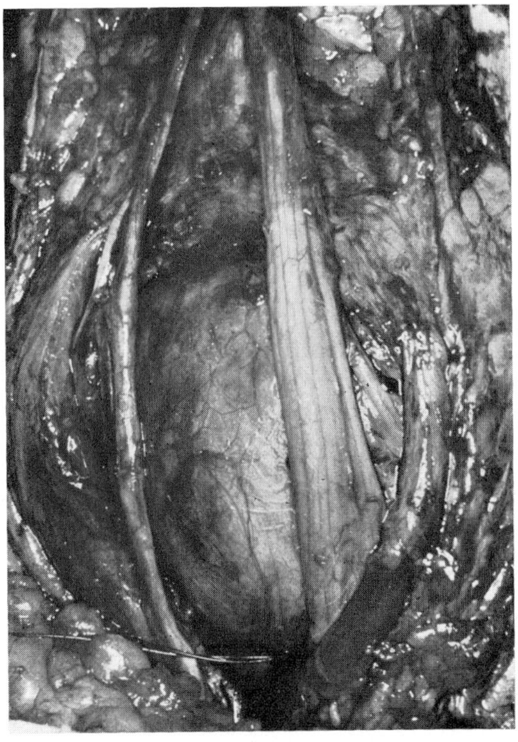

**Fig. 3.** Exposure of the mycotic popliteal aneurysm in Case 5 at operation.

**Table I.** *Cases of mycotic aneurysm treated surgically*

| *Year reported* | *Author* | *Age* | *Sex* | *Artery involved* | *Procedure* | *Result* |
|---|---|---|---|---|---|---|
| 1908 | Clutton and Dudgeon | 78 | M | Femoral | Proximal ligation; incision and drainage | Good, 3 mo. follow-up |
| 1908 | Stern | 20 | | Superior mesenteric | Ligation above and below; evacuation and packing | Died 6 wk. later from second aneurysm |
| 1909 | Lewis and Schrager | 43 | M | Brachial | Proximal ligation | Died 7 mo. later |
| 1929 | Osius | 28* | M | Popliteal | Excision | Amputation 3 days later |
| 1934 | Gage | 18 | F | Common iliac | Proximal ligation | Alive 3 mo. later, limb survived |
| 1939 | Rogers | | M | Radial | Excision | Died later, cardiac failure |
| 1943 | Martorell and Serra | 32 | M | Common femoral | (1) Ligation external iliac; (2) ligation and excision | Died of subacute bacterial endocarditis in 3 mo. |
| 1946 | Klein and Crowell | 22 | M | Ulnar | Excision | Cure |
| 1947 | Blakemore | 39 | F | Common femoral | Vitallium tube vein graft | Good over 1 year |
| 1948 | Hurwitz and Arst | 20 | M | Brachial | Excision | Cure |
| 1948 | Julian | 27 | M | Femoral | Sympathectomy, excision | Good, 8 mo. follow-up |
| 1949 | Goadby et al. | 35 | M | Femoral | Ligation, excision | Good, died of subacute bacterial endocarditis 7 mo. later |
| 1950 | Demirleau | 27 | F | Common femoral | Endoaneurysmorrhaphy | Good, 8 mo. follow-up |
| 1951 | Gerner and Fischer | 30 | F | Femoral | Ligation, excision | Good, developed intra-abdominal aneurysm 2 yr. later |
| 1951 | Rogers | 23 | M | Femoral | Sympathectomy, aneurysmorrhaphy | Good |
| 1952 | Fernbach et al. | 10 | F | Common iliac | Proximal and distal ligation | Good, 2 mo. follow-up |
| 1953 | Harrison and Desmond | 45 | F | Popliteal | Proximal ligation | Well more than 1 yr. later |
| 1953 | Tresidder and Warren | 25 | F | Posterior tibial (bilateral) | Excision (bilateral) | Good |
| 1953 | De Bakey and Cooley | 27 | F | Superior mesenteric | Resection | Well, 3½ yr. later |
| 1954 | Shnider and Cotsona | 45 | M | Ulnar | Ligation, excision | Good |
| 1954 | Barker | 24 | M | Deep femoral (bilateral) | Ligation, excision | Good, 3 mo. follow-up |
| 1954 | West | 23* | F | Common iliac | Ligation, partial excision | Good, follow-up 43 days |
| 1954 | West | 23* | F | Superior mesenteric | Restorative aneurysmorrhaphy | Good, follow-up 26 days |
| 1955 | Moore and Telling | 21 | F | Common iliac | Bifurcation homograft; aneurysm not resected | Good, 3 yr. follow-up |
| 1955 | Shea et al. | 58 | M | Common carotid | Excision with end-to-end anastomosis | Good, 1½ yr. follow-up |
| 1955 | Rogers | 29 | M | Femoral (bilateral) | Hunterian ligation of external iliacs | Good |
| 1956 | Hankins and Yeager | 76 | M | Superficial femoral | Ligation and excision | Good, follow-up several months |

*Probably mycotic, but lacking positive identification.

**Table I.** *Cont'd*

| *Year reported* | *Author* | *Age* | *Sex* | *Artery involved* | *Procedure* | *Result* |
|---|---|---|---|---|---|---|
| 1957 | Katz and Jacobson | 21 | F | Superior mesenteric | Ligation, excision, small bowel resection | Good, 8 mo. later |
| 1957 | Sullivan and Mangiardi | 26 | M | Brachial | Excision with end-to-end anastomosis | Good, follow-up 6 mo. |
| 1957 | Smith and Hutchinson | 78 | M | Superficial femoral | Excision of sac, repair of artery | Good, death from myocardial infarction 6 mo. later |
| 1957 | Smith and Hutchinson | 46* | M | Common carotid | Excision of sac, repair of artery | Good, 3 yr. follow-up |
| 1958 | Zak | 58 | M | Femoral | Excision with arterial homograft | Recurrent hemorrhages from operative site, died of coronary thrombosis 1 yr. later |
| 1958 | Zak | 55 | M | Femoral | Excision with arterial homograft | Unknown |
| 1958 | Zak | 61 | M | Abdominal aorta | Excision of ruptured aneurysm, arterial homograft | Death, 2 weeks |
| 1958 | Lovezzola | 34 | M | Mesenteric artery | Excision | Good, 2 yr. follow-up |
| 1959 | Horton | 31 | M | Ileocaecal branch superior mesenteric artery | Excision with right hemicolectomy | Good |
| 1960 | Authors | 31* | F | Abdominal aorta | Proximal sclerosing band | Good, 11 yr. follow-up |
| 1960 | Authors | 25 | M | Lateral circumflex femoral | Excision | Good, 1½ yr. |
| 1960 | Authors | 80 | M | Superficial femoral | (1) Excision with arterial homograft; (2) removal of graft, proximal and distal ligation | Initially good, amputation 5 mo. later |
| 1960 | Authors | 30 | F | Popliteal | Excision, plastic graft (Teflon) | Good, over 2 yr. |

In an effort to achieve optimum function as well as viability, various arterial reconstructive methods have been used in the treatment of mycotic aneurysms (Table II). Endoaneurysmorrhaphy, although successfully used in 3 reported instances, carries the undesirable feature of leaving an infected aneurysmal sac in situ.[6, 19, 26] Furthermore, an inflamed and frequently necrotic aneurysm may make the procedure technically impossible. Excision of the sac with lateral repair of the artery was used successfully in 2 cases by Smith and Hutchinson[22] in treating mycotic aneurysm of the femoral and carotid arteries. This method is most applicable if the communication between artery and aneurysm is small and the remaining arterial wall appears to be normal. In instances in which an appreciable part of the circumference or length of the arterial channel is involved in the infective process, excision of the artery is necessary and restoration of arterial flow is only possible by end-to-end anastomosis or the interposition of an arterial graft. In Case 5 an arterial homograft was used to re-establish arterial flow after excision of a mycotic aneurysm (Salmonella) of the superficial femoral artery. In this instance disruption of the proximal anastomosis resulted from infection of the graft and required removal of the graft. Zak[28] has called attention to the syndrome of rupture of previously diseased large arteries in the course of enterobacterial

**Table II.** *Reconstructive surgical procedures used in the treatment of mycotic aneurysms*

| *Procedure* | *No. of operations* | *Results* |
|---|---|---|
| *Without graft* | | |
| Restorative aneurysmorrhaphy | 3 | Good |
| Excision with end-to-end anastomosis | 2 | Good |
| Excision with lateral repair of artery | 2 | Good |
| *With graft* | | |
| Excision with Vitallium tube vein graft | 1 | Good* |
| Excision with arterial homograft | 5 | 1 good, 2 disrupted, 2 unknown |
| Excision with plastic prosthesis (Teflon) | 1 | Good |

*Graft occluded after 1 year.

(Salmonella) infections. He reported 3 instances in which the site of arterial infection was treated by excision and insertion of an arterial homograft. One of the cases in a femoral artery was followed by 8 episodes of massive hemorrhage from the operative site that necessitated regrafting operations. The fate of the other grafts was not stated. The undesirability of introducing a segment of nonviable organic material into an infected field is apparent.

That the plastic arterial prostheses are more acceptable grafts in the presence of infection is attested to by the experiments of Foster and associates.[4] After the deliberate infection of the retroperitoneal area of dogs with a suspension of canine feces, these investigators replaced segments of the abdominal aorta with arterial homografts and synthetic prostheses (nylon). All animals were given antibiotic drugs. Sixty-four per cent of the animals with plastic prostheses survived with functioning aortic substitutes as opposed to 17 per cent in the homograft series. However, there was evidence of residual and persistent infection around the synthetic tube in 5 of 25 long-term survivors. Harrison,[7] in an experimental study, found Teflon grafts to be preferable to homografts in the presence of infection or contamination. Case 5 illustrates the successful use of plastic prostheses (Teflon) after excision of a mycotic popliteal aneurysm (streptococcus).

Existing experimental and clinical studies have evaluated homograft and synthetic replacements in the presence of infection. Although on the basis of such studies the synthetic grafts appear to be superior, it is to be wondered if an autogenous vein graft might not be a very satisfactory replacement by virtue of the absence of foreign-body or antigenic reaction.

## SUMMARY

1. Personal experiences with the surgical management of 5 cases of mycotic aneurysm have been presented.

2. All reports of surgically treated mycotic aneurysms have been reviewed.

3. The conclusions made were (a) excision with proximal and distal arterial ligation is the treatment of choice for a mycotic aneurysm located in a noncritical artery, (b) excision with either end-to-end anastomosis or lateral arterial repair is a very satisfactory means of treating a mycotic aneurysm located in a critical artery, and (c) On the basis of existing evidence a plastic prosthesis appears to be a more acceptable graft than a homograft for use in a contaminated or infected field (a successful case of Teflon graft replacement is reported). The comparative suitability of autogenous vein grafts under such conditions cannot be positively stated at this time.

We wish to acknowledge the permission of Dr. Arthur H. Blakemore, New York, New York, for the inclusion of Case 1 in this series.

## REFERENCES

1. Barker, W.: Mycotic aneurysm, Ann. Surg. **139:** 84, 1954.
2. De Bakey, M. E., and Cooley, D. A.: Successful resection of mycotic aneurysm of superior mesenteric artery, Am. Surgeon **2:** 202, 1953.
3. Fernbach, P. A., Berman, L., and Cohen, B.: Intraperitoneal rupture of iliac aneurysm with survival following surgical treatment, Ann. Surg. **135:** 570, 1952.

4. Foster, J. H., Talivaldis, B., and Scott, H. W.: Experimental study of arterial replacement in presence of bacterial infection, Surg. Gynec. & Obst. **108:** 141, 1959.
5. Goadby, H. K., McSwiney, R. R., and Rob, C. G.: Mycotic aneurysm, St. Thomas's Hosp. Rep. **5:** 44, 1949.
6. Hankins, J. R., and Yeager, G. H.: Primary mycotic aneurysm, SURGERY **40:** 747, 1956.
7. Harrison, J. H.: Influence of infection on homografts and synthetic (Teflon) grafts, A. M. A. Arch. Surg. **76:** 67, 1957.
8. Hurwitz, A., and Arst, D. B.: Mycotic aneurysm of the brachial artery after cure of bacterial endocarditis, New England J. Med. **238:** 903, 1948.
9. Julian, O. C.: Peripheral arterial obstruction, S. Clin. North America **28:** 154, 1948.
10. Katz, B., and Jacobson, L. F.: Aneurysm of the superior mesenteric artery successfully treated, SURGERY **41:** 613, 1957.
11. Klein, J. J., and Crowell, D.: Mycotic aneurysm of the ulnar artery, J. A. M. A. **130:** 1220, 1946.
12. Lewis, D., and Schrager, V. L.: Embolomycotic aneurysms, J. A. M. A. **53:** 1808, 1909.
13. Lovezzola, M. M.: Resection of mycotic aneurysm of the small-bowel mesentery, New England J. Med. **259:** 1076, 1958.
14. Matorell, F., and Serra, J. V.: Aspecto quirugico de los aneursmas micoticos de las arterias perifericas, Rev. clín. españ. **9:** 331, 1943.
15. Moore, H. D., and Telling, M.: Resection of the aortic bifurcation for relief of a mycotic aneurysm of the left common iliac artery, and its replacement by a preserved arterial graft, Brit. J. Surg. **42:** 420, 1955.
16. Nicholson, G. H. B.: Coarctation of the aorta in a child with arrested subacute bacterial endarteritis and a calcified mycotic aneurysm at the seat of stricture, Am. Heart J. **20:** 357, 1940.
17. Osius, E. A.: A case report, J. Michigan M. Soc. **28:** 874, 1929.
18. Osler, W.: The Gulstonian lectures on malignant endocarditis, Brit. M. J. **1:** 467, 1885.
19. Rogers, L.: Mycotic aneurysms and their treatment, Ann. Roy. Coll. Surgeons **19:** 257, 1956.
20. Shnider, B. I., and Cotsona, N. J.: Embolic mycotic aneurysms. Complications of bacterial endocarditis, Am. J. Med. **16:** 246, 1954.
21. Shea, P. C., Lamar, F. G., Reid, W. A., and Harland, A.: Anastomosis of common and internal carotid arteries following excision of mycotic aneurysm, SURGERY **37:** 829, 1955.
22. Smith, G., and Hutchinson, H. E.: Lymph borne infection and aneurysm formation, Surg. Gynec. & Obst. **104:** 722, 1957.
23. Stern, K.: Operation eines Aneurysma embolo-mycoticum einer Mesenterialarterie, Beitr. klin. Chir. **57:** 315, 1908.
24. Sullivan, J. J., and Mangiardi, J. L.: Surgical management of mycotic aneurysms, Ann. Surg. **148:** 119, 1958.
25. Tresidder, G. C., and Warren, R. P.: A case of bilateral mycotic aneurysm of the posterior tibial artery treated successfully by excision, Brit. J. Surg. **41:** 333, 1953-1954.
26. West, J. P.: Aneurysm of the superior mesenteric artery successfully treated by restorative aneurysmorrhaphy, Ann. Surg. **140:** 882, 1954.
27. Wilcox, L. D., and Fisher, J. H.: Mycotic aneurysm of abdominal aorta complicating subacute bacterial endocarditis, Canad. M. A. J. **68:** 217, 1953.
28. Zak, F. G., Strauss, L., and Saphra, I.: Rupture of diseased large arteries in course of enterobacterial (Salmonella) infections, New England J. Med. **258:** 824, 1958.

# The second-look procedure in the management of ovarian malignancies and pseudomyxoma peritonei

BENJAMIN T. SANTORO, M.D.
WARD O. GRIFFEN, JR., M.D.
OWEN H. WANGENSTEEN, M.D.
MINNEAPOLIS, MINN.
*From the Department of Surgery, University of Minnesota Medical School*

Cancer of the ovary occurs with relative frequency. In most series the peak incidence obtains in patients in their fifth and sixth decades. A completely satisfactory histopathologic classification of ovarian tumors remains an unsolved problem. The systems offered by Novak and Kottmeier[2, 3] probably have the widest acceptance. More distressing, of course, is the need for improved diagnostic and therapeutic measures. The magnitude of this need is made evident in the survival experience data presented at the Fourth National Cancer Conference.[1]

It is not our purpose to debate the indications for or optimal utilization of combined surgical and radiation therapy for cure of ovarian malignancy and related disease. A strengthened armamentarium permits more physiologic management after extensive surgical procedures. The need for extended and repetitive excisions follows from the great frequency with which local extension, lymph node metastasis, and even peritoneal implantation are found at the initial exploration. Moreover, cystadenocarcinoma and pseudomucinous cystadenocarcinoma of the ovary are relatively slowly growing tumors, a circumstance which fully justifies a vigorous surgical approach to their control and cure. A similar rationale of management is applicable to pseudomyxoma peritonei in association with carcinoma of the appendix or ovary.

Received for publication March 24, 1961.

Since the institution in this clinic of systematic use of secondary operations after the original excision of a visceral cancer,[4] 14 patients (Table I) have been managed in the framework of the "second-look" program. The results have been such that an interim report is warranted.

## PLAN OF MANAGEMENT

The concept of re-exploration for patients with visceral malignancy during an asymptomatic phase evolved from an experience with treatment of a carcinoma of the colon in a female patient. She underwent a series of operative procedures during the period from 1942 to 1951. These were carried out, however, only when recurrent disease was causing symptoms. The course of this patient made reasonable the planned program of re-operation during the asymptomatic interval, before the reassertion of symptoms, embodied in the second-look program begun in this clinic in 1949.

Details of the principles of this program have been given in a number of previous communications. Suffice it to say here that re-operation is carried out in patients known to be asymptomatic and without clinical evidence of cancer approximately 6 months after original excision of malignancies with gross or microscopic evidence of spread beyond the primary site. If possible, residual or recurrent tumor is removed in its entirety. Additional "looks" are employed, if necessary, to render the patient free of cancer.

In the event that painstaking exploration and biopsies at any of the secondary operations fail to show evidence of the disease, the systematic re-exploration at 6-month intervals is discontinued and further surgical effort is made only in the event of recurrence or in selected cases in which the original lesion was widespread.

## RESULTS

Twelve of the 14 patients in this group had adenocarcinoma of the ovary and 1 a malignant ovarian teratoma. An additional patient had pseudomucinous involvement of the ovaries. The appendix was the probable primary site. The latter patient and 2 of the 12 patients with adenocarcinomas of the ovary had associated pseudomyxoma peritonei (Table I).

Two patients had no cancer at their first reoperation and are living and well. Two patients (C. H. and P. T.) with 2 or more positive looks are living and well without evidence of cancer. Two patients (E. Y. and M. D.) are living and well and are awaiting further operations since they had residual disease at their last look. An additional patient (B. O.) is living with carcinosis 5 years after a procedure thought to have effected conversion to the cancer-free state. Despite widespread metastases, she continued to lead an active and useful life until 1 month prior to this writing. Five patients died at intervals of from 19 to 50 months after their primary operations. There have been 2 postoperative deaths in this series.

## CASE REPORTS

The following cases are illustrative of a program of systematic reoperation and the gratifying results that such an approach may achieve.

**Case 1.** C. H., a 41-year-old woman, was first operated upon in this hospital on Oct. 27, 1948. At that time, she had a huge cancer which involved both ovaries and the entire pelvic peritoneum, and had metastases to the mesentery of the small bowel. The patient underwent a complete excision of pelvic viscera except for the bladder, omentectomy, and a partial jejunectomy along with removal of the involved mesentery. She was then given to postoperative irradiation. She remained well for 10 years. However, in the early part of 1958, she returned with a history of hematuria and lower abdominal pain. On March 10, 1958, she again underwent exploratory operation and was found to have tumor in the right side of the pelvis which infiltrated the right ureter, the bladder and the wall of the rectum. There were metastases to the right external iliac nodes. There was no evidence of hepatic metastases. Excision of the tumor mass, partial cystectomy, right ureterectomy with right cutaneous ureterostomy and subtotal colectomy with inversion of rectal pouch, and descending colostomy were performed.

Subsequent to this operation, the woman developed an ileal fistula and a rectovaginal fistula as well as a transverse colon fistula. The latter fistulas were treated with an additional colostomy proximal to the 2 lesions and the ileal fistula was left alone.

On Oct. 29, 1958, another exploratory operation was performed. It was our purpose to carry out another look as well as close the multiple fistulas. Results of multiple biopsies were negative for cancer. The patient underwent closure of the colocutaneous fistula as well as the rectovaginal and vesicovaginal fistulas and resection of the terminal ileum with an ileoascending colostomy. A loop ileostomy proximal to the anastomosis was performed as well as a ureterostomy, cystostomy, and drainage of the rectal pouch. She developed recurrent fistulas but remained relatively well.

She was readmitted to the hospital on Feb. 22, 1960, for another attempt to close the fistulas. Because of an active duodenal ulcer, further surgical intervention was deferred. She has continued to do well despite the fistulas and is to come in shortly for closure of the various fistulous tracts.

**Case 2.** P. T., a 36-year-old white woman, was found on Nov. 20, 1957, to have a malignancy involving the right ovary and appendix with evidence of pelvic peritoneal implantation. Total hysterectomy, right salpingo-oophorectomy, appendectomy, and excision of the tumor implants were carried out. Histologically, the lesions were determined to be pseudomucinous adenocarcinoma of the ovary with pseudomyxoma peritonei. The woman was seen at the University of Minnesota Hospitals for the first time in December, 1958, and was found to be asymptomatic and without clinical evidence of recurrent or residual carcinoma.

Nevertheless, a second-look operation was performed on Dec. 11, 1958. There were multiple areas of recurrence in the pelvis with tumor adherent to the terminal portions of both ureters. In addition, a 6 by 7 by 3 cm. mass and several smaller nodules were present in the right subphrenic space. All visible tumor was excised. The patient did well in the postoperative period.

**Table I.** *Second-look results in cases of ovarian neoplasm*

| *Status* | *Patient* | *Diagnosis* | *Age at and date of first operation* | *Course* |
|---|---|---|---|---|
| Living and well, negative second look | F. B. | Papillary cystadenocarcinoma | 47, Aug. 6, 1952 | Negative look Feb. 13, 1953; also negative at cholecystectomy Nov. 18, 1953 |
| | G. O. | Cystadenocarcinoma | 48, Jan. 7, 1959 | Negative look July 8, 1959 |
| Living and well, converted | C. H. | Cystadenocarcinoma | 41, Oct. 27, 1948 | Positive look March 10, 1958; positive look; negative look; Oct. 29, 1958 |
| | P. T. | Pseudomucinous cystadenocarcinoma (pseudomyxoma peritonei) | 36, Nov. 20, 1957 | Positive look, positive look, negative look |
| Living and well, awaiting another look | E. Y. | Adenocarcinoma (mesonephroma type) | 54, April 15, 1957 | Positive look Nov. 26, 1958 |
| | M. D. | Papillary cystadenocarcinoma | 57, Sept. 10, 1958 | Negative look May 10, 1959; positive look Feb. 1, 1961 |
| Living with residual disease | B. O. | Pseudomyxoma peritonei, ovary or appendix probable primary site | 40, July 6, 1944 | 4 positive looks; negative look in 1955; carcinomatosis Oct., 1960 |
| Dead of cancer | E. W. | Malignant teratoma | 34, Jan. 2, 1949 | 7 positive looks; died in March, 1952 |
| | S. K. | Cystadenocarcinoma | 47, Sept. 12, 1949 | 2 positive looks; died in July, 1951 |
| | M. Z. | Cystadenocarcinoma | 57, June 7, 1950 | Positive look Oct. 27, 1951; negative look Jan. 21, 1952; carcinosis Oct. 16, 1952; died in April, 1953 |
| | L. S. | Papillary cystadenocarcinoma | 49, May 20, 1954 | 4 positive looks; died in March, 1956 |
| | S. L. | Serous cystadenocarcinoma | 50, March 5, 1946 | 3 positive looks; died in October, 1951 |
| Postoperative deaths | K. D. | Pseudomucinous cystadenocarcinoma (pseudomyxoma peritonei) | 76, Nov. 24, 1954 | Carcinomatosis at look Aug. 1, 1955; died during convalescence |
| | T. B. | Papillary cystadenocarcinoma | 51, July 16, 1958 | Carcinomatosis at look Jan. 22, 1959; died during convalescence |

Upon admission to the hospital in October, 1959, she was again without symptoms or evidence of residual or recurrent carcinoma. At operation in October, 1959, carcinoma was found in the subhepatic space, omentum, left perirenal fat, and near the hilum of the spleen. Splenectomy and omenectomy and excision of all visible tumor were carried out. There was microscopic evidence of carcinoma in 17 of 32 submitted specimens.

On September 26, 1960, she again underwent exploratory operation. Multiple biopsy specimens were taken throughout the peritoneal cavity. The final pathologic report indicated no evidence of residual carcinoma. The patient remains well.

**Case 3.** E. Y. was a 57-year-old woman. At another hospital on April 15, 1957, she underwent a total hysterectomy and bilateral salpingo-oophorectomy, with removal of a very large fluid-filled cyst. The pathologic diagnosis was adenocarcinoma of the ovary, mesonephroma type. On Nov. 26, 1958, the patient came to this hospital. She was completely asymptomatic. Exploratory operation showed only cholelithiasis. There was no gross evidence of recurrence. However, a periaortic lymph node dissection was performed in addition to cholecystectomy and appendectomy. Two of 6 periaortic nodes contained carcinoma. In addition, a small nodule in the remainder of the left broad ligament was also positive for recurrent disease. The patient has remained entirely well.

Our experience with this disease has been such that on several occasions we have suggested that her consent to undergo another exploratory operation would be in her best interest. She has to date been unable to accept this recommendation, but recently suggested she will consent to the operation.

**Case 4.** In July, 1944, B. O., a 40-year-old woman, had a gelatinous periumbilical mass removed at another hospital. The specimen was said to show "low-grade adenocarcinoma." In February, 1952, she underwent a second exploratory operation and copious amounts of mucogelatinous material were removed. The pathologic diagnosis was pseudomyxoma peritonei. The patient first came to the University of Minnesota Hospitals in February, 1954. She complained of abdominal distention, constipation, and diarrhea. On Feb. 26, 1954, she was operated upon and was found to have 3 L. of gelatinous material in the abdomen. The appendix was removed and was found to show adenocarcinoma. There were also extensive pelvic peritoneal metastases. It was believed that this was a palliative procedure and the patient therefore received postoperative radiation therapy.

On June 9, 1954, during an asymptomatic period, she again underwent exploratory operation. She had a massive tumor in the pelvis attached to the anterior surface of the rectum, filling the cul-de-sac, and adherent to the uterus and urinary bladder. The parietal peritoneum, lateral and anterior abdominal walls, the capsule of the right lobe of the liver, and the serosal surface of the small bowel were found to contain metastatic tumor. A total hysterectomy, left salpingo-oophorectomy, resection of pelvic peritoneum and all palpable tumor, and a left transverse colostomy were performed at that time. She then remained well until December, 1954. At that time she returned during an asymptomatic phase and underwent another exploratory procedure. No malignant cells were found on exploration, but semiadherent mucinous material was distributed over portions of the jejunum, the cecum, the pelvic colon, the pelvic portion of the left ureter, and in the area of the gall bladder. Multiple biopsy specimens were taken and 5 of 15 were positive for mucin. Therefore, on Oct. 13, 1955, again during an asymptomatic phase, the patient underwent exploratory operation. The remaining appendical stump was removed and 19 biopsy specimens taken. Pathologic examination showed residual mucinous adenocarcinoma in the appendical stump. The other specimens, including liver biopsy material, were negative for carcinoma. The woman was followed closely in the clinic.

In August, 1960, she returned because of the appearance of an enlarging mass just above the symphysis pubis due to a recurrence in the anterior abdominal wall. Roentgen examination of the chest showed widespread pulmonary metastases. The mass was excised and proved to be recurrent adenocarcinoma. The patient had, in addition, such extensive intraperitoneal carcinosis that any further attempt at excision was precluded. She received radiation therapy after convalescence. At this time she has reached the terminal stages of the disease.

**Case 5.** M. D., a 57-year-old woman, was first operated upon at the University of Minnesota Hospitals on Sept. 6, 1958. Total hysterectomy and bilateral salpingo-oophorectomy were performed with removal of a papillary cystadenocarcinoma which involved both ovaries. There were extensive metastases along the entire length of the ovarian vessels up to the site of their origins. These were removed and periaortic and peri–vena cava lymph node dissections were carried out. A second-look procedure was carried out on May 10, 1959. Biopsy specimens from the pelvis, small bowel mesentery, porta hepatis, and retroduodenal area were negative for recurrence.

The patient continued to do well. Because of the disappointing experience with B. O., and because of the extent of the disease in this patient at the first operation, she was urged to undergo another exploration. On Feb. 1, 1961, 22 months after a "negative look" and while she was completely asymptomatic, the woman underwent another exploratory operation. There was recurrent tumor overlying the right internal iliac vein and in the perirenal fat pad near the inferior pole of the left kidney. These were excised and a splenectomy and wide dissection of both lateral parietes were carried out. Another look will be undertaken after 2 years, to which suggestion the patient already has assented.

## DISCUSSION

Recent data show that if all stages of the disease are considered, 20 to 25 per cent of patients treated for carcinoma of the ovary will survive for 5 years or more. Of those with cancer confined to the ovary at the time of diagnosis and institution of treatment, 60 to 65 per cent will be alive for 5 years.

Unfortunately, approximately 50 per cent

of ovarian cancers are found to have spread beyond the primary site at the time of original exploratory operation. The failure of radical primary operation to achieve cure in these cases continues to plague those concerned. Moreover, the combination of surgical and radiation therapy and adjunctive chemotherapy has not effected significant improvement in cure rate.

The accomplishment in many of the patients with extensive cancer has been gratifying. It is fair to say that a program of systematic secondary operation has served to alter the prognosis of patients "converted" by repeated surgical intervention. Prolongation of life has been achieved in a number of patients in whom resection of metastatic cancer prevented imminent death due to gastrointestinal or urinary tract obstruction.

The information obtained through application of these principles of management is of value to physicians and patients alike. The findings at the time of first re-operation has lent support to a widely recognized need for change in the initial operative procedure for some cancers. In addition, the experiences with 2 patients who have been declared cancer-free only to develop recurrences—one in whom the disease was "caught" in time, the other with disease out of hand at the time of exploration, indicate that some of these lesions are relatively slow-growing tumors. When a patient has been rid of very extensive disease through the second-look procedure, an additional delayed look, perhaps 2 years after one negative look, is in order to consolidate the gain.

## SUMMARY

The experience with the second-look procedure in the management of ovarian malignancies and pseudomyxoma peritonei is reviewed. Four of 13 patients with ovarian carcinomas, including one with associated pseudomyxoma peritonei, are alive and well after intervals of from 2 to 12 years after the initial operative procedure. Two of these 4 are considered to have been converted to the cancer-free state after 3 looks, while 2 who are probably converted are awaiting another look.

The second-look procedure appears to have merit in the management of ovarian malignancies and pseudomyxoma peritonei.

## REFERENCES

1. Fourth National Cancer Conference Proceedings, Philadelphia, J. B. Lippincott Company, in press.
2. Kottmeier, H. L.: Carcinoma of the female genitalia, Baltimore, 1953, Williams & Wilkins Company.
3. Novak, E., and Novak, E. R.: Gynecologic and obstetric pathology, Philadelphia, 1958, W. B. Saunders Company, ed. 4.
4. Wangensteen, O. H.: Cancer of the colon and rectum with special reference to (1) earlier recognition of alimentary tract malignancy; (2) secondary delayed re-entry of the abdomen in patients exhibiting lymph node involvement; (3) subtotal excision of the colon; (4) operation in obstruction, Wisconsin M. J. **48:** 591-597, 1949.

# Pathologic lesions in experimental hypernatremia induced by extracorporeal dialysis

BENJAMIN F. RUSH, JR., M.D.
LAURENCE FINBERG, M.D.
GEORGE F. DAVIGLUS, M.D.
CHE-SUN CHEUNG, M.D.
BALTIMORE, MD.
*From the Departments of Surgery and Pediatrics, The Johns Hopkins Hospital, The Baltimore City Hospitals and The Johns Hopkins University School of Medicine*

Hypernatremia will be encountered in any clinical situation in which the balance of water and sodium in a patient results in a persistent gain of sodium in relation to water. This may result either from losses of water in excess of losses of sodium, or from excess of sodium intake in relation to water intake, or from a combination of these events.

While hypernatremia is not observed so commonly by the surgeon as is hyponatremia, it is not a rare electrolyte disturbance, and has been found in infants with diarrhea,[7, 14, 15] in patients with heat stroke,[2] in association with intracranial lesions,[6, 16, 17] after neurosurgery,[16, 18] in the diuretic phase after renal failure,[12] in uncontrolled diabetes insipidus,[6] and during treatment of diabetes mellitus.[4] It has also been described in association with gastrointestinal bleeding,[3] and with overenthusiastic feedings of high caloric–high solute diets by nasogastric tube.[5] The mechanism which contributes to the increasing concentration of sodium in these various clinical situations differs somewhat, but the ultimate serum electrolyte pattern achieved is the same.

Supported in part by Public Health Service Grants No. A2029, B1409, and H2825.

Received for publication Oct. 3, 1960.

Hypernatremia is more often found in the very young and in the very old, or in patients with impaired renal function.[20] In all of these instances renal concentrating power is decreased, a more dilute urine excreted, and the tendency to accumulate sodium in excess of water is enhanced.

The clinical syndrome which accompanies hypernatremia is marked by malaise, restlessness, confusion, hallucinations, and convulsions.[7, 13, 20] These symptoms have drawn attention to the central nervous system, and an increasing body of clinical and experimental data indicate that definite subdural and intracranial lesions may accompany the hypernatremic state.[13, 14, 20]

Some clinical reports have suggested that renal damage also occurs,[2, 12] but the causal mechanism of the renal lesions observed is confused by the fact that most of the patients with these changes have been in shock for some time before death, or were the victims of overdoses of sulfonamide drugs.

Experimental studies of hypernatremia in the past have involved significant changes in the fluid volume of the subject, either by overhydration or by dehydration (and usually both, sequentially). Such volume changes have been necessarily accompanied by circulatory changes which are also seen in physiologic disturbances which do not involve hypernatremia. This has made analysis of the resultant pathologic process difficult in that some of the changes could well have been circulatory in origin. The present study had as one of its goals the inducement of hypernatremia without changing body water volume and without permitting changes in concentration of extracellular ions other than sodium and chloride. This report describes the use of extracorporeal dialysis as an experimental tool, and presents some of the results obtained.

## MATERIALS AND METHOD

Mongrel female dogs which weighed 18 to 20 kilograms were used. The dogs were anesthetized with a combination of sodium pentobarbital, 10 mg. per kilogram, and gallamine triethiodide (Flaxedil), 2 mg. per kilogram, given intravenously. After the initial use of pentobarbital, the animals were maintained entirely with gallamine triethiodide throughout the several hours of the experiment. The total dose amounted to approximately 2 mg. per kilogram per hour. After induction of the anesthesia an endotracheal tube was inserted and respirations were maintained by a piston respirator at a rate of 400 c.c. of room air per kilogram per minute.

The dogs were placed on an infant scale with a large pan. The femoral artery and vein of both legs were exposed. The artery and vein on one side were connected to the appropriate arterial and venous sides of a Kolff disposable coil artificial kidney. The artery of the other leg was connected to a mercury manometer, and the vein was connected to an infusion bottle. The animal was given no heparin directly, but approximately 50 mg. of heparin per 500 ml. was added to the priming blood in the disposable coil.

Electrolytes were added to the 100 L. of fluid in the artificial kidney bath to give a concentration approximating the extracellular fluid concentration of electrolytes in the dog—sodium 150, chloride 126, carbon dioxide 27, magnesium 2.1, calcium 7.2, and potassium 4 mEq. per liter. The pH was maintained at 7.4 by bubbling 5 per cent carbon dioxide through the bath. The total osmolality of the solution was 315 milliosmols per kilogram of water. This solution will be referred to as the normal bath. Creatinine was added to the bath to give a concentration of 5.8 mg. per cent. The infusion which the dog received in the contralateral vein contained a similar concentration of sodium, chloride, and carbon dioxide. A No. 14 Fr. Foley catheter, with a 5 c.c. bag, was placed in the dog's bladder. The bag was inflated and the catheter led to a graduated cylinder. The arrangement of the experiment is illustrated in Fig. 1.

After this preparation, the animals designated as controls were dialized against the normal bath for periods of from 5 to 7 hours. Since the Kolff disposable coil has 2 parallel units of dialysis tubing, 2 dogs were usually dialyzed against the same bath during each experiment. Blood flow was maintained between 200 and 300 ml. per minute. Blood and urine samples were taken before the dialysis started, and usually each hour during the experiment. Plasma was promptly separated from cells and stored under oil. These samples were analyzed for osmolality by a Fiske osmometer, for chloride by a Cotlove chloridimeter, for sodium and potassium by an internal standard flame photometer, for creatinine by the method of Hare and Hare,[11] for total proteins by the method of Greenberg,[10] and for plasma urea nitrogen by the method of Archibald.[1] Plasma water was determined by weighing an aliquot and drying to constant weight. Electrolyte concentrations are expressed in milliequivalents per liter of plasma water, corrected by a Donnan factor of 0.96. Hematocrits were also obtained at intervals by the method of Wintrobe.[19]

In some of our early experiments it was found that there was difficulty with a sudden drop of the dog's blood pressure during the initial period of the dialysis. This was reflected in a drop in the dog's glomerular filtration rate and urinary output. Two modifications in our techniques succeeded in eliminating this difficulty. One was the use of gallamine triethiodide to maintain the animal throughout the experiment, after pentobarbital anesthesia during the initial manipulations. The second was scrupulous care in preventing or compensating for fluid losses from the body while the dog was being dialyzed. Although the Kolff coil is semi-rigid, its volume does tend to increase somewhat as the blood flow through the coil is increased. This will be reflected in the first 10 or 15 minutes of dialysis by a drop in the blood pressure of the dog and a decrease in the dog's weight. By our technique, this shift of blood from dog to coil could be completely avoided. Prior to dialysis, the coil was primed with the arterial and venous cannulae connected together and the flow rate through the coil was adjusted during this priming period to the level planned for use during the experiment. With this method, the coil takes up a maximum amount of priming blood, usually 750 ml. to each half of the coil, or a total of 1,500 ml. When dialysis was started, the flow rate was slowly increased to the expected maximum over the first 10 or 15 minutes, and the dog's weight was carefully watched. Any weight loss over this period was promptly corrected by infusion of additional blood into the coil. An additional 100 to 200 ml. of blood may be required.

A second source for fluid loss is the ultrafiltration through the semirigid Kolff coil. This amounts to approximately 220 ml. per hour, per dog, at the flow rates used. A portion of this loss is probably also due to osmotic shifts between the plasma in the coil and the hypertonic bath solution, since the loss per hour decreases somewhat in the later hours of the dialysis. The third major source for fluid loss is urine formation. The last 2 sources of loss are reflected in a slow loss of weight of the animal over the course of the experiment. This is easily obviated by maintaining a stable weight with an intravenous infusion. For experimental purposes the infusion can be stopped, and any degree of dehydration can be superimposed on the electrolyte pattern maintained by the concentration of the artificial kidney bath.

A total of 51 dogs were studied by this method. Eighteen of these were treated as

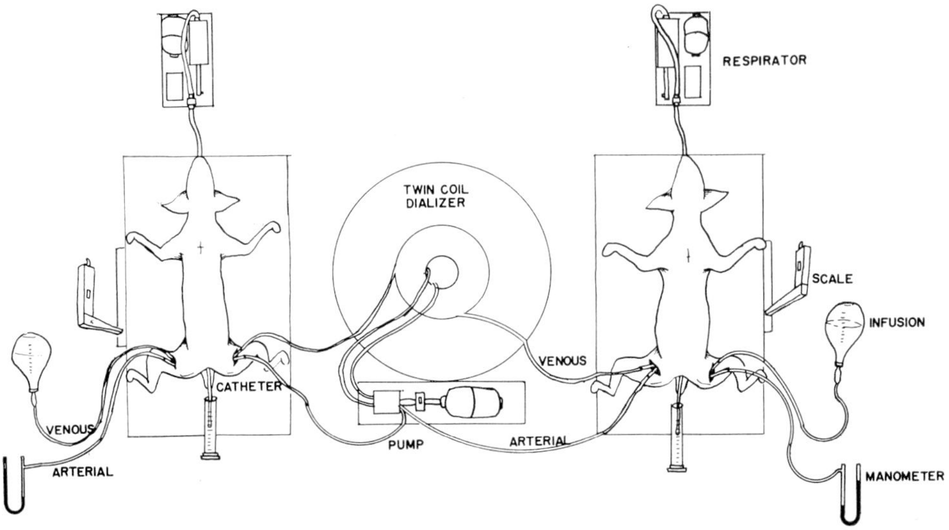


**Fig. 1.** The experimental setup used. In essence, the extracellular fluids of the dog have been increased by the volume of the extracorporeal system, an added 100 L. Once the extracellular compartment of the dog is in equilibrium with the concentration of solutes in the bath, the level of concentration is very stable, and, despite maximal effort on the part of the kidney or other mechanisms of compensation, the level of hyperosmolality is maintained in the animals dialyzed against hyperosmolar fluids.

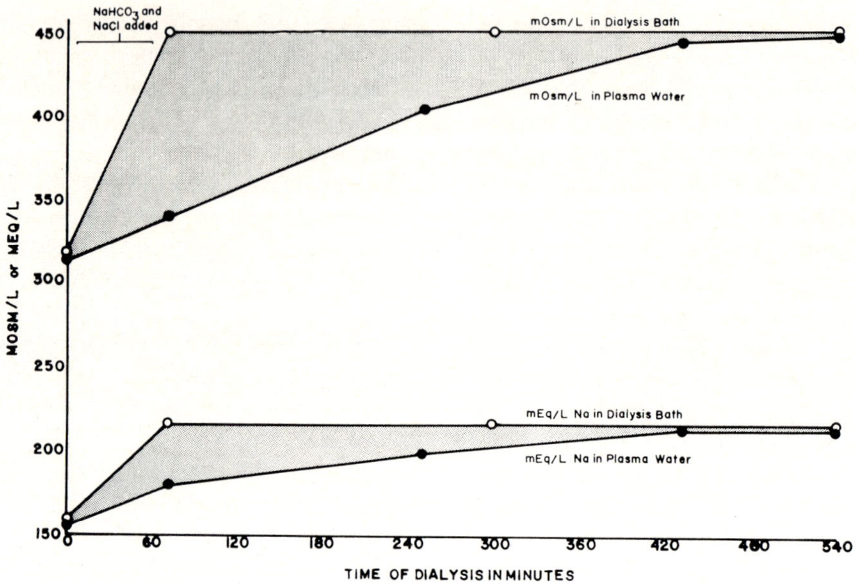


**Fig. 2.** Diagram illustrates the increase of osmolality and sodium concentration in the plasma water, compared to the concentrations in the dialysate solution. More solute was added in the first hour. Concentrations in the dialysate solution and plasma water were in near equilibrium by the end of the fourth hour after the addition of solute.

controls and dialyzed against the normal bath. Twenty-seven were dialyzed against the normal bath initially, and then sodium chloride and sodium bicarbonate were added gradually over a 1-hour period to the bath to raise the concentration of sodium to 205 mEq. per liter and of chloride to 165 mEq. per liter. The total osmolality was thus raised from 315 to 430 miliosmols per kilogram of water. The animals were dialyzed against this bath for from 5 to 8 hours. In 6 additional animals the concentration of electrolytes in the bath was left unchanged, but the osmolality was raised to 415 milliosmols per kilogram by the addition of urea to the bath.

Microscopic examination of tissue was carried out in 20 dogs. Eight of the dogs were dialyzed against the hypernatremic bath. Seven of the dogs were dialyzed against the control bath and 5 were dialyzed against the urea bath. Of the 8 animals dialyzed against the hyponatremic bath, all were dialyzed in pairs, as previously described. One animal of each pair was maintained at a constant weight, and the other was allowed to become somewhat dehydrated, to the extent of 5 to 8 per cent of its body weight, in order to better duplicate the conditions of clinical hypernatremic dehydration.

## RESULTS

After the addition of sodium chloride and sodium bicarbonate to the control bath to raise the concentrations of sodium and chloride, the sodium and chloride levels in the plasma of the dogs rose rapidly to approach the concentration in the bath. This is illustrated in Fig. 2. With allowance for the Donnan factor, the concentration of electrolytes in the plasma water of the dog approaches closely the concentration of electrolytes in the bath over the period of the dialysis. With the increasing concentration of electrolyte and osmolality in the plasma of the dogs, urinary excretion increased markedly in animals maintained at a constant weight. While urinary volume increased, sodium concentration in the urine dropped markedly until it reached a level at or below plasma levels of sodium. In animals in which dehydration was superimposed on hypernatremia, sodium concentration in the urine likewise fell, though not so far, and urine volume was concomitantly reduced. These and other renal functional changes will be discussed elsewhere.[8]

At autopsy the most striking gross findings were extensive subdural and subarachnoid hemorrhages over the cortex of the brain. These varied in size, but were usually quite extensive, often involving an entire hemisphere. The brain was noted to be shrunken, often contracted 1 cm. or more away from the overlying bone. This shrinking of the brain was noted in all animals with hypernatremia. In 7 of the 8 animals with hypernatremia, moderate to marked hemorrhages were found.

In the animals dialyzed against the control bath, no hemorrhages were found and the brain appeared to be of normal size. In the animals dialyzed against the hyperosmolar urea bath, the brains also showed some shrinkage, although this seemed to be of a lesser degree than that found in the hypernatremic animals. Subdural and arachnoid hemorrhages were not found in the brains of any of the 5 uremic dogs, although in one the brain was somewhat hyperemic. Another gross pathologic finding in both the hypernatremic and uremic dogs was multiple petechiae scattered over the parietal and visceral peritoneum. These also occurred occasionally in the control dogs, although to a much lesser degree.

Microscopic evidence of renal tubular necrosis was found in 6 of the 8 hypernatremic dogs. This was characterized (Fig. 3) by intensely eosinophilic, granular alteration of epithelial cells of the convoluted tubules, certainly proximal and possibly distal. The nuclei of these cells showed striking karyorrhexis. The latter seemed to occur first since it was often present before evident alteration of the cytoplasm.

An additional change (Fig. 4) was seen in 4 hypernatremic animals with and one without frank epithelial cell necrosis. Large, poorly defined vacuoles collected in the basal part of the convoluted tubular epithelial cells adjacent to their nuclei. In the most extreme development of this change, cleavage occurred at this level, so that the major distal portions of adjacent cells were cast into the lumen in sheets, leaving occasional nuclei and cytoplasmic shreds adherent to the basement membrane. Even a modicum of caution makes us regard this striking alteration as an artefact. We believe, however,

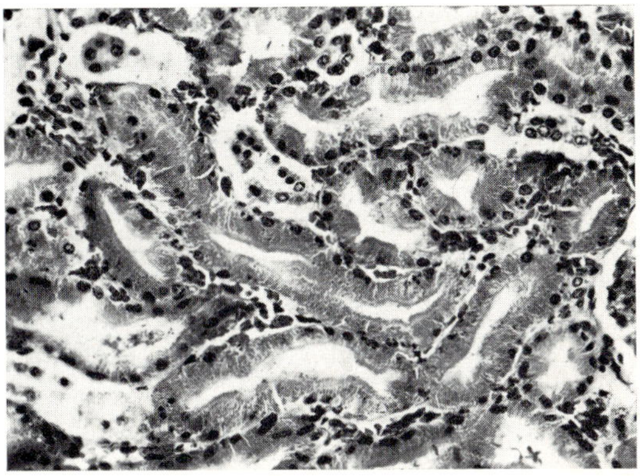

**Fig. 3.** Photomicrograph shows the acute tubular necrosis which occurred in one of the dogs made hypernatremic. The period of hypernatremia was 6 hours, with the maximum hypernatremia maintained over the last 2 hours. The marked disintegration of tubular cells is readily apparent in the tubules in the center. Granularity, loss of cellular detail, and pyknotic and fragmented nuclei are seen. (×350; reduced 4/11.)

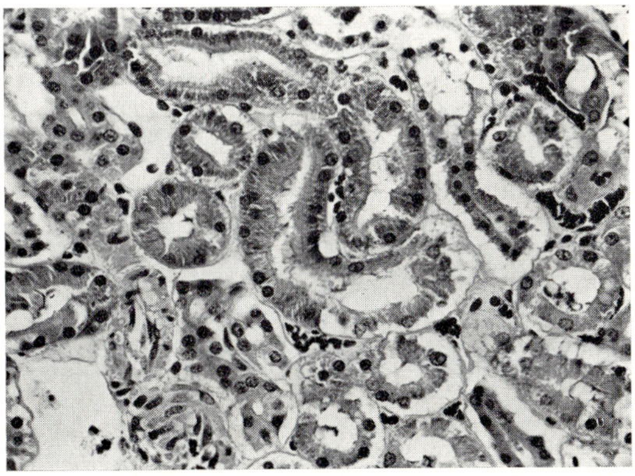

**Fig. 4.** Photomicrograph of sections of renal tissue from another dog with hypernatremia. Again marked necrosis of tubular cells is seen with pyknotic and fragmented nuclei and granular disintegrating cytoplasm. Vacuolation of tubular cells is clearly seen. (×350; reduced 4/11.)

that this may be an artefact which is preconditioned by an unusual intravital collection of fluid in the basal segments of the convoluted epithelial cells. Thus, 7 of the 8 animals showed some pathologic change within the tubular cells. The glomeruli of all of the kidneys appeared normal and without evidence of acute pathologic change on hematoxylin and eosin staining after formalin fixation.

It was interesting to note that the glomerular filtration rate, as reflected by the creatinine clearance, remained unchanged during the course of the experiment. None of the changes described were observed in any of the animals of the control series or in any of the animals in the urea series. In addition, the kidneys of 6 normal dogs, sacrificed for other reasons in the laboratory, were examined as an additional control group. In none of these animals were the changes described found.

## DISCUSSION

The results suggest that the clinical finding of renal failure and acute tubular necrosis in patients with hypernatremia may be related to the electrolyte disturbance itself. In the experimental animals of this study, the renal lesions induced in the animals which were normovolemic and hypernatremic were of approximately the same degree and type as in those which were hypovolemic and hypernatremic. Thus the entire group of 8 animals has been considered as a single group, and it is believed that the renal changes were due primarily to the increased sodium and chloride concentration of the extracellular fluid. These ions which are excluded from the interior of the cell bear the chief responsibility for the distribution of water on either side of the cell membrane. When an increase in extracellular osmolality of an equivalent degree was created by a diffusable osmol such as urea, no lesions were induced in the tubular cells. This suggests that the cellular damage was due to a marked increase in osmolality by effectively nondiffusible, or only partly diffusible, ions on one side of the cell membrane. The intracellular necrosis observed might be related to a marked intracellular dehydration as water was drawn out of the cell by the hyperosmotic extracellular fluids. It has been suggested by some[8] that there are also alterations in the chemical anatomy within the cell which produce "idiogenic osmols." The changes in chemical anatomy may represent a prenecrotic stage of cellular desiccation.

The significance of the vacuolation seen in the tubular cells is unknown, but this change appears to be related to the hypernatremic state, since it was not found in the controls, the urea treated animals, or in the untreated dogs. The gross hemorrhages found in the subdural and subarachnoid spaces of the hypernatremic dogs duplicate similar lesions found clinically in hypernatremic infants,[13] and experimentally in cats and rats made hypernatremic by intraperitoneal injections of saline and urea solutions.[14] It is likely that evidence of acute tubular necrosis found in patients with hypernatremia may be related, at least in part, to the hypernatremia per se, as well as to other complicating clinical factors.

The clinical implications of these findings are clear. Hypernatremia in the range of 200 milliosmols per liter may be lethal, through the induction of severe cellular damage to the brain and kidneys. This damage, once it has occurred, is not immediately reparable simply by returning the electrolyte balance to normal. Once the presence of hypernatremia has been discovered in a patient every effort should be made to return electrolyte balance to normal and avoid cellular damage. In the presence of severe hypernatremia, the urine produced is frequently of low osmolality and renal excretion of salt is low. Thus urinary excretion is not only unable to correct the sodium imbalance, but may actually make it worse. The only source for correction of this state is the intake of exogenous water. This would seem to be best provided by infusions of 5 per cent dextrose in water, although therapy must be individualized in accordance with the nature of the whole physiologic disturbance. At the some time, the factors which led the patient to his hypernatremic state must be corrected, if possible.

## SUMMARY AND CONCLUSIONS

With an artificial kidney, a steady state of severe hypernatremia of approximately 200 mEq. per liter was created in 8 dogs for periods of 5 to 8 hours. In 4 of these animals body water volume was held constant. In 5 animals, by the same technique, hyperosmolality without hypernatremia was created by the use of urea. Seven animals were dialyzed on the artificial kidney against a bath of normal electrolyte composition. The last 2 groups of animals served as controls for the first group.

Subarachnoid and subdural hemorrhages occurred in 7 of the 8 hypernatremic dogs. These changes did not occur in the urea-treated dogs, or in the dogs dialyzed against a normal bath.

Seven of the 8 hypernatremic dogs showed changes in the renal tubular epithelium. These changes consisted of scattered areas of acute tubular necrosis in the proximal and distal tubules. Several animals demonstrated an accompanying finding of large vacuoles in the tubular cells. The glomerular capillaries showed no change. No changes were seen in the renal tubules of the control animals or the urea-treated animals.

Severe degrees of hypernatremia, without accompanying circulatory disturbance, can induce definite histologic damage in the cerebral and renal tissues. It would not be expected that these changes, once they occur, could be corrected by returning the electrolyte pattern to normal.

The authors wish to acknowledge the assistance of Dr. Abou D. Pollack in reviewing and interpreting the histologic material.

### REFERENCES

1. Archibald, R. N.: Colorimetric determination of urea, J. Biol. Chem. **157:** 507, 1945.
2. Baxter, C. R., and Teschan, P. E.: Atypical heat stroke with hypernatremia, acute renal failure and fulminating potassium intoxication, Research Report No. 3, United States Army Surgical Research Unit, Brooke Army Medical Corps, Fort Sam Houston, Texas, March, 1958.
3. Borst, J. G. G.: The cause of hyperchloremia and hyperazotemia in patients with recurrent massive hemorrhage from peptic ulcer, Acta med. scandinav. **97:** 68, 1938.
4. Danowski, T. S., Peters, J. H., Rathbun, I. C., Quashnock, J. M., and Greenman, L.: Studies in diabetic acidosis and coma with particular emphasis on the retention of administered potassium, J. Clin. Invest. **28:** 1, 1949.
5. Engel, F. L., and Jaeger, C.: Dehydration with hypernatremia, hyperchloremia and azotemia complicating nasogastric tube feeding, Am. J. Med. **17:** 196, 1954.
6. Engstrom, W. W., and Liebman, A.: Chronic hyperosmolarity of the body fluids with a cerebral lesion causing diabetes insipidus and anterior pituitary insufficiency, Am. J. Med. **15:** 180, 1953.
7. Finberg, L., and Harrison, H. E.: Hypernatremia in infants, an evaluation of the clinical and urological findings accompanying this state, Pediatrics **16:** 1, 1955.
8. Finberg, L., Luttrell, C., and Redd, H.: Pathogenesis of lesions in the nervous system in hypernatremic states, Pediatrics **23:** 1, 1959.
9. Finberg, L., Rush, B. F., and Cheung, C. S.: Experimental studies of renal function during hypernatremia, A. M. A. J. Dis. Child. **100:** 504, 1960.
10. Greenberg, D. M.: The colorimetric determination of the serum proteins, J. Biol. Chem. **82:** 545, 1929.
11. Hare, R. S., and Hare, K.: Determinations of creatinine in blood and urine, Fed. Proc. **8:** 68, 1949.
12. Luetscher, J. A., Jr., and Blackman, J. J., Jr.: Severe injury to kidneys and brain following sulfathiazole administration: high serum sodium and chloride levels and persistent cerebral damage, Ann. Int. Med. **18:** 741, 1943.
13. Luttrell, C. N., and Finberg, L.: Hemorrhagic encephalopathy induced by hypernatremia. I. Clinical, laboratory and pathological observations, A. M. A. Arch. Neurol. & Psychiat. **81:** 425, 1959.
14. Luttrell, C. N., Finberg, L., and Drawdy, L. P.: Hemorrhagic encephalopathy induced by hypernatremia. II. Experimental observations on hyperosmolarity in cats, A. M. A. Arch. Neurol. **1:** 153, 1959.
15. Rapaport, S.: Hyperosmolarity and hyperelectrolytemia in pathological conditions of childhood, Am. J. Dis. Child. **74:** 682, 1947.
16. Schoolman, H. M., Dubin, A., and Hoffman,

W. S.: Clinical syndromes associated with hyponotremia, A. M. A. Arch. Int. Med. **95:** 15, 1955.

17. Sweet, W. H., Cotzigs, G. C., Seed, J., and Yakovlev, P.: Gastrointestinal hemorrhages, hyperglycemia, azotemia, hyperchloremia and hypernatremia following lesions of the frontal lobe in man, Arch. Nerv. & Ment. Dis. **27:** 790, 1948.

18. Welt, L. G., Selden, D. W., Nelson, W. P., III, German, W. J., and Peters, J. P.: Role of the central nervous system in the metabolism of electrolytes and water, A. M. A. Arch. Int. Med. **90:** 355, 1952.

19. Wintrobe, M. M.: Clinical hematology, Philadelphia, 1942, Lea & Febiger.

20. Zieler, K. I.: Hyperosmolarity in adults: a critical review, J. Chronic Dis. **7:** 1, 1958.

# Experimental wound infections: contamination versus surgical technique

JOHN D. CONDIE, M.D.
DONALD J. FERGUSON, M.D., PH.D.*
MINNEAPOLIS, MINN.
*From the Surgical Department, Veterans Administration Hospital, and the University of Minnesota*

It is customary in some quarters to attribute wound infections primarily to faults of asepsis. It is also widely believed that the incidence of wound infection depends in some degree on the surgical competence with which the wound is handled. We have attempted to clarify this problem by asking, "Will wounds regularly tolerate heavy contamination without becoming infected if surgical technique is otherwise strictly in accord with certain recognized principles?" An experiment based on this question was designed to test various aspects of wound closure in dogs in the presence of heavy contamination with cultures of staphylococci obtained from infected wounds.

## METHODS

The dogs were anesthetized with pentobarbital. Bilateral transverse wounds were made through the abdominal wall, with standard aseptic technique. A few dogs in preliminary experiments had 3 or 4 wounds. The external and internal oblique muscles were cut, as was a portion of the rectus. The wounds were 5 to 10 cm. long, depending on size of the animal. Ligatures of No. 4-0 chromic catgut were used for hemostasis. The peritoneum and transverse layer were closed together with a running suture before contamination.

A trial group of experiments showed that interrupted cutaneous sutures nearly always became infected superficially while a continuous subcuticular suture did not. The latter type was used in all subsequent experiments. Other procedures to be studied differed on the two sides.

The contaminating staphylococci were hemolytic, coagulase positive, and phage type 53-75-77, a pattern found in some human surgical wound infections. The original culture came from a patient's infected wound and subsequent cultures were obtained from the wounds of experimental animals. No stock cultures were kept in vitro for more than 1 month. Preliminary experiments in dogs showed that a subcutaneous injection of 800 million bacteria regularly produced abscesses. Bacterial counts were carried out on all contaminating cultures and showed 80 million to 800 million staphylococci in each 2.5 ml. Virulence of the material was verified by the fact that every culture produced some wound infections. Wounds were contaminated by instillation of 2.5 ml. of fluid from a broth culture. After contamination, wounds were covered with a gauze sponge and left undisturbed for from 5 to 15 minutes. Some preliminary work was done with purulent discharge from wounds infected with staphylococci. This was used in place of the broth culture and invariably caused a severe reaction and early breakdown of the wound. Cultures were used in the experiments reported subsequently, When wounds were irrigated, a total of 250 ml. of saline solution

Received for publication Jan. 19, 1961.

*Present address: Department of Surgery, University of Chicago, Chicago 37, Ill.

**Table I.** *Comparison of 4-layer with 7-layer closure of contaminated wounds*

| *Closure* | *No. of wounds* | *No. infected* |
|---|---|---|
| 4-layer | 12 | 11 |
| 7-layer | 12 | 3 |

**Table II.** *Comparison of No. 4-0 monofilament nylon with No. 4-0 braided silk in closure of contaminated wounds*

| *Suture* | *No. of wounds* | *No. infected* |
|---|---|---|
| Silk | 12 | 10 |
| Nylon | 12 | 4 |

was used. All visible clot and debris was flushed from crevices before closure of the next layer.

Wounds were evaluated by daily inspection, by culture, and by studies of multiple cross sections after the animals had been sacrificed. Infections for the most part were obvious, but occasionally there was only a drop or two of serous drainage. If this material drained for 2 days the wound was considered infected. Fluctuation without discharge was also observed and classed as an infection. All such wounds gave a pure culture of the original staphylococci. Open wounds, on the other hand, showed the presence of micro-aerophilic streptococci and other organisms in addition to staphylococci.

## RESULTS

Our total experience in 96 dogs is analyzed with respect to the significance of natural resistance to staphylococcal infection in the experimental animals. Eighty-eight per cent of the animals had at least 1 wound infection and 70 per cent of wounds were infected. In 31 of the 96 dogs, wound infections were unilateral. In this group, at least, it is possible that natural resistance or susceptibility did not predominate over the technical factor being studied. In some of the remaining animals there were significant differences in severity of lesions between the two sides, even though both were infected. This will be be brought out in the description of individual experiments.

The first experiment concerned with the problem of the potential dead space. One wound was closed in 4 accurately matched layers with a running suture of No. 5-0 nylon passed through the fascia or muscle at 3 mm. intervals, about 3 mm. from the edge. No attempt was made to obliterate the potential spaces between layers. The scanty subcutaneous tissue was not separately sutured. In the other wound, 7 layers were sutured, including the subcutaneous tissues. The fasciae of either side of the internal and external oblique muscles were sutured separately, and sutures included the subjacent layer in such a way that all potential dead space was nearly obliterated. All wounds were washed beginning 5 minutes after they were contaminated. Closure took approximately 1 hour, even after some experience. The side with 7 layers was more indurated than the other when the operation was completed. Table I shows data from 12 dogs. The 3 infections of the 7-layer closure were minimal. On the 4-layer side, 2 wounds completely separated, 4 had a large amount of drainage, and 5 remained fluctuant without drainage for a period of 3 to 7 days. An example of the appearance of these wounds is shown in Fig. 1. Cross sections of the wounds showed occasional small pockets in the subcutaneous tissue of the 7-layer wounds. Dead spaces were noted throughout the layers on the 4-layer side and these often extended the entire length of the wound.

**Table III.** *Comparison of No. 4-0 braided Dacron with No. 4-0 braided silk in closure of contaminated wounds*

| *Suture* | *No. of wounds* | *No. infected* |
|---|---|---|
| Dacron | 12 | 11 |
| Silk | 12 | 12 |

**Table IV.** *Effect of washing contaminated wounds with 250 ml. of saline solution during closure*

| *Treatment* | *No. of wounds* | *No. infected* |
|---|---|---|
| Washing | 12 | 9 |
| None | 12 | 10 |

There were 8 wounds that showed no evidence of infection, though the presence of infected wounds on the opposite sides of the same animals established their susceptibility.

In a second experiment nylon and silk sutures were compared (Table II). All wounds were closed with No. 4-0 suture in 5 layers with each layer being sutured to the one beneath. (Note that in the 4-layer closures in the previous experiment the layers were not approximated to each other.) In 4 nylon-sutured wounds there was minimal infection. The silk-sutured wounds showed complete separation in 3 cases and considerable discharge in the other 7. In these wounds the difference in inflammatory response (Fig. 2) was also noted on all cross sections of the two types of wounds, except in 2 dogs which had complete healing of both wounds.

After observation of the probable superiority of monofilament nylon, the question arose as to whether composition of structure of the sutures was responsible for the difference. Since braided nylon was not available, No. 4-0 braided Dacron was compared with No. 4-0 silk. Data in Table III show that there was no difference in the results with the 2 types of suture.

The effect of washing with 250 ml. of saline solution beginning 15 minutes after contamination was also studied. Bilateral wounds were treated in an identical fashion except for the washing of 1 wound. A 5-layer closure was made with No. 4-0 nylon. Contamination consisted of a dose of approximately 800 million bacteria.

Data in Table IV show no decrease in the incidence of infection with this amount of washing. Two dogs had complete healing of both wounds. Cross sections of wounds showed little difference in the two wound types. This experiment is not directly comparable with the other, because of heavier contamination and longer waiting period before washing.

## DISCUSSION

The complete obliteration of the dead space involves considerable increase in suture

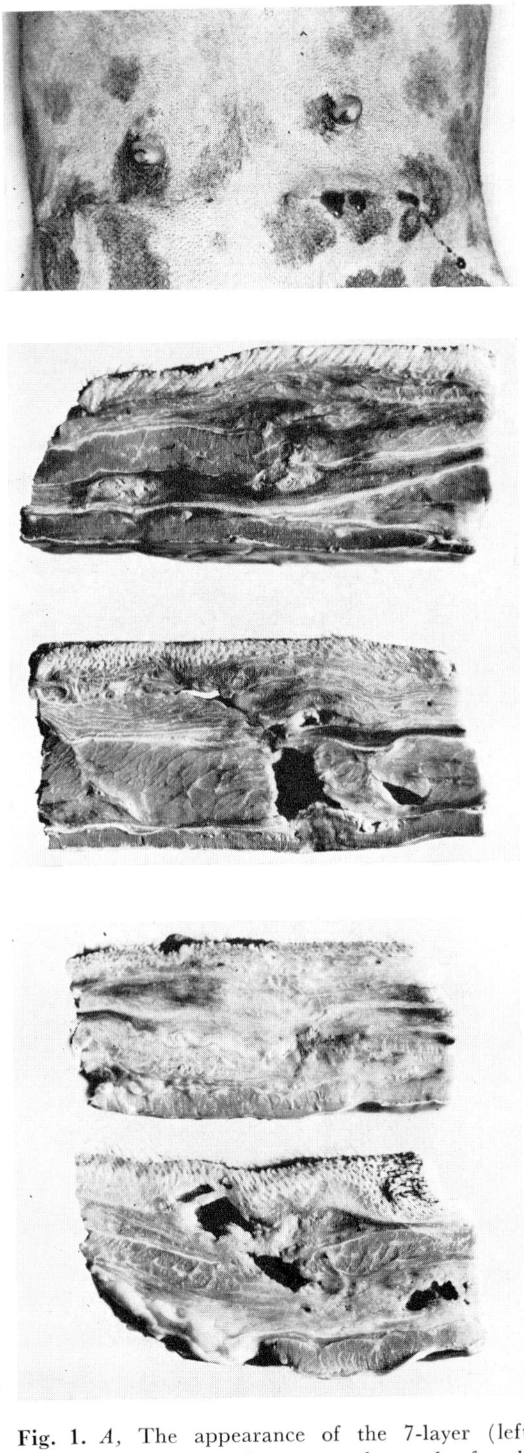

A

B

C

**Fig. 1.** *A,* The appearance of the 7-layer (left side) and draining 4-layer wounds on the fourth postoperative day. *B,* A cross section of wounds which was made on the fifth postoperative day. The upper section is the 7-layer closure. *C,* Similar sections which were taken from another animal on the sixth postoperative day.

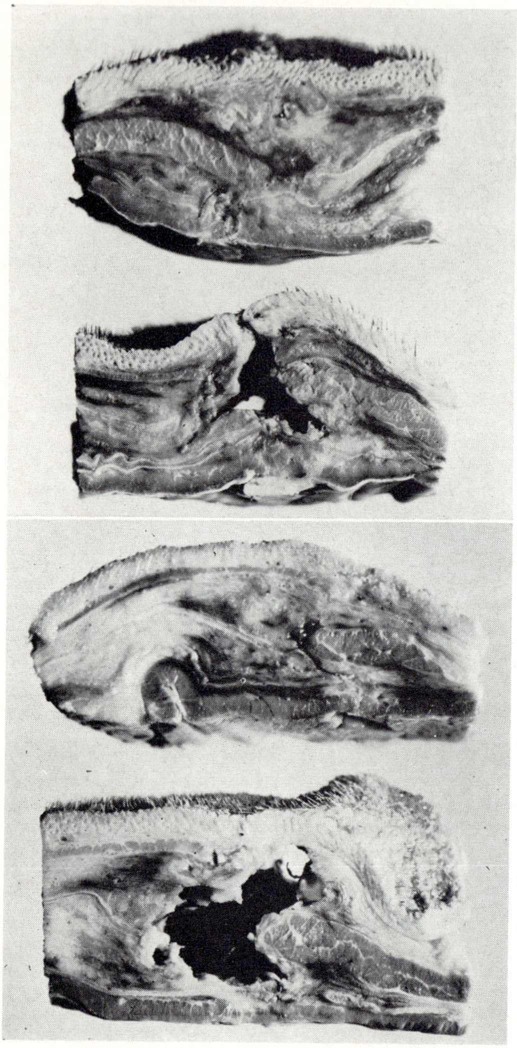

A

B

**Fig. 2.** *A,* Cross sections of wounds closed with nylon (top) and silk (bottom) on the eighth postoperative day. *B,* Similar sections from another animal on the seventh postoperative day.

material and more trauma to the tissues in the placement of sutures. Therefore, the extent to which this practice is desirable is questionable. Experimental results indicated that the increased amount of suture material and trauma was of less consequence than potential dead space in the genesis of wound infections. Thus, one item of surgical technique, the painstaking obliteration by suture of all potential dead space, appreciably reduced the occurrence of wound infections in the presence of virulent contamination.

At the same time, the use of braided sutures (whether silk or Dacron) in heavily contaminated wounds was once again shown to be deleterious, and success with the 7-layer closure was undoubtedly due in part to use of monofilament nylon. Elek[1] estimated that silk suture in a wound enhances the virulence of staphylococci by a factor of 10,000. The use of monofilament nylon in general surgery has been relatively infrequent, partly because of difficulties with knotting such slippery material. If additional evidence substantiates the apparent benignity of nylon as a running suture, even in the presence of infection, it may find considerable use clinically in that form. It is stronger, smoother, and more durable than catgut, and is easier to handle than wire.

In the experiments with washing wounds, we found no consistent effect. However, there is no doubt that washing removes both the bacteria and the blood clot, dead tissue, and so forth, on which they grow. It may be assumed that either more thorough washing or less heavy contamination might have brought out a difference, as it has in other experiments.[2] In all our groups, contamination was far in excess of anything that could occur in normal operations with clean wounds.

Surgical technique in relation to wound healing can be guided by a single principle —the assurance of maximum blood supply to all healing tissue. Concordance with this principle implies elimination of actual or potential dead space and accurate matching of tissue layers, so that all cells are directly nourished from both sides of the wound. It implies minimal ligature and suture material, devitalized tissue, and hematoma in the wound. It implies all that is technically necessary for uncomplicated wound healing, except for asepsis. The principle of asepsis, at least with respect to staphylococci, seems to be necessary in proportion with neglect of the other principle. Of course no one would willingly do without the additional safeguard of asepsis, however perfect his technique. Nevertheless, the occurrence of a staphylococcal wound infection seems more likely to be a reflection of poor technique than of unusual contamination.

## CONCLUSIONS

1. In experimental wounds contaminated by staphylococci maximum attention to obliteration of potential dead spaces by suture reduces the likelihood of infection.

2. Monofilament nylon as a continuous suture is preferable to braided Dacron or silk in these wounds.

## REFERENCES

1. Elek, S. D., and Conen, P. E.: The virulence of staphylococcus pyogenes for man, Brit. J. Exper. Path. **38:** 573, 1957.
2. Peterson, L. W.: Prophylaxis of wound infection, Arch. Surg. **50:** 177, 1945.

# Prolonged hypothermia below 25° C. for periods over 20 hours: influence of therapy and technique on survival

PETER J. CONNAUGHTON, M.D.
GORDON HOLT, B.S.
F. JOHN LEWIS, M.D.
CHICAGO, ILL.
*From the Department of Surgery, Northwestern University Medical School*

The use of hypothermia as a clinical and experimental adjunct has received much attention in the past 2 decades. Although short-term hypothermia of a few hours' duration has been the subject of most observations and has received the most clinical use, prolonged hypothermia has been investigated intermittently.

The first notable clinical use of prolonged hypothermia was reported by Smith and Fay[25] in 1939 and was applied to the treatment of cancer. In 1941, schizophrenic patients were treated by prolonged refrigeration by Dill and Forbes[6] and Talbott.[27] In 1951, Laufman[18] reported the survival of a woman exposed to –7° C. for approximately 11 hours after a heavy consumption of alcohol; body temperature was 16° C. In 1953 and 1954, Horvath's group[16, 26] reported survival in a few dogs after 20 hours of body temperature below 25° C. In 1955, Fisher and associates[12] evaluated this problem and later made additional observations on metabolic changes,[9] pathologic and histochemical changes,[8] and cardiovascular changes[7] of dogs subjected to body temperatures below 25° C. Even by 12 hours at this temperature, serious physiologic changes and a formidable mortality rate were observed. In 1957, Gray[14] cooled dogs for 72 hours at body temperatures between 26° and 30° C. and observed that the few animals which survived rewarming never regained consciousness. In 1958, MacPhee and Gray[22] reaffirmed these findings.

Most investigators who use prolonged hypothermia have sounded warnings of its dangers. Yet, there are many aspects of the problem which have not been thoroughly explored. The use of an efficient automatic respirator, proper positioning of the subject during the hypothermic period, and the effect of various therapies on survival have not been investigated. It is still not certain whether the time limits of hypothermia are contingent more on the inherent limitations of the subject or on the methods of inducing and maintaining it. The hibernator is living proof that cold is not harmful to mammals over long periods.

We have studied prolonged hypothermia for several reasons. First, it has clinical usefulness as a treatment for gravely ill, febrile patients.[19] Second, the effect of hypothermia in protecting against lethal radiation dosages[1, 15] combined with its elimination of the need for food and water may make this the ideal modality for space travel. Third, body temperatures lower than Smith and Fay[25] were able to achieve, maintained over a prolonged time, may be more beneficial in the treatment of cancer. Fourth, a thorough investigation of prolonged hypothermia would magnify any inherent dangers of short-term

Supported in part by United States Public Health Service Grant No. H-2879 and United States Air Force Grant No. AF29(600)-1729.

Received for publication March 9, 1961.

hypothermia and, by focusing attention on these danger points, would make this frequently used clinical adjunct even safer.

## METHODS AND MATERIALS

Ninety-eight mongrel dogs which weighed from 8 to 18 kilograms were studied. Anesthesia was induced by thiopental sodium, or pentobarbital sodium, 30 mg. per kilogram, with additional increments of pentobarbital sodium, thiopental sodium, or ether given as needed during the induction of hypothermia. After intubation, the dog was connected to an open-system mechanical respirator with a respiratory mixture either of room air or of 5 per cent carbon dioxide and 95 per cent oxygen. The femoral artery and vein were then cannulated and cooling was induced by wrapping in a rubber refrigeration blanket which was connected to a cooling machine. In the earlier experiments, a standard Therm-O-Rite* machine was preset to keep a constant temperature of 22° to 24° C., while in later experiments, an Autotherm† cooling apparatus was used. The latter was preset to the desired body temperature and automatically cooled or heated, depending on the reading of the electrical thermistor thermometer inserted in the dog's esophagus. It was accurate in keeping the body temperature within 0.5° C. of the preset temperature. All dogs were kept at body temperatures below 25° C. for 20 hours or longer. Cooling to 25° C. took 2.5 to 3 hours and rewarming to 35° C. approximately the same time.

Mean blood pressure was read directly from an aneroid manometer attached to the femoral artery cannula, while venous pressure was read directly from a saline manometer calibrated in centimeters of water and attached to the cannula in the femoral vein. Blood samples drawn for hematocrits from the arterial line were centrifuged for 30 minutes at 3,000 r.p.m. in Wintrobe tubes. Determinations of pH from arterial and venous samples were read from a Beckman model G pH meter (an anaerobic determination with external blood electrodes). The reading was corrected to the body temperature of the animal at the time of sampling. Serum sodium and potassium were determined by the Beckman flame photometer. Arterial and venous carbon dioxide and blood oxygen content and capacity were measured by a Van Slyke apparatus with the manometric method.

Blood and plasma volume determinations were carried out with Evans blue dye. This was injected into the femoral vein and removed 10 minutes later from the femoral artery. Electrocardiographic recordings were made with the Sanborn Poly-Viso machine. Autopsies were performed on all animals. Histologic sections from the liver, kidney, adrenal glands, lung, spleen, and intestine were taken from several animals with hematoxylin and eosin staining technique.

Twelve groups of dogs were studied. Dogs in Groups I through X had intermittent positive-pressure respiration of 15 to 20 mm. Hg while lying on their side. Group I included 9 dogs which received no medication or fluids. Group II included 12 dogs that had no medication or fluids but had a respiratory mixture of 5 per cent carbon dioxide and 95 per cent oxygen. Group III was composed of 11 dogs that received 800 ml. of saline solution or Ringer's lactate during the hypothermic period. Two of these received respiratory mixture of 5 per cent carbon dioxide and 95 per cent oxygen. Group IV included 18 dogs that received 1 to 10 mg. per kilogram of heparin in 500 ml. of saline solution or Ringer's lactate. In 7 of these the 5 per cent carbon dioxide mixture was used. Group V was composed of 6 dogs that had partial exsanguination of 200 to 400 ml. of blood 1 week prior to cooling. Group VI was composed of 4 dogs which were subjected to splenectomy 2 weeks prior to cooling and given the 5 per cent carbon dioxide mixture during cooling. Group VII was composed of 5 dogs which received a continuous drip of 40 to 80 mg. of Vasoxyl, a sympathomimetic agent, in 800

*Therm-O-Rite Products Corp., 17 Main Street, Buffalo, N. Y.

†Autotherm Corp., P.O. Box 25122, West Los Angeles 25, Calif.

ml. of saline solution during the hypothermic period. Group VIII was composed of 7 dogs which received 150 to 300 mg. of chlorpromazine and quantities of saline solution up to 2,000 ml. during the hypothermic period. Group IX was composed of 7 dogs which received Dibenzylene, a sympatholytic agent, 0.5 to 1.0 mg. per kilogram in 300 ml. of saline solution prior to and during cooling. Group X consisted of 7 dogs that received cortisone, 15 mg. per kilogram 4 times a day for the 4 days before cooling.

Dogs in Groups XI and XII had intermittent positive-pressure respiration, less than 12 mm. Hg, with an inspiratory-expiratory ratio of 1 to 5, and were cooled while in a prone position. The prevention of shivering by deep anesthesia during induction of hypothermia was a prominent feature, and the trachea was frequently aspirated during rewarming. Group XI was composed of 5 dogs which received 0.05 to 0.25 mg. per kilogram of reserpine, a hypotensive agent, before cooling. Sodium bicarbonate, 25 mEq., was given prior to rewarming. Group XII was composed of 7 dogs that received the same treatment as Group XI except for omission of reserpine.

## RESULTS

**Cold narcosis.** During the hypothermic period, additional anesthesia was not needed. The critical temperature was slightly different for each dog but tended to be approximately 22° to 24° C. Below this temperature, the dog would remain quiet and immobile with no shivering for the entire hypothermic period. If this critical temperature was exceeded by even 0.5° C., the dog would shiver slightly and make swallowing movements. These motions would cease when the temperature was again lowered. During the hypothermic period the pupils were pin point and nonreactive to light and the nictitating membrane was frequently drawn across the eye.

**Survival.** Of the 98 dogs studied, 54 (55 per cent) survived the 20-hour period of hypothermia. The dangers of rewarming were amply illustrated by the subsequent fate of 23 of these dogs which died during rewarming to 35° C. This left only 31 (32 per cent) of the 98 dogs that survived all phases of prolonged hypothermia. The subsequent fate of these 31 dogs deserves comment. A few never regained full consciousness and evidenced uncoordinated movements. In early experiments, hind-leg paralysis was noted in a few dogs. Thirteen (42 per cent) of the 31 survivors died within 24 hours after rewarming to 35° C., 3 (9 per cent) died within 48 hours, 2 (7 per cent) died within 1 week, and only 13 of the 31 survived indefinitely with no demonstrable sequelae.

The survival results in each of the 12 groups are presented in Table I. Statistical analysis of these groups by the chi-square method showed only 2 groups that had significantly increased survival rates compared to the controls in Group I. In both of the groups, shivering was carefully prevented by multiple frequent injections of pentobarbital; in both, the prone position rather than a lateral position was used, and the trachea was frequently aspirated. In addition, both received sodium bicarbonate prior to rewarming. The 5 dogs in Group XI, which received reserpine in addition to the changes in technique, all survived rewarming ($p = 0.0001$). Five of the 7 dogs in Group XII in which reserpine was omitted also survived rewarming to 35° C. ($p = 0.046$). Since these 2 groups did not differ significantly from each other, the possible value of reserpine cannot be commented upon with such small groups, and the increased survival appears to be due to the changes in technique which both groups received.

Although results in the groups in which Dibenzylene or carbon dioxide was used were somewhat better than the control results, the differences were not significant. The use of saline solution, heparin, partial exsanguination, prior splenectomy, or chlorpromazine did not affect ultimate survival in any fashion. The use of Vasoxyl or cortisone, however, was attended by a consistent mortality rate.

To determine whether any of the therapies

**Table I.** *Survival after hypothermia below 25° C. for 20 hours*

| Groups | Survivors | Died during rewarming | Died during hypothermia | Total |
|---|---|---|---|---|
| I. Controls | 2 | 1 | 6 | 9 |
| II. Carbon dioxide | 6 | 2 | 4 | 12 |
| III. Saline | 2 | 5 | 4 | 11 |
| IV. Heparin | 4 | 7 | 7 | 18 |
| V. Exsanguination | 2 | 1 | 3 | 6 |
| VI. Splenectomy | 1 | 2 | 1 | 4 |
| VII. Vasoxyl | – | – | 5 | 5 |
| VIII. Chlorpromazine | 1 | 2 | 4 | 7 |
| IX. Dibenzylene | 3 | 1 | 3 | 7 |
| X. Cortisone | – | 1 | 6 | 7 |
| XI. Reserpine and technical changes | 5 | – | – | 5 |
| XII. Technical changes | 5 | 1 | 1 | 7 |
| All dogs | 31 (32%) | 23 (23%) | 44 (45%) | 98 |

mentioned might have been effective in keeping the dog alive during the 20-hour hypothermic period, though not during rewarming, the data were rearranged to include as survivors all those that lived until rewarming began. As can be seen from Table I, the addition of dogs which died during rewarming to the survivor columns resulted in a more substantial survival rate, especially with saline, heparin, and prior splenectomy. In none, however, except Groups XI and XII, was there a significant difference in comparison to the controls. Therefore, even during the hypothermic period alone, only the previously mentioned changes in technique and possibly the addition of reserpine were significant factors in increasing survival rate.

**Hematocrit.** The 79 dogs in which hematocrits were studied showed a definite, constant, progressive increase in hematocrit. The average per cent increase at 4 hours in all dogs was 19.5 per cent; at 12 hours this increased to 30.8 per cent; and by 20 hours it had increased to 53.6 per cent. During rewarming, at approximately 30° C., the hematocrit dropped slightly to an increase of 51 per cent. The difference in per cent increase of hematocrit between survivors and dogs which died during cooling or rewarming is shown graphically in Fig. 1. The survivors had a smaller rise than nonsurvivors. At 4 hours, while the increase was only 11.4 per cent in the survivors, it was 24.5 per cent in the dogs which died during rewarming ($p = 0.0102$). At 12 hours, a similar disparity existed with survivors having a 24.6 per cent increase and dogs which died during rewarming a 39.2 per cent increase ($p = 0.0375$). At 20 hours the gap was even greater—46.4 per cent and 69 per cent, respectively ($p = 0.0131$). Dogs that died during the hypothermic period had a middle course, and did not differ statistically from survivors or dogs which died during rewarming.

During rewarming, while the survivors' hematocrit tended to stay at the same level, dogs which died during rewarming showed a progressive increase to 82 per cent. Measurements were made in only 3 of the latter and the difference was not statistically significant. The initial hematocrit reading was of no prognostic value as related to survival. In general, these changes in hematocrit are consistent with the findings of Fisher's group[10, 11] in dogs subjected to prolonged hypothermia. Even natural hibernators were shown to have a rise in hematocrit during the hibernation period.[21]

**Plasma volume.** Plasma volume studied in 13 dogs decreased 30.4 per cent by 20 hours. There was no significant correlation with survival, perhaps because of the small number of dogs. D'Amato and Hegnauer[5] have noted a decrease in plasma volume of 12 per cent when dogs were cooled to 20° C. for shorter periods.

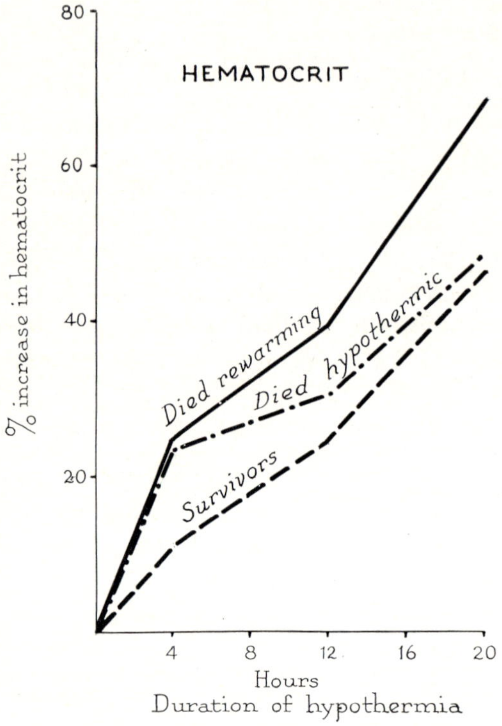


**Fig. 1.** Changes in hematocrit during prolonged hypothermia.

**Heart rate.** Changes in heart rate in 34 dogs during the hypothermic period are illustrated in Fig. 2. There was no significant correlation between changes in heart rate and survival.

**Blood pressure.** The average changes in arterial pressure in 68 dogs are also shown in Fig. 2. By 4 hours the arterial pressure had decreased to 70 mm. Hg and by 20 hours there was a further small drop to 65 mm. Hg. With Vasoxyl and cortisone, these decreases in blood pressure were avoided and the arterial pressure was maintained. However, this artificially elevated pressure seemed to have a deleterious effect, as it was associated with a 100 per cent mortality rate. Fig. 3 shows a comparison of arterial pressure changes between dogs given Vasoxyl and those given cortisone and between survivors and dogs which died during cooling and rewarming. It can clearly be seen that there is a tendency for the arterial pressure of survivors to increase slightly over the 4-hour value while dogs that die become more hypotensive. At 20 hours the difference in arterial pressure between survivors and dogs which died during rewarming ($p = 0.0088$) and survivors and dogs which died during hypothermia ($p = 0.0193$) is significant. Venous pressures showed no consistent changes and tended to remain at precooling values.

**pH.** The changes encountered in arterial pH differed considerably depending upon whether the respiratory mixture was room air or 5 per cent carbon dioxide in oxygen. The average initial pH was quite low in all dogs—7.25 in dogs given carbon dioxide and 7.32 in those given air.

Fig. 4 shows a comparison of the average changes during the hypothermic period in all dogs given room air and carbon dioxide. The general pattern in both is the same. The dogs respired with room air had a sharp rise to 7.51, probably due to hyperventilation, and then a tapering-off to 7.39 at 20 hours with no severe acidosis. In the dogs respired with 5 per cent carbon dioxide in oxygen, however, there is a slight increase to 7.29 at 4 hours, and by 12 hours this dropped to 7.15 and remained at this low level at 20 hours. There was no significant correlation found between changes in pH and survival.

The trend, then, in prolonged hypothermia, appears to be one of relatively increasing acidosis in comparison to the earlier values. Fisher[12] also found an acidosis, but the drop in pH occurred in the early hours and was not progressive. However, the dogs he studied were breathing spontaneously while the dogs in this study had artificial respiration which may have deferred the onset of the acidosis.

**Carbon dioxide content.** In one dog given a 5 per cent carbon dioxide in oxygen respiratory mixture, the carbon dioxide content remained at 50 vol. per cent throughout the entire period. The 7 dogs respired with room air had a lower initial value of 30 vol. per cent and remained at that level throughout the hypothermic period. There was no correlation between carbon dioxide content and survival. Fisher,[12] however, noted a drop in carbon dioxide content.

**Carbon dioxide tension.** In 8 dogs studied for changes in carbon dioxide tension, fairly constant levels were noted throughout the hypothermic period. There were higher constant levels when a carbon dioxide respiratory mixture was used. Again, no correlation with survival was found.

**Oxygen saturation.** The arterial and venous oxygen saturation was studied in 9 dogs. The average arterial oxygen saturation never changed appreciably and remained about 93 per cent during the hypothermic and rewarming periods. Fig. 5 illustrates the profound changes which occurred in venous saturation. Though rising above the initial value to 91 per cent at 4 hours, it had dropped to 35 per cent by 20 hours, and during rewarming dropped further to 30 per cent. These changes from initial values were statistically significant, both at 20 hours and during rewarming ($p = <0.0001$). There was no difference between survivors and nonsurvivors in this respect.

Decrease in content of venous oxygen was noted by Fisher and associates[11] to begin by 14 hours, probably secondary to the decrease in cardiac output. The stagnant anoxemia and marked increase in coefficient of oxygen utilization which result from decreased cardiac output evidently decrease the venous oxygen content.

**Plasma hemoglobin.** Twenty-seven dogs were studied for changes in plasma hemoglobin. The average initial value for all dogs was 27 mg. per cent; by 20 hours it had increased to 145 mg. per cent. Fig. 6 shows a comparison of the increases in survivors with those in dogs which died during cooling and rewarming. The greatest increase occurred in the survivors and the least in the dogs which died during hypothermia. There was a significant difference between the former and

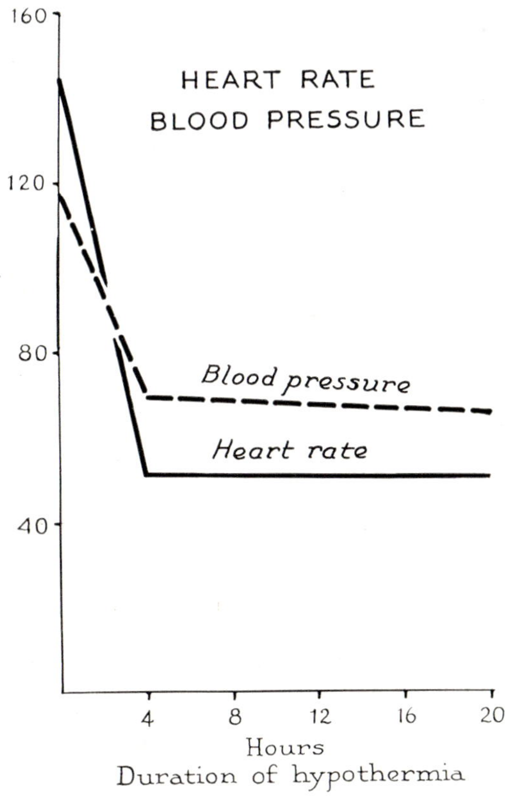


**Fig. 2.** Heart rate and arterial pressure during prolonged hypothermia.

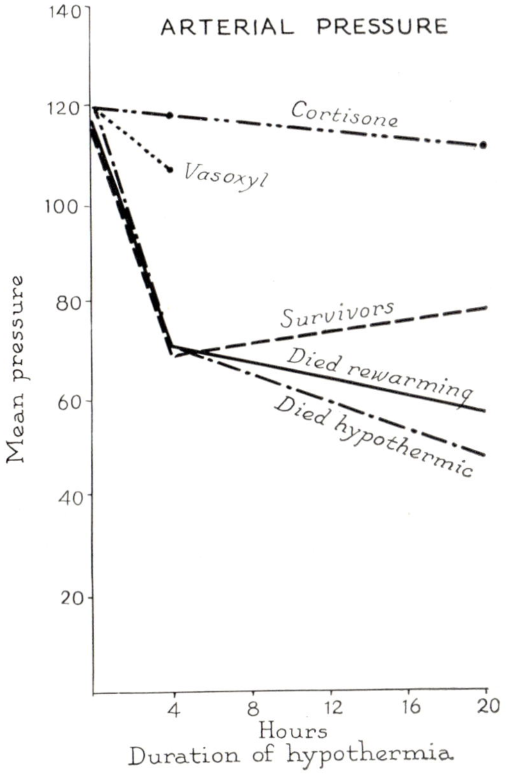


**Fig. 3.** Relation of arterial pressure to survival in prolonged hypothermia.

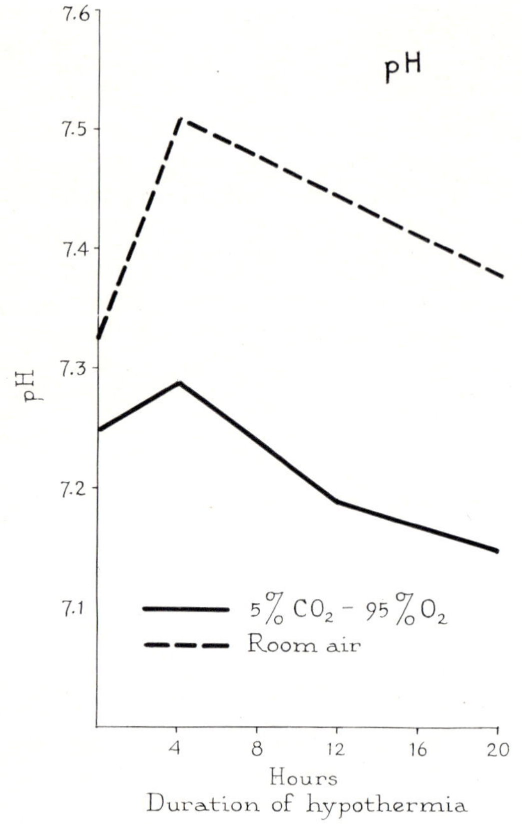


**Fig. 4.** Arterial pH with room air and carbon dioxide respiration during prolonged hypothermia.

the latter (p = 0.0203) and between dogs which died during rewarming and those which died during hypothermia (p = < 0.0001). It may be that the hemolysis occurs in all dogs but is less apparent in those that die in the cooling period because their circulation is impaired so markedly that it cannot reabsorb the hemolyzed blood from a sequestered site.

**Electrolytes.** Studies on sodium and potassium were performed only in 4 dogs. No changes from initial values were noted at 20 hours, a finding similar to that of Fisher and colleagues.[12]

**Electrocardiogram.** With progressive cooling the electrocardiogram showed gradual development of a sinus tachycardia with some prolongation of the P-R interval and QRS complex and lengthening of the Q-T segment, though findings were variable in most dogs. In addition, other changes not ordinarily associated with a slow rate were seen in the S-T segment and in the T-wave, which became diphasic and then deeply and bizarrely inverted as body temperature was lowered. Sometimes these changes did not appear until after relatively long periods of hypothermia.

The presence of a secondary wave which closely followed the ventricular complex and frequently impinged upon it was seen in some tracings. Boba[3] stated that a definite correlation exists between the appearance of this wave and the incidence of ventricular fibrillation. This wave was observed in these studies frequently in animals that subsequently died. In agreement with Fisher and his group, however, this wave cannot be interpreted uniformly as an ominous sign of impending ventricular fibrillation, since it was also seen in some survivors.

**Pathology.** Autopsy in dogs which died during the experiment showed varying degrees of congestion and hemorrhage of the bowel mucosa. These changes were frequently seen in survivors which died within 24 hours, but were not seen in survivors sacrificed later than this. Petecchial hemorrhages were found in subendothelial layers of the ventricles in the heart. Scarring from these lesions was occasionally seen in dogs which survived. Sarajas[23] has commented on the frequency of this finding after hypothermia. Pulmonary changes varied, animals which received large amounts of saline solution often showing pulmonary edema. Atelectasis of a lobe was a common finding, and on several occasions both lungs were atelectatic and were the main cause of death within 24 hours of rewarming. The liver was frequently congested and often appeared somewhat friable. No other gross findings were frequent or typical. Microscopic sections from a few animals showed congestion of the liver, spleen, and intestine. A slight vacuolation of hepatic central zone cells was seen in some animals.

## DISCUSSION

The physiologic effects of prolonged hypothermia are not trivial. A state of somnolence similar to deep anesthesia is present at low temperatures. The changes in hematocrit are profound and consistent and are correlated with survival. The decreased plasma volume further reflects the hemoconcentration present. The decreased heart rate and arterial pressure may not necessarily represent physiologic impairment, but perhaps physiologic alterations requisite for the needs of the body. An early low arterial pressure is compatible with survival as long as further decreases do not occur during the hypothermic period. Artificial methods of elevating it to a normothermic level are associated with a consistently high mortality rate. Except for the tendency of the pH to become relatively more acid during hypothermia, other indices of acid-base balance such as carbon dioxide tension and carbon dioxide content do not change with the increased duration of hypothermia.

The decreased oxygen saturation, however, may indicate a detrimental feature of prolonged cooling. Increasing cardiac output to prevent stagnant anoxemia could prevent this. On the other hand, survivors also have uniformly shown low venous oxygen saturation, and its importance is not clear. Electrolytes are not appreciably altered. The electrocardiogram shows no consistent significant changes which can be attributed to cold, except for its reflection of bradycardia at these temperatures.

In Lillihei's[20] investigation of endotoxin shock, a listing of the ensuing physiologic changes almost duplicates the changes found in this study of prolonged hypothermia. There is a decrease in plasma volume, the hematocrit increases, and the plasma hemoglobin increases. When the animal died from irreversible shock, it had congestion and hemorrhagic necrosis of the bowel and a congested liver. Even the subendothelial hemorrhages in the ventricles of the heart, which Sarajas[23] associates with hypothermia, were found in the animal which died in irreversible shock. Furthermore, the changes are not limited to endotoxin shock, but are found in irreversible hemorrhagic shock and chronic epinephrine shock.[13, 20] These pathologic findings are almost identical to what

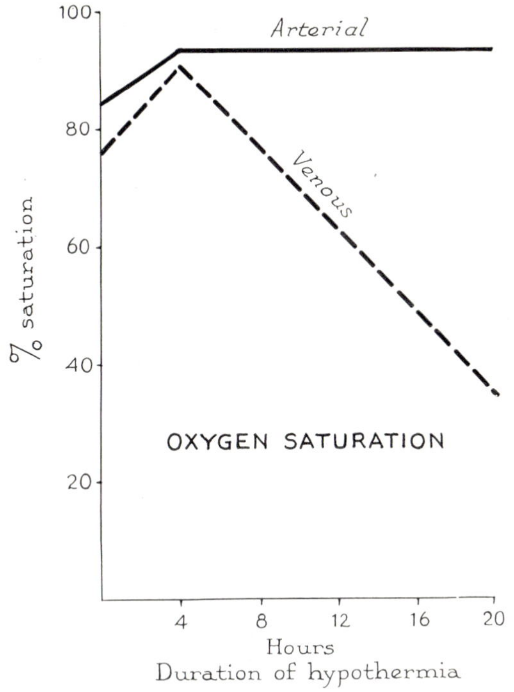


**Fig. 5.** Changes in oxygen saturation during prolonged hypothermia.

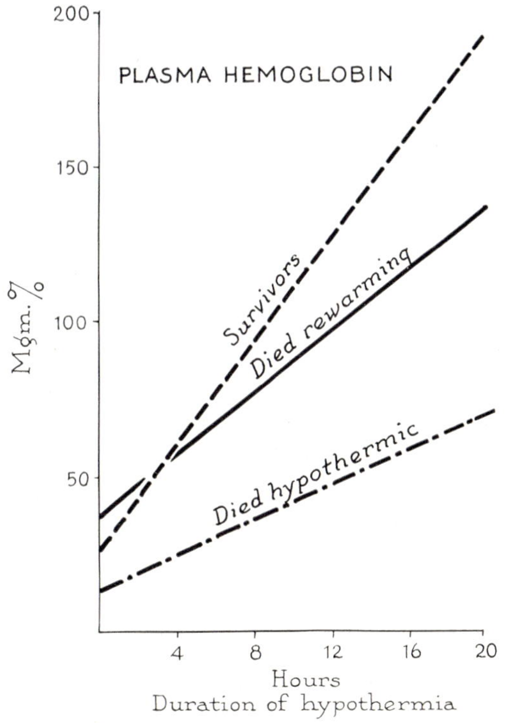


**Fig. 6.** Relation of plasma hemoglobin levels to survival during prolonged hypothermia.

is observed in the animals which die in prolonged hypothermia.

A look at the only 2 groups in which survival significantly increased in comparison to survival in the control group may shed some light on the cause of death. In Groups XI and XII, several conditions differed from those in the previous 10 groups. The control of shivering, the adoption of the prone position, the administration of sodium bicarbonate immediately prior to rewarming, the careful tracheal aspiration during rewarming, and the use of the short inspiratory phase and low pressure intermittent positive-pressure respiration are factors difficult to evaluate. The fact that these 2 groups did not differ significantly in survival from each other infers that the variation in techniques may be more pertinent than the addition of reserpine. The failure of chlorpromazine- and Dibenzylene-treated dogs to have a significantly higher survival rate also lends support to the importance of technical changes.

Whether or not it is important to control shivering during induction of hypothermia is a subject that has received much attention. If one is trying to achieve imitation of hibernators, no shivering should be allowed. The hibernator cools to 5° C. with no shivering, but uses shivering extensively as a major source of heat production in awakening and regaining normal body temperature.[21] Shivering during induction of hypothermia is not harmless. It has been noted to increase venous pressure. It also increases oxygen consumption, markedly if violent[6, 11] and slightly if it is only a fine tremor.[2] It depletes glycogen in the liver,[4, 6] probably through the release of epinephrine. Exactly the opposite occurs in hibernators, which have no depletion of liver glycogen during cooling but do have depletion of liver glycogen during arousal.[4] If, in addition to shivering, the animal is partially awake because of inadequate anesthesia during induction, it struggles violently with dilated pupils and increased respiration. This emotional response is an adequate stimulus for the increased secretion of norepinephrine.[13]

The selective depression of sympathoadrenal stimulation during induction of hypothermia may be extremely important. Whether or not there is any stress reaction during exposure to cold and hypothermia is a controversial point. Hume,[17] in measuring secretion of corticoids and catecholamines in the adrenal vein, found no increase in the anesthetized or unanesthetized animal. However, others have reported histologic evidence of stress during hypothermia. Even more pertinent to this study, pentobarbital was found to selectively depress this stress reaction in comparison to ether or nitrous oxide.[24] The lethal effects of administration of norepinephrine during endotoxin shock,[20] and the uniform mortality rate that occurred in the present study when Vasoxyl was administered, tend to bear out the concept of the pernicious effects of sympathoadrenal stimulation.

The failure of Dibenzylene to increase survival rate significantly is difficult to explain, but these dogs received none of the ancillary changes in technique enumerated for the last 2 groups. The consistent mortality rate noted when cortisone was used is also inexplicable at present. The dogs treated with chlorpromazine received up to 2,000 ml. of saline solution, and many died of pulmonary edema. Consequently, an adequate trial of chlorpromazine alone cannot be commented upon.

From these studies we can conclude that definite physiologic changes are related directly to the duration of hypothermia below 25° C. The encouraging survival rates noted with the addition of the techniques described certainly demand further investigation. Although prolonged hypothermia may still be the ideal modality for space travel, as well as a desirable technique to evaluate in the treatment of carcinoma, its present dangerous status would preclude any present clinical application without additional study.

## SUMMARY

In this study, we have tried to evaluate the physiologic alterations which occur in prolonged hypothermia and the effect of technique and therapy upon survival. Several features, such as the control of shivering during induction and the use of the prone position seem to be important technical details. The use of 5 per cent carbon dioxide in oxygen as a respiratory mixture, splenectomy, saline solution, partial exsanguination, chlorpromazine, heparin, or Dibenzylene did not significantly increase survival over that of the controls. The use of Vasoxyl or cortisone was attended by a uniform mortality rate. Treatment with reserpine was followed by consistent survival, but control dogs with similar changes in technique of cooling also had a high survival rate, which suggests that the change in technique may be more important than the addition of reserpine. In its present state of development, prolonged hypothermia below 25° C. is too dangerous to recommend for clinical use without further study.

## REFERENCES

1. Benvenuto, R., and Lewis, F. J.: Influence of deep hypothermia upon sensitivity of rats to x-irradiation, S. Forum **10:** 558, 1960.
2. Bigelow, W. G., Lindsay, W. K., Harrison, K. C., Gordon, R. A., and Greenwood, W. F.: Oxygen transport and utilization in dogs at low body temperatures, Am. J. Physiol. **160:** 125, 1950.
3. Boba, A.: An abnormal electrocardiogram and its relation to ventricular fibrillation, Am. Heart J. **57:** 255, 1959.
4. Brauer, R. W., Holloway, R. J., Krebs, J. S., Leong, G. F., and Carroll, H. W.: The liver in hypothermia. Ann. New York Acad. Sc. **80:** 395, 1959.
5. D'Amato, H. E., and Hegnauer, A. H.: Blood volume in the hypothermic dog, Am. J. Physiol. **173:** 100, 1953.
6. Dill, D. B., and Forbes, W. H.: Respiratory and metabolic effects of hypothermia, Am. J. Physiol. **132:** 685, 1941.
7. Fedor, E., and Fisher, B.: Rewarming following hypothermia of two to twelve hours. I. Cardiovascular effects, Ann. Surg. **147:** 515, 1958.
8. Fisher, E. R., Fedor, E. J., and Fisher, B.: Pathologic and histochemical observations in experimental hypothermia, A. M. A. Arch. Surg. **75:** 817, 1957.
9. Fisher, B., Fedor, E. J., and Lee, S. H.: Rewarming following hypothermia for two to twelve hours. II. Some metabolic effects, Ann. Surg. **148:** 1, 1958.
10. Fisher, B., Fedor, E. J., Lee, S. H., Wentzel, W. K., Selker, R. G., and Russ, C.: Some physiologic effects of short and long term hypothermia upon the liver, SURGERY, **40:** 862, 1956.
11. Fisher, B., Russ, C., and Fedor, E. J.: Effect of hypothermia of two to twenty-four hours on oxygen consumption and cardiac output in the dog, Am. J. Physiol. **188:** 473, 1957.
12. Fisher, B., Russ, C., Fedor, E., Wilde, R., Engstrom, R., Happel, J., and Prendergast, P.: Experimental evaluation of prolonged hypothermia, A. M. A. Arch. Surg. **71:** 431, 1955.
13. Freeman, N. E.: Decrease in blood volume after prolonged hyperactivity of the sympathetic nervous system, Am. J. Physiol. **103:** 185, 1933.
14. Gray, T. C.: Reflections in circulatory control, Lancet **1:** 383, 1957.
15. Hornsey, S.: Protection from whole body irradiation afforded to adult mice by reducing body temperature, Nature **178:** 87, 1956.
16. Horvath, S. M., Hutt, B. K., Spurr, G. B., and Stevens, G. E.: Some metabolic responses of dogs having low body temperatures, Science **118:** 100, 1953.
17. Hume, D. M., and Egdahl, R. H.: Effect of hypothermia and of cold exposure on adrenal cortical and medullary secretion, Ann. New York Acad. Sc. **80:** 435, 1959.
18. Laufman, H.: Profound accidental hypothermia, J. A. M. A. **147:** 1201, 1951.
19. Lewis, F. J.: Hypothermia in surgery, J. Nat. M. A. **48:** 317, 1956.
20. Lillihei, R. C., and McLean, D.: The intestinal factor in irreversible endotoxin shock, Ann. Surg. **148:** 513, 1958.
21. Lyman, C. P., and Chatfield, P. O.: Physiology of hibernation in mammals, Physiol. Rev. **35:** 403, 1955.
22. MacPhee, I., Gray, C. T., and Davis, S.: Effects of hypothermia on adrenocortical response to operation, Lancet **2:** 1196, 1958.
23. Sarajas, H. S.: Evidence for heart damage in association with systemic hypothermia in dogs, Am. Heart J. **51:** 298, 1956.
24. Sarajas, H. S., Nyholm, P., and Suomalainen, P.: Stress in hypothermia, Nature **181:** 612, 1958.
25. Smith, L. W., and Fay, T.: Temperature factors in cancer and embryonal cell growth, J. A. M. A. **113:** 653, 1939.
26. Spurr, G. B., Hutt, B. K., and Horvath, S. M.: Prolonged hypothermia in the dog, Am. J. Physiol. **178:** 275, 1954.
27. Talbott, J. H., Consalazio, W. V., and Pecora, L. J.: Hypothermia, Arch. Int. Med. **68:** 1120, 1941.

# The coating of intravascular plastic prostheses with colloidal graphite

VINCENT L. GOTT, M.D.
DONALD E. KOEPKE, M.D.
RONALD L. DAGGETT, B.S., M.S.M.E.
WILLIAM ZARNSTORFF, B.S.E.E.
WILLIAM P. YOUNG, M.D.
MADISON, WIS.
*From the Department of Surgery and the McArdle Cardiovascular Laboratory, University of Wisconsin Medical School*

At the present time there are several types of prosthetic valves that are available for placement in the canine and human heart. Most of these valves are constructed of plastic with the cusp, flap, or ball valve principle used in their design. Many of these prosthetic units have been evaluated in mechanical valve testers over long periods of time and appear to be extremely satisfactory from a hemodynamic and functional standpoint; however, their successful use in the canine and human heart has been markedly impeded by the very serious problem of thrombus formation on the valve unit. At the recent Public Health Symposium "Prosthetic Valves for Cardiac Surgery," there were only a few reported cases of long-term survival of dogs after placement of valvular prostheses.[2, 4-6] In almost every instance, dogs that survived the immediate postoperative period soon died as a result of thrombosis on the prosthesis. Valve design and valve material did not seem to alter these results in the canine heart. Ross and associates[7] studied clotting on plastic probes in the superior vena cava of the dog, and found that all plastics tested were the site of thrombus formation within 30 minutes. Even with Teflon there was moderate clot formation after 22 minutes. Frater and Ellis[2] found that all types of valves, constructed of several different plastics, clotted after insertion in the canine heart. The clotting seemed to occur even in the presence of prolonged heparinization. Kolff[4] reported equally discouraging results. He noted the occurrence of thrombi on several types of plastic valves and intracardiac plastic patches even while systemic fibrinolysin was used. Muller and Littlefield[6] reported the experience at the University of Virginia with a Teflon fabric cusp valve in the aortic area. The valve was placed in 50 animals and there were no long-term survivals. Long and his group[5] reported the experience at the University of Minnesota with a bicuspid silastic valve in the mitral and tricuspid area. This valve was placed in 25 dogs and the longest survival was 19 days. Again clotting was a serious problem. Many other investigators have had equally discouraging results in canine studies. Although it is generally agreed that clot formation on valve prostheses is not as serious a factor in the human heart, the severity of the problem in the canine heart has made it very difficult to adequately evaluate valve designs prior to clinical use.

At the University of Wisconsin many different valve designs have been evaluated. We have had the greatest experience, however, with a flap valve constructed of a rigid

Supported by United States Public Health Service Grant H-4162 and by funds from the Wisconsin Heart Association and the Wisconsin Alumni Research Foundation.
Received for publication April 21, 1960.

plastic housing and a flexible butterfly-wing leaflet. This type of valve performs well in the pulse duplicator, opens with a minimum of pressure, and produces no measurable pressure gradient across the valve. This valve has been constructed of several different thermoplastic materials and in almost every instance thrombosis on the prosthesis has led to early death of the dog.

In an attempt to find a more satisfactory material for valve prostheses, the authors initiated a study of the clot-producing characteristics of several plastic materials and coating substances. It was believed that a severe test of clot prevention would be the placement of a prosthesis in the venous stream in a manner similar to that employed by Ross.[7] Rather than placing plastic probes in the vena cava as Ross did, we elected to utilize tubular plastic rings which were somewhat analogous to the rigid valve housing used for the flap valve. It was decided to construct these rings of several different rigid plastic materials and also to coat some of them with substances that might aid in clot prevention. We also elected to evaluate the factor of electric charge as related to clot formation on the plastic rings.

It has long been known that white blood cells, red blood cells, fibrinogen, and other protein components of the blood are negatively charged at the normal pH of blood. In an electrophoretic cell, Abramson[1] was able to demonstrate that the white blood cells migrate to the positive pole of the cell. It was also shown that washed platelets migrate to the positive pole of an electrophoretic cell. In 1953 Sawyer and colleagues[8, 9] demonstrated that the normal potential difference across a blood vessel wall was 1 to 5 mv. with the blood or intima relatively negative with respect to the adventitia. These authors reported that injury to the intima altered the normal potential difference and when the transmural polarity was reversed, making the blood or intima relatively positive with respect to the adventitia, thrombosis frequently occurred. More recently, several additional studies have been reported which show the influence of electric charge on clotting in blood vessels. Williams, and his group[12] demonstrated that if negatively and positively charged platinum electrodes were externally placed on opposite sides of the canine jugular vein, a moderate clot developed on the vein wall nearest the positive electrode (5 Ma. current for 1 hour). Long-term studies with a low voltage circuit led these authors to conclude that it was tissue damage from current flow rather than regional electropositivity that caused the thrombosis. Schwartz,[11] in a similar study of intravascular clotting, observed that clotting occurred in an occluded femoral vein enclosed in a positively charged platinum sheath but not in a vein enclosed in a negatively charged platinum sheath. Heparin prevented clotting from occurring within the positive field, and dicumarol did not offer this protection. The difference in effectiveness of the two drugs was partially attributed to the extreme negative charge of heparin. Sawyer and associates[10] studied the effects of small electrical currents on clotting in the mesenteric vessels of the rat and noted that thrombosis seemed to occur first on the vessel wall nearest the positive electrode. With regard to intravascular prostheses, it has been noted that an epicardial-endocardial electrode placed in the canine heart for chronic heart block was usually free of clot when the endocardial plate carried the negative charge.[3] Also, Ross and colleagues,[7] in evaluating the clot formation on different plastics and other substances, believed that the best results were obtained with coatings of sulfonated or sulfated polysaccharides which possessed a high negative charge.

The evidence of the several investigators mentioned seems to indicate a significant relationship between electrical charge and intravascular clotting. Although the present study was originally planned as an investigation of the clot propagating properties of plastic materials, it was believed that this would afford a good opportunity to further evaluate the factor of electrical charge as related to clotting on intravascular prostheses.

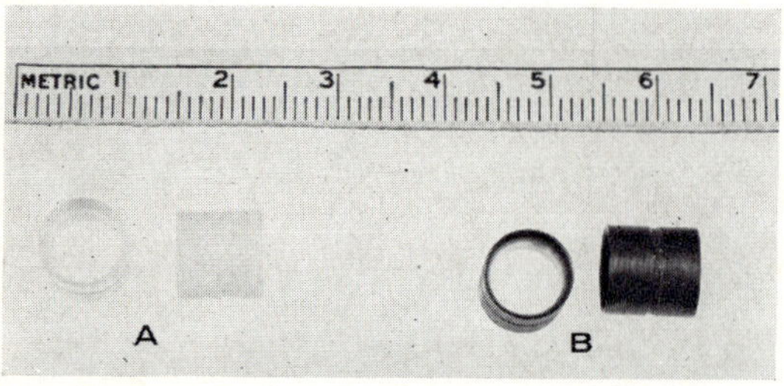


Fig. 1. *A,* A pair of Kel-F rings which show design and size of the plastic rings used in this study. *B,* Plastic rings coated with colloidal graphite.

## METHODS

Rigid plastic rings were designed with a 7 mm. internal diameter and a 0.5 mm. wall thickness. The rings were 8 mm. long and had sharp leading and trailing edges (Fig. 1, *A*). All rings were molded except for those of methyl methacrylate and tetrafluoroethylene (Teflon) which were machined from a rod stock and highly polished. This was necessary because of difficulty in molding satisfactory rings of the latter 2 plastics. Rings of acetal (Delrin), polycarbonate (Lexan), polypropylene, both intermediate and high density polyethylene, and trifluorochloroethylene (Kel-F) were injection-molded in suitable dies. Polyvinyl chloride rings were also molded with a rigid plastisol formulation by modified injection techniques. Polyurethane and silicone rubber, which have been used in making flexible valve constructions and leaflets, were not tested because we were principally interested in materials suitable for rigid valve housings.

A siliconized surface was tested, however, by coating methyl methacrylate rings with Dow Corning silicone No. 200 (350 centistrokes viscosity). This is a silicone solution designed for application to plastic and was baked on at 130° F.

Methyl methacrylate rings were also coated with conductive colloidal graphite* (Fig. 1, *B*.) In 1 series of 5 rings the graphite was painted on the methyl methacrylate; however, brush application left several tiny uncoated areas. A second series of 5 methyl methacrylate rings were therefore dipped in a graphite solution and evaluated for clot propagation. It was found that the ideal solution for dip-coating was a colloidal graphite solution diluted 3 to 1 with 95 per cent ethanol. This solution was thin enough to permit dipping yet appeared to provide an adequate coating of graphite. Each ring was initially dipped in plain ethanol for the purpose of cleaning and pretreating the plastic surface. This permitted a better bond between the plastic and the colloidal graphite. Some rings were dipped 2 or 3 times in the graphite solution for a better coating. Most of the rings were placed in a forced-draft oven at 130° F. for 72 hours in order to remove all diluting solvents.

In another series of graphite-coated rings, an insulated wire was connected to the prosthesis (Fig. 2) so that an electrical charge could be applied by use of a dry cell battery.

Healthy dogs which weighed 7 to 10 kilograms were anesthetized with Nembutal and placed on a respirator which utilized compressed air. A right thoracotomy was performed through the fifth intercostal space, the superior and inferior venae cavae were carefully dissected from surrounding tissue, and tapes were passed around these vessels as far from the heart as possible. A purse-string suture was placed in the right atrial wall. With very short periods of inflow stasis, a plastic ring was inserted through a right atriotomy into one of the exposed caval vessels and immediately wrapped with a piece of Teflon fabric. The Teflon fabric was placed around the vein so that there was no cul-de-sac between the prosthesis and vein wall. There was virtually no discrepancy in size between the plastic rings and the venae cavae in animals of this weight range. The rings were examined at 1 hour and rings with a patent lumen were placed back in the vena cava and examined again at the end of 2 hours. Each vena cava was utilized for the testing of only 1 prosthetic ring and there was no apparent difference in clotting between the superior and inferior venae

*Dag 154 colloidal graphite manufactured by the Acheson Colloids Company, Port Huron, Mich.

cavae. Systemic anticoagulation was not used; however, the rings were rinsed initially in a dilute solution of heparinized saline in order to minimize clotting during the placement with inflow stasis.

The wired graphite rings were placed in the superior vena cava and the wire connected to 1 pole of a 9 V. nickel cadmium battery. A 2,200 ohm resistor was placed in series with the battery and the circuit completed by placement of a wire between the battery and the latissimus dorsi (Fig. 2). Voltages across the resistor and the conductive graphite ring were approximately 6 and 3 V., respectively, with the average current being 3 Ma. The wired rings were evaluated with both a positive charge and a negative charge. Five rings of each of the plastics and coatings were placed in the vena cava for evaluation.

## RESULTS

The data on clot formation in the different types of rings are depicted in Figs. 3 and 4. The clot in each ring is depicted diagrammatically.

**Uncoated plastic rings.** It may be noted that all of the Delrin rings were completely clotted within 1 hour. Rings of Lexan, polyvinyl chloride, polypropylene, and medium density polyethylene were severely clotted in 1 hour and all of these rings were completely occluded at the end of 2 hours. High density polyethylene and Kel-F rings provided the best results of all the uncoated plastic prostheses tested. In each of the last 2 groups, 1 ring was clotted at 1 hour and a second ring was clotted or almost clotted after 2 hours. All of the Teflon rings were severely clotted after 2 hours in the vena cava.

**Silicone-coated methyl methacrylate rings.** A silicone coating on the highly polished, machined rings of methyl methacrylate significantly improved the clot-repelling qualities of these rings, as might be expected. We were surprised to observe, however, that 1 ring was completely occluded and a second ring was nearly occluded after 2 hours in the vena cava (Figs. 3 and 5).

**Graphite-coated methyl methacrylate rings (brush application).** Four of the 5 methyl methacrylate rings painted with colloidal graphite were relatively clean after a

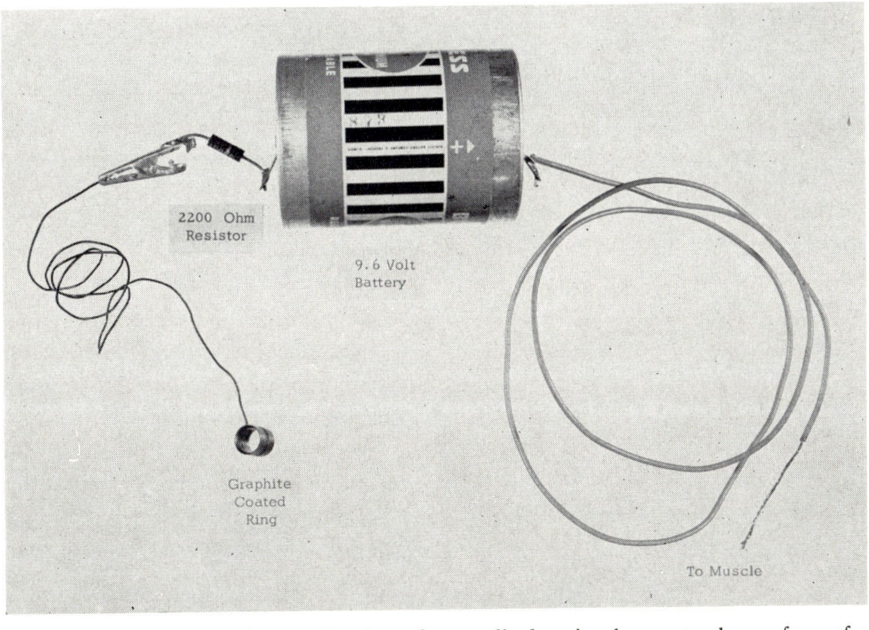


**Fig. 2.** The technique for application of a small electric charge to the surface of a graphite-coated plastic ring.

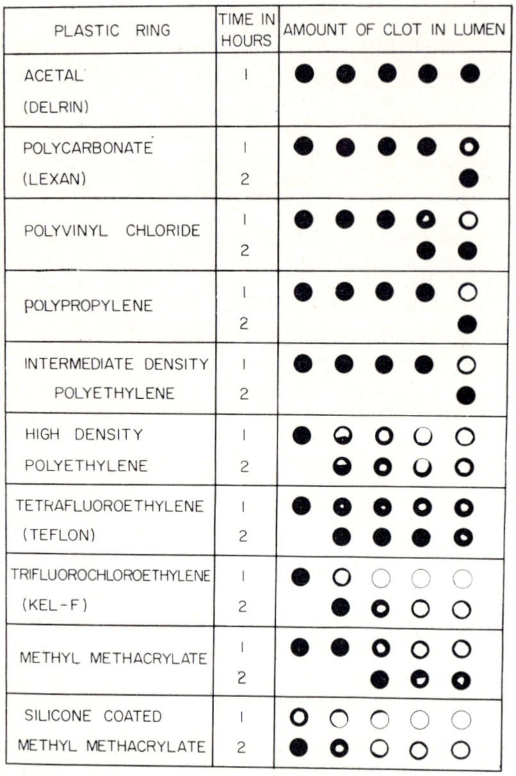


**Fig. 3.** The clot formation in different types of plastic rings as depicted diagrammatically. Rings that had a patent lumen at the end of 1 hour were replaced in the same vessel for an additional hour.

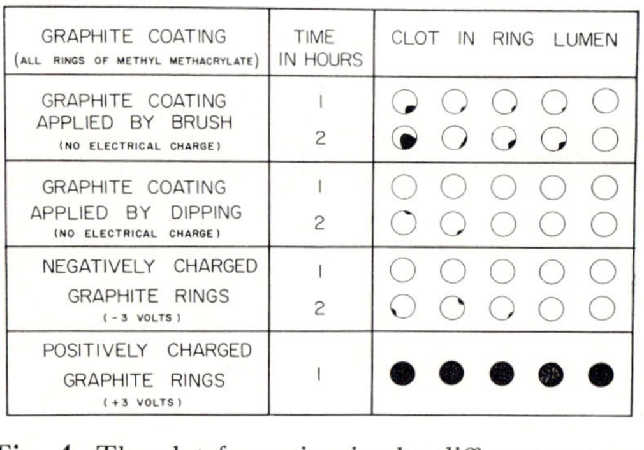


**Fig. 4.** The clot formation in the different groups of graphite-coated plastic rings.

2-hour placement in the vena cava. The fifth ring had a moderate clot at 2 hours. This was one of the first rings which had been painted with colloidal graphite, and it was interesting to note that the clot originated from a small area of methyl methacrylate which was not coated with graphite. The clear area was the result of a brush mark. Care was then taken to cover the methyl methacrylate rings as thoroughly as possible with graphite, but in 3 rings there were tiny clots which originated from minute, clear areas of methyl methacrylate. The fifth ring was completely clean at 2 hours.

**Graphite-coated methyl methacrylate rings (dip application).** In order to obviate the occurrence of microscopic and macroscopic clear areas that resulted from brush marks, 5 rings were dipped in a diluted colloidal graphite solution. All 5 rings were completely clean at 1 hour and 2 rings had 0.5 mm. particles of thrombus at 2 hours (Figs. 4 and 6). Three rings which had been dipped in graphite were completely clean after 2 hours in the vena cava.

**Graphite-coated methyl methacrylate rings with electrical charge.** Five graphite-coated rings with a negative charge of approximately 3 V. were as free of clot as rings without a charge. Five graphite-coated rings with a positive charge of approximately 3 V. were completely clotted within 1 hour. Pressure recordings in the jugular vein during some of the latter experiments showed complete thrombotic occlusion within 30 minutes.

## DISCUSSION

The placement of a prosthesis in the vena cava is an extremely severe test for any plastic material. The poor results obtained with the plastic rings in our study need not incriminate these materials for use in prosthetic valves in a high velocity blood stream. It was believed, however, that this type of study would provide information on the relative clot-repelling ability of different plastic materials and coating substances.

A comparative analysis of the pure plastic rings indicates that Kel-F and high density polyethylene resisted clotting to a better degree than any of the other plastics. It is possible that molded (as opposed to machined) Teflon rings would have performed as well as or better than Kel-F rings because of the close similarity of these plastics; however, we found that Kel-F was much easier to mold than Teflon and provided extremely clean castings. The silicone coating certainly improved the performance of the methyl methacrylate rings, as might be anticipated.

The data obtained on the graphite-coated rings, with and without small electrical charges, are particularly interesting. At the inception of the study it was believed that a graphite coating with a negative charge might offer some protection against clotting. We were encouraged, therefore, to observe that the negatively charged graphite rings were extremely clean after 2 hours in the venous stream. It was of interest also that the positively charged rings had severe clot formation in less than 1 hour, and the clots were much more firmly attached than those which occurred in the lumina of the pure plastic rings. It is obviously not desirable to connect a wire and a battery to an intracardiac prosthetic valve unit in order to prevent the formation of thrombus. There could be interference with myocardial conduction and other readily apparent problems. We were pleased to note, therefore, that the graphite-dipped rings without an externally applied negative charge were also relatively free of clot after 2 hours in the vena cava.

Colloidal graphite was chosen as the conductive coating for this study because it could be easily applied to a flexible or hard plastic prosthesis. Graphite is elemental carbon in the form of laminar hexagonal crystals. It is a nonmetallic conductor and has been used extensively in electrical circuits. In the colloidal form (Dag 154), extremely fine particles of graphite are suspended in a vehicle which consists mainly of isopropyl alcohol. The particles are separated for the most part as crystal aggregates and the mass mean particle size is between 1 and 2 $\mu$. There are a very few flocculant particles present, ranging in size up to 8 $\mu$ in diameter. When Dag 154 is applied to plastic the solvent evaporates and leaves the graphite crystals in a small amount of cellulosic plastic binder. The graphite adheres very well to most plastics,* forms an extremely smooth surface, and, like Teflon, is slightly waxy to touch. It is the latter quality that has led to the extensive use of graphite as a dry lubricant in industry.

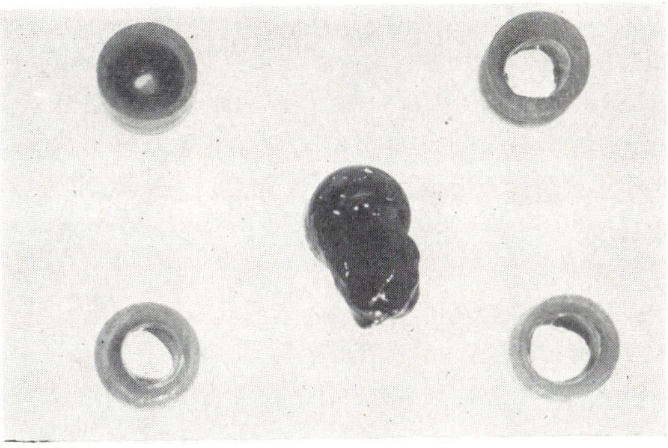

**Fig. 5.** The clot formation in 5 silicone-coated methyl methacrylate rings. All of these were placed in the vena cava for 2 hours.

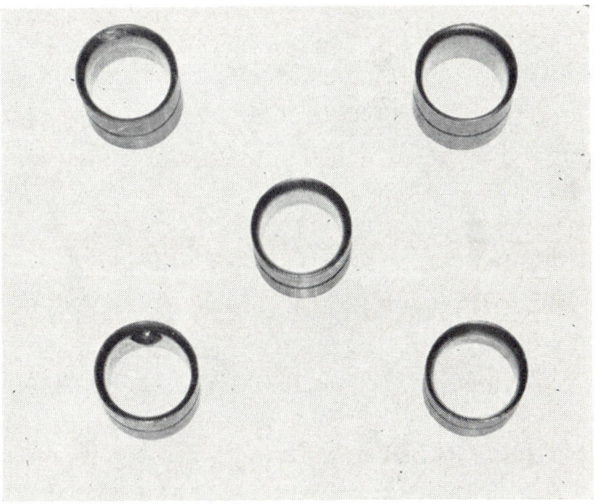

**Fig. 6.** The appearance of 5 graphite-coated plastic rings after 2-hour placement in the vena cava. The 2 rings on the left have small particles of thrombus on the upper edge.

We believe that the encouraging results obtained with the graphite-coated rings may be related to several factors. The graphite appears to fill in and cover microscopic and macroscopic defects in the plastic and thus provide an extremely smooth

*The colloidal graphite does not adhere well to silicone rubber.

surface. Also, the graphite coating is conductive, which may be of some importance. It is conceivable that a nonconductive prosthesis of plastic material accumulates a positive electrostatic charge as a result of the friction of the negatively charged blood elements flowing over the surface. When a positive static charge builds up on the plastic prosthesis, the negatively charged blood elements are attracted to it with resultant early clot formation. There are several analogous examples of this problem of electrostatic charge in industry and commerce. The friction of the air stream flowing over the surface of an airplane wing permits the accummulation of an electrostatic charge on the wing surface. Because of the hazard of explosion from this electrostatic charge, short segments of sash cord dipped in colloidal graphite are attached to the trailing edge of the wing. The slightly frayed end of the sash cord provides hundreds of fine points for dispersion of the electrostatic charge from the wing surface. Thus, in the case of the graphite-coated rings, it may have been the ability of the conductive graphite crystals to dissipate a positive electrostatic charge that contributed to the successful performance of these rings. Certainly this is only one of several major factors in clot prevention. Chemical reactivity of a foreign surface is of extreme importance in clot formation. Other factors, such as nonwettability of a surface, are of questionable importance.[7] Comparative in vitro studies on wettability and chemical reactivity of graphite and other coating substances are presently being carried out and will be reported in the near future.

Long-term studies of graphite-coated prostheses have not been completed. Several graphite-coated rings have been examined after a 1-week placement in the vena cava and most of these rings are free of clot. Also, several graphite-coated rings have been examined after a 2-month placement in the thoracic aorta. These rings were covered with a thin layer of endothelium and there was no destruction of the graphite surface. There was no adverse reaction around the graphite-coated ring in the blood vessel or in the surrounding tissue. Toxicity tests are now in progress. It is believed that graphite (as elemental carbon) will be well tolerated by the body tissues.

A few graphite-coated flap valves have been placed in the canine heart and at this early date the results are encouraging. Considerable work still has to be done with regard to application of the graphite and its solvents to the thin plastic films used for valve leaflets. There is no problem in the application of colloidal graphite to a rigid plastic valve housing, but some solvents can be detrimental to certain plastic films and care has to be exercised in the coating of these materials. Also, some flexibility is lost when graphite is applied to a plastic film and thinner materials must be used. The use of films of conductive plastic for the flexible leaflet appears promising.

Studies are also progressing on the use of graphite coatings in several additional areas. Teflon grafts have been coated with graphite for replacement of vena caval and small-lumen arterial segments. Results to date in these studies are also encouraging and will be the subject of reports in the future.

## CONCLUSIONS

1. Rigid plastic rings were constructed of 9 different plastic materials and placed in the canine vena cava for evaluation of clot formation. With the exception of rings constructed of Kel-F and high density polyethylene, all rings were severely clotted within 2 hours.

2. A silicone coating on methyl methacrylate rings reduced the clot formation on these prostheses very significantly; however, there was severe clotting on 2 of 5 siliconized rings after 2 hours in the vena cava.

3. Methyl methacrylate rings coated with conductive colloidal graphite (by a dipping process) were virtually free of clot after 2 hours in the vena cava. Application of a small negative charge to the conductive graphite surface did not alter these results; however, application of a positive charge to the graphite surface produced a severe

thrombosis within a 1-hour period.

4. It is postulated that satisfactory results were obtained with the graphite-coated rings because this material provides an extremely smooth surface which may dissipate a positive electrostatic charge from the prosthesis. This would minimize the attraction of negatively charged blood elements to the prosthesis.

5. Early results with graphite-coated flap valves and graphite-coated vascular grafts have been encouraging.

The authors wish to thank Dr. Charles W. Crumpton, Director of the McArdle Cardiovascular Laboratories for his assistance and co-operation during the course of this project. We would also like to thank Mr. Francis McMahan, Mr. Mark Mergen, and Mr. Marcus Ravnan for their technical assistance in the performance of these studies, and Dr. Harold J. Dawe and Mr. Arthur J. Stock of the Acheson Colloids Company for supplying technical data on the graphite materials.

## REFERENCES

1. Abramson, H. A.: The influence of a low electromotive force on the electrophoresis of lymphocytes of different ages, J. Exper. Med. **41:** 445, 1925.
2. Frater, R. W. M., and Ellis, F. H., Jr.: Problems in the development of a mitral valve prosthesis. *In* Prosthetic valves for cardiac surgery, Springfield, Ill., 1961, Charles C Thomas, Publisher, p. 244.
3. Gott, V. L., Sellers, R. D., and Lillehei, C. W.: The development of an epicardial-endocardial electrode for permanent placement in Stokes-Adams Disease, S. Forum **11:** 250, 1960.
4. Kolff, W. J., Seidel, W., Akutsu, T., Mirkovitch, V., and Hindberg, J. R.: Studies of thrombosis on artificial heart valves. *In* Prosthetic valves for cardiac surgery, Springfield, Ill., 1961, Charles C Thomas, Publisher, p. 199.
5. Long, D. M., Gott, V. L., Sterns, L. P., Finsterbusch, W., Mehre, N., Varco, R. L., and Lillehei, C. W.: Reconstruction and replacement of the mitral valve with plastic prostheses. *In* Prosthetic valves for cardiac surgery, Springfield, Ill., 1961, Charles C Thomas, Publisher, p. 385.
6. Muller, W. H., Jr., Littlefield, J. B., and Dammann, J. F., Jr.: Prosthetic replacement of the aortic valve. *In* Prosthetic valves for cardiac surgery, Springfield, Ill., 1961, Charles C Thomas, Publisher, p. 493.
7. Ross, J., Jr., Greenfield, L. J., Bowman, R. L., and Morrow, A. G.: The chemical structure and surface properties of certain synthetic polymers and their relationship to thrombosis. *In* Prosthetic valves for cardiac surgery, Springfield, Ill., 1961, Charles C Thomas, Publisher, p. 212.
8. Sawyer, P. N., and Pate, J. W.: Bioelectric phenomena as an etiologic factor in intravascular thrombosis, Am. J. Physiol. **175:** 103, 1953.
9. Sawyer, P. N., Pate, J. W., and Weldon, C. S.: Relations of abnormal and injury electric potential differences to intravascular thrombosis, Am. J. Physiol. **175:** 108, 1953.
10. Sawyer, P. N., Suckling, E. E., and Wesolowski, S. A.: Effect of small electric currents on intravascular thrombosis in the visualized rat mesentary, Am. J. Physiol. **198:** 1006, 1960.
11. Schwartz, S. I.: Prevention and production of thrombosis by alterations in electric environment, Surg. Gynec. & Obst. **108:** 533, 1959.
12. Williams, R. D., and Carey, L. C.: Studies in the production of standard venous thrombosis, Ann. Surg. **149:** 381, 1959.

## ADDENDUM

Further studies on the colloidal graphite surfaces show some additional factors which may be of value in minimizing clot formation. There may be a very minimal negative charge on the unwired graphite surface which could be of value. We have not been able to measure this directly but some indirect evidence suggests that this is true. A second factor that may play a role in the effectiveness of graphite is the adsorption from the blood stream of heparinlike mucopolysaccharides by the graphite surface. Attempts are presently being made to elute the surface of some of the graphite-coated rings that have been in the vena cava and aorta for several weeks and to try to determine the nature of the eluate. A third factor of questionable importance is the extreme nonwettability of a graphite surface. Additional experience in coating various plastic surfaces shows that the best results are obtained with plastics that are slightly attacked by the diluting solvents in the colloidal graphite. The best coating results to date have been obtained on polycarbonate (Lexan), polyvinyl, and methyl methacrylate.

# Effect of hypothermia on blood ammonia formation

HAROLD F. WELCH, M.D.
RASHEED AFFIFI, M.D.
CARMEN L. ROSANO, M.S.
ALBANY, N. Y.
*From the Department of Surgery, Albany Medical College, and General Medical Research Laboratory, Veterans Administration Hospital*

Hypothermia has been suggested as an adjunct to the surgical operation of portacaval shunting in the treatment of acute hemorrhage from esophageal varices.[4, 11] Since one of the sequelae of bleeding into the gastrointestinal tract in patients with cirrhosis of the liver is ammonia intoxication, it seemed important to determine the effect of hypothermia on ammonia formation.

It is well known that bacterial metabolism and growth are temperature dependent. The general effect of increasing temperature upon a given chemical reaction is an increase in the rate of that reaction, and conversely, cooling will, within limits, slow the velocity. Since ammonia is formed mainly by the action of bacterial enzymes within the bowel, it would be expected that both enzymatic action and bacterial growth would be slowed by general hypothermia and if the magnitude of this change is sufficient, then hypothermia might be of clinical value in the treatment of ammonia intoxication in the bleeding cirrhotic patient.

In this study the effect of hypothermia on blood ammonia formation was investigated by determination of the effect of lowering the incubation temperature to 30° C. on fecal cultures and by notation of the effect of general hypothermia on dogs subjected to cooling to 30° C.

Supported in part by United States Public Health Service Grant A708.

Received for publication Oct. 10, 1960.

## MATERIALS AND METHODS

**Determination of effect of temperature change on ammonia production by fecal cultures.** Fresh stools were obtained from 3 dogs fed normal kennel rations. The stool specimens were diluted with saline solution 1 to 10 and 0.3 ml. aliquots of this mixture were incubated at 37.5° and 30° C. in closed containers. A total of 28 such aliquots from the saline and fecal mixture were incubated at each temperature. After 60 minutes of incubation, 1.4 ml. of 20 per cent chilled trichloroacetic acid was added to each sample which was then thoroughly mixed and centrifuged. A 0.25 ml. aliquot of the supernatant solution was used for ammonia determination according to the method of Nathan and Rodkey.[9] Zero time was established by the addition of trichloroacetic acid at the time saline solution was added to the fecal mixture.

**Investigation of effect of hypothermia on blood ammonia levels of dogs cooled to 30° C.** Fourteen dogs were anesthetized with pentobarbital and cooled to 30° C. with cooling blankets. This was accomplished in 2 to 3 hours. Temperatures were measured with an esophageal thermometer. Blood for ammonia determination was taken from the inferior mesenteric vein through a catheter threaded into the small branch of this vein. Care was taken to avoid any obvious congestion of the inferior mesenteric vein. The terminal ileum and low sigmoid colon were ligated in an effort to keep the source of ammonia relatively constant during the experiment. In 9 of the animals concomitant arterial ammonia levels were measured from the femoral artery. In 6 animals, peripheral venous samples were taken from the femoral vein. The final ammonia level was determined as soon as the temperature fell to 30° C. The ammonia determinations were made by a modification of the Conway method[8] with a 10-minute diffusion time. Because of the possible effect of temperature on diffusion in the Conway technique, the results of this method were compared in 2 dogs in which the method of Nathan and Rodkey[9] was also used. The changes produced by hypothermia appeared consistent with either technique and consequently the Conway method was used for the remainder of the project because of the comparative simplicity of its performance.

Controls were established on 5 dogs which were anesthetized for a similar period of time but were not cooled. Blood was taken from the inferior mesenteric vein and femoral vein and artery in the same manner as in dogs which underwent hypothermia.

Because of the known effect of changes in pH and carbon dioxide tension on blood ammonia levels,[7] pH and carbon dioxide tension in addition to blood ammonia levels were determined in 5 of the dogs subjected to hypothermia. The plasma carbon dioxide was determined according to the method of Van Slyke and Neill[12] and conversion to carbon dioxide tension was made with solubility coefficients and pK changes in reference to temperature.[3]

## RESULTS

**Determination of temperature coefficient of ammonia production.** The reduction in ammonia formation resulting from incubation of the 3 stool specimens at the lower temperature (30° C.) was found to be 88, 64, and 46 per cent, as noted in Table I. The average reduction with combination of all 28 aliquots so incubated at this temperature was 66 per cent. The effect of reduction of the temperature upon the growth rate of bacteria was not measured in this experiment.

**Measurement of blood ammonia changes which resulted from cooling to 30° C.** The changes in the ammonia content of the inferior mesenteric vein, femoral vein, and femoral artery upon cooling to 30° C. are recorded in Table II. The average ammonia level in the inferior mesenteric vein before cooling was 793 mcg. per cent. This value varied considerably depending on the contents of the colon and the proximity of the tip of the catheter to the main portal flow. The average reduction in the inferior mesenteric vein ammonia level produced by cooling was 463 mcg. per cent or 58 per cent of the original value. In the 14 dogs, there were only 4 in which the drop was less than 50 per cent. The lowest reduction was 25 per cent of the original value. Upon rewarming, the ammonia levels in the inferior mesenteric vein rose rapidly to precooling levels or higher. As evidenced in Table II, the arterial and peripheral venous levels rose in most instances during cooling. In the 9 dogs in which arterial ammonia level was

**Table I.** *Effect of temperature change on ammonia production of fecal cultures*

| *Fecal culture* | *Incubation temperature (C.)* | *No. of determinations* | *Average mcg. % ammonia produced* | *% decrease in ammonia production* | *Average % decrease* |
|---|---|---|---|---|---|
| I | 37.5° | 8 | 174 | | |
| | 30.0° | 8 | 94 | 46 | — |
| II | 37.5° | 10 | 787 | | |
| | 30.0° | 10 | 282 | 64 | 66 |
| III | 37.5° | 10 | 1,440 | | |
| | 30.0° | 10 | 160 | 88 | — |

**Table II.** *Effect of general hypothermia to 30° C. on blood ammonia*

| | *Inferior mesenteric vein ammonia level (mcg. %)* | | *Femoral artery ammonia level (mcg. %)* | | *Femoral venous ammonia level (mcg. %)* | |
|---|---|---|---|---|---|---|
| | *37.5° C.* | *30.0° C.* | *37.5° C.* | *30.0° C.* | *37.5° C.* | *30.0° C.* |
| | 1,320 | 515 | — | — | — | — |
| | 250 | 150 | — | — | — | — |
| | 1,348 | 323 | — | — | — | — |
| | 560 | 122 | — | — | — | — |
| | 862 | 238 | — | — | — | — |
| | 656 | 214 | 52 | 111 | — | — |
| | 803 | 186 | 37 | 67 | — | — |
| | 629 | 246 | 69 | 76 | — | — |
| | 715 | 261 | 63 | 119 | 38 | 79 |
| | 564 | 156 | 60 | 107 | 38 | 153 |
| | 763 | 437 | 61 | 153 | 38 | 114 |
| | 610 | 359 | 76 | 61 | 61 | 91 |
| | 482 | 289 | 133 | 52 | 111 | 97 |
| | 1,583 | 1,172 | 53 | 61 | 61 | 80 |
| Average % increase in blood ammonia level | | 0 | | 77 (7 dogs) | | 75 (5 dogs) |
| Average % decrease in blood ammonia level | | 51.8 (14 dogs) | | 46 (2 dogs) | | 12 (1 dog) |

**Table III.** *Effect of 3-hour anesthesia on blood ammonia level without hypothermia*

| | *Inferior mesenteric vein ammonia level (mcg. %)* | | *Femoral artery ammonia level (mcg. %)* | | *Femoral venous ammonia level (mcg. %)* | |
|---|---|---|---|---|---|---|
| | *Initial* | *Final* | *Initial* | *Final* | *Initial* | *Final* |
| | 552 | 522 | 90 | 79 | 61 | 54 |
| | 910 | 880 | 84 | 69 | 61 | 53 |
| | 354 | 369 | 69 | 77 | 40 | 47 |
| | 225 | 376 | 38 | 61 | 46 | 61 |
| | 378 | 401 | 45 | 60 | 61 | 69 |
| Average % increase in blood ammonia level | | 29 (2 dogs) | | 40 (2 dogs) | | 16 (2 dogs) |
| Average % decrease in blood ammonia level | | 4 (3 dogs) | | 14 (3 dogs) | | 11 (3 dogs) |

measured, it rose in 7 animals and was reduced in 2. In the 6 dogs in which peripheral venous ammonia level was measured, it rose in 5 and was reduced in 1. However, this rise in ammonia level in the peripheral circulation, when compared with the controls (Table III), failed to be statistically significant at 0.05 level with "F" tables. This may be the result of the small number of animals in these groups.

The 5 dogs under hypothermia, in which the pH and carbon dioxide tension were measured, showed varying degrees of acidosis. As noted in Table IV, the carbon dioxide tension was reduced slightly in all 5 animals. There did not appear to be any definite correlation with the degree of elevation of the peripheral ammonia levels and the degree of acidosis, other than the general observation that a reduction in pH was associated with an elevation in the ammonia content of arterial and femoral venous blood in most of the dogs.

## DISCUSSION

Protein decomposition by enzymatic action of ammonia-forming organisms in the bowel is believed to be the main source of the ammonia found in the blood. The action of these enzymes, largely urease and amino acid oxidase, is temperature-dependent as are all chemical reactions. It is of interest that Poland[10] found the temperature coefficient for plant urease to be 1.49 for the temperature interval of 30° to 40° C. Although the effect of temperature upon the growth rate of bacteria was not measured in this experiment, with the data established by Barber[1] in 1908 on *Escherichia coli,* the temperature coefficient for total rate of cell formation for the temperature interval 30° to 37° C. is approximately 1.7.

It is acknowledged that the reduction in ammonia formation afforded by incubation of fecal cultures at lower temperatures is dependent on many variables, such as the amount of substrate in the stool and the number and type of viable organisms. However, we believe hypothermia will reduce the ammonia formation significantly in each instance as demonstrated in this experiment with random fecal specimens without regard to these variables.

Lawrence and associates,[7] in their study on the effect of varying pH on total ammonia levels, found a small but consistent increase in plasma ammonia level with a decrease in pH. The converse occurred with an elevation of pH. The means employed to produce these changes in pH seemed to have little bearing on these changes in total ammonia.[7] These investigators found this elevation in ammonia level in the portal as well as arterial and peripheral venous blood. It is unlikely, therefore, in our study that the changes in blood ammonia levels under hypothermia are due entirely to pH changes; for with cooling to 30° C. the arterial and peripheral venous levels rose in most instances as expected with a decrease in pH, but the inferior mesenteric vein ammonia level was consistently reduced. It was noted, however, during the course of the experiment that the ammonia level in the inferior mesenteric vein tended to rise slightly during shivering and varied with the respiratory rate. An unexpected finding was a consistent rise in the ammonia content of the inferior mesenteric vein when mechanical ventilation with positive-pressure breathing was used. The mechanism for the latter phenomenon is not clear.

The tendency toward elevation of the peripheral venous and arterial ammonia levels may be due to the interplay of many factors; influence of blood-tissue pH gradient, decreased utilization by the liver, increased production by the kidney, or increased shunting around the liver. Regardless, these elevations in the peripheral ammonia levels should be viewed in light of the fact that the "free ammonia" expressed as $pNH_3$ or partial pressure of ammonia will be reduced in the animals cooled to 30° C. because of

**Table IV.** *Effect of hypothermia (30° C.) on ammonia, carbon dioxide tension, and pH*

| *Ammonia (mcg. %)* | | *$pCO_2$ (mm. Hg)* | | *pH* | |
|---|---|---|---|---|---|
| *37.5° C.* | *30° C.* | *37.5° C.* | *30° C.* | *37.5° C.* | *30° C.* |
| *Inferior mesenteric vein* | | | | | |
| 763 | 437 | 60.2 | 77.6 | 7.31 | 7.01 |
| 610 | 359 | 60.2 | 54.4 | 7.49 | 7.30 |
| 482 | 289 | 64.3 | 54.5 | 7.30 | 7.24 |
| 1,583 | 1,172 | 59.7 | 54.5 | 7.43 | 7.42 |
| 564 | 156 | 65.1 | 56.4 | 7.31 | 7.05 |
| *Femoral artery* | | | | | |
| 61 | 153 | 56.2 | 72.2 | 7.41 | 6.99 |
| 76 | 61 | 58.0 | 51.7 | 7.56 | 7.36 |
| 133 | 52 | 56.6 | 51.3 | 7.38 | 7.26 |
| 53 | 61 | 54.3 | 49.2 | 7.52 | 7.49 |
| 60 | 107 | 55.8 | 50.1 | 7.35 | 7.21 |

the reduction in pH and temperature. The ratio between nonionized or free ammonia and the ionized form of ammonia is fixed by the pH and pK of the plasma as expressed by the Henderson-Hasselbach equation.[6] It has been reported that the correlation between the "free ammonia" and symptoms of ammonia intoxication is closer than with the total ammonia concentration and that the free ammonia as expressed by $pNH_3$ is the more toxic and significant form of ammonia.[6]

Many of the data reported on the effect of hypothermia on the liver are relative to the protective influence of the reduced metabolic needs of the cooled liver in regard to hypoxia.[2] Whether this reduced metabolism of the liver of the cirrhotic patient under hypothermia would also interfere with the detoxification of ammonia to the extent that it would offset any reduction afforded in the formation of ammonia is a problem which needs study. However, the increasing number of reports[4, 11] suggesting the use of hypothermia as an adjunct at the time of portacaval shunt operation tend to sustain experimental evidence that hypothermia of moderate duration (12 hours) has no detrimental effect on liver function.[5] The results of our study suggest that hypothermia may be of benefit to the patient with ammonia intoxication in 2 ways, first by reducing the partial pressure of ammonia with consequent amelioration of symptoms and second by the reduction of the actual formation of ammonia within the bowel.

## SUMMARY

1. Hypothermia will decrease the production of ammonia. Fecal samples incubated at 30° C. showed a marked decrease in ammonia formation when compared with similar samples incubated at 37.5° C.

2. The inferior mesenteric vein blood ammonia level in dogs cooled to 30° C. was consistently reduced. The average reduction in 14 dogs was 58 per cent of the original value. The peripheral venous and arterial blood ammonia levels rose in most dogs subjected to hypothermia. This rise, however, was not significant.

### REFERENCES

1. Barber, M. A.: The rate of multiplication of *Bacillus coli* at different temperatures, J. Infect. Dis. **5:** 379, 1908.
2. Bernhard, W. F., Cahill, G. F., Jr., and Curtis, G. W.: The rationale of surgery under hypothermia in certain patients with severe hepatocellular disease, Ann. Surg. **145:** 289, 1957.
3. Bradley, A. F., Stupfel, M., and Severinghaus, J. W.: Effect of temperature on $pCO_2$ and $pO_2$ of blood in vitro, J. Appl. Physiol. **9:** 201, 1956.
4. Clauss, R. H., Junker, R. D., Browning, L. D., and MacFee, W. F.: Hypothermia for portacaval shunts, Ann. Surg. **150:** 99, 1959.
5. Fisher, B., Fedor, E. J., Lee, S. H., Weitzel, W. K., Selker, R., and Russ, C.: Some physiologic effects of short- and long-term hypothermia upon the liver, SURGERY **40:** 862, 1956.
6. Jacquez, J. A., Poppell, J. W., Lawrence, W., Jr., and Roberts, K. E.: Clinical significance of the partial pressure of Ammonia ($pNH_3$) in patients with ammonia toxicity, Clin. Res. Proc. **5:** 20, 1957.
7. Lawrence, W., Jr., Jacquez, J. A., Dienst, S. G., Poppell, J. W., Randall, H. T., and Roberts, K. E.: The effect of changes in blood pH on the plasma total ammonia level, SURGERY **42:** 50, 1957.
8. McDermott, W. V., and Adams, R. D.: Episodic stupor associated with an Eck fistula in the human with particular reference to the metabolism of Ammonia, J. Clin. Invest. **33:** 1, 1954.
9. Nathan, D. G., and Rodkey, F. L.: A colorimetric procedure for determination of blood ammonia, J. Lab. & Clin. Med. **49:** 779, 1957.
10. Poland, L. O., *in* Sumner, J. B., and Somers, G. F., editors: Chemistry and methods of enzymes, New York, 1943, Academic Press, Inc., p. 14.
11. Postlethwait, R. W., Shingleton, W. W., Stephen, C. R., and Anlyan, W. G.: Portacaval shunts, A. M. A. Arch. Surg. **80:** 125, 1960.
12. Van Slyke, D. D., and Neill, J. M.: Determination of gases in blood and other solutions by vacuum extraction and manometric measurement, J. Biol. Chem. **61:** 523, 1924.

# Cancer cells in the blood in simulated colon cancer, resectable and unresectable: effect of fibrinolysin and heparin on growth potential

EUGENE E. CLIFFTON, M.D.
DOMENICO AGOSTINO, V.M.D.
NEW YORK, N. Y.
*From the Division of Experimental Surgery and Physiology and Division of Experimental Pathology, Sloan-Kettering Institute; and the Department of Surgery, Cornell University Medical College*

Cancer cells are found in the circulating blood of many patients with primary resectable neoplasms.[5] This fact has resulted in renewed interest in the mechanisms whereby tumors spread and in the significance of the circulating cancer cells. The demonstration of cancer cells in the venous drainage of human colon cancers has led to the suggestions that early ligation of the vascular pedicle is essential and that chemotherapeutic agents be used at the time of operation.[3, 4] It seems important that methods be developed whereby controlled experiments may determine the effectiveness of different agents in controlling metastases via the bloodstream. Also requiring investigation are the conditions which may affect the viability and ability of the circulating cancer cells to produce metastases. Fibrin formation and clumping of cells might be expected to affect fixation of the cancer cells.

Pulmonary metastases of the $VX_2$ carcinoma of the rabbit were reported to be decreased by large amounts of heparin.[9] The thromboplastic nature of the $VX_2$ carcinoma was first thought to explain this phenomenon. It seemed wise to extend the studies of the influence of clotting factors to other tumors and to other materials which affect the clotting mechanism. Human fibrinolysin was found to be effective in greatly diminishing and preventing pulmonary metastases after intravenous inoculation of the $VX_2$ carcinoma, and of hepatic metastases after inoculation of the Brown-Pearce tumor in rabbits.[2] With the Walker 256 carcinosarcoma, a similar result was obtained when human fibrinolysin was given to rats prior to intravenous inoculation. In the control group there were 81 per cent pulmonary metastases, while in the treated group there were only 25 per cent pulmonary metastases. Other studies of the fate and survival of intravenously inoculated Walker 256 carcinosarcoma cells have been reported and are being studied.[7, 8]

The introduction of large numbers of cancer cells in 1 injection is of value in studying the methods of metastasis, but is certainly unlike any clinical situation. It was believed that a method should be used which is more in keeping with the usual clinical situation in which a tumor is explored and perhaps resected. This would be more likely to yield results applicable to cases in human beings. Such a method of producing a transplanted colon cancer in the rat has permitted the study of the spread of cancer by both lymphatic and vascular routes.[1] It provides a tumor that is satisfactory for the evaluation of hemodynamic and coagulation factors in the spread of cancer. The first purpose of this study was to correlate the presence of tumor cells in the blood with resectability of

Supported by Grants No. C-3817, National Cancer Institute, No. H-5055 of the National Heart Institute, and institutional funds.

Received for publication Oct. 8, 1960. Resubmitted Dec. 30, 1960.

a simulated colon cancer in the rat, and to determine whether or not manipulation of the tumor altered the pattern of spread of the tumor cells. The second purpose was to determine whether alterations in blood coagulability would affect the vascular spread of tumor emboli when this type of tumor transplant was used.

## MATERIALS AND METHODS

**Materials.** Two hundred forty adult female rats from the Charles River Farm of 150 to 200 grams each were used. The Walker 256 carcinosarcoma, which has been carried in solid form and in the peritoneum of rats in our laboratory for over 3 years, was employed. Heparin* (aqueous), 50 USP units, was injected intravenously and human fibrinolysin† (Cohn, fraction III-3), activated with streptokinase, 6,000 units per kilogram of body weight, was given intravenously prior to manipulation of the tumor.

**Method.** The simulated colon cancer was produced in the rats by a previously reported technique.[1] A piece of solid Walker 256 carcinosarcoma in a gelatin capsule was inverted into the cecal wall at the cecal appendical junction.

Two weeks after the implantation, all animals were re-explored and were divided into 1 group with resectable and another group with unresectable tumor, according to the size and degree of spread of the tumor. If the tumor was localized to the cecal pouch and was less than 1.5 cm. in diameter and there were no grossly palpable lymph node metastases or other gross evidence of spread, it was considered resectable. If the tumor was 1.6 cm. or more in size or lymph node metastases, ascites, or peritoneal implants were present, it was considered unresectable.

At the time of re-exploration blood samples were drawn from the portal vein, vena cava, femoral vein, jugular vein, and aorta (not all in the same animal), and the blood studied for tumor cells (Seal's[10] technique).

*Liquaemin, Organon Inc., West Orange, N. J.
†Thrombolysin, Merck Sharp & Dohme, West Point, Pa.

Blood from these sites was also inoculated into weanling rats to determine the viability and the transmissibility of cancer cells in the blood. Twenty-five recipient (weanling) animals were used for each donor animal.

In both, animals with resectable and those with unresectable tumor, the effect of a 1-minute digital massage of the cecal tumor on the number and transmissibility of cancer cells in the blood was studied. In approximately half of the animals in the group of rats with tumor considered resectable, the cecal tumor was removed after massage. In alternate animals of each group, saline solution, heparin, or human fibrinolysin was infused either before or after massage.

The recipient (weanling) rats which had received the subcutaneous injection of blood were observed for 9 weeks. If there was no obvious growth of tumor at 9 weeks, they were subjected to massage of the implantation site and laparotomy at 9, 11, 13, and 15 weeks, and were then observed to a total of 18 weeks after the injection of the blood. They were then sacrificed, and a careful postmortem examination was made.

## RESULTS

All the animals (100 per cent) with tumor implanted in the cecal pouch developed a neoplasm in the bowel wall. Of the animals explored at 2 weeks after implantation, 38 per cent were considered to have resectable tumor, and 62 per cent had unresectable tumor by the established criteria.

Histologic study of a branch of the mesenteric vein in several rats with unresectable tumor showed tumor emboli in the lumen.

**Group with resectable tumor (38 per cent).** Samples of blood were taken from the portal vein, vena cava, and aorta. No free cells were found in any of these vessels in the control group. When the cecal tumor was massaged for 1 minute, tumor cells were found in the blood samples of all the control animals with resectable tumor. After resection of the tumor, the cells disappeared in most cases (Fig. 1). When blood from the vena cava was injected into the recipient (weanling) rats at the time of massage, 1 of

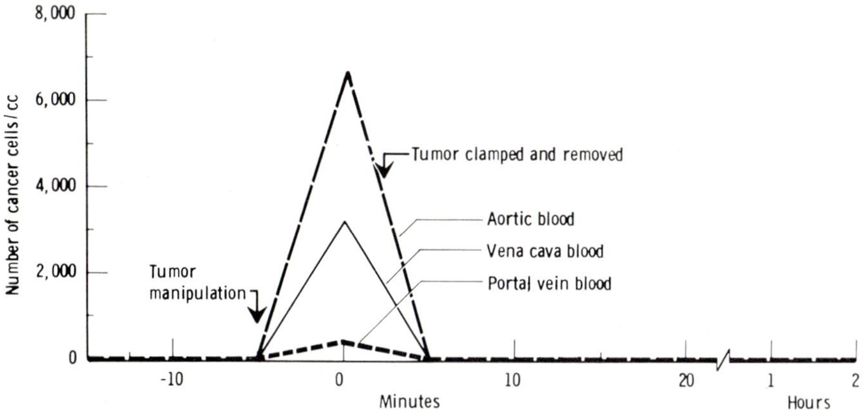


**Fig. 1.** A study of aortic, portal, and vena caval blood of animals with resectable tumor. Note shower of cancer cells at time of massage of tumor. Cancer cells disappeared from circulating blood after 5 minutes even if tumor was not removed.

25 rats (4 per cent) showed growth at 9 weeks (Table I). When the 24 remaining recipient rats were subjected to repeated laparotomies and massage of the subcutaneous implant sites, 6 or 25 per cent developed tumor at the implant site by 18 weeks.

With aortic blood from rats with resectable tumor, subcutaneous inoculation resulted in tumor growth in 2 or 8 per cent of the 25 rats at 9 weeks. When the remaining 23 recipient rats were subjected to laparotomies and massage of the tumor, 8 or 35 per cent had subcutaneous tumor growth by 18 weeks (Table II).

**Group with unresectable tumor (62 per cent).** Study of the rats in the group considered to have unresectable tumor showed a different picture. All animals showed tumor cells in blood from the portal vein, vena cava, and aorta. Under control (preoperative) conditions, there were approximately 42 cells per milliliter in the blood from the portal vein. With manipulation of the tumor, there was a temporary increase to an average of 296 cells per milliliter followed by a return to the preoperative level. Many more tumor cells were noted in blood from the vena cava and the aorta (Fig. 2) than in blood from the portal vein. Cells were not only present under control circumstances, but also increased markedly in number with massage of the tumor. It should be noted that in these rats with unresectable tumor, no cells were found from the jugular vein or the femoral vein prior to manipulation. However, after massage of the tumor in rats from group with unresectable tumor, large numbers of cells were found in blood from the jugular and femoral veins (approximately 3,000 cells per milliliter).

In all cases, whether the tumor was resectable or unresectable, increase of cells in the blood was marked after manipulation.

When the blood from the vena cava or aorta of animals with unresectable tumor at time of massage was injected into donor (weanling) rats, tumor growth occurred in 100 per cent of the animals at 9 weeks (Table II). This was in contrast to the very low rate of tumor growth at 9 weeks in the animals with resectable tumor.

**The effect of heparin and fibrinolysin in animals with resectable tumor.** It has already been noted that control animals with resectable tumor showed no free cells in the blood prior to manipulation. Significant numbers of cells appeared (up to 6,000 per milliliter) after manipulation, but there was a rapid decrease to no cells after resection (Fig. 1). It also was shown that even with tumor cells in the blood at the time of tumor massage, only 1 or 2 out of 25 recipient rats would develop tumors subcutaneously. With repeated massage, tumor growth was found in 25 to 35 per cent (of the recipient) at 18 weeks after injection of the blood taken from

**Table I.** *Vena cava blood injected subcutaneously in groups of 25 rats*

| | |
|---|---|
| *Resectable* | |
| No. of rats injected subcutaneously with approximately 6,000 t.c. (1 minute after manipulation) | 25 |
| No. of takes | 1 |
| Per cent takes | 4 |
| Repeated laparotomies and manipulation of site of implant | 24 |
| No. of takes | 6 |
| Per cent takes | 25 |
| *Unresectable* | |
| No. of rats injected subcutaneously with approximately 19,000 t.c. (1 minute after manipulation) | 25 |
| No. of takes | 25 |
| Per cent takes | 100 |

**Table II.** *Aortic blood injected subcutaneously in groups of 25 rats*

| | |
|---|---|
| *Resectable* | |
| No. of rats injected subcutaneously with approximately 6,000 t.c. (1 minute after manipulation) | 25 |
| No. of takes | 2 |
| Per cent takes | 8 |
| Repeated laparotomies and manipulation of site of implant | 23 |
| No. of takes | 8 |
| Per cent takes | 35 |
| *Unresectable* | |
| No. of rats injected subcutaneously with approximately 14,000 t.c. (1 minute after manipulation) | 25 |
| No. of takes | 25 |
| Per cent takes | 100 |

**Table III.** *Vena caval blood (1 ml.) injected subcutaneously in groups of 25 rats*

| | *No. of rats* | *No. of takes* | % |
|---|---|---|---|
| Control | 25 | 25 | 100 |
| Fibrinolysin (6,000 U./Kg.) | 25 | 5 | 20 |
| Heparin (50 USP units) | 25 | 4 | 16 |

the animals with resectable tumor at the time of manipulation (Tables I and II).

When 50 USP units of heparin was injected intravenously just prior to manipulation of the primary tumor, fewer cells were found in the blood after manipulation than in the control group (Fig. 3). However, cells could be found in the circulation for 2 hours, in contrast to their presence for only 5 minutes in the controls.

A similar result was noted with infusion of fibrinolysin prior to manipulation (Fig. 3).

**Group with unresectable tumor treated with heparin and fibrinolysin.** In the control animals with unresectable tumor, many tumor cells were present in blood from the vena cava and the aorta, and after manipulation there was a significant rise to high levels in blood from the vena cava and aorta (Fig. 4). When heparin was injected intravenously before manipulation, the number of cells in the vena caval blood decreased. At the time of manipulation there was only a slight rise (Fig. 4) instead of the marked rise seen in the controls (Fig. 2). After this slight rise, the decline in number of cells continued and the effect lasted for at least 2 hours. Blood from these same animals with unresectable tumor injected with heparin prior to manipulation produced subcutaneous tumors in only 4 of the 25 donor animals (16 per cent) compared with the 25 or 100 per cent takes in the controls (Table III).

When human fibrinolysin (6,000 U. per kilogram) was injected intravenously 5 minutes before manipulation of the tumor and blood from the vena cava was studied, it was found that the number of cancer cells fell to low levels and remained there for 2 hours despite the manipulation. There was a minimal rise in the number of circulating cancer cells at the time of manipulation (Fig. 4). Furthermore, subcutaneous injection of vena caval blood resulted in tumor growth at 9 weeks in only 5 or 20 per cent of the 25 donor animals (Table III).

When human fibrinolysin was injected intravenously after tumor manipulation, the number of cells in the portal vein blood decreased to a level below that seen prior to manipulation. In these same animals the cancer cells disappeared from the aortic blood for at least 4 hours. In animals not injected with fibrinolysin, the number of cells in the blood from the aorta returned to the premanipulation level after the peak which followed manipulation of the tumor. Unfor-

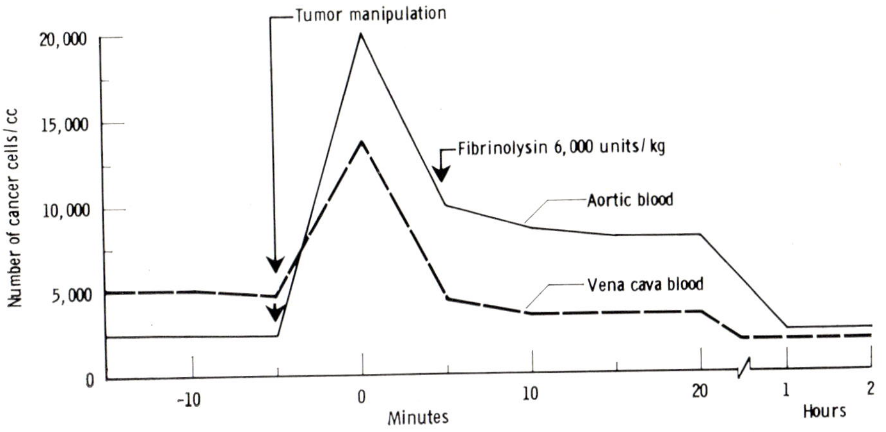


**Fig. 2.** Study of aortic and vena caval blood of animals with unresectable tumor. Note presence of cancer cells before manipulation of the tumor, rapid increase at time of massage, and then fall to the original control level in one-half hour. Note different scales of Figs. 1 and 2.

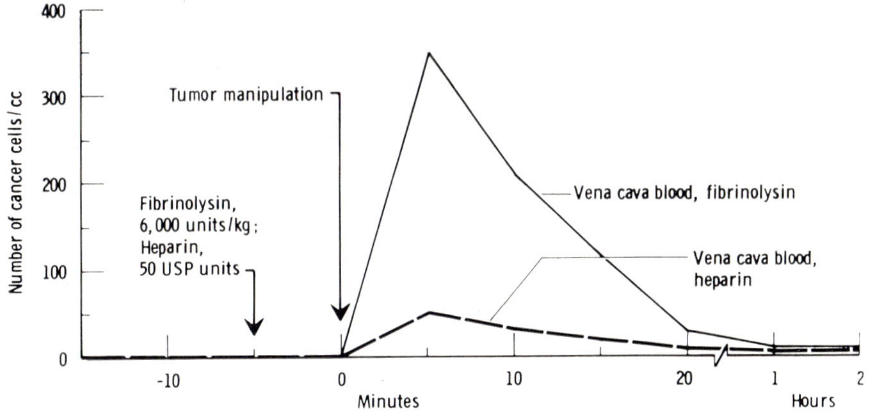


**Fig. 3.** Study of vena caval blood of animals with resectable tumor treated with heparin and fibrinolysin prior to manipulation of the tumor. Note the decrease in number of cells found immediately, but their prolonged presence.

tunately there are no data concerning the growth in donor animals under these circumstances, but it should be noted that in no instance has there been growth in any recipient animal without obvious tumor cells in the blood.

## DISCUSSION

It is probably significant that in this series of animals the rats with resectable tumor did not have detectable tumor cells in the blood, while all of the animals with unresectable tumor had a large number of circulating tumor cells in blood from the portal vein, vena cava, and aorta. Also significant is the finding that after massage of the resectable tumor, a number of tumor cells were found in the blood of the portal vein, vena cava, and aorta. The tumor cells remained in the circulation for 5 minutes whether or not the tumor was removed (Fig. 3). This demonstrates the very rapid removal of the tumor cells from the circulation in animals with small resectable tumors. The method of removal is of sufficient importance to warrant active investigation.

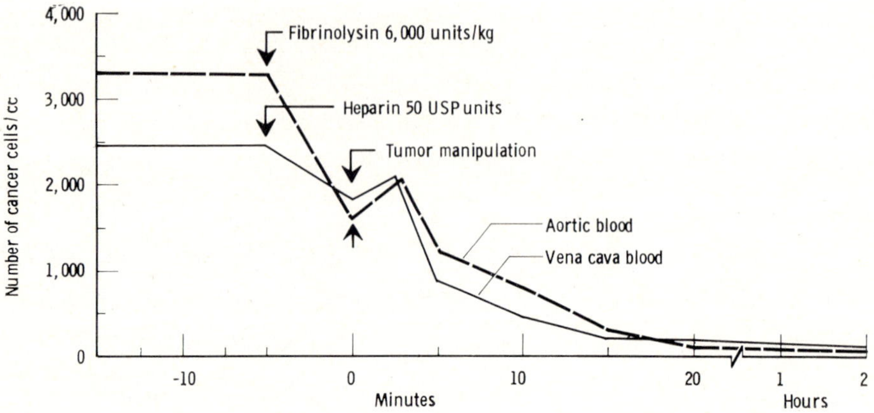


**Fig. 4.** A study of vena caval and aortic blood of animals with unresectable tumor. Note effect of heparin and fibrinolysin in lowering control cell count and decreasing markedly the rise after manipulation. The number of cancer cells continues to fall to almost zero within 30 minutes.

After manipulation of the unresectable tumors, there was a marked increase in the number of cells, but the intriguing finding was that the greatest number of cells were found in blood from the vena cava and aorta, but not in that from the portal vein. This might be attributable to spillage of tumor cells into the systemic circulation, but when one considers that this observation was made also in the animals with tumors considered resectable, this does not seem likely. It seems more logical to suspect that once the tumor cells pass through the liver, they remain in the systemic circulation for a much longer period of time. This finding is similar to an observation we made with infused tumor cells.[8] When the cells were injected into the femoral or the jugular vein, large numbers of cells were found in the vena cava and aorta, but none in the portal vein.

It is possible that in the present case cells which are spilled into the portal system pass through the liver and then continue to circulate. A large number are flowing through the aorta at all times, but are probably filtered out in the splanchnic bed. Another possibility is that massage increases the number of cells in the systemic circulation by opening portal systemic shunts with abnormally high portal pressures through the liver or elsewhere.

The effect of heparin and fibrinolysin on the circulating cancer cells is difficult to explain. With both agents, the number of cells present in animals with unresectable tumor is decreased and the rise after manipulation is minimal. They also decrease the number of tumor cells found in the blood after manipulation of the resectable tumors. In the treated group with resectable tumor, however, the cells continue to circulate for a longer period of time.

The results of the growth of tumor in the recipient animals are particularly interesting. The presence of dormant tumor cells is indicated by the increased take from 8 to 25 or 35 per cent when the tumor site was massaged and repeated laparotomies were performed. This is similar to the observations of Fisher and Fisher with hepatic metastases.[6]

The effect of heparin and fibrinolysin on animals in the group with tumor considered unresectable is very significant. Under control circumstances, blood from those animals produced 100 per cent takes in the recipients. When heparin or fibrinolysin was infused just prior to massage of the tumor, only 16 to 20 per cent of the recipient rats developed tumors at 9 weeks. These findings confirm the results of studies carried out with tumor cells injected intravenously, thus indicating that fibrinolytic enzymes or heparin have an effect on the number of circulating cells and the viability or transmissibility of the cancer cells circulating in the blood. The reason for this decrease in the number of cells in the circulation and the decrease in transplantability of cells present in the circulation is still a subject for speculation. It might be necessary for the cells to group or clump and to be fixed by some kind of fibrin film before they can begin to grow either in the capillaries of the lung or other organs or in the subcutaneous tissues of the recipient rats. Heparin or fibrinolysin could prevent this fibrin from accumulating. It is possible that heparin and fibrinolysin affect the tumor cells themselves, but in previous studies, fibrinolysin in vitro failed to alter the transmissibility of the Walker 256 carcinosarcoma.[7] The same has been shown to be true of heparin (unpublished data). It is also conceivable that fibrin coating of the cancer cells protects them from destructive elements in the animal's blood.

These two agents have only one thing in common—they alter the clotting mechanism. And they accomplish even this by different means. Heparin prevents clotting by altering the thrombin-fibrinogen reaction to produce fibrin, and fibrinolysin alters clotting by digesting fibrinogen or lysing the clot after it is formed.

Additional investigations of the effect of fibrin formation or clotting on metastases and growth of malignant tumors are obviously needed. These should include studies of the effects of other anticoagulants on the growth and metastasis of tumor. The effect of alterations of the mechanism by fibrin formation or clotting must also be investigated.

## CONCLUSIONS

In rats with small tumors considered resectable and without evidence of local extension or distant spread, no cancer cells were found in the blood. At the time of manipulation of the local tumor, cells were found in the blood stream, but they disappeared within 5 minutes. These tumor cells were transmissible subcutaneously in a small percentage of recipient animals. Manipulation of the donor sites increased the rate of growth. In rats bearing tumors considered unresectable, cancer cells were found in the circulating blood under control circumstances, and there was a sharp rise in the number of tumor cells at the time of manipulation and for a few minutes thereafter. There was 100 per cent take of tumors in the recipient animals under control circumstances. Injection of human fibrinolysin or heparin resulted in a marked diminution in the number of tumor cells in the blood of animals with unresectable tumors and a decrease in the number of cells at the time of manipulation in animals with both resectable and unresectable tumors. There was a marked decrease in the number of tumor growths in recipient animals.

## REFERENCES

1. Agostino, D., Seal, S. H., and Nickson, J. J.: Capsule implantation: method for establishing simulated colon carcinoma in rats, Proc. Soc. Exper. Biol. & Med. **100:** 717, 1959.
2. Cliffton, E. E., and Grossi, C. E.: Effect of human plasmin on the toxic effects and growth of blood borne metastasis of the Brown-Pearce carcinoma and the $VX_2$ carcinoma of the rabbit, Cancer **9:** 1147, 1956.
3. Cole, W. H., Packard, D., and Southwick, H. W.: Carcinoma of the colon with special reference to prevention and recurrence, J.A. M.A. **155:** 1549, 1954.
4. Cole, W. H., Robert, S., McDonald, G. O., and Watne, A. L.: Current trends in treatment of cancer, Postgrad. Med. **23:** 231, 1958.
5. Engell, H. C.: Cancer cells in the circulating blood, Acta chir. scandinav., vol. 1, suppl. 201, 1955.
6. Fisher, B., and Fisher, R. E.: Experimental evidence in support of the dormant tumor cells, Science **130:** 918, 1959.
7. Grossi, C. E., Agostino, D., and Cliffton, E. E.: The effect of human fibrinolysin on pulmonary metastasis of Walker 256 carcinosarcoma, Cancer Res. **20:** 505, 1960.
8. Grossi, C. E., Agostino, D., Melamed, M., and Cliffton, E. E.: The effect of human fibrinolysin on survival of Waker 256 carcinosarcoma cells in the blood. Cancer. In press.
9. Lawrence, E. A., Bowman, D. E., Moore, D. B., and Bernstein, G. I.: A thromboplastic property of neoplasms, S. Forum (1952), pp. 694-698, 1953.
10. Seal, S. H.: Silicone flotation: simple quantitative method for isolation of free-floating cancer cells from blood, Cancer **12:** 590, 1959.

# A venous cannula for use in experimental animals

WILLIAM G. PACE, M.D.
COLUMBUS, OHIO
*From the Department of Surgery, The Ohio State University Health Center*

It is difficult to obtain multiple samples of portal blood or of blood from other inaccessible deep veins in the course of investigations in the ambulatory experimental animal. Expensive guides machined from stainless steel have been described which accomplish this purpose to some degree. These devices utilize the principle of directing the needle to the entrapped vein. Although the steel devices usually function satisfactorily, they have definite limitations. A more simple and inexpensive device with greater flexibility should be available.

Teflon* in the solid form can easily be made into a slightly flexible, nonreactive cannula without special machinery. Teflon rod, used in industry in the manufacture of bearings, was found to be ideal for the fabrication. The physical characteristics of this material[2] make it ideal for permanent implantation in living tissues. It is slippery to touch, completely nonwetting, and nonreactive. It may be shaped without difficulty with a scalpel blade for any minor changes in contour. The material is readily available from plastic dealers as rod stock in any diameter and in any length.

In the cannula construction, an open funneled end is made to receive the aspirating needle (Fig. 1, *A*). A tunnel is formed at the opposite end which may be opened and then closed over the vein to be aspirated (Fig. 1, *B*). The tunnel is formed first from the rough rod before shaping is started. A hole the size of the vein to be aspirated is drilled perpendicularly through the rod. The distance of the hole from the funnel end of the cannula is determined by the average depth of the vein beneath the skin of the animal. The rod is then cut off distal to the hole and shaped by hand trimming to remove the rough corners around the vein tunnel. Access is made to the tunnel by cutting along the lateral aspect (Fig. 1, *C*) and placing 2 small holes (Fig. 1, *D*) for reapproximation of the tunnel around the vein. Two small sutures are used for this closure, and the flexibility of the plastic allows for an indefinite number of openings and closings without damage to the cannula.

The shaft of the cannula is then shaped to the contour shown in Fig. 1. This allows fixation of the cannula in the fascia beneath the skin of the animal. The funnel end remains the same size as the diameter of the original rod stock. The taper of the inside of the funnel is long enough so that insertion of a needle is easy. The needle tunnel (Fig. 1, *E*) at the apex of the funnel is drilled to fit an 18 gauge needle.

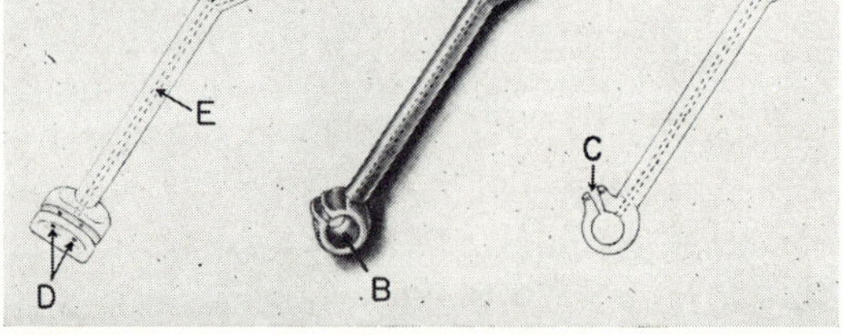


**Fig. 1**

Received for publication Sept. 29, 1960.

*Polytetrafluoroethylene.

This cannula may be made in various sizes. It can be left in the animal for an indefinite period without local reaction. There is a low incidence of thrombosis of the vessel under study if small, sharp needles are used and if care is exercised in the aspiration of the sample. Samples have been drawn from the same vein as often as every 15 minutes without thrombosis.

## SUMMARY

A Teflon vessel cannula has been described. The use of solid rod Teflon allows the fabrication of a device which is effective, inexpensive, and easily adaptable to a wide variety of applications. The material is nonreactive in living tissues. The relative softness of this plastic makes it ideal for fabrication without special tools and minor variations can readily be made at any time. The cannula can be boiled or steam autoclaved or soaked in sterilizing solutions without deterioration.

## REFERENCES

1. Government specifications on Teflon (polytetrafluoroethylene), Military Pamphlet 14078, Army Ordinance.
2. Government specifications on Teflon (polytetrafluoroethylene), United States Navy Pamphlet 19468.

# The use of fascial grafts in experimental bladder wall defects: preliminary report on application in the repair of exstrophy of the bladder


FRANK G. DeLUCA, M.D.
ORVAR SWENSON, M.D.
BOSTON, MASS., AND CHICAGO, ILL.


Exstrophy of the bladder can be repaired by means of various surgical procedures. A large number of procedures, both experimental and clinical, have been described in the literature, but none is entirely satisfactory. At the moment it appears that primary repair of the bladder is the best. One of the problems encountered with this operation is that when the bladder is small, it has proved difficult and at times impossible to achieve a primary repair. One method of solving this problem would be to use a graft to enlarge and close the bladder.

We became interested in determining experimentally whether a "free fascial graft" would "take" in the presence of bladder mucosa and whether such grafts would interfere with normal bladder function and growth. When our experimental studies on dogs proved to be successful, the same surgical procedure was performed clinically and a fascial graft was used for the repair of exstrophy of the bladder in 2 children.

## METHOD

Ten adult mongrel male and female dogs weighing from 18 to 25 pounds were selected for the experiments. There were no preoperative preparations. The first 2 experiments were performed on male dogs and because difficulty was encountered in urethral catheterization, female dogs were used for the other 8 experiments. Sterile technique was used for all procedures. Anterior rectus fascia, which is well developed and easily accessible, was the source of our grafts.

After anesthetization with intravenously administered Nembutal, a suprapubic longitudinal incision was made and the subcutaneous tissue dissected from the anterior rectus fascia. The anterior sheath of the rectus fascia was dissected from the anterior rectus muscle (Fig. 1). The size of the graft averaged 3.5 by 5 cm. The peritoneum was incised and bladder and ureters identified. In the first 2 experiments approximately 2 by 3 cm. of bladder wall was excised. The defect was repaired with a 2 by 2 cm. graft. In the remaining 8 experiments all of the bladder wall but 1 cm. above each ureteral orifice was excised (Fig. 2). The bleeders were clamped and ligated with No. 5-0 plain catgut. The fascial graft in this series averaged 3 by 5 cm. This was approximated to the bladder mucosa with interrupted No. 5-0 plain catgut sutures. The muscular layer was approximated to the fascia with inter-


Supported in part by United States Public Health Grant No. A-4185.

Received for publication Nov. 19, 1960.

rupted No. 5-0 chromic catgut (Fig. 3). The bladder was filled with sterile saline and examined for leakage. The bladder area was not drained and the urethral catheter was removed at the end of the procedure. The edges of the defect of rectus fascia were approximated with No. 5-0 interrupted silk sutures. The dogs were placed in special cages which permitted the accurate collection of urine. The urine volumes were charted daily for the first 5 days. The dogs were checked for residual urine at monthly intervals. Intravenous pyelograms and cystograms were performed at the end of the first, third, and sixth months after operation. Blood urea nitrogen, sodium, potassium, chloride, and carbon dioxide levels were determined prior to operation and at the third postoperative month. Urine cultures and colony counts were performed prior to operation and at monthly intervals postoperatively. Histologic sections of bladder wall and fascial grafts were taken at various intervals postoperatively.

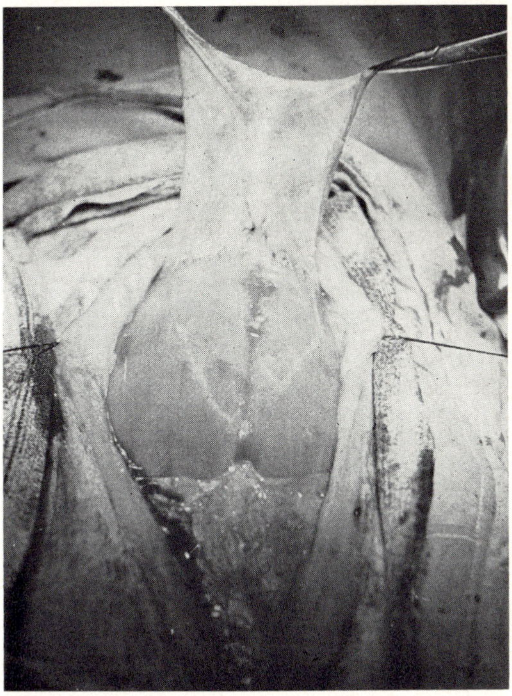

**Fig. 1.** Anterior layer of rectus sheath dissected from rectus muscle of dog No. 506.

## RESULTS

There were no postoperative deaths or fistula formations in the 10 experiments. During the first 3 postoperative days, the dogs voided frequently. The amount of urine voided each time gradually increased during the first 2 weeks. Residual urine measurements were obtained immediately after the animals voided and the volume never exceeded 5 ml.

One month after operation urine cultures were negative in 8 animals and in the remaining 2 there was a *Staphylococcus aureus* growth of one-half million per milliliter. The results of urine cultures were negative in all animals at the end of the third month.

After operation the blood urea nitrogen, as well as the serum sodium, potassium, chloride, and carbon dioxide levels remained unchanged from preoperative levels. In all experiments, the upper urinary tracts were radiographically normal. Cystograms performed 1 month after operation outlined a small urinary bladder with irregular contours at the site of the fascial graft. Sanguineous urine was observed after the insertion of a Foley catheter. After 2 months the bladders were enlarged and the contours were smooth. The urine was clear after catheterization. Three months after operation cystograms showed normal bladders (Fig. 4).

Bladder function was evaluated by measurement of residual urine and by artificial stimulation of the bladder. At operation prior to the excision of a large segment of bladder, we were able to simulate a sustained detrusor contraction by attaching electrodes bilaterally to the pelvic nerves and applying a 6 v. stimulus. The intraluminal bladder pressure was increased from 15 cm. $H_2O$ to 45 cm. $H_2O$. The same procedure was repeated at a subsequent operation after the final gross examination of the bladder graft site. The increase in the intraluminal bladder pressure at this time was approximately the same as that recorded from the intact bladder prior to grafting.

By the end of the first month, the graft was less than half of its original size and

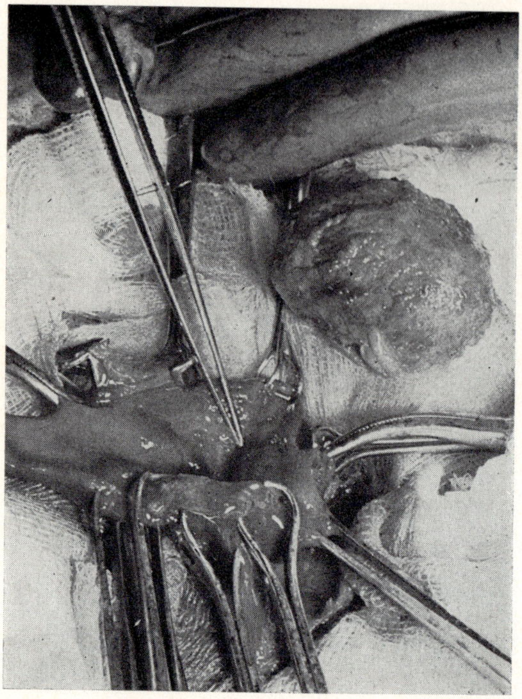

**Fig. 2.** Bladder remnant of dog with approximately 1 cm. of bladder wall above each ureteral orifice. Forceps points to left ureteral orifice. The excised portion of bladder is located in the upper part of photograph.

the bladder was normal in shape. Its internal surface was smooth except for the fascial graft, which was covered by healthy granulation tissue. By the end of the third month, the fascial graft was reduced to less than 1 cm. in width and 2 cm. in length. The external surface of the graft was smooth, glistening, and firm (Fig. 5). In all experiments the bladder mucosa covered the fascial graft completely (Fig. 6). An incision through the graft site showed it to be gritty, firm, and thickest at its most central portion (Fig. 7). After a period of 6 months, no calculi could be observed in any of the bladders.

Transitional epithelium covered the fascial remnant completely (Fig. 8). This remnant consisted of thick connective tissue. In 3 of the 10 experiments there were small foci of ectopic bone. This is a finding also reported by Baret and associates.[1] The bladder wall surrounding the graft appeared normal.

## DISCUSSION AND CONCLUSIONS

In 1953 Baret and his colleagues[1] used a rectus fascia and muscle graft in the experimental repair of bladder wall defects in dogs. They reported a high incidence of fistula formation which was attributed to inadequate bladder drainage. We believe that the muscle and fascia graft combination may have contributed to the formation of fistulas. Suturing of the muscle makes it permeable. The muscle portion of the graft, without an intact vascular supply, must have undergone necrosis. The combination of necrotic tissue and urine leakage must have contributed significantly to fistula formation.

In the present study rectus fascia without muscle was used to repair the defect in the bladder wall. There was no fistula formation in any of the 10 dogs. Furthermore, all studies of renal and bladder function yielded normal results after operation. With the fascial grafts the blood chemistry studies showed no significant changes like those that occurred with absorbing mucosal grafts. All of the fascial remnant was eventually completely covered with normal bladder mucosa. The fascia did not inhibit the rapid regeneration of bladder mucosa.

At the end of 3 months, cystograms showed a bladder, normal in size and shape, without ureterovesical backflow. We believe that reflux was absent because the ureterovesical trigone was not disturbed and also because prolonged elevations of intravesical pressure and chronic bladder infection were lacking.

The fascial graft did not interfere with complete bladder emptying as demonstrated by the negligible amount of residual urine. The bladder remnant not only maintained its resiliency and adaptability to increasing bladder pressure, but also exhibited an efficient emptying detrusor mechanism. The integrity of the bladder muscle was further demonstrated by the fact that an adequate sustained contraction was obtained on stimulation of the pelvic nerves.

The gross anatomic and histologic studies confirmed the ability of the bladder remnant to enlarge its size by gradually adapting itself to increasing volumes and pressures. The results of histologic studies left no doubt of the complete regeneration of the transitional epithelium. The microscopic bony spicule formation was probably due to the direct effect of bladder mucosa when it was in contact with the fascia. As soon as the entire surface of fascia was covered with the neouroepithelium, the ectopic bone formation was arrested. The ectopic bone did not interfere with bladder function.

A fascial graft is a worth-while adjunct in the primary repair of exstrophy of the bladder. In some patients the bladder remnant is so small that it cannot be turned into a viscus and in others it is so small that it can not accommodate a catheter for drainage. Moreover, in such cases attempted closure under tension will cause the bladder wound to break down and a fistula to develop. The problem is further aggravated by the postoperative mucosal edema. In our series of 29 patients with primary closure of the bladder, 6 had no urinary output for from 48 to 72 hours after the repair. One additional patient had no urinary output for the first 5 days after the operation and an elevation of serum potassium to 6.7 mEq. per liter. The formation of a small bladder by primary closure and superimposed postoperative mucosal edema may cause an elevation of the intraureteral pressure to levels above those compatible with proper functioning of the kidneys and the ureters. This favors the development of severe urinary infection. The additional problem of fistula formation may also originate during this period. The complications of this period may be avoided by the use of a fascial graft which will adequately enlarge the bladder reservoir.

Our experiments have demonstrated the easy accessibility and sufficient pliability of a fascial graft. The blood supply to the graft is not jeopardized with a fascial graft as it is with a seromuscular graft or loop of ileum or rectum.

Shoemaker and Marcucci[2] in 1956 had hoped that their seromuscular graft would

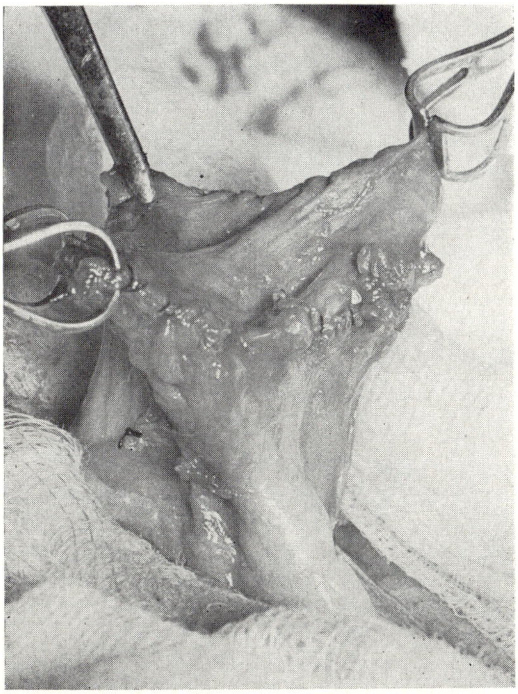

**Fig. 3.** The fascial graft, measuring 3.5 by 5 cm., sutured to the dog's bladder remnant.

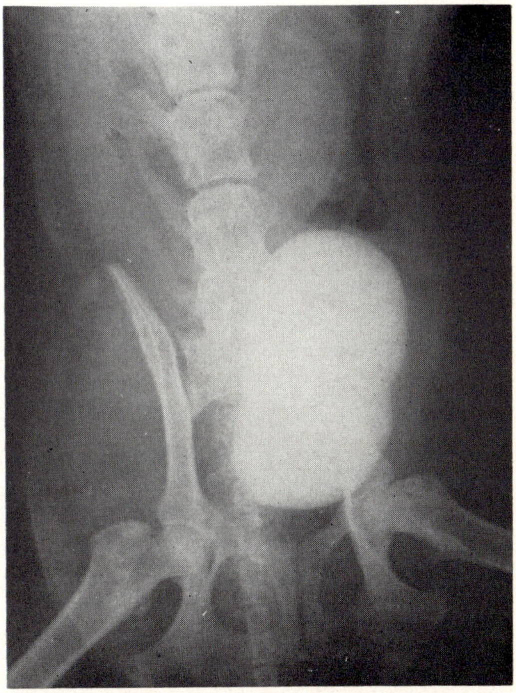

**Fig. 4.** A cystogram performed on the dog 3 months postoperatively outlines a bladder normal in size and shape.

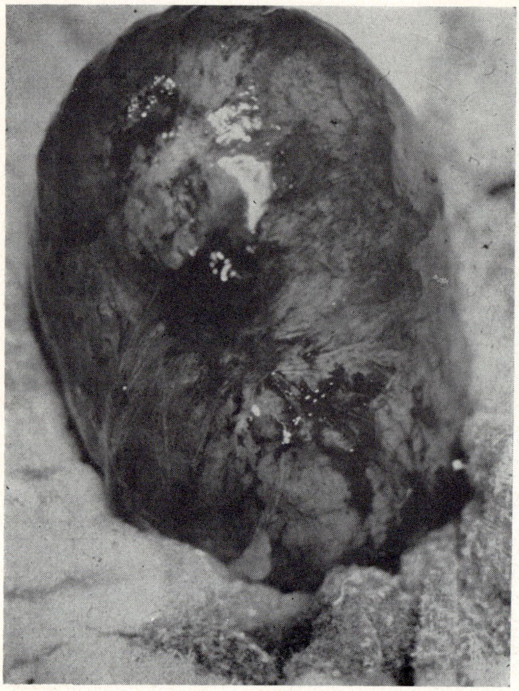

**Fig. 5.** The external surface of dog's bladder, 3 months after operation, is smooth and soft. Fascial graft is reduced to less than one-third of its original size.

function as an integral unit of the bladder. We believe that this is impossible because the stimulus which acts upon the bladder muscle has no way of being transmitted to the seromuscular graft. This graft simply helps to form a part of the bladder wall. A seromuscular graft will interfere with sustained detrusor contraction because it has no way of contracting simultaneously with the bladder remnant. The graft will allow some loss of emptying power because it will expand with the increased intraluminal pressure and act as a bladder diverticulum. The fascial graft affords an adequate bladder reservoir initially. As the bladder wall enlarges and the mucosa regenerates, the graft shrinks proportionately. The fascia is not distensible and allows the entire bladder remnant to expand. It is the latter process which makes possible the gradual enlargement of the bladder remnant and shrinkage of the graft after it has fulfilled its usefulness.

Influenced by the results with experimental fascial grafts, we have employed rectus fascia autografts in 2 patients for primary closure of exstrophy of the bladder.

## CASE REPORTS

**Case 1.** M. R. was a girl, 2 years and 10 months of age. The bladder remnant measured 3 by 3 cm. and the mucosa was friable and hypertrophied. Excretory urograms showed large dilated ureters bilaterally. Ureteral peristalsis was poor bilaterally. Urine culture and colony count showed that there were over 3 million *Aerobacter aerogenes* per milliliter. The child was treated with a specific antibiotic for 5 days and then underwent bilateral iliac osteotomies.

Three days later a primary closure of the bladder was performed. The redundant folds of mucosa were excised and the bladder mucosa was approximated with interrupted plain catgut sutures. An incision was made around the periphery of the bladder and cephalad the peritoneum was separated by blunt dissection. Laterally, the bladder wall was separated from the rectus muscle by sharp dissection. The bladder neck and urethra were freed sufficiently to allow the mucosal edges to be brought together without tension. The urethral mucosa was approximated with interrupted No. 5-0 plain catgut sutures. The approximation was carried out to about 1 cm. beyond the bladder neck. In the region of the bladder neck, the mucosal suture line was reinforced with flaps of fibrous tissue. No urethral splint was used.

A transverse incision was made in the left upper quadrant of the abdomen and a 2.5 by 2.5 cm. portion of anterior rectus fascia was excised. The fascial defect was repaired with interrupted No. 5-0 silk sutures. The skin incision was closed with a continuous No. 5-0 plain catgut subcuticular suture. The fascial graft was sutured to the bladder mucosa with interrupted No. 5-0 plain catgut sutures. The muscular layer was then sutured to the fascia with interrupted No. 4-0 chromic catgut sutures. A No. 12 Malecot catheter was inserted through an incision made in the dome of the bladder wall and fixed to it with a No. 5-0 chromic catgut suture. The pubic bones were approximated with 3 interrupted No. 2-0 chromic catgut sutures and the medial borders of the rectus muscles were sutured together with interrupted No. 4-0 chromic catgut sutures. The skin was approximated with interrupted No. 5-0 silk sutures.

Within 24 hours after operation, the urinary output was normal. The postoperative course was uneventful and the suprapubic catheter was removed on the fourteenth postoperative day. Six

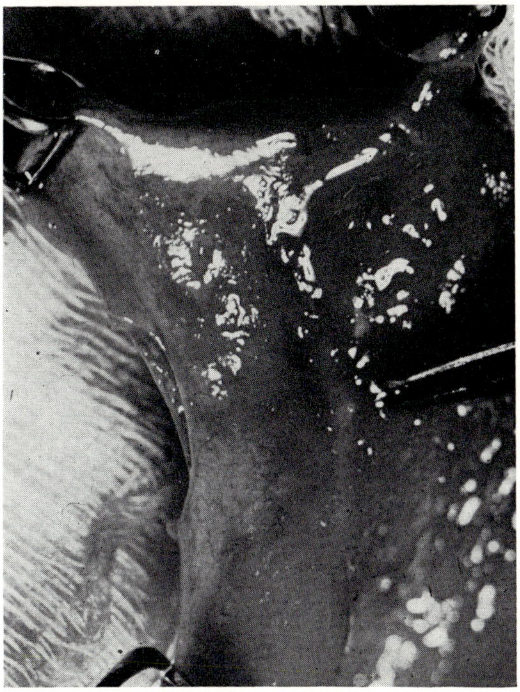

**Fig. 6.** The internal surface of dog's bladder 3 months after operation indicates normal appearance of the bladder mucosa. To left of forceps is fascial graft covered with bladder mucosa.

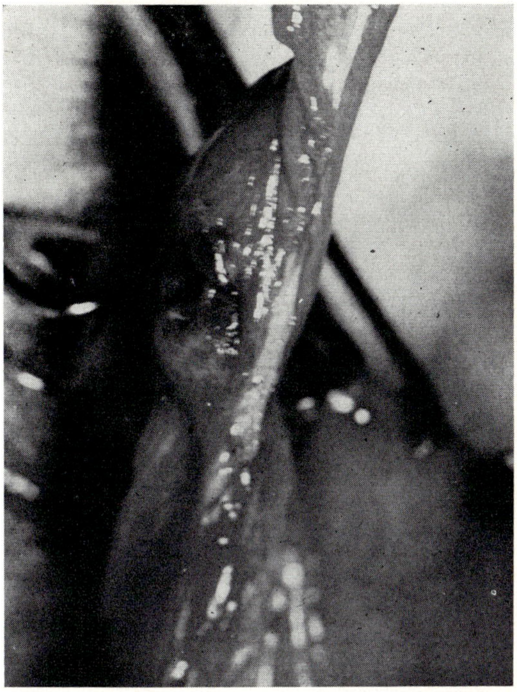

**Fig. 7.** An incision through the fascial graft site of dog's bladder after 3 months demonstrates that grossly the graft is reduced in size and completely covered by bladder mucosa.

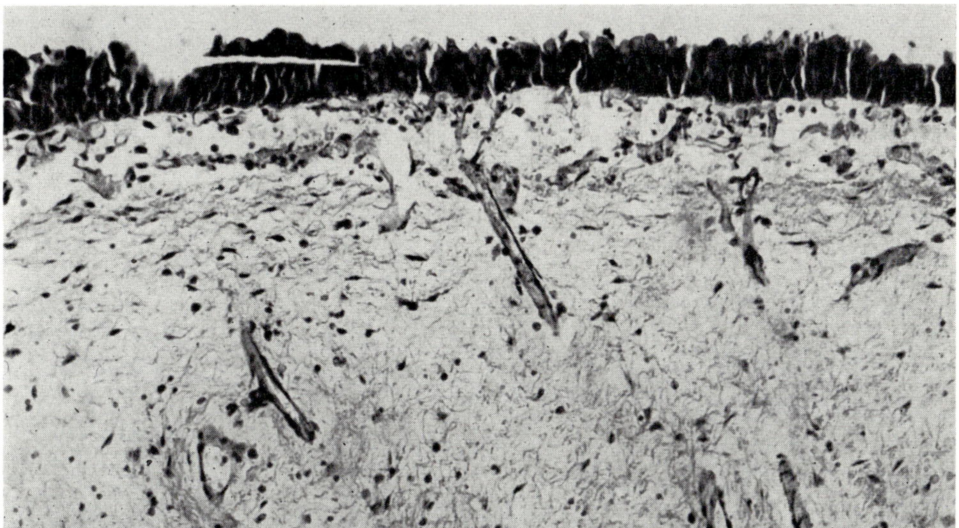

**Fig. 8.** A thin layer of transitional uroepithelium overlying the fascial remnant in a dog 3 months after operation.

months after the repair, the patient was admitted to the hospital and a cystogram was performed which showed a bladder normal in shape. The bladder capacity was 45 ml.

**Case 2.** L. R. was a 5-day-old white boy who was admitted to the hospital because of bladder exstrophy. The bladder remnant measured approximately 2.5 by 2.5 cm. The urine contained over 2 million *E. coli* per milliliter. Ureteral peristalsis was normal in the right ureter and irregular and infrequent in the left ureter. The intravenous pyelogram outlined a dilated upper urinary tract bilaterally. The urinary tract infection was treated with a specific antibiotic for 6 days. Bilateral iliac osteotomies were performed and 3 days later the primary closure of the bladder remnant was carried out. The bladder remnant was small and the same procedure as described in Case 1 was performed, except that the corpora cavernosa were freed up to their attachments to the pubic bones. The corpora were approximated with interrupted No. 4-0 chromic catgut sutures over the newly formed urethra. The urinary output was satisfactory within 24 hours. Three weeks after the bladder repair, the suprapubic catheter was removed and the patient was discharged. Seven months later he was admitted to the hospital for the repair of bilateral inguinal hernias. During this admission the urine contained 3 million *Aerobacter aerogenes* per milliliter and specific antibiotic therapy was continued for 6 days. A cystogram outlined an oval-shaped bladder with a capacity of 30 ml. The patient has had a negative colony count since his last admission.

The use of the fascial grafts in the 2 patients confirms their usefulness in primary closure of bladder exstrophy. Without a graft of this nature, we would have had to perform a procedure for urine diversion in the 2 patients. We believe that the use of a fascial graft allowed for an enlarged bladder reservoir which did not interfere with the urine flow to the bladder.

## SUMMARY

Rectus fascia autografts were used successfully to repair experimental bladder wall defects in 10 dogs. Repeated gross and histologic studies of the reconstructed bladder demonstrated the remnant to be expanding and growing concomitantly with regression of the fascial graft.

Normal bladder function and capacity were obtained. Biochemical studies of the blood as well as intravenous pyelograms showed normal renal function.

Postoperative wound complications were not encountered.

The practical application of the fascial graft in 2 children with exstrophy of the bladder is described. The preliminary early results are satisfactory and encouraging. However, sufficient time has not elapsed for evaluation of the late results of the fascial graft with respect to the development of the bladder and renal function.

### REFERENCES

1. Baret, A. C., DeMuth, W., Murphy, J., and Muir, M.: Experimental repair of exstrophy of bladder without cystectomy by using a free fascial graft, Surg. Gynec. & Obst. **97:** 633, 1953.
2. Shoemaker, W. C., and Marcucci, H. D.: Experimental use of seromuscular grafts in bladder reconstruction. J. Urol. **73:** 2, 1955.

# Vesicoileosigmoidostomy in the treatment of exstrophy of the bladder

DANIEL M. HAYS, M.D.
TRACY O. POWELL, M.D.
LOS ANGELES, CALIF.
*From the Urological and General Surgical Divisions, Department of Surgery, Los Angeles Childrens Hospital*

In a previous publication from the Los Angeles Childrens Hospital,[3] the use of different intestinal segments to enlarge the exstrophied bladder was described. The utilization of isolated loops of ileum and sigmoid colon as urinary conduits distal to the reconstructed bladder was studied in 11 patients.* The combined use of both of these intestinal elements as a conduit, that is, vesicoileosigmoidostomy (Fig. 1), has been discussed in a previous report.[5]

Six children with exstrophy in whom previous reconstructive procedures had proved unsuccessful have been operated upon by this procedure with a uniform technique.

## HISTORIES OF 6 PATIENTS WHO UNDERWENT VESICOILEOSIGMOIDOSTOMY FOR EXSTROPHY

Five of the children were girls and 1 was a boy. The average age at the time of this procedure was 5 years (range 16 months to 7 years, 6 months).

In 3 patients, exstrophy was associated with additional major upper urinary tract disease. Renal agenesis (left) had been suspected in the patient in Case 1 from the date of the initial excretory studies and was confirmed at laparotomy. Ureterectasis without structural ureterovesical obstruction had been observed in the patient in Case 2 prior to the initial operative procedures. It may represent neurogenic megaloureter. Unilateral ureterectasis without obstruction developed in the patient in Case 6 during the course of the series of plastic procedures performed (Table I).

Imperforate anus, noted in Case 1, was of the membranous type (Ladd type II), apparently readily corrected on the second day of life. Other congenital defects included an infantile rectal prolapse (Case 5) which was sufficiently severe to prompt operative correction when the patient was 6 months old. The absence of digits was noted in 1 patient.

All patients had undergone at least 1 previous surgical procedure for the correction of exstrophy (in this or other institutions). In 2, there had been 4 prior operations for this anomaly (Table I).

**Types of previous surgical procedures.** Anterior reconstruction of the bladder and abdominal wall with techniques similar to those described by Young,[10] Sweetser,[8] and Swenson,[9] were initially employed in all except one of these patients (3 in other institutions). Two such attempts were made in 1 child, and 3 (anterior reconstructions) in 2 others. These procedures resulted (except in 1 instance) in the formation of a solid, cosmetically satisfactory anterior abdominal wall over the reconstructed bladder. True continence, however, was never achieved and partial continence only when accompanied by some degree of bladder outlet obstruction.

Received for publication Oct. 13, 1960.

*Four of these patients are included in the present study (Table I, Nos. 2, 4, 5, and 6.)

**Table I.** *Vesicoileosigmoidostomy in exstrophy of the bladder*

| *Sex and present age* | *Associated anomalies* | *Previous operations for exstrophy (age)* |
|---|---|---|
| Case 1,* female, 2 yr. | Left renal agenesis, imperforate anus, absent digit (prematurity) | Plastic reconstruction of "urethra" (only), 6 months |
| Case 2, female, 4 yr. | Ureterectasis (right) noted on initial urogram at 18 mo., "megaloureter" | Anterior plastic reconstruction, 18 mo.; bladder enlargement with isolated ileal segment and anterior reconstruction, 3 yr. |
| Case 3, female, 6½ yr. | None | Anterior plastic reconstruction, 2½ yr.; anterior plastic reconstruction, 3½ yr.; anterior plastic reconstruction, 4½ yr. |
| Case 4, female, 5 yr. | None | Bladder enlargement with isolated ileal segment, 3 yr.; anterior plastic reconstruction, 4 yr. |
| Case 5, female, 7½ yr. | Rectal prolapse from age 3 wk. | Anterior plastic reconstruction; 2½ yr.; bladder enlargement with isolated colon segment, 4½ yr.; anterior plastic reconstruction, 5½ yr.; anterior plastic reconstruction, 6½ yr. |
| Case 6, male, 6 yr. | None | Anterior plastic reconstruction, 9 mo.; bladder enlargement with isolated colon segment, 2½ yr.; anterior plastic reconstruction, 3½ yr.; anterior plastic reconstruction, 5 yr. |

*Cases 1, 2, and 3 have been referred to in a prior publication.[5]
†Serum chloride determination 119 mEq./L. at 2 months, decreased to 102 mEq./L. at 6 months postoperatively.

In addition to anterior reconstruction, in 4 patients the rudimentary bladder had previously been enlarged with isolated intestinal segments. In 2 of these, ileal segments had been employed. In 2 others, a segment of sigmoid colon had been used to enlarge the bladder and form a conduit to the perineum.[3] In the latter, stenosis of the distal end of the sigmoid conduit had occurred.

In 1 case an attempt to form an anterior urethra with a pedunculated flap of bladder wall, as a preliminary step toward vesical closure, had been the only prior procedure utilized.

The growth curves (height and weight) in 3 of the children were within the normal range.* In 3 others, including 2 of those with additional major genitourinary tract disease, a regularly ascending growth curve was found, but with a low starting point and a maintained depression, largely below the second percentile.

Completely satisfactory control of defecation had been achieved in all but one, the youngest (Case 1), including the girl with early rectal prolapse. After the anterior plastic procedures noted, the children were no longer subject to the constant irritation

*State University of Iowa standard curves.

| *Preoperative status* | *Age at time of this procedure* | *Postoperative status* |
|---|---|---|
| Bladder interior exposed; prompt excretion (right) slight ureterovesical narrowing (right) on I.V.P.; NPN 27 mg.%; no abnormalities of serum electrolytes | 15 mo. | Anterior bladder closure intact; urinary (and fecal) continence satisfactory for age; I.V.P. unchanged (1, 2, and 6 mo.); NPN not elevated (1, 2, and 6 mo.); serum electrolytes unchanged (1, 2,† and 6 mo.) |
| Bladder interior exposed, anemia secondary to chronic blood loss; prompt excretion ureterectasia (bilateral), no obstruction on I.V.P.; NPN 35 mg.%; no alteration in serum electrolytes | 3 yr., 9 mo. | Anterior bladder closure intact; partial urinary continence; I.V.P. unchanged (1 and 3 mo.); no NPN elevation (1 and 3 mo.); serum electrolyte levels unchanged (1 and 3 mo.) |
| Anterior bladder closure intact; total urinary incontinence; prompt excretion, normal structure of upper tract on I.V.P.; NPN 30 mg.%; no alterations in serum electrolytes | 6 yr., 6 mo. | Anterior bladder closure intact; urinary continence at night (daytime stress incontinence); I.V.P. unchanged (1 mo.); NPN not elevated (1 and 3 mo.); serum electrolyte levels unchanged (1 and 3 mo.) |
| Anterior bladder closure intact; total urinary incontinence; prompt excretion, normal structure of upper urinary tract on I.V.P.; NPN 17 mg. %; no alterations in serum electrolytes | 5 yr. | Anterior bladder closure intact; urinary continence complete; I.V.P. unchanged (1 mo.); NPN 14 mg.% (1 mo.); serum electrolyte levels unchanged (1 mo.) |
| Anterior bladder closure intact; total urinary incontinence; prompt excretion, normal structure of upper urinary tract on I.V.P.; NPN 21 mg.%; no alterations in serum electrolytes | 7 yr., 6 mo. | Anterior bladder closure intact with anterior vesical fistula; rectal continence for urine and feces satisfactory; I.V.P. unchanged (1 mo.); NPN 20 mg.% (1 mo.); serum electrolyte levels unchanged (1 mo.) |
| Anterior bladder closure intact; total urinary incontinence; prompt excretion (bilateral), calyectasis and ureterectasis without obstruction (right) on I.V.P.; NPN 22 mg.%; no alterations in serum electrolytes | 6 yr. | Anterior bladder closure intact; urinary continence satisfactory; I.V.P. unchanged (1 mo.); NPN 25 mg.% (1 mo.); serum electrolytes unchanged (1 mo.) |

of an exposed bladder surface, and from the point of view of the parent, their only real disability was urinary incontinence.

Three of the patients (Cases 1, 2, and 6) had grossly abnormal excretory urograms. Two had been noted from the time of initial examinations and the third had developed during the course of previous anterior reconstructions (Table I). In addition, in Case 1, the right ureteropelvic junction seemed slightly narrowed in studies performed immediately prior to the definitive procedure. Each of the remaining patients had serial intravenous pyelograms performed before, during, and after the preliminary operative procedures described (Table I) with normal excretion demonstrated and no alterations in the structure of the upper urinary tract.

Determinations of serum nonprotein nitrogen and electrolyte concentrations (sodium, potassium, chloride, and carbon dioxide) were within the usual range in all of the children prior to operation.

## TECHNIQUE OF THE OPERATIVE PROCEDURE

The operation was performed through 2 incisions, (1) an initial superior transperitoneal approach and (2) a secondary, extra-

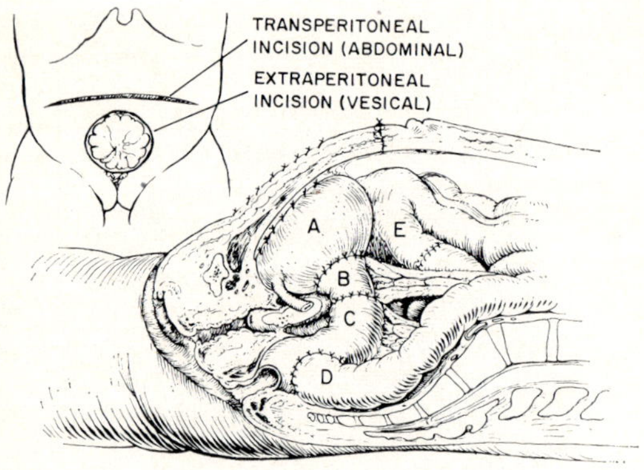


**Fig. 1.** Vesicoileosigmoidostomy. *A,* Urinary bladder after anterior closure. *B,* Isolated ileal segment with anastomosis to the bladder and colon. *C,* Sigmoid colon segment utilized as a urinary conduit. *D,* Sigmoid colon (functional intestinal tract). *E,* The terminal ileum after end-to-end anastomosis.

peritoneal dissection about the rudimentary bladder.

In only one of the present cases was the exstrophy in an approximately natural state, and the form of the second (vesical) incision depended upon the type of previous procedure employed. In all, however, the bladder was widely opened anteriorly (if not open), and an extensive mobilization of lateral vesical walls performed.

The superior approach was made uniformly through a wide, transverse lower abdominal incision with division of both rectus muscles. This operative field was kept separate from, and lay 2 to 3 cm. superior to, the incision about the exstrophied bladder (or its reconstruction).

The intra-abdominal procedure may be divided into 4 steps, (1) separation of the colon to form divided fecal and urinary conduits, (2) isolation of an ileal segment, (3) connection of the "urinary" colon conduit and ileal segment utilizing a valve-like (ileal "nipple") anastomosis, and (4) connection of the ileal segment to the posterior wall of the bladder.

The initial step was accomplished by transection of the colon approximately 10 cm. above the pelvic floor. The proximal end of the divided colon was then brought down to a position immediately above the peritoneal reflexion where an end-to-side anastomosis was performed between the end of the proximal segment and the side of the distal colon. A routine 2-layer anastomosis by an "open" technique with internal, continuous absorbable sutures supported externally by interrupted nonabsorbable sutures was employed. This provided a diverticular intestinal segment for use as a urinary conduit.

The second step consisted of isolation of a segment of terminal ileum with intact mesentery by the usual techniques. This segment should be 8 to 10 cm. in length, and lie approximately 10 cm. proximal to the ileocecal junction. Intestinal continuity was re-established by end-to-end anastomosis.

In the third step the distal end of the isolated ileal segment was opened and the serosa removed or scarified for 2 cm. from the distal margin of transection. The mucosa and submucosa were then everted and sutured to the margin of the intact serosa proximally with fine absorbable sutures. This formed a "nipple" of mucosa-covered ileum, 1 cm. in length. This technique is similar to that used in forming an ileostomy stoma on the anterior abdominal wall. The nipple of ileum was then introduced into the open end of the distal colon segment where it projected into the lumen for approximately 1 cm. (Fig. 2). A serosa-to-serosa closure between ileum and colon was formed around the base of the ileal nipple with nonabsorbable sutures.

The fourth step was performed through both the abdominal and the vesical incisions. It was preceded by reflexion of the peritoneum from the posterior vesical wall and mobilization of the superior and posterior aspects of the bladder. The ureters were identified and dissection carried between them. An opening was made in the pelvic peritoneum and in the base of the left broad ligament (in the female) for the passage of the conduit to the bladder.

Anastomosis between the proximal end of the ileal segment and the vesical wall was begun within the bladder. A vertical incision was made in the posterior wall between the ureteral orifices, extending superiorly for approximately 2 cm. Into this opening the proximal end of the isolated ileal segment was inserted. The ileal mucosal layer was sutured to the vesical mucosal and muscular wall with fine, interrupted absorbable sutures placed throughout the circumference of the bladder opening (Fig. 3). Through the peritoneal incision, the ileal seromuscular surface was then approximated to the advential wall of the bladder with interrupted nonabsorbable sutures. The margins of the peritoneum were also sutured to the ileal wall where the latter passes through the peritoneum toward the vesical anastomosis.

The final phase began with completion of the mobilization of the exstrophied bladder wall. If not previously accomplished, a division of the skin margins was continued inferiorly about the edge of the bladder mucosa. The full thickness of bladder wall was then freed from surrounding tissues both laterally and inferiorly (the superior and posterior aspects had been previously elevated). Only the vascular pedicles about the ureteral openings remained after this dissection. The bladder was then closed anteriorly and inferiorly with a double row of absorbable sutures. This was facilitated by the relaxation which results from the introduction of the ileal segment into the posterior wall. If the bladder mucosal area is quite small, it may be necessary to enlarge it with an intestinal segment as a preliminary operative procedure.[3] A large catheter was passed from the side of the reconstructed bladder through the anterior abdominal wall.

The abdominal procedure was completed by the closure of the 2 mesenteric defects (ileal and colonic) and approximation of the combined ileocolonic segment to posterior peritoneal surfaces. It may be possible to place all or a part of the conduit segment (ileum and colon) in an extraperitoneal space posterior and superior to the bladder.

Abdominal closure was made in layers. The peritoneum was usually intact and could be closed with continuous sutures. The fascial layers of both incisions were approximated with interrupted sutures of steel wire (No. 30) and the subcutaneous fascia with absorbable sutures. In the female the cli-

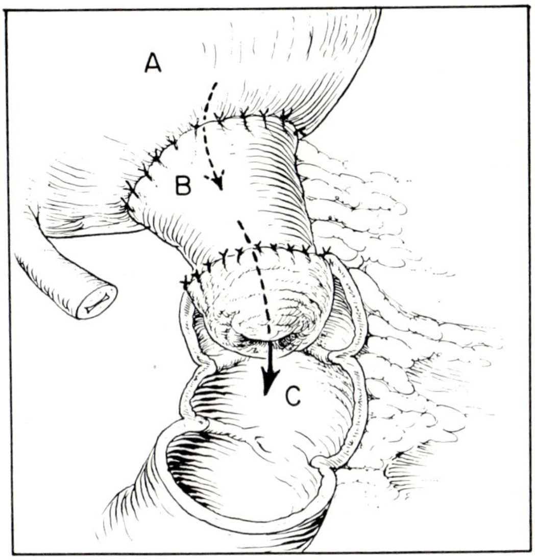


**Fig. 2.** Detailed study of the ileal nipple formed at the anastomosis between the isolated ileal segment *(B)* and sigmoid urinary conduit *(C)*. The ileal segment is shortened for diagrammatic clarity. Its actual length after eversion of the distal end to form the nipple is 6 to 7 cm.

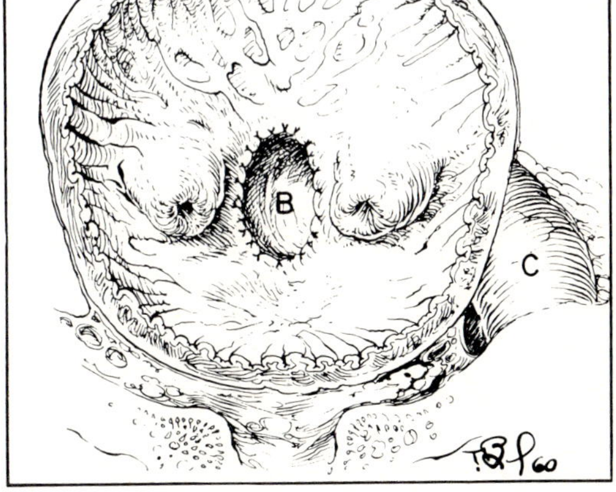


**Fig. 3.** Anterior view of the interior of the bladder after anastomosis of the isolated ileal segment *(B)* to the vesical wall between the ureteral orifices. *C,* Sigmoid colon.

toris was formed by uniting its 2 halves in the midline and the vulva was further reconstructed by mobilization and closure of laterally placed tissues. In the male the genital openings were left intact for subsequent penial reconstruction.

Preoperative preparation for this procedure has included a regimen of orally administered neomycin, catharsis, and enemas for 2 days. Bladder drainage by anterior abdominal wall catheters has been maintained for 2 weeks postoperatively in all patients.

## IMMEDIATE AND SHORT-TERM EVALUATION OF EFFECTS OF VESICOILEOSIGMOIDOSTOMY

There has been no death associated with this procedure. The postoperative period of study of these patients has been short, averaging 3 months, with the longest of 8 months' duration.

Temporary anterior vesical fistulas have developed in 2 children. One has closed spontaneously.

In addition to exstrophy, 3 patients upon whom this procedure was employed had major structural alterations in the upper urinary tract, unilateral renal agenesis and ureterectasia (possible megaloureter), without mechanical obstruction in 2. These patients were not azotemic, and their postoperative status was not altered in this regard. Azotemia and hyperchloremia were reported to have developed in Patient 1 during a severe febrile illness in another city 4 months after operation. There was no laboratory evidence of either state when the patient was evaluated subsequently in this institution. An elevation of serum chloride levels to 119 mEq. per liter was noted in the same patient 2 months after our operation, but a normal level (102 mEq. per liter) was found 4 months later.

In the remaining patients, intravenous pyelography has shown no alteration in excretory function or structure of the upper urinary tract and results of nonprotein nitrogen determinations have always been within normal limits. No evidence of hyperchloremia or other deviations from expected serum electrolyte concentrations have been observed.

As might be anticipated from the results obtained in children with ureterointestinal transplants, the voluntary control of urinary outflow through the rectum has been generally, although not completely, satisfactory. The youngest child (Case 1), age 2 years, is the only patient in the series in whom partial control is still in doubt.

Cystograms performed in 3 patients after operation showed a prompt passage of contrast material to the rectum. In one, a delay in emptying was followed by a sudden and complete bladder evacuation, possibly secondary to a bladder contraction.

A barium enema study in 2 patients showed apparent competence of the ileosigmoid anastomosis to the barium solution, as the pressures employed were sufficient to cause filling of the colon diverticulum (and the remaining colon), but not of the bladder (Fig. 4). The ileal nipple may be viewed with a proctoscope and the bladder catheterized.

## DISCUSSION

Upon review of the procedures employed by American and European surgeons for exstrophy prior to the adoption of ureterointestinal transplants, it seems that every conceivable anastomotic arrangement of the ureters, bladder, colon, rectum, and ileum had been attempted. The technique described here (vesicoileosigmoidostomy) includes some elements of operations originally reported as early as 1903 (Borelius[2]) and 1907 (Berg[1]) with adaptation described as recently as 1958 (Snyder[7]). To credit even major contributors in this field of lower urinary tract reconstruction would require monograph form.[6, 10] The combined features of the vesicoileosigmoidostomy technique, however, have apparently not been previously employed.

The rationale behind the adoption of this complicated operative technique was based on the apparent desirability of including certain features in the reconstruction of the

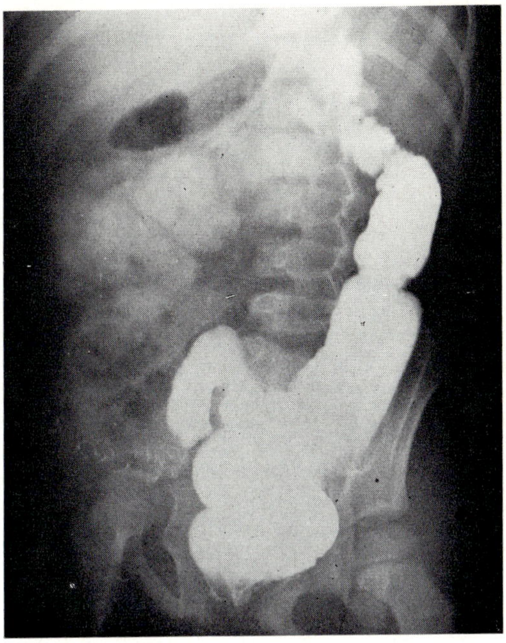

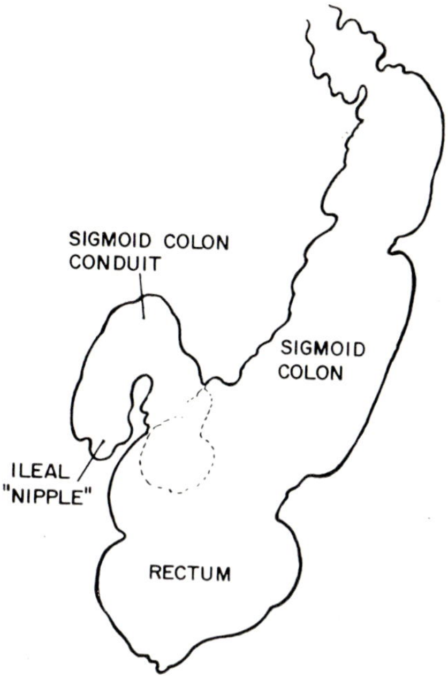


**Fig. 4.** Roentgenographic study with barium emulsion under usual pressure (36 inches) passing into the colon and urinary conduit, but not into the ileal segment or bladder.

bladder and its outflow tract. These included (1) preservation of the ureterovesical junctions, (2) anterior vesical closure to form a urinary reservoir, and (3) formation of a conduit between the reconstructed bladder and the rectum, with sufficient valve-like activity to prevent gross fecal contamination of the vesical cavity.

It has been regarded as advantageous to preserve the ureterovesical junction as a deterrent to ascending infection in the urinary tract. Theoretically, the bladder is a more desirable urinary reservoir than the rectum or colon because of the absence of absorptive activity in the mucosa. Under these circumstances, unfortunately, it may also act as a source of stasis and recurrent infection, although this has not been apparent in our series to date.

Whether the bladder will actually function as a reservoir or simply as a conduit when connected by the operative technique described is uncertain.

The conduit between the bladder and the rectum has been formed from 2 intestinal segments, ileum and sigmoid colon, in order to minimize the length of ileum utilized and facilitate construction of a valve-like anastomosis which would keep solid fecal material in the colon segment. The "valve" is simply a projection or nipple of ileum which protrudes into the colon lumen. This was placed in a colon diverticulum rather than in the sigmoid colon itself to avoid the intestinal complications of partial obstruction or intussusception.

It is recognized that the worth of an innovation such as this in the treatment of exstrophy must be determined by an assessment of its effectiveness over several decades. Specifically, one wonders if it can provide more protection to the renal reserve of the child than does standard sigmoid ureterointestinal anastomosis. Although theoretical arguments as to why it may, or may not, provide protection from renal infection of intestinal origin are of interest, there is probably no way to determine the answer to this question except by clinical study.

This basic procedure might be modified to include the transplantation of the ureters to the ileal segment in the management of vesical carcinoma, and so forth, when cystectomy is required.

## SUMMARY

A technique of bladder reconstruction and formation of a vesical outflow tract to the rectum for the management of exstrophy is described. In this procedure an isolated ileal segment and a partially divided sigmoid colon conduit are utilized. The union of the ileal and colonic elements of the urinary drainage tract is made in a valve-like anastomosis to minimze fecal regurgitation into the re-formed bladder. Six patients in whom this technique has been employed have shown no evidence of renal impairment or significant alterations in serum electrolyte concentrations during the immediate postoperative period. They appear to have a high degree of urinary continence. A long-term evaluation of this procedure as a substitute for ureterointestinal anastomosis in patients with exstrophy of the bladder seems warranted.

### REFERENCES

1. Berg, J.: Über die Behandlung der Ectopia vesicae, Nord. Med. Ark., Stockholm **7:** 1, 1907.
2. Borelius, J.: Eine neue Modification de Maydlschen Operationsmethode bei Angeborener Blasenektopie, Zentralbl. f. Chir. Leipz. **30:** 780, 1903.
3. Hays, D. M., and Powell, T. O.: Various intestinal segments utilized for bladder enlargement in pediatric patients with reference to the management of exstrophy, SURGERY **47:** 999, 1960.
4. Hinman, F., and Weyrauch, H. M., Jr.: A critical study of the different principles of surgery which have been used in ureterointestinal implantation, Int. Abst. Surg. **64:** 313, 1937.
5. Powell, T. O., and Hays, D. M.: An improved surgical procedure for exstrophy of the bladder, West. J. Surg. In press.
6. Sorrentino, F. M., and Leonetti, P.: Terapia della estrofia vesicale. Relazione Ufficiale al XXXI Congresso della Societa' Italiana di Urologia., 1958.
7. Snyder, C. C.: A new therapeutic concept of the exstrophied bladder, Plast. & Reconstruct. Surg. **22:** 1, 1958.
8. Sweetser, T. H., Chisholm, T. C., and Thompson, W.: Exstrophy of the urinary bladder, its treatment by plastic surgery, J. Urol. **75:** 448, 1956.
9. Swenson, O.: Changing trends in the management of exstrophy of the bladder, SURGERY **42:** 61, 1957.
10. Young, H. H.: Exstrophy of the bladder. The first case in which a normal bladder and urinary control have been obtained by plastic operations, Surg. Gynec. & Obst. **74:** 729, 1942.

# Surgical treatment of bowel and bladder dysfunction in a case of spina bifida with meningomyelocele

PATRICK C. DEVINE, M.D.
FRANK N. BILISOLY, M.D.
E. IDE SMITH, M.D.
NORFOLK, VA.

Congenital and acquired lesions of the lumbosacral spine may result in incapacitating bowel and bladder dysfunction in addition to the more obvious musculoskeletal deformities. The most common congenital lesion which affects the lumbosacral nerve roots is spina bifida cystica. Spina bifida is said to occur once in every 1,500 births.[6] Disturbances of the lumbosacral nerve roots usually produce bowel and bladder symptoms recognizable in infancy, but, as in diastematomyelia, patients may experience no dysfunction until linear growth advances to such a degree that traction produces neural injury. Trauma or neoplasia similarly may result in the onset of symptoms.

The consequences of these neurological disturbances on both micturition and defecation have been well documented. Urologic problems associated with spastic paraplegia have been discussed by Bors,[1-3] Bors and Comarr,[4] and by Hutch,[12] while those associated with flaccid paraplegia of spina bifida have been summarized by Kennedy and Hodges[14] and by McCarthy and Lindsay.[15] Stolov[21] and Bumpus and associates[5] have reviewed the urologic complications which result from spinal injuries.

The influence of spinal abnormalities on rectal function and the evacuation reflex were summarized by Guttman[11] in a symposium on rectal incontinence. Swenson[22] has pointed out the possible importance of a lack of normal sacral sensation in the constipation seen in patients with meningomyelocele. The experimental evidence of the relationship of sacral neurological lesions to bowel dysfunction has been shown by the work of Scott,[18] Schlitt,[17] and Denny-Brown.[8] Experimental studies relating these lesions to bladder dysfunction have been reported by Jacobson[13] and by Shoemaker.[19, 20]

The possible operative approaches to the problems have been discussed by Gross,[10] Emmett,[9] and Thompson.[23] Permanent diversion of either the urinary or the fecal stream has been considered as only a last resort.

Since World War II much has been written concerning the management of the visceral dysfunction of spastic paraplegia of military and of civilian patients.[16] An aggressive and coordinated approach can be applied also to the treatment of the visceral dysfunctions associated with flaccid paraplegia, particularly since many of the individuals with this condition are of normal mental development.[10]

A case history is presented as illustrative of the rewarding outcome of such a coordinated and aggressive approach.

## CASE REPORT

G. B. M., a 15-year-old white male high school student was first seen with gross hematuria associated with suprapubic pain of 24 hours' duration.

The patient had been the product of a full term, uncomplicated pregnancy with spontaneous delivery. At birth he was found to have a lumbosacral spina bifida cystica. A neurosurgical con-

Supported by a grant from the Rotary Research Foundation of Norfolk, Va.
Received for publication Jan. 1, 1961.

sultant advised then, and later, that exploratory operation was not indicated. The patient was in a hip spica from the age of 20 months to 24 months for reduction of a congenital dislocation of the left hip, with a satisfactory result. Prior to this he was said to have had spontaneous bowel movements, but subsequently obstipation developed which necessitated enemas 2 to 3 times per week. Over the next 12 years the regular enemas became progressively more arduous until 2 to 5 hours was required to accomplish each irrigation and often the evacuation was not completed until several hours later. There was otherwise no fecal soiling.

Diapers had been necessary throughout the patient's life because of total urinary incontinence. There had been a single episode of urinary tract infection when he was 3 years of age, but otherwise there had been no symptoms of urinary tract disease. The patient had apparently had normal erections and emissions since the onset of puberty.

Mental development had been excellent and the patient's academic accomplishment had been superior despite his physical handicaps.

There was no family history of congenital deformity or of neuromuscular disease, and the one younger male sibling was normal. When admitted, the patient had recently undergone a triple arthrodesis and tendon transplantation for correction of an equinovarus deformity of the left foot, with good functional result.

**Physical examination.** The blood pressure was 110/80 mm. Hg. The abdomen was unremarkable except for an enlargement of the bladder extending midway to the umbilicus. On the back, beneath an area of hypertrichosis, a soft 12 by 14 cm. mass was present, overlying the sacrum and left gluteal regions. The genitals were normal. Slight tone was present in the external anal sphincter. The ampulla was filled with firm feces. The prostate gland and seminal vesicles were normal. Bimanual examination confirmed the enlargement of the urinary bladder. Good voluntary levator ani muscle contraction was present.

**Neurological examination.** The gait was abnormal with a marked limp in favor of the shortened left leg. Results of the Romberg test were negative. The musculature of the trunk, superficial abdominal reflexes, and trunk sensation were normal. In the left leg, which was shorter than the right leg by a half inch, there was marked atrophy of all muscle groups. The thigh muscles on the left were involved to a greater extent than the muscles of the lower leg and foot, and there was marked underdevelopment of the left gluteal group. The knee jerks were active and equal. The ankle jerks were absent. There was complete anesthesia and analgesia involving the perianal area and the posterior aspect of the right thigh to the popliteal space. A wide band of hypesthesia and hypalgesia extended across the left buttock and down the entire posterior surface of the left leg and over the lateral dorsum of the foot.

**Laboratory tests.** The hemoglobin was 13.0 Gm., white blood cells 12,500, polymorphonuclear neutrophils 77, eosinophils 1, and lymphocytes 22. Urinalysis showed the urine to be red in color. Its character was cloudy, specific gravity 1.020, pH 7.5, and albumin 4+. Sugar was negative, red blood cells innumerable, white blood cells innumerable, and there were no casts. *B. proteus,* sensitive to chloramphenicol, chlortetracycline, oxytetracycline, and nitrofurantoin, was cultured from the urine. The nonprotein nitrogen was 30 mg. per cent.

**Roentgenographic reports.** No calculi were noted on the excretory urogram. There was an abnormality of the lumbar spine and sacrum. Bilateral ureteropyelocalycectasis was present. Cystography showed a contracted bladder with a marked degree of trabeculation with deep cellules throughout. No vesicoureteral regurgitation was demonstrated.

**Hospital course.**

*First admission.* At the time of entry to the hospital the residual urine was equal to the total bladder capacity of 200 ml. and an inlying urethral catheter was left for straight drainage. The urinary infection was treated with nitrofurantoin. Cystoscopy under anesthesia disclosed a normal vesical neck and ureteral orifices. There was no apparent ureteral efflux. A cystometrogram was consistent with an autonomous neurogenic bladder with a voluntary voiding effort on 90 mm. Hg of Credé pressure.

A transurethral resection of the vesical neck was carried out under general anesthesia with the hope of reducing the outflow resistance and relieving the urinary retention and overflow incontinence. The urethral catheter was removed on the third postoperative day. There was slight dribbling of urine for 24 hours, but the patient has since voided a good stream with Credé compression and has remained completely continent of urine.

Initial bowel investigation was begun during this hospitalization and the patient was discharged on the eleventh postoperative day in good condition and voiding well.

*Second admission.* On the fifteenth postoperative day the patient was readmitted with urinary tract bleeding which was controlled by inlying catheter drainage.

*Third admission.* Fluoroscopy of the colon with barium enema showed normal peristalsis of the transverse colon, but a lack of peristalsis throughout the left colon, which was dilated. There was no "spastic area" to suggest an aganglionic mega-

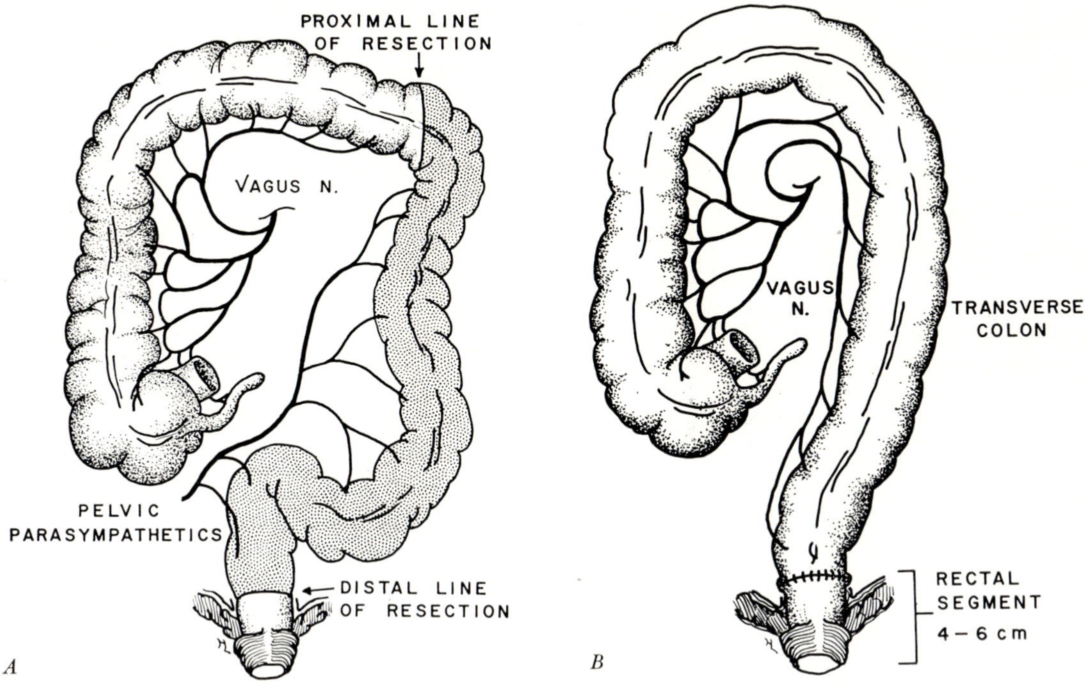


**Fig. 1.** *A,* Preresection and *B,* postresection diagrams of colon which show limits of resection for elimination of the sacrally innervated colon. Only a 4 to 6 cm. rectal segment is left.

colon or Hirschsprung's disease, but rather a general hypotonia of the left colon and rectum with no coordinated propulsion. Balloon studies demonstrated normal peristaltic activity in the transverse colon, but little spontaneous activity in the sigmoid or rectum. With distention of the balloon discomfort was experienced only in the transverse colon, with complete absence of a sensation of fullness in the sigmoid and descending colon. A diminished but definite contraction of the external anal sphincter was elicited. Levator ani contraction was strong. A trial of medical management, consisting of Prostigmine and pentolinium tartrate (Ansolysen) administration and enemas, was initiated. This and other systems of medical therapy, which were carried out at the patient's home over the next 3 to 4 months, were unsuccessful in eliminating the need for regular and prolonged enemas.

*Fourth admission.* The patient was readmitted for left colon resection. The bowel was prepared with saline irrigations, succinylsulfathiazole, and neomycin. On visualization the left colon appeared abnormal. It was tubular, thickened, and uniform in size. Peristaltic waves were absent on stimulation. Peristaltic activity of the transverse colon, by contrast, was normal. The left colon was resected beyond the last arcade from the superior mesenteric artery, and a pull-through rectocolic anastomosis was performed, preserving the last 4 to 6 cm. of the rectum (Figs. 1 and 2). The resection was performed proximal to the level of resection usual in a Swenson procedure in order to compensate for the deficient external anal sphincter. Microscopic examination of the 32 cm. resected segment of colon and rectum showed ganglion cells to be present throughout the specimen.

After a rectal irrigation on the fourth postoperative day, the patient defecated involuntarily for the next 6 days. Fecal continence, with only periodic soiling, began on the tenth postoperative day. Voluntary control, without soiling, was attained over the next 4 weeks.

Postoperative urinary retention was managed by inlying catheter drainage for 1 week. After the removal of the catheter, attempted evacuation of either the bowel or the bladder resulted in simultaneous evacuation of both. Differential control was attained gradually over a 6-week period.

Over the $2\frac{1}{2}$-year period during which the patient has been followed after colonic resection, the bowel function has remained very satisfactory. During the past year he has passed 1 to 2 stools per day without any complicating impactions. He attended school without difficulty, and soiled only once or twice during the entire year. For approximately 1 year he employed a small saline irrigation in the morning to facilitate a bowel

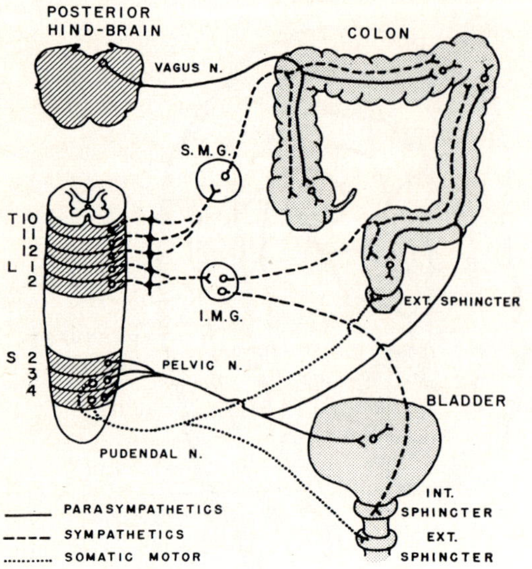


**Fig. 2.** Autonomic and somatic motor innervation of the lower bowel and bladder.

movement before school, but has found that even this is no longer necessary. A roentgenogram taken after a barium enema 1 year after resection showed no dilatation of the colon above the anastomosis. With the exception of an occasional episode of cystitis, readily controlled with chemotherapy, the patient has had no urinary difficulties. He carries no residual urine, and a recent intravenous pyelogram shows the kidneys to be normal.

The improvement in this patient's personal outlook and his release from a dependency upon his parents has been particularly impressive. Although he has not been given normal function of bowel or bladder, the improvement has been unquestionably beneficial.

## DISCUSSION

A combined evaluation and therapeutic approach to conditions of this type by the many disciplines concerned offers maximal possibilities for rehabilitation. As shown in Fig. 3, the left colon and the rectum, the bladder, and the sphincters of the urinary and the gastrointestinal tract depend upon intact innervation from the sacral region. Lesions in this area may result in widely varying dysfunction. The resulting failure of either the lower gastrointestinal tract or the urinary tract to function normally leads to a proximal decompensation. If function is to be restored toward normal, the defectively innervated portion must be repaired, bypassed, excised, or replaced with a normally innervated substitute.

Management of the urinary tract depends upon a thorough assessment of the structural condition of all of the component parts of the urinary system as well as the functional integrity of the entire system. If decompensation has occurred, a period of drainage which is sufficient to allow restoration of optimal renal function is necessary before definitive correction can be initiated.

Procedures to decrease outflow resistance as utilized in our patient are effective only if the detrusor force of the defectively innervated bladder, and increased intra-abdominal pressure, will produce voluntary bladder emptying. Measures to increase detrusor force should be combined with reduction of the outflow resistance. When a segment of bowel is used for detrusor force in a cystoplasty, it must be normally innervated, and use of the left colon may be contraindicated in cases in which sacral neurological deficit exists. Apparent incontinence should not necessarily contraindicate operation to reduce outflow resistance.

The bowel dysfunction secondary to sacral nerve defects can in most instances be managed well by thorough and persistent nonoperative measures (daily enemas or colonic irrigations, diet, and use of suppositories), all of which aim at the development of regular and complete emptying of the colon. In some instances, as in our case, these measures fail to evacuate the colon or become so involved and time consuming as to pose a serious handicap to the patient. In this case excision of the defectively innervated colon improved function considerably. While improvement after such a resection may be related to the increased liquidity of the stool passed, as Davis[7] suggests in advising resection for dolichocolon, it appears in this case that the ability of the bowel to respond to stimuli and to have more normal propulsive force is of equal or greater importance. To our knowledge the possibilities of such resection of the defectively innervated colon in this group of patients have not been previously realized. Even if colonic irrigations were necessary, the advantages of dealing with a normally responsive bowel as contrasted with an inert one are obvious. Improvement of continence with a marginally functioning sphincter muscle is greatly enhanced, as in our case, with the elimination of impaction and "fecal decompensation." As with the urinary tract, permanent diversion should be reserved for failures of a more direct approach.

## SUMMARY

In patients with bladder and bowel dysfunction resulting from lumbosacral neurological deficits, an aggressive and dynamic attempt should be made to secure the maximal improvement toward normal. Many of the patients with normal to superior intelligence are crippled primarily by the limitations imposed by bowel or bladder dysfunction. In such patients the lower urinary tract and the left colon, which derive their innervation from the diseased spinal area, lack normal sensation and motor innervation to varying degrees. Although conservative nonoperative management may suffice, when decompensation occurs or if nonoperative management imposes crippling limitations, surgical approaches are indicated. Resection of the defectively innervated colon can be performed, and a normally innervated segment of colon anastomosed to the rectum. Reduction of outflow resistance in the urinary bladder by transurethral resection or vesical neck revision allows for more adequate bladder emptying by detrusor force and Credé pressure. With these measures, utilization of available structures is attempted for a more anatomic means of improving function.

Such a program appeared necessary in the case of a 15-year-old boy with a lumbosacral myelomeningocele with a lifelong history of obstipation and urinary dribbling. The dramatic changes in bowel function and urinary function have changed this patient's outlook and adjustment to society.

## REFERENCES


1. Bors, E.: Bladder disturbances and the management of patients with injury to the spinal cord, J. Internat. Coll. Surgeons **21:** 513, 1954.
2. Bors, E.: Neurogenic bladder, Urol. Survey **7:** 177, 1957.
3. Bors, E.: Some new myologic and neurologic concepts of the human urinary bladder, J. Internat. Coll. Surgeons **30:** 324, 1958.
4. Bors, E., and Comarr, A. E.: Vesico-ureteral reflux in paraplegic patients, J. Urol. **68:** 691, 1952.
5. Bumpus, H. C., Jr., Nourse, M. H., and Thompson, G. J.: Urologic complications in injury of the spinal cord, J. A. M. A. **133:** 366, 1947.
6. Campbell, M.: Clinical pediatric urology, Philadelphia, 1951, W. B. Saunders Company.
7. Davis, D. A.: Personal communication, 1958.
8. Denny-Brown, D. E., and Robertson, E. G.: Investigation of nervous control of defecation, Brain **58:** 256, 1935.
9. Emmett, J. L., and Simon, H. B.: Transurethral resection in infants and children for congenital obstruction of the vesical neck and myelodysplasia, J. Urol. **76:** 595, 1956.
10. Gross, R. E., Holcomb, G. W., Jr., and Swan, H.: Treatment of neurogenic urinary and fecal incontinence, A. M. A. Arch. Surg. **66:** 143, 1953.
11. Guttman, L.: The regulation of rectal function in spinal paraplegia, Proc. Roy. Soc. Med. **52:** 86, 1959.
12. Hutch, J. A.: Vesico-ureteral reflux in paraplegic: cause and correction, J. Urol. **68:** 457, 1952.
13. Jacobson, C. E., Jr.: Neurogenic vesical dysfunction: an experimental study, J. Urol. **53:** 670, 1945.
14. Kennedy, B. C., and Hodges, C. V.: Urologic problems in spina bifida, Tr. West. Sect. Am.. Urol. A. **23:** 72, 1956.
15. MacCarthy, D., and Lindsay, M.: Discussion on the problems of spina bifida cystica, Proc. Roy. Soc. Med. **50:** 737, 1957.
16. Munro, D.: Care of civilians rendered paraplegic by an injury to the spinal cord or cauda equina, New England J. Med. **261:** 833, 1959.
17. Schlitt, R. J., McNally, J. J., and Hinton, J. W.: Response of the distal colon to external stimuli in relation to autonomic nerve section for ulcerative colitis, Surg. Gynec. & Obst. **92:** 223, 1951.
18. Scott, H. W., and Cantrell, J. R.: Colonmetrographic studies of the effects of section of the parasympathetic nerves of the colon, Bull. Johns Hopkins Hosp. **35:** 310, 1949.

19. Shoemaker, W. C., Long, D. M., Jr.: Functional studies on transplanted intestinal smooth muscle grafts used to reconstruct the denervated canine bladder, Surg. Gynec. & Obst. **108:** 523, 1959.
20. Shoemaker, W. C., Long, D. M., Jr.: Experimental studies on the reconstruction of the neurogenic bladder; a preliminary report, J. Urol. **76:** 150, 1956.
21. Stolov, W. C.: Rehabilitation of the bladder in injuries of the spinal cord, Arch. Phys. Med. **40:** 467, 1959.
22. Swenson, O.: Classification and treatment of children with severe chronic constipation, Am. J. Surg. **86:** 497, 1953.
23. Thompson, G. J., Jacobson, C. E., Jr.: Neurogenic vesical dysfunction due to spina bifida and myelodysplasia. Treatment by transurethral resection of the vesical neck, Am. J. Surg. **61:** 224, 1943.

*Conducted by* CLARENCE DENNIS, M.D., AND ALFRED HURWITZ, M.D.

# Duodenal closure after gastrectomy for duodenal ulcer

PHILIP COOPER, M.D.
NEW YORK, N. Y.
*From the Bronx Veterans Administration Hospital and Albert Einstein College of Medicine*

In February, 1956, we reported preliminary results of a method for duodenal closure after gastrectomy for the large ulcer of the posterior wall of the first part of the duodenum.[1] This was a modification of a method recommended by Nissen[3] for the duodenal closure when a pancreatic duct entered the base of the ulcer. When there was no pancreatic duct opening, Nissen used both the proximal and distal margins of the ulcer for the closure. With our method the distal margin is not utilized and it has not been found necessary, in many cases, to use the proximal margin of the ulcer. When the duodenal wall is absent, sutures are placed in the pancreatic capsule and scar tissue adjacent to the ulcer edge. This method requires a fairly pliable, well-vascularized anterior duodenal wall.

With this technique, as the dissection is carried posteriorly distal to the pylorus, the ulcer may be intentionally entered and the contiguous duodenal wall trimmed and excised as indicated. Thick, indurated, and edematous duodenal wall proximal and adjacent to the ulcer may be removed as long as the duodenal wall along the upper and lower borders of the duodenum is retained. Enough anterior wall should be left to permit easy closure without undue tension (Fig. 1, *A*).

The closure is accomplished with 2 or 3 layers of interrupted No. 4-0 silk. The sutures on the pancreatic side are placed superficially in a Lembert fashion. Adequate bulk of tissue for proper support can be obtained by taking multiple bites in a diagonal fashion as shown in Fig. 1, *B* and *C*. Near the ulcer crater, the seromuscular layer of the duodenal wall may be incorporated in the sutures. Frequently, near the upper and lower borders, the posterior sutures can be placed in the duodenal wall alone. By placement of the sutures superficially into the pancreas, the hazard of deep penetration into the head of the pancreas is avoided. On the anterior duodenal side, Lembert or Cushing mattress sutures have been used, depending on the width of the wall which has to be turned into the lumen. Frequently a more satisfactory closure is made when the sutures in the anterior wall are seromuscular rather than full-thickness. If a bleeding vessel is present in the base of the ulcer it is secured by figure-of-eight sutures of No. 2-0 silk.

It is obvious that this method of duodenal closure is not necessary when the ulcer is on the anterior surface of the pancreas and adequate length of duodenal wall is present beyond the ulcer which can be readily freed without dissection into pancreatic tissue. In that situation the ulcer can be exteriorized.

Since the original publication, use of the special technique for duodenal closure has been continued at the Providence Veterans Administration Hospital and has been introduced at the Bronx Veterans Administration

Received for publication Oct. 3, 1960.

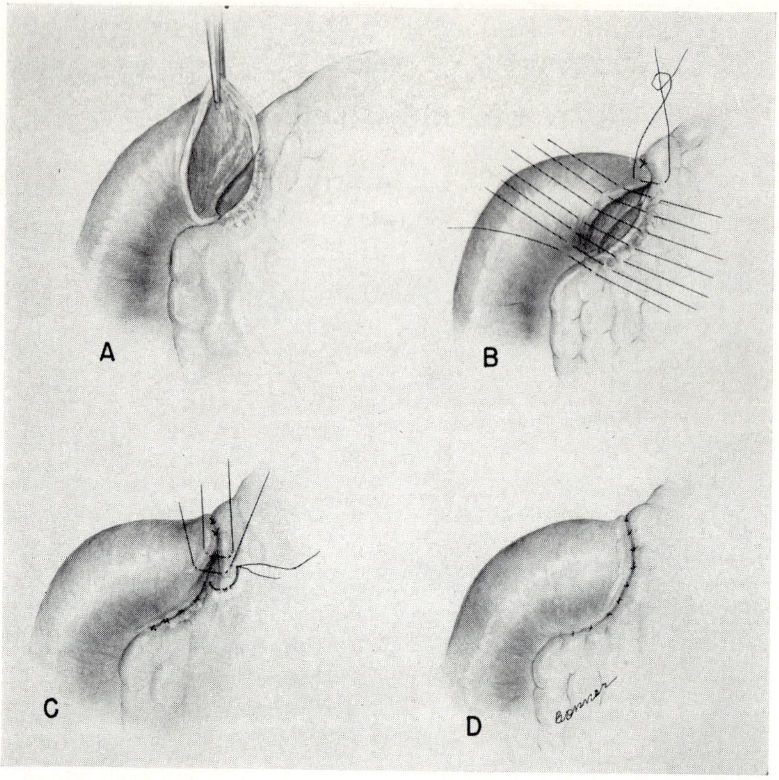


**Fig. 1.** *A*, Ulcer crater is entered and the posterior and anterior wall of the duodenum excised as indicated. *B*, First layer of sutures is inserted. *C*, Second layer of sutures is being inserted. Note diagonal placement of suture with multiple bites of tissue. *D*, Completed closure.

Hospital. At the former hospital[2] it has been found advisable to utilize this method in 109 of 699 duodenal closures. There was only 1 duodenal complication in the 109 cases. This occurred when the duodenum was extensively involved with ulcer and the anterior duodenal wall was thickened. The duodenal fistula closed spontaneously. At the Bronx Veterans Administration Hospital the method has been used on approximately 25 occasions with no duodenal stump complications.

This method allows a safe and rapid dissection of the duodenum and incision of or trauma to the pancreas is avoided. The dissection must be carried out meticulously and adequate blood supply of the duodenal wall retained. If one is concerned about the security of the closure a Penrose drain may be inserted near the duodenum. As one gains experience with this method the drain is rarely utilized.

## CONCLUSION

The technique and results of a method for duodenal closure after gastrectomy for the large posterior ulcer of the first part of the duodenum are reviewed. This method has been found to be safe and secure if performed according to the recommended technique.

### REFERENCES

1. Cooper, P., and Pecora, D.: The problem of duodenal closure after gastrectomy for duodenal ulcer, Am. J. Surg. **91:** 231, 1956.
2. Harrower, H.: Personal communication.
3. Nissen, R.: Duodenal and jejunal peptic ulcer —technique of resection, New York, 1945, Grune & Stratton, Inc.

# Historical views of the ideal surgeon

DAVID CHAS. SCHECHTER, M.D.
HENRY SWAN, M.D.
DENVER, COLO.
*From the Department of Surgery, University of Colorado Medical Center*

There have been but few instances in history when the medical community has been in as glaring a limelight as it is at present. Divested of much of the semiprotective veneer of mysticism with which it was formerly cloaked, it is now under close scrutiny from both within and without. Those who would see organized medicine as we know it flourish recognize that this is only possible by providing an ever-demanding laity with physicians of the first rank, both in training and comportment. In an age when the Decalogue of Mount Sinai and the Golden Rule are relegated to the Sunday school, the reaffirmation of basic principles becomes essential for survival. Educators have become more keenly aware that the student of medicine, who is exposed to a formal course of medical ethics only under unusual circumstances, and pledges his troth to mankind and his profession merely by a monotone recitation of the Oath of Hippocrates at graduation, may require more intensive inculcation. Hence, there has been a recent resurgent concern and promulgation by several regional and national medical associations of diverse codes of ethics and requirements of aptitude and behavior.

It is interesting to review the opinions of some of the early fathers of Surgery concerning the precepts governing the ideal practitioner of their craft. These concepts went much further than to require of him the oft-quoted "eye of an eagle, heart of a lion, and hand of a woman."

One can start with the Hindu surgeons, Sushruta and Charaka. They lived in the period of Indian history called the Vedic epoch after the four *Vedas,* or sacred writings, of the ancient East which constitute the glory of Sanskrit language and literature. Sushruta and Charaka wrote extensive treatises on surgery and medicine called *Samhitas.*

The *Sushruta-Samhita,* circa 600 B.C., states, "Surgery is the first and highest division of the healing art, least liable to fallacy, pure in itself, perpetual in its applicability, the worthy product of heaven, the sure source of fame on earth."

But it stresses the value of all-around training and knowledge of Medicine, and of study as well as factual practice when it says, "He who knows only one branch is like a bird with one wing . . . but he who combines reading with experience proceeds safely and surely like a chariot on two wheels."

There is a chapter in the *Sushruta-Samhita,* entitled "Instruction in Surgical Operations," which describes the training procedures without which the surgeon's education would be left wanting.

> The preceptor should see that his disciple attends the practice of surgery even if he has already thoroughly mastered the several branches of the science of medicine, or has perused it in its entirety. In all acts connected with surgical operations of incision . . . and injection of oil . . . the pupil should be fully instructed as regards the channels along or into which the operations or applications are to be made. A pupil, otherwise

well read, but uninitiated into the practice of surgery is not competent to take in hand the medical or surgical treatment of a disease. The art of making specific forms of incision should be taught by making cuts in the body of a gourd, watermelon, cucumber. . . . The art of making cuts either in the upward or downward direction should be similarly taught. The art of making incisions should be practically demonstrated by making openings in the body of a full water bag, or in the bladder of a dead animal, or in the side of a leather pouch full of slime or water. The art of scraping should be instructed on a piece of skin on which the hair has been allowed to remain. The art of venesection should be taught on the vein of a dead animal or with the help of a lotus stem. The art of probing and stuffing should be taught on worm-eaten wood, or on the reed of a bamboo, or on the mouth of a dried gourd. The art of extracting should be taught by withdrawing seeds from the kernel of a Jack fruit, as well as by extracting teeth from the jaws of a dead animal. The act of secreting or evacuating should be taught on the surface of a plank covered over with a coat of beeswax, and suturing on pieces of cloth, skin or hide. Similarly, the art of bandaging or ligaturing should be practically learned by tying bandages around the specific limbs and members of a full-sized doll made of stuffed linen. The art of tying up a severed ear lobe should be practically demonstrated on a soft muscle or on flesh, or with the stem of a lotus lilly. The art of cauterizing or applying caustics should be demonstrated on a piece of soft flesh; and, lastly, the art of inserting syringes and injecting enemas into the region of the bladder, or into an ulcerated channel, should be taught by asking the pupil to insert a tube into a lateral fissure of a pitcher, full of water, or into the mouth of a gourd.

An intelligent physician who has tried his prentice hand in surgery, or has learnt the art with the help of things as stated above, or has been instructed in the art of cauterization or blistering by experimenting on things which are most akin, or similar to the parts of members of the human body they are usually applied to, will never lose his presence of mind in his professional practice.

The *Sushruta-Samhita* prescribes, moreover, that after satisfactory initiation of the disciple, he is to be addressed by his preceptor:

Thou shalt renounce lust, anger, greed, ignorance, vanity, egotistic feelings, envy, harshness, parsimony, falsehood, idleness, nay all acts that soil the good name of a man. In proper season thou shalt pare thy nails and clip thy hair and put on the sacred cloth, dyed brownish-yellow, live the life of a truthful self-controlled anchorite, and be obedient and respectful toward thy preceptor. In sleep, in rest, or while moving about—while at meals or in study, and in all acts thou shalt be guided by my directions. . . . Thou shalt help thy professional skill and knowledge, the Brahmanas, thy elders, preceptors and friends, the indigent, the honest, the anchorites, the helpless and those who shall come to thee from a distance, or those who shall live close by, as well as thy relations and kinsmen, to the best of thy knowledge and ability, and thou shalt give them medicine without charging for it any remuneration whatever, and God will bless thee for that. Thou shalt not treat medicinally a professional hunter, a fowler, a habitual sinner, or him who has been degraded in life; and even by so doing thou shalt acquire friends, fame, piety, wealth and all wished-for objects in life, and thy knowledge shall gain publicity.

The training program suggested by Charaka is similar to that of Sushruta. In addition, Charaka urges the young surgeon, "Not for self, not for the fulfillment of any earthly desire or gain, but solely for the good of suffering humanity should you treat your patients, and so excel all."

Another one of Charaka's precepts, "Thou should'st never give out the practices of the patient's house," is evidently an injunction to keep professional secrets.

It is possible that, unlike the Oath of Maimonedes, which is a highly individual statement of creed, the so-called Hippocratic Oath may be more correctly ascribed to have been a pledge taken by members of the School at Cos and the Grecian Temples of Health in the fourth century B.C. It remains one of the most cherished documents in medical heritage. More pertinent from the surgeon's standpoint, however, are the prosaic but exacting passages in the writings of Hippocrates which treat of the requirements of a surgeon. The section "On the Surgery" is illustrative.

It is the business of the physician to know, in the first place, things similar and things dissimilar; those connected with things most important, most easily known, and in anywise known; which are to be seen, touched, and heard; which are to be perceived in the sight, and the touch, and the hearing, and the nose, and the tongue, and the understanding; which are to be known by all the means we know other things.

The things relating to surgery, are—the patient; the operator; the assistants; the instruments; the light, where and how; how many things, and how; where the body, and the instruments; the time; the manner; the place.

The operator is either sitting or standing, conveniently for himself, for the person operated upon, for the light. There are two kinds of light, the common and the artificial; the common is not at our disposal, the artificial is at our disposal . . . we must turn the part to be operated upon to that which is most brilliant of present and convenient lights . . . thus, the part that is operated upon should be opposite the light, and the operator opposite the part operated upon, except in so far as he does not stand in his own light; for in this case the operator will indeed see, but the thing operated upon will not be seen. With regard to himself: when sitting, his feet should be raised to a direct line with his knees, and nearly in contact with one another; the knees a little higher than the groins, and at some distance from one another, for the elbows to rest upon them. The robe, in a neat and orderly manner, is to be thrown over the elbows and shoulders equally and proportionally. . . . When standing, he must make his inspection, resting firmly and equally on both feet; but he must operate while supporting himself upon either leg, and not the one on the same side with the hand which he makes use of; the knee being raised to the height of the groins as while sitting; and the other measures in like manner. The person operated upon should accommodate the operator with regard to the other parts of his body, either standing, sitting, or lying; so as that he may continue to preserve his figure, avoid sinking down, shrinking from, turning away; and may maintain the figure and position of the part operated upon, during the act of presentation, during the operation, and in the subsequent position.

The nails should be neither longer nor shorter than the points of the fingers; and the surgeon should practice with the extremities of the fingers, the index-finger being usually turned to the thumb; when using the entire hand, it should be prone; when both hands, they should be opposed to one another. It greatly promotes a dextrous use of the fingers when the space between them is large, and when the thumb is opposed to the index. But it is clearly a disease when the thumb is impaired from birth, or when, from a habit contracted during the time of nursing, it is impeded in its motions by the fingers. One should practice all sorts of work with either of them, and with both together (for they are both alike), endeavoring to do them well, elegantly, quickly, without trouble, neatly, and promptly.

The instruments, and when and how they should be prepared, will be treated of afterwards; so that they may not impede the work, and that there may be no difficulty in taking hold of them, with the part of the body which operates. But if another gives them, he must be ready a little beforehand, and do as you direct.

Those about the patient must present the part to be operated upon as may seem proper, and they must hold the rest of body steady, in silence, and listening to the commands of the operator.

One could discuss at great length the many features mentioned in this writing by Hippocrates, and indeed they have been the subject of innumerable commentaries from the time of Galen on. Suffice it to say only that one marvels at how various clauses, from specifications as to the length of the fingernails to posture and decorum while operating, are defined graphically.

Aurelius Cornelius Celsus (25 B.C. to A.D. 50), the Roman physician whose epochal *De Medecina* is one of the most important reference sources of the Greek and Alexandrian Schools, wrote:

Now a surgeon ought to be young, or at all events, not much advanced in years; possessed of a hand that is firm, steady, uniformly devoid of tremor; he should be able to use both hands with equal dexterity; his sight should be penetrating and clear; with a mind undaunted, he should retain so much compassion as may lead him to wish for his patient's recovery, without being so far moved by his shrieks as to induce him to make unnecessary haste, or to cut less than is absolutely expedient; but he ought to complete his operation, in all respects, as though the cries of the sufferer gave rise to no emotion. . . . For my own part, I conceive that the same person may be capable of practicing all the three branches (regimen, drugs, and surgery); but since a division has been effected, I laud that man whose range of information is the most extensive.

Abu Yaqub Ishaq Sulaynam al Israïli, better known as Isaac Judaeus, a surgeon of the tenth century, served under several Egyptian rulers. In his book, *The Guide of Physicians,* many aphorisms are found:

The majority of diseases are cured by nature.

It is in keeping with the character of the physician that he should, in his mode of life, be content with well prepared food in moderation and be no glutton. Also, it is a shame that he should suffer from a long-drawn-out disease, else the vulgar will say: "If he cannot cure himself, how can he cure others?"

Let not thy mouth condemn, if an accusation be made against a physician, for to every man comes his hour. Let thy deeds be thy praise, rather than find honor in another man's shame.

If the patient does not follow thy directions, or his servants and household do not carry out thy orders with dispatch or treat thee with respect, relinquish the treatment.

Demand thy fee of the patient when his illness is increasing or at its height; when he is healed he forgets what thou hast done for him. The more thou demandest for thy treatment, the more highly thou esteemest thy cure, the higher will thou stand in the eyes of the people. The art will be held of no account only by those whom thou treatest gratuitously.

Visit not the patient too often, nor remain too long with him, unless the treatment demand it, for it is only the fresh encounter which gives pleasure.

Note the recommendation that the physician abstain from derogatory comments against a confrere, an exhortation reiterated frequently in later writings.

Abu'l Qasim Zahrawi, or Albucasis (1013 to 1106), Arabian physician of Cordova in Moorish Spain, authored an encyclopedia on the healing art called *Altasrif,* consisting of some 30 volumes, 3 of which are on surgery. In one of these he remarks:

Surgery is no longer in honor in our country. In its actual decadence, it has disappeared, almost without leaving traces. There remain some vestiges in the writings of the Ancients, but they have corrupted the transcriptions; error and confusion have overrun them, in a manner to render them unintelligible and useless. . . . You know, my children, that surgical operations are divided into two classes: those that benefit the patient, and those that more often kill. . . . It is necessary to be prudent and to abstain from dangerous operations, not to give the ignorant cause for malevolent comment. Conduct yourselves with reserve and caution: have gentleness and perseverance for the patients; follow the good road which leads to favorable and happy outcomes. Abstain from undertaking dangerous and difficult treatments. Avoid that which might injure your honor or your welfare; it is the better part for your reputation and more consistent with your interests in this world and the other.

The archives of the School of Salerno are replete with common-sense advice (such as the *Regimen*), to medical practitioners. A tract of general guidance on manners in Medicine was written around 1100 A.D. by one Archimathaeus, a surgeon about whose life history little is known. A passage from this pamphlet concerns protocol to be observed at the initial visit to a patient:

When you are called to a patient, may the name of God be your help, and may the angel who walked with Tobias be the companion of your mind and body. At your entrance inquire of him who greets you from what disease the sick man suffers and how his illness progresses; this is advisable in order that you come to him not entirely uninformed as to the illness. . . . Again when you reach the house and before you see him, ask if he has seen his confessor, and if he has not done this, arrange for him to do so, or have him promise to do so, for if the sick man hears talk on this subject after he has been examined and the signs of his illness studied, he will begin to despair of it. Entering the sick-room you should have neither proud nor greedy countenance; you should repeat the greeting of those who rise as you enter, and with a gesture seat yourself when they sit down. Next, you may resume the conversation with a few remarks in which you praise the neighborhood, commend the arrangements of the house, if it seems appropriate, or compliment the liberality of the family.

Then turning to the patient you may ask how it goes with him, and have him put out his arm. At first there may be differences, between your own state and that of the patient, either because he is excited at your arrival, or because he is worried about the size of your fee, so that you find the pulse rather confusing; therefore you should consider the pulse only after the patient has become steadier. Take care that he does not lie upon his side nor has his finger over-extended or flexed against his palm. Support his arm with your left hand and observe the pulse for at least 100 beats in order to feel all its variations, and thus you will be able to satisfy the expectant bystanders with words which they are glad to hear.

Next you have the urine brought to you, that the sick man may see you study his illnesses not only from the pulse but from the urine. When examining the urine you should observe its color, substance, quantity, and content; after which you may promise the patient that with the help of God you will cure him. As you go away, however, you should say to his servants that he is in a very bad way, because if he recovers you will receive great credit and praise, and if he dies, they will remember that you despaired of his health from the beginning. Meanwhile, I urge you not to turn a lingering eye upon his wife, his daughter, or his maid-servant, for this sort of thing blinds the eye of the doctor, averts the favor of God, and makes the doctor abhorrent to the patient and less confident in himself. Be therefore careful in speech, respectable in conduct, attentively seeking Divine aid. If the people of the house invite you to a meal, as often happens, do not seem too much gratified, and do not seek the first place at the table, although it is the custom to give this to the priest or the doctor. Do not criticize the food or drink, and when in the country do not show distaste for country food, for example millet bread, even though you can scarcely control your stomach.

While you eat you may inquire as to the conditions of the patient from anyone who is present, for in this way the sick man will confide in you all the more, since he sees that you do not forget him while seeking your own comfort. When you rise from the table you may mention that you have been well looked after; this too will give pleasure to the patient.

William of Saliceto (1210 to 1277), professor of Surgery at Bologna and later at Verona, wrote similar counsel, with the added admonition, "A wise surgeon will refrain from stealing while he is actually in attendance upon a patient."

Lanfranchi of Milan (1250 to 1315), Saliceto's ablest pupil, was a Surgeon of the Long Robe, and associated with the college of St. Come. Lanfranchi deplored the separation of Medicine from Surgery, a dichotomy which had existed since Avicenna's time.

Good God, why this abandoning of operations by physicians to lay persons, disdaining surgery because they do not know how to operate, an abuse which has reached such a point that the vulgar begin to think the same man cannot know both surgery and medicine? I say, however, that no man can be a good physician who has no knowledge of operative surgery, a knowledge of both branches is essential.

In this stand he was supported by another surgeon, John of Mirfield, who wrote:

Long ago, unless I mistake, physicians used to practice surgery, but nowadays there is a great distinction between surgery and medicine, and this, I fear arises from pride, because physicians disdain to work with their hands, though, indeed, I myself have a suspicion that it is because they do not know how to perform particular operations; and this unfortunate usage has led the public to believe that a man cannot know both subjects, but the well informed are aware that he cannot be a good physician who neglects every part of surgery, and, on the other hand, a surgeon is good for nothing who is without knowledge of medicine.

Lanfranchi's *Cyrurgia Magna* (1296) has the following passage:

It is necessary that a surgeon should have a temperate and moderate disposition, that he should have well-formed fingers, a strong body, not inclined to tremble and with all his members trained to the capable fulfillment of the wishes of his mind. He should be of deep intelligence and of a simple, humble, brave but not audacious disposition. He should be well-grounded in natural science, and should know not only medicine, but every part of philosophy, should know logic well, so as to be able to understand what is written, to talk properly, and to support what he has to say by good reasons.

Henri de Mondeville (1260 to 1320) studied at Montpellier. Graduates from its school of medicine included such celebrities as Arnold of Villanova, John of Arderne, and Guy de Chauliac. De Mondeville achieved eminence in surgery. He was an implacable enemy of charlatanism and empiricism. The following excerpts are from his writings:

A surgeon ought to be fairly bold. He should not quarrel before the laity and although he should operate wisely and prudently he should not undertake any dangerous operation unless he is sure that it is the only way to avoid a greater danger. His limbs, and especially his hands, should be well-shaped with long, delicate and supple fingers which must not be tremulous. He ought to promise a cure to every patient but should tell the parents or friends if there is any danger. He should refuse as far as possible all difficult cases and never interfere with the desperate ones. He may give advice to the poor for the love of God only, but the rich should be made to pay well. He should neither praise himself nor blame others and he should not hate any of his colleagues. He ought to sympathize with his patients in their distress and fall in with their lawful requests so far as they do not interfere with the treatment. Patients, on the other hand, should obey their surgeon implicitly in everything appertaining to their cure. The surgeon's assistants must be loyal to their master and friendly to his patients. They ought not to tell the patient what the surgeon says unless the news is pleasant and they should always appear cheerful. They should not be constantly grumbling, because this inspires fear and doubt in the patient.

Many more surgeons know how to cause suppuration than how to heal a wound. Keep your needles sharp and clean or they will infect the wound. Surgery is an integral part of medicine for it is in reality a method of treatment.

Take care to regulate the whole regimen of the patient's life for joy and happiness by promising that he will soon be well, by allowing his relatives and special friends to cheer him and by having someone to tell him jokes, and let him be solaced also by music on the viol or psaltery.

You, then surgeons, if you have operated conscientiously on the rich for a suitable fee, and on the poor for charity, you need not fear fire, rain or wind, you have no need to go into religion, to make pilgrimages, or other acts of the sort, because by your science you have been able to save your souls, live without poverty and die in your homes, live in peace . . . and exult because reward is great in the Heavens. . . .

For good measure, de Mondeville interjected a few items of "horse-sense" reminiscent of the essays of Chalmers Da Costa:

Never dine with a patient who is in your debt, but get your dinner at an inn. Otherwise, he will deduct the cost of his hospitality from your fee.

I have never found anyone so rich, or even so honest . . . who was ready to pay what he had promised unless obligated and convicted.

He also reprimanded surgeons who lacked originality and did not make use of their own initiative and intellect, preferring only to quote their preceptors. He exclaimed contemptuously, "God did not exhaust all His creative powers in making Galen!"

The teachings of Guy de Chauliac (1300 to 1368), Prince of French Surgery during the mediaeval epoch and physician to several Popes, were of greatest authority for a considerable period. His chief work was the *Chirurgia,* written in 1363, in which he enumerates attributes desirable in a surgeon.

The prerequisites of a Surgeon are four in number: first, that he be lettered, second, expert, third, ingenious, fourth, well schooled in Ethics. It is thus required from the start that the Surgeon be lettered, not only in the principles of Surgery, but also of Medicine, both in theory as well as practice. He should be bold in sure things, fearful in hazardous ones, fleeing from bad cures or practices. He should be gracious to patients, benevolent towards his colleagues, sage in his predictions. He should be chaste, sober, compassionate and merciful: neither coveter nor extortionist of money: but receiving moderate stipend, according to his work, the ability of the patient, the quality of the issue or event, and his dignity.

The most prominent British surgeon in Chaucer's time was John of Arderne, or Arden (1307 to 1380), who referred to himself as "chirurgicus inter medicos," a surgeon among physicians. He was the first to revive the healing art of Surgery in England. One of his most famous articles, entitled *Of ye manere of ye leche,* expounds on the methods whereby a surgical practice may be conducted properly. Its influence was far-reaching in that critical period of surgical history. The principles laid down by John of Arderne for the guidance of the leech (physician) in regard to his patients as well as in his dealings with his colleagues cannot be held in too high esteem. It would surely be well if we could at all times act in the same gentle manner towards our brethren in the profession, and answer courteously when asked about them, "I learned nought nor have I heard of him but good and honest."

First, it behooves him that will profit in his craft, that he set God afore evermore in all his works, and evermore call meekly with heart and mouth His help. He should sometime visit of his own willingness poor men in his midst, that they by their prayers may get him grace of the Holy Ghost. He should not be found rash or boastful in his speech or his deeds. He should abstain from much speech, especially among great men. He should answer warily to things asked, that he be not mistaken in his words. For, if his works be oft time known, if he discord from his words and his promises, he shall be unworthy and blemish his own good fame: whereupon says a verse, "Work overcome thy word, for boasting lessens good report." A leech should not laugh or play too much. And also, as much as he may without harm, he should flee the fellowship of knaves and of disreputable persons. He should evermore be occupied in things that pertain to his craft. He should either read, or study, or write, or pray, for a leech worships the exercise of books; for which he shall both be esteemed and be more wise. Above all this, it will profit him to be found evermore sober, for drunkenness destroys all virtue and brings it to nought; as says a wise man,

"Drunkenness breaks what wisdom touches." Be he content in strange places of meats and drinks that he finds, using measure in all things; for the wise man says, "As it profits to put measure in all things that are, so without measure perish all things that are." Scorn he no man, for of that it is said, "He that scorns other men shall not go away unscorned." If there be made speech to him of any leech, neither set he at him, nor praise him too much or commend him, but thus may he courteously answer, "I have not any knowledge of him; but I learned nought nor have I heard of him but good and honest;" and of this shall honor and thankings of each party increase and multiply to him; after this, honor is in the honorant and not in the honored. Consider he not over-openly the lady or the daughters or other fair women in great men's houses, nor proffer to kiss, or touch, neither privately nor openly, their breasts or their hands or their hair, that he run not into the indignation of the lord nor of none of his household. Inasmuch as he may, grieve he no servants, but get he their love and their good will. He should abstain from harlotry in words as well as in deeds in every place, for if he becomes used to harlotry in private places, sometime in open place, there may fall to him habit of evil usage.

When sick men, or any of their relatives, come to the leech to ask help or counsel of him, he should not be overfriendly or overfamiliar, but act in bearing according to the requirements of the persons, to some reverently, to some commonly, for according to wise men," over-familiarity breeds despising." Also, it is of advantage that he have proper excuses, that he may not incline to their asking, without slighting or causing indignation of some great man or friend. Feign he hurt or illness, or some other convenient cause by which he may likely be excused. Therefore if he will favor to any man's asking, make he covenant for his travail and take it before hand. But the leech should take care that he give no certain answer in any case before seeing first the sickness and its nature; and when he has seen and assayed it, although it may seem to him that the sick person may be healed, nevertheless he shall make prognostication to the patient the perils to come if the cure be deferred. . . .

And if the patients or their friends or servants ask by how much time he hopes to heal it, always let the leech name the double of what he estimates. That is, if the leech hopes to heal the patient by twenty weeks, which is the common course of curing, add he so many more; for it is better that the term be lengthened than the cure; for prolongation of the cure gives cause of despairing to the patients, when trust in the leech is most hope of health. And if the patient consider or wonder or ask, why that he put him so long a time of curing, since he healed him by half? Answer he, it was because the patient was strong-hearted and suffered well sharp things, and that he was of good complexion, and had able flesh to heal, and feign he other causes pleasable to the patient, for patients of such words are proud and delighted.

Also, it disposes a leech that in clothes and other apparel he be honest, not likening himself in apparel or bearing to minstrels, but in clothing and bearing follow the manner of clerks; for it seems any discreet man clad with clerks' clothing is worthy to occupy gentlemen's boards. The leech should also have clean hands, and well-shaped nails cleansed from all blackness and filth. He should be courteous at lord's boards, and not displease in words or deeds the guests sitting by. He should hear many things but speak little, for as a wise man said, "It benefits more to use the ears than the tongue." And in another place, "If thou had been still, thou would have been thought a philosopher." And when he shall speak, be the words short, and as much as he may, fair and reasonable and without swearing. Beware that there never be found double words in his mouth; for if he be found true in his words, few or none shall doubt in his deeds.

The book of Jerome of Brunswick (1450 to 1533) has the distinction of being the first illustrated treatise on surgery of its kind printed in the English language. Jerome was an unrelenting foe of the barber-surgeons. In the prologue, Jerome's summing up of the value of the consultation bears repeating:

First, you learn by chance things that you seldom or never have seen before. Secondarily, if ought in your hands happen to misfortune, that you may quickly amend it. Thirdly, that the wounded person have less grudge or mistrust in you. Fourthly, when the cure has good speed, then you be partaker of all the honour thereof; and if misfortune fall between your hands, then every man is bound to bear the charge of your hinder and losses which would be too much for you alone. Fifthly, for this wise deed you be praised of all them that be discrete or learned men, who will speak of you saying you desire to learn, and will not that any man should be by you negligently spilt or perished. And thus may you come to your purpose with honesty and pleasure, which else might turn to your great shame and displeasure.

Heinrich von Pfolspeundt was a notable Bavarian army surgeon of the mid-fifteenth century. His *Buch der Bundth-Ertznei* is the oldest surgical book in the German language. Pfolspeundt must have had a flair for the sacerdotal in surgery:

Firstly, I advise anyone who wishes to work in this art and to heal, that he should not go to a wounded or sick person in the early morning or treat him before he has heard Mass, so far as is possible, unless there is great need, but he shall pray to the Good Lord to bless the wounds, to say a Pater Noster and an Ave Maria and confess his faith, so that strength and wisdome be given him to heal the people. . . .

And he should guard himself against drunkenness when he is to treat patients, for because of it they may easily be neglected, and the doctor would be guilty of that and be punished by God. And especially, he should guard himself, if he has eaten onions or beans, or slept the previous night with an unclean woman . . . against breathing into anyone's wound. Also, he should bind with clean white cloths, for if they are not clean, harm results. He should also wash his hands before he treats anyone. Also he should love healing for the sake of God, if he is able; also if the doctor knows himself to be unclean, he should not look actively into the wounds . . . else mischief and harm arises. . . . And keep people protected, or you will have to do penance before God, if you are to blame."

Felix Wirtz (1510? to 1580), an itinerant Swiss surgeon, was an admirer of Paracelsus and, like him, was an "angry young man" of Surgery. Although he was not exactly a burner of books, as Paracelsus, he had the courage to explode publicly to students, "What do you suppose I care whether Galen's or Avicenna's or Guy de Chauliac's opinion does or does not agree with mine?"

Moreover, unlike Paracelsus, whose writings were imbued with necromancy and metaphysics, Wirtz was almost brutally practical. He was scornful on matters of surgical theory, remarking tartly, "Surgery depends more on dexterity than on twaddle."

Ambroise Paré (1510 to 1590), paragon of surgeons in the Renaissance, is probably second only to John Hunter for his role in raising surgery to loftier terrain than it had been previously. He carved for himself a niche in immortality with the modest words, "Je l'ay pansé, Dieu le guarit." The introduction of his tome, *A la Chirurgie,* contains various topics defining the integral role of surgery in medicine. He also stated: "As for me, I am of the same opinion as Celsus, who urges the Surgeon to be assured of his tasks, and not be timid and afraid; so that when he operates with his hands, he should heed neither the clamor of the patient nor the assistants, slowed down no more than avoidable, and not hastening unnecessarily, but accomplishing his purpose without regard for those who in their ignorance despise the Surgeon. . . ."

Juan Rodrigo de Castel-Branco, or Amatus Lusitanus (1536 to 1614), was a Portuguese Jewish surgeon who fled the Inquisition from his native country, only to be summoned as consultant during the illness of Pope Julius III. The Oath of Amatus, published in his *Centuriae,* is similar to the Maimonedic Oath in its personal theme. It is one of the noblest compositions in the annals of surgical literature, and should be in print more frequently than it has been.

I swear by the Eternal God and by His ten most holy commandments, which were given on Mount Sinai through Moses as lawgiver after the people had been freed from their bondage in Egypt, that I have never, at any time, done anything in these my treatments save what inviolate faith handed down to posterity; that I have never feigned anything, added anything or changed anything for the sake of gain; that I have always striven after this one thing, namely, that benefit might spread forth to mankind; that I have praised no one, and censured no one merely to indulge in private passions, unless zeal for truth demanded this. If I lie, may I incur the eternal wrath of God and his angel Raphael, and may I not succeed according to my intent in any of my medical work.

Concerning the remuneration, furthermore, which is commonly given to physicians, I have not been anxious for this, but I have treated many, not only zealously, but even without pay; and have unselfishly and unswervingly refused several rewards offered by many people; and have rather sought that the sick might, by my care and diligence, recover their lost health than that I might become richer by their liberality. All men have been considered equal by me of whatever religion they were, whether Hebrews, Christians, or the followers of the Moslem faith.

As concerns loftiness of station, that has never been a matter of concern to me, and I have accorded the same care to the poor as to those born in exalted rank. I have never brought about sickness; in diagnosis I have always said what I thought to be true. I have unduly favored no vendors of drugs, except perhaps those whom I knew to surpass the others by reason of their skill in their art or because of their natural qualities of mind. In prescribing drugs I have exercised moderation in proportion as the powers of the sick man allowed. I have revealed to no one a secret entrusted to me; I have given no one a fatal draught. No woman has ever brought about an abortion by my aid; nothing base has been committed by me in my house where I was practicing; in short, nothing has been done by me which might be considered unbecoming an excellent and famous physician.

I have always held up to myself Hippocrates and Galen, the fathers of the medical art, as examples worthy of being followed by me, and the records of many other excellent men in the medical art have not been scorned by me. In my method of studying, I have been so eager that no task, however difficult, could lead me away from the reading of good authors, neither the loss of private fortune, nor frequent journeys, nor yet exile, which, as befits a philosopher, I have thus far borne with calm and invincible courage. And the many students which I have thus far had I have always considered my sons, have taught them very frankly, and have urged them to strive to conduct themselves like good men.

I have published my books on medical matters with no desire for profit, but I have had regard for this one thing, namely, that I might, in some measure, provide for the health of mankind. Whether I have succeeded in this, I leave to the judgment of others, At all events, I have held this always before me, and have given it chief place in my prayers.

William Bulleine, educated at Cambridge, was a London surgeon during the reign of King Henry VIII. He died in 1576, 14 years after publishing his interesting monograph, *A little dialogue between two men, the one called Sorenes and the other Chirurgi: concernyng Apostumacions and Woundes their causes and also their cures*. His notion of a worthy surgeon was expressed as follows:

Eight things or properties of a good Chirurgeon. He must begin first in youth with good learning, and exercise in this noble art; he must also be cleanly, nimble-handed, sharp-sighted, pregnant-witted, bold-spirted, cleanly-appareled, pitiful-hearted, but not womanly-affectionated to weep or tremble when he sees broken bones or bloody wounds, neither must he give place to cry of his sore Patient, for soft Chirurgeons make foul sores. On the other hand, he may not play the part of a Butcher to cut, rend, or tear the body of mankind. For although it be frail, sore, and weak, yet it is the pleasure of God to call it his Temple, his Instrument, and dwelling-place, and the Philosopher does call it Orbiculus, that is, a little world. That is, Nature is the worker, the Physician is but his minister. Therefore the Chirurgical Physician is Nature's Servant.

Thomas Gale (1507 to 1587), was a contemporary of William Bulleine and Ambroise Paré. He saw much service as a military surgeon, greatly lamented the state of the profession in his day, and was a prime moving spirit in demanding legislation to curb effectively the practicing of surgery by unitiated and unschooled individuals. In 1563 he published the treatise, *An institution of a Chirurgian conteyning the sure Groundes and Principles of Chirurgiry moste necessary and mete for all those that will attayne the arte perfectly*. This was a well-digested work intended to ground the young student in ethics, and to expose that empirical kind of practice which busied itself with the mere collection of forms of therapy, without adequate knowledge of their proper application. The situation prevailing in this period of the reign of the Tudors is deplored by Gale:

The greater number of Chirurgeons (I mean those that are there unto lawfully called), are so rude and unskilful in their art because they have no method, no exact way, or yet order in learning the grounds and principles of Chirurgery. . . . So that they are confused in their studies and make rather a rude chaos than a perfect art of Chirurgery. For now it is come to this point, that if they can get this receipt (prescription) and that receipt, as they term it, they think they need no further study. So that the more receipts he has, the greater a Chirurgeon he thinks himself to be; such ignorance now reigns that receipts bear the bell; theory of Chirurgery is quite forsaken or not regarded. . . .

Gale also gives an account of the qualifications and tenets which should be inherent in the model surgeon. The Guido he alludes to was Guido Guidi, or Vidius, a coeval educator who was Italy's leading surgeon, and after whom the Vidian canal and nerve are named.

Guido requires four things in him that is or would be a Chirurgeon. First, that he should be lettered, secondly, that he should be expert, thirdly, that he be ingenious, and last, that he be virtuous and well-mannered. . . . And touching these four points, note first when Guido says he must be lettered, he does mean that he should be learned, and that chiefly in such doctrine as is in his art requisite. That is at the least, that he can write, read, and understand the mind of Latin authours. If he had knowledge in geometry for making his incision, for curing fractures and luxations, and also in curing malignant ulcers; knowing what figure would most speedily unite, and join the lips of the ulcer; it would be very commendable. Natural Philosophy is a goodly adornment to the Chirurgeon, for it shows him what results when diverse and sundry simples are mixed together. But I will go to the second point, he must be expert, that is he must be garnished with much and long experience, which is excogitated by firm and certain reasons and by them also confirmed; otherwise he is to be accompted rude, and an empiric, if he has no reason annexed and joined to his experience.

Thirdly, says Guido, he must be ingenious, unto which there are five things principally required. First, is the ready and good conceiving; then, a firm and sure memory; next, a sound and right judgement; after, an easy calling things to mind which we have heard or seen; and last, a lively and sharp readiness in finding and inventing remedies.

The manners which Guido would have in a Chirurgeon are reckoned of Hippocrates and Celsus, which briefly I will number; he must be bold and without fear in such cures as are without peril, and which necessity requires. Also in cures that be doubtful, not too risky and hasty, to be gentle and courteous toward the sick patient, to be friendly and loving toward those of his profession. Also wise and circumspect in prognostications. Last of all, he must be chaste and temperate of body, merciful toward the poor, and not too greedy of money. And this is sufficient touching the description of he that must be admitted in Chirurgery.

In relation to the patient, Gale observes:

The Chirurgeon must also in these his operations observe six things principally. First, that he does it safely, and without hurt and damage to the patient. Secondly, that he does not detract time or let sleep good occasions offered in working, but with such speed as art shall suffer, let him finish his cure. Thirdly, that he would gently, courteously, and with as little pain to the patient as conveniently he may, and not roughly, butcherly, rudely. . . . Fourthly, that he be as free from craftiness and deceit in all his workings as the East is from the West. Fifthly, that he take no cure in hand for lucre or gains-sake only, but rather for an honest and competent reward with a godly affection to do his diligence. Last of all, that he make no warranty of such sicknesses as are incurable, as to cure a cancer not ulcerated, or elephantiasis confirmed; but circumspectly to consider what the effect is, and promise no more than art can perform. . . .

This compilation, then, presents exemplary ideas of great men during the infancy of surgery. They constitute part of our legacy and are worthy of recapitulation. Many of the tenets and wisdom expressed therein are as relevant in our day as when they were penned; for, in the words of a Chinese proverb, "The ancients saw not the modern moon, but the modern moon shone on the ancients."

## ERRATUM

In the paper "Duplication of the Stomach," by George Abrami, M.B., Ch.B., and Wallace M. Dennison, M.D., in the June, 1961, issue of SURGERY, Figs. 5 and 6 were reversed. The legend appearing under Fig. 5 should be with Fig. 6 and vice versa.

Volume 50 Number 3

SURGERY

SEPTEMBER, 1961

Clinical surgery

# Hemorrhagic tendency after massive transfusion of preserved blood

TERUTAKE SUNADA, M.D.
HIROSHI SUGIHARA, M.D.
KUNSO SATO, M.D.
MITSUAKI SAKATA, M.D.
TORU SATO, M.D.
OKAYAMA, JAPAN
*From the Department of Surgery, Okayama University Medical School*

Patients who receive massive blood transfusion are on the increase because of the recent progress in surgical procedures and in blood supply facilities. The hemorrhagic tendency associated with this has raised challenging questions, which have been discussed and studied for the past several years.[2, 4, 6, 9, 12, 24, 25, 28]

We have had 8 patients (5 underwent pulmonary operations and 3 underwent gastric and esophageal resections) who developed such hemorrhagic tendency in our clinic in the past 4 years. They represent 0.7 per cent of the total number of blood-receiving patients in this period.

The causes of the hemorrhagic tendency and the therapeutic problems are still far from being completely understood. In this article the results of our clinical and experimental research for the past 4 years are given.

Received for publication Nov. 3, 1960.

## MATERIALS AND METHODS

In addition to our clinical experiences, experimental studies were performed with dogs and rabbits. Compatible preserved blood amounting to from 0.8 to 2.0 times the estimated circulating blood volume was infused, while the proportional amount of blood was being drawn out under general inhalation anesthesia. The blood had been prepared in 250 ml. bottles containing acid citrate dextrose solution and was stored at 4° to 6° C. for 2 or 3 weeks.

Observations were made of bleeding time, clotting time, platelet count, platelet fragility, platelet adhesiveness,[14] platelet factor III (thromboplastinogenase), platelet serotonin level,[26] and distribution of platelets after blood transfusion (by $P^{32}$-tagged platelets). Electromicroscopic and phase-contrast microscopic observations were made of platelets.[10] Thrombopoiesis was observed by tissue culture of the bone marrow. Determinations were also made of clot

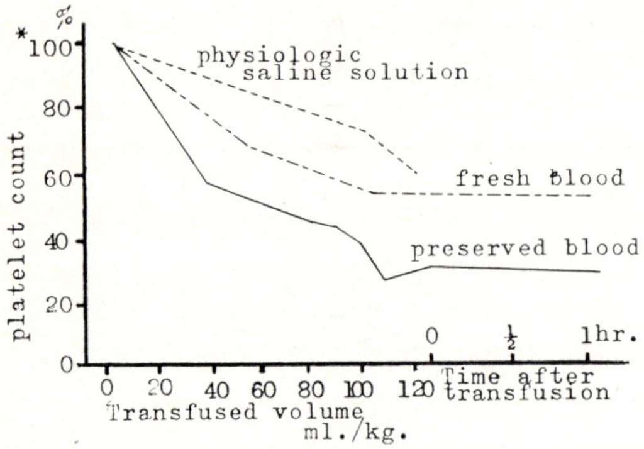


**Fig. 1.** Decrease in platelet count during and after transfusion (average value in per cent). A value of 100 per cent (*) corresponds to pretransfusion level.

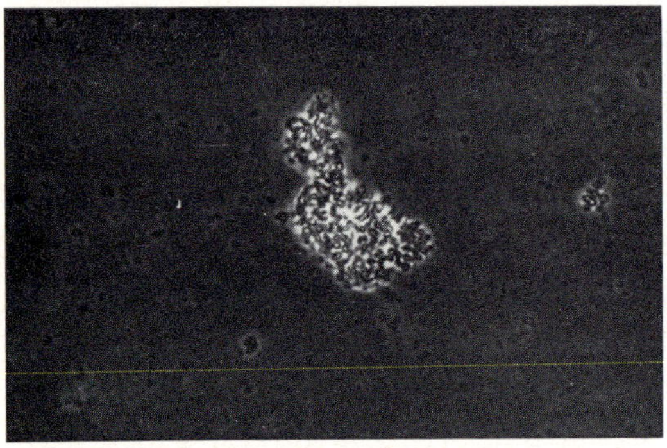

**Fig. 2.** Platelet clump formation.

**Table I.** *Platelet clump formation activity in recipient's plasma after transfusion of preserved blood (80 to 100 ml. per kilogram)*

| | *Before transfusion* | *After transfusion* |
|---|---|---|
| Total No. of patients | 32 | 32 |
| Cases of clump formation | 4 | 24 |
| Per cent | 12.5 | 75.0 |

retraction, recalcification time, thromboplastin generation, prothrombin (one-stage Quick method and two-stage Ware-Seegers method), fibrinogen level, fibrinolytic activity, fibrinolysin level, antifibrinolysin level, and antithrombin activity. Assays were made of heparin and thrombelastograms were taken. Capillary resistance was determined by the modified negative pressure method of Robson,[17] and serum calcium and citric acid levels[7] were also studied.

Except for several special determinations, for which separate references are given, we used methods described in the chapter on laboratory methods in *Hemorrhagic Diseases* by A. J. Quick.[16]

## RESULTS AND COMMENT

**Factors which cause the bleeding tendency.**

*Mechanism of a decrease in platelet count.* The decreased platelet count which always appears after the massive transfusion of preserved blood is considered to be one of the factors which cause the bleeding tendency.[12, 24, 25] Several theories[2, 4, 5, 12, 15, 22] have been presented concerning the mechanism of this deficiency, but none of these is authoritative. In our experiments, platelets in the preserved blood show marked destruction at the third day of preservation. However, dilution with the platelet-poor plasma has a small effect on this phenomenon, and the platelet count decreases much more than can be attributed to the effect of dilution with the infusion of the preserved plasma (Fig. 1).

The appearance of platelet antibodies and agglutinins in the preserved blood is very rare, and thus cannot be the cause of the deficient platelet count which occurs in almost every case.

Studying the function of platelet formation in the bone marrow, we did not notice any abnormalities of megakaryocytes immediately or 24 hours after massive transfusion of preserved blood. Also, changes in the distribution of platelets were observed in dogs which had received the blood transfusion after reinfusion of $P^{32}$-tagged platelets. The platelet levels decreased markedly in the peripheral venous blood and showed a marked increase in the lung and bone marrow in comparison with the levels in control animals which received an infusion of physiologic saline solution. These facts are thought to show that the abnormal

**Table II.** *Morphologic platelet changes seen with an electron microscope after transfusion and incubation of preserved plasma (frequency of forms I to V)*

| | *I* | *II* | *III* | *IV* | *V* |
|---|---|---|---|---|---|
| Before transfusion (normal) | 19% | 20% | 38% | 11% | 12% |
| After transfusion of preserved blood, 120 ml. per kilogram | 9 | 10 | 9 | 44 | 28 |
| After incubation in preserved plasma (37° C., 30 min.) | 14 | 10 | 16 | 37 | 23 |

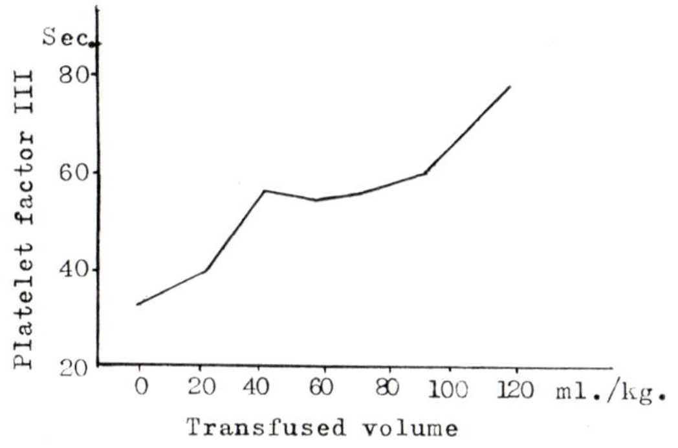


**Fig. 3.** Decrease of platelet factor III which occurs during the transfusion of preserved blood (average value).

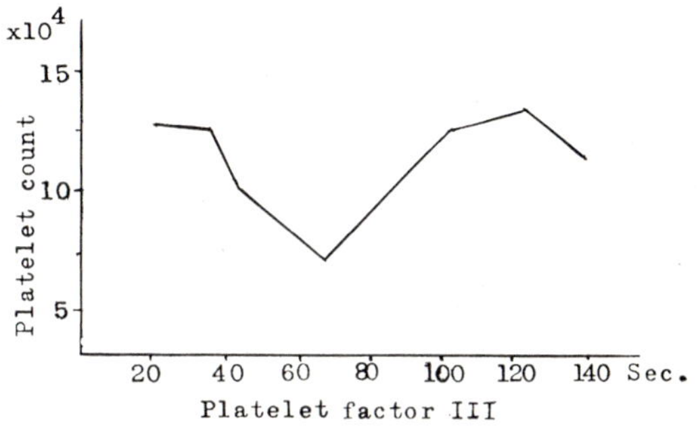


**Fig. 4.** Relation between platelet count and platelet factor III during transfusion of preserved blood (average value).

distribution of platelets which occurs after the blood transfusion is due to some unknown mechanism. This mechanism is still under investigation, and we will present a summary of the results which seem to be most interesting at present. When normal platelets were incubated in the compatible plasma in A-B-O system from a recipient who had received a transfusion of preserved blood, platelet clump formation appeared among the scattered platelets (Fig. 2). This phenomenon is observed in few recipients' plasma before blood is transfused (Table I). The same platelet clump formation is observed when platelets are incubated in the preserved blood. These phenomena still await further investigation, but are useful in explaining the cause of thrombocytopenia and the abnormal distribution of platelets in the body which is noted for a relatively short time after the transfusion of preserved blood.

*Qualitative and morphologic platelet changes.* After massive blood transfusion, in addition to the deficient platelet count, there are observed qualitative or functional changes. These include a decrease of platelet factor III (Fig. 3), which is not in proportion to the decrease of platelet count (Fig. 4); a slight increase of platelet fragility; a 20 to 50 per cent decrease of platelet adhesiveness (Fig. 5); and a decrease of the serotonin level in the platelets and of clot retraction, which is not proportional to the decrease of the platelet count (Fig. 6).

Morphologic observation with an electron microscope shows that normal platelets, in

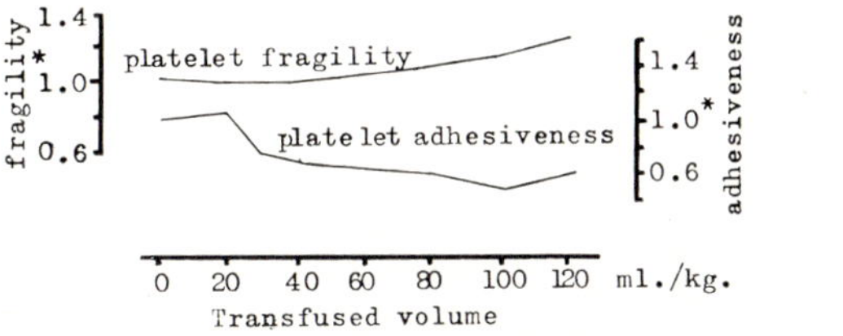


**Fig. 5.** Platelet fragility and adhesiveness during transfusion of preserved blood (average value).

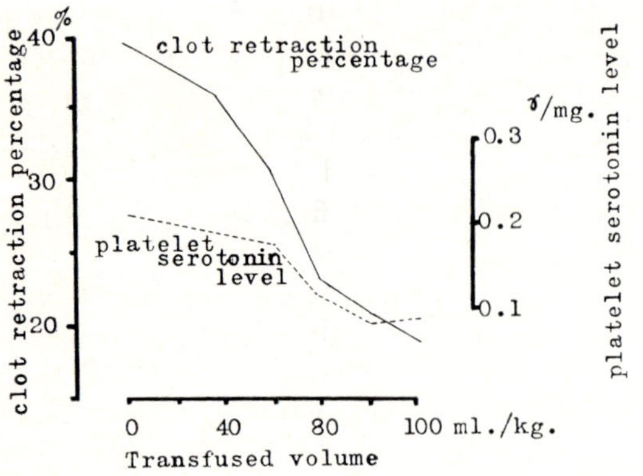


**Fig. 6.** Platelet serotonin level and clot retraction during transfusion of preserved blood (average value).

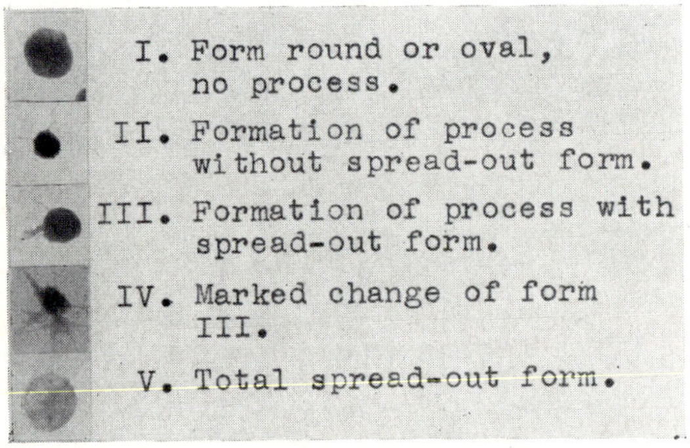


**Fig. 7.** Classification of morphologies of platelets by study with electron microscope.

most cases, have many processes and few take the spread-out form, while few platelets have processes and most of them are in the spread-out form after the preserved blood transfusion. Some ghost cells appear also. According to a platelet form classification of I, II, III, IV, and V (Fig. 7),[11] increased IV and V forms are observed after the transfusion of preserved blood (Table II). This phenomenon is very similar to that which occurs when normal platelets are incubated in preserved plasma at 37° C. for 30 minutes.

These results suggest that massive transfusion of the preserved blood causes not only a deficiency in the quantity of platelets, but also causes changes in morphology or quality.

*Other factors which cause platelet disturbance.* Research was carried out on other factors which are supposed to cause platelet deficiency.[27] These factors, such as operative procedures, hemorrhagic shock, and anoxia, except for fibrinolysis which will be mentioned later, were proved to have little influence on the platelet factor. When patients who received transfusion alone were compared with those who received transfusion during an operative procedure, hemorrhagic shock, or anoxia, there were no conspicuous differences in platelet deficiency (Fig. 8).

Thus, we can conclude that the transfusion of preserved blood itself is the main cause of platelet deficiency.

*Vascular disturbance.* In our experimental observations with an apparatus for measurement of capillary resistance of the mesentery, in most cases a decrease of capillary resistance was noted in proportion to the amount of blood transfused. However, the degree was slight, in general, and the phenomenon was not marked even in cases of accompanying oozing (Fig. 9). Other factors, such as operative procedure, hemorrhagic shock, or

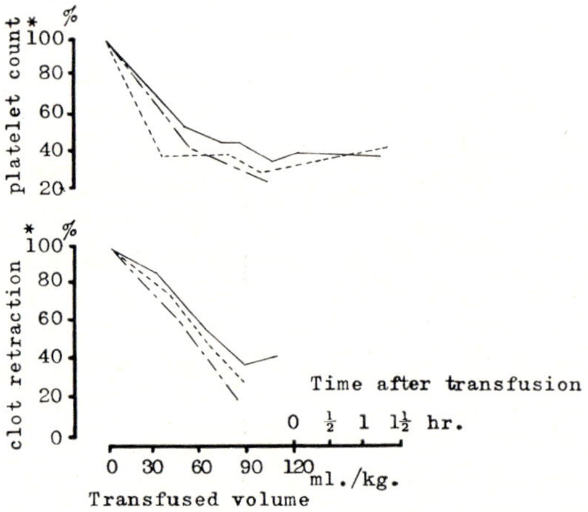


**Fig. 8.** Influences of operative procedure or hemorrhagic shock on platelet deficiency (average values in per cent). A value of 100 per cent (*) corresponds to pretransfusion level. Solid line, transfusion of preserved blood alone; dotted line, transfusion of preserved blood with operative procedure; and dot-dash line, transfusion of preserved blood with hemorrhagic shock.

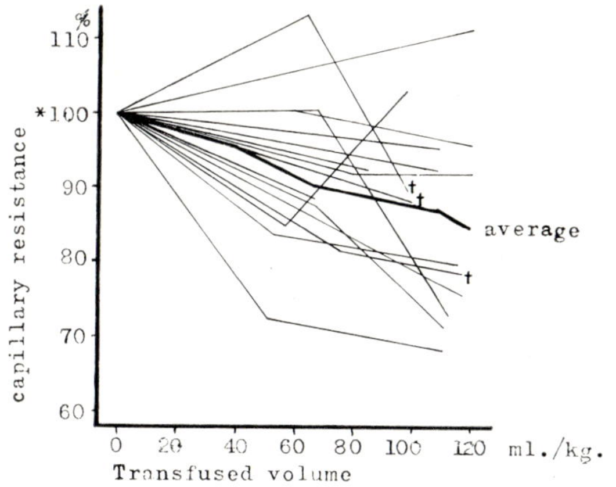


**Fig. 9.** Decrease of capillary resistance during transfusion of preserved blood. A value of 100 per cent (*) corresponds to pretransfusion level. Daggers indicate cases in which oozing appeared.

anoxia, have little influence on the disturbance of the vascular factors (Fig. 10). The preserved blood itself is thought to be the main cause.

*Changes in the clotting mechanism.* Seen most frequently after massive transfusion of preserved blood are disturbances of thromboplastin generation due to the decrease in number and qualitative deficiency of platelets, and the disturbance of thrombin generation due to decreases of prothrombin and of its conversion accelerator, especially a labile factor.[19, 28] On a thrombelastogram they are shown as prolonged r and k and decreased ma. However, these disturbances of clotting factors are not strong enough to cause bleeding as in other hemorrhagic maladies. Also, in most cases they are conspicuous about 12 hours after blood transfusion, when the deficiencies of platelet and vascular factors are already improving (Fig. 11).

Clotting factors are more strongly impaired when the massive transfusion is accompanied with other factors such as major operative procedures, hemorrhagic shock,[20] anoxia, and liver damage.[21] Liver damage initiates a vicious cycle. It causes the disturbance of clotting factors which causes more and more bleeding. Transfusion to restore the blood level in turn causes poorer liver function. Clotting factors are also strongly impaired when fibrinolysis appears.

*Occurrence of fibrinolysis.* Fibrinolysis can be the main cause of hemorrhagic tendency after preserved blood transfusion. We have had 4 patients with fibrinolysis, 1 of whom had gastric carcinoma and 3 of whom had pulmonary disease, out of the 8 who developed hemorrhagic disorders during operation.

Partial fibrinolysis which did not lead to the appearance of the hemorrhagic tendency was encountered relatively often, especially in pulmonary operations. The degree of fibrinolysis (total or partial) did

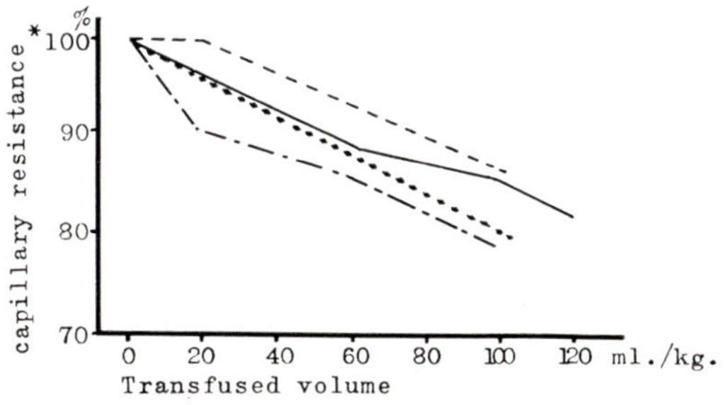


**Fig. 10.** Influences of operative procedure, hemorrhagic shock, or anoxia on capillary resistance (average value in per cent). A value of 100 per cent (*) corresponds to pretransfusion level. Solid line, transfusion of preserved blood alone; dotted line, transfusion of preserved blood with operative procedure; dot-dash line, transfusion of preserved blood with hemorrhagic shock; and dash line, transfusion of preserved blood with anoxia.

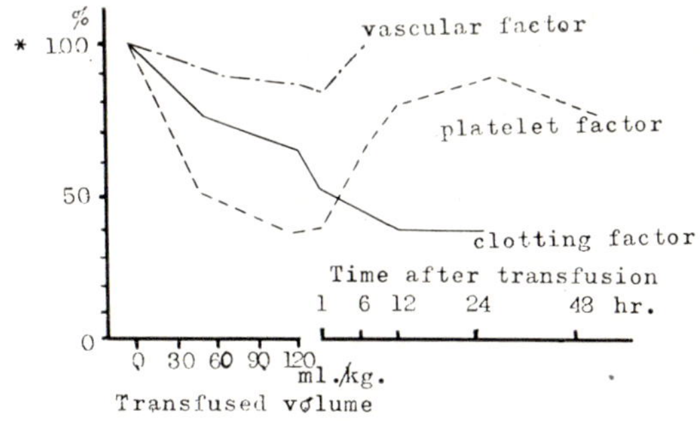


**Fig. 11.** Transition of the 3 factors during and after transfusion of preserved blood (average values). A value of 100 per cent (*) corresponds to pretransfusion level.

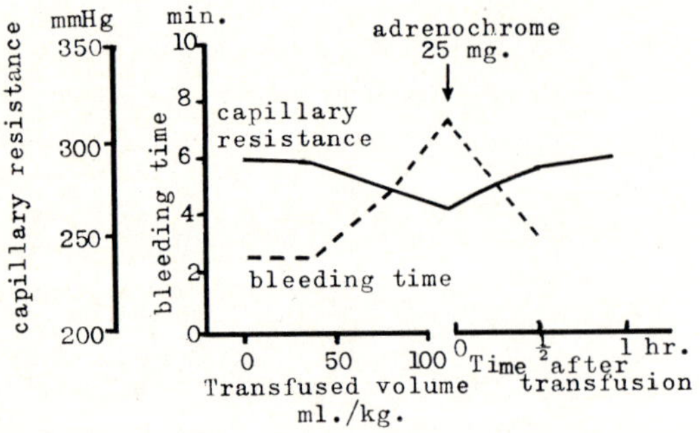


**Fig. 12.** Effect of intravenous administration of adrenochrome on vascular factors.

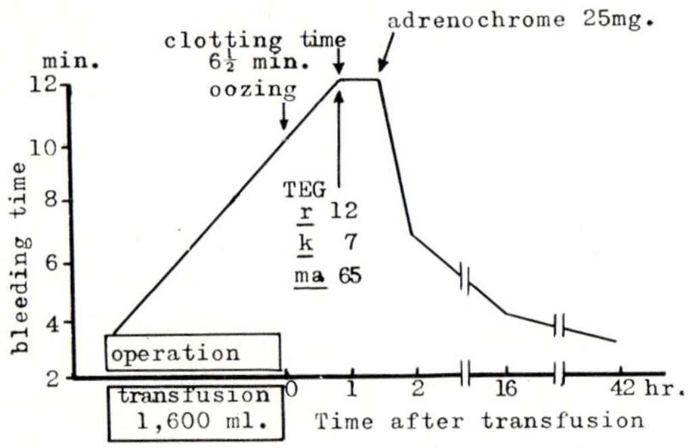


**Fig. 13.** Hemostatic effect of intravenous administration of adrenocrome in a clinical case (58-year-old man with stomach carcinoma).

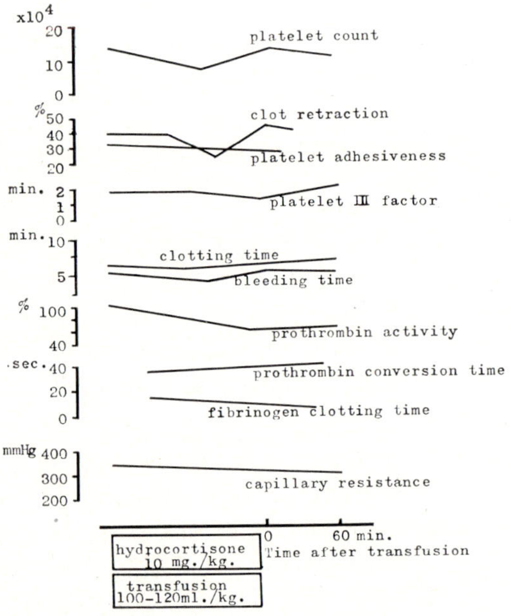


**Fig. 14.** Effects of intravenous drip infusion of hydrocortisone.

not correlate with the amount of transfused blood. Marked fibrinolysis was produced with operations on the lung or pancreas and in cases of hemorrhagic shock. Neither activation nor increase of fibrinolysin was noticed in the preserved blood. No decrease of the antifibrinolysin level was observed in the serum of recipients of preserved blood. Accordingly, we can impute fibrinolysis to such factors as hemorrhagic shock, surgical trauma, the specific locations of operations, and poor physical condition of patients, rather than to the preserved blood transfusion per se. Once fibrinolysis develops, it can induce hemorrhagic tendency in cooperation with many other factors involved.

*Increases of circulating anticoagulants.* In our experiments, neither heparin nor antithrombin levels increased in the serum of recipients of preserved blood. But, in clinical cases or in combination with major surgical trauma, these levels were proved to be much increased and probably became one of the causes of impaired coagulation.

*Increased citric acid level.* We recognized no remarkable decrease in the serum calcium level, despite a rapid rise of citric acid level in serum after massive blood transfusion, probably because of the release of tissue calcium into the blood.

Although the cause of a rapid drop of blood pressure followed by death, produced experimentally by citric acid intoxication, was thought to be an abnormality of electrolytes in cardiac muscle, a hemorrhagic tendency due to decreased calcium level was not produced by massive citrated blood transfusion.

**Therapy and prophylaxis for the bleeding tendency.** As mentioned previously, we cannot attribute the bleeding tendency after massive transfusion of preserved blood to the blood transfusion per se. The bleeding tendency varies in severity and character in each case in correlation with many other factors. Therefore, once the bleeding tendency appears, we should try to use an adequate combination of various agents which are effective for platelet, vascular, or clotting factors or fibrinolysis.

To select adequate agents, we made several observations to evaluate the effects of various agents and procedures on impaired platelet, vascular, or clotting factors in experimental cases of massive transfusion of preserved blood.

*Thromboplastin preparation.* Concerning platelet factors, thromboplastin preparation does improve somewhat the action of thromboplastinogenase or act as its substitute. It also shortens clotting time when thromboplastin generation is impaired. Thromboplastin preparation also increases capillary resistance approximately 40 per cent and shortens bleeding time.

*Adrenochrome.* Adrenochrome is effective in cases of impaired vascular factors (Fig. 12). It causes a hemostatic effect which strengthens resistance of the vascular wall. It proved useful in a case of bleeding time prolonged for over 10 minutes during operation (Fig. 13).

*Intravenous drip infusion of hydrocortisone.* There have been many opinions on the effectiveness of hydrocortisone.[3, 12, 18] In fact, there is a considerable variation in its effectiveness, depending upon amount and method of its administration. For example, our experiments show that hydrocortisone is more effective when it is used in continuous drip administration, all through the duration of blood transfusion, than when the same dose is administered only during the first half or latter half of the blood transfusion or after it.

When 10 mg. per kilogram of hydrocortisone is administered continuously by intravenous drip throughout massive transfusion of preserved blood, it can markedly reduce impairment of platelet, clotting, and vascular factors (Fig. 14). Thus, it reduces bleeding and decreases the amount of blood to be transfused.

*ACTH and DOCA.*[3] When 1 U. per kilogram of ACTH or 0.5 mg. per kilogram of DOCA is given before blood transfusion, it decreases platelet deficiency but has little effect on prothrombin activity or vascular factors.

*Platelet transfusion.*[8, 23] Platelet transfusion decreased the impairment of platelet factors, that is, it increases platelet count and improves platelet function (Fig. 15). It improves thromboplastin generation impaired by the transfusion of preserved blood

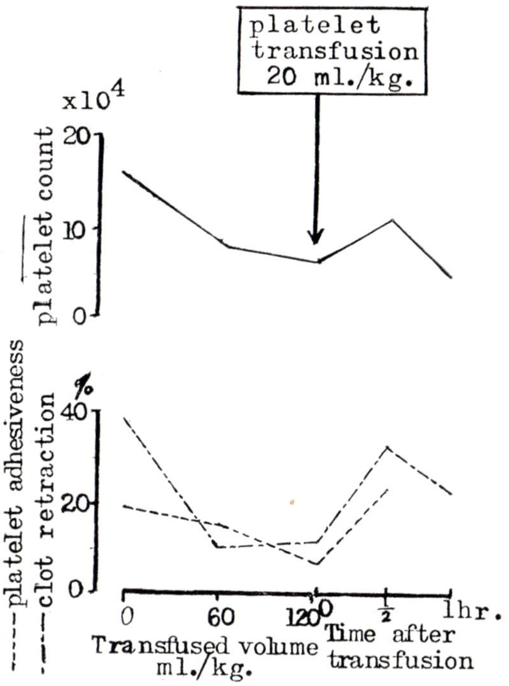


**Fig. 15.** Effect of platelet transfusion on platelet factor impaired by massive transfusion of preserved blood.

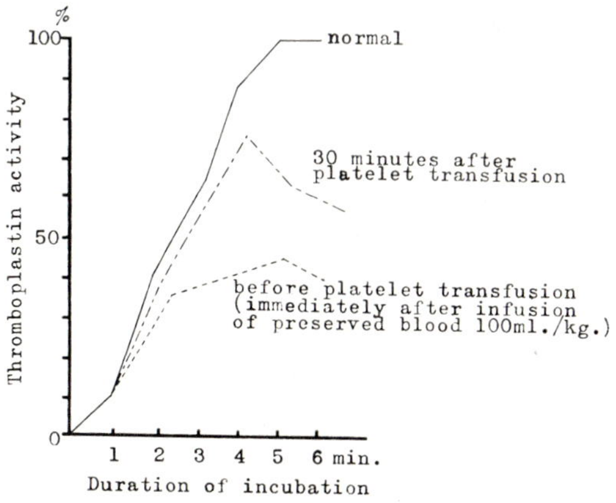


**Fig. 16.** Effect of platelet transfusion on thromboplastin generation impaired by massive transfusion of preserved blood. (Thromboplastin generation test: normal serum plus normal plasma plus recipient's platelet suspension.)

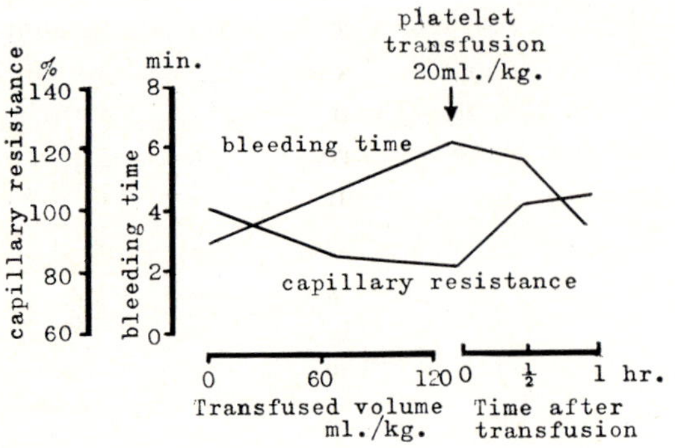


**Fig. 17.** Effect of platelet transfusion on vascular factors impaired by massive transfusion of preserved blood.

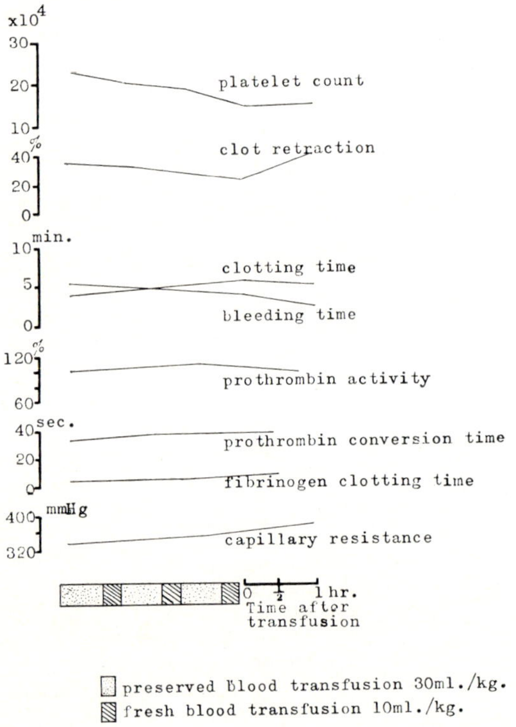


**Fig. 18.** Transition of various deficiencies when fresh blood is given alternately with preserved blood.

(Fig. 16) and is also effective for vascular factors (Fig. 17). However, these effects are all transient, and we have practical difficulties in collecting platelets and repeating their administration easily enough to meet an emergency need, although we have plenty of time with chronic bleeding diseases.

*Fresh blood transfusion.*[1, 4] When fresh blood was given with nonwettable instruments after transfusion of preserved blood, we noticed increases of platelet count, of platelet factor III, of platelet adhesiveness, and of clot retraction. Fresh blood transfusion had a good effect on clotting factors. It improved thromboplastin generation and prothrombin activity, and also strengthened capillary resistance. These effects, however, were not marked.

When fresh blood was given alternately with preserved blood, for example, 10 ml. per kilogram of fresh blood given alternately with 30 ml. per kilogram of preserved blood, it was more effective in controlling impairment of platelet, clotting, and vascular factors, and worked better in preventing a bleeding tendency than when the same total amount of fresh blood was given at one time (Fig. 18).

*Therapeutic agents for fibrinolysis.* The most effective agents for fibrinolysis are hydrocortisone given intravenously,[13] ε-aminocaproic acid given intravenously, or a combination of both. In our experiments, we had many cases in which fibrinolysis was quickly controlled with the intravenous administration of hydrocortisone or ε-aminocaproic acid (Fig. 19).

In our clinical experience, also, hydrocortisone, ε-aminocaproic acid, or a combination was successful in suppressing fibrinolysis in pulmonary and other operations.

## CONCLUSION

**Causes of the bleeding tendency after massive transfusion of preserved blood.** Bleeding tendency cannot be caused by a single factor. Combinations of deficiency in number and function of platelets and impaired vascular factors caused by massive transfusion of preserved blood brought about hemorrhage in combination with local factors such as physical stimulation. Clotting disturbance, promoted by other factors such as hemorrhagic shock, anoxia, poor physical condition, major surgical trauma, and fibrinolysis, prolongs bleeding and leads to uncontrolled bleeding, that is, the bleeding tendency.

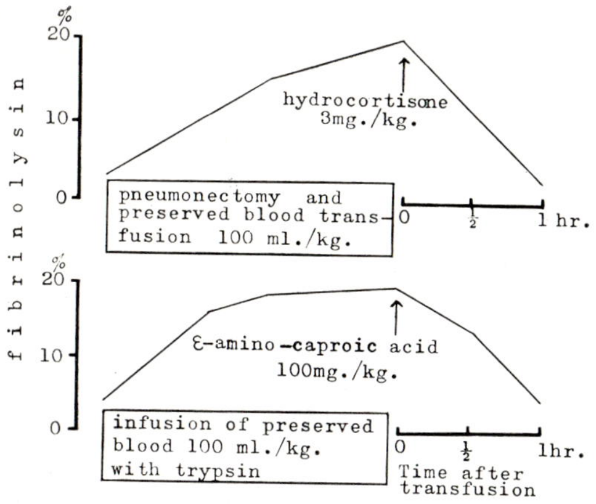


Fig. 19. Correction of fibrinolysis by intravenous administration of hydrocortisone or ε-aminocaproic acid.

**Therapy and prophylaxis for the bleeding tendency after massive transfusion of preserved blood.** In our experience, it was impossible in most cases to determine the causative factor with screening tests at the moment of difficulty. For this reason, we needed various kinds and large doses of drugs to control the bleeding tendency which had already developed. Nevertheless, we cannot always expect complete success.

In our opinion, the emphasis should be on prevention. When it is expected that a massive blood transfusion will be given especially when causal factors such as hemorrhagic shock, anoxia, liver damage, and so forth are present, we should always take complete prophylactic precautions as early as possible.

Our methods include (1) administration of ε-aminocaproic acid for prevention of fibrinolysis, (2) continuous intravenous drip instillation of hydrocortisone, (3) alternating transfusions of fresh and preserved blood, and (4) administration of an adequate combination of adrenochrome, thromboplastin preparations, and calcium. Also, close attention should be paid to the factors which impair the coagulation system.

## SUMMARY

The bleeding tendency after massive transfusion of preserved blood is caused by intrinsic and extrinsic factors such as hemorrhagic shock, anoxia, liver damage, and so forth, rather than the blood transfused per se. The best approach to this problem is prevention and the methods described were found to be effective.

The authors wish to express their appreciation to Dr. Bruce L. Douglas, Fulbright exchange professor, Okayama University Medical School, for his editorial assistance in the preparation of this manuscript.

## REFERENCES

1. Artz, C. P.: Massive transfusion in the severely wounded, Surgery **37:** 469, 1955.
2. Bell, W. N.: The clinical use of the coagulogram, M. Clin. North America **37:** 1843, 1953.
3. Bernard, M., and Jacobson, M.: Effects of cortisone and corticotropin on prolonged bleeding time; treatment in certain hemorrhagic states, A. M. A. Arch. Int. Med. **92:** 471, 1953.
4. Cliffton, E. E., Grossi, C., and Siegel, M.: Hemorrhage during and after operation secondary to changes in the clotting mechanism, Surgery **45:** 37, 1956.
5. Crosby, W. H., and Howard, J. M.: The hematologic response to wounding and to resuscitation accomplished by large transfusion of stored blood, Blood **9:** 439, 1954.
6. Crosby, W. H., and Stefanini, M.: Pathogenesis of the plasma transfusion reaction with special reference to the blood coagulation system, J. Lab. & Clin. Med. **40:** 374, 1952.
7. Ettinger, R. H., Galdbaum, L. R., and Smith, L. H.: Simplified photometric method for determination of citric acid in biological fluids, J. Biol. Chem. **199:** 531, 1952.
8. Gardner, F. H., Howell, D., and Hirsch, E. D.: Platelet transfusion utilizing plastic equipment, J. Lab. & Clin. Med. **43:** 196, 1954.
9. Gollub, S., Ulin, A. W., Winchell, H. S., Ehrlich, E., and Weiss, W.: Hemorrhagic diathesis associated with massive whole blood transfusion, J. A. M. A. **159:** 171, 1955.
10. Haydon, G. B.: Electron microscopic observation of blood platelet and fibrin formation, A. M. A. Arch. Path. **64:** 393, 1957.
11. Igarashi, C.: Electron microscopic study of human blood platelets, Toho Igakkai Zasshi (Japan) **4:** 31, 1957.
12. Krevans, J. R., and Jackson, D. P.: Hemorrhagic disorder following massive blood transfusion, J. A. M. A. **159:** 171, 1955.
13. Kwaan, H. C., and McFadjean, A. J. S.:

Inhibition of clot lysis by corticotropin, Lancet **1:** 136, 1956.
14. Moolten, S. E., and Vroman, L.: The adhesiveness of blood platelets in thromboembolism and hemorrhagic disorders, Am. J. Clin. Path. **19:** 701, 1949.
15. Mustard, J. F.: The Effect of stored blood transfusion on the platelet levels in patients undergoing surgical procedures, Acta haemat. **18:** 80, 1957.
16. Quick, A. J.: Hemorrhagic diseases, Philadelphia, 1957, Lea & Febiger.
17. Robson, H. N., and Duthie, J. R.: Capillary resistance and adrenocortical activity, Brit. M. J. **1:** 971, 1950.
18. Robson, H. N., and Duthie, J. R.: Further observation on capillary resistance and adrenocortical activity, Brit. M. J. **10:** 994, 1952.
19. Scott, R., and Crosby, W. H.: Changes in the coagulation mechanism following wounding and resuscitation with stored blood; a study of battle casualties in Korea, Blood **6:** 609, 1954.
20. Scott, R., and Crosby, W. H.: The hemostatic response to injury; a study of the Korean battle casualty, Ann. Surg. **141:** 347, 1955.
21. Stefanini, M.: Hemorrhagic diasthesis of liver dysfunction and obstructive jaundice, Proc. 3rd Internat. Cong. Internat. Soc. Hemat. New York, 1951.
22. Stefanini, M., and Chatterjea, J. B.: Studies on platelets. IV. A thrombocytopenic factor in normal human blood, plasma or serum, Proc. Soc. Exper. Biol. & Med. **79:** 623, 1952.
23. Stefanini, M., and Dameshek, W.: Collection, preservation and transfusion of platelets with special reference to clinical effectiveness of transfused platelets, New England J. Med. **248:** 797, 1953.
24. Sunada, T.: Hemorrhagic tendency following massive blood transfusion, Jap. M. J. **1733:** 3, 1957.
25. Sunada, T.: Untoward effects of massive blood transfusion, Fukuoka Igakkai Zasshi (Japan) **48:** 457, 1957.
26. Udenfriend, S., Weissbach, H., and Clark, C. T.: The estimation of 5-hydroxytryptamine in biological tissue, J. Biol. Chem. **215:** 337, 1955.
27. William, J. A., and Warren, R.: Endocrine factors in the alternations of the blood coagulation mechanism following surgery, J. Lab. & Clin. Med. **50:** 373, 1957.
28. Zucker, M. B., Siegel, M., Cliffton, E. E., Bellville, J. M., Howland, W. S., and Grossi, C. E.: Generalized excessive Oozing in patients undergoing major surgery and receiving multiple blood transfusion, J. Lab. & Clin. Med. **50:** 849, 1957.

# 5-Hydroxytryptamine and antidiuresis after operation

M. H. FRICK, M.D.
L. VIRKKULA, M.D.
M. K. PAASONEN, M.D.
HELSINKI, FINLAND
*From the Wihuri Research Institute and the Departments of Thoracic Surgery and Pharmacology, University of Helsinki*

Despite intensive research, some facets of postoperative renal function still lack proper understanding. Current concepts of renal disorders after trauma have focused attention on the importance of glomerular filtration,[13] and the earlier view of tubular dysfunction as the primary cause of traumatic renal failure may have to be revised.[25] The changes in the electrolyte balance after operation are in a rather good correlation with the known actions of adrenocortical hormones, especially aldosterone, and with the behavior of body cells as osmotic regulators. However, water retention in excess of electrolytes, although the renal function may otherwise be normal, is one of the subtle features of the postoperative renal function.[31]

Besides renal pathologic changes, humoral agents, especially the antidiuretic hormone (ADH), have received attention. Postoperatively urine possesses antidiuretic activity which indubitably is in relation to an increased ADH secretion.[8] The role of ADH in postoperative oliguria is also confirmed by observations in patients with diabetes insipidus,[31] but the common occurrence of a persistent oliguric phase shows that ADH is not the complete solution of the problem.

Platelets, the most fragile cellular blood elements, are known to contain 5-hydroxytryptamine (5-HT, serotonin),[16, 32] a substance with antidiuretic properties. Previously it has been suggested that the 5-HT released from disintegrated platelets during extracorporeal circulation[24] has a certain influence on the renal function during cardiopulmonary bypass operations.[11] The present study was made in an attempt to clarify whether or not 5-HT bears any relationship to postoperative water retention.

Received for publication Nov. 4, 1960.

## MATERIAL AND METHODS

Thirteen patients, aged 32 to 61 years, who underwent intrathoracic operations without a heart-lung machine, were studied. The daily urine output was measured pre- and postoperatively with an accuracy of 5 ml. The postoperative measurement was begun the moment the patient was returned to bed from the operating room. The urinary excretion of 5-hydroxyindolacetic acid (5-HIAA),* the main metabolic derivative of 5-HT, was determined spectrophotometrically[28] on 2 consecutive preoperative days and 7 times after the operation over a postoperative period of 10 days. The platelet count and hematocrit were determined by routine techniques. In 5 patients the 5-HT of whole blood was determined after acetone extraction[3] with the rat stomach preparation[29] on 2 preoperative days and 5 times after the operation. The recoveries of 5-HT added to blood have been approximately 40 per cent. No values have been adjusted for rate of recovery.

Siliconized glassware and needles† were

*5-HIAA was supplied by The Upjohn Company, Kalamazoo, Mich.

†Desicoute, Beckman Instruments, Inc., Fullerton, Calif.

**Table I.** *5-HT and 5-HIAA values and other data on main collection days (mean and range)*

| | *Preoperative days* | | *Postoperative days* | | | | |
|---|---|---|---|---|---|---|---|
| | *2* | *1* | *1* | *2* | *4* | *6* | *9* |
| Platelets ($\times 10^3$/ml.) | 335<br>220-470 | 345<br>231-500 | 271<br>39-490 | 304<br>205-450 | 346<br>239-490 | 353<br>233-487 | 346<br>232-411 |
| 5-HT (ng.*/ml.) | 47<br>24-110 | 34<br>17-60 | 45<br>13-106 | 29<br>12-80 | 32<br>20-40 | 37<br>32-45 | 30<br>12-60 |
| 5-HIAA (mg./24 hr.) | 3.7<br>1.9-9.3 | 3.0<br>1.9-7.6 | 5.4<br>2.5-9.0 | 4.3<br>2.2-9.3 | 4.1<br>2.2-7.7 | 3.9<br>2.1-8.9 | 4.0<br>1.5-7.2 |
| Hematocrit (vol. %) | 46<br>41-49 | 43<br>36-47 | 45<br>43-50 | 46<br>44-48 | 44<br>35-50 | 38<br>33-42 | 40<br>34-50 |
| Urine output (ml./24 hr.) | 1,141<br>715-1,575 | 1,144<br>435-2,010 | 644<br>210-1,200 | 512<br>155-675 | 657<br>250-950 | 874<br>720-1,220 | 910<br>450-1,355 |
| Specific gravity (+ 1,000) | 20<br>15-26 | 20<br>14-27 | 30<br>26-35 | 29<br>24-35 | 28<br>23-33 | 25<br>15-30 | 19<br>5-29 |

*Nanogram equals $10^{-3}\mu g$.

used throughout the study. The urine and blood-acetone samples were kept at –20° C. before determinations. Reserpine compounds, chlorpromazine, and banana feeding were avoided. The usual surgical regime with premedications and transfusions was not changed.

## RESULTS

The principal findings are recorded in Table I. Increase of the specific gravity paralleled the familiar restriction of the urine output. The daily urine flow reached approximately the preoperative level on the ninth day after operation. In the mean values of 5-HT, no clear-cut decrease became evident. The mean values, however, do not show the whole truth, since the individual values of 5-HT followed the platelet count, in which the drop was equally distributed to the first and second postoperative days. For example, in 1 patient the platelets decreased from a preoperative level of 257,000 to 39,000 per milliliter on the first day after operation and the 5-HT from 30 to 13 ng.* per milliliter, respectively. In one other illustrative case the changes in platelets were from 360,000 to 277,000 per milliliter on the second postoperative day and changes in the 5-HT were from 46 to 12 ng. per milliliter, respectively. If there was no noteworthy change in the platelet count, the 5-HT values did not show a decreasing trend. Fig. 1 demonstrates the amounts of 5-HIAA excreted and the urine output in the periods in question. The significance of the mean differences of the 5-HIAA excretion was analyzed by use of the t test. The mean of the 2 preoperative values of each patient was used as the control figure. There was a significant increase in the excretion on the first and second postoperative days ($p < 0.01$) and also on the fourth day ($p < 0.02$). Under basal conditions the 5-HIAA excretion remains rather constant in the same individual.[28] The variation from day to day in our laboratories has not, as a rule, exceeded 20 per cent. The 5-HIAA values necessitate, however, an interpretation against this range. When it is taken into account, only the values on the first 2 postoperative days exceeded the preoperative level. This occurred in 7 patients, whereas in 6 patients the excretion was unaffected by the operation. The hematocrit for the most part remained unchanged.

*Nanogram equals $10^{-3}$ $\mu g$.

## DISCUSSION

The response of the platelet count to a major operation is usually an initial depression followed by an elevation to preoperative levels and above. During the second postoperative week the platelet count may be 2 or 3 times the preoperative level.[17] This elevation has been of particular interest, since it coincides with the peak occurrence of thrombotic complications. The initial depression, which can reach considerable dimensions by even 2 hours after the operation,[19] is also associated with a shortened bleeding time.[30] It is due, at least in part, to an increased platelet conglutination, and to disintegration of platelets in the operative field and local hemorrhages. This local factor is nicely illustrated by the observation that the drop can be prevented by rinsing the wound edges with heparin and epinephrine.[19]

When the initial decrease in the platelet count occurred in the present series it was associated with a decrease in the whole blood 5-HT and an elevation in the urinary excretion of 5-HIAA. Theoretically, the blood transfusions given to the patients can be held responsible for the changes observed. However, stored blood, unless specially handled, contains only a few viable platelets[12] and it has been demonstrated that 5-HT is oxidized in human serum.[20]

In a study of the value of 5-HIAA excretion as an indication of impending thrombotic complications after operation (including open-heart operations) in a group of patients, the 5-HIAA values were not elevated during the first postoperative days.[27] This difference from the present findings is probably due to the amount of renal suppression. The decreased glomerular filtration rate and renal blood flow usually recover after operation, but this might be delayed after cardiopulmonary bypass operations. The finding of a decreased 5-HIAA excretion during operation is in accord with other reports.[11, 24] The excretion of 5-HIAA is due to an active tubular excretion[7, 21] and is uninfluenced by the urinary pH.[21] According to these concepts the urinary 5-HIAA ought to be independent of the urine flow per se, but it is certainly affected by a decreased renal blood flow and renal pathologic changes. In such states, as has been pointed out earlier,[11] 5-HIAA values may give an unreliable impression unless the 5-HT values of the blood are measured simultaneously.

The rise in the specific gravity after operation indicates that we are not dealing with postoperative renal failure. Admittedly, no significant renal pathologic changes can be suspected to exist in the present series.

The antidiuretic effect of 5-HT has been demonstrated in all the usual laboratory animals[1, 5, 9, 10, 23, 26] and in man.[4, 14, 15] Divergent opinions exist on the mode of this action. Perfusion experiments have shown a strong vasoconstrictor response in the renal vessels,[6, 22] but several studies with renal clearance measurements have presented evidence that the antidiuretic action of 5-HT is due to an increased water reabsorption from the tubules.[23, 26] The finding that 5-HT contracts the ureteral muscle[2] makes a decision no easier. An intact posterior lobe of the hypophysis is not essential in 5-HT antidiuresis[1, 5] and 5-HT antidiuresis has also been demonstrated in patients with diabetes insipidus.[4] This pathway, however, must be taken into account because it has been observed that 5-HT decreases the amount of neurosecretory substance in the posterior pituitary gland.[18]

In view of the data given, suggestive evidence is found that 5-HT, a substance with antidiuretic properties, is released into plasma after major operations. The question

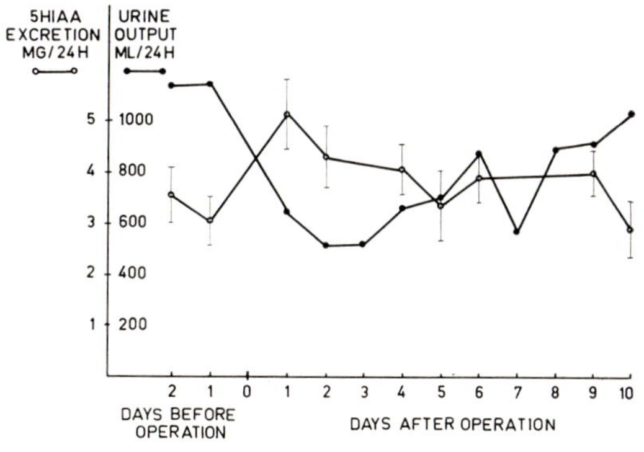


**Fig. 1.** The mean urine output and excretion of 5-hydroxyindolacetic acid (± standard error of the mean) of 13 patients before and after operation.

of the extent of its responsibility for the antidiuresis cannot be answered. Restriction of the postoperative urine output occurred also in patients without evidence of 5-HT release. The present findings confirm, however, the assumption that humoral vasoconstrictors play a part in the pathogenesis of posttraumatic renal function.[25]

## SUMMARY

Thirteen patients were studied after major operations to find out whether or not the typical pattern of the postoperative platelet count was associated with alterations in the amount of 5-hydroxytryptamine in the blood. It was found that in patients with a drop in the platelet count on the first 2 postoperative days the 5-hydroxytryptamine content of whole blood was correspondingly decreased, and a simultaneous increase occurred in the urinary excretion of 5-hydroxyindolacetic acid. In view of the antidiuretic properties of 5-hydroxytryptamine, it is suggested that this humoral agent participates in postoperative antidiuresis.

### REFERENCES

1. Abrahams, V. C., and Pickford, M.: The effect of 5-hydroxytryptamine on the excretion of water in conscious dog, Brit. J. Pharmacol. **11:** 35, 1956.
2. Abrahams, V. C., and Pickford, M.: The effect of 5-hydroxytryptamine on the ureter and on the blood pressure of dogs; and of adrenaline, noradrenaline and posterior pituitary extracts on the ureter, Brit. J. Pharmacol. **11:** 44, 1956.
3. Amin, A. H., Crawford, T. B., and Gaddum, J. H.: The distribution of substance P and 5-hydroxytryptamine in the central nervous system of the dog, J. Physiol. **126:** 596, 1954.
4. Annoni, G., Lucchelli, P. D., and Barbiera, G.: L'azione della 5-idrossitriptamina (enteramina-serotonina) sulla diuresi nell'uomo, Farmaco ed. sci. **10:** 306, 1955.
5. Barac, G.: Recherches sur la brûlure. Sur l'effect antidiurétique de la 5-hydroxytryptamine chez le chien, Arch. internat. physiol. **61:** 403, 1953.
6. Cerletti, A., Carpi, A., and Rothlin, E.: Über die Wirkung von 5-Oxytryptamin (Serotonin) auf Diurese und Nierendurchblutung, Helvet. physiol. acta **13:** C 8, 1955.
7. Despopoulos, A., and Weissbach, H.: Renal metabolism of 5-hydroxyindoleacetic acid, Am. J. Physiol. **189:** 548, 1957.
8. Eisen, V. D., and Lewis, A. A. G.: Antidiuretic activity of human urine after surgical operation, Lancet **2:** 361, 1954.
9. Erspamer, V.: Pharmacology of indolealkylamines, Pharmacol. Rev. **6:** 425, 1954.
10. Erspamer, V., and Ottolenghi, A.: Pharmacological studies on enteramine. VIII. Action of enteramine on the diuresis and the renal circulation of the rat, Arch. internat. pharmacodyn. et thérap. **93:** 177, 1953.
11. Frick, M. H.: Influence of 5-hydroxytryptamine on renal function in extracorporeal circulation, Nature **187:** 609, 1960.
12. Gardner, F. H., and Cohen, P.: The value of platelet transfusions, M. Clin. North Amer. **44:** 1425, 1960.
13. Graber, I. G., and Sevitt, S.: Renal function in burned patients and its relationship to morphological changes, J. Clin. Path. **12:** 25, 1959.
14. Hollander, W., and Michelson, A. L.: Effects of serotonin and antiserotonins in hypertensive man, J. Clin. Invest. **35:** 712, 1956.
15. Hollander, W., Michelson, A. L., and Wilkins, R. W.: Serotonin and antiserotonins. I. Their circulatory, respiratory, and renal effects in man, Circulation **16:** 246, 1957.
16. Humphrey, J. H., and Jaques, R.: The histamine and serotonin content of the platelets and polymorphonuclear leucocytes of various species, J. Physiol. **124:** 305, 1954.
17. Jamieson, R. A., and Kay, A. W.: Textbook of surgical physiology, Edinburgh and London, 1959, E. & S. Livingstone, p. 258.
18. Kivalo, E., Rinne, U. K., and Marjanen, P.: Response of the neurohypophysis to serotonin, reserpine, and chlorpromazine, Ann. med. int. Fenniae **46:** 191, 1957.
19. Lenggenhager, K. *In* Hellner, H., Nissen, R., and Vosschulte, K.: Lehrbuch der Chirurgie, Stuttgart, 1958, Georg Thieme, p. 120.
20. Martin, G., Eriksen, N., and Benditt, E. P.: Oxidation of 5-hydroxytryptamine by human serum and its inhibition by iproniazid, Fed. Proc. **17:** 477, 1958.
21. Milne, M. D., Crawford, M. A., Cirão, C. B., and Loughridge, L.: The excretion of indolylacetic acid and related indolic acids in man and the rat, Clin. Sc. **19:** 165, 1960.
22. Page, I. H., and McCubbin, J. W.: Renal vascular and systemic arterial pressure responses to nervous and chemical stimulation of the kidney, Am. J. Physiol. **173:** 411, 1953.
23. Sala, G., and Castegnaro, E.: Influence of enteramine (5-hydroxytryptamine) on renal function of the dog, Proc. Soc. Exper. Biol. & Med. **82:** 621, 1953.

24. Sarajas, H. S. S., Kristoffersson, R., and Frick, M. H.: Release of 5-hydroxytryptamine and adenosinetriphosphate in extracorporeal circulatory systems as a result of corpuscular blood trauma, Am. J. Physiol. **197:** 1195, 1959.
25. Sevitt, S.: Pathogenesis of traumatic uraemia, Lancet **2:** 135, 1959.
26. Spinazzola, A. J., and Sherrod, T. R.: The effects of serotonin (5-hydroxytryptamine) on renal hemodynamics, J. Pharmacol. & Exper. Therap. **119:** 114, 1957.
27. Sullenberger, J. W., Anlyan, W. G., and Weaver, W. T.: Serotonin in intravascular thrombosis, SURGERY **46:** 22, 1959.
28. Udenfriend, S., Titus, E., and Weissbach, H.: The identification of 5-hydroxy-3-indolacetic acid in normal urine and a method for its assay, J. Biol. Chem. **216:** 499, 1955.
29. Vane, J. R.: A sensitive method for the assay of 5-hydroxytryptamine, Brit. J. Pharmacol. **12:** 344, 1957.
30. Von Kaulla, N.: Zur Frage der postoperativen Gerinnungsbeschleunigung, Deutsche Ztschr. Chir. **256:** 74, 1942.
31. Wynn, V.: Some problems of water metabolism following surgery. *In* the biochemical response to injury, Oxford, 1960, Blackwell Scientific Publications, p. 291.
32. Zucker, M. B., and Borrelli, J.: Quantity, assay, and release of serotonin in human platelets, J. Appl. Physiol. **7:** 425, 1955.

# Intravenous l-norepinephrine as a cause of reduced plasma volume

KARL J. SCHMUTZER, M.D.
EKKEHART RASCHKE, M.D.
JAMES V. MALONEY, JR., M.D.*
LOS ANGELES, CALIF.
*From the Department of Surgery, University of California Medical Center*

Ten years ago, intravenous l-norepinephrine was first shown by Goldenberg and co-workers[6] to be of value in the clinical management of certain hypotensive states. Since that time, the drug has been found useful in a variety of surgical and medical emergencies. It has become apparent, however, that sudden withdrawal of the drug after its prolonged administration is frequently accompanied by an immediate fall of the arterial blood pressure to such low levels as to endanger the life of the patient. It is common clinical practice to decrease the rate of administration of l-norepinephrine slowly and progressively in an effort to prevent the occurrence of this phenomenon. Incidental observations in the course of other studies on shock[8] suggested that patients who receive l-norepinephrine show a steadily decreasing plasma volume. The purpose of the present investigation was to determine the effect of the intravenous administration of l-norepinephrine on plasma volume in dogs. During the course of this study, a method was evolved to permit instantaneous discontinuation of the drug without the occurrence of the commonly observed secondary hypotension.

The investigations of von Euler,[11, 12] Holtz,[7] and others evaluated the physiologic and biochemical properties of l-norepinephrine and established its significance as a vasopressor agent. It was not until 1949, when clinical application of the drug began, that reports appeared regarding complications which occurred with its use. The majority of these publications stressed the necrotizing effect of the drug on the tissues at the site of injection.[3] Early case reports show that sudden withdrawal of l-norepinephrine may result in severe hypotension and shock. It has, therefore, been recommended that the rate of administration be reduced gradually.[9] Saave[10] reported 3 instances. In one, the patient died after unintentional sudden discontinuation of l-norepinephrine and in the other two, withdrawal of the drug was accompanied by a steady fall of arterial blood pressure and a deterioration of the patients' condition. After adequate blood transfusions both of the patients recovered.

This paper will present a physiologic explanation for the secondary hypotension described in the literature and encountered by the authors in the clinical use of l-norepinephrine.

## METHODS

Thirty-four healthy fasting mongrel dogs which ranged from 10.0 to 20.3 kilograms in body weight were employed for these studies. All animals were splenectomized at least 3 days prior to the experiment because of the well-recognized lability of splenic blood volume in the dog. Anesthesia was induced by the intravenous administration

Supported by a grant-in-aid from the American Heart Association.

Received for publication Nov. 10, 1960.

*Dr. Maloney's work was supported in part by the Scholar Program of the John and Mary R. Markle Foundation.

of pentobarbital sodium, 30 mg. per kilogram of body weight. One femoral artery was cannulated and connected to a strain gauge manometer for continuous recording of arterial blood pressure. The other femoral artery was exposed to facilitate repeated puncture for sampling of arterial blood. One femoral vein was cannulated for the intravenous administration of a continuous drip of l-norepinephrine.* The contralateral femoral vein was used for the injection of dye for blood volume determination.

The blue dye method with acetone extraction, as modified by Chinard,[2] was adopted for the blood volume studies. A sample of arterial blood was drawn to provide a plasma blank for the spectrophotometer. An accurately weighed amount of Evans blue dye† was injected intravenously. After an interval of 10 minutes, an arterial sample was withdrawn. The concentration of the dye was determined in plasma with the use of a Beckman spectrophotometer at a wave length of 620 $\mu$ employing cuvettes with a 10 mm. layer. The blank plasma sample obtained before the injection of the dye was first read against distilled water. After conversion of percentage transmission into values for optical density, the plasma volume was calculated. Hematocrit was determined by centrifugation of a specimen for 20 minutes at 3,000 r.p.m. and was corrected for plasma trapping by a factor of 0.96. Blood volume was calculated by the formula:

$$BV = \frac{PV}{100\text{-}H \times F\ \text{cells}} \times 100$$

where BV is blood volume, PV is plasma volume, and H is corrected hematocrit. F cells is a factor of 0.88 to correct peripheral to total body hematocrit.

**Procedure.** An initial determination of blood pressure and blood volume was made. Immediately thereafter, a continuous infusion of l-norepinephrine in the amount of 4.0 mcg. per kilogram of body weight per

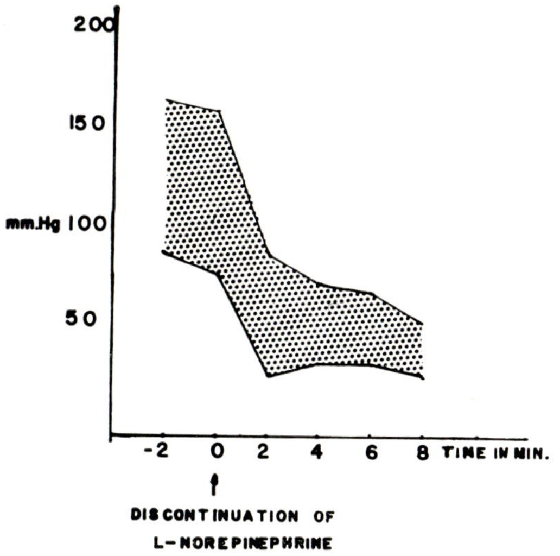


**Fig. 1.** Mean change in arterial blood pressure in 8 animals after discontinuation of l-norepinephrine is illustrated. Severe hypotension results from the administration of the drug to these normal anesthetized animals.

minute was begun. The infusion was continued for a period of 100 minutes. Ninety minutes after the beginning of the l-norepinephrine administration, a second sample of arterial blood was drawn, and Evan's blue dye injected. At 100 minutes, the final plasma volume determination was carried out and the l-norepinephrine discontinued.

In a group of 10 animals, arterial blood pressure was monitored continuously before, during, and after a 100-minute period of l-norepinephrine administration (4 mcg. per kilogram of body weight per minute). Eight minutes after discontinuation of the drug, blood pressure fell from the hypertensive levels maintained by l-norepinephrine to a mean of 54/28 mm. Hg (Fig. 1). Two animals in this group showed a progressive diminution in arterial blood pressure and died within 2 hours after completion of the experiment. An illustration of this severe hypotensive response in a single dog is given in Fig. 2.

In pilot experiments on a preliminary series of 8 animals, an average decrease in plasma volume of 29.3 ± 12.5 per cent was noted. However, in these animals a volume of 400 to 800 ml. of saline solution was employed as a vehicle in the administration of

*Levophed, Winthrop Laboratories, New York 18, N. Y.
†Supplied through the courtesy of Eli Lilly & Company, Indianapolis, Ind.

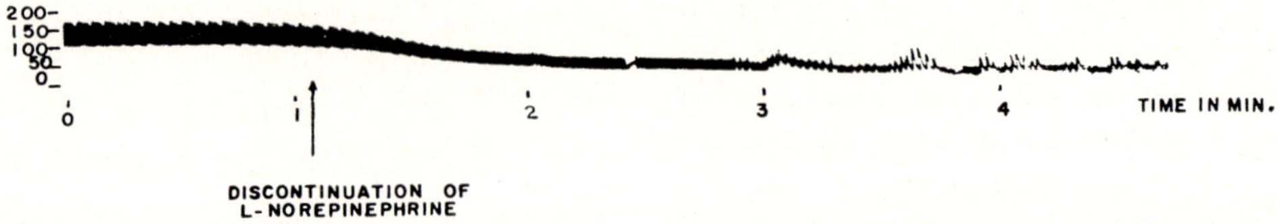


**Fig. 2.** Severe hypotension occurs in a normal anesthetized dog on withdrawal of l-norepinephrine after a 100-minute infusion at 4 mcg. per kilogram per minute.

l-norepinephrine. The hematocrit of these animals decreased by an average of 4.6 per cent. It was apparent that the large volume of saline solution administered may have had a physiologic effect independent of the effect of the drug.

In another series of 8 animals, the experimental protocol was modified by elimination of the large amounts of saline solution which were used as a vehicle for the l-norepinephrine. In each experiment, the total dose of the drug was carried in 30 ml. of normal saline solution. Changes in plasma volume in this series of animals are presented in Table I. It is noted that there was a mean decrease in plasma volume of 26.8 ± 18.5 per cent. Associated with this decrease was a mean increase in hematocrit

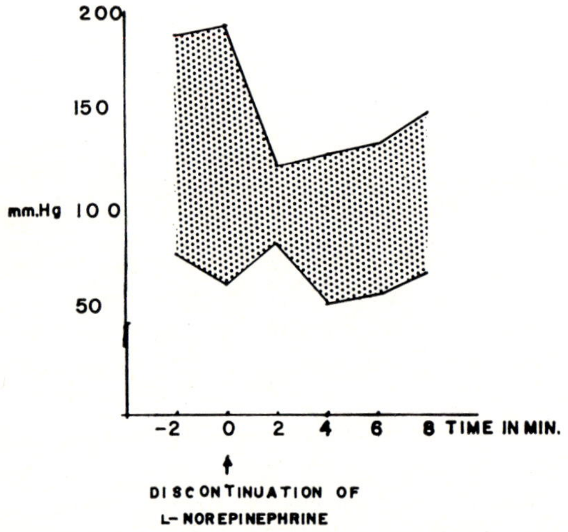


**Fig. 3.** When the l-norepinephrine infusion was discontinued in these 8 animals, an amount of dextran equal to 15 per cent of estimated blood volume was rapidly infused intravenously. In contrast to results illustrated in Fig. 2, the arterial blood pressure was maintained at normal levels in these animals.

of 4.2 per cent. Calculated total blood volume diminished on an average of 21.2 ± 23.0 per cent.

All animals showed an elevation in arterial pressure with the beginning of the l-norepinephrine infusion. At the end of the infusion, a volume of dextran equal to 15 per cent of estimated blood volume was infused intravenously within 2 to 3 minutes. In contrast to the previously described animals (Fig. 1), these animals did not develop a secondary hypotension. Blood pressure returned from the hypertensive levels maintained by the drug to normal and remained there (Figs. 3 and 4).

**Control experiments.** Six animals were employed in several types of control experiment. When the infusion did not contain l-norepinephrine, there was no significant change in either plasma volume or hematocrit (Table I). Since l-norepinephrine had been demonstrated to produce hypovolemia in normal dogs, it was decided to test the drug in the presence of shock due to hemorrhage. Although the drug elevated arterial blood pressure in the presence of hemorrhagic shock, it caused an average loss of plasma volume of 18.8 per cent in addition to that already lost by hemorrhage.

These control experiments were interpreted as indicating that factors in the protocol other than the l-norepinephrine did not produce the observed changes in plasma volume. They also indicate that l-norepinephrine causes the same loss in plasma volume in dogs in hemorrhagic shock as it does in normal anesthetized dogs.

## DISCUSSION

These experiments on the effect of intravenous l-norepinephrine in the normal dog show a striking diminution in plasma volume. The mechanism of this decrease in plasma volume is not definitively demonstrated in this study. A possible explanation may lie in the diminished volume of the peripheral vascular bed caused by the intense vasoconstriction. Such vasoconstriction might be postulated to "squeeze" fluid from the intravascular to the extravascular space. Some support of this theory is seen in the changes that were noted in hematocrit. The hemoconcentration that occurred during the experimental infusion (Table I) does suggest that fluid is leaving the intravascular compartment. The well-recognized discrepancy in peripheral hematocrit and total body hematocrit makes it difficult to correlate quantitatively the loss of plasma and the rise in hematocrit. Calculation of red blood cell volume changes from the data in Table I shows a mean decrease of 13.1 per cent. However, this does not represent a statistically significant change from the volume present before l-norepinephrine administration.

It was clearly demonstrated that in animals in which severe hypotension occurred on discontinuation of the drug, normal arterial pressure could be restored by the rapid infusion of dextran or whole blood. This is presumptive evidence that in at least some clinical situations, the hypotension seen after discontinuation of l-norepinephrine may be due to the drug itself, rather than to the underlying disease for which the drug was originally administered.

This experimental study is not completely analogous to the clinical situation, since each of the animals had a relatively normal cardiovascular status before the administration of the drug. It can only be presumed that the hypovolemia-inducing action of l-norepinephrine demonstrated in normal animals would be present also in clinical situations in which the drug is used. It was demonstrated that hypovolemia due to hemorrhage could be further aggravated by the intravenous administration of l-norepinephrine. Despite the fact that blood pressure was maintained at more normal levels after hemorrhage, administration of the drug caused a further diminution of plasma volume.

The results of this study have been applied clinically in a limited number of patients. Because of the emergency nature of situations which require the intravenous administration of l-norepinephrine, it has not been possible to obtain blood volume measurements under controlled conditions in patients, despite several attempts. During the course of this study, there were 6 surgical patients in whom l-norepinephrine was employed as a temporary measure to maintain arterial pressure and in whom attempts to reduce the rate of administration of the drug in a stepwise fashion resulted in progressive hypotension. In each patient, the effort to discontinue the drug was made only after it was considered that the underlying cause of the patient's initial hypotension had been corrected. In these 6 patients, it was possible to discontinue instantaneously the administration of l-norepinephrine by the rapid intravenous injection (3 to 5 minutes) of from 300 to 500 ml. of blood or dextran.

It should be pointed out that in clinical practice the volume of blood or plasma expander infused is less than that demonstrated to be lost in the present experimental study. Smaller volumes have been found adequate

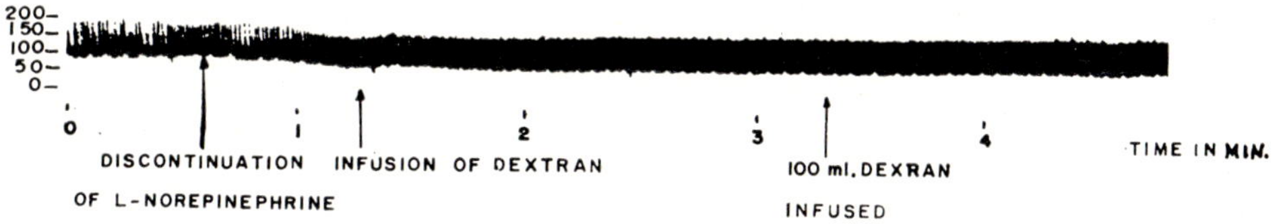


**Fig. 4.** When arterial blood pressure began to decline 1 minute after cessation of l-norepinephrine infusion, dextran infusion restored blood volume and prevented hypotension.

**Table I.** *Changes in plasma volume, blood volume, and hematocrit after l-norepinephrine infusion*

| *Experiment No.* | *Weight* | *Plasma volume* | | | *Blood volume* | | | *Hematocrit* | | |
|---|---|---|---|---|---|---|---|---|---|---|
| | | *Before* | *After* | *% change* | *Before* | *After* | *% change* | *Before* | *After* | *% change* |
| 1 | 18.3 | 950 | 588 | -38 | 1,610 | 1,030 | -36 | 46.1 | 48.0 | +1.9 |
| 2 | 17.0 | 956 | 924 | - 3 | 1,630 | 1,700 | + 4 | 46.1 | 51.8 | +5.7 |
| 3 | 18.0 | 1,128 | 745 | -34 | 1,950 | 1,330 | -32 | 48.0 | 49.8 | +1.8 |
| 4 | 20.3 | 1,445 | 772 | -47 | 2,220 | 1,230 | -45 | 39.8 | 42.2 | +2.4 |
| 5 | 17.0 | 812 | 661 | -19 | 1,440 | 1,210 | -16 | 49.9 | 51.8 | +1.9 |
| 6 | 12.0 | 657 | 644 | - 2 | 1,120 | 1,280 | +14 | 47.0 | 56.6 | +9.6 |
| 7 | 12.5 | 465 | 232 | -50 | 930 | 478 | -49 | 56.7 | 58.5 | +1.8 |
| 8 | 13.0 | 547 | 433 | -21 | 910 | 822 | -10 | 45.2 | 53.8 | +8.6 |
| Average | | | | -26.8 ± 18.5 (S.D.)* | | | -21.2 ± 23.0 (S.D.)* | | | +4.2 ± 3.2 (S.D.)* |
| *Controls* | | | | | | | | | | |
| 1 | 17.5 | 517 | 508 | - 2 | 1,050 | 1,030 | - 2 | 56 | 56 | 0 |
| 2 | 9.7 | 464 | 462 | 0 | 1,080 | 1,050 | - 3 | 49 | 50 | +1 |
| Average | | | | - 1.0 | | | - 2.5 | | | +0.5 |

*A statistically significant change.

and appear to reduce the danger of hypervolemia. Many clinical situations have been encountered in which this rapid infusion would not permit the discontinuation of l-norepinephrine. In these circumstances, it is considered that the hypotension is due not to the hypovolemia caused by l-norepinephrine, but rather to the underlying circulatory disorder which originally necessitated the administration of the drug.

The findings of this investigation are not surprising if one considers the fact that l-norepinephrine is, in its properties and effects, closely related to epinephrine. In dog experiments, Bainbridge and Trevan[1] found that sudden discontinuation of epinephrine infused intravenously resulted in shock. Similar observations are recorded by Freeman and associates who demonstrated that the intravenous administration of epinephrine resulted in hypovolemia. The latter investigators found an average decrease in plasma volume of 30.6 per cent after a 90-minute infusion of epinephrine, a result which is strikingly similar to the results of the present study with l-norepinephrine. They found evidence that at least part of the fluid loss with epinephrine is into the lumen of the intestinal tract.

It is interesting to recall the history of epinephrine which, after its discovery, was heralded as a panacea for shock. Within a short time, it was proved to be contraindicated in the treatment of this condition. Epinephrine itself produces hypovolemic shock. The initial enthusiasm which many physicians had for l-norepinephrine waned when it was realized how few patients survive its administration. The present study demonstrates that l-norepinephrine, like epinephrine, produces hypovolemic shock. We do not wish to take a position regarding the relative indications for, and merits of, epinephrine and l-norepinephrine. Rather, we wish to point out the interesting historical and physiologic parallel between the two drugs for thoughtful consideration.

## SUMMARY

A study of the effects of l-norepinephrine on arterial pressure and plasma volume has been carried out in a series of 34 anesthetized, splenectomized dogs.

1. After sudden discontinuation of the drug, a decline in arterial blood pressure to hypotensive levels may occur. This observation confirms clinical experience.

2. The intravenous administration of l-norepinephrine (4 mcg. per kilogram of body weight per minute) for a period of 100 minutes in a series of 8 dogs resulted in an average decrease in plasma volume of 26.8 per cent.

3. These data demonstrate that the hypo-

tension encountered with the sudden discontinuation of l-norepinephrine may be due to hypovolemia caused by the drug. This secondary hypotension may be prevented by rapid infusion of blood or dextran (15 per cent of estimated blood volume) immediately after withdrawal of l-norepinephrine. Clinical confirmation of this observation has been obtained.

## REFERENCES

1. Bainbridge, F. A., and Trevan, J. W.: Memorandom upon surgical shock and some allied conditions, Brit. M. J. **1:** 381, 1917.
2. Chinard, F. P.: Estimation of plasma volume by dye dilution method, Chicago, 1951, The Year Book Publishers, Inc., p. 38.
3. Crawford, E. S., and Haynes, B. W., Jr.: The use of norepinephrine in the treatment of hypotension associated with common surgical conditions, Am. Surgeon **19:** 191, 1953.
4. Freeman, N. E.: Decrease in blood volume after prolonged hyperactivity of the sympathetic nervous system, Am. J. Physiol. **103:** 185, 1933.
5. Freeman, N. E., Freeman, H., and Miller, C. C.: The production of shock by the prolonged continuous injection of adrenaline in unanesthetized dogs, Am. J. Physiol. **131:** 545, 1941.
6. Goldenberg, M., Apgar, V., Deterling, R., and Pines, K. L.: Norepinephrine (Arterenol, Sympathin N) as a pressor drug, J. A. M. A. **140:** 776, 1949.
7. Holtz, P.: Die Wirkstoffe des sympathiko-adrenalen Systems; zum 50 jährigen Jubilaüm der ersten Hormonsynthese, Deutsche med. Wchnschr. **80:** 2, 1955.
8. Maloney, J. V., Jr., Elam, J. O., Handford, S. W., Balla, G. A., Eastwood, D. W., Brown, E. S., and Ten Pas, R. H.: Importance of negative pressure phase in mechanical respirators, J. A. M. A. **152:** 212, 1953.
9. Ritchie, H. D.: Acute peripheral circulatory failure in surgical cases; treatment with l-noradrenaline, Brit. M. J. **1:** 371, 1956.
10. Saave, J. J.: Surgical injury and peripheral circulatory failure, M. J. Australia **43:** 97, 1956.
11. Von Euler, U. S.: Noradrenaline in hypotensive states and shock; physiological aspects, Lancet **2:** 151, 1955.
12. Von Euler, U. S.: Physiologic basis for the clinical use of noradrenaline, Ann. Int. Med. **41:** 699, 1954.

# Treatment of malignant retroperitoneal sarcomas with use of the second-look approach

WARD O. GRIFFEN, JR., M.D.
CONRAD B. JENSON, M.D.
STUART W. ARHELGER, M.D.
OWEN H. WANGENSTEEN, M.D.
MINNEAPOLIS, MINN.
*From the Department of Surgery, University of Minnesota Medical School*

The most effective treatment for primary retroperitoneal tumors is surgical excision. Obviously, the earlier the diagnosis is made and operation carried out, the better the results. Unfortunately, since most of the sarcomas are slow-growing tumors, they are quite large at the time of their initial finding. The recurrences of these tumors are also slow growing and often reach enormous size before the recurrence is suspected and operative treatment is again undertaken. It is a well-known fact, however, that soft-tissue tumors which occur on the extremities can be treated effectively and for a long period of time with multiple excisions as the recurrences are noted.

In 1949, because of the disparity in accomplishment in lymph-node positive and lymph-node negative patients, the idea of performing reoperation on the lymph-node positive patients with cancer of the stomach, colon, or rectum from 4 to 9 months after the original procedure was suggested.[2] The second operation was carried out at a time when the patient was asymptomatic. It has been found that approximately 50 per cent of the lymph-node positive cancer patients still harbored residual tumor at the occasion of the first re-entry of the abdomen. Some successes with this method suggested the possibility that the second-look procedure might be employed to increase the number of survivors in patients with large retroperitoneal sarcomas in which the cure rate, at least in our experience, was negligible. In fact, the records of this hospital failed to show any cures in patients operated upon for sarcomatous retroperitoneal tumors prior to employment of second-look procedures.

Our plan of treatment of retroperitoneal sarcoma with the second-look approach is essentially the same as that for the visceral cancers. Because of the slow growth of most of these tumors, the interval between "looks" had been lengthened to 10 to 18 months. In addition, some of the reoperations have been carried out because of signs and symptoms of recurrence.

## RESULTS

To date 8 patients have been treated according to the second-look principle (Table I) and of these 8 patients, 2 are alive and well over 5 years since the original procedure. Two patients are living and well 7 and 8 years, respectively, since the primary procedures, although the last look in both cases was positive. There is 1 patient who died 11 years after the original operation and 1 year after his last look, which had been negative. One patient died of the sarcoma after 11 years and the other 2 patients died of their disease in less than 5 years.

## CASE REPORTS

**Case 1.** On March 22, 1948, Mrs. N. H., a 63-year-old woman had an excision of a large

The Second-Look Program is sponsored by the Minnesota Division of the American Cancer Society and the Malignant Disease Research Fund.

Received for publication Oct. 10, 1960.

rhabdomyosarcoma which involved the left ovary and retroperitoneal space. In addition, the tumor was intimately adherent to the sigmoid colon and a loop of ileum. The uterus and left tube and ovary were excised but no intestine was removed. Postoperatively, deep x-ray therapy was given to the area. Eight months later, on Nov. 8, 1948, the patient returned to the hospital with small bowel obstruction due to a residual tumor mass located at the ileocecal junction and involving the tissues at the level of the bifurcation of the inferior vena cava. The terminal ileum and cecum were excised, along with the neoplasm, after which deep x-ray treatment again was given. Another exploratory operation was performed on July 15, 1949, at a time when the patient was

**Table I**

| *Patient* | *Age at onset* | *Sex* | *Type of sarcoma* | *Original operation* | *Status at reoperations and date** | *Present status* | *Length of survival after original procedure (yr.)* |
|---|---|---|---|---|---|---|---|
| N. H. | 63 | F | Rhabdomyosarcoma | Excision of mass with adherent left ovary, tube, and overus (1948) | Positive, 1948; negative, 1949 | Living and well | 12 |
| G. C. | 54 | M | Fibrosarcoma | Excision of original retroperitoneal tumor (1950) | Positive, 1953; positive, 1953; positive, 1953; positive, 1953; negative, 1953 | Living and well | 10 |
| R. E. | 18 | M | Myxochondrosarcoma | Subtotal excision of tumor involving right ilium (1953) | Hemipelvectomy, 1954; positive, 1954; positive, 1955; positive, 1955; positive, 1956; negative, excision of recurrence in 1959 and again in 1960 | Living | 7 |
| E. N. | 47 | M | Liposarcoma | Removal of tumor from left retroperitoneal area and left nephrectomy (1952) | Positive, 1955; negative, 1956; positive, 1957; positive, 1959 | Living and well | 8 |
| E. H. | 42 | F | Myxosarcoma | Excision presacral myxosarcoma (1947) | Positive, 1954; positive, 1955 | Dead of sarcoma | 11 |
| M. S. | 63 | M | Fibrosarcoma | Excision of mass from left perirenal area (1947) | Positive, 1956; negative, 1957 | Dead, no sarcoma at autopsy | 11 |
| I. Z. | 64 | F | Leiomyosarcoma | Excision of large tumor from pelvis (1955) | Positive, 1957; positive, 1957 | Dead of sarcoma | 4 |
| J. P. | 53 | M | Fibrosarcoma | Removal of 6 Kg. mass along with the right kidney | Positive, 1958; positive, 1958 | Dead postoperatively without recurrence | 1 |

*As of Oct. 1, 1960.

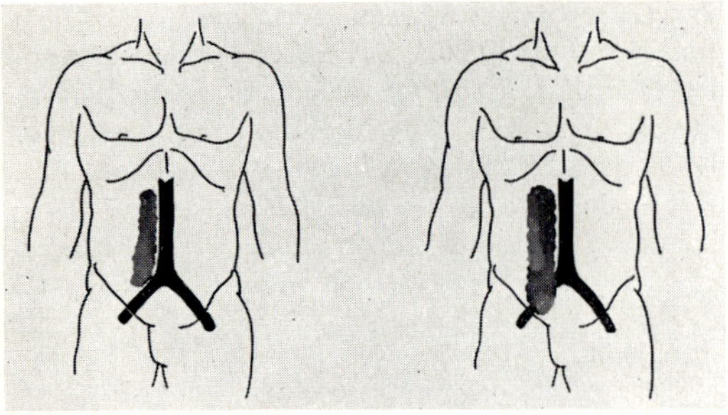

*A* *B*

**Fig. 1.** Case 2. Schematic representation of first 2 procedures performed at another hospital. *A,* First operation, July, 1950 (excision of retroperitoneal fibrosarcoma). *B,* Second operation, February, 1953 (partial excision of symptomatic residual tumor).

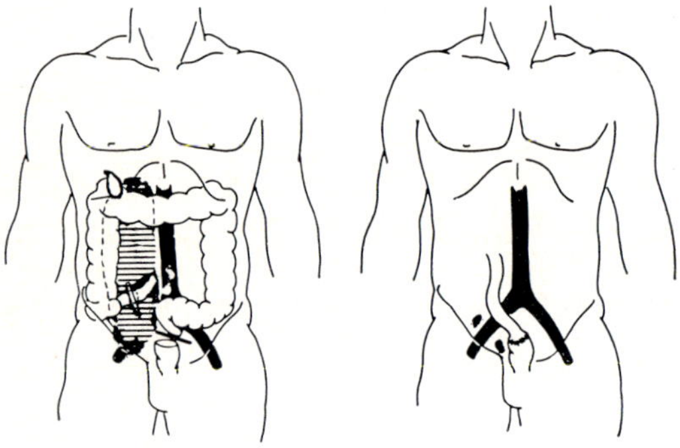

*A* *B*

**Fig. 2.** Case 2. First 2 operations performed at University of Minnesota Hospitals. *A,* Third operation, May, 1953 (excision of all gross residual tumor). *B,* Fourth operation, December, 1953 (second look).

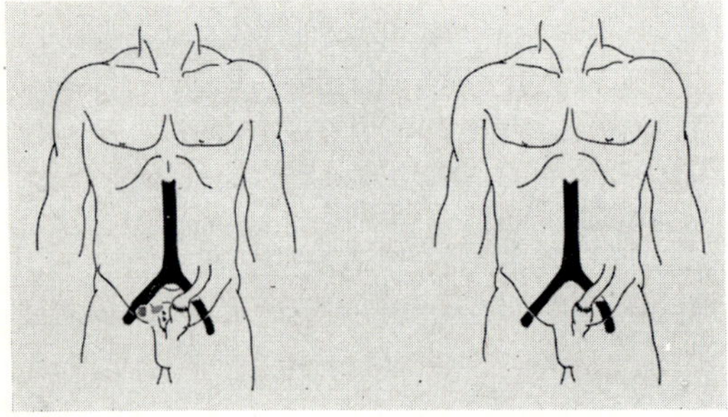

*A* *B*

**Fig. 3.** Case 2. Eventual attainment of a cancer-free state at sixth operation. *A,* Fifth operation, June, 1954 (third look). *B,* Sixth operation, June, 1955 (fourth look, negative).

completely asymptomatic and without clinical evidence of recurrence. At this time, no residual tumor was found. This patient was last seen in August, 1960, 12 years, 5 months, after the original procedure, and 11 years, 1 month, after the last negative look. At this time, she has no clinical signs of residual tumor and appears completely well. The last look was negative.

**Case 2.** On Aug. 3, 1950, Mr. G. C., a 54-year-old white man, underwent an exploratory laparotomy, at which time a large retroperitoneal sarcoma was removed. The patient remained well until March, 1953, when an enlarging abdominal mass was again noted along with urinary symptoms. Subtotal resection of the mass was carried out and the patient was then referred here for more definitive therapy. At the time of his first admission to this hospital, he had evidence of local recurrence of a tumor, but no evidence of distant spread. On May 13, 1953, the patient underwent excision of a huge fibrosarcoma (6.4 Kg.) which extended from the level of the gall bladder and liver to the deep pelvis. The entire colon and 75 cm. of the terminal ileum were removed, along with the tumor. Intestinal continuity was established by ileoproctostomy.

On Dec. 16, 1953, a second-look procedure was carried out while the patient was asymptomatic. Two small nodules of recurrence at the lateral aspect of the right common iliac artery and over the second sacral vertebra were found and removed. The patient remained well and on June 28, 1954, another exploratory procedure was carried out. At this time, 1 lymph node medial to the right common iliac vein was positive, although many biopsies gave negative results. On June 2, 1955, the patient underwent exploratory operation and no recurrence was found in the 16 specimens of tissue removed for histologic examination. The patient, when last seen in August, 1960, was completely free of symptoms and without clinical evidence or recurrence. He does have persistent diarrhea because of extensive loss of ileum and colon.

**Case 3.** On. Oct. 15, 1953, R. E., an 18-year-old man, underwent palliative excision of a myxochondrosarcoma which involved the inner aspect of the right ileum. Eight months later, the right femoral nerve became paralyzed by massive tumor recurrence which involved the right wing of the ileum and right pelvis. At this time, he was referred to the University of Minnesota Medical Center. No evidence of pulmonary metastasis was observed on roentgenographic examination. On May 24, 1954, a right hemipelvectomy was performed. Postoperatively, he did well and 5 months later, on Oct. 26, 1954, during an asymptomatic phase, a second-look operation was performed. At this time, 3 fairly well circumscribed masses of tumor were present. One was located in the pelvis, fixed between the tissues of the rectum and the base of the bladder; another was adherent to the descending colon; and a third mass was encountered at the inferior margin of the right kidney. All these nodules were excised, without sacrifice of any organs.

Five months later, on April 5, 1955, when the patient was without evidence of clinical recurrence, a third look was performed. At this time, the only evidence of tumor was limited to two 3 cm. nodules to the right of the urinary bladder. These were excised without sacrifice of the organ. Eight months later, in December, 1955, a fourth look was carried out at a time when the patient was asymptomatic. Two small tumor nodules were found opposite the second and third lumbar vertebrae and these were removed. In addition, a number of additional biopsy specimens were taken, all of which were negative. Finally, on May 31, 1956, during an asymptomatic period, the patient underwent a fifth look and no evidence of cancer was found grossly. Two biopsies of suspicious areas yielded negative histologic results.

The patient remained well until October, 1959, when he developed a swelling at the hemipelvectomy site. At a sixth look he was found to have a recurrence arising from the amputated ilium which intimately involved the mesocolon on the right side of the abdomen. The ilium was re-resected and the right colon and its mesentery were excised with re-establishment of intestinal continuity. The patient has returned since with recurrence in the right ilium treated by complete removal of the remaining ilium.

**Case 4.** On October 27, 1952, Mr. E. N., 47-year-old man, had excision of a liposarcoma of the left retroperitoneal area along with a left nephrectomy. He remained well until 3 years later, when a left lower quadrant mass was noted. The patient was referred to the University of Minnesota Medical Center for excision of the mass. On Nov. 8, 1955, at a second exploratory operation, a 4.5 Kg. mass of recurrent liposarcoma was removed. On Aug. 7, 1956, the patient was clinically well and without evidence of recurrence. At that time, a third look failed to reveal any recurrent cancer.

However, in June of 1957, the patient returned with a large left upper quadrant mass and partial large bowel obstruction. On June 21, 1957, an 8 cm. tumor of the left upper quadrant, along with 2 smaller masses located on the left diaphragm and several smaller tumors in the retropancreatic area were removed. They proved to be liposarcoma. Postoperatively, irradiation was given to the patient. He remained well until May, 1959, when he returned because of a mobile right upper quadrant mass. An intravenous pyelogram showed an upward displacement of the right kidney. At operation on May 27, 1959, a 10 by 15 by 20 cm. recurrent mass arising from the perirenal fat was excised. In addition, 2 other suspicious areas, one in the anterior abdominal wall of the left upper quadrant and the other in the sigmoid mesocolon, were removed. These were negative for malignancy on microscopic study. The patient continues to be well without evidence of recurrence and has returned to work. The last look was positive.

**Case 5.** Mrs. E. H., a 42-year-old woman, had undergone excision of a presacral myxosarcoma in 1947. She was then well for 5½ years, and then the abdomen began to enlarge markedly. She was first seen here in December, 1954, at which time a recurrence of the mass was obvious. Roentgenographic examination failed to show any evidence of distant metastases and on Dec. 24, 1954, a 3 Kg. tumor was excised, along with a portion of the terminal ileum and colon.

The patient remained well until August, 1955, when a left suprapubic mass was noted. Exploratory operation on Aug. 25, 1955, confirmed the presence of a large 8 cm. tumor mass adherent to the bladder, abdominal wall, and the small bowel in several areas. In addition, there were 7 smaller tumor nodules attached to the small bowel and 5 similar nodules on the liver surface, none of which invaded more than 1 cm. in depth. All these nodules were excised along with a 62 cm. segment of ileum which was densely adherent to the main tumor mass. The patient refused the proposal of an additional look procedure in March, 1956. On Feb. 4, 1958, the patient died after a steadily worsening course from residual sarcoma.

**Case 6.** Mr. M. S., a 63-year-old man, was operated upon in 1947 for a left upper quadrant tumor which was partially excised. The pathologic diagnosis at that time was hypernephroma. Irradiation of the area followed the operation and the patient was without medical aid until July, 1956, when he noted an abdominal mass and left upper quadrant discomfort associated with anorexia. The patient then saw his own physician, who advised a second course of irradiation, and he was then referred to the University of Minnesota Medical Center.

On physical examination, there was a large, hard, fixed left abdominal mass. Laboratory tests at that time showed a slight anemia and a small left pleural effusion with no function of the left kidney on intravenous pyelogram, although the right appeared to function normally. On review of the slides originally taken, the opinion of the pathologist was that the lesion was a fibrosarcoma. Prior to operation a tap of the pleural effusion was negative for tumor cells.

On Aug. 14, 1956, the patient again underwent exploratory operation and a 10 Kg. retroperitoneal fibrosarcoma was excised along with the left kidney, left colon, a portion of the duodenum, and the left adrenal gland. A paravertebral and periaortic node dissection was also performed.

He was then followed closely and had gained 20 pounds and felt well when he was admitted early in 1957 for a second look. On Feb. 8, 1957, the patient again underwent exploratory operation and no tumor was found although 9 biopsy specimens were taken. The patient was last seen here 8 months after the operation (October, 1957) at which time he was feeling well and had gained some weight. A chest roentgenogram taken at that time was negative for metastases. The patient died suddenly on Jan. 10, 1958, and autopsy failed to disclose the cause of death. No residual tumor was found.

**Case 7.** On Jan. 6, 1955, Mrs. I. Z., a 64-year-old woman, sought medical advice with regard to an obvious pelvic tumor. A 13 by 14 by 12.5 cm. mass was removed from the deep pelvis and a pathologic diagnosis of a leiomyosarcoma was made. The patient remained well until March, 1957, when a mass in the upper abdomen again was noted. Physical examination at this admission showed the upper abdominal mass and also a recurrence of the pelvic mass. Consequently, on April 8, 1957, the pelvic mass was excised and the woman was well until August, 1957, when a right upper quadrant mass was noted. On Sept. 18, 1957, a 30 by 20 by 9 cm. tumor attached to the right lobe of the liver was excised along with a portion of the liver. A smaller right lower quadrant tumor was also removed. The patient was given cobalt therapy postoperatively. She did well, was gaining weight, and was admitted for a second look in the fall of 1958. On physical examination, a right upper quadrant mass was found. Chest roentgenogram and planigrams showed bilateral pulmonary metastases. The patient was not operated upon. On March 22, 1959, the patient died from the leiomyosarcoma.

**Case 8.** On Oct. 23, 1957, J. P., 53-year-old man, noted right upper quadrant pain and an abdominal mass of relatively short duration. On Nov. 6, 1957, a large fibrosarcoma which weighed 6 Kg., involved the edge and inferior surface of the liver, surrounded the right kidney, involved the adventitia of the aorta and iliac vessels, and extended into the pelvis, was removed. The patient remained well until 3 weeks prior to a second admission on Feb. 10, 1958, at which time an enlarging right upper quadrant mass was palpated. Excision was performed and the patient received cobalt radiotherapy postoperatively. Five months later, the patient was re-admitted with right upper quadrant pain and bilateral lower extremity edema. While in hospital the patient became jaundiced; partial bowel obstruction at the level of the duodenum also was present. On July 18, 1958, exploratory operation was carried out and massive recurrence throughout the abdomen was found. The larger of these recurrences was removed in order to relieve the obstruction of the upper jejunum. The patient's jaundice relented somewhat postoperatively, but *Candida albicans* septicemia supervened and the patient died with residual neoplasm Aug. 7, 1958.

## DISCUSSION

Pack and his associates[1] state that retroperitoneal tumors are famous for their propensity to recur after radical excision. In many of the studies of retroperitoneal tumors in the literature, the average 5-year survival rate is less than 10 per cent and the 10-year survival rate is even more discouraging. It was the poor results in this hospital with these neoplasms that persuaded one of us (O. H. W.) to implement the second-look procedure in these cases.

The general plan of treatment has been the same as with the second-look procedure for abdominal visceral cancers. The one exception has been that since the sarcomatous lesions are slow growing, the interval between operations has been longer, ranging from 12 to 18 months. Also, because of the fact that large tumors in this area are often resectable even when symptomatic, there have been a number of so-called second-looks performed at a time when the patient had obvious recurrent disease.

Fourteen of the 25 repeat exploratory procedures performed in the 8 cases reported were undertaken during a symptomatic phase. However, only patients who underwent such procedures when asymptomatic are living and well today! In fact, two of these patients have been declared "negative" at a final look and are without clinical evidence of disease more than 10 years since the original operation. One hospital death occurred after operation in this group of patients, a mortality rate of 12.5 per cent by patient and 4 per cent by operation.

## SUMMARY

The experience with use of the second-look program for large retroperitoneal sarcomas suggests definitely that this method of treatment has merit in the surgical attack upon such tumors. The high salvage rate obtained is heartening and warrants the attention of the profession.

## ADDENDUM

Since this report was written, 2 patients (Cases 3 and 4) have undergone additional operations. The patient in Case 3 was operated upon on March 1, 1961, and recurrent tumor in the right ilium was removed as well as a segment of involved small bowel. He was examined in June, 1961, at which time he was well and without evidence of recurrence. The patient in Case 4 returned in late October, 1960, with bowel obstruction. Re-exploration of the abdomen on Nov. 4, 1960, showed far-advanced disease which was the cause of the obstruction. He died on Dec. 18, 1960, after discharge from the hospital.

## REFERENCES

1. Pack, G. T., and Tabak, E. J.: Collective review; primary retroperitoneal tumors, Surg. Gynec. & Obst. **99:** 209, 313, 1954.
2. Wangensteen, O. H.: Cancer of the colon and rectum, Wisconsin M. J. **48:** 591, 1949.

# Paper electrophoresis of extracts from normal and malignant human breast tissue

W. W. SLACK, B.M., B.CH. (OXON), F.R.C.S. (ENG.)
With the technical assistance of E. T. Hoppe
CHICAGO, ILL.
*From the Department of Surgery, University of Illinois College of Medicine*

Electrophoresis of the serum in patients with cancer has been carried out by many workers and no specific changes in the protein spectrum have been found. There is usually a diminished amount of albumin and an alteration in the alpha component of the globulin fraction, but these are both changes that are found in other diseases marked by debilitation and tissue breakdown.

The protein content of both normal and malignant tissues has been studied in animals and human beings, but there have been practically no reports on the electrophoretic pattern of proteins extracted from human malignant tissue. This paper will describe a method to show that there is a difference in protein structure between normal and malignant tissue in at least 1 human organ.

Barry,[2] working with rat fibrosarcoma extracts, produced electrophoretic patterns which were reproducible from one preparation to another. Miller and associates[4] demonstrated marked differences in the electrophoretic pattern between normal muscle and rhabdomyosarcoma in mice. Abrams and Cohen,[1] working with normal human tonsillar tissue, produced patterns from the tissue extract which had some similarities to those of human serum.

## MATERIALS AND METHODS

The normal and malignant tissues were obtained from specimens that had been removed surgically. The tissue was stored at +4° C. until it was analyzed. The analysis was always performed on the day the specimen was removed from the patient. One gram of carcinoma or 1 Gm. of normal breast tissue from which as much fat as possible was removed was cut into small pieces with scissors and washed twice with 0.89 per cent saline solution to remove as much blood and lymph as possible. The tissue was then mixed with fine sand (sand flour, 325 mesh) and 3 ml. of 0.89 per cent saline solution and was ground with a mortar and pestle. The resulting mixture was then centrifuged at a relative centrifugal force of 620 for 20 minutes, and the supernatant fluid was submitted to electrophoretic analysis with Beckman's Spinco apparatus. A Veronal buffer of pH 8.6 and ionic strength 0.075 was used; a sample of 0.05 ml. was applied to the paper strip and a constant current of 2.5 Ma. was connected for 16 hours. The paper strips were then stained by the alcoholic bromphenol blue method and scanned by an Analytrol.

## RESULTS

Thirteen portions of carcinoma of the breast and 13 portions of normal breast tissue have been studied. In 11 cases the carcinoma and the sample of normal tissue were obtained from the same patient. In the malignant tissue extract the average albumin content according to electrophoretic analysis was 19.62 per cent compared to 80.38 per cent globulin. In the normal breast tissue the albumin content was 51.82 per cent

Supported by Grant No. 3482 from the United States Public Health Service.
Received for publication Oct. 24, 1960.

compared to 48.28 per cent globulin (Table I). The globulin portion was divided into fractions with similar mobilities to serum globulin fractions and there was found to be no great difference in the proportions of the globulin fractions between the malignant and normal tissues (Table II). It was possible to estimate the percentages in only 8 of the 13 normal portions of tissue, as there was no distinct dividing mark between the various fractions in the other 5. Alpha$_1$ and alpha$_2$ were estimated together, as any division of the two would have been arbitrary.

## DISCUSSION

By the use of paper electrophoresis it has been shown that there is approximately 4 times as much globulin as albumin in malignant breast tissue, and approximately equal proportions in normal breast tissue. Other

**Table I.** *The percentage of albumin and globulin in malignant and normal breast tissue*

| Case No. | Age (yr.) | Histologic grading of tumor | Carcinoma | | Normal tissue | |
|---|---|---|---|---|---|---|
| | | | Albumin | Globulin | Albumin | Globulin |
| 1 | 48 | Well differentiated | 18.8 | 81.7 | 51.5 | 48.5 |
| 2 | 52 | Average | 15.7 | 84.3 | 52.6 | 47.4 |
| 3 | 44 | Average | 3.6 | 96.4 | 50.4 | 49.6 |
| 4 | 56 | Average | 21.3 | 78.7 | 59.1 | 40.9 |
| 5 | 32 | Undifferentiated | 23.3 | 76.7 | 64.5 | 35.5 |
| 6 | 71 | Well differentiated | 32.6 | 67.4 | 46.2 | 53.8 |
| 7 | 71 | Undifferentiated | 26.2 | 73.8 | — | — |
| 8 | 58 | Average | 21.4 | 78.6 | 47.3 | 52.7 |
| 9 | 64 | Average | 11.5 | 88.5 | 66.7 | 33.3 |
| 10 | 77 | Well differentiated | 33.3 | 66.7 | 50.0 | 50.0 |
| 11 | 79 | Average | 17.7 | 82.3 | 46.2 | 53.8 |
| 12 | 53 | Average | 15.1 | 74.9 | — | — |
| 13 | 58 | Average | 14.5 | 85.5 | 41.5 | 58.5 |
| 14 | 21 | — | — | — | 42.5 | 57.5 |
| 15 | — | — | — | — | 55.2 | 44.8 |
| | | Mean | 19.6 | 80.4 | 51.8 | 48.2 |

**Table II.** *The percentage of the different globulins in malignant and normal breast tissue*

| Case No. | Carcinoma | | | Normal tissue | | |
|---|---|---|---|---|---|---|
| | Alpha$_1$ and alpha$_2$ | Beta | Gamma | Alpha$_1$ and alpha$_2$ | Beta | Gamma |
| 1 | 24.3 | 21.1 | 54.6 | 25.0 | 25.0 | 50.0 |
| 2 | 22.7 | 22.7 | 54.6 | — | — | — |
| 3 | 18.2 | 39.5 | 42.3 | 32.2 | 25.4 | 42.4 |
| 4 | 24.6 | 22.2 | 53.2 | 37.2 | 23.3 | 39.5 |
| 5 | 23.2 | 23.2 | 54.6 | — | — | — |
| 6 | 20.7 | 22.4 | 56.9 | 27.8 | 30.6 | 41.6 |
| 7 | 34.2 | 25.0 | 40.8 | — | — | — |
| 8 | 15.2 | 54.5 | 30.3 | 24.1 | 34.5 | 41.4 |
| 9 | 25.9 | 33.4 | 40.7 | — | — | — |
| 10 | 23.8 | 35.7 | 40.5 | 28.5 | 34.3 | 37.2 |
| 11 | 26.2 | 22.6 | 55.2 | — | — | — |
| 12 | 22.2 | 33.0 | 44.8 | — | — | — |
| 13 | 30.0 | 28.3 | 41.7 | — | — | — |
| 14 | — | — | — | 22.0 | 28.0 | 50.0 |
| 15 | — | — | — | 34.6 | 19.2 | 46.2 |
| Mean | 24.1 | 33.4 | 42.5 | 27.5 | 31.3 | 41.2 |

normal and malignant tissues, including stomach and colon, were also studied, but no such significant differences were found. Both the normal and the malignant tissues gave an electrophoretic pattern which tended to resemble the pattern of malignant breast tissue. This suggests that human tumor extracts may have similar electrophoretic patterns, but that normal tissues show considerable variation, as has been shown by Greenstein[3] in animals. Degree of histologic differentiation did not appear to exert any influence on the type of electrophoretic pattern.

## CONCLUSIONS

By the use of paper electrophoresis it has been shown that there is 4 times as much globulin as albumin in human breast carcinomas, whereas normal breast tissue contains approximately equal proportions of the two proteins. However, the relative amounts of the various globulin fractions in both the malignant and normal breast tissue are not significantly different.

### REFERENCES

1. Abrams, A., and Cohen, P. P.: Electrophoretic and chemical characterization of human lymphoid tissue and calf thymus, J. Biol. Chem. **177:** 439, 1949.
2. Barry, G. T.: Cytoplasmic proteins. A partial physical and chemical characterization of cytoplasmic proteins, Cancer Res. **10:** 694, 1950.
3. Greenstein, J. P.: Biochemistry of cancer, New York, 1954, Academic Press, Inc., p. 461.
4. Miller, G. L., Green, E. U., Miller, E. E., and Kolb, J. J.: Studies on the proteins of rhabdomyosarcoma and normal muscle of mice. II. Electrophoretic and viscerometric measurements, Cancer Res. **10:** 148, 1950.

# Observations on the isolated ileal loop as a substitute in urinary tract operations

A. C. ABBOTT, M.D.
T. K. GOODHAND, M.D.
W. J. McCORD, M.D.
J. T. MacDOUGALL, M.D.
WINNIPEG, MANITOBA
*From the Departments of Surgery, University of Manitoba and St. Boniface Hospital, and The Abbott Clinic*

The advent of radical pelvic surgery has, in the past decade or more, been an impetus to urologists to find newer and better methods of preserving kidney function. We are now truly living in the age of spare parts. Two years ago, we presented a series of experiments which illustrated total replacement of the ureter by a loop of ileum.[3] A dog with a solitary kidney and an ileal ureter remained in good health with normal electrolyte balance for 1 year. Fig. 1 is an actual photograph of a solitary kidney, ileal ureter, and normal dog bladder in one of our animals.

Our original idea was conceived as a possible method of total replacement of the ureter in children with adynamic ureters. Swenson has used approximately the same procedure, but decreased the size of the ileum by resecting the antimesenteric portion of the ileum throughout its length to reduce the absorptive surface. He advised its use only in unilateral cases when repeated tests had proved that there was no peristalsis. All patients had been repeatedly checked before this procedure was embarked upon. No patients with bilateral disease would be treated until those with unilateral disease had been observed for several years. He favored and performed a one-stage procedure.[4] It could be a valuable method in cases in which ureteropyeloplasty has failed. Postoperative strictures would be less likely to occur because of the similarity in size of the ileum and pelvis.

The practical application of this procedure, slightly modified, is shown in Fig. 2. This is a drawing of the kidney in a young girl, 21 years of age, with a solitary adynamic hydronephrotic kidney. Two attempts to reconstruct the pelviureteral junction had failed. Pyuria was constant and uncontrollable, in spite of all forms of medication. We believed that the persistent pyuria was due to pooling of the infected urine in the lower dilated calyx.

A loop of ileum 12 inches long was anastomosed to the lower calyx. This was done retroperitoneally behind the ascending colon. The distal end of the ileal loop was anastomosed end-to-side to the bladder. It is now 3 years since this procedure was carried out. The urine is negative except for an occasional pus cell. The electrolyte determinations taken on June 17 were blood urea nitrogen, 16.8 mg. per cent; serum chlorides, 100 mEq. per liter; serum potassium, 3.92 mEq. per liter; and serum sodium, 142 mEq. per liter. The patient is in exceedingly good health.[1]

Partial replacement must not be forgotten. It is an excellent procedure for replacing the lower part of the ureter that has been destroyed or damaged after radical pelvic op-

Supported by grant from the Banting Research Foundation.
Presented at The Canadian Urological Associated Meeting, Banff Springs Hotel, Banff, Alberta, July 1-3, 1960.
Received for publication Oct. 28, 1960.

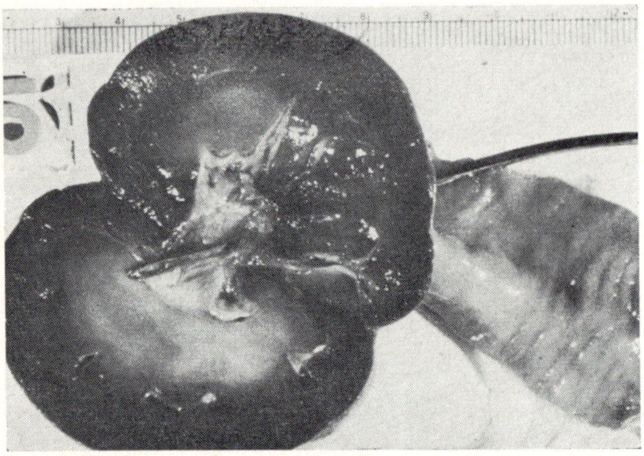

**Fig. 1.** The solitary kidney from one of our animals has been bisected and the ileal ureter opened. Note the normal appearance of the kidney and ureter. A probe has been passed from the ileal ureter into the kidney pelvis.

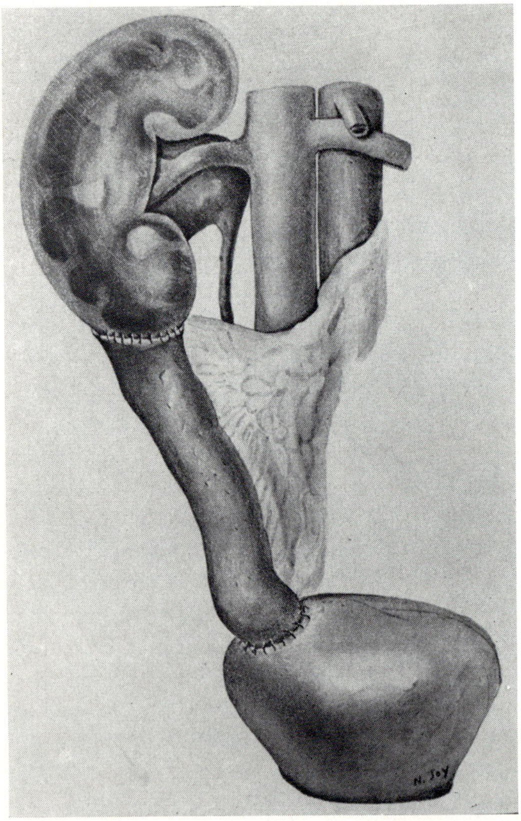

**Fig. 2.** Drawing of solitary adynamic hydronephrotic kidney of 21-year-old girl. Dependant drainage has been established by a calycoileoneocystostomy. The ureter was left as a safety valve. Before the procedure, pyuria had been constant.

erations, trauma from stones, inflammatory lesions, and obstruction due to fibrosis after radiation. Fig. 3 illustrates a case in which the lower end of the ureter was partially constricted after irradiation for carcinoma of the cervix. Hydronephrosis was present. A loop of ileum 6 inches long was inserted between the distal end of the ureter and the bladder. It is interesting to note that 18 months were required for this kidney to completely recover its original condition.

Bricker[2] and many others have used a loop of ileum to replace the bladder. The distal end of the ileal loop is brought out through the abdominal wall as a urinary fistula. This necessitates the wearing of some form of receptacle to catch the urine. We conceived the idea of inserting the distal end of the ileal loop into the sigmoid, thus eliminating the external urinary fistula. The peristaltic action of the ileum might protect the kidney against ascending infection, which occurs so frequently, when the ureters are transplanted directly into the sigmoid. If ascending infection were prevented, the electrolyte balance might still be a problem because of the increase in absorptive area due to the use of the sigmoid for drainage. We were unaware of the work of Turnbull and Higgins[5] at the Cleveland Clinic, a report of which was published just prior to the time we began our study.

We conducted a series of experiments on dogs to test the feasibility of the procedure. Our approach to the subject changed as we proceeded with each experiment. Five experiments were performed.

## METHODS

**Experiment 1.** In a one-stage procedure, a loop of ileum 6 inches long was isolated. The proximal end was closed. A valve was fashioned at the distal end and inserted into the sigmoid, just above the peritoneal reflection, after the method of Turnbull. Both ureters were transplanted into the ileum. All animals died within 4 days. Three deaths were considered to be due to anesthesia. The remaining 5 dogs died with symptoms suggestive of uremia. No gross pathologic lesion was found at postmortem examination. Histologic studies showed a protein exudate into Bowman's capsule and the proximal tubules.

A staged procedure seemed advisable. In the original procedure of Turnbull and Higgins[5] the ileal bladder was decompressed temporarily by a Foley catheter inserted into the proximal end of the ileal loop. In our first experiment, edema in the valve due to operative trauma and possibly mild constriction at the junction with the sigmoid may have in reality formed a closed loop. If the ileal loop were formed as a first step and time allowed for edema to subside and proper drainage of the loop into the sigmoid to become established, the outcome might be different.

**Experiment 2.** In a three-stage procedure, an isolated loop of ileum was formed as in Experiment 1, and inserted into the sigmoid. After 1 month, as a minimum, the right ureter was transplanted into the ileal loop. The loop was observed to be draining well. The animals did well and had no fever. No electrolyte imbalance occurred. Intravenous pyelograms were normal. The question arose as to whether the animals would survive if we performed a left nephrectomy. This would make them comparable to our animals which lived with one kidney and an ileal ureter. In our original experiment, the urine drained into the bladder, while in the latter the urine drained into the sigmoid. A left nephrectomy was performed in 2 dogs as a third stage.

In our first dog, the blood urea level rose to 240 mg. per cent in 7 days and 270 mg. per cent in 10 days. The animal gradually developed loss of appetite, muscular twitching, nausea, vomiting, and loss of weight. It died on the tenth day. The second dog followed an identical course. The electrolytes otherwise remained normal. Postmortem examination showed no gross pathologic lesion. Fig. 4 is a postmortem photograph of the solitary kidney which was taken from the second dog. Histologic studies of the solitary kidney from both animals showed only a protein exudate into Bowman's capsule (Fig. 5). In the tubules there was also a protein exudate and well-marked vacuolation (Fig. 6).

**Experiment 3.** In a three-stage procedure, an isolated ileal loop was formed and in-

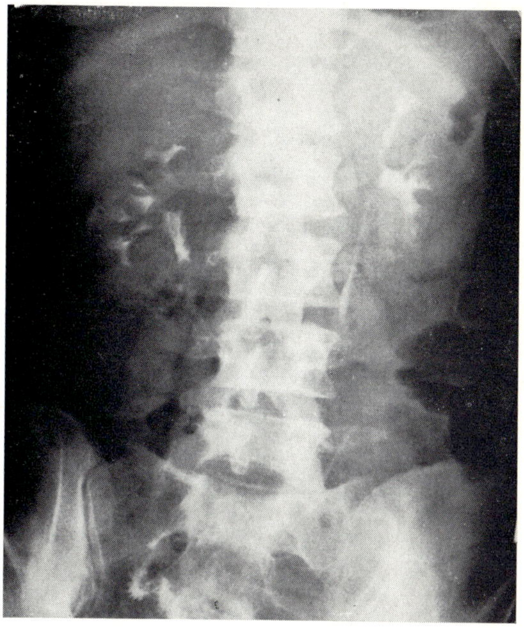

**Fig. 3.** An intravenous pyelogram, 18 months after replacement of the lower third of the ureter with an isolated loop of ileum. Thirty minutes after injection of Skiodan the patient voided and film was taken. The ileal ureter is faintly visualized. Note excellent cupping in minor calyces.

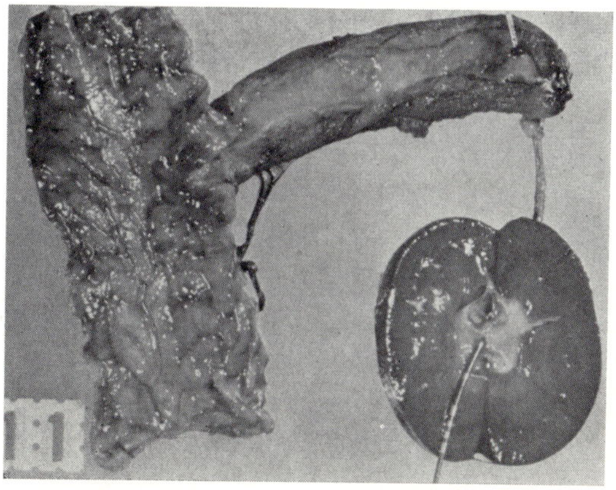


**Fig. 4.** On bisection of the kidney, no gross pathologic process was visible. The pelvis was normal. A probe is shown passed from the kidney down the normal ureter into the ileal bladder.

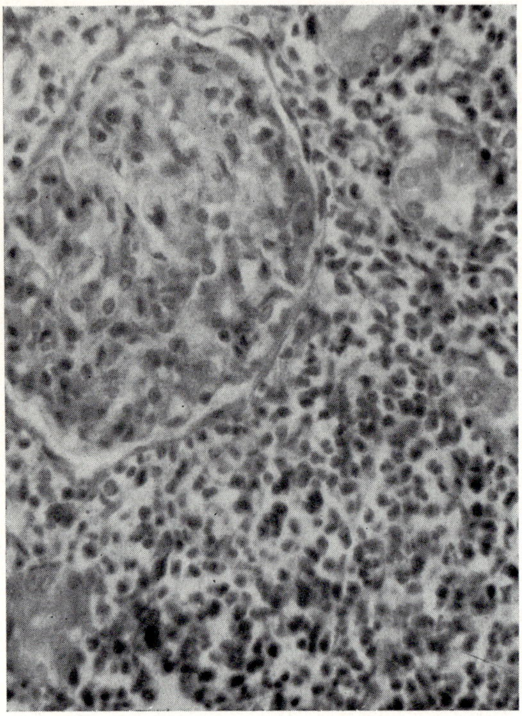

**Fig. 5.** Membranous glomerulitis. The capillaries have thickened walls. The surrounding stroma contains chronic inflammatory infiltrate. (×400; reduced ⅔.)

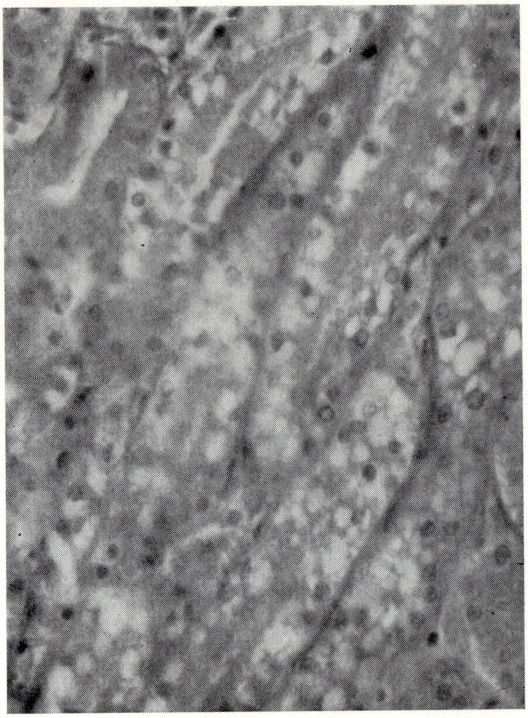

**Fig. 6.** Renal tubular changes. There is vacuolation of the tubular epithelium and protein material within the tubular lumina. (×400; reduced ⅔.)

serted into the sigmoid. The right and left ureters were transplanted into the ileal loop at monthly intervals.

The first dog (No. 12) died in 7 days. The changes in the electrolyte levels from the time of the second transplantation were blood urea nitrogen (BUN), 18 to 169 mg. per cent; serum chlorides, 110 to 109 mEq. per liter; serum sodium, 142 to 145 mEq. per liter; serum potassium, 3.6 to 3.1 mEq. per liter; and carbon dioxide combining power, 21 to 19 mEq. per liter.

The second animal lived 28 days. The electrolyte changes were BUN, 20 to 330 mg. per cent; serum chlorides, 127 to 83 mEq. per liter; serum sodium, 156 to 119 mEq. per liter; and carbon dioxide combining power, 21 to 6 mEq. per liter.

The pathologic reports on the 2 dogs were quite different. In Dog 12 a stricture of the right ureter was found, 1 inch long, close to the ileal loop. The kidney was one-half the size of the opposite kidney. Pathologic section showed protein tubular casts in the kidney and a chronic periureteritis partially obliterating the lower end of the ureter. Dog 14 had an acute bilateral necrotizing papillitis, acute pyelonephritis, and acute ureteritis (Figs. 7 and 8).

**Experiment 4.** Our fourth experiment was a two-stage procedure. An ileal loop was isolated as in the previous experiment. One month or more later, both ureters were transplanted into the ileal loop. In 7 animals the postoperative course was similar. The blood urea nitrogen rose gradually, but not as fast or as high as when the ureters were transplanted at different stages. The serum chloride and serum sodium levels remained normal. Serum potassium levels fell to a low normal. Carbon dioxide combining power fell in all cases and the average was 13.8 mEq. per liter. The average life of these animals was 23 days postoperatively.

The eighth dog followed a different pattern. There was an interval of 7 weeks be-

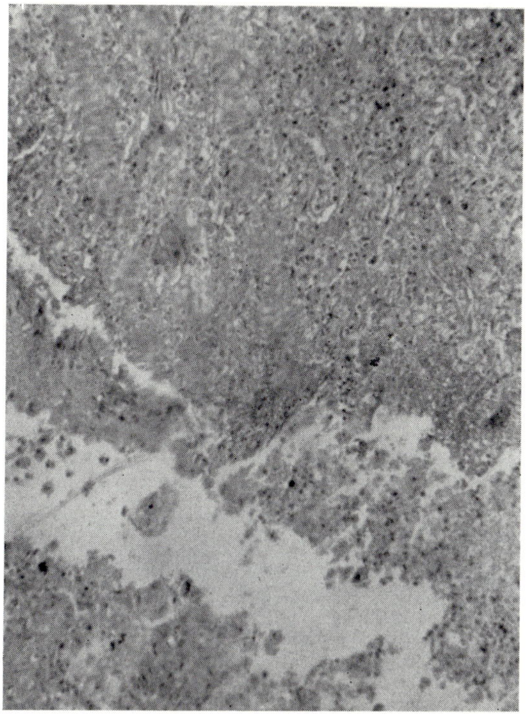

**Fig. 7.** Necrotizing papillitis. Note the ulceration of the renal papillae and the acute inflammatory reaction present. (×150; reduced 2/9.)

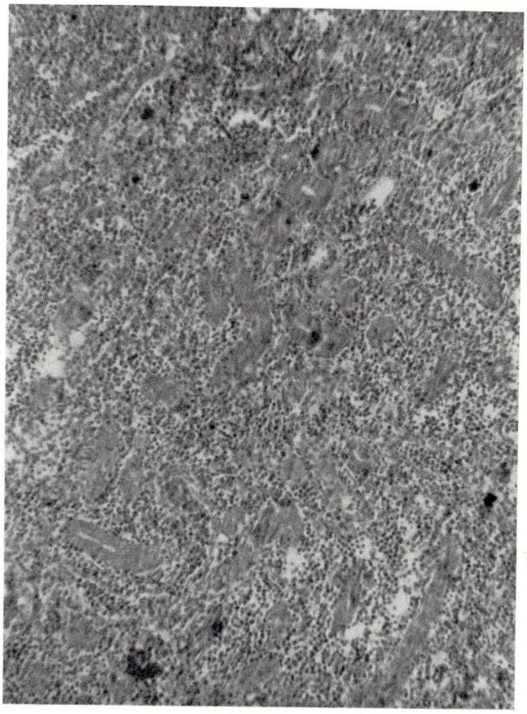

**Fig. 8.** Acute pyelonephritis. The interstitial tissues are diffusely infiltrated by acute inflammatory cells. (×150; reduced 2/9.)

tween the ureteral transplants. The BUN at the first stage was 11 mg. per cent, and 20 mg. per cent at the second stage. Weekly BUN determinations were taken for 6 weeks, and the results were 26, 50, 52, 42, 36, and 32 mg. per cent. The carbon dioxide combining power fell as the BUN rose, and rose as it fell. The animal began gaining weight, looked better, and ate better. We discontinued our electrolyte studies temporarily, and the animal died suddenly, 2½ months after the ureteral transplant. Postmortem examination showed an incomplete stricture at the lower end of the right ureter. Histologic section of the right kidney showed an acute pyelitis and ureteritis. On the left side there was a huge hydroureter and a chronic pyelitis and ureteritis.

**Experiment 5.** On Nov. 17, 1959, we formed an ileal loop attached to the sigmoid in animal (No. 21). Bilateral ureteral transplants of both ureters were carried out on December 22. The animal weighed 22 pounds. December 28, the BUN was 50 mg. per cent. Repeat electrolyte studies were performed on January 18 and were BUN, 76 mg. per cent; serum potassium, 3.9 mEq. per liter; serum sodium, 145 mEq. per liter; serum chlorides 120 mEq. per liter; and carbon dioxide combining power, 13 mEq. per liter, the animal weighed 18 pounds and was in poor condition. On January 19, we again operated on this dog, disconnected the ileal loop from the sigmoid, and performed an end-to-side anastomosis of the ileal loop to the bladder. On March 30, 1960, the animal had regained its normal weight. The BUN had fallen to 28 mg. per cent. The animal looked well. On June 25, the BUN was 22 mg. per cent and the animal weighed 23 pounds.

## SUMMARY

This is a preliminary report. We are aware that our series is not large enough to allow us to draw definite conclusions. We do believe that some pertinent observations are in order.

1. A loop of ileum acting as a urinary conduit between the ureter or kidney and bladder is compatible with a normal existence in animals and human beings. The electrolyte balance is not disturbed.

2. A loop of ileum used as a urinary conduit between the ureters and sigmoid has 3 disadvantages, (1) the reabsorptive area is greatly increased (ileal loop and sigmoid), (2) the urinary tract is exposed to an ascending infection from the sigmoid, and (3) the pressure in the urinary tract is increased because the pressure in the sigmoid is greater than that normally found in the urinary tract.

3. The active peristalsis in the isolated ileal loop does not prevent ascending infection.

4. A valve at the distal end of the ileum does not prevent ascending infection but appears to prevent regurgitation of fecal content into the ileal loop.

5. A valve at the distal end of the ileum appears to at least temporarily add an obstructive element to the free flow of urine from the ileal loop into the sigmoid.

6. Transplantation of the ileal loop into the sigmoid is followed by infection of various degrees in the ureter, kidney pelvis, and kidney. This tends to electrolyte imbalance and a rapid and great rise in the BUN, and terminated in death in all our animals.

7. The process can be reversed by disconnection of the ileal loop from the sigmoid and re-insertion of it into the urinary bladder. The animal regains its health and electrolyte balance is re-established.

8. It appears that diverting urine by way of an ileal conduit to the sigmoid is not a satisfactory procedure.

9. Formation of the ileal bladder as a first stage and allowing time for all edema to subside appeared to increase the life span of our experimental animals.

The biochemical, bacteriologic, and pathologic studies were graciously carried out gratis by the Departments of Biochemistry, Bacteriology, and Pathology at the St. Boniface Hospital. All photographic work was done by Mr. Stanford, in the Photographic Department at the St. Boniface Hospital. Miss Nancy Joy, medical artist from the School of Medicine, made the diagram for our case of calycoileoneocystostomy. Johnson & Johnson donated suture material to help us with our project. We are grateful to a number of anaesthetists, particularly Dr. Joseph Hayakawa, who donated their services for our operations.

## REFERENCES

1. Abbott, A. C., Goodhand, T. K., and MacDougall, J. T.: Hydronephrosis in a solitary kidney—its treatment by nephro-ileoneocystostomy, J. Urol. **84:** 505, 1960.
2. Bricker, E. M.: Substitution for the urinary bladder by the use of isolated ileal loops, S. Clin. North America **36:** 1117, 1130, 1956.
3. Goodhand, T. K., Abbott, W. E., Abbott, A. C., MacDougall, J. T., and Anderson, E. N.: The use of an isolated ileal loop for total replacement of the ureter, Canad. J. Surg. **3:** 24, 1959.
4. Swenson, O.: Personal communication, Feb. 4, 1958.
5. Turnbull, R. B., and Higgins, C. C.: Ileal valve pouch for urinary tract diversion, Cleveland Clin. Quart. **24:** 187, 1957.

# The percutaneous transhepatic approach of the portal vein in man in the determination of patency of splenorenal shunts

LUCIANO DE CASTRO SILVA, M.D.
JOÃO BAPTISTA SÃO THIAGO, M.D.
ERMETTIS FERRARINI, M.D.
FÁBIO SCHMIDT GOFFI, M.D.
SÃO PAULO, BRAZIL
*From the Department of Surgery, Hospital das Clínicas, University of São Paulo*

A great advance was achieved in the treatment of portal hypertension with the introduction of portacaval shunts. With the aid of splenoportography, we can easily determine the patency of a portacaval shunt, but for the splenorenal shunt we have to rely upon operative portography. This is one argument voiced by those who are opposed to the use of splenorenal shunts. We cannot demonstrate the patency of the splenorenal shunt with the same ease as we demonstrate that of the portacaval shunt. Bierman and his group[2] in 1952 presented the percutaneous transhepatic puncture of the portal vein and in 1955[1] performed catheterization of the portal vein, but they concluded that catheterization was inadequate for portography because of the small caliber of the catheter that had to be used. Since 1958,[3] we have been performing the percutaneous transhepatic puncture of the portal and hepatic veins in all cases of portal hypertension in order to determine the portal and hepatic pressures and draw blood for biochemical studies. The rationale of the percutaneous transhepatic approach of the portal or hepatic veins is that the portal vein branches after entering the liver, with one branch for the right lobe and the other for the left. In a transverse cross section which passes through the xiphoid process, the largest branches of the portal vein are seen to lie to the right of the midline in an angle which varies from 10 to 45 degrees (Fig. 1). At this point the liver is in direct contact with the anterior abdominal wall, so that no organ is interposed between. If at this point a long needle is inserted through the skin at an angle of 20 degrees to the right, one of the branches of the portal vein will probably be entered. If the needle is inserted 5 to 10 degrees cranially and 10 to 15 degrees to the right, one of the hepatic veins may be entered. In 17 patients with splenorenal shunts a percutaneous transhepatic approach of the portal vein was tried and portography was performed either directly through the needle or after catheterization of the portal vein.

## TECHNIQUE

The patient, in a fasting condition, was well sedated with a mixture of 100 mg. of Demerol, 25 mg. of chlorpromazine, and 50 mg. of promethazine given intramuscularly 45 minutes before the procedure. The patient was then placed in a supine position on the x-ray table with the hands under the head and the skin was prepared with an antiseptic solution. An infiltration of all the planes of the abdominal wall was carried out with a solution of 1 per cent procaine at the site of puncture which was just to the right of the xiphoid process. The needle, which has to be long and proper for catheterization, was made by one of us. It was

Received for publication Nov. 4, 1960.

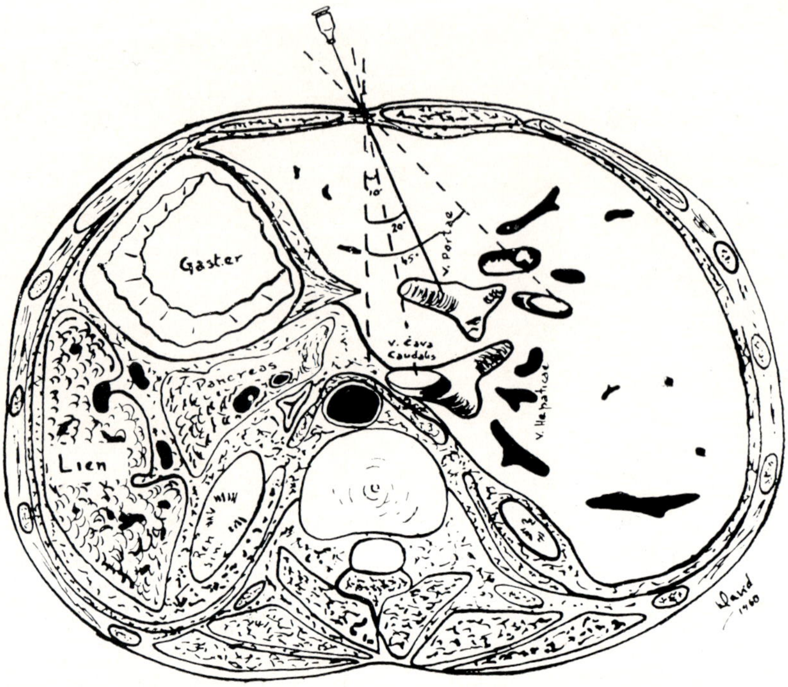


**Fig. 1.** A transverse cross section through the xiphoid process which shows the positions of the large blood vessels in the liver.

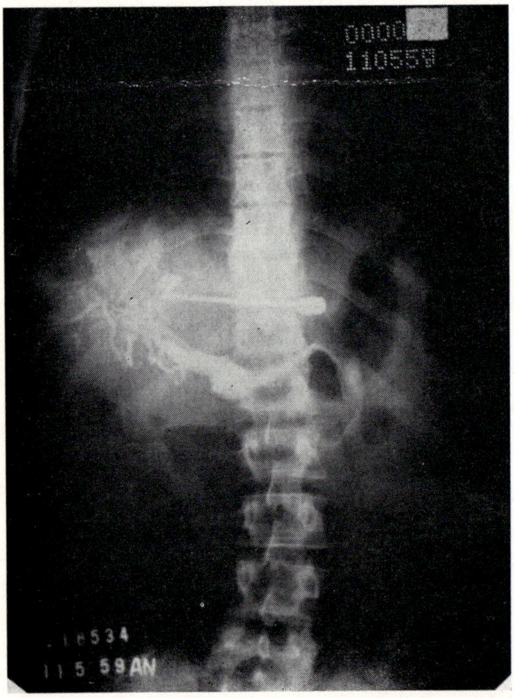

**Fig. 2.** The first film, taken immediately after injection of contrast medium (20 ml.) through polyethylene tube.

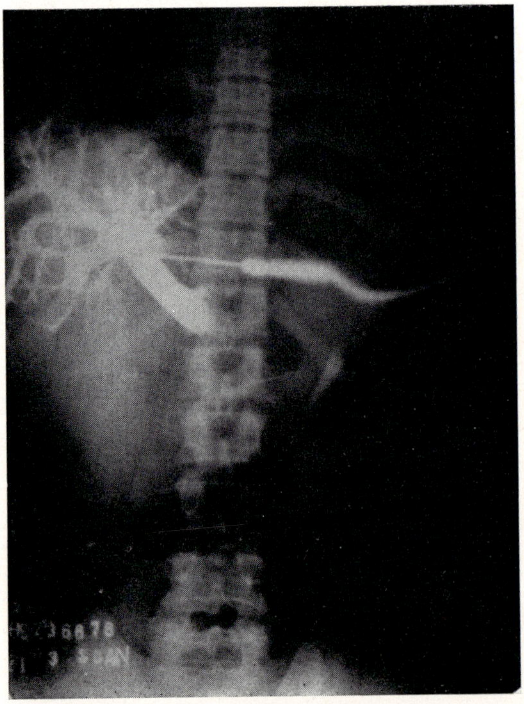

**Fig. 3.** The film taken after the contrast medium had been injected directly through the needle. There has been no backflow to splenic vein.

18 cm. long, 1.8 mm. in diameter, and had a well-curved Huber point. Thus, a catheter threaded through the needle would come out through the point which was already angled to permit progression of the catheter into the vein. Without this posterior curving of the needle point it would not be possible to thread a catheter of sufficient width through the needle into the vein. A No. 60 polyethylene catheter was used. The needle was inserted completely into the liver mass at an angle of 20 degrees to the right. A syringe was adapted to the needle and the needle then slowly pulled back while the syringe was being aspirated. Blood flowing into the syringe indicated that the needle had penetrated a vein, probably one of the branches of the portal vein. When blood flowed freely in and out of the syringe, it meant that the opening of the needle was in a good position in the vein. Before threading the catheter we had to be sure that the vein punctured was the portal vein. This was very easy to confirm in patients with portal hypertension, even in those who had a splenorenal shunt, since the portal pressure in these cases is much higher than the hepatic pressure. We found the hepatic pressure to vary from 60 to 120 mm. $H_2O$ and was rarely higher than 150 mm. $H_2O$, considering the base line at the posterior axillary line. However, if we were still in doubt venography was performed by injection of a small amount of contrast medium (5 to 10 ml.). The polyethylene tube was then threaded through the needle and easily advanced, down the portal vein, generally going to the splenic vein. Twenty milliliters of contrast medium, such as Opacoron 400, was then injected rapidly through the polyethylene tube with a 20 ml. syringe and the first film was taken just at the end of the injection (Fig. 2). The catheter was then removed and a syringe with an intermediate rubber tube adapted to the needle. Thirty milliliters of the contrast medium was rapidly injected for the second film. The reason that 2 films should be taken is that if the contrast medium is injected directly into the needle, it will not always flow back against

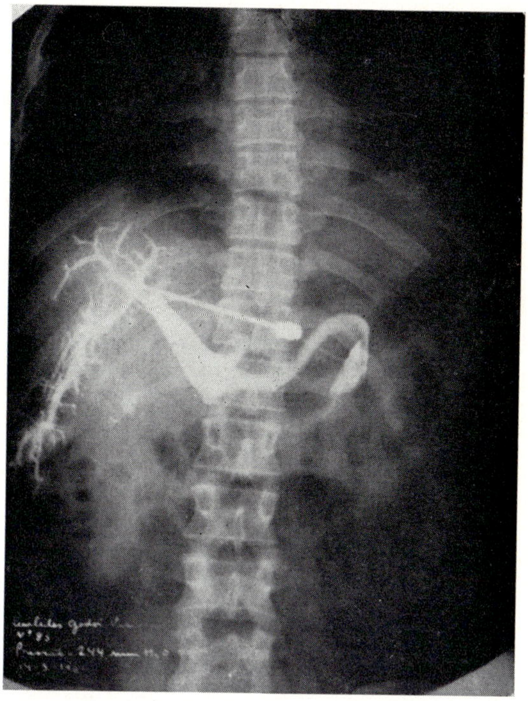

**Fig. 4.** In this instance the contrast medium has been injected through the polyethylene catheter.

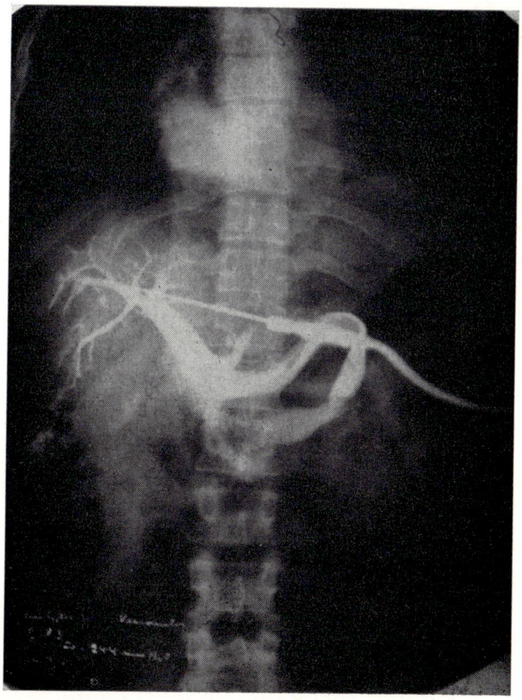

**Fig. 5.** Same patient as in Fig. 4. Contrast medium was injected directly into needle. Portal vein, splenic vein, left renal vein, inferior vena cava, and right atrium of the heart can be seen.

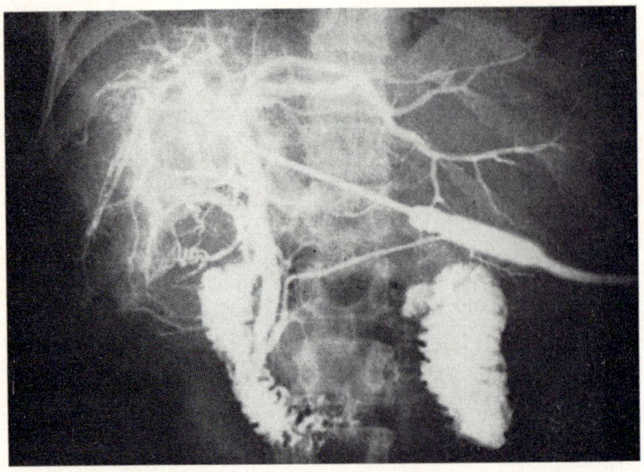

**Fig. 6.** Contrast medium inadvertently injected into biliary tract.

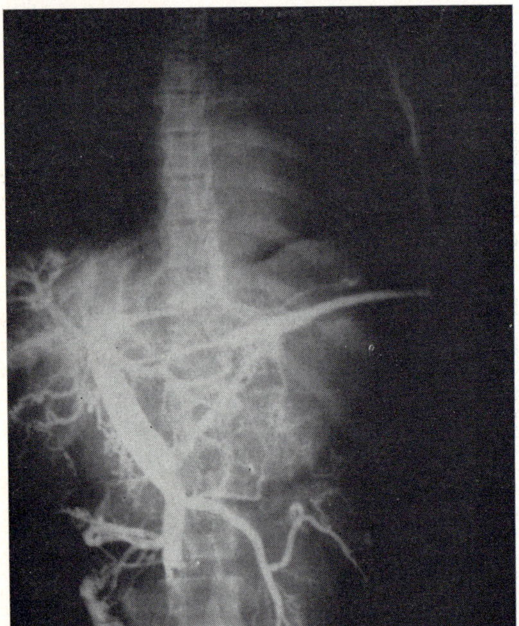

**Fig. 7.** Case in which shunt was thrombosed.

the blood stream in the portal vein to the splenic vein (Fig. 3). If the contrast medium goes by this way through the portal vein to the splenic vein the picture will be much clearer than the one obtained by injection of contrast medium through the polyethylene tube because the relatively small size of the tube will not permit a rapid introduction of the contrast medium (Figs. 4 and 5).

If the portal vein cannot be punctured with the angulation recommended, other angulations can be tried. There will be no harm in performing several punctures while trying to locate the right vein.

## RESULTS

We attempted to demonstrate the splenorenal shunt roentgenographically in 17 patients. In 2 cases we failed to puncture the portal vein. Of the 15 cases in which the portal vein was punctured, catheterization was not attempted in 1 and in 6 cases our catheterization efforts failed, probably because of the small caliber of the vein that was punctured. In these 6 cases venography was performed directly through the needle. In one there was no backflow of the contrast medium along the portal vein to the splenic vein and in the other, the biliary tract was incidentally shown (Fig. 6). In the patient in whom catheterization was not attempted, the introduction of the contrast medium directly through the needle showed a portal vein with many collaterals, such as the left gastric vein, with a venous plexus going to the esophagus, and the superior and inferior mesenteric veins denoting thrombosis of the shunt (Fig. 7). Of the 8 patients catheterized, in 4 the catheter went into the splenic vein and in all of them radiography showed the shunt to be patent. In 1 case the roentgenogram showed the catheter to have entered the biliary tract, and in the remaining 3 cases the shunt was thrombosed. Therefore, of the 17 cases presented, the splenorenal shunt was shown to be patent in 4, it was thrombosed in 6, and in the remaining 7 cases either the portal vein could not be punctured, or it was punctured but could not be catheterized, or the biliary tract was punctured inadvertently.

## DISCUSSION

This method is relatively simple and safe for the patient. There is no serious risk of internal bleeding either due to rupture of the liver substance or bleeding from the tract of the needle in the liver. Bierman[1] refers to 144 punctures without a single accident. We performed 86 punctures with a large needle and no serious bleeding occurred. We have performed punctures of the portal and hepatic veins in the same patient and sometimes have had to make several attempts before the desired vein was punctured. In the few cases in which the patient underwent operation on the day after the puncture, a certain amount of blood was found in the abdominal cavity varying roughly from 50 to 150 ml., but because splenoportography had been performed at the same time in these patients, we could not determine exactly how much of the blood was from the liver and how much was from the spleen. Four patients of the 86 mentioned had small hematemesis after the punctures when they returned to the ward. We attributed this small amount of bleeding to a traumatic hemobiliary fistula caused by the needle. None of them needed blood transfusion, had fall of blood pressure, or had a rise of the pulse rate. None of them experienced bleeding after repeat puncture later in the postoperative period. None of the 17 patients discussed in this paper had any accident. The patients should breathe smoothly and if they have nausea or vomiting the needle should promptly be removed to prevent any possible rupture of the liver substance.

There is no danger of bile peritonitis as long as there is no obstruction to the free flow of bile.

With the patients well sedated as we recommend the puncture is well tolerated and most of them remain practically asleep.

## SUMMARY

We wish to call attention to the fact that one of the arguments against the splenorenal shunt is the fact that one cannot demonstrate the patency of the shunt unless a laparotomy is performed. Using the percutaneous transhepatic puncture of the portal vein complemented with catheterization, we were able to demonstrate the splenorenal shunt by means of roentgenograms. In 17 cases, the patency of the shunt could be demonstrated in 4, the shunt was thrombosed in 6, and in the remaining 7 either the portal vein could not be punctured or catheterized or the biliary tract was inadvertently punctured. The method is a simple and safe one.

### REFERENCES

1. Bierman, H. R., Kelly, K. H., White, L. P., Coblentz, A., and Fisher, A.: Transhepatic venous catheterization and venography, J. A. M. A. **158:** 1331, 1955.
2. Bierman, H. R., Steinbach, H. L., White, L. P., and Kelly, K. H.: Portal venipuncture. A percutaneous transhepatic approach. Proc. Soc. Exper. Biol. & Med. **79:** 550, 1952.
3. de Castro Silva, L., São Thiago, J. B., Ferrarini, E., and Goffi, F. S.: Percutaneous transhepatic puncture of the portal vein. Portographies. Presented at the Meeting of the Department of Surgery of the São Paulo Medical Association, São Paulo, Brazil, April 10, 1958.

# The relation of blood pH to the movement of ammonia into cerebral and peripheral tissues during hypothermia

SAMUEL P. BESSMAN, M.D.
FRIEDA RUDO, B.S.
R ADAMS COWLEY, M.D.
BALTIMORE, MD.
*From the Departments of Pediatrics and Surgery, University of Maryland School of Medicine*

A mechanism for the role of ammonia in hepatic coma has been proposed on the basis of the fact that ammonia is taken up by the peripheral and cerebral tissues as the level of ammonia rises in the blood.[3, 6] The ammonia that enters the brain tissue is considered to react with the alpha-ketoglutarate of the Krebs's cycle to form glutamate. This process depletes the Krebs's cycle of intermediates, which results in the inability of the brain to oxidize substrate and generate energy, and this in turn causes coma. A considerable amount of evidence has now been adduced to support this theory.[1, 2, 4, 7, 8] This mechanism offers an explanation of the toxic intracellular action of ammonia. It was assumed that diffusion over a gradient from blood to tissue was the primary factor in the movement of ammonia into the cells. Another mechanism which stimulates the uptake of ammonia by tissues has been proposed.[17, 23] This is based on the well-known fact that the ammonium ion cannot penetrate tissues, but that unionized ammonia can pass through the cell membrane.[13] It is also known that the proportion of unionized ammonia is increased with alkalinity, and is decreased under acid conditions. It has therefore been suggested that the hyperventilation associated with hepatic coma causes an alkalosis which stimulates the movement of ammonia from the blood into the tissues, thus aggravating the coma.[12] An opportunity to test this attractive hypothesis was offered by a series of observations which we have been making on the events which transpire during refrigeration anesthesia.[10] Over periods of up to 7 hours we have measured the pH and ammonia content of arterial, peripheral venous, and jugular blood, and can therefore correlate arterial-venous differences with the pH of the blood at the moment. Long-term fluctuations of blood pH up to 0.50 U. have been observed, and the concomitant changes in ammonia have been recorded.

Supported by grants from the National Science Foundation, The National Institutes of Health, and No. DA-49-007-MD-674, Office of the Surgeon General, Department of the Army, Washington, D. C.

Received for publication Oct. 10, 1960.

## METHODS

A catheter was threaded through the femoral vein to the bifurcation of the vena cava, well below the renal outflow, to obtain venous blood and arterial blood was sampled through a catheter in the common carotid artery. The jugular bulb blood was sampled through a catheter threaded through the superior vena cava after the chest was opened. Ammonia was measured by a modification of Seligson's procedure[19] in duplicate. The maximum difference from the mean of any pair of observations reported was 0.06 gamma per milliliter. The pH was measured anaerobically at 37° C. by means of a Leeds-Northrop pH meter with a special blood electrode. The patients were put into a hypothermic state by immersion in ice water, about 30 minutes after the first observation. Rectal temperatures of 28° to 32° C. were maintained. Eleven patients were studied. Only data on simultaneously drawn samples of blood are compared, and no values are included which represent the first 2 minutes after release of occlusion of cerebral vessels in view of marked and transient pH variation seen during this period.[5]

## RESULTS

Fig. 1 shows the relation between arterial level of ammonia, arteriovenous difference of ammonia, and pH of the arterial blood. The pH of arterial blood is recorded because this has been proposed as the critical factor in the movement of ammonia into the tissues.[20] The arteriovenous difference of the extremity, in this case the lower limb, varied between a positive value of 0.63 gamma per milliliter and a negative value of approximately 0.15 gamma per milliliter. During the same period the pH of the blood varied between 7.30 and 7.50. The data have been so plotted that if the curves parallel each other, they indicate a positive correlation. It can be seen from Fig. 1 that there is no significant correlation between the fluctuations in peripheral arteriovenous difference of ammonia and the variations in arterial pH. On the other hand, there is a clear correlation between the arterial level and the peripheral arteriovenous difference of ammonia. Fig. 2 is another set of observations which shows a lack of correlation between arterial pH and arteriovenous difference at the same time that a remarkably good correlation can be seen between arterial level and arteriovenous difference. It is also of interest that alteration in the ammonia economy of the extremity covered the range between a positive difference of 0.3 gamma per milliliter to a negative difference of 0.7 gamma per milliliter, so that, as in the first case, a shift in direction of movement of ammonia into the tissues occurred during a time when the arterial pH fluctuated only minimally. The arterial ammonia level which correlated with these shifts varied over a range of approximately 50 per cent.

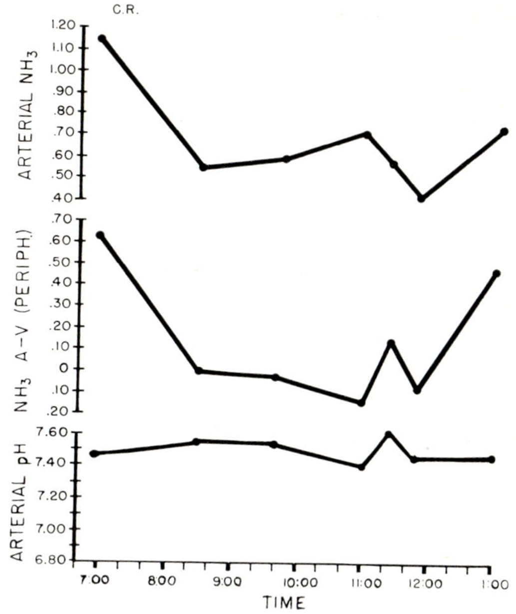


**Fig. 1.** Arterial pH, ammonium concentration, and arteriovenous difference of ammonium across the lower extremity in Patient C. R.

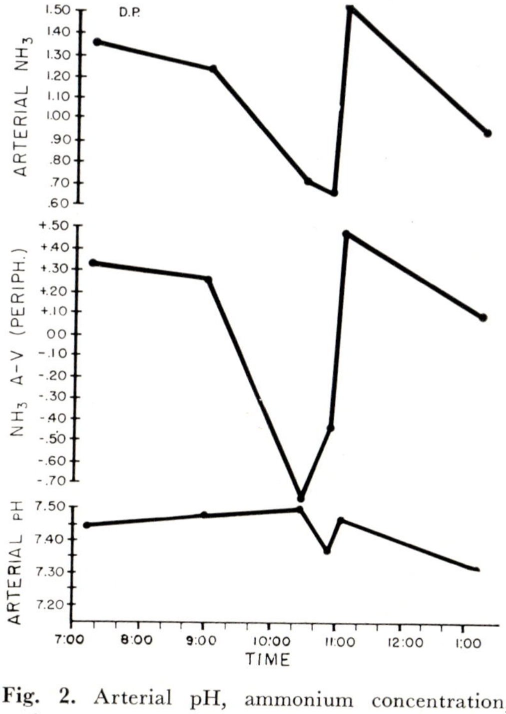


**Fig. 2.** Arterial pH, ammonium concentration, and arteriovenous difference of ammonium across the lower extremity in Patient D. P.

**Table I.** *Protocol for Patient J. P., 7-year-old boy, on Oct. 11, 1957*

| *Time* | *Source* | *pH* | $NH_4$ | *Temperature (C.)* |
|---|---|---|---|---|
| 7:52 A.M. | Femoral artery | – | 2.18 | 37.6° |
| 7:59 | Inferior vena cava | 7.36 | 2.17 | |
| | (hypothermia) | | | |
| 11:06 | Femoral artery | 7.64 | 0.66 | 28.0° |
| | Inferior vena cava | 7.52 | 0.59 | |
| | Jugular vein | 7.32 | 1.06 | |
| 11:20 | Clamp on inferior vena cava | | | |
| | Clamp on superior vena cava | | | |
| 11:22 | Femoral artery | 7.66 | 0.80 | 28.5° |
| | Inferior vena cava | 7.54 | 1.21 | |
| | Jugular vein | – | 1.24 | |
| 11:28 | Removal of both clamps | | | |
| | Jugular vein | 7.54 | 0.91 | |
| 11:32 | Femoral artery | 7.48 | 1.00 | 28.5° |
| | Inferior vena cava | 7.52 | 0.95 | |
| | Jugular vein | 7.58 | 0.95 | |
| 11:38 | Femoral artery | 7.50 | 1.09 | 28.5° |
| | Inferior vena cava | 7.38 | 0.62 | |
| | Jugular vein | 7.48 | 1.03 | |
| 11:44 | Femoral artery | 7.61 | 0.74 | 28.5° |
| | Inferior vena cava | 7.54 | 0.76 | |
| | Jugular vein | 7.50 | 0.86 | |
| 11:49 | Femoral artery | 7.54 | 0.79 | 29.5° |
| | Inferior vena cava | 7.55 | 0.77 | |
| | Jugular vein | 7.50 | 0.54 | |
| | (return to normal temperature) | | | |
| 5:00 P.M. | Femoral artery | – | 0.83 | 37.0° |
| | Inferior vena cava | – | 0.77 | |

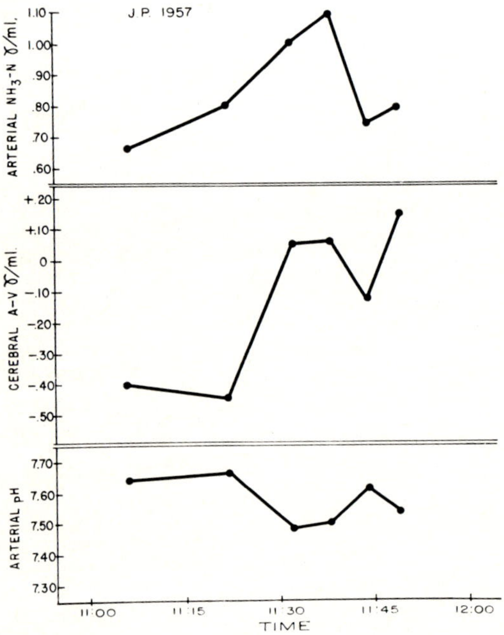


**Fig. 3.** Arterial pH, ammonium concentration, and arterial-jugular difference in Patient J. P.

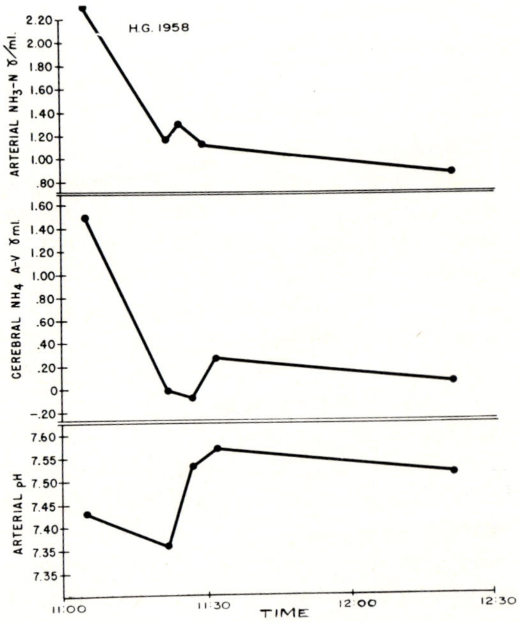


**Fig. 4.** Arterial pH, ammonium concentration, and arterial-jugular difference in Patient H. G.

Fig. 3 shows observations on the cerebral arteriovenous difference of ammonia in relation to arterial level and jugular pH. Again there is a good correlation between arterial level and arteriovenous difference. In this case there is somewhat better correlation between arterial pH and cerebral uptake than there was between peripheral uptake of ammonia and pH in Figs. 1 and 2. On the other hand, the general trend (increase or decrease) of arteriovenous difference of ammonia parallels the course of variation of arterial level better than it fits the variation of arterial pH. The greatest change in pH is associated with the least alteration in arteriovenous difference. The protocol which was used for this typical experiment is given in Table I.

Fig. 4 shows the cerebral arteriovenous differences of ammonia in another patient and a clear inverse relation can be seen between pH and variation of arteriovenous difference across the brain. This covers a sufficient number of points to make the relation more than fortuitous. The fluctuations in arteriovenous difference across the brain are closely related to the arterial ammonia changes. Every change in uptake vector is in the same direction as arterial vector change.

Fig. 5 is a scattergram of arterial pH values versus arteriovenous difference taken from 11 cases. There are 62 values for peripheral and 34 values for cerebral arteriovenous difference. No positive correlation can be seen between the arteriovenous difference, either cerebral or peripheral, and the pH of the blood. Table II gives the correlation coefficients for Fig. 5, and for Figs. 6 and 7 which show the relation between arterial ammonia level and peripheral and cerebral arteriovenous difference, respectively. A negligible negative correlation exists between arterial pH and peripheral arteriovenous difference of ammonia, but the negative correlation between cerebral pH and cerebral arteriovenous difference may be significant. The positive correlations between arterial level and cerebral and peripheral arteriovenous difference of ammonia are significant at the 0.0001 and 0.02 probability levels.

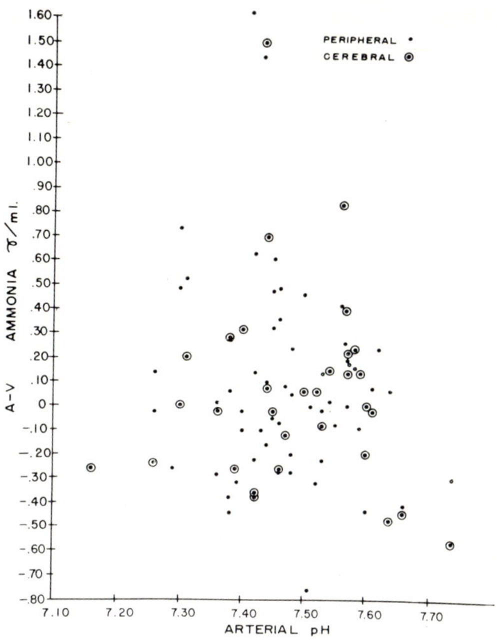


**Fig. 5.** Lack of relation between arterial pH and cerebral or peripheral arteriovenous difference of ammonium.

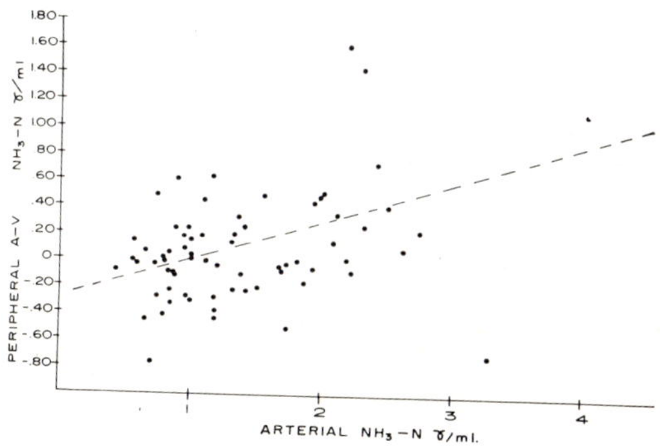


**Fig. 6.** Peripheral (lower extremity) arteriovenous difference of ammonium as a function of arterial level of ammonium.

It should be noted at this point that plots of venous pH data showed the same trends as the arterial data given. Fig. 8 shows the lack of correlation between venous pH and arteriovenous difference.

## DISCUSSION

These data, and more fragmentary observations on a number of other patients,

**Table II.** *Correlation coefficients for cerebral and peripheral uptake of ammonia*

| | $n$ | $r$ | $p$ |
|---|---|---|---|
| pH (peripheral uptake) | 62 | -0.19 | $> 0.10$ |
| pH (cerebral uptake) | 34 | -0.50 | $< 0.005$ |
| Arterial ammonia (peripheral uptake) | 62 | +0.31 | $< 0.02$ |
| Arterial ammonia (cerebral uptake) | 34 | +0.61 | $< 0.0001$ |

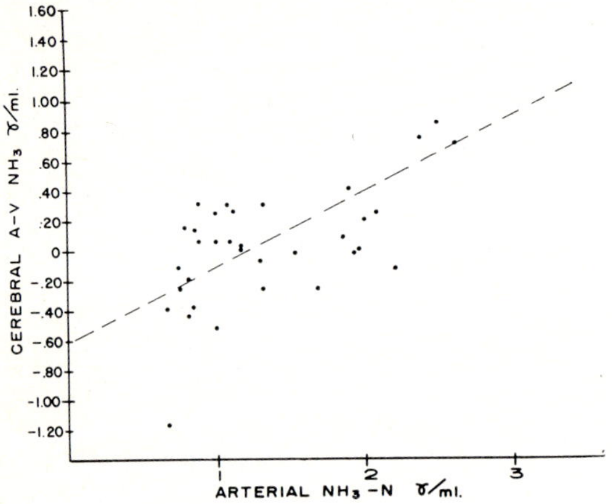


**Fig. 7.** The cerebral arteriovenous difference of ammonium as a function of the arterial ammonium level.

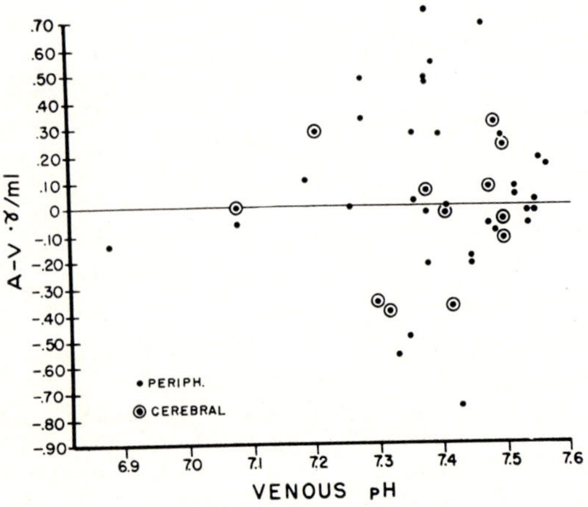


**Fig. 8.** Lack of correlation between venous pH and peripheral and cerebral arteriovenous difference of ammonium.

suggest that there is little effect of the pH of the blood upon the arteriovenous difference of ammonia across tissues. The experiments of Jacobs and Parpart[13] showed indirectly (as indicated by osmotic swelling) an increase in red cell ammonia in vitro as the medium was made more alkaline, but no direct measurements of this phenomenon have been reported. The work of Jacquez and others[11, 18] on the vapor pressure of ammonia in vivo leaves no doubt as to the effect of pH in altering the proportion of ammonia in the gaseous or diffusible form. Our own experiments[21] with distribution of ammonia between red blood cells and plasma suggest a slight effect of pH, but cannot account for the fall in blood ammonia seen clinically on alkalization and the rise seen in acidosis. Lawrence and associates[16] demonstrated alterations in the blood ammonia of dogs infused with acid or alkali or subjected to hyperventilation. When the pH of the blood was made strongly acid, the blood ammonia level was considerably higher than when the pH of the blood was alkaline. This was cited as evidence that the ammonia had moved into or out of the tissues under the circumstances of the experiment. Examination of the data, however, shows the interesting fact that the peripheral arteriovenous difference at acid pH was the same for comparable total ammonia levels as the difference at an alkaline pH. In other words, the only data which might indicate actual movement of ammonia into the tissues in the experiments of these authors were not influenced by the pH. The arterial level of ammonia was inversely related to the pH, and this is a different matter. It suggests that a general mechanism of removal of ammonia from the arterial blood may be affected by the pH of the blood; that is, the removal of ammonia by hepatic formation of urea was probably impaired by the acidity of the blood. This is illuminated by experiments reported from Krebs's laboratory.[15]

It was shown, in measuring the formation of urea from ammonia by liver slices in vitro, that both the pH of the medium and the bicarbonate content had a remarkable influence upon the rate of urea synthesis; that alkaline conditions favored synthesis of urea and acid conditions inhibited it. These effects were manifest within the physiologic range of pH. The recent demonstration by Jones and Lipmann[14] that carbamyl phosphate synthesis, the first step in the incorporation of ammonia into urea, is at a maximum at approximately pH 8 may identify the pH-sensitive enzymatic step which is implied in Krebs's experiments. The effect, therefore, of pH upon the level of blood ammonia demonstrated by Lawrence and colleagues[16] is not an effect of pH on the movement of ammonia into the tissues, but is more likely an effect of pH upon the synthesis of urea by the liver. The negative correlation between pH and arteriovenous difference which can be observed is consistent with this interpretation. When the pH is acidic, urea synthesis slows down, the blood ammonia level rises, and tissues take up ammonia. When the pH rises, urea synthesis improves, the arterial ammonia level falls, and less ammonia is taken up by tissues. The conversion of even the equivalent of 5 gamma of ammonia per milliliter of blood, a formidable amount, to urea would raise the blood urea nitrogen by 0.5 mg. per 100 ml., a negligible, and probably undetectable, difference. The only reference to blood urea nitrogen changes during pH manipulations is by Stabenau and his group[20] who say that there was "no striking difference in rate of BUN elevation," but give no data. The therapeutic benefits reported from the use of acidifying measures probably can be attributed to the fact that alkalosis in general is deleterious to neural function and tends to aggravate neurological signs.

We appreciate the fact that alterations in acidity of the blood might affect ammoniagenic coma, as suggested by the Sloan-Kettering group. We take issue merely with the interpretation of the results, and believe that a more physiologic interpretation can be derived than that the effect of acidification is upon the movement of ammonia into tissues. In reality the movement of ammonia into tissues is apparently governed

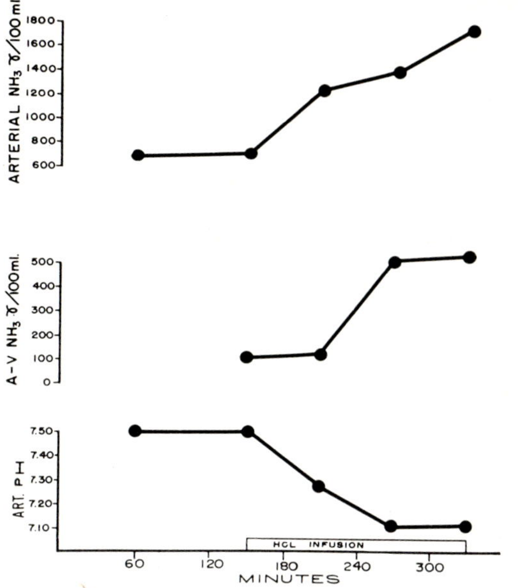


**Fig. 9.** Relation of peripheral arteriovenous difference of ammonium to arterial concentration and pH of arterial blood plotted from Table IV of Stabenau and associates[20] (Dog 1).

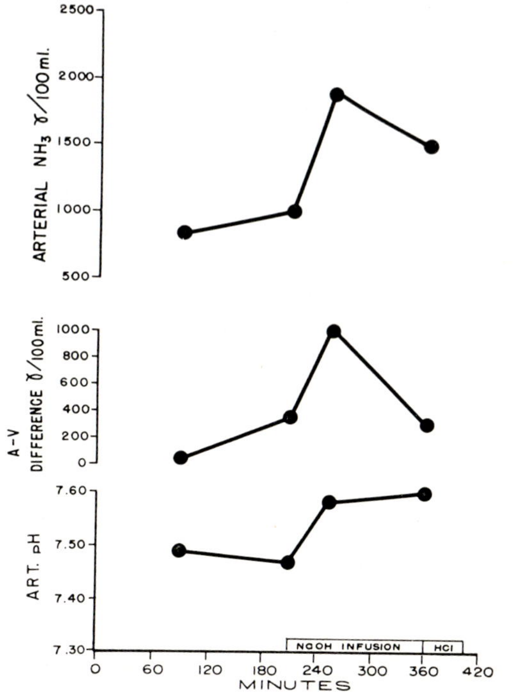


**Fig. 10.** Relation of peripheral arteriovenous difference of ammonium to arterial concentration and pH of arterial blood plotted from Table IV of Stabenau and associates[20] (Dog 3).

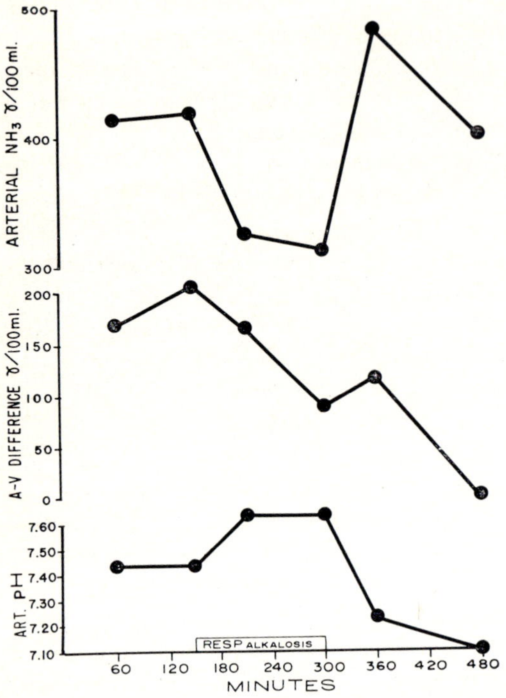


**Fig. 11.** Relation of peripheral arteriovenous difference of ammonium to arterial concentration and pH of arterial blood plotted from Table IV of Stabenau and associates[20] (Dog 4).

mainly by the arterial level of ammonia. This is not to say that there is a particular level of ammonia which stimulates a particular rate of movement into the tissues. This again is conditioned by many factors, including, perhaps significantly, the actual level of ammonia within the tissues at the time. In the same patient, however, followed over a long period of time, the movement of ammonia into the tissues is related to the arterial level of ammonia, not to the pH of the blood. The experiments[20, 24, 25] in which overwhelming amounts of ammonium salts were administered to animals and wide deviations of pH were instituted do not appear to be germane to the problem of the role of pH under physiologic or even pathologic conditions. The fact that enormous levels of ammonia appeared in the brain tissue at high blood pH is expected from the experiments of Jacobs. Similar results can be obtained by performance of diffusion experiments across semipermeable membranes.

The problem at hand is not whether or not ammonium salts ionize. The problem is whether the movement of ammonia into tissues is determined mainly by arterial pH or by arterial level of ammonia. Obviously it would be preferable to have measurements of blood flow to make a quantitative decision. Nevertheless, there appear to be sufficient data at hand to make a fair conclusion possible.

Since there is material in the literature which purports to show a significant effect of pH upon movement of ammonia into tissues, it is necessary to determine whether the proffered data actually support this hypothesis. Stabenau and colleagues[20] report a relation between tissue distribution and blood pH, and the figures presented seem to bear this out. Closer scrutiny of Fig. 2 in their report shows that the data of their Table IV have not been included. When they are included, the relation between pH of blood and muscle-blood distribution becomes considerably less significant. The same question can be raised for their Fig. 3 which loses its significance in demonstrating an effect of pH upon brain-blood distribution when the data of their Table IV are added to it. Table III shows that muscle content of ammonia is the same in respiratory acidosis as in metabolic alkalosis; even in respiratory alkalosis there is no significant difference from the controls in muscle content of ammonia.

The information on tissue and blood concentration is presented mainly as ratios. The only absolute values, Table VI, show a number of discrepancies between data and discussion which are worth considering. The sodium hydroxide infusion produces a higher blood ammonia level than hydrochloric acid infusion (against the hypothesis) at the same time as an apparent change in the "right" (according to hypothesis) direction occurs for brain and muscle concentration. Furthermore, respiratory alkalosis results in a blood level which falls even as the tissue levels also fall (but they should rise if the ammonia which left the blood entered the tissues).

It is instructive to plot the arteriovenous differences which can be calculated from the data presented in this paper (Table IV) as we have plotted ours. Figs. 9, 10, and 11 have been so plotted and show a remarkable resemblance to our data, demonstrating that, in fact, the observations on the dogs studied by Stabenau and associates agree with our observations on human beings. The only difference is in presentation of data and interpretation. For further clarification of this problem we can examine the report by Warren and Nathan[25] which deals directly with toxicity of ammonium salts and the ammonia concentrations found in the brains of mice. Table I of this paper shows little difference among the brain levels of ammonium produced by L.D.$_{50}$ doses of acid or neutral ammonium salts, but there is a considerably lower level of ammonia in brain after an L.D.$_{50}$ dose of ammonium carbonate, and the lowest level after ammonium hydroxide. This is remarkable, because if the death of the animals was caused by ammonium being forced into the brain because of alkaline pH, the brain levels should have been the same or higher than those found with an L.D.$_{50}$ of acid salts. These data are compatible with the concept that alkalosis increases the lethality of ammonium, which was proposed by Roberts and her group,[17, 23] but not with the further proposition that this increased lethality is due to increased movement of ammonium into the brain. Table II of the paper by Warren and Nathan[25] also shows that severe alkalosis does not increase the level of ammonia in the brain, but actually decreases it. This is consistent with most of the data of the paper by Stabenau and associates, and if we look merely at the data without any preconceived notion about transport across membranes, we are forced to the conclusion that alkalosis does not drive ammonia into the brain.

It is obvious that tissue uptake is the product of blood flow and arteriovenous difference, but it requires a rather gymnastic approach to the data presented in this paper[25] and to that graphed by Stabenau and colleagues[20] to propose that the inverse relation seen between blood pH and arteriovenous difference may be counterbalanced at all times by a hypothetical alteration in blood flow. No conceivable alteration in blood flow could account for the change from positive to negative arteriovenous difference seen in our Figs. 1 and 2 and in Table I. These values were taken at close enough intervals that the inertia of the blood flow through the extremity or brain would not have given these results. For example, in Fig. 2 the very low arterial ammonia level persisted over a 10-minute period, and 2 consecutive observations, allowing even for a mean transit time of ammonia of 10 minutes through the extremity, clearly show this reversal of arteriovenous difference in direct relation to the arterial level. The data of Table I and Figs. 1 through 4 show little acute change in pH of blood passing through the tissues, although fairly wide ranges of pH were traversed. The pH and ammonia values appear to follow a regular pattern and do not oscillate significantly. All of the curves are relatively monophasic over fairly long periods. The parellel between arterial level and arteriovenous difference in all of the data must be given some weight.

The data of our Figs. 5 and 6 underline the above proposition, and show no correlation between arterial pH and arteriovenous difference, but a clear correlation between arterial level and arteriovenous difference. This is consistent with previous data from our laboratory and from that of Webster and Gabuzda.[26] It should also be noted that although Fazekas and his co-workers[9] are often quoted as showing no relation between arterial level and uptake of ammonia by brain, their actual conclusion is that in cirrhosis there is no greater uptake of ammonia by brain in comatose patients than in noncomatose patients. A plot of their data for arteriovenous differences versus arterial level of ammonia shows the same relation between blood level and cerebral arteriovenous difference that we have reported. Summerskill and associates[22] show that there is occasionally no cerebral uptake of ammonia in hepatic coma. Nevertheless, their data also reveal the same general trend of increasing arteriovenous difference with arterial level.

The patients described in our report were under many different conditions of body temperature and were undergoing operation. The samples were taken at least 2 minutes after occlusion of the vessels was released, allowing time for "washout" of the circulation. Venous pH values had returned to preocclusion levels, which suggested a return of tissue pH to normal. The extreme tissue acidosis which must occur during occlusion[5] should stimulate tissue uptake of ammonia unless arterial pH drops remarkably. This phenomenon was not seen in the patients studied. It is the very point of our data, particularly of Figs. 5 and 6, that under a variety of circumstances the arteriovenous difference is proportional to the arterial level and is not related to the pH.

Let us interject at this point a plea for analysis of the data for its own sake rather than from the standpoint of a theoretical bias. There is no doubt that the pH of an ammonium solution influences the quantity of diffusible species present. This is no proof that the role of pH in movement of ammonia into tissues under physiologic conditions is more than trivial. Experiments in which animals are drowned in floods of intermediates do no more than demonstrate physicochemical phenomena, predictable from physical data. Their physiologic significance is questionable. The remarkable fact is that living organisms confound these experiments by demonstrating, frequently, disparate results. These cannot be tossed aside lightly, for they show that the physical principles invoked as mechanism are trivial in comparison to the physiologic phenomena which are at play. In regard to ammonium uptake by tissues, it is apparent that although pH may theoretically affect it significantly when the quantities involved are beyond the physiologic and pathologic range, it also appears that the pH effect is insignificant in proportion to the chemical mass action effect of arterial concentration.

## SUMMARY AND CONCLUSIONS

Serial observations of arterial pH and arteriovenous difference of ammonia have been made on 11 patients undergoing hypothermia and cardiac operation over a prolonged period. The fluctuations in the arteriovenous differences of ammonia, both peripheral and cerebral, did not correspond to the fluctuations in pH, but corresponded remarkably closely to alterations in the arterial level of ammonia. It is therefore concluded that in a particular individual, the movement of ammonia into or out of the tissues is a function primarily of the arterial level of ammonia, rather than of the arterial or venous pH of the blood. An analysis of data reported from other laboratories also supports this view. An explanation of the experimental observations relating blood level of ammonia and pH can be obtained from the reported effects of pH upon the synthesis of urea.

### REFERENCES

1. Bessman, S. P.: Ammoniagenic coma, the chemistry of an endogenous intoxication, Proc. Fourth Internat. Cong. Biochem., Vienna, 141, 1958.
2. Bessman, S. P., and Bessman, A. N.: Ammonia poisoning of hepatic coma-cerebral arteriovenous amino acid levels, Fed. Proc. **13:** 336, 1954.
3. Bessman, S. P., and Bessman, A. N.: The cerebral and peripheral uptake of ammonia in liver disease with an hypothesis for the mechanism of hepatic coma, J. Clin. Invest. **34:** 4, 1955.
4. Bessman, S. P., and Bradley, J. E.: Uptake of ammonia by muscle: its implications in ammoniagenic coma, New England J. Med. **253:** 1143, 1955.
5. Bessman, S. P., and Cowley, R. A.: Biochemical changes in human beings during refrigeration anesthesia, Ann. New York Acad. Sc. **80:** 540, 1959.
6. Bessman, S. P., Fazekas, J. F., Bessman, A. N.: Uptake of Ammonia by the brain in hepatic coma, Proc. Soc. Exper. Biol. & Med. **85:** 66, 1954.
7. Clark, G. M., and Eiseman, B.: Studies in ammonia metabolism. IV. Biochemical

changes in brain tissue of dogs during ammonia induced coma, New England J. Med. **259:** 178, 1958.
8. Eiseman, B., Fowler, W. G., White, P. J., and Clark, G. M.: The role of ammonia in the production of hepatic coma, S. Forum **6:** 369, 1955.
9. Fazekas, J. F., Ticktin, H. E., Ehrmentraut, W. R., and Alman, R. W.: Cerebral metabolism in hepatic insufficiency, Am. J. Med. **21:** 843, 1956.
10. Hankins, J., Bessman, S. P., Mansberger, A., and Cowley, R. A.: The origin and utilization of ammonia in shock: a comparison of the levels of blood ammonia in the portal and systemic circulation during shock induced by the Fine technique, Bull. Soc. Internat. Chir. **1:** 1, 1959.
11. Jacquez, J. A., Poppell, J. W., and Jeltsch, R.: Partial pressure of ammonia in alveolar air, Science **129:** 269, 1959.
12. Jacquez, J. A., Poppell, J. N., Lawrence, W., Jr., and Roberts, K. E.: Clinical significance of the partial pressure of ammonia ($PNH_3$) in patients with ammonium toxicity, Clin. Res. Proc. **5:** 20, 1957.
13. Jacobs, M. H., and Parpart, A. K.: Osmotic properties of the erythrocyte X: on the permeability of the erythrocyte to ammonia and the ammonia ion, J. Cell. & Comp. Physiol. **11:** 175, 1938.
14. Jones, M. E., Spector, L., and Lipmann, F.: Carbamyl phosphate, the carbamyl donor in citrulline synthesis, J. Am. Chem. Soc. **77:** 821, 1955.
15. Krebs, H. A., and Henseleit, K.: Untersuchungen über die Harnstoffbildung im Tierkörper, J. Physiol. Chem. **201:** 33, 1932.
16. Lawrence, W., Jr., Jacquez, J. A., Dienst, S. G., Poppell, J. W., Randall, H. T., and Roberts, K. E.: The effect of changes in blood pH on the plasma total ammonia level, Surgery **42:** 50, 1957.
17. Roberts, K. E., Thompson, F. G., III, Poppell, J. N., and Vanamee, P.: Respiratory alkalosis accompanying ammonium toxicity, J. Appl. Physiol. **9:** 367, 1956.
18. Robin, E. D., Travis, D. M., Bromberg, P. A., Forkner, C. E., Jr., and Tyler, J. M.: Ammonia excretion by mammalian lung, Science **129:** 270, 1959.
19. Seligson, D., and Seligson, H.: A microdiffusion method for the measurement of nitrogen liberated as ammonia, J. Lab. & Clin. Med. **38:** 324, 1951.
20. Stabenau, J. R., Warren, K. S., and Rall, D. P.: The role of pH gradient in the distribution of ammonia between blood and cerebrospinal fluid, brain and muscle, J. Clin. Invest. **38:** 373, 1959.
21. Stauffer, J., and Bessman, S. P.: Unpublished data.
22. Summerskill, W. H. J., Wolfe, S. J., and Davidson, C. S.: The metabolism of ammonia and alpha keto acids in liver disease and hepatic coma, J. Clin. Invest. **36:** 361, 1957.
23. Vanamee, P., Poppell, J. W., Glicksman, A. S., Randall, H. T., and Roberts, K. E.: Respiratory alkalosis in hepatic coma, A. M. A. Arch. Int. Med. **97:** 762, 1956.
24. Warren, K. S.: The differential toxicity of ammonium salts, J. Clin. Invest. **37:** 497, 1958.
25. Warren, K. S., and Nathan, D. G.: The passage of ammonia across the blood-brain barrier and its relation to blood pH, J. Clin. Invest. **37:** 1724, 1958.
26. Webster, L. T., Jr., and Gabuzda, G. J.: Ammonium uptake by the extremities and brain in hepatic coma, J. Clin. Invest. **37:** 414, 1958.

# Mechanism of declamping shock in operations on the abdominal aorta

D. E. STRANDNESS, JR., M.D.*
D. G. PARRISH, B.S.
J. W. BELL, M.D.
SEATTLE, WASH.
*From the Department of Surgery, Seattle Veterans Administration Hospital and University of Washington School of Medicine*

A common problem encountered in the resection of abdominal aortic aneurysms is the marked drop in blood pressure which may occur when the clamps are removed.[1, 2, 4, 6] In our experience the magnitude of the drop is quite variable, ranging from 10 to 130 mm. Hg in 23 cases studied. The etiology of this pressure drop has been presumed to be a form of normovolemic shock in which blood is pooled transiently in the areas distal to the clamp.[3] An experimental study was designed to investigate this hypothesis and possible methods of prevention of the hypotension.

## METHODS

Mongrel dogs were used in this study. The anesthesia employed was pentobarbital sodium, 30 mg. per kilogram. The dogs were divided into 2 groups.

**Group 1.** In 17 dogs the aorta just distal to the left renal vein was clamped for 1 hour. During the clamping period 8 animals received 200 ml. of whole blood; the remainder received an equivalent volume of 6 per cent dextran in isotonic sodium chloride.

**Group 2.** In 13 dogs the effects of duration of occlusion were observed by changing the clamping period to 15 minutes and subsequently to 1 to 2 minutes.

Four parameters were studied—central aortic pressure, cardiac output, leg volume changes, and femoral arterial pressures.

**Central aortic pressure.** A No. 205 polyethylene catheter was inserted into the aorta via the left brachial artery. Pressures were measured by a Statham pressure transducer and Sanborn Twin-Viso amplifier and recorder.

**Cardiac output.** Cardiac outputs were measured in animals in Group 1 before clamping, at the end of the clamping period, and within 1 to 2 minutes of declamping. To measure cardiac output, 20 to 50 $\mu$c of $I^{131}$ was injected into the inferior vena cava. The sampling site was the central aorta. An automatic pipetting machine* was utilized which sampled 0.5 ml. per second and delivered this volume into a multiple fraction collector. Cardiac outputs were calculated from the obtained dye-dilution curve.

**Leg volume changes.** Changes in both foreleg and hindleg volume were monitored by a mercury strain gauge plethysmograph.[7] Particular attention was paid to the volume shifts which occurred with clamping and declamping.

**Femoral arterial pressures.** In Group 2 animals, femoral arterial pressures were monitored with a No. 90 polyethylene catheter inserted so as not to obstruct arterial inflow to the extremity.

Received for publication Oct. 28, 1960.
*United States Public Health Service Research Fellow (Grant No. HF-9583), Seattle Veterans Administration Hospital.

*Filamatic Duplex Automatic Pipetter, Model DAB, National Instrument Company, Baltimore, Md.

After base-line responses were obtained on animals in Group 2, two studies were performed to modify or eliminate the pressure drop. (1) In 8 animals, 60 to 320 mcg. of levarterenol* was injected distal to the clamp immediately prior to declamping. (2) In 5 animals, 60 to 240 mcg. of levarterenol was injected proximal to the clamp into the central arterial circulation prior to declamping.

## RESULTS

**Group 1.** When the aorta was clamped just distal to the left renal vein there was an immediate increase in the average mean pressure from 101 to 109 mm. Hg, a 7.4 per cent rise. During the hour of clamping the mean pressure gradually increased to 123 mm. Hg, a 17 per cent rise from base line. This increase was probably the result of the 200 ml. infusion of whole blood or dextran during this time.

When the clamp was removed the mean aortic pressure dropped an average of 23 per cent, from 117 to 90 mm. Hg. There was essentially no difference in the animals which received whole blood and those which received the dextran. The cardiac output dropped an average of 21 per cent, from 1,350 to 1,060 ml. per minute when the clamp was removed (Table I).

The hindleg volume rapidly decreased, with aortic occlusion reaching a plateau within 30 seconds (Fig. 1). When the clamp was removed, leg volume increased and reached its maximal level in approximately 30 to 60 seconds. The leg volume then gradually decreased toward the preclamping values.

**Group 2.** In these animals the magnitude of the pressure drop did not vary significantly regardless of the duration of occlusion. The average gradient of pressure as reflected in the difference between aortic and femoral arterial pressure across the clamp at the time of declamping was also essentially the same.

*Levophed, Winthrop Laboratories, Inc., New York, N. Y.

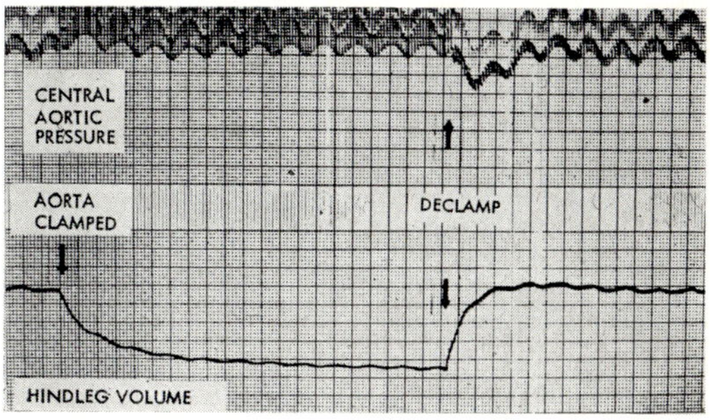


**Fig. 1.** Plethysmographic record which shows rapid decrease in hindleg volume with aortic clamping. Acute increase in leg volume with declamping coincides with pressure drop.

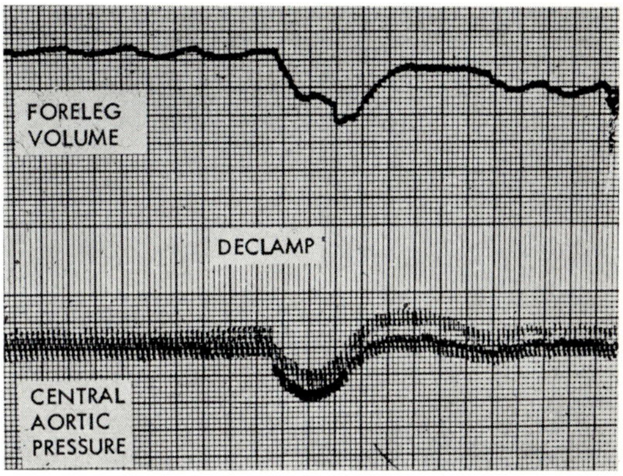


**Fig. 2.** Foreleg volume decreases simultaneously with drop in central aortic pressure at declamping.

The hindleg volume changes were the same as those noted in Group 1. The displacement of upper extremity blood volume with aortic declamping coincided almost exactly with the central aortic pressure drop (Fig. 2). As the central blood volume is translocated, the foreleg volume decreases. Thus, an inverse relation between foreleg and hindleg volume changes was observed at the time of declamping (Fig. 3).

The rapid injection of levarterenol distal to the clamp prior to removal was the most effective measure employed in reducing or eliminating the pressure drop (Table II). The clamp was removed when the maximal femoral arterial pressure was attained. In the group with 15-minute occlusion, the pressure drop was reduced from an average

**Table I.** *Results of varying the duration of aortic occlusion*

| *Occlusion time* | *Average mean aortic pressure (mm. Hg)* | | *Average pressure gradient at declamping (mm. Hg)* | *Average cardiac output (ml./min.)* | |
|---|---|---|---|---|---|
| | *Before declamping* | *After declamping* | | *Before declamping* | *After declamping* |
| 1 to 2 min. (7 animals, 14 occlusions) | 126 | 100 (21% decrease) | 89 | — | — |
| 15 min. (13 animals, 13 occlusions) | 139 | 107 (23% decrease) | 91 | — | — |
| 1 hr. (17 animals, 17 occlusions) | 117 | 90 (23% decrease) | — | 1,350 | 1,060 (21% decrease) |

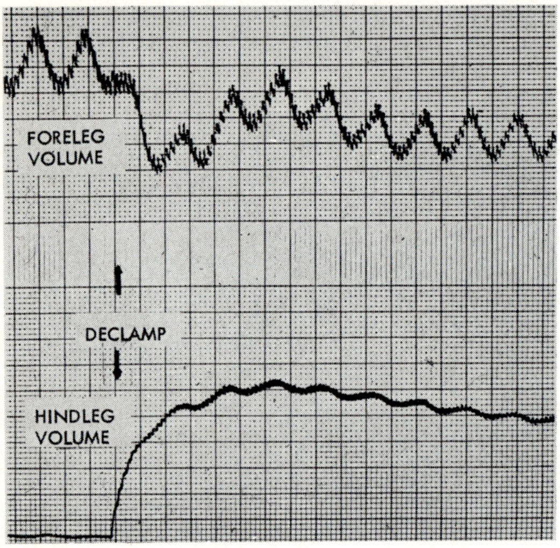


**Fig. 3.** Inverse relation between foreleg and hindleg volume at declamping.

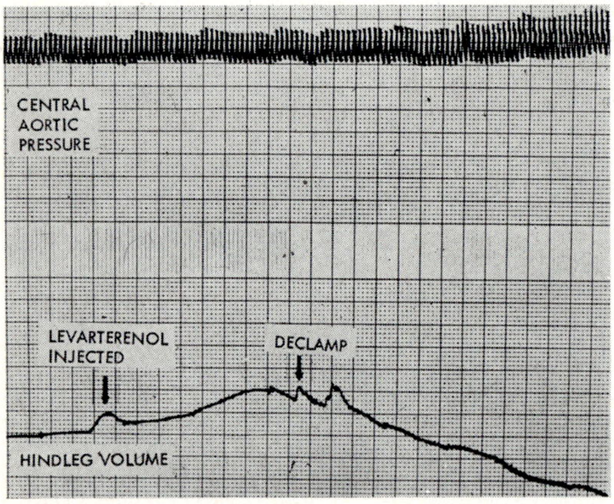


**Fig. 4.** Effect of 60 mcg. of levarterenol injected distal to clamp. Hindleg volume increases as blood pools on arterial side. When peak leg volume was reached, declamping resulted in no change in central aortic pressure.

of 23 to 5 per cent. In the group with 1- to 2-minute occlusion, the response was reduced from 21 to 8 per cent. In each instance the gradient of pressure across the clamp was greatly reduced.

When levarterenol was injected distal to the clamp, the increase in hindleg volume was greatly minimized or did not occur, depending upon the magnitude of the pressure drop (Fig. 4). If no drop in pressure occurred, no sudden increase in hindleg volume was recorded. Similarly, the decrease in foreleg volume was greatly reduced or abolished, depending on the amount of blood volume shift to the hindleg.

The rapid injection of levarterenol into the central arterial circulation proximal to the clamp did not alter the response to declamping in the 5 animals tested (Table II). The foreleg and hindleg volume shifts still occurred in these animals.

## DISCUSSION

An average decrease in mean aortic pressure of 23 per cent after clamp release in animals subjected to 1 hour of aortic occlusion without significant blood loss suggests that this shock is indeed a redistribution phenomenon. The decrease in cardiac output (average 21 per cent) was accompanied by a corresponding increase in hindleg volume, which also suggests a normovolemic shift.

In the Group 2 animals the aortic pressure drops at 1- to 2-minute and 15-minute occlusion were essentially the same as drops for the 1-hour occlusion–21 and 23 per cent, respectively. The independence of pressure-time relationship is apparent in these experiments.

The magnitude of the pressure drop appears to be related to the gradient of pressure across the clamp and the extremity blood volume at the time of declamping. Since the vascular bed is elastic, the greater the pressure head to which it is suddenly subjected upon declamping, the greater will be the volume displaced into it.

The most effective method employed to minimize or prevent the pressure drop was to inject levarterenol distal to the clamp immediately prior to declamping. Levarterenol infusion results in an increase in femoral arterial mean pressure and an initial increase in limb volume followed by a decrease. Shadle and associates[5] believe the initial volume increase is the result of arteriolar constriction which impounds blood on the arterial side. As arterial pressure increases and overcomes arteriolar resistance, an increased amount of drug is presented to the veins. This results in venous constriction which increases venous return and decreases the limb volume. This finding is substantiated by the plethysmographic data (Fig. 5). Thus, increased arteriolar resistance seems to be the most important factor in preventing the volume shift and subsequent hypotension, since the clamp may be removed before the venous constriction phase and the drop in pressure will not occur (Fig. 4). However, the vasopressor continues to be effective in preventing the volume shift and hypotension during the venous constriction phase (Fig. 6).

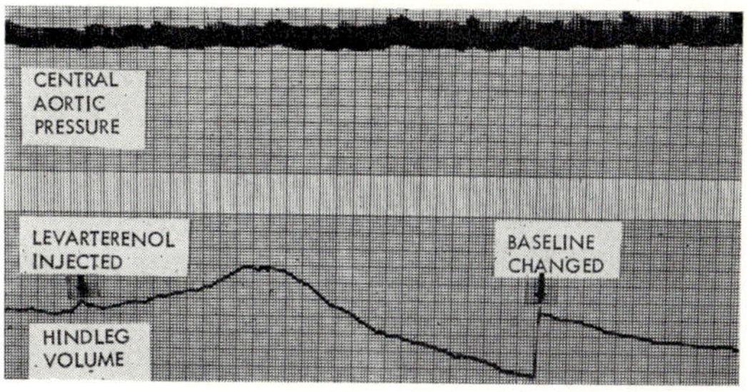


**Fig. 5.** After distal injection of levarterenol, hindleg volume increase is followed by rapid decrease as the vasopressor reaches the venules and veins, constricting them and increasing venous return.

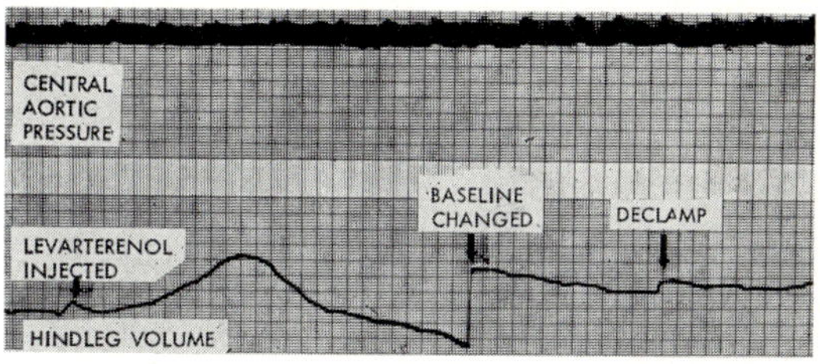


**Fig. 6.** Effect of vasopressor in preventing hypotension during venous constriction phase. Clamp removal was approximately 1 minute after hindleg volume began to decrease.

Any measure which tended to increase the central pressure alone or in greater proportion to the distal pressure would tend to increase the drop in pressure. Although the injection of levarterenol proximal to the aortic clamp did not increase the drop in

**Table II.** *Effect of levarterenol on the magnitude of the pressure drop*

| *Occlusion time* | *Average central aortic mean pressure (mm. Hg)* | | *Average pressure gradient at declamping (mm. Hg)* |
|---|---|---|---|
| | *Before declamping* | *After declamping* | |
| *Levarterenol (60 to 320 mcg.) injected distal to clamp immediately prior to declamping* | | | |
| 1 to 2 min. (4 animals, 8 occlusions) | 129 | 118 (8% decrease) | 60 |
| 15 min. (7 animals, 7 occlusions) | 139 | 133 (5% decrease) | 53 |
| *Levarterenol (60 to 240 mcg.) injected proximal to clamp immediately prior to declamping* | | | |
| 1 to 2 min. (5 animals, 7 occlusions) | 133 | 102 (23% decrease) | — |

pressure, it certainly did not reduce it. The drop was not increased because the distal pressure was also elevated and tended to keep the gradient about the same.

There is one major difference between the experimental situation and that encountered clinically. In the clinical situation, there is frequently a fair amount of bleeding from the anastomoses. This will tend to add the problem of hypovolemic shock to the already existing redistributional shock.

## SUMMARY

The acute drop in blood pressure which occurs at the end of temporary abdominal aortic occlusion is the result of translocation of blood into the vascular bed distal to the clamp and is independent of the duration of clamping if blood volume is unchanged. The gradient of pressure across the clamp at the time of release of occlusion appears to be the most important factor determining the magnitude of the blood volume shift and resultant drop in pressure.

The rapid injection of levarterenol distal to the clamp immediately prior to removal is effective in eliminating or minimizing the drop. This vasopressor drug rapidly raises arteriolar resistance and prevents displacement of blood to the distensible venous bed.

## REFERENCES

1. Deterling, R. A.: Discussion of aneurysm and occlusive diseases of aorta, International Symposium, Henry Ford Hospital, Philadelphia, 1955, W. B. Saunders Company, p. 493.
2. Eliot, J. A., McKenzie, A. D., and Chung, W. B.: Ruptured abdominal aneurysm, SURGERY **46:** 605, 1959.
3. Gross, R. E.: Technical consideration in surgical therapy for coarctation of the aorta, SURGERY **20:** 1, 1946.
4. Mavor, G. E., Davidson, L. D., and Clark, C. G.: The ruptured abdominal aortic aneurysm and its treatment, Brit. J. Surg. **47:** 292, 1959.
5. Shadle, O. W., Zukof, M., and Diana, J.: Translocation of blood from the isolated dog's hindlimb during levarterenol infusion and sciatic nerve stimulation, Circulation Res. **6:** 326, 1958.
6. Szilagyi, D. E., Smith, R. F., and Whitcomb, J. G.: The kidneys in surgery of the abdominal aorta, A. M. A. Arch. Surg. **79:** 252, 1959.
7. Whitney, R. J.: The measurement of volume changes in human limbs, J. Physiol. **12:** 1, 1953.

# Thrombogenic properties at the site of vascular anastomoses studied by a new technique for measuring platelet adherence

KIYOSHI INOKUCHI, M.D., D.SC.
TETSURO KONISHI, M.D.
HIROSHI YAGI, M.D.
TERUHISA NAKAMURA, M.D.
MASAAKI SAKAGUCHI, M.D.
NOZOMU NAKAMURA, M.D.
FUKUOKA, JAPAN
*From the Second Department of Surgery, Kyushu University Faculty of Medicine*

The uninjured intimal surface of blood vessels is endowed with the property of preventing blood coagulation. However, when the intima is injured, it no longer retains this anticoagulative property, and the streaming blood tends to clot at the site of the injury. In this sense, the injured intima may be said to be predisposed toward thrombus formation. Many reports concerning the reparative process of the injured blood vessel wall have been published since the last century, but information bearing on the thrombogenic condition of the injured intima is very scant.

We have recently developed a new method for measuring the degree of predisposition of the intima toward thrombus formation.[3, 4] This involves measurement of the degree of adherence of radioactively labeled blood platelets at the surface of the intima. In the present series of experiments the method was applied to study changes in the state of the intima during the healing process at sites where vessels had been sutured or anastomosed. It was found that at such sites the risk of thrombosis is greatest on the fifth or sixth day after operation. The technique which was used to study these changes and the results of the experiments are discussed.

Received for publication Oct. 18, 1960.

## EXPERIMENTAL METHOD

One hundred and forty-three dogs were used. After anesthesia (Orlopan given intravenously) had been induced, the abdomen was opened and the 4 operations were carried out, (1) end-to-end anastomosis of the transected abdominal aorta by Carrel's manual suture technique, (2) closure of the longitudinally slit abdominal aorta by continuous manual suture, (3) end-to-end anastomosis of the transected inferior vena cava by the Carrel technique, and (4) end-to-end anastomosis of the transected abdominal aorta with the suturing apparatus devised by one of us (K. I.).[5, 6]

When suturing was done by hand, No. 4-0 silk thread and an atraumatic needle were employed. No anticoagulants were used. After varying periods of time, the dogs were sacrificed and the vessel specimens were removed with approximately 2 cm. left on each side of the anastomotic site.

Canine blood platelets, separated by centrifugation, were suspended in physiologic saline solution, incubated with $P^{32}$ for 2 hours at 37° C, according to the method of Julliard,[7] and washed with saline solution until no further decrease appeared in the radioactivity of the supernatant. The concentration of the platelets was adjusted to about 2 times $10^5$ per cubic millimeter.

The specimen was cut open lengthwise

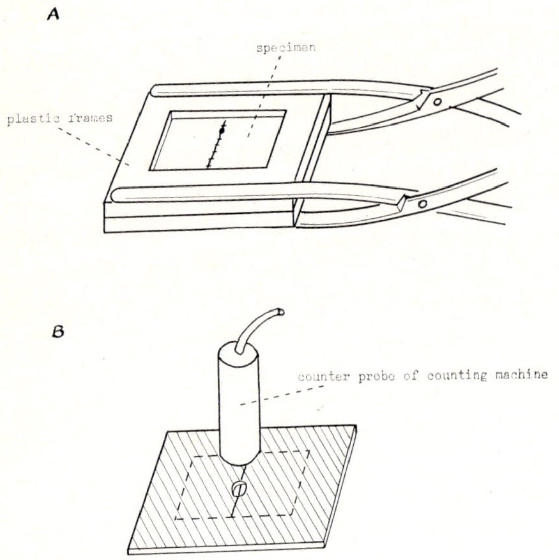


**Fig. 1.** Schematic illustration of procedure for measuring the adherence of radiolabeled platelets onto the intimal surface of blood vessel specimen. The vessel specimen is set in a pair of plastic frames and allowed to remain in contact with the radiolabeled platelet suspension for a measured period of time (*A*). The specimen is detached from the frames and the radioactivity on the intimal surface is measured (*B*).

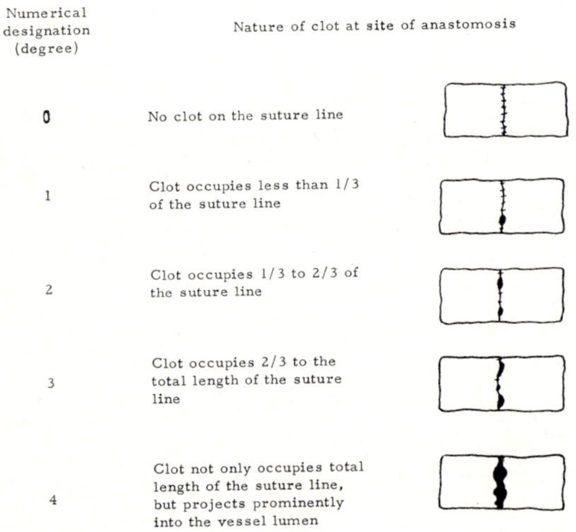


**Fig. 2.** Arbitrary classification of the extent of clot attached to the anastomotic site. Degrees of clot attached to the suture line in Figs. 3 through 5 and 7 are taken as the average values of the numerical designation of each case.

and set in a pair of plastic frames as shown in Fig. 1. These frames, 3 mm. in thickness and with an opening of 3.0 by 0.9 cm., were so made that when fastened together with clamps, no leakage occurred at the lines of contact with the specimen. Thus, the intima of the specimen to be tested formed the bottom of a shallow tray. The seal of the tray was tested for 5 minutes with saline solution. Then, 2 ml. of the platelet suspension was poured into the tray, and allowed contact with the intimal surface for 5 minutes at room temperature. After this procedure, the tray was upset to throw away the platelet suspension, and rinsed in saline solution for 30 seconds. Then the specimen was detached from the frames and the degree of radioactivity on the intimal surface was measured with a Geiger-Müller counter. A lead shield with a circular opening 5 mm. in diameter was used for selecting the desired portion of the specimen. This was placed over the suture line at the point where there was the least amount of clotting. The same procedure was carried out on a segment of normal thoracic aorta from the same dog, and the level of radioactivity thus measured was used as a control value. The rate of adherence of blood platelets onto the intima was defined as:

$$R = \frac{I_a - N}{I_c - N}$$

R is the rate of adherence, $I_a$ the counts per minute on the anastomosed portion, $I_c$ the counts per minute on the normal intimal surface, and N the background counts per minute for the counting machine. The measurements were made 4 times at each site, and the average values were taken.

Attention was paid to the size of the clot adhering to the intima, and also to the extent to which the newly growing intima covered the anastomotic site on successive days after operation. Both gross and microscopic examinations were made. The arbitrary classification shown in Fig. 2 was used to indicate the size of the attached clot.

## EXPERIMENTAL RESULTS

**Group 1. End-to-end anastomosis of abdominal aorta with Carrel's method.** Fifty-two dogs were used in these experiments. Macroscopically, clot was seen at the anastomotic site in almost all the specimens from the first to the eighth postoperative day. The clot increased in amount gradually as time elapsed, and attained a maximum on the fifth day, while on the sixth to the eighth day the clot began to decrease. The clots shortly after operation were generally red or red brown with a smooth surface, while those after about the sixth postoperative day were dark red or brown with a somewhat rough surface.

After 9 days had elapsed, macroscopic observation showed a thin, glistening layer covering the suture site in almost all specimens, while 6 to 8 days after the operation the anastomotic line was seen to be covered by newly growing tissue in some specimens, but not in others. Macroscopic findings indicated that the development of intima began on about the sixth day and was complete on approximately the tenth day after operation.

New intima tended to develop more poorly over clotted than over clot-free surface. In specimens from approximately 2 weeks to 7 weeks after operation, the inner layer at the anastomotic site projected slightly above the surface of the surrounding intima. This disappeared by the fourteenth week.

It was seen that the platelet adherence rate on the clot-free surface, which was 4.8 on the first postoperative day, generally increased until it reached a maximum of 6.6 on about the fifth day and then decreased rather steeply to about 3.0 on the eighth to ninth day, gradually approaching the normal level after 100 days or more. Adherence at the surface of the clot followed a similar pattern, though the values in the latter case were approximately 15 per cent higher. These results are shown in Fig. 3.

**Group 2. End-to-end anastomosis of inferior vena cava with Carrel's method.** Thirty-one dogs were used in these experiments. Immediately after operation, the platelet adherence rate increased and reached a maximum of 7.2 on the sixth postoperative day. Thereafter the rate decreased sharply, leaving a marked peak in the curve. The size of the clot, still small

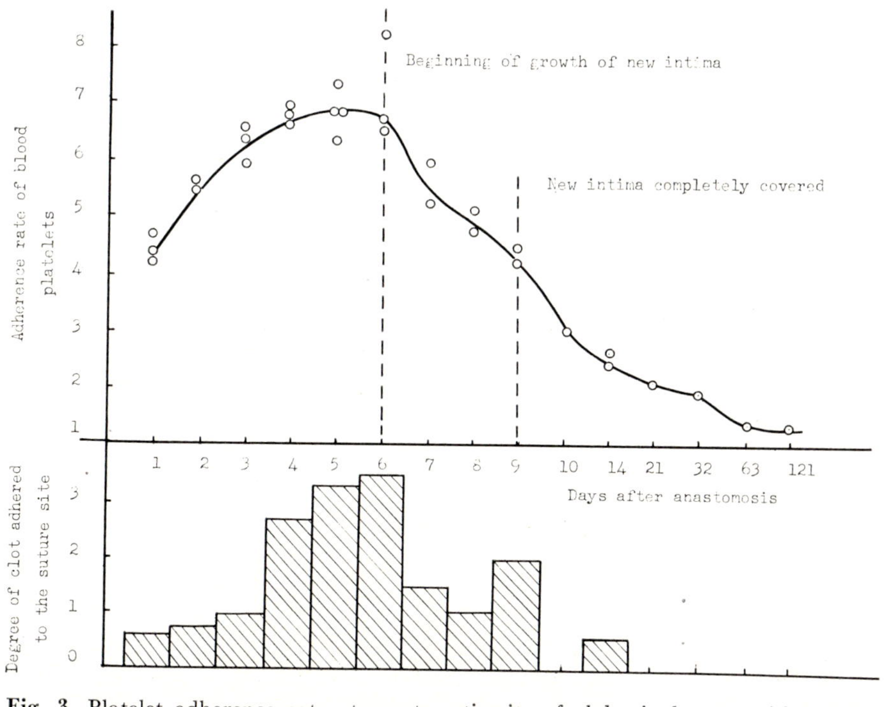


**Fig. 3.** Platelet adherence rate at anastomotic site of abdominal aorta with Carrel's method

on the third postoperative day, increased rather sharply on the fourth to the sixth postoperative day, and then decreased again on the eighth to the ninth day. Intimal development was seen to begin on about the sixth day and was complete on the ninth day. The surface of the intima was rough in specimens excised during the first 30 days, while in those taken after 60 days it had become smooth and hardly distinguishable from the original intima. The behavior is shown in Fig. 4.

**Group 3. Continuous hand suture of longitudinally slit abdominal aorta.** Thirty-two dogs were used in these experiments. The platelet adherence curve, which began at 2.5 on the first postoperative day, increased steeply to 5.2 on the fourth day, and then decreased gradually to about 2.0 on the tenth day. The size of the clot attached to the anastomotic site was maximal on the fifth day, though the size was generally lower than in Groups 1 and 2. It was observed that the newly growing intima began to develop on the sixth postoperative day and completely covered the suture line on the ninth postoperative day. This is shown in Fig. 5.

**Group 4. End-to-end anastomosis of abdominal aorta with the suturing apparatus.** Twenty-eight dogs were used in this group. Only 3 specimens, taken on the fifth, seventh, and ninth days, showed clotting, and even in these cases the extent of the clot was small (1 degree or less). In other specimens, no clot was observed. Fig. 6 shows a comparison of the appearance of abdominal aorta segments anastomosed by apparatus and by hand. Whereas the specimen 4 days after being anastomosed by hand suture shows an appreciable clot, the mechanically sutured specimen showed very little clot. The platelet adherence rate, 2.3 on the first postoperative day, passes through a maximum of 3.5 on the fifth day, drops to 2.0 by the fourteenth day, and then gradually decreases to the normal level. It will be noticed that these values are only about one-third those obtained with Carrel's method. The newly growing intima was seen to begin to develop on the fifth postoperative day by manual suturing technique. With

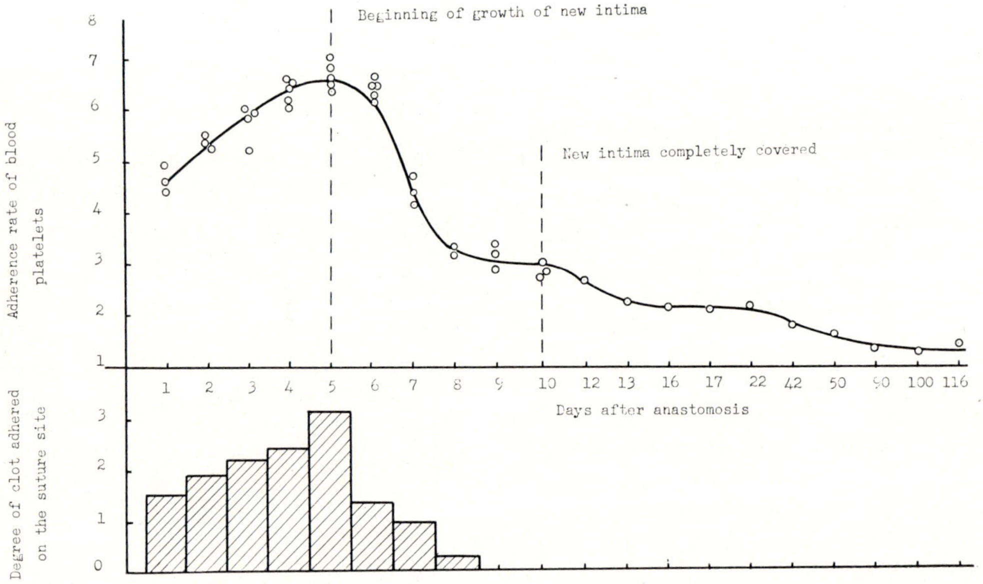


**Fig. 4.** Platelet adherence rate at the anastomotic site of inferior vena cava with Carrel's hand suture method.

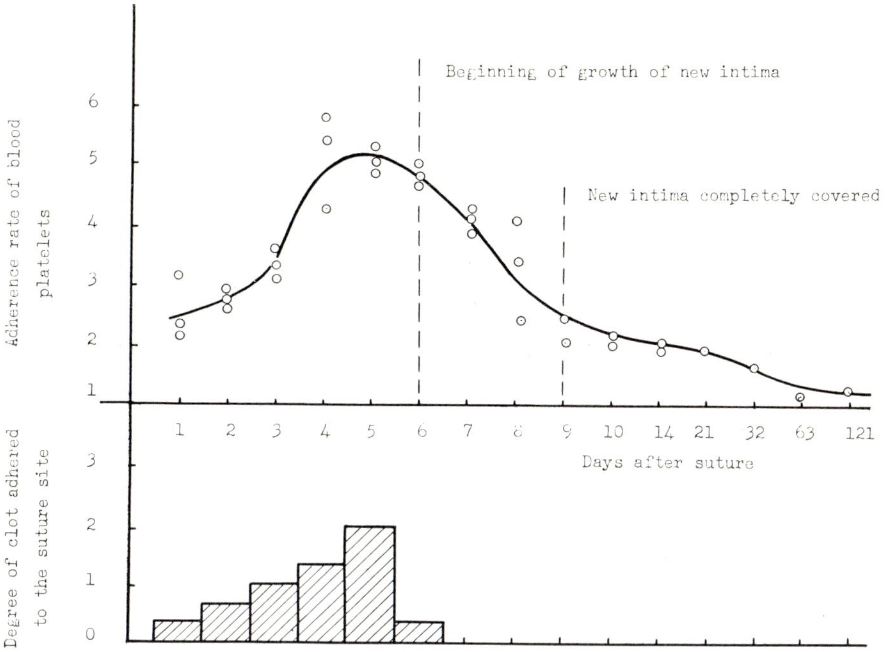


**Fig. 5.** Platelet adherence rate at the site of continuous hand suture of longitudinally slit abdominal aorta.

mechanical anastomosis, intimal formation began on about the seventh day, and was complete on approximately the tenth day. These results are shown in Fig. 7.

## DISCUSSION

It generally has been recognized that the aggregation of blood platelets constitutes the initial stage in thrombus formation. Bizzozero[1] and Eberth and Schimmelbusch[2] reported that platelets in streaming blood tend to adhere to the injured portions of blood vessels. In addition, recent papers by O'Neil,[10] Moolton,[8] and Samuels[11] deal with the adherence of platelets to the injured intima. Previous studies at this laboratory[3, 4, 9, 12] have recently shown that radiolabeled platelets strongly adhered to the damaged intima of excised specimens of blood vessels as well as onto freshly clotted surface. Moreover, these experiments have shown that the adherence of platelets takes place in advance of macroscopic evidence of thrombosis.

In the present study, platelet adherence at the anastomosed or sutured site was studied on successive days after operation. Significant correlation between clot size and the platelet adherence rate at the clot-free surface was found. These facts lead us to conclude that the rate of platelet adherence at the intimal surface may be a good index

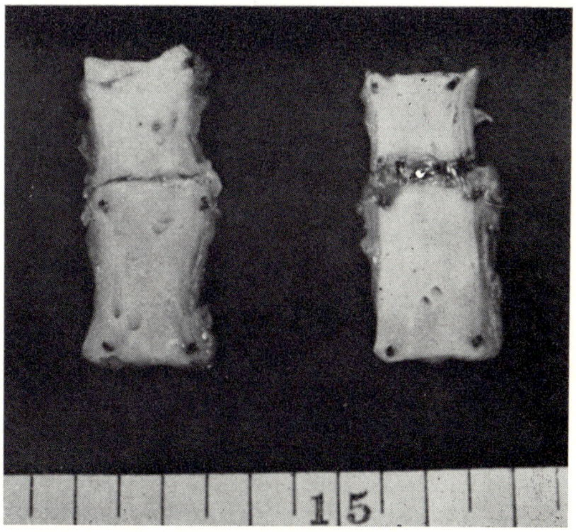

**Fig. 6.** Comparison of the intimal surface of anastomotic sites of dog's abdominal aorta with mechanical suture *(A)* and hand suture *(B)*. No clot with mechanical suture is seen.

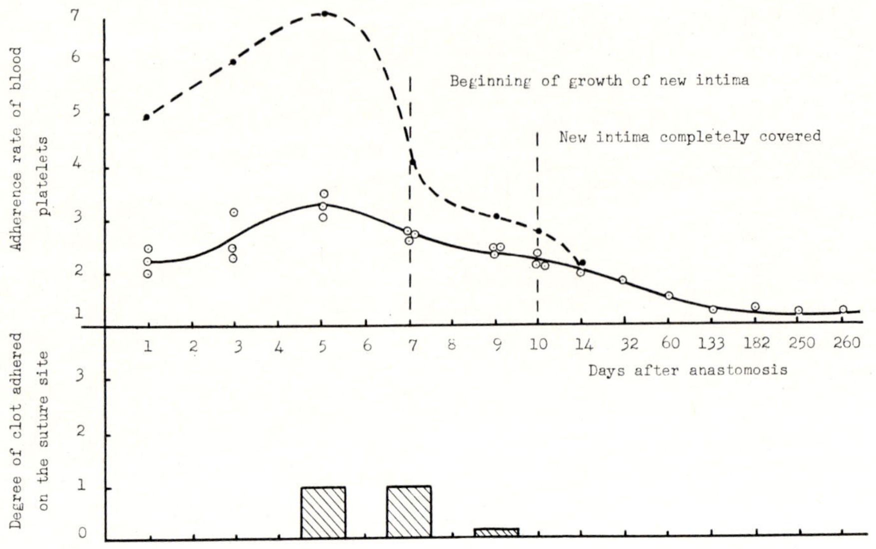


**Fig. 7.** Platelet adherence rate at the anastomotic site of abdominal aorta with Inokuchi's mechanical suturing apparatus (solid line). Broken line indicates the rate by hand suture. Apparent low values with the mechanical suture are noted.

for the evaluation of the predisposition of the intima toward clot formation.

In the specimens in the present study, peak adherence of platelets occurred on approximately the fifth postoperative day. This was true regardless of the type of vessel anastomosed (abdominal aorta or inferior vena cava), or the technique used (manual or mechanical), or the kind of anastomosis performed (end-to-end anastomosis or closure of longitudinal slit in vessel wall). In all cases the extent of the clot was also greatest on about the sixth postoperative day. This seems to indicate that the intimal surface at the anastomotic site is temporarily especially prone to thrombus formation on about the fifth postoperative day.

It would be interesting to know how long it takes for the intima to regain its normal condition. In these experiments it took 2 to 3 weeks for the platelet adherence rate to fall to twice the control level and more than 10 weeks for it to drop to control levels. It is difficult to determine the exact stage at which the condition of the intima is no longer conducive to thrombus formation because the actual development of a thrombus depends not only on the condition of the intima but also on such secondary factors as vessel size, speed of blood flow, coagulability of blood, and so forth. However, it is clear that the condition of the intima is most favorable for thrombus formation on about the fifth postoperative day and that it takes some weeks for it to return to normal.

Dates of initiation and completion of new intimal development (determined by macroscopic inspection of the suture line) varied little with different types of experiments and were sixth and ninth days for the longitudinally slit abdominal aorta closed with a continuous hand suture, fifth and tenth days for the severed abdominal aorta anastomosed by Carrel's hand suture method, sixth and ninth days for the inferior vena cava anastomosed by Carrel's method, and seventh and tenth days for the abdominal aorta anastomosed mechanically. The period of development of intima corresponds to the decreasing slope of the platelet adherence curve, which falls to about 3.0 after new intima has covered the suture line. It will be seen that new intima begins to develop at a time when platelet adherence is close to its peak value.

In the case of anastomoses with Inokuchi's

suturing apparatus, there is much less platelet adherence and the clot at the anastomotic site is much smaller. It is apparent that this apparatus minimizes the risk of thrombosis after operation. It should be a particularly desirable instrument in anastomosing vessels of small caliber and veins, in which the difficulties inherent in manual technique ordinarily produce a high incidence of thrombosis.

Finally, it should be noted that our results have been obtained after operations on normal vessels in animals. In diseased vessels in human beings, the course of the reparative process may be somewhat different. The present paper, however, may be worthwhile in that it has demonstrated the basic pattern of the healing process from the standpoint of the thrombogenicity of blood vessels operated upon. Moreover, it seems to us that experimental methods of the type mentioned in this paper may yield still more information about the thrombogenic property of blood vessels than the studies reported here.

## SUMMARY

In order to obtain greater understanding of the reparative process of the surface of the injured intima of blood vessels, anastomotic sites of abdominal aorta and inferior vena cava in dogs were studied by the technique of measuring the extent of adherence of $P^{32}$-labeled blood platelets onto the surface of the intima to be tested. The results obtained were: (1) platelet adherence was found to be related to the size of the clot and to the state of development of the intima at the anastomotic site, (2) platelet adherence at the anastomotic site reached a maximum on approximately the fifth postoperative day, and after the peak it took several weeks for degree of adherence to return to the normal preoperative level, (3) after anastomosis with Inokuchi's suturing apparatus, there was much less platelet adherence than after anastomosis by Carrel's manual suture method, (4) consequently, it might be deduced that the risk of thrombosis is greatest at about the fifth postoperative day, and that this risk can be minimized by use of the suturing apparatus.

The authors wish to express their thanks to Prof. M. Tomoda for his helpful encouragement throughout this work.

## REFERENCES

1. Bizzozero, J.: Über einen neuen Formbestandteil des Blutes und dessen Rolle bei der Thrombose und der Blutgerinnung, Arch. path. Anat. **90:** 261, 1882.
2. Eberth, J. C., and Schimmelbusch, C.: Experimentelle Untersuchungen über Thrombose, Arch. path. Anat. **103:** 39, 1886.
3. Inokuchi, K.: Ein neuer Gefässanastomosenapparat, Zentralbl. Chir. **84:** 419, 1959.
4. Inokuchi, K.: A new type of vessel-suturing apparatus, A. M. A. Arch. Surg. **77:** 954, 1958.
5. Inokuchi, K., and Yagi, H.: A preliminary report on the etiological mechanism of thrombosis by means of radioactively labelled blood platelets with $P^{32}$, with special reference to the surface properties of the intima, Kyushu J. M. Sc. **7:** 192, 1956.
6. Inokuchi, K., and Yagi, H.: Rapport préliminaire sur le méchanisme étiologique de la thrombose étudié au moyen des plaquettes sanguines marqués par le P-32, en considérant plus particulièrement les propriétés de surface de l'intima, Sang **28:** 855, 1957.
7. Julliard, J.: Premiers essais de transfusion a l'nomme de leucocytes et de plaquettes marquées en radiophosphore, Presse méd. **60:** 518, 1952.
8. Moolton, S. E., and Vroman, L.: Role of blood platelets in thromboembolism, Arch. Int. Med. **84:** 667, 1949.
9. Nakamura, T.: An experimental study on the mechanism of thrombus formation with radioactive platelets, with special reference to the phenomenon of dissolution of platelets on the injured intima, Acta med. Jap. **30:** 38, 1960.
10. O'Neil, J. F.: The effect on venous endothelium of alternations in blood flow through blood vessels, in vein walls, and possible relation to thrombosis, Ann. Surg. **126:** 270, 1947.
11. Samuels, F. B., and Websters, D. R.: The role of venous endothelium in the inception of thrombosis, Ann. Surg. **136:** 422, 1952.
12. Yagi, H.: Study on thrombus by means of radioactively labelled blood platelets with $P^{32}$ with special reference to the selectivity of blood platelets onto the intima surface of the injured blood vessel, Acta med. Jap. **28:** 3522, 1958.

# The removal of a wire lodged in the interventricular septum of the heart

LEROY J. KLEINSASSER, M.D.
DALLAS, TEXAS
*From Baylor University Hospital Medical Center*

The widespread use of the rotary lawn mower has resulted not only in direct injuries, but also in more serious trauma from missiles hurled by the whirling blade. This report concerns such an injury by a fragment of heavy wire 18 mm. long which penetrated the heart and lodged in the interventricular septum. A problem of accurate location of the foreign body, a veritable "needle in the haystack," arose since this was a prerequisite for its successful removal. It is the purpose of this report to describe the indications for the removal of such a foreign body, to restate the value of angiocardiography, to emphasize the use of temporary cardiopulmonary bypass of the heart to provide a relatively dry field for the removal of a small foreign body, and to call attention to the use of the Berman Locator.

## CASE REPORT

G. D. H., a 30-year-old man, while mowing his lawn with a rotary mower on May 13, 1960, heard a loud explosion and felt a sudden pain in his chest. He was able to walk to his car, but fainted while on the way to see his physician, Dr. Frank Rainone. He soon regained consciousness and although he was hypotensive at first, his blood pressure soon returned to a normal level. He was hospitalized at the Flow Memorial Hospital in Denton, Texas, and was given intravenous fluids, antibiotics, and tetanus toxoid. The chest pain persisted. Roentgenograms of the chest showed what appeared to be a piece of bailing wire present in the region of the right ventricle. He was transferred to Baylor University Medical Center in Dallas on May 14, 1960, for removal of the foreign body. The wire had entered the chest in the fifth intercostal space, 4 cm. to the right of the midline, and the opening appeared to be 8 mm. in diameter. There were some nonspecific changes in the electrocardiogram which were definitely abnormal. Roentgenograms of the chest taken after a barium swallow showed the wire to be anterior, in the midline, and probably in the right ventricle projecting from the interventricular septum. On fluoroscopy, the wire was seen to move with each heartbeat, and appeared to be imbedded in the septum with the other end moving freely in the right ventricle. Angiocardiography confirmed the location (Figs. 1 and 2).

The patient was operated upon on May 19, 1960, through a median sternotomy after a roentgenogram of the chest had been taken on the operating table to be certain the foreign body had not moved. One hundred fifty milliliters of old and fresh liquid blood was found on opening the pericardium and there appeared to have been no clotting. The wire had entered the right ventricle anteriorly and inferiorly near the atrioventricular groove without injury to the right coronary artery and the point of entry was covered with a fibrin plug. The heart was examined digitally through the right atrial appendage, but the wire could not be felt. It seemed unwise to pursue this manipulation energetically for fear of dislodging the foreign body. The patient was prepared for total cardiopulmonary bypass with a Pemco Kay-Cross pump-oxygenator by administration of heparin and insertion of catheters into the right femoral artery and into the vena cava for siphon drainage. The Berman Locator was then used and although it appeared to locate the wire in the right ventricle, it gave a false reaction when in the metallic field of the sternal rib spreader. Upon opening of the right ventricle and evacuation of the blood, the foreign body, covered with fibrin, could be seen projecting from the interventricular septum, penetrating one of the chordae tendineae of the septal leaflet of the tricuspid valve. The wire was grasped and removed, leaving no apparent defect in the septum, and the ventriculotomy closed. The vessels were decannulated after 15 minutes of bypass and the cardiac activity remained vigorous and effective. The pericardium was closed loosely, chest tubes

Received for publication Oct. 31, 1960.

inserted for drainage, and the sternum approximated with stainless steel wire. The femoral and brachial arteries were repaired.

This patient's recovery after operation was excellent. He was given antibiotics and digitalized. The chest tubes were removed by March 22, 1960, and roentgenograms of the chest showed good lung expansion. The incision was healing well and the sutures were removed on June 1, 1960, and the patient discharged. The patient was last seen Oct. 17, 1960, after having gone back to work in August, 1960. His blood pressure was 120/80, no cardiac murmurs could be heard, and his condition is excellent with a complete recovery.

## DISCUSSION

Foreign bodies may enter the heart directly or from a vessel proximal to a heart chamber. If the patient recovers from the initial injury, the problem is what to do with a patient who may or may not have symptoms and is discovered to have a retained metallic foreign body in the wall or chamber of the heart. The arguments advanced for the removal of cardiac foreign bodies[4] are (1) to prevent embolism of the foreign body or an associated clot, (2) to reduce the danger of bacterial endocarditis, (3) to prevent recurrent pericardial effusions, and (4) to diminish the incidence of myocardial damage with ventricular aneurysm and rupture.

On the other hand, many patients with foreign bodies in the heart have been described who were essentially asymptomatic for periods varying from months to years after their intial injury. Not everyone agrees that the hazards of retained foreign bodies are great. Fritz and associates,[3] performed experimental studies of foreign bodies in 62 dogs by introducing foreign bodies directly into the heart. They concluded that the majority of foreign bodies retained in and around the heart, as long as they do not produce symptoms or signs of cardiac dysfunction, may be permitted to remain undisturbed. However, a large number introduced directly into the chamber embolized unless they were caught in the chordae. It appears that foreign bodies may behave differently depending upon their location within the heart. Foreign bodies free in a chamber have a strong tendency for early embolism. Those entirely within the myocardium, which are not infected, will soon become enclosed in a fibrous capsule and will not tend to migrate or injure adjacent myocardium, while those which are in such a position that the myocardium or valve leaflet impinges upon them during cardiac systole tend to cause erosion and produce bacterial invasion and myocardial obstruction.[6] Decker,[1] after a review of 109 cases, stated that foreign bodies should not be removed simply because of their presence. "No emergency exists in those patients

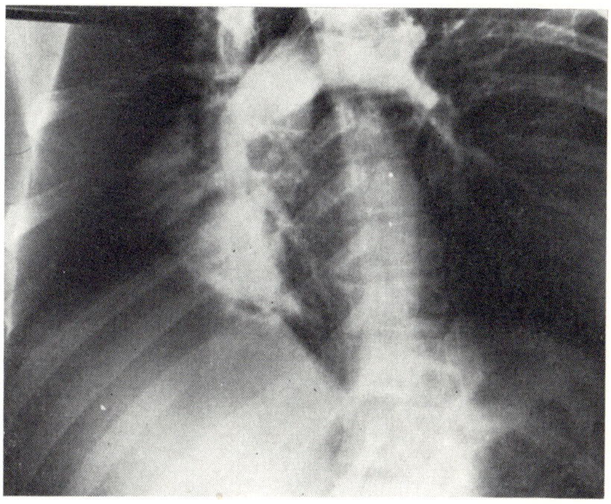

**Fig. 1.** Left anterior oblique angiocardiogram which shows the foreign body in the chamber of the right ventricle.

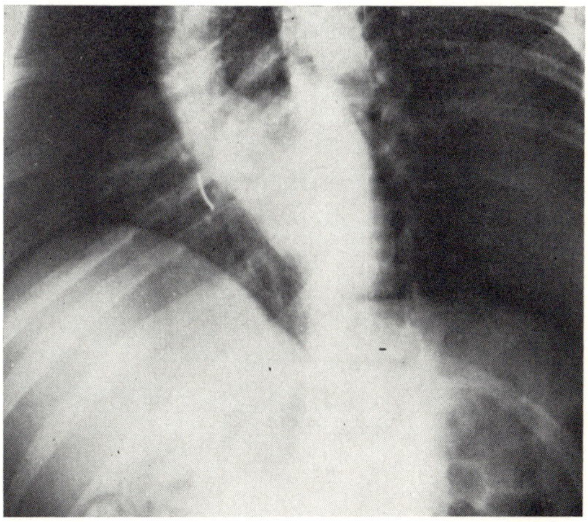

**Fig. 2.** Left anterior oblique angiocardiogram which shows the foreign body outside the cavity of the left ventricle with one end in the interventricular septum.

who survive the original trauma, unless one chooses to consider that free cavity bodies, sharp needle-like bodies and large objects need immediate or early surgery." The prominent subjective symptoms in these cases were pain, dyspnea on exertion, asthenia, and neurotic manifestations. In 2 of the cases reviewed the patients had involvement of the interventricular septum. This appears to be the rarest location. Magnan, in 1911, reported a needle three-fourths of an inch long in the interventricular septum which had been present 29 years and was not removed, but found at autopsy.[1]

Partial review of the literature indicates several deliberate attempts to remove foreign bodies in the interventricular septum. Swan and his group,[6] in 1952, reported 2 cases of foreign bodies in the interventricular septum. One, 1 cm. by 4 mm. in size, was wholly within the septum and there appeared to be no indication for its removal. The second was a shell fragment which was partially imbedded in the midpoint of the interventricular septum and protruded into the chamber of the right ventricle. There was pericardial effusion. Electrocardiogram showed a pattern of pericarditis with a right bundle branch block. The fragment was removed through an anterior bilateral sternum—dividing thoracotomy during inflow vena caval occlusion of 1 minute and 40 seconds through a right ventriculotomy. Valle,[7] in 1955, reviewed 117 injuries of the heart and pericardium which occurred in 2,811 casualties of the Korean conflict listed at the Tokyo Army Hospital. Nineteen had foreign bodies in the myocardium and these were removed successfully by closed methods except in 3 cases in which the foreign bodies were lodged in the interventricular septum. Efforts to remove these were unsuccessful. Flick,[2] in 1960, reported the removal of an embolic .22 caliber bullet trapped beneath the chordae tendineae of the tricuspid valve within the right ventricle. This was successfully accomplished in a 9-year-old boy by a closed method through the right ventricular wall. However, the foreign body could be palpated through the intact wall of the right ventricle.

The presence of a foreign body imbedded in the heart presents a difficult problem. The danger of allowing it to remain with the attendent consequences must be balanced against the hazard of removal. In the present report, the principal indications for the removal of the wire were the danger of bacterial endocarditis, embolization, and possible injury to the interventricular septum if the foreign body were allowed to remain. The patient's desire to be rid of a foreign body in his heart is of considerable psychological importance, but this presents no real indication for operation. Once the decision is made to remove the foreign body every effort should be made to locate it so that no time will be lost in seeking it. Cardiac fluoroscopy and angiocardiography should be used. Angiocardiography in the left anterior oblique view which outlines the interventricular septum is best for location of missiles in or near the ventricles. This is demonstrated by Figs. 1 and 2 in which it will be noted that the wire is outside the lumen of the left ventricle, but is in the region of the right ventricle. This was first emphasized by Swan and associates.[6] The foreign body in the interventricular septum is best removed during total cardiopulmonary bypass and the hazard of the cardiotomy in the otherwise healthy heart is considered to be minimal. This allows a relatively dry field and time for deliberate location and removal of the foreign body. The Berman Locator, which was successfully utilized by Simpson[5] in locating a foreign body in the sulcus between the right atrium and the right ventricle just to the left of the right coronary artery, emits a high-pitched noise when near metal, and was employed in this case. Although it appeared to locate the wire in the right ventricle, a false reaction was given when the probe was in the field of the sternum-splitting retractor. It seems advisable to remove all metallic objects from the immediate field if the use of the locator becomes critical.

## SUMMARY

The successful removal of a fragment of baling wire which, propelled by a rotary lawn mower, had penetrated the heart and lodged in the interventricular septum with one end free in the right ventricle is reported. This was accomplished during total cardiopulmonary bypass. The indications for the removal of foreign bodies located in the interventricular septum are reviewed. The accurate location by roentgenograms, fluoroscopy, and angiocardiography is stressed as a requirement for the successful removal of small foreign bodies in the heart.

## REFERENCES

1. Decker, H. R.: Foreign bodies in the heart and pericardium—should they be removed? J. Thoracic Surg. **9:** 62, 1939.
2. Flick, J. B., Jr.: Right ventriculotomy for removal of intracardiac bullet, Ann. Surg. **151:** 231, 1960.
3. Fritz, J. M., Newman, M. M., Jampolis, R. W., and Adams, W. E.: Fate of cardiac foreign bodies, Surgery **25:** 869, 1949.
4. Harken, D. E., and Zoll, P. M.: Foreign bodies in and in relation to the thoracic blood vessels and heart. III. Indications for the removal of intracardiac foreign bodies and the behavior of the heart during manipulation, Am. Heart J. **32:** 1, 1946.
5. Simpson, J.: Foreign body of embolic origin in the right ventricle of the heart removed with successful result, A. M. A. Arch. Surg. **65:** 926, 1952.
6. Swan, H., Forsee, J. H., and Goyette, E. M.: Foreign bodies in the heart, indications for and technique of removal with temporary interruption of cardiac blood flow, Ann. Surg. **135:** 314, 1952.
7. Valle, A. R.: War injuries of heart and mediastinum, A. M. A. Arch. Surg. **70:** 398, 1955.

# Gelatin sealing to prevent blood loss from knitted arterial grafts

JOHN U. BASCOM, M.D.
MINNEAPOLIS, MINN.
*From the experimental laboratories, Minneapolis General Hospital Research Foundation, Inc.*

Early use of fabric arterial grafts was attended by serious hemorrhage when flow was re-established after surgical placement. Efforts to control blood loss by reducing pore size have been successful but as pore size has become smaller, fabric grafts have tended to resemble solid-wall tubes. Edwards[3] showed in 1957 that tubes with solid walls were unsuitable for use as arterial grafts because the solid walls delayed or prevented healing of the inner fibrin lining and thrombosis occurred frequently. After pondering the question of how to provide walls solid enough to be leakproof, yet porous enough to heal, we thought the answer might be a porous graft coated with an impervious material which would be slowly absorbed by the body. Gelatin film, known to be absorbable with minimal reaction, appeared to be a logical coating material. In the course of our experiments a flexible gelatin coating was developed and tested which controlled blood loss from fabric grafts while causing only a minimal delay in normal healing.

## EXPERIMENTAL PROCEDURE

Sixty-nine arterial grafts, each measuring 5 cm. in length, were thoroughly impregnated with a gelatin solution. The experimental series consisted of 57 grafts of coarsely knitted Teflon, 9 grafts of coarsely knitted Dacron, and 3 grafts of braided nylon. A control graft of identical material was prepared for each gelatin-treated graft, giving a total of 138 grafts that were placed in animals.

The grafts were packaged in test tubes and each gelatin-coated graft paired with its control graft. The 69 pairs of grafts in their tubes were baked for 4 hours at 140° C. (284° F.) in a laboratory drying oven. The baked gelatin-coated grafts and their controls were then inserted into a series of mongrel dogs. The dogs were of small to moderate size, weighing an average of 14.5 kilograms. Most (42) of the pairs of treated and control grafts were used to bypass ligated segments of the right and left carotid arteries. Some (22) of the treated grafts were sewn end-to-end to their controls, and the paired grafts inserted to replace an excised segment of the abdominal aorta. The control graft was placed proximally in some animals and distally in others. A few femoral bypasses were attempted.

Each dog served as its own control and had treated and control grafts inserted into the same, or symmetrical, arterial sites on the same day. Animals were sacrificed at intervals and the grafts removed for evaluation. The grafts were examined, sketched, photographed, fixed in formalin, and sectioned. In an effort to overcome any bias, grafts were compared and evaluated before they were identified as gelatin treated or control.

Supported by National Heart Institute Training Grant No. HTS-5376 and the Cargill Foundation.

Abridged from a thesis submitted to the Graduate School of the University of Minnesota in partial fulfillment of the requirements for the degree of Doctor of Philosophy in Surgery, June, 1960.

Received for publication Nov. 7, 1960.

## PREPARATION OF GELATINIZED PROSTHETIC GRAFTS

In this study the first attempts at sealing Teflon arterial grafts were made with commercially available Teflon tubing.* The grafts were one-fourth inch in diameter and were designated as 1040T knitted Teflon tubing. They were made of 400 denier, 60 filament yarn with 1 twist per inch and knitted at 60 courses per inch into crimped tubes. It was impossible to successfully coat this material with gelatin.

Close inspection of a graft showed that it had been partially sealed after knitting with Kel-F which prevented adherence of the gelatin. The manufacturer kindly provided uncoated grafts that were otherwise identical and these were readily sealed with gelatin. From this it was learned that all preliminary coatings on Teflon yarn must be avoided and gelatin must be applied directly to the raw fabric.

The Teflon grafts coated with Kel-F also had been treated by the calendering process whereby pore size was partially reduced. The flattening of the yarn during calendering may also have interfered with the bonding of the gelatin. Gelatin coating probably will be most successful on grafts that retain their original porosity as they come from the knitting machine.

The raw gelatin used as the sealing solution was USP pigskin gelatin† taken from the stock of raw materials used in the manufacture of gelatin film (Gelfilm) and gelatin foam sponges (Gelfoam). After experimenting with solutions of various concentrations maintained at various temperatures, we found the most satisfactory preparation to be a 7 per cent gelatin solution warmed to 70° C. in a water bath. During saturation of the material with the gelatin all air bubbles had to be carefully worked out of the fabric. Excess gelatin solution was drained from the fabric. Care was necessary to avoid stripping the drained graft between the fingers or squeezing it in the hand, for this led to leaks. An experiment demonstrated that drying the grafts in room air at normal temperatures by suspending them with a mild amount of weight on one end prevented adherence of adjacent ridges of the crimped fabric. This controlled the leaks that had appeared after separation of adherent ridges on the early gelatin-coated grafts. The initial drying in room air is important because the subsequent baking process will convert a moist jelled coating back into a warm liquid that will drain free of the graft when it is placed in the oven.

Baking is an essential part of the preparation, for it denatures the gelatin to render it less soluble in warm blood and more resistant to absorption by the tissues. Baking was accomplished by placing the grafts in a laboratory drying oven for 4 hours at 140° C. (284° F.). Aluminum containers were found to turn the grafts a very unattractive dark gray color during baking. Glass and some paper containers are more satisfactory. The baking process renders the grafts sterile and they can be maintained in this condition by storage in the closed containers in which they were baked. However, sterilization immediately prior to implantation in the animal or patient can be accomplished also by autoclaving for 5 minutes at 140° C.

Rough handling of the dry or baked grafts will crack the gelatin seal. Once the graft is remoistened, however, the gelatin coating becomes flexible and the graft can be handled freely at the operating table. It should be noted that excessive handling in a rough manner as well as sharp crimping of the material may lead to breaks in the continuity of the film and an unsatisfactory result.

As one extreme test of the sealing properties of gelatin a transparent gelatin tube was prepared by dipping a cylinder of nylon net into gelatin solution. The net openings were 2 mm. in diameter. The tube was used to replace a segment of aorta. Defective areas in the transparent tube began to leak within less than 1 minute, but it appeared that

*Furnished by the United States Catheter & Instrument Corp., Glens Falls, N. Y.

†Furnished by The Upjohn Company, Kalamazoo, Mich.

elimination of bubbles in the gelatin film might have given a stable and durable preparation. Such a tube of gelatin, supported by fabric net, might be used in experiments to help define the effect of variable porosity on graft healing.

## RESULTS

**Blood loss.** The gelatin coating successfully controlled blood loss. In 77 per cent of the graft pairs the blood loss from the coated graft was prevented completely or reduced to a minimal ooze. Table I shows the blood loss experience. In every instance blood loss was less severe from the gelatin-coated graft than from the untreated control. While this data was being accumulated various concentrations of gelatin and various methods of preparation were being tried. If only the perfected preparations were included, the data would be even more conclusive. On the basis of this experience it appears that blood loss through fabric graft material which is quite porous can be completely prevented by gelatin treatment of the fabric.

The terms "heavy" and "minimal" used in Table I are relative and require further definition. Attempts to measured blood loss by weighing sponges were unsuccessful. Minor errors in fashioning the anastomosis had a greater influence on the blood loss than did the presence or absence of a gelatin coating on the graft—though gelatin-treated grafts in general showed less leakage along the suture line. An acute experiment was performed which helped to define degrees of blood loss.

The femoral artery of a dog was divided and plastic catheters were tied into the proximal and distal segments of the vessel. The catheter ends were joined by a 5 cm. segment of the graft being tested. Femoral flow was re-established via these catheters through the graft. Blood loss through graft pores was measured. Imperfect though they were, early gelatin coatings permitted total losses of only 50 and 75 ml. when, with no intermittent reclamping, these imperfectly coated grafts were made a part of the femoral circulation. This loss was characterized as "moderate." Loss through the control grafts was so severe under similar circumstances (700 ml.) that the dog went into shock and would have died of exsanguination had the clamps not been reapplied. This and similar losses were characterized as "heavy."

**Table I.** *Blood loss from arterial grafts*

| | *Gelatin coated* | | *Control* | |
|---|---|---|---|---|
| | *No.* | *%* | *No.* | *%* |
| Heavy | 1 | 1 | 52 | 75 |
| Moderate | 15 | 22 | 17 | 25 |
| Minimal | 26 | 38 | 0 | 0 |
| None | 27 | 39 | 0 | 0 |

**Thrombosis.** There was no evidence that gelatin coating increased or enhanced thrombosis of grafts. The knowledge that gelatin foam sponges are in common use as hemostatic agents suggested that gelatin might have thrombogenic properties and be unsuitable as a material to be applied to vascular grafts. An acute experiment was set up to investigate the possibility.

Test tubes for the performance of Lee-White clotting time determinations were carefully cleaned. The determinations were then performed in control tubes and in tubes that had previously been coated with silicone, paraffin, and baked gelatin. As Table II shows, a baked gelatin lining was nearly as effective as a silicone lining in delaying clotting. This demonstrated that gelatin is not thrombogenic in vitro.

The results of animal experiments confirmed the impression that a gelatin film is not thrombogenic. Grafts that did clot in dogs were divided into (1) grafts that thrombosed within the first 24 hours after implantation and (2) grafts that thrombosed later in the postoperative course. This was considered an important division on a theoretical basis for, as Harrison[5] and Szilagyi[10] have pointed out, early thrombosis is often a result of shortcomings in operative technique while later thrombosis usually reflects undesirable characteristics of the graft material. All grafts which showed evidence of gross infection were excluded from this portion of the study.

With regard to the acute thrombosis encountered in carotid grafts (that is, thrombosis more likely to be due to poor operative technique) the results in the 2 groups were identical. There were 3 acute failures in 50 gelatin-coated grafts and 3 acute failures in 50 control grafts.

Late thrombosis (that is, thrombosis more apt to be influenced by the presence of a gelatin coating) was also as frequent among control grafts as among gelatin-coated grafts. In the 26 pairs of carotid grafts in which valid comparisons could be made, 3 gelatin-coated grafts and 3 control grafts showed late thrombosis. (Excluded from consideration were 27 animals with grafts other than carotid, 6 animals with carotid grafts that clotted within one day, 4 animals sacrificed on the first postoperative day, 4 animals with infected grafts, and 2 in which there had been technical errors.)

This experience with late thrombosis is of critical importance for 2 reasons. First, it establishes gelatin as a sealing material that can be used without fear of increased thrombosis. Second, this experience demonstrates that dog carotid arteries or other such vessels averaging 4 mm. in diameter can be successfully bypassed by fabric arterial grafts. Previous workers have abandoned carotid arteries as a useful implantation site because of thrombosis rates approaching 100 per cent. The success obtained in this experiment is probably due to the use of end-to-side anastomoses, careful operative technique, and the use of seamless tubes.

The similarity of treated and control grafts in their tendency to form thrombi is further evidenced by the 6 carotid grafts which became thrombosed 24 hours or more postoperatively. Bilateral thrombosis of carotid grafts in 2 dogs accounted for 4 of the 6 thrombosed grafts (2 gelatin-coated and 2 control grafts). Two other dogs developed late thrombosis in 1 of the 2 carotid grafts, 1 in a treated graft and 1 in a control graft. In both dogs the lining of the patent graft, opposite the thrombosed graft, consisted of unusually heavy fibrin which partially occluded the lumen. These linings were much heavier than those found in any other patent grafts in the series. Thus in each of the 6 instances of late thrombosis in carotid grafts there was evidence of a similar excessive fibrin deposit in both treated and control grafts. This indicates that the presence or absence of the gelatin coating was a factor of less magnitude in graft failure than the characteristics of the animal which received the grafts.

**Table II.** *Lee-White clotting time determinations (venous dog blood)*

| *Tube lining* | *Determinations* | *Average (min.)* | *Range (min.)* |
|---|---|---|---|
| Clean glass | 4 | 10.0 | 7.5-11.5 |
| Paraffin | 2 | 10.7 | 10.0-11.5 |
| Gelatin | 4 | 14.7 | 14.0-15.5 |
| Silicone | 2 | 16.5 | 13.5-19.5 |

**Infection.** In the 53 pairs of grafts which were valid for comparison with respect to infection, 75 per cent of the treated grafts were free of infection and 70 per cent of the control grafts were free of infection. Though treated grafts appear to be slightly superior to the controls, the difference was not significant.

**Hematoma formation.** Delayed leakage with hematoma formation about the graft was not a problem with either the treated or the control grafts.

**Fibrin accumulation.** Teflon grafts were selected for their property of accumulating only minimal amounts of fibrin—a property emphasized by Harrison[5] and Edwards.[4] It was found that these minimal accumulations were slightly increased by the application of a gelatin sealing coat. On the uneven surface of a crimped Teflon graft with minimal fibrin, the true thickness of fibrin is difficult to measure. By approximation it seemed that gelatin treatment increased the fibrin coat to 0.85 or 0.9 mm. in experimental grafts as compared to an average of 0.8 mm. in control grafts. However, variations in fibrin thickness from animal to animal were greater than the variations in fibrin thickness between treated and control grafts. It should be noted that, while the small in-

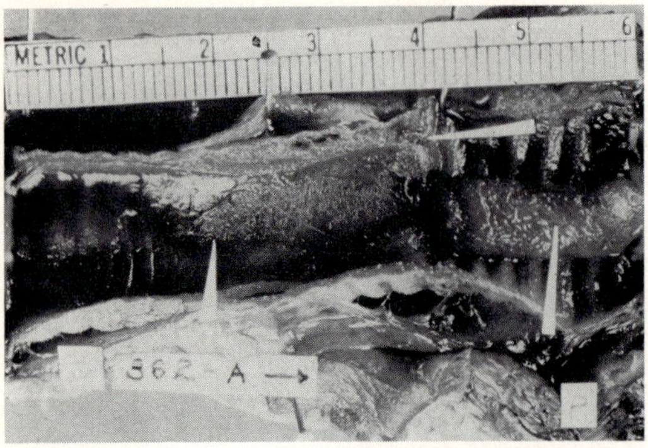


**Fig. 1.** Aortic graft. The horizontal arrow indicates the suture line joining the gelatin-coated segment on the left to the control segment on the right. The control segment is occluded by a solid fibrin plug which is sharply confined to that segment.

crease in fibrin in treated grafts is reported for the sake of completeness and accuracy, the increase was of no final importance since it was quite small and it did not lead to an increased thrombosis rate in gelatin coated grafts.

Results with aortic grafts indicated that the gelatin coating may actually retard or prevent heavy fibrin accumulations in some instances. There is no statistical evidence of this in the series, but close inspection of 3 aortic grafts that did thrombose suggested this conclusion. Recall that each abdominal aortic replacement graft consisted of a segment of gelatin-treated graft sewed end-to-end to its control graft. In some replacements the treated graft was placed distally and in others it was placed proximally. In Fig. 1 an aortic graft is shown which was occluded by a short cylinder of firm, pink fibrin. The fibrin had formed within the control graft only. By contrast, the treated segment had no fibrin plug but only a smooth, thin, 1 mm. lining of fibrin. Two other thrombosed aortic grafts showed a similar but less striking picture. They both had a pink clot in the control segment and a dark red clot in the gelatin-coated segment of the graft. The pink clots in the control segment were presumably formed by slow accumulation on the graft walls of fibrin in which very few red cells were trapped. When this fibrin in the control segment became thick enough, it slowed and finally stopped blood flow through the grafts. Blood in the adjacent gelatin-coated segment and the distal aorta then clotted abruptly with entrapment of red cells and formation of the uniform dark red clot. Thus, it seemed that the control segments and the pink clots found within them were responsible for thrombosis of the aorta and for the formation of the fresh dark red clots within the treated segments.

In the aortic grafts described, some process which was responsible for slow fibrin accumulation on the walls of control segments seems to have been repressed or inhibited in the gelatin-coated segments. Almost immediately after re-establishment of blood flow both treated and control segments of each of these aortic grafts must have been coated with a thin layer of fibrin deposited out of the flowing blood. From that moment on the physical and chemical characteristics of the linings of the treated and control segments should have been the same. Yet through some mechanism that continued to exert its effect through the thin fibrin barriers, the control segment accumulated fibrin to the point of occlusion while the fibrin deposits in the treated segment remained thin. The key to a fundamental understanding of processes at work in grafts that become thrombosed might lie hidden in these 3 aortic grafts. It could be that orientation of fibrin molecules absorbed into the gelatin, with respect to the electrical charges such fibrin molecules present to the moving stream of blood, might be a factor. The interested reader is referred to an excellent article by Sawyer and associates[9] concerning the electrical fields which are found about damaged vessels and their influence upon the clotting patterns within those vessels.

**Disappearance of gelatin.** Gelatin was deposited on grafts in a thin layer only one twentieth to one fiftieth as thick as the graft fabric. In Teflon grafts the gelatin filled the major pores and coated the fabric but it did not work its way around each individual

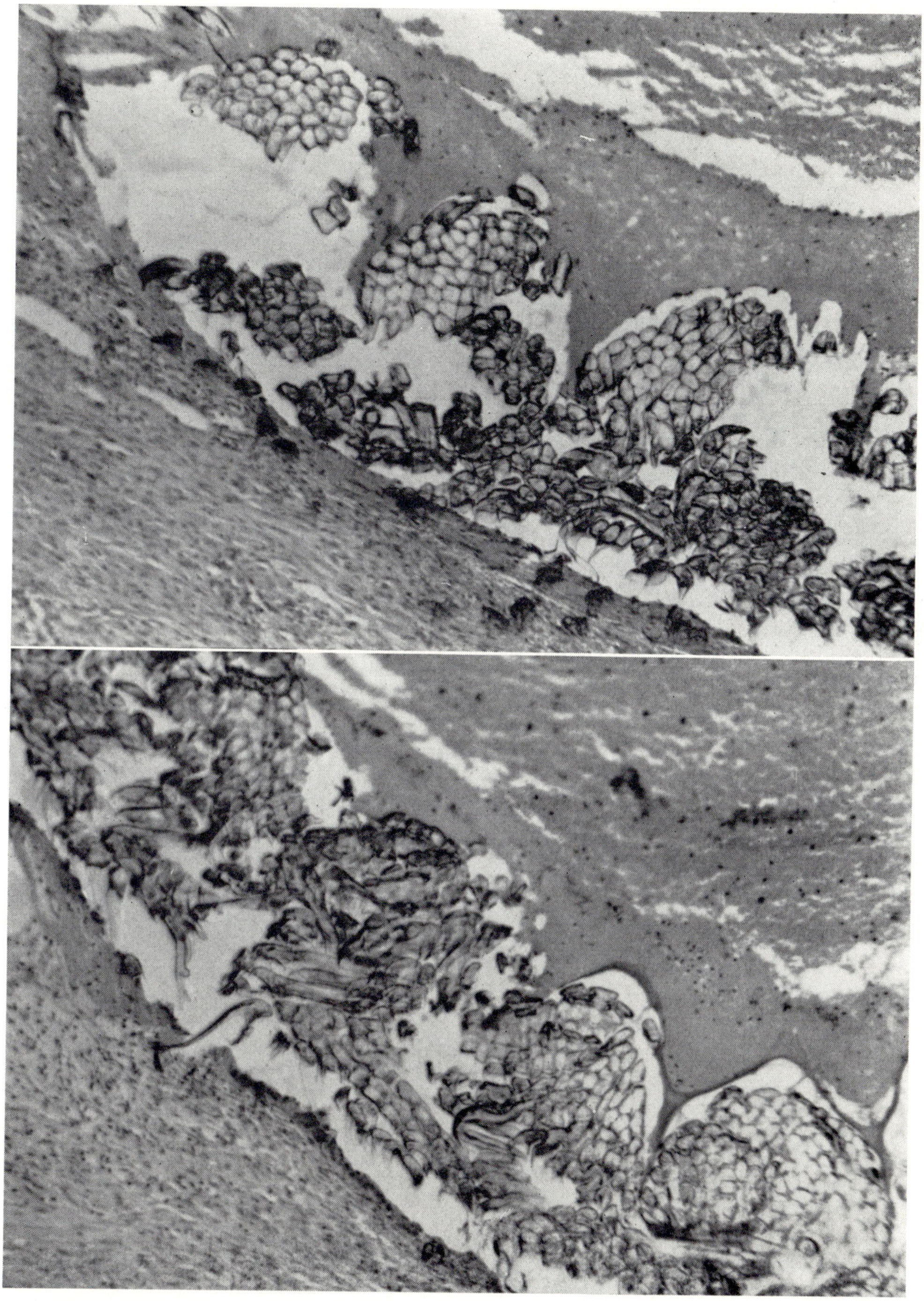

A

B

**Fig. 2.** A pair of Teflon carotid grafts which were removed on the twelfth postoperative day. *A,* The control graft. *B,* The graft coated with gelatin which appears as a dark line at the base of the fibrin lining of the graft. Note that there are nearly identical adventitial responses in the 2 specimens.

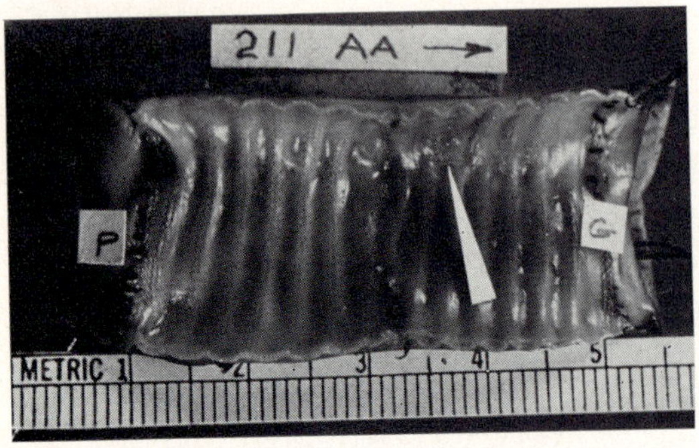


**Fig. 3.** An abdominal aortic graft removed 4½ months after implantation. The control graft is to the left (proximal) and the gelatin-coated graft is on the right. The arrow indicates a small area of minimal fibrin roughening still to be converted to fibrous tissue in the gelatin segment of the graft.

fiber. Such a gelatin coat appears in Fig. 2, *B*. On Dacron grafts the gelatin closed major pores but it also surrounded each fiber of the strands of yarn. This difference between the way Teflon and Dacron hold the gelatin coating seemed of no mechanical or biologic importance on gross or microscopic examination. Presumably the difference was due to the fact that Dacron fibers have a wettable surface and Teflon fibers have a nonwettable surface.

Teflon causes less reaction in surrounding tissue than any other graft material in common use. Teflon was selected for most of this experiment since tissue reaction was never severe enough to mask even mild adverse tissue reactions to gelatin.

In the experimental animals all traces of gelatin were gone completely by the twentieth postoperative day. Microscopic sections of a typical pair of grafts removed on the twelfth postoperative day are shown in Fig. 2. Tissue reactions about control grafts and gelatin-coated grafts are virtually identical grossly and microscopically at all stages of healing. Gelatin was absorbed by the body without accumulation of giant cells and with no greater number of macrophages or polymorphonuclear leukocytes present than were required to absorb and organize the fibrin deposited about control grafts. There was no evidence that the temporary presence of gelatin influenced in any way the amount of fibrous tissue deposited about the healed grafts.

**Rate of healing.** The gelatin coating did retard the rate of healing by 10 per cent. Early healing seems to begin by vigorous ingrowth of fibrous tissue and endothelium from the adjacent vessel ends. Early healing of this nature was not delayed by the gelatin coating.

Later healing takes place by fibrous replacement of the fibrin which lines the midportion of the graft. For this stage of healing it appeared necessary that fibroblasts grow in through the pores of the fabric. When gelatin temporarily sealed the pores, ingrowth of fibroblasts appeared to be slightly delayed. The delay amounted to 10 per cent of total healing time. Fig. 3 shows a pair of grafts removed 4½ months after implantation. Gross and microscopic patterns of healing in the gelatin-treated grafts and the control grafts are identical except for this slight delay in the healing time of treated grafts. Here again the differences between animals exceeded the differences in any one animal between a treated graft and its control.

## DISCUSSION

Gelatin is believed to be a safe material for graft sealing. This conclusion is based on the demonstrated inertness of gelatin foam sponges which have been used clinically for years as hemostatic agents. Antigen-antibody reactions have not been a problem with the use of gelatin foam sponges or with repeated intravenous administration of gelatin.[7] It therefore appears unlikely that gelatin graft coatings would present any hazard to patients, even when used repeatedly.

From recent studies, the degree of porosity of vascular prosthetic grafts appears to be an important consideration in their ultimate successful use. Edwards[3] has shown the necessity for pores that will permit fibroblasts to grow into the lumen of the graft, organize the fibrin, and heal the graft in place. Best results are obtained when the fibroblasts can penetrate the interstices of graft material into the inner fibrin lining from their source in the surrounding tissue. Other investigators[1, 2, 8] suspect that infections are a greater problem with impervious grafts than with porous grafts. However, substantial proof for this impression is lacking as yet.

Coincident with the need for an as yet unspecified degree of porosity in the graft material to permit maximum healing is the need to control hemorrhage and prevent undue blood loss at the time flow is re-established through the vascular prosthesis. Of the many different methods which have been tried to solve this problem, those in use at the present time include (1) the use of fuzzy or untwisted yarns to fabricate grafts, (2) the development of tightly knitted materials, (3) the development of extremely tight weaves, (4) heavy calendering of fabrics, (5) preclotting of the graft material with the patient's blood prior to implantation of the graft, (6) sequential opening and closing of the flow through the implanted graft at the time of re-establishment of flow to permit the deposition of fibrin in the interstices, and (7) partial sealing of the pores of the grafts with such nonabsorbable materials as Kel-F, silicone, Silastic, and microscopic fragments of the parent fiber. Extremely tight weaves have been particularly successful in solving the problem of immediate blood loss since these weaves are not only blood tight but also are very nearly air tight. However, the virtual complete loss of porosity in these materials may well lead to the same degree of poor healing as has previously been noted in grafts made of compressed Ivalon sponge.[6]

The use of permanent and nonabsorbable materials to fill the pores of a loosely knitted material simply converts the desirably porous material into a solid tube that would lead to the disadvantages mentioned. These studies have shown perfect healing of the gelatin-coated grafts at the end of 4 months with no evidence of gelatin remaining in the tissues. Though slightly delayed, the healing process is otherwise equal in every respect to that seen in the control grafts untreated with gelatin. The final comparison of gelatin sealing to other methods of treating grafts for blood loss awaits further trial. On the basis of this experimental work, an extensive clinical trial of this method seemed indicated and is underway at Minneapolis General Hospital.

## SUMMARY

The problem of preventing excessive blood loss through the pores of knitted vascular prosthetic grafts has been approached in our laboratories with a technique of impregnating the graft with an impervious film of baked gelatin. The baked gelatin film has sharply limited or prevented blood loss from porous knitted grafts without producing any detrimental side effects in the experimental animals. In a carefully controlled series, 138 grafts have been implanted into 69 dogs as controlled pairs. The gelatin-coated grafts have been distinguishable from the untreated grafts only in terms of a 10 per cent delay in the total healing time. The gelatin has been absorbed within 20 days and there have been no untoward side effects such as increased thrombosis in the grafts or increased inflammatory reactions in the tissues about the grafts. A clinical trial on an expanded basis appears necessary now to determine the effectiveness of this method in clinical surgery.

### REFERENCES

1. Creech, O., Jr.: Personal communication.
2. Deterling, R. A., Jr.: Personal communication.
3. Edwards, W. S.: The effect of porosity on solid plastic artery grafts, S. Forum **8:** 446, 1957.
4. Edwards, W. S.: Progress in synthetic graft development—an improved crimped graft of Teflon, SURGERY **45:** 298, 1959.
5. Harrison, J. H.: Synthetic materials as vascular prostheses. I. Comparative study in small vessels of nylon, Dacron, Orlon, Ivalon sponge, and Teflon, Am. J. Surg. **95:** 3, 1958.
6. Hitchcock, C. R.: Personal communication.
7. Parkins, W. M., Koop, C. E., Riegel, C., Vars, H. M., and Lockwood, J. S.: Gelatin as a plasma substitute: with particular refer-

ence to experimental hemorrhage and burn shock, Ann. Surg. **118:** 193, 1943.
8. Perry, John F., Jr.: Personal communication.
9. Sawyer, P. N., Deutch, B., Harshaw, D. W., and Duchdala, G.: The effect of induced periaortic infection on the potential difference measured across the aortic wall, SURGERY **38:** 342, 1955.
10. Szilagyi, D. E.: in discussion of Dale, W. A., and Niguidula, F. N.: Study of elasticized Dacron as arterial prosthesis, A. M. A. Arch. Surg. **78:** 259, 1959.

# The silicone-foam diagnostic enema. I. An assessment with surgical specimens of human sigmoid colon

GALEN B. COOK, M.D.
ALEXANDER R. MARGULIS, M.D.
ST. LOUIS, MO.
*From the Department of Surgery and The Edward Mallinckrodt Institute of Radiology, Washington University School of Medicine*

This presentation is the first in a series which will describe the development of a diagnostic technique designed for the discovery of small abnormalities in the mucosa of the human large intestine. The investigation is particularly concerned with the midsigmoid colon because it is beyond the range of the sigmoidoscope and is frequently difficult to study roentgenographically.

The need for a reliable and thorough method for the examination of the interior of the large intestine can be appreciated after a review of the diverse and inventive approaches which have evolved in the history of colon diagnosis. Radiography of the colon began with the radiopaque enema.[11] This was followed by the double-contrast enema,[8] the use of semitransparent media,[14] the addition of overexposed roentgenographic films,[19] and high-voltage technique.[10] Subsequently, chemicals such as tannic acid[20] and isatin[22] were added to the barium sulfate, and later external bag compression, filling of the urinary bladder,[3] and the Chassard-Lapine[18] and cephalad-oblique-prone projections[7] were introduced. Proctosigmoidoscopy was begun with the introduction of the proctosigmoidoscope. The technique was extended by lengthening the barrel, by coloscopy through colotomies,[6] and by use of the traction sigmoidoscope,[17] the suction-lavage sigmoidoscope,[21] the lucite Y tube,[9] and, most recently, the flexible coloscope.[13] The third avenue of approach has been cytologic study of material obtained by bulb pipetting,[16] sigmoidoscopic aspiration,[23] enema washing,[15] direct tissue smearing,[5] and millipore filtration of colonic washings.[12]

From this array of techniques useful combinations have emerged and are applied today regularly. The reliability of any combination, however, is not absolute, nor is the applicability universal for the discovery of small sessile cancers of the large intestine—especially when they are located in the region of the sigmoid colon. A recent evaluation of the accuracy of cytologic study of material collected above the reach of the sigmoidoscope showed only 4.3 per cent reliability.[4] Even with sigmoidoscopes of advanced design, the sigmoid colons of 25 per cent of patients could not be satisfactorily examined because of anatomic peculiarities.[17] Coloscopy is attended by an appreciable risk of secondary wound infection[2] and is not satisfactory for the examination of the colonic flexures. The accuracy of the barium enema, with all of its modifications, has seldom exceeded 90 per cent; in fact, reliabilities as low as 28 per cent have been reported.[1]

Because of these limitations attempts were made to find a method for making retrievable mucosal molds which have accurate de-

The latter phase of this study was supported in part by a University Institutional Grant from the American Cancer Society.

Received for publication April 17, 1961.

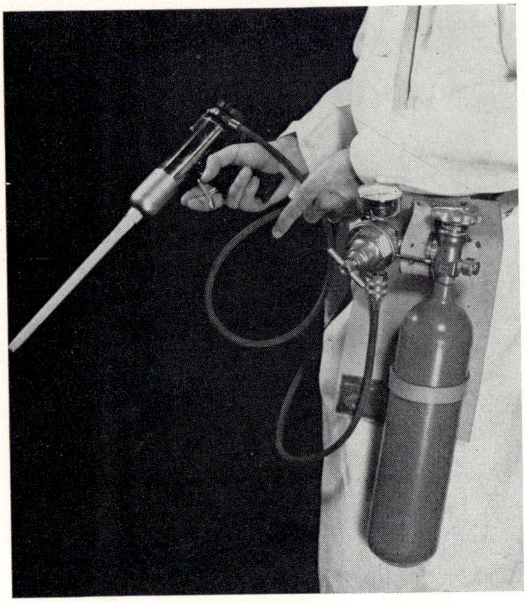

**Fig. 1.** Semco industrial sealant gun used for injection of silicone foam.

tails of mucosal relief and retain sufficient numbers of mucosal cells to permit accurately located cytologic sampling in the colons of living persons.

The requirements for such a mold are that it be (1) a liquid capable of being converted to an elastic, compressible, readily extrudable solid; (2) non-toxic in both the liquid and solid states; (3) available in quantity, easily handled, and inexpensive; (4) a material (in the liquid phase) with a low viscosity and a high miscibility with radiopaque media; (5) converted from liquid to solid in the bowel rapidly, predictably, and endothermically; and (6) a material (in the solid phase) that is spongy, cohesive, and freely and atraumatically separable from the mucous membrane.

Several sol-gel systems and many plastics were tried and eventually the criteria were met by silicone elastomers. Through the cooperation of the Dow Corning Center for Aid to Medical Research a silicone rubber (Silastic RTV 502*) was selected as the basic component. The molecule of this polymer is a chain of several thousand alternate silicon and oxygen atoms with side branches of short aliphatic radicals (predominately methyl groups):

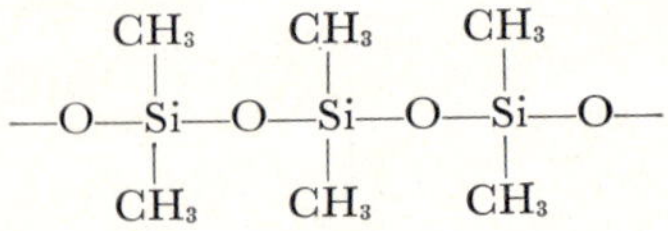

Polymerization occurs at room temperature and is effected with stannous octoate by a crosslinking of opposing methyl groups at intervals of several hundred monomer units. This reaction converts the liquid prepolymer into a synthetic rubber in from 3 to 10 minutes, depending upon the amount of the octoate added to it. To provide compressibility in the polymer, a silicone rubber foam (Silastic Q-3-0030*) was added to the Silastic RTV 502. This intumescent releases hydrogen gas (0.4 moles per 100 Gm. of Q-3-0030) during polymerization and this gas renders the polymerized mixture spongy. The addition of this hydrogen-evolving silicone does not significantly affect the surface impression detail nor does it impair the cohesiveness of the final product. It does, however, greatly increase the compressibility of the polymer and thereby increases the ease of extrusion. Stannous octoate is also the polymerizing agent for this compound.

The viscosity of a mixture of these two silicones in their prepolymeric phase ranges from 6,000 to 50,000 centistokes, depending upon the proportions of Silastic RTV 502 and Silastic Q-3-0030 added. However, with any combination of these two silicone prepolymers, a relatively viscous fluid is produced. By the addition of a cyclic dimethyl polysiloxane (Silicone Fluid 200, 20 centistokes*) to such mixtures the viscosity may be appreciably reduced. This facilitates giving the fluid as an enema. The character of the polymerized elastomers is not significantly altered if Silicone Fluid 200 represents less than 30 per cent of the prepolymer mixture. Being cyclic, Silicone Fluid 200 does not crosslink and therefore needs no polymerizing agent.

As a final step in the compounding of the

*Dow Corning Corporation, Midland, Mich.

*Dow Corning Corporation, Midland, Mich.

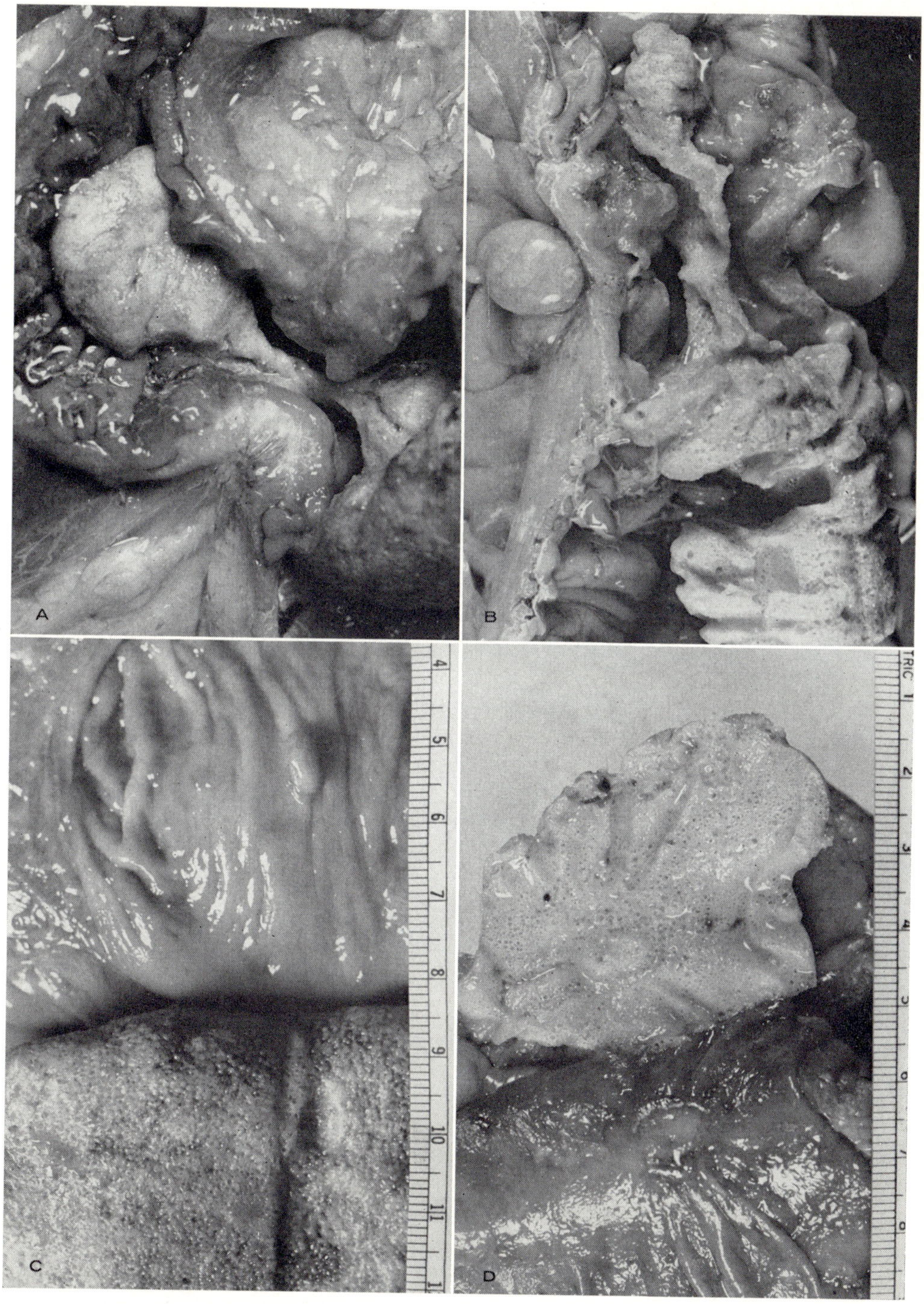


**Fig. 2.** *A* and *B*, Specimens of constricting adenocarcinoma of the colon with silicone-foam molds within the lumina. *C*, Mucosal polyp of the colon adjacent to silicone-foam impression of the lesion. *D*, Small ulcerating carcinoma of the colon with facsimile of the lesion imprinted on silicone foam.

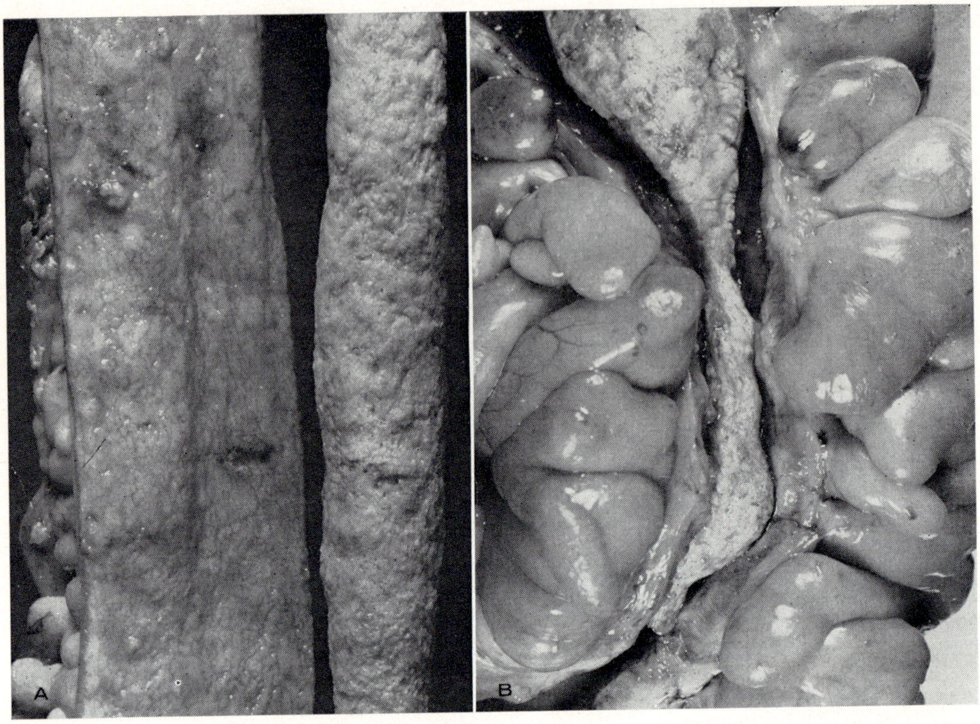

**Fig. 3.** *A,* Mucosal surface of colon involved with ulcerative colitis (left), and intraluminal silicone-foam mold of same region (right). *B,* Surgical specimen of colon with ulcerative colitis and signet-ring cell carcinoma containing intraluminal silicone-foam mold.

enema, a radiopaque material was added to the silicones so that the inflow could be observed fluoroscopically and the extent of the filling controlled safely and with certainty. Diatrizoate sodium (Hypaque*) was chosen empirically.

Various combinations of the 5 agents were compounded and the mixture finally selected for experimental use was Silastic RTV 502, 50 Gm.; Silastic Q-3-0030, 50 Gm.; Silicone Fluid 200 (20 centistokes), 10 Gm.; diatrizoate sodium, 25 Gm. in 20 ml. water; and stannous octoate catalyst, 2 ml.

First it was introduced into washed pieces of resected human colons. The distal line of resection was opened and through it the bowel was filled with the silicone-foam mixture administered from an industrial sealant gun† (Fig. 1). This apparatus contained the silicone fluid in a disposable polyethylene cartridge and extruded it at a uniform rate by a pressure of 5 pounds air per square inch. The specimens were filled completely but were not distended beyond their natural dimensions. Polymerization required approximately 10 minutes; during this period the bowel was massaged gently to simulate peristalsis.

Upon completion of polymerization, the specimens were carefully opened along the antimesenteric borders. Incisions into the rubber mold and, in specimens with tumors, incisions into the tumor were avoided. Photographs were made with the molds in place and they were then removed from the specimens, suspended in Hartman's solution, agitated, and dried for study of imprint detail. Cellular suspensions were taken to the Cytological Laboratory of Barnes Hospital for centrifugation and microscopic examination.

## RESULTS

Five surgical specimens of the sigmoid colon, each containing advanced, constricting

*Winthrop Laboratories, New York, N. Y.

†Semco Sales and Service, Inc., Inglewood, Calif.

adenocarcinomas, were studied (Fig. 2). In one of these specimens an adenomatous polyp was also found—its greatest dimension was less than 1 cm. (Fig. 2, *C*). In another specimen, a second carcinoma attended the major lesion (Fig. 2, *D*). The smaller malignancy remained occult until the silicone mold was studied. Upon recognition of it, the mold was transected so that the silicone reproduction of both the major and minor lesions could be submitted separately for cytologic study.

Two colons involved with advanced ulcerative colitis were examined (Fig. 3). The second specimen contained a signet-ring cell carcinoma in addition to colitis.

The cytologic examination of the cellular debris in every malignant lesion gave positive indications of carcinomatous cells (Fig. 4).

An even better appreciation of the precision with which the silicone-foam mixture records surface details can be obtained by observing a mold of the human palm (Fig. 5). Here the relief is more intricate and also more familiar than the mucosal surface of the large intestine.

## DISCUSSION

It is evident from a study of these molds that silicone elastomers, as combined here, record minute variations on any surface they contact and consequently give information that is more discrete and more precise than that yielded by radiographic methods.

Silicone elastomers are produced commercially and are readily available. Their cost, when used in the quantities described in this study, does not exceed 1 dollar per examination. With the accessory equipment used by us, the bowel is easily filled.

The physiologic inertness of silicone compounds has been their most attractive characteristic for medical application. Toxicity data are presented in a subsequent report.

The credibility of any technique based on direct removal of malignant cells from an occult region is statistically suspect. For this reason, the 100 per cent recovery of malignant cells recorded in this report is not meant to predict a similar recovery rate clinically. The mold's excursion may denude it of some, or perhaps all, of the cells attached at the site of impression. A clinical trial will expose this difference.

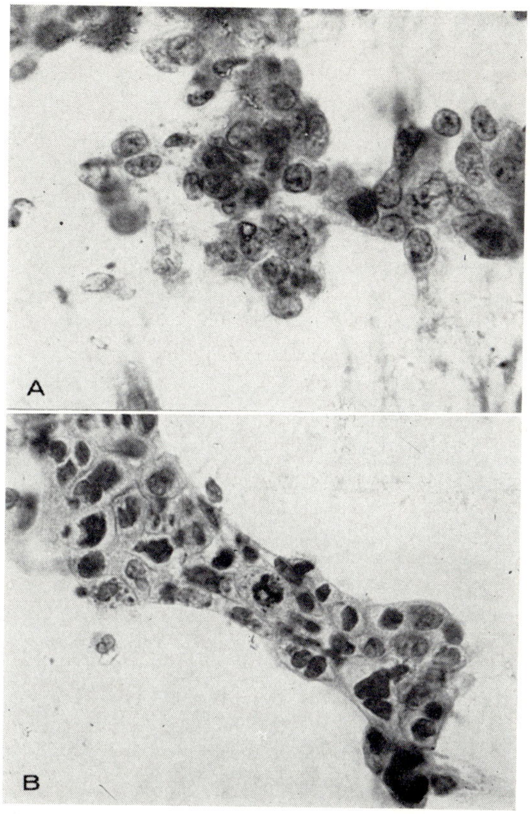


**Fig. 4.** *A* and *B*, Malignant cells obtained from Hartman's solution suspension of silicone-foam molds.

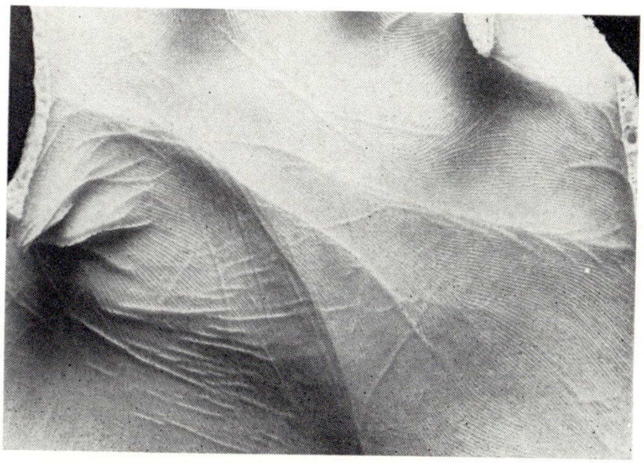

**Fig. 5.** Photograph of a silicone-foam impression of the human hand to demonstrate the fine detail which the material records.

## SUMMARY

A newly conceived technique for the diagnosis of disease in the sigmoid colon is introduced. The method is based on the proposition that a retrievable foam rubber intraluminal mold of the distal intestine would be useful in an assessment of the character of its mucosal surface. A mixture of silicone elastomers which can be converted at body temperature from a liquid prepolymer to a foamed polymer is presented. The results in reproducing surface abnormalities and recovering malignant cells from human surgical specimens are recorded.

The authors wish to thank Dr. William F. Newton for his support in this study.

### REFERENCES

1. Ascherman, S. W.: Carcinoma of the colon and rectum, A. M. A. Arch. Surg. **66:** 208, 1952.
2. Barden, R. P., and Stayman, J. W., Jr.: The continuing problem of polyps of the colon, Am. Surgeon **25:** 86, 1959.
3. Billing, L.: Zur Technik der Kontrastuntersuchung des Colon Sigmoideum, Acta Radiol. **25:** 418, 1944.
4. Cameron, A. S., and Knoernschild, H. E.: The value of cytologic study during proctosigmoidoscopy for the detection of carcinoma of the colon, S. Forum **11:** 77, 1960.
5. Cantor, A. J.: Diagnosis of carcinoma of rectum by cytologic study, Rev. Gastroenterol. **16:** 582, 1949.
6. Deddish, M. F., and Fairweather, W. H.: Colotomy and coloscopy, Cancer **6:** 1021, 1953.
7. Ettinger, A., and Elkin, M.: Study of the sigmoid by special roentgenographic views, Am. J. Roentgenol. **72:** 199, 1954.
8. Fischer, A. W.: Über eine neue roentgenologische Untersuchungsmethod des Dickdarms, Klin. Wchnschr. **2:** 1595, 1923.
9. Gerwig, W. H.: Transabdominal operative visualization of the mucosal surface of the large bowel, Am. J. Surg. **101:** 78, 1961.
10. Gianturco, C.: High-voltage technique in the diagnosis of polypoid growths of the colon, Radiology **55:** 27, 1950.
11. Groedel, F. M.: Recent advances in the roentgen diagnosis of diseases of the stomach and bowels, Arch. Roentgen Ray **15:** 51, 1910-1911.
12. Knoernschild, H. E., Cameron, A. B., and Zollinger, R. M.: Millipore filtration of colonic washings in malignant lesions of the large bowel, Am. J. Surg. **101:** 20, 1961.
13. Kreel, I., Lyons, A. S., and Turrell, R.: Aids in finding adenomas at laparotomy, Am. J. Surg. **101:** 81, 1961.
14. Ledoux-Lebard, R., and Garcia-Calderon, J.: Les techniques d'examen de la muqueuse du gros intestin, J. radiol. et électro. **17:** 429, 1933.
15. Loeb, R. A., and Scapier, J.: Rectal washings, technique for cytologic study of rectosigmoid; a preliminary report, Am. J. Surg. **81:** 298, 1951.
16. Mackenzie, L. L., and Hecht, E. L.: A case of carcinoma of rectum diagnosed by the cytologic method, Rev. Gastroenterol. **15:** 915, 1948.
17. Moore, A. E.: Traction sigmoidoscopy, S. Clin. North America **37:** 1283, 1957.
18. Raap, G.: Position of value in studying the pelvis and its contents, South. M. J. **44:** 95, 1951.
19. Rigler, L. G., and Eriksen, L. G.: Benign tumors of the stomach, Radiology **26:** 6, 1936.
20. Sackett, G. L., quoted by Hamilton, J. B.: The use of tannic acid in barium enemas, Am. J. Roentgenol. **56:** 101, 1946.
21. Wasserman, I. F.: New suction-lavage sigmoidoscope, J. A. M. A. **172:** 1036, 1960.
22. Welin, S.: Modern trends in diagnostic roentgenology of the colon, Brit. J. Radiol. **31:** 453, 1958.
23. Wisseman, C. L., Jr., Lemon, H. M., and Lawrence, K. B.: Cytologic diagnosis of cancer of the descending colon and rectum, Surg. Gynec. & Obst. **89:** 24, 1949.

# The silicone-foam diagnostic enema. II. An experimental evaluation in dogs

GALEN B. COOK, M.D.
ALEXANDER R. MARGULIS, M.D.
ST. LOUIS, MO.
*From the Department of Surgery and The Edward Mallinckrodt Institute of Radiology, Washington University School of Medicine*

Polysiloxane elastomers, when polymerized within segments of resected intestine, produce synthetic foam rubber molds which take true intraluminal impressions of the bowel mucosa. These elastomers have a sufficiently low viscosity to permit easy injection. They polymerize at room temperature and provide a precise and permanent record of the mucosal detail.[1]

Before such materials can be used to examine the colon of living men, it must be shown that (1) the injection of the prepolymer can be effected safely, efficiently, and painlessly, (2) the material does not injure the intestine in any way, and (3) the expulsion of the polymerized mold can proceed spontaneously, rapidly, completely, and without pain even from a bowel with polyps, diverticula, strictures, or many loops. To assess these criteria we have used the silicone-foam enema in the colons of dogs.

## MATERIALS AND METHODS

The silicone-foam enema used in these experiments is composed of Silastic RTV 502,* 20 Gm.; Silastic Q-3-0030,* 50 Gm.; Silicone fluid 200 (20 centistrokes),* 30 Gm.; diatrizoate sodium,† 25 Gm. in 20 ml. of water; and stannous octoate* 2 ml.

This mixture is somewhat different than the one previously reported.[1] It is less viscous as a prepolymer and softer as a polymer, but retains the other important characteristics of the original mixture.

**The preparation of anatomic deformities in the colon.** In order to make the straight colon of the dog resemble the human sigmoid colon, loops were made in it by sewing the serosa to form consecutive C curves. Sequences of 2 to 4 loops were made. The most caudal one was placed within 15 cm. of the anus in order to simulate the position and shape of the human sigmoid.

"Polyps" were made by incising the surface of the colon 10 cm. from the anus and preparing a 2 by 2 cm. pedicle. The pedicle was made into a serosa-lined tube and suspended in the intestinal lumen as the bowel wall was closed over it.

Diverticula were prepared by excising circles of serosa and circular muscle of 1 cm. diameter from the lateral portions of the antimesenteric surface of the colon in a zone 10 to 20 cm. from the anus. The underlying mucosa was everted through these defects and the muscular margins were secured to the intact peripheral serosa.

Strictures were produced by placing bands of vinylite, 1 cm. in width, circumferentially about the bowel and securing the resultant ring to the serosal surface with silk sutures. One to 2 weeks later these bands were removed and a partially obstructing stricture remained.

**Evaluation of the physical characteristics of the enema.** During polymerization the

The latter phase of this study was supported in part by a University Institutional Grant from the American Cancer Society.

Received for publication April 17, 1961.

*Dow Corning Corporation, Midland, Mich.

†Winthrop Laboratories, New York, N. Y.

silicone mixture expands. This of course could be dangerous. Consequently, we measured this volume change by placing the prepolymerized material in an open cylinder, measuring the height of the column, effecting polymerization, and then again measuring the column at the completion of the reaction.

The tendency for the material to push itself through small channels during polymerization was ascertained with Penrose drains (4 cm. wide) placed through a series of holes of varying diameters drilled through a rubber block 2 cm. thick. This device was designed on the premise that a human colonic tumor which had grown to completely encircle the bowel would have a longitudinal dimension of no less than 2 cm.[7] The proximal half of the drain was filled with 50 Gm. of silicone enema and sealed. Polymerization was allowed to go to completion and the weights of the polymerized rubber on each side of the constriction were compared.

One component of the enema, Silastic Q-3-0030, imparts the spongy character to the polymer by releasing hydrogen gas during the polymerization. Although much of this gas is held in the polymerized elastomer, some of it escapes. Because of the explosiveness of an oxygen-hydrogen mixture, the amount of hydrogen escaping from the polymer was measured by placing 50 Gm. of the enema mixture in a sealed condom and polymerizing it. The volume of hydrogen gas evolved from the polymer was measured by Archimedes' principle. The possible explosiveness of this gas in vivo was further appraised by giving a silicone-foam enema to an anesthetized mouse which had an empty colon. During polymerization an open flame was held to the anus. This flame was touched to the portion of the enema that extruded from the rectum as the prepolymers expanded. After polymerization, the animal was killed and the flame was held close to the intestinal loops as they were opened with scissors to allow the egress of any gases retained in them.

A deformation analysis of the polymerized elastomer was made. Tangential stress was applied with an infant's sphygomomanometer wrapped about a column of the foam 4 cm. in diameter. The strain was recorded on a centimeter scale by measuring the deflection of a pointer, the fulcrum of which rested at the edge of the pressure cuff with its proximal tip at the center of the compressed area. Longitudinal stress was measured by applying weights to the same foam column and recording strain as the reduction in height per unit added weight to an 8 cm. column of polymer. The longitudinal measurement was made with the foam column held in a lubricated polyethylene tube and also with the foam surrounded only by air.

The rise of temperature of the mixture during polymerization was measured with initial temperatures of 25, 30, and 35° C.

The tissue reaction to silicone foam was investigated by isolating a segment of dogs' colon in vivo and filling it with the enema mixture. One week later this intestine was removed and examined. Multiple biopsies were also made of the mucosa of the distal colon through a sigmoidoscope at various

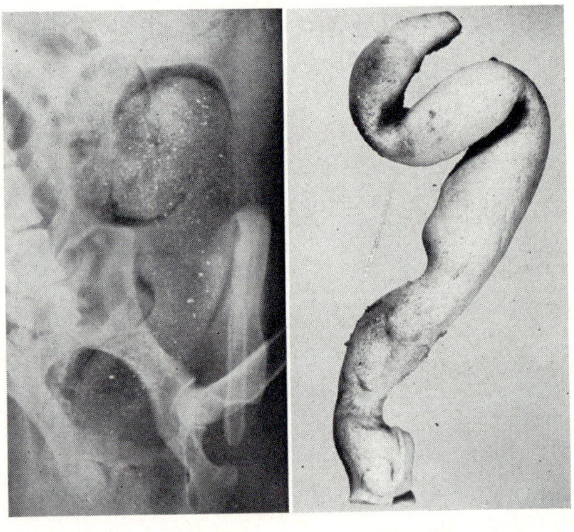

*A* *B*

**Fig. 1.** *A,* Roentgenograph of radiopaque silicone-foam enema within the colon of a dog prepared with 2 C loops. *B,* The same silicone-foam mold after expulsion shows the configurational stability of the material. It has returned to the position it held in the bowel.

intervals after exposure to the silicone-foam enema. A final study was made by injecting 60 Gm. of the enema directly into the peritoneal cavity and studying the tissue response 1 week later.

**Evaluation of the injection of the enema.** Initially the enema was released into the rectum through the nozzle of the sealant gun.[1] Later the nozzle was attached to a Foley catheter fitted with a 30 c.c. Bardex bag.*

Early in this study all animals were anesthetized during the injection, but as confidence was gained this was found unwarranted and thereafter the only pre-examination preparation was the giving of a 4.5 fluid ounce sodium phosphate/sodium biphosphate Fleet† enema.

Cineradiography was used to observe the rate and character of the injection in 3 instances. A head of pressure of 5 pounds per square inch of compressed air was used in these and all subsequent studies for expelling the prepolymerized enema from the sealant gun into the rectum.

**Evaluation of the expulsion of the enema.** Immediately after polymerization of the silicone foam (determined by observation of the material which remained in the sealant gun cartridge) the dogs were placed on a radiographic table and a right posterior-oblique scout film of the abdomen was made. The animals were then allowed to move about the room and pass the cast.

## RESULTS

**Anatomic deformities.** A silicone-foam enema was administered to a dog with the colon in the natural state. The examination was then made in dogs prepared with redundant loops (Fig. 1), a polyp (Fig. 2, *A*), diverticula (Fig. 2, *B*), and strictures (Fig. 3). The severest stricture produced had a diameter 35 per cent as great as the diameter of the uninvolved bowel cephalad to the constriction.

*Hamilton-Schmidt Surgical Co., St. Louis, Mo.

†C. P. Fleet Co., Inc., Lynchburg, Va.

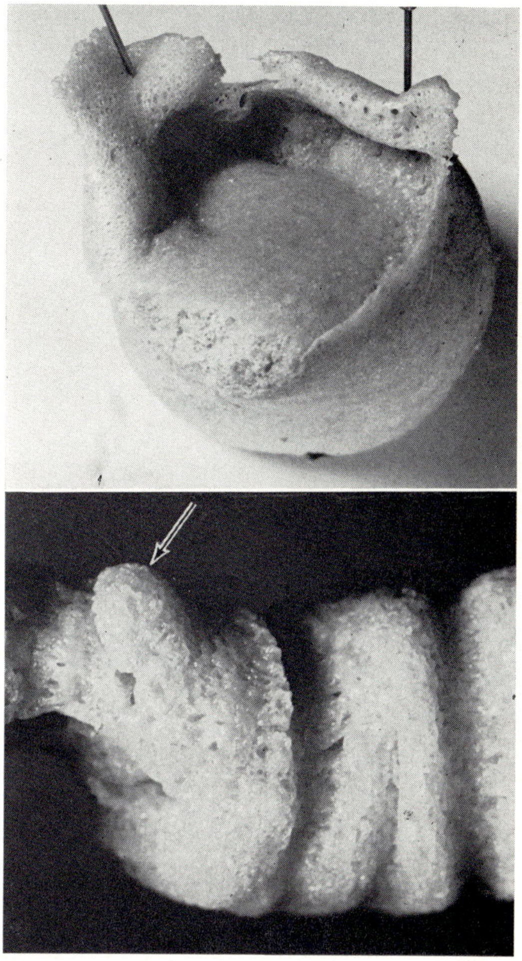

A

B

**Fig. 2.** *A,* Photograph of "pocket" in silicone-foam enema produced by experimentally prepared "polyp." This view is from the base of the "polyp" and is directed caudally. *B,* Silicone-foam impression of surgically prepared diverticulum *(arrow)*.

In every instance the mold was expelled promptly and without assistance; there were no manifestations of pain. Not all specimens, however, were passed as single units—the polyp mold and several of the stricture molds were expelled in 2 parts with the second portion following the first 4 to 8 hours later. In each case in which a fracture appeared it developed at the narrowest part of the mold. Repeat examinations in the same animals were not always attended by fracture of the mold.

Examination of the molds clearly showed

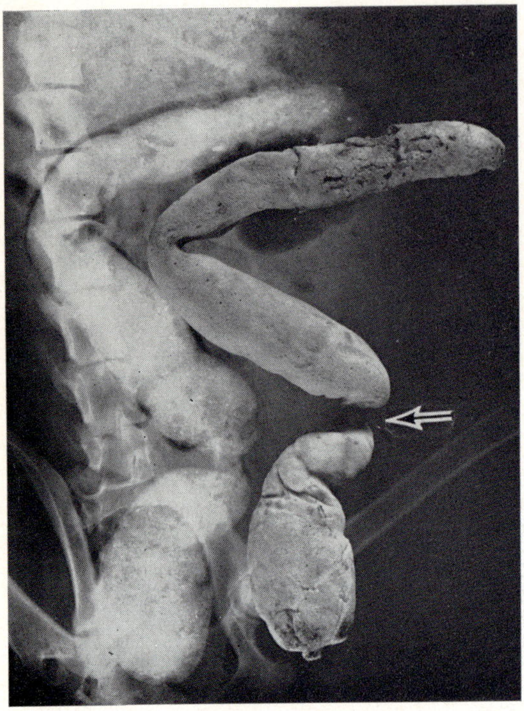

**Fig. 3.** Photograph of silicone-foam mold lying on a roentgenograph of the same mold before expulsion. The diameter of the constricted zone *(arrow)* is less than one-third that of the greatest diameter above it.

the abnormalities which had been prepared in the colons. The specimen of the 4-loop bowel provided an especially convincing demonstration of the ability of the foam to retain the geometrical configuration that was present at the time of polymerization.

**Physical characteristics of silicone foam.** The silicone-foam enema had a viscosity of 2,000 centistokes at the time of injection.[6] During polymerization the volume increased 140 per cent and the temperature rose less than 3° C. (maximum temperture rise 2.3° C.).

During polymerization, 70 cc. of free gas escaped the mold. When it was ignited in vitro a flame 5 cm. in height rose from it and burned for approximately 2 seconds; an explosion did not occur. When the flame was applied to the anus or over the incised, distended bowel of a mouse, neither an ignition nor explosion resulted.

The overflow of foam through a constriction was found to be a function of the size of the constriction being directly related to its cross-sectional area:

$$\frac{\text{cross-sectional area of constriction}}{\text{cross-sectional area of proximal lumen}} \times 100$$

compared with

$$\frac{\text{weight of silicone foam above constriction}}{\text{total weight of silicone foam administered}} \times 100$$

37.5%:39.5%
50 %:42.5%
62.5%:45.7%

The deformation analysis (Fig. 4) showed that the strength of the normal bowel (> 200 mm. Hg²) would be capable of compressing the foamed elastomer to a cross-sectional area less than 50 per cent of its prestressed size.

A tissue response attributable to the silicone was not found. The peritoneal cavity was involved with a moderate inflammatory reaction which was interpreted as an effect of bacterial contamination in view of the complete absence of response in all other material examined. The wall of the colonic pouch which had been in contact with silicone foam for 1 week, as well as the immediate and delayed rectal biopsies, showed no reaction (Fig. 5).

**Injection and expulsion of the enema.** Administration of the silicone foam through a rectal catheter identical to that used for barium enema examinations was functionally satisfactory. However, because of the relative viscosity of the prepolymer, it was found necessary to continue to employ the sealant gun instead of the traditional gravity flow technique used for barium enemas. The animals showed no signs of pain during the injection or during the expansion of the material as it polymerized.

In these studies, as in all examinations of the colon, mucosal cleanliness is essential. Without exception, the Fleet enema prepared the lower colon so that a satisfactory examination could be performed.

Cineradiographic observations of the injection showed a steady, controlled inflow of the silicone foam. The Hypaque concentration was satisfactory for good visualization at all times.

Expulsion of the molds began 1 to 5 minutes after the animals were allowed to stand. It was complete 3 to 10 seconds later. There were no manifestations of pain.

## DISCUSSION

Our attempted simulations of human polyps, diverticula, strictures, and redundant loops in the colons of dogs are admittedly crude. However, they did serve to demonstrate that the silicone foam is capable of accurately recording the forms. In addition, they demonstrated that the silicone mold is sufficiently pliable to prevent injury to any part of the bowel during extrusion. We believe that it can be safely introduced into man and will provide a very accurate and permanent record of the structural details of the colon of living persons. The value of such records is obvious.

Although we could not demonstrate that the hydrogen evolved during polymerization would burn or produce an explosive mixture in vivo, we still believe that this constitutes a potential hazard and consequently warrants the taking of care to avoid flame or sparks. All fluoroscopic and electrical radiographic equipment must be well insulated.

That no mucosal injury occurred during the silicone-foam enema was expected because the exposure of the gastrointestinal tract to other polysiloxanes for long periods produced none.[3, 4] The short time that the silicone-foam enema remains in the colon is insignificant compared to the lengths of time that silicone elastomers have been left subcutaneously, intramuscularly, and intraperitoneally without producing discernible changes in the tissues contacting them.[5]

The use of a Foley catheter to introduce the enema into the rectum serves to protect the area from the rigid polyethylene nozzle of the sealant gun and prevents overfilling the rectal ampulla with the polymer. However, this method of introducing the silicones is cumbersome and expensive and therefore we are now attempting to overcome these problems with a flexible, disposable apparatus.

Our experience with the silicone-foam enema in human beings is in its early stage. In 50 instances of its employment, no pain has been experienced during the introduction or polymerization of the material. The elastic casts have recorded the details of the sigmoid colons of living human beings as accurately as those of the dogs' colons.

## SUMMARY

The application of a new technique in which silicone elastomers are used for recording mucosal detail and gross anatomic configuration of the sigmoid colon of dogs

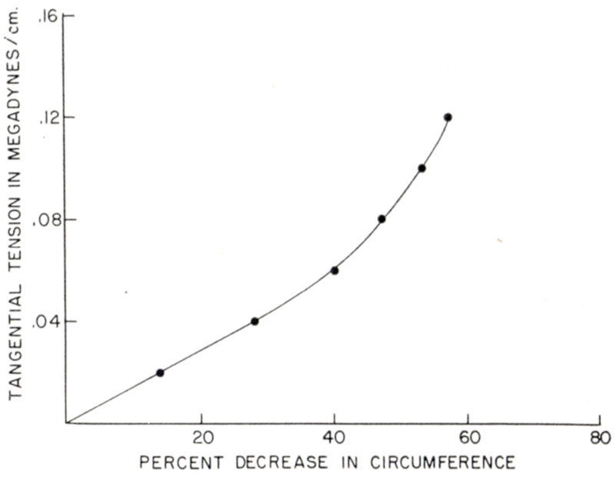


**Fig. 4.** Graph which demonstrates the compressibility (tension-circumference relationship) of the silicone-foam enema after polymerization.

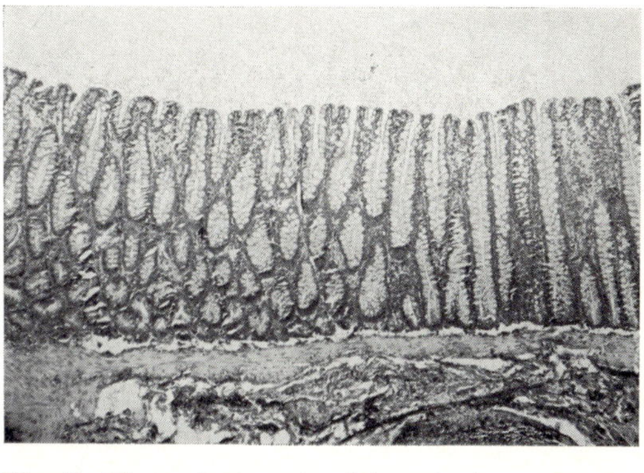

**Fig. 5.** Photomicrograph of intestinal mucosa exposed to the silicone-foam enema for 1 week in an isolated bowel segment.

in vivo is presented. The physical properties of the material and the conditions of its administration, polymerization, and evacuation have been investigated. An absence of tissue response has been encountered. Human studies, to date, closely parallel the experiences with dogs.

## REFERENCES

1. Cook, G. B., and Margulis, A. R.: The Silicone-foam diagnostic enema. I. An assessment with surgical specimens of human sigmoid colon, SURGERY **50:** 513, 1961.
2. Jackman, R. J.: Lesions of the lower bowel, Springfield, Ill., 1958, Charles C Thomas, Publisher, p. 21.
3. Kern, S. F., Anderson, R. C., and Harris, P. N.: Observations of the toxicity of methylsilicone, J. Am. Pharm. A. (Scient. Ed.) **38:** 575, 1949.
4. Polemann, G., and Froitzheim, G.: Biological compatibility of silicones, Arzneimittel-Forsch. **3:** 457, 1953.
5. Rowe, V. K., Spencer, H. S., and Bass, S. L.: Toxicological studies on certain commercial silicones and hydrolyzable silane intermediates, J. Indust. Hyg. & Toxicol. **30:** 332, 1948.
6. Silicone Notes, 3-106a, January, 1959, Dow Corning Corporation, Midland, Mich.
7. Spratt, J. S., Jr.: Personal communication.

# The healing wound in experimental diabetes

RICHARD G. ROSEN, M.D.
IRVING F. ENQUIST, M.D.
BROOKLYN, N. Y.
*From the Department of Surgery, State University of New York Downstate Medical Center*

Patients with diabetes are subject to some diseases for which they must undergo operation more frequently than the population at large, but as clinical knowledge and surgical techniques improve, diabetes is becoming less of a barrier to elective surgical procedures. Because the aging of the population brings with it an increase in the incidence of diabetes, a proper understanding of the effect of diabetes on surgical procedures and wound physiology assumes a greater importance than ever before.

Statements regarding the relationship between diabetes and wound healing can be found frequently in the literature. Eagleton,[2] writing in 1904 before the introduction of insulin, observed that even in the absence of infection diabetic wounds were slow to granulate and to heal. More recently it has been stated that there is no retardation of healing if therapy is adequate, and that diabetes has no effect on wound healing in the absence of infection.[9] Unfortunately, there are very few reports of a well-controlled clinical or experimental investigation to substantiate these opinions. Bennet,[1] of the Mayo Foundation, was one of the few to look into this problem critically. He examined standard abdominal incisions in dogs after total pancreatectomy and without insulin supplementation, using normal dogs as controls. He found that healing proceeded in an abnormal fashion in the diabetic dogs. The tissues were edematous, fibrin deposits were delayed and decreased in amount, the cellular reaction was excessive, blood vessel formation was slow, and thromboses were increased. Although he answered many questions about the method of healing in diabetes, he left unanswered the essential point—do diabetic patients heal as rapidly and as completely as normal persons, and if not, does control with insulin influence the result? The present study is an attempt to provide some additional information on this subject.

Supported by Grant No. A-3609, National Institute of Arthritis and Metabolic Diseases, United States Public Health Service.

Received for publication Nov. 7, 1960.

## METHODS AND RESULTS

White male albino Wistar rats were used. Diabetes was induced by subcutaneous or intraperitoneal injection of alloxan, 150 mg. per kilogram, in rats which had been fasting for 48 hours. Each animal had received 0.25 U. of regular insulin 1 hour prior to the alloxan administration. Diabetic rats were given 1.5 U. of protamine zinc insulin (PZI) subcutaneously daily to prevent cachexia and dehydration. Blood sugar levels in this group remained over 300 mg. per cent. A second group was made diabetic in a similar manner, but after the diabetes was well established they were given 7 to 9 U. of PZI daily. This was sufficient to maintain the blood sugar levels in the normal range of 65 to 135 mg. per cent. This group is referred to as insulin controls. A third group of normal rats of the same colony which never received alloxan was also used.

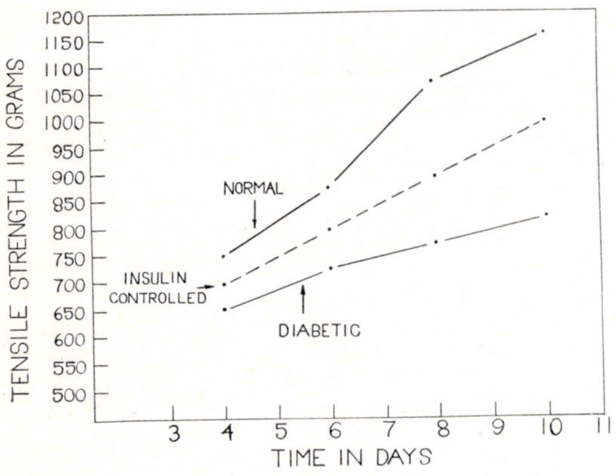


**Fig. 1.** Gain in tensile strength of sutured incised wounds.

**Incised wounds.** Rats which weighed between 200 and 250 grams were anesthetized intraperitoneally with pentobarbital. Under sterile conditions, the skin and subcutaneous tissue of the upper abdomen were incised in the midline. A 4 cm. vertical incision through the musculofascial layer, including peritoneum, was then made in the left upper quadrant of the abdomen. This incision was then repaired with 7 interrupted simple sutures of No. 4-0 silk. These sutures were placed exactly 0.5 cm. apart and 0.5 cm. from the ends of the incision. Each suture took in the entire musculofascial wall, including peritoneum but excluding subcutaneous tissue and skin. Each suture was tied with a square knot and another squared throw, and the ends cut 1 mm. from the knot. The skin was then closed with a continuous silk suture.

The surviving rats were sacrificed on the fourth, sixth, eighth, and tenth postoperative days. The abdominal skin was removed and the remainder of the abdominal wall excised. Three strips were cut from the wound, each strip 1 cm. wide and containing 2 of the previously placed sutures. All 3 strips were tested for tensile strength on a motor-driven tensiometer, calibrated to read the breaking force to the nearest 5 Gm. Most, but not all, of the specimens broke at the suture line. The results are summarized in Table I and are plotted graphically in Fig. 1. Parabolas were constructed for each of the 3 groups and the algebraic equivalents determined. An F test on the residual variation of the parabolas indicated that the 3 parabolas differed significantly from each other ($p < 0.001$) and that this difference lies in the level rather than the slope of the curve.

**Open wounds.** Rats weighing between 160 and 210 grams were used. Under intraperitoneal pentobarbital anesthesia the right flank was shaved and a square full-thickness skin defect, 2 by 2 cm., created. Sterility was not observed. Hemostasis was established and the wound left undressed. The wound was inspected daily until full healing occurred. The absence of any visible granulation tissue was used as the end point of healing.

Again, 3 separate groups of animals were studied—diabetic rats, insulin controls, and normal rats. The results are presented in Table II. There is no significant difference between any 2 of the 3 groups, despite the fact that the diabetes was so severe that the diabetic rats gained an average of only 1.5 grams per day compared to 4.7 grams in the normal group and 3.7 grams in the insulin control group. Wound infections were most common in the diabetic group, but could be noted to some degree in all groups. Fungus

**Table I.** *Tensile strength of sutured incised wounds*

| *Day of sacrifice* | *Study group* | *No. of animals* | *Average tensile strength of wounds (Gm.)* | *Standard deviation* |
|---|---|---|---|---|
| 4 | Normal | 11 | 741 | 73 |
| 4 | Insulin control | 11 | 700 | 64 |
| 4 | Diabetic | 15 | 645 | 77 |
| 6 | Normal | 11 | 873 | 73 |
| 6 | Insulin control | 11 | 794 | 93 |
| 6 | Diabetic | 10 | 732 | 52 |
| 8 | Normal | 11 | 1,088 | 69 |
| 8 | Insulin control | 10 | 900 | 131 |
| 8 | Diabetic | 11 | 789 | 101 |
| 10 | Normal | 11 | 1,161 | 83 |
| 10 | Insulin control | 10 | 1,003 | 126 |
| 10 | Diabetic | 11 | 884 | 112 |

Table II. *Healing time of open granulating wounds*

| Study group | No. of animals | Average weight gain (Gm./day) | Range of healing time (days) | Average healing time (days) | Standard deviation |
|---|---|---|---|---|---|
| Normal | 27 | 4.4 | 12-20 | 15.9 | 2.3 |
| Insulin control | 19 | 3.5 | 13-28 | 17.1 | 3.9 |
| Diabetic | 29 | 1.5 | 13-21 | 15.8 | 2.2 |

infection occurred in 3 of the diabetic animals but in none of the others.

## DISCUSSION

Diabetes alters the healing of wounds in a number of ways, not all of which are simulated by alloxan injection in the experimental animals. The main metabolic difference between alloxan diabetes and clinical diabetes is in the relatively frequent occurrence of ketosis in the latter condition. There are some microscopic differences also. The pancreatic beta cells are absent or markedly reduced in number in the alloxan form, while in the clinical type the decrease in the number of beta cells is not as marked, although with special stains, 60 per cent of diabetics can be shown to have a partial or complete degranulation of the cells.

The similarities between the 2 forms, however, are greater than the dissimilarities. Hyperglycemia, glycosuria, insulin deficiency, and hyperlipemia are common to both. Both are aggravated by thyroxin and ACTH, while both are ameliorated by adrenalectomy, fasting, high-fat diet and insulin. Some authors even believe that alloxan plays a part in clinical diabetes. Loubatieres[7] was able to isolate alloxan and its metabolites in greater amount from the blood of diabetic patients than from nondiabetic control subjects. The vascular changes which are associated with well-established diabetes probably did not occur in our experimental animals in which the diabetes was of short duration. In all other important respects, the experimental situation is probably comparable to the clinical.

It is pertinent that all 3 curves in Fig. 1 have the same slope. In other words, the rate of healing from the fourth to the tenth day does not differ significantly from group to group. This is confirmed in the second part of the study, in which rate (the time factor) was the only variant investigated. Experimentally, almost all tissues studied (cornea,[4] skin, fascia, muscle, stomach, and so forth[6]) have the same rate of healing. It is not surprising that the same tissues from diabetic and nondiabetic animals of the same species should also heal at the same rate. Nevertheless, the curves in Fig. 1 do differ significantly from one another in height. The amount, or strength, of healing differs; for example, a healed corneal wound is never as strong as a healed skin or fascial wound.

The mechanisms by which wounds heal are still only imperfectly understood, and the reasons why they heal are even more conjectural. It is not surprising, therefore, that we have few hints as to the reason for the difference in healing between diabetic and nondiabetic patients. Bennet implied that this difference was due, in part, to the differences in sugar content of the local tissues. He quoted Trimble and Carey,[8] who found that the true sugar content of skin and muscle was roughly proportional to the blood sugar level. The skin and muscle sugar levels in diabetic patients were approximately twice those of nondiabetic patients. Greene and associates[5] analyzed the infection rate and rate of healing of the wounds of 324 diabetic patients, and related these rates to the strictness of control of the diabetes as evidenced by the blood sugar levels. They could find no apparent relationship between the blood sugar level and wound infections or delayed wound healing. Forscher and Cecil[3] have shown that tissue levels of tyrosine, desoxyribonucleic acid, and acid-soluble organic phosphorus increased in the wounds of normal rats but failed to increase in the wounds of diabetic rats, while the rate of increase in tissue glycogen was greater in the wounds of diabetic rats. They implied that altered wound healing in diabetic patients was due to these differences from the normal. In our study the group of insulin controls had normal blood sugar levels but had altered healing, although the healing was more nearly normal than in the rats with uncontrolled diabetes.

## SUMMARY AND CONCLUSIONS

1. The healing of sutured incised wounds and open granulating wounds has been studied in rats with alloxan diabetes.

2. The healing of sutured incised wounds is impaired in severely diabetic animals; this impairment is partially ameliorated by strict control of the diabetic state.

3. The healing of open granulating wounds appears to proceed at a normal rate in rats with well-controlled and poorly-controlled diabetes.

### REFERENCES

1. Bennet, R. J., Jr.: An experimental study of wound healing after pancreatectomy. Thesis submitted to Graduate School of the University of Minnesota, 1932.
2. Eagleton, W. P.: Influence of old age, diabetes, arteriosclerosis, and gout on the healing of wounds, Am. Med. **7:** 898, 1904.
3. Forscher, B. K., and Cecil, H. C.: Some effects of alloxan diabetes on acute inflammation, J. Appl. Physiol. **13:** 278, 1958.
4. Gliedman, M. L., and Karlson, K. E.: Wound healing and wound strength of sutured limbal wounds, Am. J. Ophth. **39:** 859, 1955.
5. Greene, J. A., Swanson, L. W., and Jacobs, C. A.: Control of diabetes mellitus: relation to the healing of clean and infected wounds and to the incidences of infection in clean wounds, J. A. M. A. **115:** 1518, 1940.
6. Howes, E. L., Sooey, J. W., and Harvey, S. C.: The healing of wounds as determined by their tensile strength, J. A. M. A. **92:** 42, 1929.
7. Loubatieres, A.: Does alloxan play a part in the pathogenesis of diabetes mellitus? *In* Experimental diabetes and its relation to the clinical disease, Oxford, 1954, Blackwell Scientific Publications.
8. Trimble, H. C., and Carey, B. W., Jr.: On the true sugar content of skin and of muscle in diabetic and non-diabetic persons, J. Biol. Chem. **90:** 655, 1931.
9. Wheelock, F. C., Jr., and Root, H. F.: Surgery and diabetes. *In* Joslin, E. P., Root, H. F., Pricilla, and Marble, A.: The treatment of diabetes mellitus, Philadelphia, 1959, Lea & Febiger, ed. 10.

# Paradoxical variation of the femoral pulse in occlusion of the iliac artery

F. WILLIAM BLAISDELL, M.D.
PETER J. GAUDER, M.D.
SAN FRANCISCO, CALIF.
*From the Surgical Service of the San Francisco Veterans Administration Hospital*

Presence or absence of the femoral pulse is an important guide to the evaluation of a patient suspected of having arterial occlusive disease of the lower extremities. A weak or absent femoral pulse denotes a proximal occlusive lesion, and if a reconstructive operation is indicated the precise location of the lesion may be verified by aortography. A strong femoral pulse is often interpreted as an indication that no significant proximal lesion exists. Routine aortography in patients with good femoral pulses, however, will demonstrate that many do have proximal lesions of the aorta or iliac arteries. Although these arteries may not be completely obstructed, an appreciable number will be found to have a marked stenosis of a degree greater than might be expected from the good character of the femoral pulse. In this situation, surgical relief of a distal occlusive lesion in the leg may fail immediately because of inadequate proximal blood flow or at a later date because of progression of the proximal lesion with reocclusion of the distal operative area.

The occurrence of a good femoral pulse below a significant occlusion in the absence of distal obstructive lesions is seen only rarely, usually in patients in the younger age group. In these patients, large collateral channels can be demonstrated by physical examination or arteriography.

The association of proximal iliac lesions with occlusive lesions of the femoral artery has been seen occasionally with good femoral pulses and has raised the question as to what effect multiple occlusive lesions have on the intervening pulse. A series of experiments was carried out in animals with the production of simultaneous iliac and femoral obstructions in an attempt to answer this question.

## METHOD

Four mongrel dogs, which varied in weight from 15 to 20 kilograms were subjected to laparotomy under intravenous pentobarbital anesthesia. The aortic trifurcation and the entire iliac artery on one side were exposed and the iliac artery mobilized from the aorta to the inguinal ligament. All branches except for the pudendoepigastric trunk were ligated and divided. This left a system which simulated the human external iliac artery and common femoral artery with its bifurcation into superficial and profunda branches. The iliac artery in these dogs averaged 4 mm. in diameter at its upper portion and 3 mm. in diameter below the pudendoepigastric branch. The latter averaged 2.5 mm. in diameter. A No. 20 needle was inserted into the midportion of the iliac artery and this was connected by polyethylene tubing to a Statham transducer. Pressures were transcribed on a Sanborn 350 recorder. Base line or control pressures were then recorded and a screw clamp applied gradually to the iliac artery at its origin from the aorta. Sufficient progressive constriction was applied to convert the pulsatile pressure distal to the clamp to a flat, dampened pressure but not enough to produce complete occlusion.

Received for publication June 13, 1961.

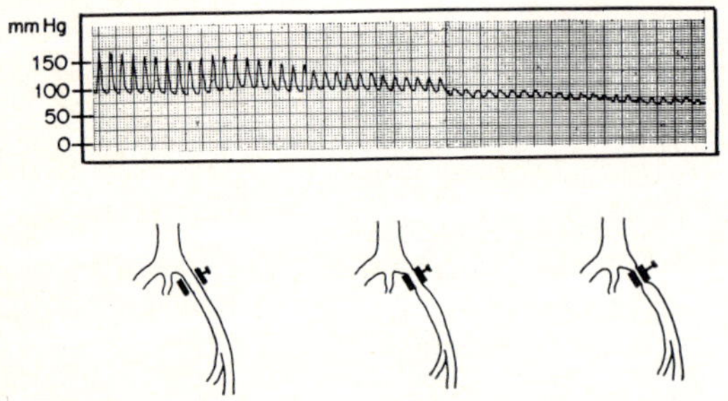


**Fig. 1.** Application of progressive occlusion to the proximal portion of the iliac artery until dampening of the distal pressure tracing occurs.

In the first portion of each experiment a vascular clamp was then applied to the distal iliac artery to produce complete obstruction. This clamp was alternately removed and applied at intervals of 10 seconds to 2 minutes as pressures were recorded in the artery just above.

In the second stage of the experiment, a bulldog clamp was applied to the distal iliac artery beyond the pudendoepigastric trunk and this was followed by the application of another occlusive bulldog clamp to the pudendoepigastric vessel.

In the third stage of the experiment, a screw clamp was also applied to the distal iliac artery and progressive occlusion produced, then released. Pressures were measured continuously as described.

During each of the portions of the experiment in the 4 animals the proximal occluding clamp was not touched and the upper block remained the same.

## RESULTS

The findings in all the animals were similar and are illustrated in representative tracings. The initial, or control, blood pressure was first recorded. The pressure was then noted during progressive proximal occlusion until a pulse pressure well below 15 mm. Hg was obtained (Fig. 1).

Fig. 2 illustrates the first portion of the experiment in which the distal occluding clamp was applied for 10-second periods and released. Application of the distal occluding clamp uniformly resulted in the return of definite pulsatile pressure in the segment above. This pulse pressure was equal to that obtained in the unobstructed artery at the start of the experiment.

Fig. 3 demonstrates the findings in the second portion of the experiment. With the application of the bulldog clamp to the femoral artery the pressure became pulsatile with a pulse pressure averaging 69 per cent of the control value. With the application of an additional bulldog clamp to the pudendoepigastric branch, the pressure rose to normal control levels.

Fig. 4 illustrates the findings in the third portion of the experiment. With the application of the screw clamp distally, the pulsatile pressure gradually returned in the segment above, reaching a peak with complete occlusion of the vessel. As the clamp was again opened the proximal pressure fell and pulse pressure returned to 5 to 10 mm. Hg.

## DISCUSSION

These experiments indicated that the dampening effect on the pressure produced by a proximal iliac stenosis could be negated by the production of a distal occlusion. Complete distal occlusion at a level corresponding to the femoral bifurcation uniformly restored proximal pulsatile pressure in the common femoral artery to the control level. The presence of 1 main collateral leaving the obstructed segment was still associated with the return of a pulsatile pressure (Fig. 3), although this pressure amounted to roughly two-thirds of the control pressure. This would correspond to the clinical sit-

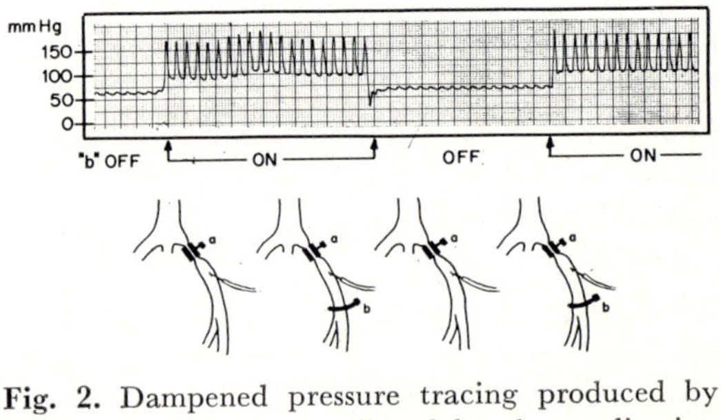


**Fig. 2.** Dampened pressure tracing produced by the proximal stenosis, relieved by the application of a distal occluding bulldog clamp.

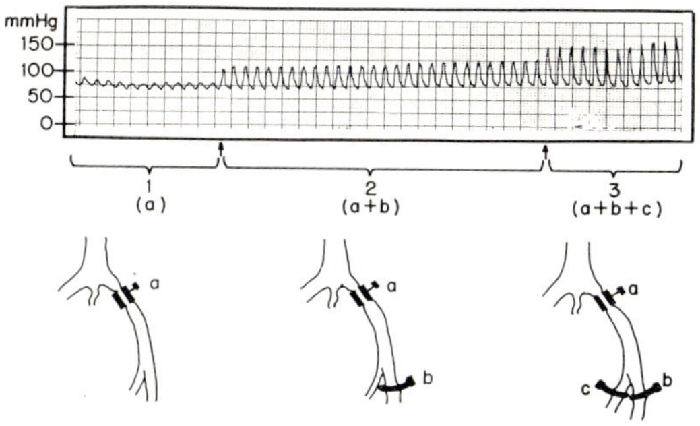


**Fig. 3.** Dampened pressure tracing produced by the proximal stenosis partially relieved by the application of a bulldog clamp to the superficial femoral artery, then completely relieved by the application of another bulldog clamp to the pudendoepigastric (profunda) branch.

uation in which proximal iliac stenosis existed with superficial femoral occlusion and the profunda femoris represented the only open vessel. Because the quantitation of a palpable pulse is difficult, the pulse pressure was taken as the alternative measurement. In these animals it was noted that a pulse pressure in excess of 20 mm. Hg was associated with a good palpable pulse, and a pulse pressure under 15 mm. Hg with a weak or absent pulse. Thus, complete distal occlusion always resulted in the return of the proximal pulse to the control levels. The degree of occlusion required to restore the pulse was not quantitated, but a collateral branch half the size of the proximal partially occluded artery still permitted the return of the pulse upon occlusion of the distal main vessel.

The explanation for this apparent paradox can be found by the application of Pascal's law, which states that pressure exerted anywhere on a confined liquid is transmitted undiminished to every portion of the interior of the containing vessel. For fluid in motion this law may well not apply, but when, as in the first experiment (Fig. 2), a distal occluding clamp is applied, the segment of artery above is converted into a closed system communicating with the pulsatile pressure in the aorta through the small opening of the proximal occlusion. There is an analogy between the transmission of a pulsatile pressure through the small catheter into the transducer which was used to record pressures in this experiment and the similar transmission of pulsatile pressure through a proximal stenosis into a distally occluded segment of vessel. This simulates a profound obstructive state which is not seen clinically without thrombosis in the segment of vessel in which stasis of blood occurs.

With the use of the screw clamps in this experiment, precise calibration of the size of the block was not possible, although the number of turns required to open the clamp after complete occlusion could be used as a rough guide. Precise determinations of the relative size of the occlusions required to do this are now underway and will be reported at a later date. However, it was our impression in the third experiment (Fig. 4) that even though the distal occluding clamp was gradually opened, the pressure in the vessel just above remained pulsatile until the distal opening was larger than the proximal opening. Thus, it is postulated that when the opening in the distal block becomes larger than that in the proximal block, the pressure in the segment above will rapidly drop off until, with further distal release of the occlusion, the flat pulse tracing secondary to proximal block again occurs.

The results of these experiments, particularly that illustrated in Fig. 3, which comes closest to simulating the clinical situation,

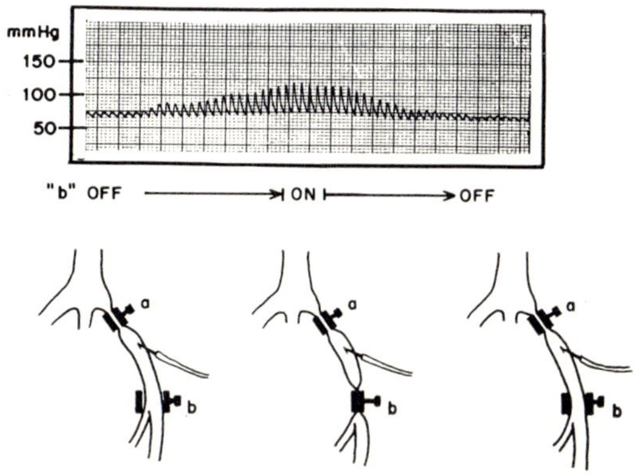


**Fig. 4.** Dampened pressure tracing produced by the proximal stenosis, relieved by the progressive application of a screw clamp. Gradual release of clamp results in return of dampened pressure.

show that under certain circumstances distal occlusive lesions may augment or restore the pulse which otherwise would be dampened by a proximal occluding lesion. The clinical state in which a weak or absent femoral pulse due to an iliac stenosis may be augmented to a moderate or strong pulse by extensive distal femoral occlusive disease may exist much oftener than has been suspected. This is not to decry the value of the femoral or any other pulse in the assessment of arterial occlusive disease, but to point out that in certain instances, particularly those in which there is associated distal occlusive disease, the pulse may be deceiving. Thus, the presence of a good femoral pulse does not in itself rule out significant proximal stenosis. Complete arteriography is required to evaluate the proximal aorto-iliac tree properly when significant femoral occlusive disease exists.

## SUMMARY AND CONCLUSIONS

The concept that strong femoral pulses rule out significant proximal arterial occlusive disease is questioned. In experiments performed on dogs, stenotic lesions were produced in the iliac arteries which were sufficient to obliterate the distal pulse. The restoration of a normal pulse in the femoral area was accomplished by the production of a complete distal obstruction. In addition, clamping of the superficial femoral artery in the dog was also sufficient to restore a good pulse in the common femoral artery even though the profunda femoris remained patent.

This suggests that a palpable femoral pulse in association with severe distal occlusive disease of the superficial femoral artery and profunda femoris in man does not necessarily signify lack of proximal disease. Aortography would be indicated routinely in these patients prior to the performance of reconstructive procedures in the legs because the distal operation may fail immediately or be compromised soon thereafter by an unsuspected aortic or iliac occlusive lesion.

# Effect of removal of adventitia from arteries: an experimental study

ELMER V. DAHL, M.D.*
ERIC C. EDWARDS, M.D.
JOHN H. GRINDLAY, M.D.
JESSE E. EDWARDS, M.D.
ROCHESTER, MINN.
*From the Mayo Clinic and Mayo Foundation*

During the course of experiments concerned with alteration of arterial structure, it became necessary for us to know what changes, if any, could be attributed to the surgical removal of adventitia from the wall of an artery. Little information was available on this subject, and for that reason it seemed desirable for us to record our observations. Knowledge concerning the reaction of an artery to removal of its adventitia is of interest not only to investigators who manipulate blood vessels experimentally, but also to surgeons who perform operations in which arteries are stripped, such as radical operation for cancer, or in which arteries are removed from their usual bed, such as procedures to augment the coronary circulation of the heart.[3]

There is general agreement that the metabolic needs of the walls of large arteries are supplied both by means of the vasa vasorum, which are present in the adventitia and send branches into the media, and by diffusion from the blood within the lumen of the artery.[1, 2, 5] The effect on the arterial wall of destruction of the adventitial source of nutriment has been the subject of a number of investigations. In 1871, Durante mechanically removed as much of the adventitia as he could from the carotid arteries of rabbits and subsequently studied those vessels histologically. He concluded that, with the adventitial blood supply removed, the arteries disintegrated despite continuous flow of blood through them. His investigations were complicated by the occurrence of infection and mural thrombosis.

Lange removed as much of the adventitia as possible from 1.5 cm. lengths of aorta and from carotid and renal arteries in rabbits, and then he surrounded the vessels with a sheath of lanolin and beeswax. Thickening of the intima within the sheathed part of the vessel occurred in less than 12 days. In the course of performing periarterial sympathectomies, Haberland removed as much adventitia as possible from unspecified lengths of major arteries in dogs and rabbits. No damage attributable to disturbances of nutrition in the walls of the vessels was apparent on microscopic examination after postoperative periods of as long as 51 days. Schilling observed intimal proliferation after removal of adventitia from arteries in rabbits, but only at sites where the media had been traumatized. In other studies in which the adventitia was cauterized by heat[19-22] or treated with caustic chemicals,[9, 10, 24] abnormalities of both media and intima were produced.

Removal of adventitia from an artery not

Supported in part by Research Grant No. H-4014 of the National Heart Institute, United States Public Health Service.

Abridgment of portion of thesis submitted by Dr. Dahl to the Faculty of the Graduate School of the University of Minnesota in partial fulfillment of the requirements for the degree of Doctor of Philosophy in Pathology.

Received for publication Oct. 18, 1960.

*On assignment from the United States Air Force. The contents of this article are the personal views of the Air Force officer and are not to be construed as statement of official Air Force policy or as Air Force endorsement of any commercial product described.

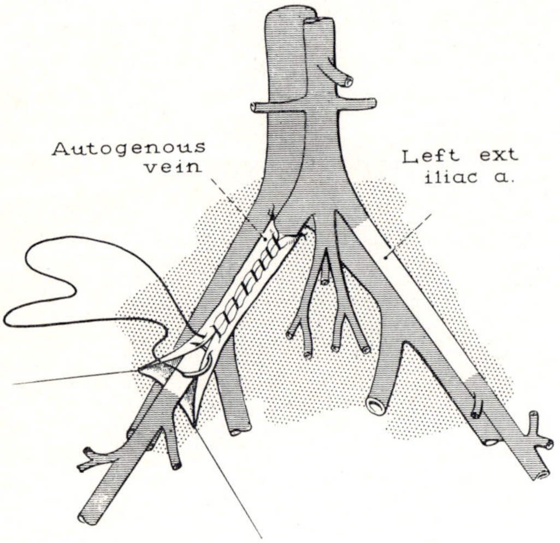


**Fig. 1.** Operative site. Each external iliac artery, from aorta to deep femoral artery, was stripped of as much adventitia as possible, and a cuff of autogenous vein was sutured about one of the arteries.

only interrupts the intrinsic vasculature of the wall, but also disturbs the innervation. That interruption of the nerves to an artery results in anatomic changes in the arterial wall has been claimed[11, 17, 25] and denied.[4, 6, 13]

None of the experiments cited provided information from which the effect of simple surgical removal of adventitia from a relatively long segment of artery could be deduced. Our purpose was to gain this information. In order to obtain, at the same time, information concerning the pathogenesis of whatever changes might be produced, we attempted to delay revascularization of the walls of the freed arteries by suturing a cuff of autogenous vein, endothelial surface outward, about one of the external iliac arteries in each animal (Fig. 1). Autogenous veins have been used surgically to avert penetration by granulation tissue in operations for repair of tendons[12] and reconstruction of nerves.[15] They were expected to function similarly in our studies.

## PROCEDURES

In 14 mongrel dogs anesthetized with pentobarbital sodium, the aortic trifurcation was exposed through a midline lower abdominal incision. The pelvic peritoneum overlying the external iliac artery on each side was incised. Each external iliac artery, from the aortic trifurcation to near the origin of the deep femoral artery, was stripped of as much of its adventitia as possible by blunt and sharp dissection. The length of the artery thus freed varied with the size of the dog and ranged from 4 to 7 cm. Preliminary dissection in anesthetized dogs (which is not discussed further in this report) indicated that a thin layer of adventitia, approximately 0.1 mm. thick, must remain on the external iliac artery. Attempts to remove this inner layer of adventitia invariably tore the artery. In each of the 14 dogs to be described in this report, a meticulous attempt was made to dissect away adventitia to the point of impending arterial rupture. The dense connective tissue of the adventitia was teased off with aneurysmal needle, fine forceps, and scalpel until the surface texture, increased translucence, and flexibility of the arterial wall indicated that further dissection would be hazardous.

An 8 cm. length of external jugular vein was removed through an incision in the neck, and the ends of the vein left in place were ligated. The excised vein was opened longitudinally and was then sutured, intimal surface outward, about a dissected external iliac artery in each dog. A continuous suture with No. 5-0 arterial silk was used. Each end of the sleeve of vein was anchored to adjacent tissue with 2 silk sutures. The opened autogenous vein, stretched to surround the artery, formed a snugly fitting sleeve over a 3 to 4 cm. length of that vessel.

All operations were performed aseptically. No anticoagulants were administered and no special postoperative care was provided. The dogs were fed the usual balanced kennel ration.

Arteriograms were made in 4 dogs for the purpose of visualizing the terminal aorta and its branches. Radiopaque medium was injected through a polyvinyl tube that had been inserted into the aorta via a common carotid artery to a point immediately proximal to the aortic trifurcation. The pertinent arteries were demonstrated by arteriography 6 months after operation and again 18 months after operation in 2 dogs, and 12 months after operation in another 2 dogs.

The dogs were killed by exsanguination under pentobarbital sodium anesthesia after postoperative intervals of 10 days (2 dogs); 20 days (1 dog); 30 days (1 dog); and 2, 4, 6, 12, and 18 months (2 dogs at each time). Immediately after death the distal portions of the aorta and the external iliac arteries were isolated from the rest of the arterial system by ligatures. They were perfused in situ for 4 hours with Bouin's fluid at a pressure equivalent to 90 mm. Hg. This procedure fixed and hardened the arteries in a configuration which more closely approached that in the living animal than does the usual, simpler method of placing an excised segment of artery in fixative. After excision and further fixation, the arteries were sectioned at 3 levels for histologic examination. Morphologic features of the right and left external iliac arteries from each experimental animal were compared with each other and with similarly perfused and prepared external iliac arteries from 14 healthy control dogs of similar size. The experimental dogs ranged in weight from 7.2 to 14.4 kilograms, and their average weight was 9.7 kilograms. The control dogs ranged in weight from 7.0 to 16.8 kilograms, with an average weight of 12.0 kilograms.

## RESULTS

In 3 of the 4 dogs in which the experimental vessels were visualized roentgenographically, the external iliac arteries that were surrounded by autogenous vein had diameters slightly smaller than the opposite uncovered arteries (Fig. 2).

Examination of histologic sections showed that a layer of adventitia approximately 0.1 mm. thick had remained on each dissected artery. Vasa vasorum which had either escaped removal or had re-formed since the operation were demonstrated within or immediately adjacent to the remaining layer of adventitia of all arteries, including those which had been surrounded by vein after dissection.

A collar of collagenous connective tissue with sparsely scattered elastic fibers rapidly formed about the dissected arteries. Collagenous tissue was especially prominent between the autogenous veins and the arteries they surrounded (Fig. 3). This layer of connective tissue had apparently caused the minor reduction in the lumen size of vessels sheathed by vein. In arteries examined after postoperative intervals longer than 1 month, the coat of collagenous tissue appeared hyaline and relatively acellular. The thickness of the collagenous neoadventitia varied greatly from dog to dog and was independent of the duration of the experimental interval. Elastic fibers, which are prominent in the adventitia of the dog's external iliac arteries, formed a minor part of the neoadventitia.

No consistent abnormalities of the intima or of the media were found in histologic sections of the experimental arteries. No differences could be demonstrated between the intima or media of the vessels from which adventitia had been removed and those of the vessels which had, in addition, been surrounded by autogenous vein.

The media in each artery appeared structurally intact except that, in an isolated

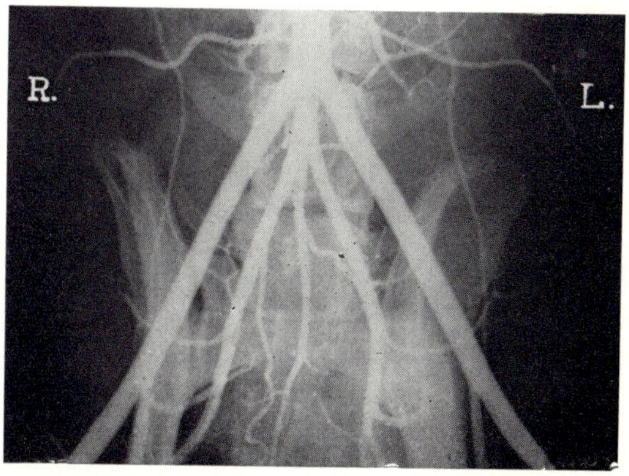


**Fig. 2.** Aortogram made 12 months after removal of adventitia from both external iliac arteries in a dog. Right external iliac artery, which was surrounded by a sleeve of vein, is slightly narrower than left.

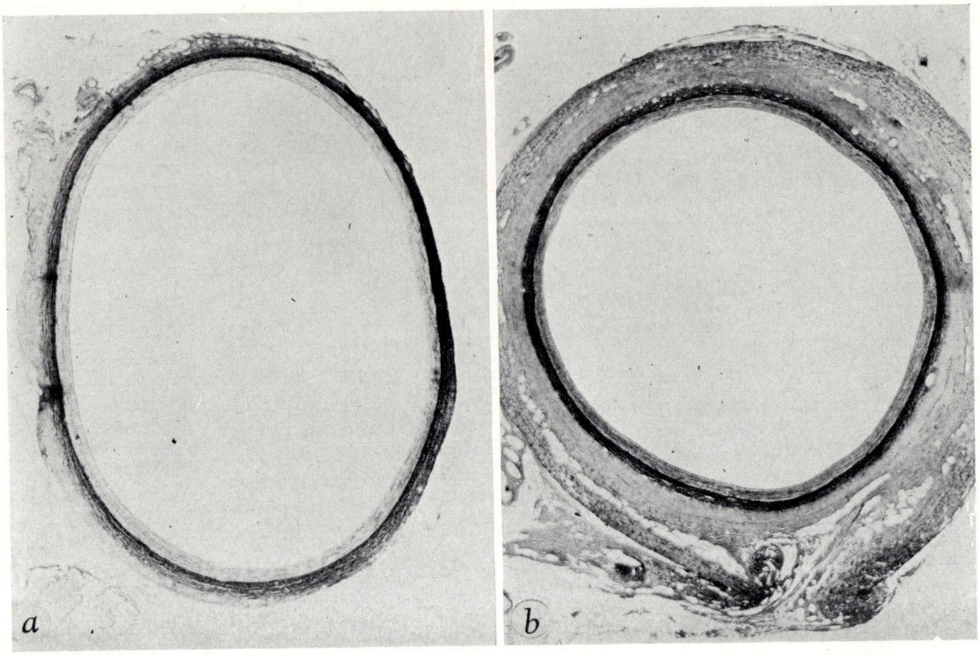

**Fig. 3.** Cross sections of left (*a*) and right (*b*) external iliac arteries of a dog 12 months after surgical removal of adventitia (*a*) and suture of a sleeve of vein about one of the arteries (*b*). These are same arteries outlined by aortogram in Fig. 2. Difference in luminal dimensions, barely apparent in aortogram, has been exaggerated by fixation. Note heavy collagenous envelope surrounding artery at right. No abnormality of media or intima is evident. (Verhoeff's elastic tissue stain counterstained with van Gieson's connective tissue stain; ×20; reduced 1/7.)

focus in each of 2 arteries, connective tissue had replaced smooth muscle. Each of these 2 defects was associated with a rupture of the adjacent inner elastic membrane and with disorganization and disappearance of elastic fibers in the media.

In order to determine whether a change had occurred in the mass of the media during the course of the study, planimetric measurements were performed and the average cross-sectional area of each artery was derived. Each of 3 histologic sections from each artery was projected at a magnification of 30 diameters. The media in the projected image of the artery was outlined on paper, and its area was determined by planimetry. The mean cross-sectional area of the media in the experimental arteries was 1.196 mm.$^2$ The mean cross-sectional area of the media in the control arteries was 1.156 mm.$^2$ The slightly larger cross-sectional area in the experimental arteries was not significant ($p = 0.38$). There was no significant difference between the cross-sectional area of the media of arteries from which adventitia had been removed (1.218 mm.$^2$) and those which had, in addition, been surrounded by autogenous vein (1.173 mm.$^2$).

The greater part of the intima was normal in all of the arteries, and the entire intima was normal in all histologic sections examined from 7 of the 28 experimental arteries from the 14 dogs (Fig. 4). Small focal lesions were observed in the intima of 21 vessels; the inner lining of these vessels otherwise retained its normal appearance, with a single layer of endothelial cells resting directly on the inner elastic membrane. Included among these focal lesions were breaks and reduplications in the inner elastic lamina, focal accumulations of collagenous connective tissue covered by endothelium and protruding into the lumen (Fig. 5), and shallow intimal crescents of proliferated connective tissue. The largest of these crescents, which was present in a dog killed 4 months after operation, is shown in Fig. 6. This lesion, which contained both collagenous and elastic tissue, was located near a discrete foreign-body reaction which surrounded a silk ligature that had been used to tie off a small branch of the autogenous vein placed around the artery. Most of the intimal lesions were associated with disruption or reduplication of the inner elastic membrane. Fibrin was demonstrated by Weigert's method in one such lesion in an artery examined 10 days after removal of adventitia.

## DISCUSSION

The focal nature of the intimal lesions found in this study and their frequent association with abnormalities of the inner elastic membrane led us to believe that these proliferations of connective tissue in the intima were the result of trauma incurred during surgical dissection of the adventitia. The presence of fibrin in 1 early lesion suggested that its origin was a small mural thrombus, perhaps at a site of minor injury. That proliferation of connective tissue occurs in the intima overlying tears in the inner elastic membrane and over traumatic lesions

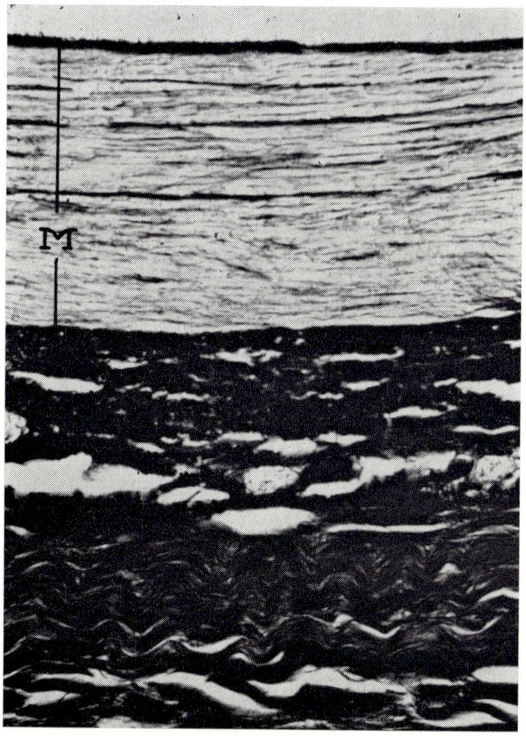


**Fig. 4.** Cross section of the external iliac artery of a dog 18 months after surgical removal of the adventitia. The lumen is at the top, adventitia is at the bottom, and the media is indicated by *M*. Nuclei of endothelial cells, which were flattened by perfusion of the vessel with fixative under pressure, are barely visible on the heavy internal elastic membrane. The intima and media appear entirely normal. Spaces which appear in the adventitia are fixation artifacts. (Verhoeff's elastic tissue stain counterstained with van Gieson's connective tissue stain; ×350.)

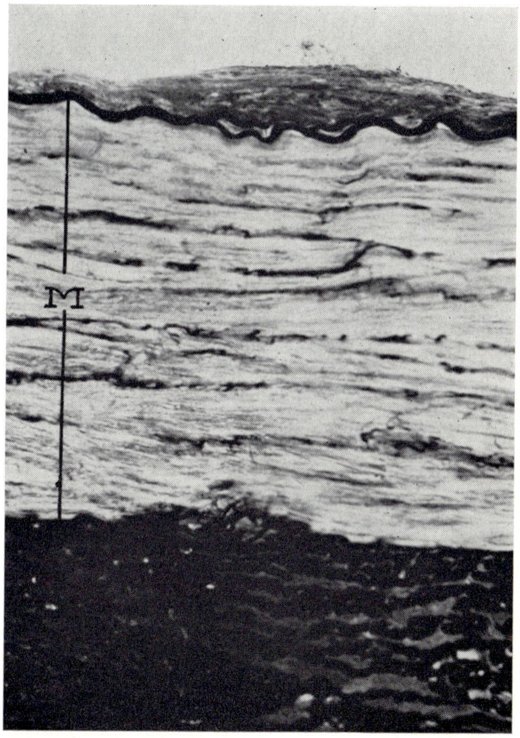


**Fig. 5.** Cross section of external iliac artery of a dog 12 months after surgical removal of adventitia. Lumen is at top, adventitia is at bottom, and media is indicated by *M*. Focal intimal lesion consists mainly of collagenous connective tissue. Fibrin was demonstrated in a similar lesion from a dog examined 10 days postoperatively which suggested that the lesion arose from a small mural thrombus. The inner elastic membrane is split at the base of the lesion. (Verhoeff's elastic tissue stain counterstained with van Gieson's connective tissue stain; ×350.) (From the Armed Forces Institute of Pathology, Washington 25, D. C.)

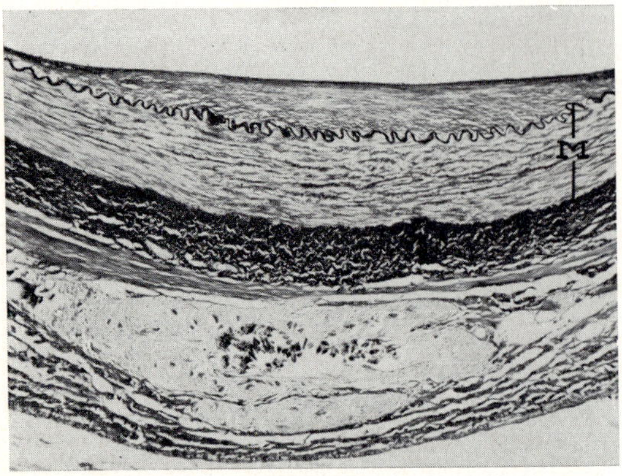


**Fig. 6.** Crescent of collagenous and elastic tissue in intima of external iliac artery of a dog 4 months after surgical removal of adventitia. Lumen is at top, adventitia is at bottom, and media is indicated by *M.* Intimal lesion overlies circumscribed foreign-body reaction about suture material near bottom of photograph. (Verhoeff's elastic tissue stain counterstained with van Gieson's connective tissue stain; ×70; reduced 3/10.) (From the Armed Forces Institute of Pathology, Washington 25, D. C.)

of the media is well known.[16, 21, 23, 26] Healing of small traumatic medial lesions may be so complete that the site of injury can later be identified only by persisting changes in the intima.

Deterling reported histologic studies of arterial autografts in which minor decreases in thickness of the media were observed in the graft. Those studies concerned carotid arterial grafts in dogs. It seems reasonable to suppose that complete, if temporary, disruption of the vasa vasorum which supply the grafted segment of artery had something to do with the loss of medial substance found by Deterling. The absence of this change and of all other consistent degenerative changes in the media of the experimental arteries observed by us may be interpreted as indicating either that (1) the surgical removal of adventitia left intact an adequate network of vasa vasorum to supply the needs of the artery wall or that (2) the metabolic needs of the walls of the arteries were supplied by diffusion from the lumen of the arteries and from surrounding tissue during the period, presumably short, required for re-establishment of an intact vasal network. In either case, the conclusion remains the same—the adventitia of the external iliac arteries of the dog may be reduced surgically to the point of impending arterial rupture without pathologic effect on the media or intima of the vessels.

## SUMMARY

Meticulous surgical removal of as much adventitia as possible from the external iliac arteries in 14 dogs caused no consistent changes in the media or intima of those arteries during periods of as long as 18 months. Focal intimal and medial lesions which were produced could be attributed to the trauma of the procedure. Wrapping the dissected arteries with segments of autogenous vein to delay revascularization of the walls of the arteries had no pathologic effect except that, in 3 of 4 animals studied by aortography, arteries surrounded by vein were slightly smaller than arteries not surrounded by vein.

### REFERENCES

1. Altschul, R.: Endothelium: its development, morphology, function, and pathology, New York, 1954, The Macmillan Company.
2. Anitschkow, N.: Das Wesen und die Entstehung der Atherosklerose, Ergebn. inn. Med. u. Kinderh. **28:** 1, 1925.
3. Bellman, S., and Frank, H. A.: Vascular channels established by implantation of a systemic artery into the myocardium, Ann. Surg. **147:** 425, 1958.
4. Benda, C.: Die Gefässe. *In* Aschoff, L.: Pathologische Anatomie, Jena, 1928, Gustav Fischer, vol. 2, pp. 54-107.
5. Benninghoff, A.: Die Arterien. *In* von Möllendorff, W.: Handbuch der mikroskopischen Anatomie des Menschen, Berlin, 1930, Julius Springer, vol. VI, pp. 49-131.
6. v. Czyhlarz, E. R., and Helbing, C.: Experimentelle Untersuchungen über die Beziehung von Nervenläsionen zu Gefässveränderungen, Centralbl. allg. Path. **8:** 849, 1897.
7. Deterling, R. A., Jr.: Blood vessels: transplantation of blood vessels. *In* Peer, L. A.: Transplantation of tissues, Baltimore, 1959, The Williams & Wilkins Company, vol. 2, pp. 313-397.
8. Durante: Untersuchungen über Entzündung der Gefässwände, Med. Jahrbuch. Wien, pp. 321-334, 1871.
9. Fabris, A.: Experimentelle Untersuchungen

über die Pathogenese der Aneurysmen, Arch. path. Anat. **165:** 439, 1901.
10. Farmachidis, C.: Quoted by Thorel, Ch.: Pathologie der Kreislauforgane des Menschen. V. Experimentelle Sklerosen des Gefässsystems, Ergebn. allg. Path. **18:** 218, 1915.
11. Fraenkel, A.: Ueber neurotische Angiosklerose, Wien. klin. Wchnschr. **9:** 170, 1896.
12. Gueukdjian, S. A.: A new method of canalizing tendon sutures with vein grafts, A. M. A. Arch. Surg. **73:** 1018, 1956.
13. Haberland, H. F. O.: Untersuchungen der Gefässwand nach der periarteriellen Sympathektomie und technische Bemerkungen zu dieser Operation, Arch. klin. Chir. **132:** 621, 1924.
14. Lange, F.: Studien zur Pathologie der Arterien, insbesondere zur Lehre von der Arteriosklerose, Arch. path. Anat. **248:** 463, 1924.
15. Lodge, W. O., and Gueukdjian, S. A.: De la paralysie faciale: modifications des opérations d'anastomose facio-hypoglosse et de plastie faciale, Presse méd. **63:** 1025, 1955.
16. Malkoff, G. M.: Ueber die Bedeutung der traumatischen Verletzungen von Arterien (Quetschung, Dehnung) für die Entwicklung der wahren Aneurysmen und der Arteriosklerose, Beitr. path. Anat. **25:** 431, 1899.
17. Manouélian, Y.: Recherches sur la pathogénie des altérations artérioscléreuses, Ann. Inst. Pasteur **27:** 19, 1913.
18. Schilling: Experimentelle Erzeugung von Intimahyperplasien, Verhandl. d. deutsch. path. Gesselsch. **20:** 154, 1925.
19. Schlichter, J. G.: Experimental medionecrosis of the aorta, Arch. Path. **42:** 182, 1946.
20. Schlichter, J. G., Katz, L. N., and Meyer, J.: The occurrence of atheromatous lesions after cauterization of the aorta followed by cholesterol administration, Am. J. M. Sc. **218:** 603, 1949.
21. Ssolowjew, A.: Experimentelle Untersuchungen über die Bedeutung von lokaler Schädigung für die Lipoidablagerung in der Arterienwand, Ztschr. ges. exper. Med. **69:** 94, 1929-1930.
22. Ssolowjew, A.: Experimentelle Untersuchungen über die Heilungsvorgänge in der Arterienwand, Beitr. path. Anat. **83:** 485, 1929.
23. Ssolowjew, A.: Über experimentell hervorgerufene Elasticarisse der Arterien und deren Bedeutung für die Lipoidablagerung, Arch. path. Anat. **283:** 213, 1932.
24. Sumikawa, P.: Ein Beitrag zur Genese der Arteriosklerose, Beitr. path. Anat. **34:** 242, 1903.
25. Todd, T. W.: Bloodvessel changes consequent on nervous lesions, J. Nerv. & Ment. Dis. **40:** 439, 1913.
26. Ziegler: Ueber traumatische Arteriitis und deren Beziehungen zur Arteriosklerose und zum Aneurysma, Centralbl. allg. Path. **9:** 844, 1898.

# Mucosal replacement of gastric explants by free autogenous grafts

FRANK G. MOODY, M.D.
CHARLES K. McSHERRY, M.D.
JOHN M. BEAL, M.D.
NEW YORK, N. Y.
*From the Department of Surgery, The New York Hospital—Cornell Medical Center*

Previous reports have described studies of replacement of gastric mucosa by a nonsecretory epithelium.[1, 2] The application of split-thickness autogenous skin grafts to the denuded gastric wall in the pig was followed by variable success, which yielded an average survival of approximately 45 per cent of the grafted skin. Additional studies have been conducted to determine the factors that may influence the fate of these skin grafts. A wedge of the greater curvature portion of the stomach with an intact pedicle was employed as an explant on the anterior abdominal wall to visualize the events that follow mucosal stripping and grafting.

## METHODS

Ten-week-old pigs which weighed 20 to 30 pounds were anesthetized intraperitoneally with Nembutal and maintained with an ether-oxygen mixture administered through an endotracheal tube. A split-thickness skin graft approximately 0.010 inches in thickness was obtained from the anterior abdominal wall of 5 pigs. Jejunal mucosa was obtained in 9 pigs by stripping the mucosa from a resected portion of the jejunum. Bladder mucosa was obtained by performing a cystotomy and stripping the transitional epithelium just above the muscularis of the urinary bladder in 3 others. The grafts were kept in a saline-soaked sponge until the gastric explant was prepared.

Supported by United States Public Health Service Grant No. A-790.

Received for publication Nov. 14, 1960.

The abdomen was entered through an upper midline incision, and a well-vascularized wedge of the greater curvature of the fundus measuring 4 by 8 cm. was excised. The gastric defect was closed with continuous inverting chromic catgut sutures and reinforced with interrupted sutures of fine silk. The explant with its intact vascular pedicle was transferred to the anterior abdominal wall. The incision was closed in layers with interrupted fine silk sutures about the vascular pedicle. The explant was secured to the abdomen at its margins and then stripped of gastric mucosa by blunt and sharp dissection just below the muscularis mucosa, a relatively avascular, filmy areolar plane (Fig. 1). Hemostasis was obtained by compression. The graft was applied and secured to the explant by interrupted fine silk sutures (Fig. 2). A bulky bolus dressing was utilized. The dressings were changed at 3- or 4-day intervals so that the progress of the graft could be observed and documented by photographs and histologic sections. Four explants were transferred into the subcutaneous tissues of the anterior abdominal wall in an attempt to secure successful jejunal mucosal grafts. In these instances the graft site was not disturbed for a period of 1 to 2 weeks.

## RESULTS

Split-thickness skin grafts which covered the gastric explant demonstrated virtually complete survival in the 5 animals at the time of sacrifice 3 weeks after application.

The sequence of healing is demonstrated in Fig. 3. A smooth, pliable surface was obtained in each instance. Though there was no evidence of shrinking of the explant for the duration of this study, the histologic sections demonstrated a dense desmoplastic scar beneath the graft (Fig. 4). Nine grafts of jejunal mucosa were performed. Two pigs died from pneumonia 3 and 4 days after operation with the grafts still intact. Six grafts survived 7 to 12 days and then sloughed. The longest graft survival was 20 days in a pig in which the explant had been transferred into the subcutaneous position rather than onto the anterior abdominal wall.

Three preparations in which urinary bladder mucosa was applied to the denuded explant were unsuccessful. Two demonstrated loss of the graft in 3 days, while the third graft survived for 11 days and was then lost.

## DISCUSSION

The replacement of gastric mucosa by nonsecretory epithelium with preservation of the storage and trituratory functions of the stomach would be a desirable adjunct to the surgical therapy of peptic ulcer disease. However, there are numerous obstacles to the practical solution of this problem. Among these has been the regeneration of gastric mucosa beneath and around the graft site in the intact stomach of some laboratory animals. This was solved in part by the use of the pig in which the mucosa can be completely stripped with ease beneath the muscularis mucosa.[2] Acid-secreting mucosa, however, remains at the margins and continually bathes the graft with gastric juice. Constant motion at the graft site from the muscular contractions of the gastric wall tend to displace the grafts as well. Attempts to secure immobilization by use of a bolus, multiple fixation sutures, or distention of the gastric lumen have met with indifferent results.

The gastric explant as employed in this study has afforded an opportunity for direct-vision study of grafts applied to a well-vascularized immobile surface, free from the effects of gastric juice. A uniform, pliable, nonsecretory surface was insured when split-thickness skin grafts were employed. The success of these preparations confirms the role of immobilization of the graft site, a principle which is basic to successful grafting in all areas of the body. The significance of establishing an acid-free environment demands additional study.

A third factor to be considered is the effect of shrinkage of the desmoplastic scar beneath the graft. Within the time period of this study, which was of short duration, there was no gross shrinkage of the explant. Longer periods of observation are necessary to determine the effects of contraction as the underlying scar in the graft bed matures.

Attempts to graft the denuded explant with epithelium other than skin were unsuccessful. Lippman[3] observed in his prep-

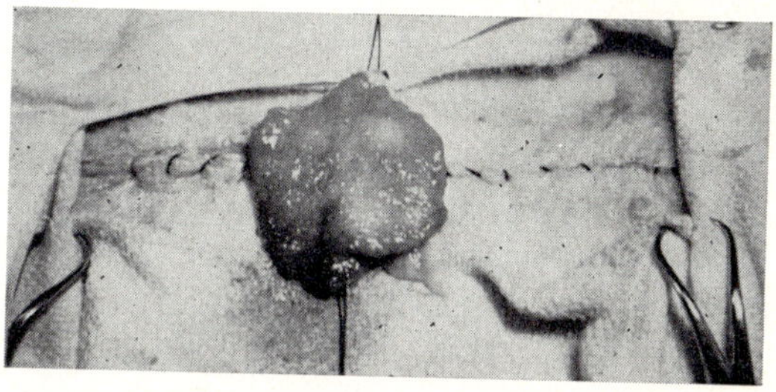

**Fig. 1.** Appearance of the gastric explant which has been formed from a section of the greater curvature of the stomach and has been stripped of the gastric mucosa.

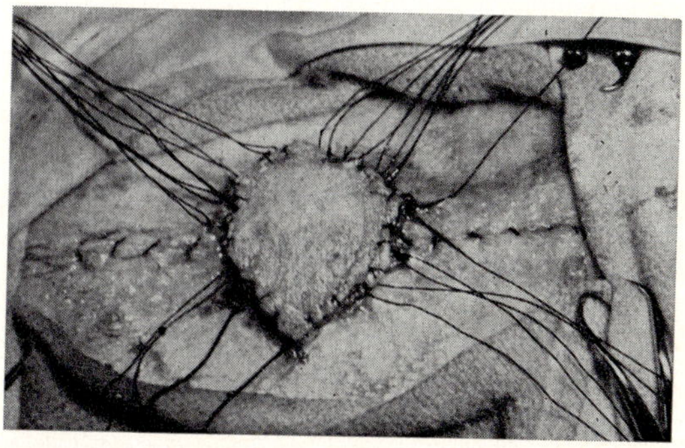

**Fig. 2.** A split-thickness autogenous skin graft has been applied to the gastric explant in a pig and the margins of the explant have been sutured to the skin of the anterior abdominal wall.

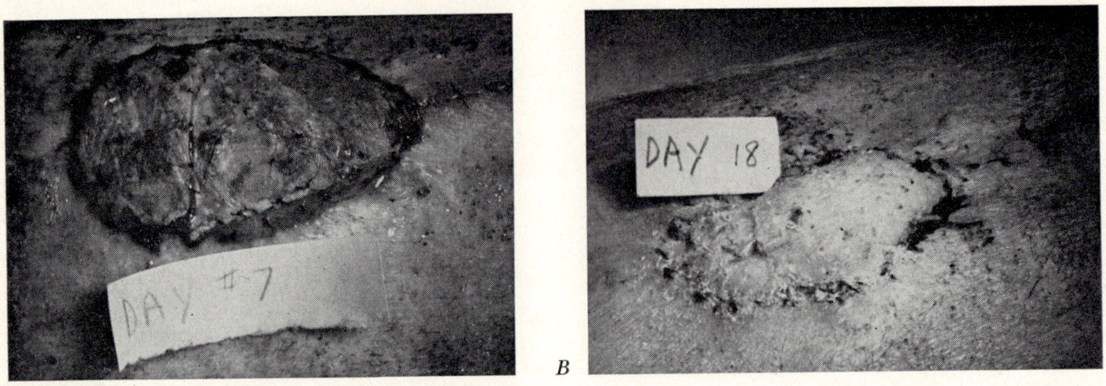


*A* *B*

**Fig. 3.** *A,* Appearance of the grafted explant 7 days after the application of the skin graft. *B,* The skin graft has taken well 18 days after application.

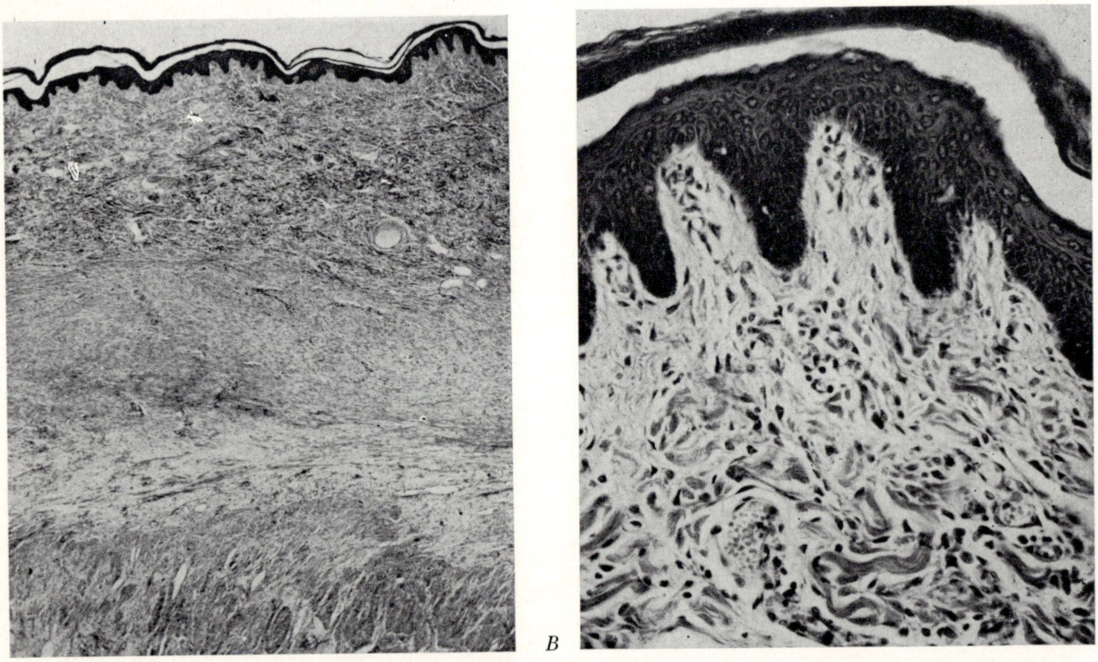

*A* *B*

**Fig. 4.** *A,* Photomicrograph of section through the grafted explant 3 weeks after application of skin (low-power view). *B,* High-power view of the same section which demonstrates the formation of scar tissue beneath the graft. (Reduced 3/10.)

arations that the jejunal mucosa for the most part undergoes necrosis, with only a few cells remaining as histologically recognizable jejunal mucosa. We judged the failure of our preparations by the gross appearance of slough, and it may be that further observation of these grafts would have demonstrated subsequent regeneration.

The failure to secure successful bladder mucosal grafts cannot be explained at this time. A chronic inflammatory reaction was observed in the explant in each instance which may have led to the rejection of the graft. The etiology of this response, however, remains obscure.

The excellent surface obtained with skin, in addition to its availability, has encouraged its continued use as an appropriate epithelium for relining the stomach. The problem centers on a method for insuring a uniform "take" of a large grafted surface in the intact stomach. The method presented in this paper was used in an attempt to study one of the factors that appears to be involved in the problem.

## SUMMARY

Free autogenous grafts have been applied to a gastric explant of the pig's stomach denuded of its mucosa. An acceptable epithelial surface of split-thickness skin was obtained. Jejunal and urinary bladder mucosal grafts were unsuccessful.

## REFERENCES

1. Dineen, J. P., Fuller, W. F., and Beal, J. M.: Application of autogenous skin grafts to the gastric wall, SURGERY **45:** 251, 1959.
2. Free, E. A., Mannix, H., Jr., and Beal, J. M.: Replacement of gastric mucosa with autogenous skin grafts, SURGERY **40:** 554, 1956.
3. Lippman, H. N., and Longmire, W. P., Jr.: Studies on the transplantation of free jejunal mucosa-submucosa autografts to the mucosa-stripped stomach of the dog, Ann. Surg. **140:** 86, 1954.

# Artificial respirator for dogs

KONRAD W. SCHEEL
NEW ORLEANS, LA.
*From the Department of Surgery, Tulane University School of Medicine*

Unless respiration is assisted by manual aid or a mechanical device, the administration of an anesthetic such as Nembutal will produce hypoventilation and may reduce the oxygen saturation of arterial blood to approximately 75 per cent. An artificial respirator is required not only for open-chest operations, but also in all experimental procedures in which organ function must be studied without the interference of anoxemia. Experiments on 10 dogs with a newly devised positive-pressure respirator have resulted in arterial blood oxygen saturation of nearly 90 per cent. Besides its effectiveness in improving ventilation and combating anoxemia, the apparatus is simple to operate and easy to control.

## DESCRIPTION

A motor-driven electric timer (Fig. 1, *TM*), which has a 2-second-on, 2-second-off cycle, activates relay $RI_1$.

During the 2-second-off cycle a negative grid bias of 4 V. is applied to thyratron tube *(V)*, keeping it cut off. In the 2-second-on position, $RL_1$ allows the charged capacitor $(C_2)$ to discharge through $R_2$, $R_3$, $R_4$, or $R_5$, resulting in a time constant of ½, 1, 1½, and 2 seconds, respectively. The discharge of $C_2$ lowers the voltage on the grid of $V$, causing the tube to conduct and energize $RL_2$. When $RL_2$ is energized, $RL_3$ is de-energized, which in turn activates the solenoid valve $(SL_2)$, through which the dog exhales. The variable time lapse between the start of the on cycle of the timer and the conduction of $V$ is the interval during which the solenoid valve, *SL,* is energized and the dog inhales (positive inhalation). The relationship between these cycles is shown in Fig. 2.

A laboratory air line is connected through a pressure regulator to the solenoid valves which, during the inspiratory cycle, allow

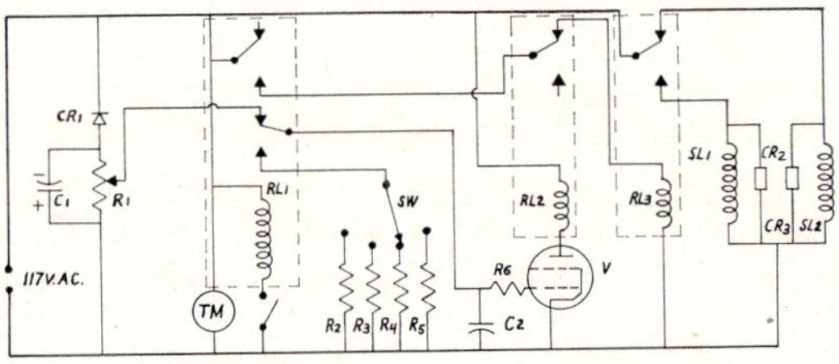


**Fig. 1.** Circuit diagram. $CR_1$, 150 Ma. selenium rectifier; $CR_2$, and $CR_3$, contact protectors, International Rectifier Corp., No. 56Y6P; $R_1$, 30 kohm, 4W potentiometer; $R_2$, 1 megohm ½ W resistor; $R_3$, 2 megohm ½ W resistor; $R_4$, 3 megohm ½ W resistor; $R_5$, 4 megohm ½ W resistor; $R_6$, 10 kohm ½ W resistor; $C_1$, 8 MFD 150 v. capacitor; $C_2$, 0.5 MFD 150 v. capacitor; $V$, 2 D 21 tube; *TM,* Industrial Timer Corp. model CMO 115/60; $RL_1$, Potter and Brumfield relay KRP11A; $RL_2$ and $RL_3$, Potter and Brumfield relay KRP5A; $SL_1$, V 5 D 6260C solenoid valve; and $SL_2$, V 5 D 1920S solenoid valve. The pressure regulator is Black, Sivalls and Bryson type 001-21.

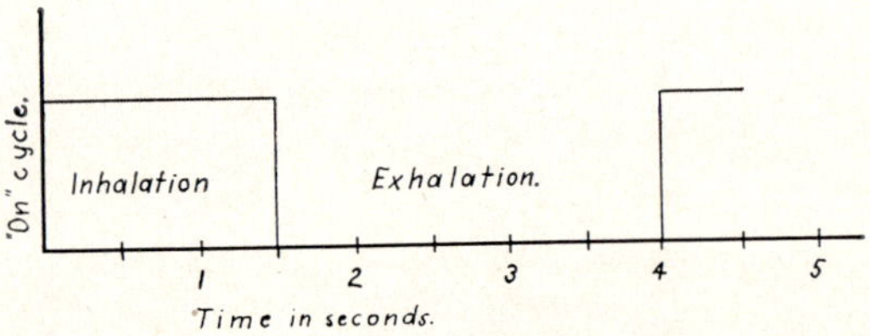


**Fig. 2.** Comparison of inhalation and exhalation time with SW in the 1.5 second position.

Received for publication Nov. 8, 1960

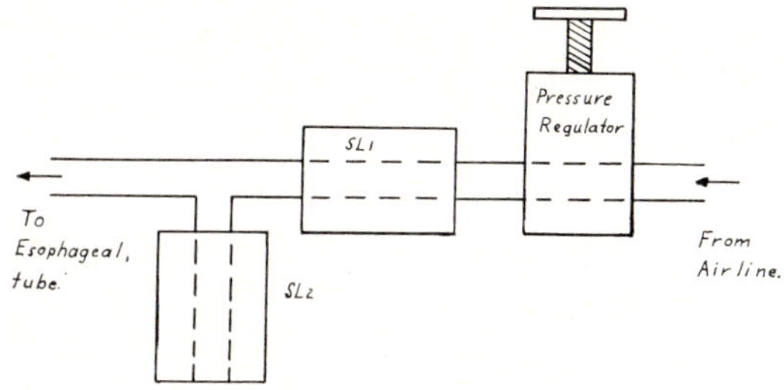


**Fig. 3.** Diagram of the air system.

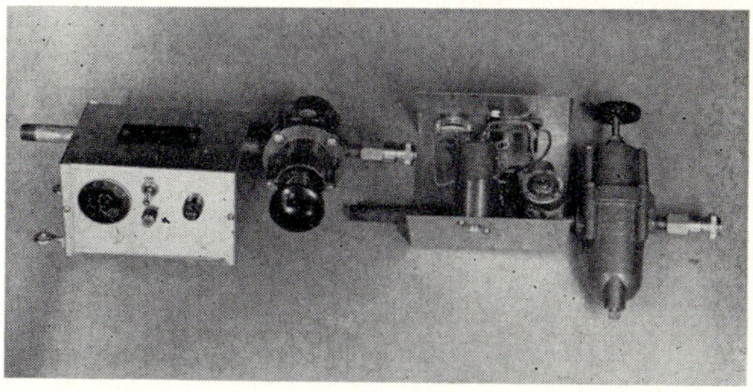

**Fig. 4.** Two remote units shown in an assembled and exploded view.

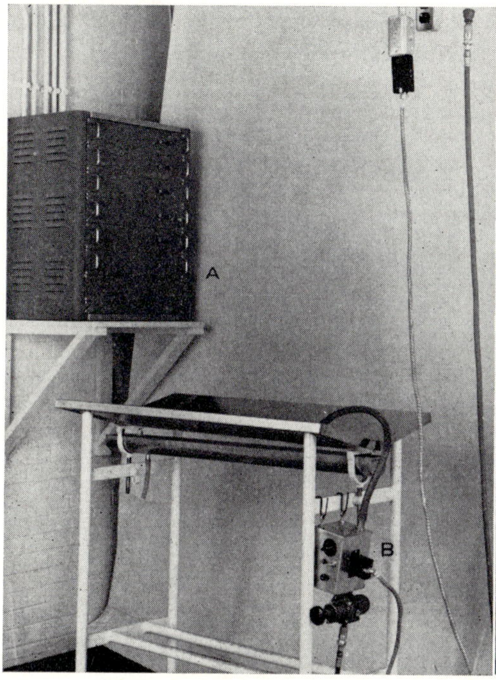


5

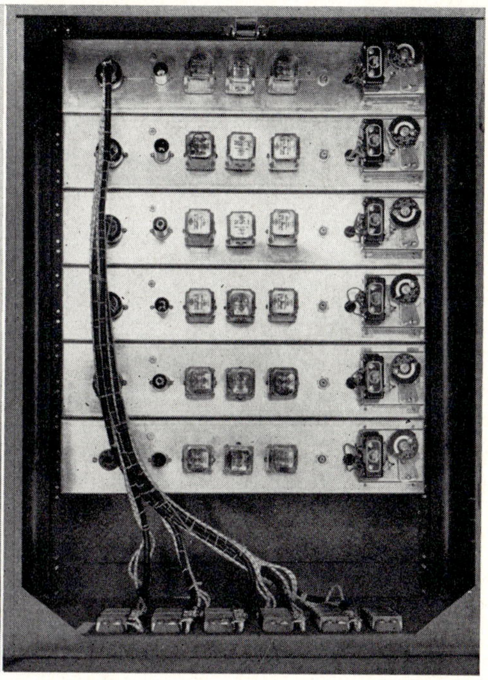

6

**Fig. 5.** *A,* Master unit containing 5 individual respirator units with 1 unit as a spare. *B,* Remote unit mounted to the operating table.

**Fig. 6.** Rear view of master unit which shows the electrical connections to the remote unit.

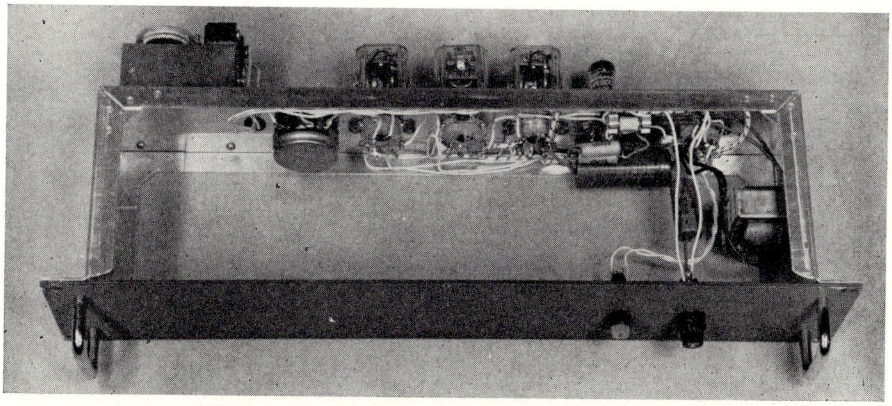

**Fig. 7.** View of individual rack-mounted unit.

the air to flow through an intertracheal tube to the lungs of the dog (Fig. 3). The large orifice of $SL_2$ allows complete exhalation. $CR_2$ and $CR_3$ are used for arc-suppression across the contacts of $RL_3$.

## SPECIAL FEATURES

The 2 solenoid valves, the pressure regulator, the on-off switch, and the tap switch (for adjusting the inspiration time) are mounted in a small aluminum box (Fig. 4). This box may be attached to the operating table usually used for animals (Fig. 5).

Electrical connections to the master unit (Fig. 6) are made via a cable and plug. The air line is connected by a quick connect-disconnect coupling that allows fast disassembly and easy storage in a crowded laboratory. Plug-in type relays are used for quick and simple servicing. The unit shown in Figs. 5, *A*, and 6 accommodates 5 separate respirators with 1 for use as a spare. All channels are rack-mounted for ready removal (Fig. 7).

## SUMMARY

The respirator described is a very simple yet reliable unit. It complies with the basic demands for 15 respirations per minute, a variable inspiration time (½ to 2 seconds), adjustable flow and pressure to the lungs, operational simplicity, and compactness. This unit can also be connected to a supply of oxygen or other gas mixtures.

The author wishes to thank Dr. Oscar Creech, Jr., Professor and Chairman of the Department of Surgery, Tulane University School of Medicine, for his cooperation in the development of this respirator. The suggestions of Professor James Cronwich of the Electrical Engineering Department of Tulane University concerning the preparation of this paper are gratefully acknowledged.

# Anomalies of the lungs associated with congenital diaphragmatic hernia

GABRIEL A. SABGA, M.D.
WILLIAM E. NEVILLE, M.D.
LOUIS R. M. DEL GUERCIO, M.D.
CLEVELAND, OHIO
*From Western Reserve University School of Medicine, Department of Surgery, Cleveland Metropolitan General Hospital*

Structural defects in the closure of the pleuroperitoneal hiatus or the formation of the hemidiaphragm account for the majority of congenital diaphragmatic hernias in infants and children.[10] Invariably, some other embryologic abnormality is associated with these diaphragmatic defects.[3] The one commonly reported is the abnormal mesenteric attachment of the small and large bowel.[5, 8, 10, 19] However, the occurrence of another anomaly accompanying congenital herniation of the abdominal viscera into the thoracic cavity, namely the ipsilateral lung, has received little attention.[3, 20] While most reports of large series of patients treated operatively fail to mention the state of the lungs at operation, others, more recently, have stressed the high incidence of accompanying pulmonary hypoplasia.[3, 20] Another uncommon pulmonary anomaly, a "lower accessory lung" or "extralobar sequestration," has been seen to accompany congenital diaphragmatic defects both at autopsy and at operation.[9, 21, 22]

The case histories of 5 patients who had congenital diaphragmatic hernias with associated pulmonary abnormalities are reported. In 2 patients, pulmonary hypoplasia of the ipsilateral lung was seen at operation, while in the third, an unsuspected "extralobar sequestration" of the lung was found during repair of the hernia and was resected. In 2 other patients with congenital diaphragmatic hernias, in whom death occurred soon after birth, autopsies were performed. In one there was definite hypoplasia of the ipsilateral lung, while in the other there was nonpneumatization of both lungs. The variety and high incidence of pulmonary anomalies encountered with congenital diaphragmatic hernias and the importance of recognizing the presence of these anomalies prompted us to report these case histories and to review the literature on the subject.

Received for publication Feb. 6, 1961.

## CASE REPORTS

**Case 1.** A 6 pound, 13 ounce baby girl was born at St. Alexis Hospital at 3:35 p.m. on Oct. 10, 1952. Respirations were spontaneous, but labored, and the baby was cyanotic. Breath sounds were absent on the left side of the chest. Roentgenograms were suggestive of the presence of a congenital diaphragmatic hernia on the left (Fig. 1). The baby was operated upon 48 hours after birth. A thoracoabdominal approach was utilized. All the abdominal organs, with the exception of the kidneys, descending colon, and rectum, were in the left hemithorax. The left hemidiaphragm was completely absent. The hernia was repaired with the left lobe of the liver used to close the communication between the pleural and peritoneal cavities. The edge of the liver was sutured to the endothoracic fascia. Repeated efforts during operation to expand the small and collapsed left lung were unsuccessful. At the time of closure, the left lung was completely collapsed against the medias-

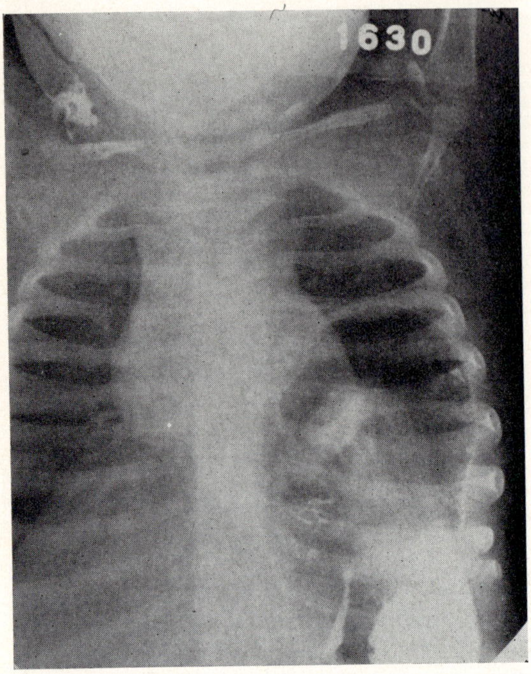

**Fig. 1.** Case 1. Preoperative chest roentgenogram after a barium swallow. Note the fundus of the stomach high in the left pleural cavity. The mediastinum is not displaced.

tinum. Postoperatively, the thoracotomy tube was attached for water-sealed drainage. Negative pressure was applied to the thoracotomy tube every 4 hours. Gradual expansion of the left lung took place. The thoracotomy tube was removed on the ninth day when roentgenograms of the chest showed the heart to be back in its normal position and both lungs to be aerating well. Eight years later the patient was doing well (Fig. 2).

**Case 2.** In December, 1952, a 24-hour-old, 7½ month premature infant was seen at Huron Road Hospital with signs of a right diaphragmatic hernia. Roentgenograms showed the stomach to be in the abdomen, but the small bowel and most of the colon were in the right hemithorax. The baby was operated upon through a right thoraco-abdominal approach in the eighth intercostal space. The right hemidiaphragm was completely absent. There was difficulty in reducing the small intestine and colon back into the abdomen because of marked distention of the bowel. The right lung was completely collapsed and proved impossible to expand. The liver was sutured to the endothoracic fascia and effectively created a barrier between the two cavities. At the conclusion of the operation, cardiac arrest occurred and the heart failed to respond to cardiac massage and other measures. No other abnormalities were seen at autopsy.

**Case 3.** A 4 pound, 3 ounce male was born on Oct. 19, 1954, at Cleveland Metropolitan General Hospital. The baby cried spontaneously at birth, but was cyanotic and had shallow, irregular breathing. His condition deteriorated rapidly and he died a few hours after birth. At autopsy, the left hemithorax was found to contain the left lobe of the liver, cecum, terminal ileum, transverse colon, and spleen. There was a hernial sac present. Both lungs were completely collapsed, were reported as showing "nonpneumatization," and were probably hypoplastic (Fig. 3).

**Case 4.** The patient was a 3½-month-old male, who, on a routine examination in the clinic for an upper respiratory infection, was found to have a shift of the mediastinum to the right. Roentgenogram of the chest (Fig. 4) was suggestive of a left diaphragmatic hernia, and the patient was admitted to the hospital. He had been born at full term at this hospital on Nov. 1, 1958, and discharged 5 days later in good condition. He ate well and developed normally. On admission the baby was in no acute distress. There was a shift of the trachea and the mediastinum to the right, and the left side of the chest showed increased tympany and depressed breath sounds. A left thoracotomy was performed through the eighth intercostal space. A defect 5 cm. in diameter was found in the posterolateral portion of the muscular diaphragm. Through this defect protruded the stomach, spleen, transverse colon, and loops of small bowel. There were 2 normal looking lobes of the left lung. However, between the lower lobe and the diaphragm a third and apparently atelectatic lobe was seen. This felt like liver. The lobe received a systemic artery which entered through the posterior rim of the diaphragm. The vein drained below the diaphragm. There were no connections with the bronchial tree or pulmonary vessels. It was attached by alveolar tissue to the hilum. The mass was recognized as a "sequestrated lobe" (Fig. 5). The hernia was repaired after the sac had been opened and its contents easily reduced into the abdomen. The sequestrated lobe was then resected. The chest cavity was drained under a water seal. The patient made an uneventful recovery. The pathologic diagnosis of the resected tissue was "consistent with a sequestrated lobe of the lung" (Fig. 6). The patient was seen 20 months later and was doing well at that time (Fig. 7).

**Case 5.** A full-term male baby was born on July 5, 1959, at Cleveland Metropolitan General Hospital. The baby weighed 2,800 grams at birth, was cyanotic and flaccid with absent corneal reflexes, and was gasping. In spite of attempts at resuscitation, the baby remained cyanotic and died soon after birth. At autopsy, congenital absence of the left hemidiaphragm was found with herniation of the stomach, pancreas, spleen, left lobe of the liver, most of the small intestine, cecum, and ascending and transverse colon into the left hemithorax. The left lung was hypoplastic (Fig. 8) and both lungs were atelectatic.

## DISCUSSION

**Pulmonary hypoplasia.** The association of hypoplasia of the lung with congenital diaphragmatic hernias has been fully described as a postmortem finding by pathologists, but it was not until recently that the condition was recognized by the surgeon at operation. Potter,[14] in her book, *The Pathology of the Foetus and the Newborn,* writes, "Any condition that reduces the capacity of the thoracic cage early in foetal life will cause hypoplasia of the lung tissue. To develop normally the lung must have adequate room for growth, and growth will be inhibited in proportion to lack of space. The most profound reduction in size of the lungs occurs with diaphragmatic herniae, especially in the lung on the side of the diaphragmatic defect."

Campanale and Rowland,[3] in 1955, were the first to call attention to the presence of pulmonary hypoplasia in patients treated surgically for congenital diaphragmatic hernias. A moderate to severe hypoplasia of the lung was seen in every one of their 5 patients, 3 of whom were operated upon. However, a review by these authors of the surgical literature of the preceding 30 years, failed to disclose a single mention of this condition by the surgeon.[3] Gross,[3] after an extensive experience with congenital diaphragmatic hernias at Children's Hospital in Boston, could not recall noting at operation a single instance of definite hypoplasia of the lung and believed that it must be rare. Other surgeons who have recorded their observations on the lungs at operation indicate that a high percentage of the lungs were hypoplastic. Roe,[20] in 1956, reviewed the hospital records and autopsy protocols for all cases of congenital diaphragmatic hernias in 11 San Francisco hospitals over a period of 20 years. A total of 47 patients were studied and analyzed. Of 24 patients operated upon, in only 5 was satisfactory lung expansion described. In 10 cases the surgeon noted that the lung remained small and collapsed, in 1 there was partial lung expansion, and in the remaining 8 no comment on the lung was made in the operative note. Autopsy observations on 21 cases indicated that in size, the lung on the hernia side was often only a small fraction of the size of the contralateral lung, with an average weight ratio of 0.39. In 2 of our patients who were operated upon,[16] the appearance of the lungs was suggestive of hypoplasia. These lungs failed to expand in spite of strong positive pressure exerted through an endotracheal tube. In Case 2 there was a persistent pneumothorax postoperatively in spite of intermittent suction through a drainage tube, which indicated that the lung was hypoplastic and incapable of rapid expansion. There was definite hypo-

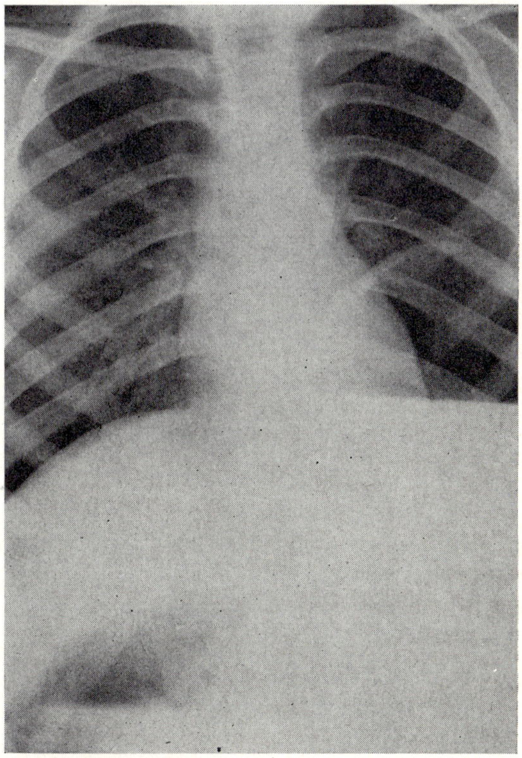

**Fig. 2.** Case 1. Chest roentgenogram 8 years postoperatively. The fundus of the stomach still appears higher than normal on the left side. The patient is asymptomatic.

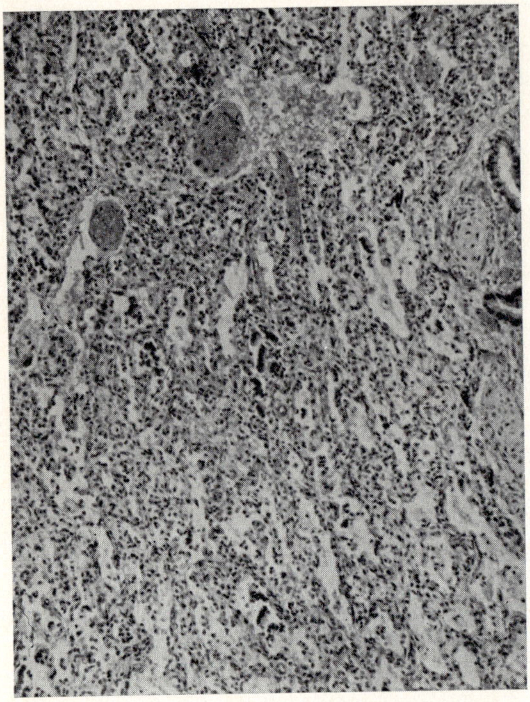

**Fig. 3.** Case 3. Photomicrograph of the left lung which shows nonpneumatization. Note few air-filled alveoli and atelectasis consistent with mild hypoplasia of the lung (×200; reduced ¼.)

plasia of the pulmonary tissue in the patient in Case 5 at autopsy.

**Extralobar sequestration.** This lung anomaly, also called "lower accessory lobe," is commonly associated with congenital diaphragmatic hernias. St. Raymond and coworkers,[21] who analyzed all cases reported in the literature up to 1956, found several characteristics common to all. These anomalies consisted of masses of lung tissue in various stages of differentiation occurring in the thorax, lower neck, or upper abdomen and not connected with the normal respiratory tree. They were not incompatible with life and were much more common on the left side. The presence of an associated defect of the diaphragm, predominantly of the left side, was not an infrequent finding. Except for an occasional rare case, the blood supply of the lower accessory lung was not associated with the pulmonary vascular system, but was derived from the aorta.[21] The venous drainage was usually to the hemiazygous system.[17] Concerning the genesis of this embryonic defect, the "traction" theory advanced by Pryce and colleagues[17] in 1947 adequately explains the developmental anomaly. In brief, they consider the abnormal blood supply of the "accessory lobe" to be the first abnormality, and sequestration to be an accidental complication. Abnormal arteries from the dorsal aorta on one side or the other of the embryo "capture" one or more "bulbous" tips of the developing lung tree. If such a "bulbous" tip of lung tissue survives, it becomes a "sequestrated" lobe. This same theory is advanced by these authors to explain the association of sequestrated lobes and diaphragmatic defects, and even the latter abnormality when present alone. According to this theory, congenital diaphragmatic defects are also the result of ischemic traction on abnormal embryonic arteries which run from the developing diaphragm to the developing lung. These are more common toward the pulmonary ligament on the left side. If a detached tip of lung tissue survives, the defect is then associated with a sequestrated lobe. Most diaphragmatic defects are not associated with sequestrated lobes because of the low survival rate of the detached pulmonary element.[17] In 1932, Guy and Rand[9] collected 34 cases of accessory lobe of the lung. Of these, 7 were associated with a congenital diaphragmatic hernia. They added an eighth case of their own. In 1947, Valle and White[22] collected 37 cases of lower accessory lungs. Of these, 29.7 per cent were associated with congenital diaphragmatic hernias. St. Raymond and his group,[21] in 1956, stated that about 40 cases of lower accessory lung had been reported. The majority of these cases were found at autopsy. St. Raymond reported the first case in which a patient with congenital diaphragmatic hernia associated with an accessory lobe was successfully operated upon. In 1947, Valle and White[22] had operated upon a similar patient who did not survive. Both patients were children with congenital diaphragmatic hernias in whom no lung anomalies had been suspected preoperatively. On exploration through a thoracic incision the accessory lobes were encountered and were resected. Our patient in Case 4 constitutes the third to be operated upon and the second reported to have survived. Similarly, in this case no lung anomaly was suspected preoperatively, and the condition was discovered at operation.

Other authors have reported the cases of patients with lower accessory lobes associated with other types of diaphragmatic defects. Claman and Ehrenhaft[4] described a patient 64 years old with an extralobar sequestration associated with a posterolateral weakness of the diaphragm. Berman[2] reported 2 cases of extralobar sequestration associated with "eventration of the diaphragm."

It thus appears that the lung anomalies, hypoplasia and extralobar sequestration, are more commonly associated with congenital diaphragmatic hernias than previously suspected. These anomalies have eluded the surgeons for several reasons. The first and most important reason may well be the great respiratory distress experienced by the newborn infant with a congenital diaphragmatic hernia in whom 1 lung is severely hypoplastic and the other compressed. Such patients rarely reach a surgeon and, understandably enough, the lesion has for a long time been not a surgical, but a postmortem finding. In Potter's[15] experience, only 1 infant with a diagnosis of congenital diaphragmatic hernia at the Chicago Lying-in Hospital survived more than 6 hours. Nevertheless, the experience of many surgeons[1, 5, 7, 10, 11, 19] has shown that not only can these babies be saved if operated upon soon after birth, but that a hypoplastic lung in the presence of a congenital diaphragmatic hernia is not incompatible with many years of life. Rakover and associates[18] reported the case of an 11-year-old boy with a congenital diaphragmatic hernia in whom the ipsilateral lung was quite hypoplastic and hardly filled one-third of the chest cavity when inflated by pressure at operation. The second cause for the lack of the surgeon's awareness of these associated

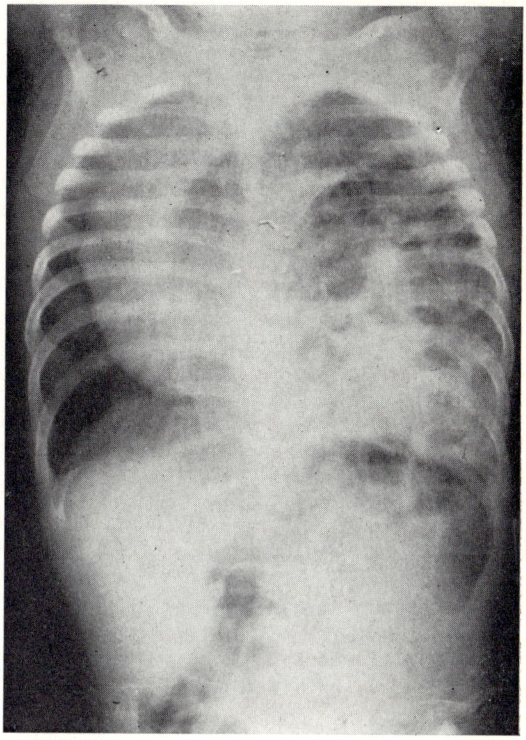

**Fig. 4.** Case 4. Preoperative posteroanterior chest roentgenogram which shows that the mediastinum is markedly displaced to the right and loops of the small bowel are filling the left hemithorax.

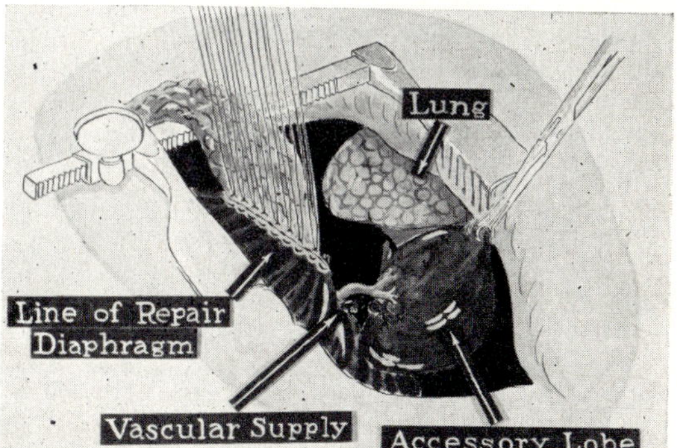


**Fig. 5.** Case 4. Drawing which shows the findings at operation (transthoracic approach). The suture line in the dome of the diaphragm is shown with the excess tissue from the redundant sac. The "extralobar sequestration" is shown with its vascular supply passing through the posterior rim of the diaphragm.

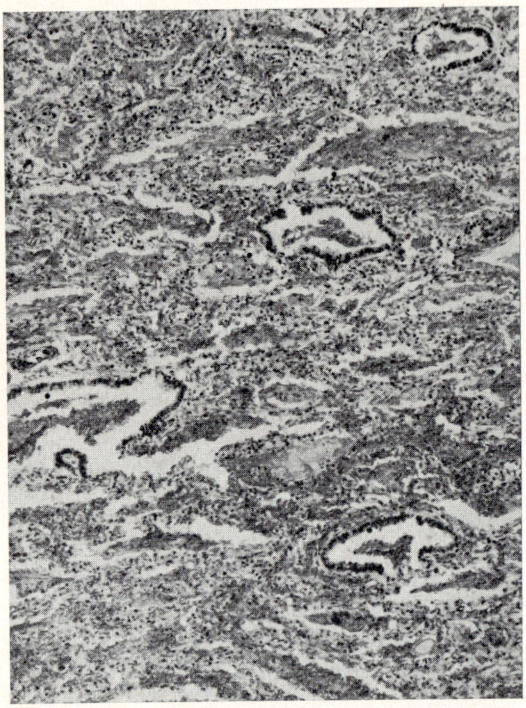

**Fig. 6.** Case 4. Photomicrograph of the resected tissue which shows cuboidal cell–lined air passages and structures like alveoli filled with blood, consistent with a "sequestrated lobe" of the lung (×200; reduced ¼.)

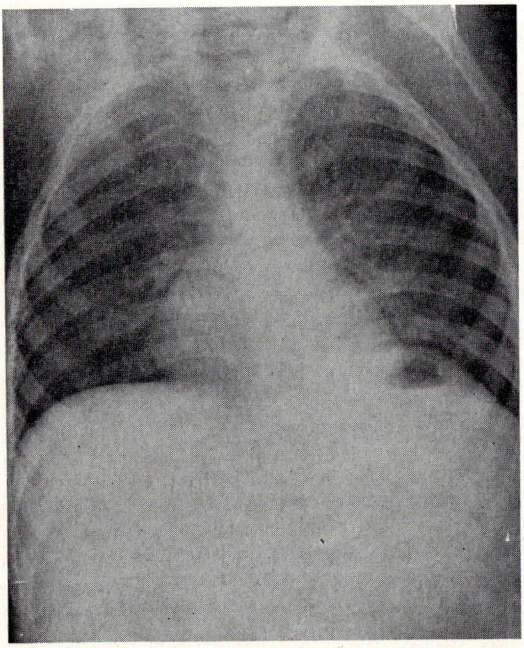

**Fig. 7.** Case 4. Postoperative roentgenogram taken 20 months later which shows a normal thoracic cavity with a normal diaphragm.

pulmonary anomalies is their failure to notice and record the presence of abnormalities of the lungs during operation. It is possible that since the majority of surgeons utilize the abdominal approach for the repair of this type of hernia,[5, 8, 10, 19] the exact state of the lungs and thoracic contents at operation remains unknown. A moderately hypoplastic lung or an extralobar sequestration may go unnoticed because the abdominal exposure precludes good visualization of the thoracic cavity.

According to Campanale and Rowland,[3] hypoplastic lungs present an anatomic and physiologic abnormality different from that of a collapsed but expandable lung. It is thus important for the surgeon not only to be aware of its frequent occurrence but also to recognize the condition when present. Forceful attempts to expand the lungs during operation with positive pressure through an endotracheal tube may be quite harmful and even fatal.[20] Furthermore, such efforts are rarely, if ever, rewarding since the hypoplastic lung is incapable of rapid expansion, as seen in 2 of our cases. The injudicious application of strong intrapleural negative pressure in an effort to "bring out the lung" can also lead to harmful effects.[3] In the presence of a poorly expandable hypoplastic lung the complete withdrawal of air will produce a mediastinal shift with cardiorespiratory embarrassment. Infants with this combination of defects have so limited a cardiorespiratory reserve to begin with that the superimposition of this added handicap can result in catastrophe.[3] It is advised that the intrapleural pressures be adjusted according to over-all clinical evaluation of cardiorespiratory function and not according to roentgenograms. Closed underwater drainage will assure gradual re-expansion of the lung to the extent possible.[3] Roe and Stephens[20] advocate intermittent gentle positive pressure to aid alveolar aeration and tracheostomy to reduce dead space in some cases. They also use closed sealed drainage to protect against tension pneumothorax and to promote gentle and gradual expansion of the hypoplastic lung.

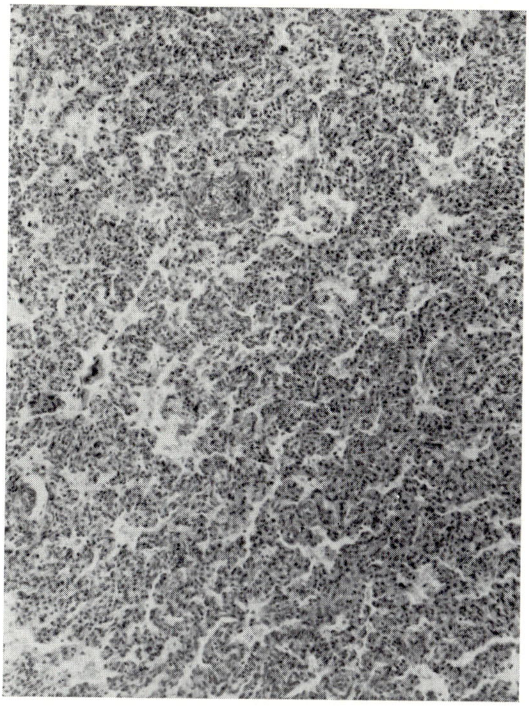

**Fig. 8.** Case 5. Photomicrograph of the left lung which shows hypoplasia. Note the poor degree of alveolar differentiation (×200; reduced ¼.)

An extralobar sequestration accompanying a congenital diaphragmatic hernia should be resected. Such a lobe can be the seat of inflammation.[6]

The routine use of a thoracic approach for the repair of congenital hernias allows easy detection of any lung anomaly. The thoracic approach has been previously advocated by Koop and Johnson.[12] These authors give as their reasons for this the immediate respiratory relief experienced by the baby on opening of the chest and relief of the intrathoracic pressure, the ease of repair of the defect, and the excellent exposure. An additional reason, in our opinion, is the high association of pulmonary malformations with these hernias. A thoracic approach affords the best opportunity for detecting and managing these abnormalities.

## SUMMARY

1. The cases of 5 patients with congenital hernias through defects in the diaphragm associated with (1) hypoplasia of the lung and (2) extralobar sequestration are reported.

2. The association of pulmonary anomalies with such congenital hernias is more common than suspected. The literature is reviewed.

3. The thoracic approach for the repair of these hernias affords an opportunity for the detection and treatment of either lung anomaly and intelligent handling of the situation in the postoperative period.

## REFERENCES

1. Baumgartner, C. J., and Scott, R. F.: Surgical emergency of diaphragmatic hernia in infancy, Arch. Surg. **61:** 170, 1950.
2. Berman, E. J.: Extralobar sequestration of the lung, A. M. A. Arch. Surg. **76:** 724, 1958.
3. Campanale, R. P., and Rowland, R. H.: Hypoplasia of the lung associated with congenital diaphragmatic hernia, Ann. Surg. **142:** 176, 1955.
4. Claman, M. A., and Ehrenhaft, J. L.: Bronchopulmonary sequestration, J. Thoracic Surg. **39:** 531, 1960.
5. Donovan, E. J.: Congenital diaphragmatic hernia, Ann. Surg. **122:** 569, 1945.
6. Freedlander, S. O., and Gebauer, P. W.: Diseases of aberrant lung tissues, J. Thoracic Surg. **8:** 581, 1939.
7. Gross, R. E.: Congenital hernia of the diaphragm, Am. J. Dis. Child. **71:** 579, 1946.
8. Gross, R. E.: Surgery of infancy and childhood, Philadelphia, 1953, W. B. Saunders Company, p. 428.
9. Guy, C. C., and Rand, G. L.: Congenital diaphragmatic hernia associated with an accessory lung, Illinois M. J. **62:** 61, 1932.
10. Harrington, S. W.: Diaphragmatic hernia of children, Ann. Surg. **115:** 705, 1942.
11. Hartzell, J. B.: Diaphragmatic hernia in children—résumé of 68 cases in children treated by operation, Am. J. Surg. **48:** 582, 1940.
12. Koop, C. E., and Johnson, J.: Transthoracic repair of diaphragmatic hernia, Ann. Surg. **136:** 1007, 1952.
13. Ladd, W. E., and Gross, R. E.: Congenital diaphragmatic hernia, New England J. Med. **223:** 917, 1940.
14. Potter, E. L.: Pathology of the fetus in the newborn, Chicago, 1952, Yearbook Publishers, Inc., p. 260.
15. Potter, E. L.: Pathology of the fetus and the newborn, Chicago, 1952, Yearbook Publishers, Inc., p. 320.
16. Neville, W. E., and Clowes, G. H. A., Jr.: Congenital absence of the hemidiaphragm

and use of a lobe of liver in its surgical correction, A. M. A. Arch. Surg. **69:** 282, 1954.
17. Pryce, D. M., Sellors, T. H., and Blair, L. G.: Intralobar sequestration of the lung associated with an abnormal pulmonary artery, Brit. J. Surg. **35:** 18, 1947.
18. Rakover, J., Milwidsky, H., and Wayl, P.: Hypoplasia of the lung in congenital diaphragmatic hernia, J. Thoracic Surg. **31:** 527, 1956.
19. Riker, W. L.: Congenital diaphragmatic hernia, A. M. A. Arch. Surg. **69:** 291, 1954.
20. Roe, B., and Stephens, H. B.: Congenital diaphragmatic hernia and hypoplastic lung, J. Thoracic Surg. **32:** 279, 1956.
21. St. Raymond, A. H., Jr., Hardy, J. D., and Robbins, S. G.: Lower accessory lung communicating with the esophagus and associated with congenital diaphragmatic hernia, J. Thoracic Surg. **31:** 354, 1956.
22. Valle, A. R., and White, M. L., Jr.: Subdiaphragmatic aberrant pulmonary tissue, Dis. Chest. **13:** 631, 1947.

# Management of recurrent or metastatic Wilms' tumor

R. T. SOPER, M.D.*
IOWA CITY, IOWA

Much has been written about Wilms' tumor since the first case was described 150 years ago.[14] The bulk of the literature concerns the primary neoplasm, its embryologic derivation, signs and symptoms, histopathologic features, treatment, and end-result studies. With improvement in the methods of diagnosis and treatment, the survival percentages have correspondingly increased. The improved mortality rate permits the survival of patients with recurrent or metastatic disease who previously would have died of the primary tumor or its therapy. This increasingly important phase of the disease has received little attention.

The 28 cases of Wilms' tumor diagnosed in the Liverpool area during the last 12 years have been reviewed. Seven of the patients had recurrent or metastatic disease which was managed with apparent success so far as eradication of the neoplasm was concerned. Although only 4 of these are long-term survivors, the principles employed for the management of metastatic Wilms' tumor might be used to draw analogies applicable to the problem in general. For these reasons, a closer scrutiny has been made of this particular fraction of the group.

## MATERIAL

The pertinent data concerning the 28 patients with histologically confirmed Wilms' tumors are recorded in Table I. The patients have all been drawn from Liverpool and its environs over the past 12 years. None of the cases has been previously reported except the 2 instances of bilateral neoplasm.[17] One of these patients has now survived 6 years free from known recurrence of the disease. Of the 9 patients who survived longer than 2 years, 4 had only the primary neoplasm and were treated for it alone. The remaining 5 patients were considered hopeless at one stage or another of the disease. Three of these are discussed at length (Cases 1, 2, and 3) and one of the others is the survivor with bilateral neoplasm alluded to previously.

In the light of the current concept that the younger the patient at diagnosis and treatment of the neoplasm, the better the prognosis, it is of interest to observe from Table I that the average age of the 2-year survivors in this series was slightly greater than that of the patients as a whole. This curious fact is not explained, except perhaps by our use of more aggressive therapeutic approach in children with recurrences than might be thought justified at other centers.

Treatment of the primary lesion, which has been largely standardized in this series, is summarized in Table II. It consists of extirpation of the neoplasm followed by deep roentgen therapy. The radiation is given during the first postoperative month to the dosage of 3,500 tumor roentgens delivered to the tumor site. In the patients treated during the past 18 months, the abdominal cavity has been irrigated with Clorpactin XCB at the conclusion of the operation, and actinomycin D has been given intravenously.

The following are the case reports of the 7 patients previously mentioned, in whom

Received for publication Jan. 3, 1961.

*Currently, Assistant Professor of Surgery, State University of Iowa College of Medicine. Formerly, Surgical Registrar to Mr. P. P. Rickham, M. S., F.R.C.S., D.C.H., Consultant Pediatric Surgeon, Alder Hey Children's Hospital, Liverpool, England.

**Table I.** *Cases of Wilms' tumor in the Liverpool area, 1948 to present*

| | |
|---|---|
| Cases | 28 |
| Location | |
| Right side | 12 |
| Left side | 14 |
| Bilateral | 2 |
| Palpable mass | 26 |
| Hematuria | |
| Gross | 5 |
| Microscopic | 9 |
| Untreated | 2 |
| Dead of neoplasm | 12 |
| Dead of other causes | 3 |
| Alive | 11 |
| 2-year survivors | 9 of 21 (42.8%) |
| Average age at diagnosis | |
| Entire series | 3 yr., 1 mo. |
| 2-year survivors | 3 yr., 5 mo. |

**Table II.** *Standard treatment of Wilms' tumor (primary)*

*Surgical*

Semiemergent, transabdominal approach, early ligature of vessels, en bloc node dissection

*Irradiation*

Begun in first postoperative week, dosage 3,500 r administered over 3 to 4 weeks

*Recent adjuncts*

Clorpactin used in surgical field and actinomycin D given intravenously, 15 mcg. per kilogram per day for 5 days

recurrent or metastatic neoplasm was successfully managed.

## CASE REPORTS

**Case 1.** L. G. was an 8-year-old boy who had undergone resection of a huge Wilms' tumor on the left side. The primary tumor measured 22 by 13 by 12 cm., and weighed 1,650 Gm. No "spill" occurred during en bloc removal of the tumor and the grossly enlarged periaortic lymph nodes. The nodes were as large as 6 cm. in diameter. On histologic examination the neoplasm was found to be anaplastic and showed venous and lymphatic invasion. The regional lymph nodes were uniformly replaced by tumor. The patient was given the routine postoperative deep roentgen therapy. He is clinically well and chest roentgenographic examination showed him to be normal 7 years later.

A technical tour de force, this case illustrates the gratifying result which meticulous en bloc dissection and irradiation can achieve even with an extremely large tumor and regional metastases. This neoplasm, highly malignant on both clinical and histologic grounds, has been eradicated and the patient apparently cured.

**Case 2.** S. S. was a 4-year-old girl who was treated for a Wilms' tumor of the left side in the previously described manner. Four months after operation a chest roentgenogram showed rounded densities in both lung fields compatible with metastatic neoplasm. These disappeared after a course of deep radiation therapy (3,000 r) administered to both lung fields. Except for mild exertional dyspnea, the patient is well 12 years after treatment. She menstruates regularly and has grossly normal secondary sex development.

The case illustrates apparent cure of widespread pulmonary metastases by irradiation alone. Patently beneficial was the careful shielding of gonadal tissue while the patient was undergoing extensive roentgen therapy to the primary tumor site.

**Case 3.** F. M. was a 6-year-old girl who underwent resection of a Wilms' tumor of the right side. The tumor was dissected away from the inferior vena cava, which was displaced medially by neoplasm. The adrenal gland and periaortic lymph nodes were removed en bloc. Postoperative routine roentgen treatment was given. Four months later a pelvic mass was palpated, and chest roentgenogram showed rounded opacities in the lower lobes of both lungs. These lesions, compatible with metastatic neoplasm, disappeared after radiation therapy (3,000 r) to lung and pelvic fields. Six months after the operation apical pulmonary tuberculosis was diagnosed by chest roentgenogram and sputum culture, and was appropriately treated. The patient remains well 6 years after diagnosis of the neoplasm.

This case demonstrates effective management of multiple metastases by radiation therapy alone. The phenomenon of tuberculosis as a sequel to pulmonary irradiation is interesting, although the two are probably not causally related.

**Case 4.** E. D. was a 5½-year-old girl who had a nephroblastoma on the left side treated by en bloc resection and postoperative radiation. Histologic examination of the surgical specimen showed venous and lymphatic invasion. The preoperative chest roentgenogram was normal, but 1 month after operation repeat films showed infiltrates in the right lower and upper lung fields. These lesions disappeared after roentgen therapy (3,500 r) to both lungs. The patient died 4 months after operation. Postmortem examination showed pulmonary edema, bronchopneumonia, and pleural effusion. There was no gross or microscopic evidence of residual neoplasm.

This case demonstrates rapid dissemination of neoplasm which was presumably related to venous invasion. Ironically, the radiation therapy which destroyed the pulmonary metastases also probably contributed to the death of the patient.

**Case 5.** P. F. was a 4-year-old girl who underwent resection of a Wilms' tumor on the left side. Postoperative roentgen therapy was administered in the routine manner. A metastasis was found in the left lung base by roentgenogram 10 months after operation which disappeared after radiation therapy (3,500 r) to the lung fields. The patient died 4 months after completion of this treatment. Postmortem examination showed bilateral pulmonary fibrosis with cor pulmonale and right-heart failure. No residual neoplasm was demonstrated by careful gross and microscopic studies.

This case again illustrates resolution of pulmonary metastases after roentgen therapy. However, the ultimate result was poor since death resulted from the cardiopulmonary changes which presumably occurred secondary to heavy pulmonary radiation.

**Case 6.** I. K. H. is a 5-year-old boy who underwent resection of a nephroblastoma on the left side at the age of 3 years. The tumor measured 18 by 11 by 8 cm., and weighed 1,080 Gm. The neoplasm had completely replaced the kidney and presented a variegated microscopic picture of anaplastic and mesenchymal elements. Routine radiation therapy was given. Eight months later chest roentgenogram showed a single "coin" lesion in the lower lobe of the right lung. In view of the noxious effects of pulmonary irradiation in the 2 previous cases, and since this metastasis appeared to be solitary, the lesion was resected. Histologic examination proved it to be a metastasis. The patient is clinically well and has no evidence of further pulmonary metastases by serial roentgenograms 20 months after resection of the lung metastasis.

This case has several interesting aspects. The primary tumor was large and presented a formidable technical problem at the time of extirpation. It contained most of the histologic variations which this pleomorphic neoplasm can assume. Finally, an apparently solitary lung metastasis was successfully managed by surgical means alone.

**Case 7.** P. P. was 7 years old when she underwent resection of a Wilms' tumor (right side) en bloc with the right renal vein, which contained a large tumor thrombus. The neoplasm had completely replaced the kidney, measured 18 by 10 by 6 cm., and on histologic examination appeared quite anaplastic. The aortic lymph nodes were microscopically free of tumor and the liver was grossly normal. Postoperatively the child was given a course of oral actinomycin D followed by the routine roentgen therapy. Ten months after operation a large epigastric mass was palpated. The patient's general condition was deteriorating. A second course of actinomycin D was administered, this time intravenously, with disappearance of the mass within 4 weeks. The patient remains well 9 months after treatment of the secondary tumor.

This case is an example of a clinically and histologically aggressive neoplasm which was effectively treated by a combination of operation, roentgen therapy, and chemotherapy. Of special interest is the response of the recurrent tumor to a second course of actinomycin D alone.

## COMMENT

Management of primary Wilms' tumor is reasonably standardized, involving surgical extirpation and irradiation of the tumor area. Differences of opinion exist regarding the order in which these modalities should be used. Gross and Neuhauser[8] and others prefer resection prior to the radiation while Flocks and Kadesky[5] and others favor the reverse order. Kinzel and associates[9] and others suggest favorable results with preoperative irradiation, nephrectomy, and postoperative irradiation. The 2-year survival rates in these series do not indicate a clear superiority of any one approach as compared to the others. Judicious selection of cases for each sequence might be entertained. Preoperative irradiation might be used for huge lesions to increase the operability rate, technically facilitate the extirpation, and perhaps reduce tumor embolism incident to operative manipulation of the neoplasm. Operation followed by irradiation might then be reserved for tumors of more modest size and when histologic diagnosis is uncertain.

The incision used may be abdominal, thoracoabdominal, or loin (Nagamatsu). It should be large enough for adequate exposure of the lesion. The choice might be influenced by such factors as the surgeon's preference, size and location of the palpable mass, and so forth. Early ligation of veins and en bloc removal of nodes extending from the undersurface of the diaphragm or liver to the bifurcation of the great vessels with sacrifice of expendable contiguous structures involved by the neoplasm are time-honored principles of cancer surgery which are applicable in these cases.

A recent technical addition to treatment

of the primary neoplasm is irrigation of the surgical field with Clorpactin XCB at the conclusion of the operation, in hope of preventing growth of spilled tumor cells.[1, 7] The period of follow-up in these cases is so short that no conclusions can be drawn regarding its effect upon the incidence of local recurrence of neoplasm. No deleterious effects have been observed other than a possible increase in wound induration and inflammation. New experimental data presented by Cole and his group[11] suggest that a buffered 0.5 per cent sodium hypochlorite solution might be safer and more effective than Clorpactin for wound irrigation.

Another recent addition has been the intravenous administration of actinomycin D, 15 mcg. per kilogram of body weight daily for 5 days, the first fraction being administered concomitantly with surgical extirpation of the primary lesion. This chemotherapeutic agent has not been used long enough for any statement to be made regarding improvement in survival rates.

The objectives of this combination of therapeutic modalities is to remove all accessible gross neoplasm, destroy viable cancer cells spilled locally during surgical manipulation, reduce the viability of neoplastic emboli and, finally, destroy residual tumor in the local and regional areas by means of radiation.

Treatment of secondary manifestations of the disease is poorly documented and standardized. There is evidence of cure of metastases after roentgen therapy alone,[3, 6, 12] a presumption which the results in Cases 2 and 3 support. However, it is apparent that this method alone is not curative in most instances. Furthermore, heavy irradiation is noxious to normal as well as neoplastic tissue. Pulmonary tissue, one of the commonest sites of metastatic Wilms' tumor,[4] is particularly susceptible to irradiation damage.[15] Such damage contributed materially to the death of 2 patients (Cases 4 and 5).

Occasionally solitary and/or localized metastases in accessible sites can be resected[10, 16] as illustrated by Case 6. Stevens[20] suggests the use of intravenous chemotherapeutic agents while metastases are being resected. If this method can protect against tumor emboli dislodged by manipulation, it might enhance the role of surgical procedures in the management of secondary nephroblastoma.

Theoretically, systemically administered chemotherapeutic agents which are effective only against autonomously growing neoplastic tissue would be the ideal approach to the treatment of recurrent or metastatic neoplasm. Such agents are not yet available. Actinomycin D is one of the newer chemotherapeutic agents which is being tested. Reports which have thus far appeared suggest that its effect on tumor is unpredictable and palliation is measured in terms of weeks even in patients who respond favorably.[13, 18] Our own experience with this agent is limited, but as Case 7 illustrates, there is promise that palliation in at least some cases of metastatic Wilms' tumor can be anticipated. The side effects of actinomycin D treatment are annoying, especially when it is combined with roentgen therapy. They include accentuation of irradiation dermatitis, pancytopenia, alopecia, and inflammation of surgical wounds. To avoid the side effects of systemic administration, the concept of isolated perfusion of the pulmonary system[2] with actinomycin D seems attractive. If the leakage factor[19] could be reduced to a reasonably low level, thereby allowing actinomycin D to be given in greater concentrations than are now considered to be safe for systemic administration, this technique would be a worthwhile adjunct to the management of metastatic Wilms' tumor.

Multiple courses of treatment with actinomycin D can be given,[21] as shown by Case 7. It is believed that progressively less tumor effect will result with successive retreatments.[18, 21]

Wilms' tumors present formidable therapeutic problems. However, the course is as unpredictable as the histologic aspect is variegated. The criteria commonly associated with short survival, such as the occurrence of hematuria, large primary tumor, extensive regional node metastases, lymphatic and/or venous invasion, histologic anaplasticity, older age of the patient, and the appearance of distant secondary lesions are not incompatible with long survival, as suggested by some of the cases discussed. Until the reasons for these inconsistencies are better understood, we must be patient and persistent in our approach to the problem and flexible in our attitude.

## SUMMARY

A review is given of 28 patients with Wilms' tumors from the Liverpool area seen during the past 12 years. The 7 cases reviewed in detail are of particular interest because of recurrent or metastatic neoplasm which was managed with some success by operation, irradiation, or chemotherapy, singly or in various combinations. Recommendations are made and discussed for treatment of primary and secondary manifestations of the disease.

I wish to express my appreciation to J. S. Fulton, Medical Director of the Liverpool Regional Radiotherapy Centre, for allowing inclusion of his cases and providing details of roentgen therapy. Also, my thanks are extended to Miss I. Forshall and Mr. P. P. Rickham, Consultant Pediatric Surgeons to Alder Hey Children's Hospital in Liverpool, for permission to use their surgical cases and their advice and assistance in the preparation of this manuscript. Finally, I am grateful to R. H. Flocks, Professor and Head of the Department of Urology, State University of Iowa College of Medicine, Iowa City, Iowa, for constructive criticism of the manuscript.

## REFERENCES

1. Bacon, H. E., and Berkley, J. W.: Refinements in prevention of recurrent carcinoma prior to and during resection of the colon and rectum: preliminary report, J. Internat. Coll. Surgeons, **30:** 539, 1958.
2. Creech, O., Krementz, E. T., Ryan, R. F., Reemtsma, K., and Winblad, J. N.: Experiences with isolation-perfusion technics in the treatment of cancer, Ann. Surg. **149:** 627, 1959.
3. Creary, C. D., and Reiner, M. P.: Wilms' tumor, Bull. Univ. Minnesota Hosp. **22:** 292, 1951.
4. Dargeon, H. W.: Tumors of childhood, New York, 1960, Paul B. Hoeber, Inc., p. 239.
5. Flocks, R. H., and Kadesky, M. C.: Malignant neoplasms of the kidney, Tr. Am. A. Genito-Urin. Surgeons **149:** 105, 1957.
6. Garrett, R. A., and Mertz, H. O.: Wilms' tumor in children, J. Urol. **70:** 684, 1953.
7. Gleidman, M., Grant, R., Rogers, C., and Karlson, K. E.: Clorpactin, a surgical adjunct, tumorcidal and antimicrobial properties, S. Forum **8:** 104, 1958.
8. Gross, R. E., and Neuhauser, E. B. D.: Treatment of mixed tumors of the kidney in childhood, Pediatrics **6:** 843, 1950.
9. Kinzel, R. E., Mills, S. D., Childs, D. S., and DeWeerd, J. H.: Wilms' tumor: a review of 47 cases, J. A. M. A. **174:** 1925, 1960.
10. Livermore, G. R.: Wilms' tumor in an adult. Discussion by Dean, A. W., and Nesbitt, R. M.: Tr. Am. A. Genito-Urin. Surgeons **44:** 18, 1952.
11. McDonald, G. O., Gines, S. M., and Cole, W. H.: Wound irrigation in cancer surgery, A. M. A. Arch. Surg. **80:** 920, 1960.
12. Ng, E., and Low-Brer, B. V. A.: Treatment of the Wilms' tumor, J. Pediat. **48:** 763, 1956.
13. Pinkel, D.: Actinomycin D in childhood cancer: a preliminary report, Pediatrics **23:** 342, 1959.
14. Rance, T. F.: A case of fungus hematoides in the kidneys, M. & Phys. J. **32:** 19, 1814.
15. Randall, A.: Advantages of pre-operative irradiation for various malignant neoplasms of the kidney, Ann. Surg. **100:** 462, 1934.
16. Richardson, W. R., *in* Cresson, S. W., and Pilling, G. P.: Renal tumors, Pediat. Clin. North America **6:** 473, 1959.
17. Rickham, P. P.: Bilateral Wilms' Tumor, Brit. J. Surg. **44:** 492, 1957.
18. Shaw, R. K., Moore, E. W., Mudler, P. S., Frei, E., and Watkin, D. M.: The effect of actinomycin D on childhood neoplasms, A. M. A. J. Dis. Child. **99:** 628, 1960.
19. Stehlin, J. S., Clarke, R. W., White, E. C., Healey, J. E., Deeney, W. C., and Beerstecher, S.: The leakage factor in regional perfusion with chemotherapeutic agents, A. M. A. Arch. Surg. **80:** 934, 1960.
20. Stevens, D.: Personal communication.
21. Tan, C. T. C., Dargeon, H. W., and Burchenal, J. H.: The effect of actinomycin D on cancer in childhood, Pediatrics **24:** 544, 1959.

# Coronary–internal mammary artery anastomosis in dogs


ROBERT J. HALL, LIEUTENANT COLONEL, MC, USA*
EDWARD M. KHOURI
DONALD E. GREGG, M.D., PH.D.
WASHINGTON, D. C.
*From the Department of Cardiorespiratory Diseases, Walter Reed Army Institute of Research*


Systemic-to-coronary artery anastomosis by various suture techniques[1, 2, 6, 8, 9] has met with only a limited degree of success in the experimental laboratory. The time required to perform suture anastomosis is such that some method of coronary perfusion is necessary to prevent ventricular fibrillation and infarction. Factors which limit successful anastomoses are the high acute surgical mortality rate and the propensity for vessels of this caliber, even in large dogs, to thrombose postoperatively. Intimal trauma, inherent in the performance of suture anastomoses, and the various techniques of coronary perfusion increase this risk of thrombosis. Carter and Roth,[4] stimulated by the success of nonsuture anastomotic techniques of Blakemore,[3] Weiss and Lam,[10] and Egdahl and Hume,[5] reported successful internal mammary–coronary artery anastomoses with polyethylene rings and a nonsuture technique. The average follow-up of their animals was 7 to 8 weeks.

This report documents the ease of the nonsuture technique and the high incidence of wide patency in a 1- to 2-year follow-up evaluation by anatomic observations and in vivo flow studies.


Presented as an exhibit at the Thirty-second Scientific Sessions of the American Heart Association, Philadelphia, Pa., Oct. 23-25, 1959.

Received for publication May 8, 1961.


*Currently Chief, Cardiology Service, Brooke General Hospital, Fort Sam Houston, Texas.

## METHOD

Thirty-three dogs, 21 mongrels and 12 greyhounds (19.9 to 36.4 kilograms average 25.2 kilograms, and 20.9 to 28.6 kilograms, average 25.5 kilograms, respectively), underwent nonsuture anastomosis of the left internal mammary artery to the circumflex branch of the left coronary artery near its origin. The anastomosis was performed under Nembutal anesthesia through a fourth left intercostal space thoracotomy, with respiration supported by a positive-pressure respirator using room air. The proximal circumflex artery was dissected from the epicardial fat for a distance of 2 cm., usually with sacrificing of 1 or 2 small descending branches. The left internal mammary artery was then dissected free and its branches tied, clamped at its origin, and transected at the level of the fourth intercostal space. Cuffs available for the anastomoses were of either nylon (for 18 dogs) or stainless steel (for 15 dogs). The cuffs had been previously machined to 4 mm. lengths, 0.15 mm. in wall thickness, and in an appropriate range of internal diameter (2.4 to 3.7 mm., average 2.9 mm.). The appropriate size for the prosthesis was chosen by micrometer measurement of both the internal mammary and circumflex arteries prior to clamping. The size selected was just larger than the external diameter of the internal mammary artery (2.0 to

3.75 mm., average 2.75 mm.) and slightly smaller than the external diameter of the circumflex artery (2.0 to 4.0 mm., average 3.2 mm.). Such snug fits did not significantly interfere with the technique. In 1 animal the diameter of the internal mammary artery at the fourth intercostal space was too small; hence, the subclavian artery was transected beyond the origin of the internal mammary artery and turned down, so that a more proximal portion of the internal mammary artery of larger diameter could be used for the anastomosis. The cut end of the internal mammary artery was then carefully everted over the cuff, with avoidance of intimal trauma, and secured with 2 circumferential fine silk ligatures (Fig. 1, *A*). The circumflex coronary artery was ligated close to its origin and the cuffed internal mammary artery was inserted into the circumflex artery distal to the ligature through an inverted T incision (Fig. 1, *B* and *C*). Flow was reestablished promptly by removal of the clamp on the internal mammary artery, which was then secured within the circumflex artery by 1 or 2 circumferential ligatures about the coronary artery, over the cuff (Fig. 1, *D*). The circumflex artery was then completely transected between the ligature and the anastomosis.

Electrocardiograms were secured preoperatively, continuously during the time of circumflex arterial occlusion, and at selected intervals postoperatively. Arteriography was performed by retrograde femoral arterial catheterization of the aorta in 8 dogs, 13 days to 5 months postoperatively. A single roentgenogram was obtained at the end of a 10 ml. hand injection of 70 per cent Diodrast near or into the ostium of the left subclavian artery.

The animals were allowed to survive 12 to 24 months before additional studies or

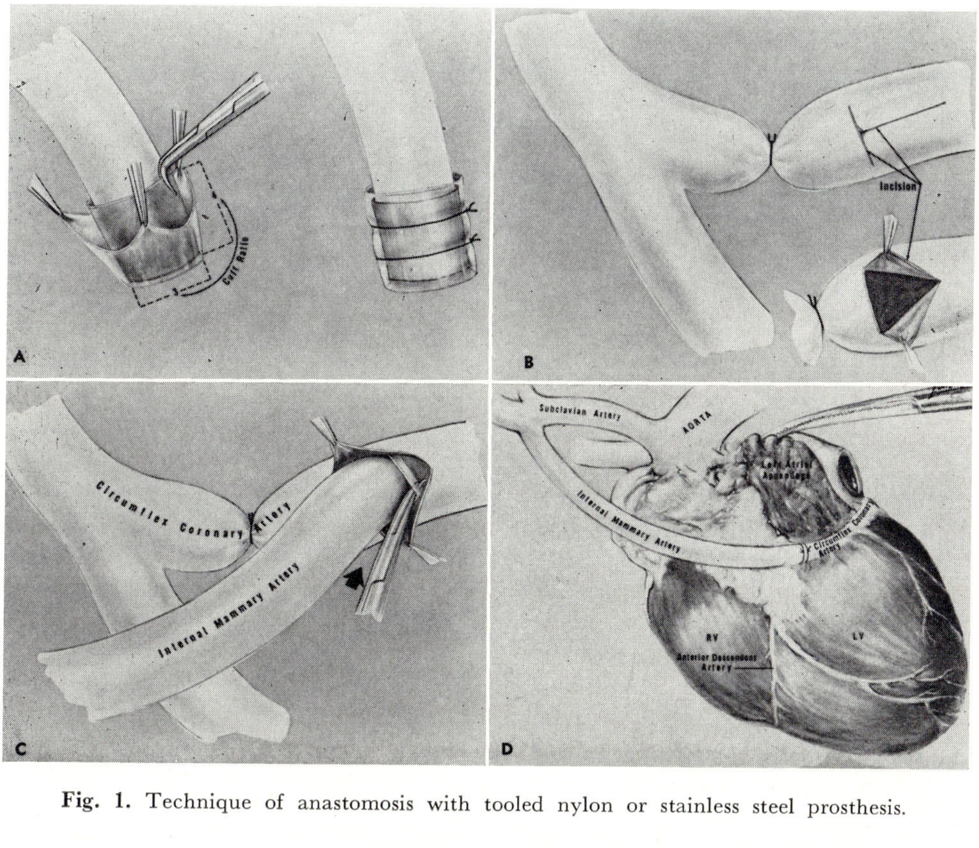


**Fig. 1.** Technique of anastomosis with tooled nylon or stainless steel prosthesis.

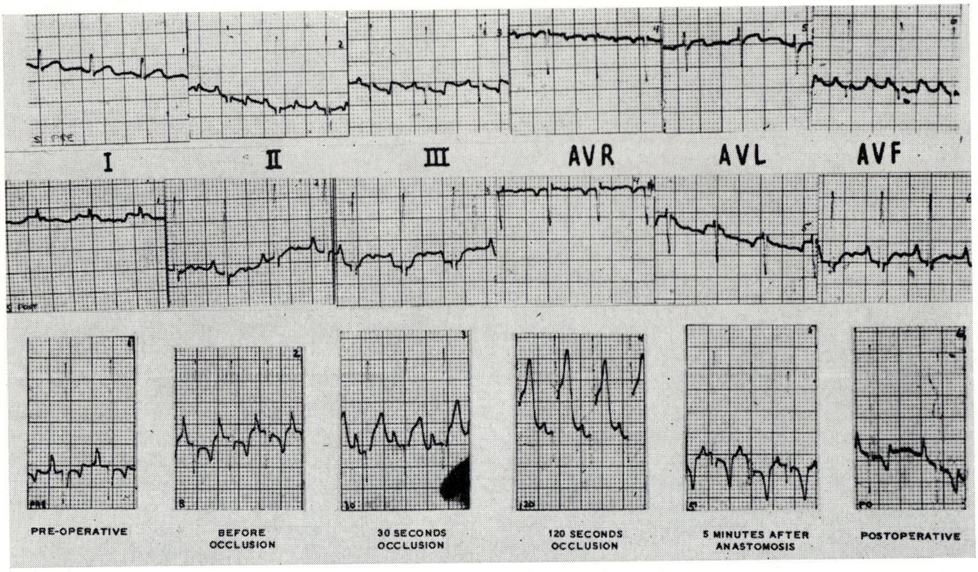


**Fig. 2.** Electrocardiogram before (top) and after (middle) anastomosis. Lead $aV_F$ (bottom) recorded continuously during period of anastomosis demonstrates marked current of injury pattern during acute occlusion of circumflex artery with prompt recovery after restoration of coronary flow.

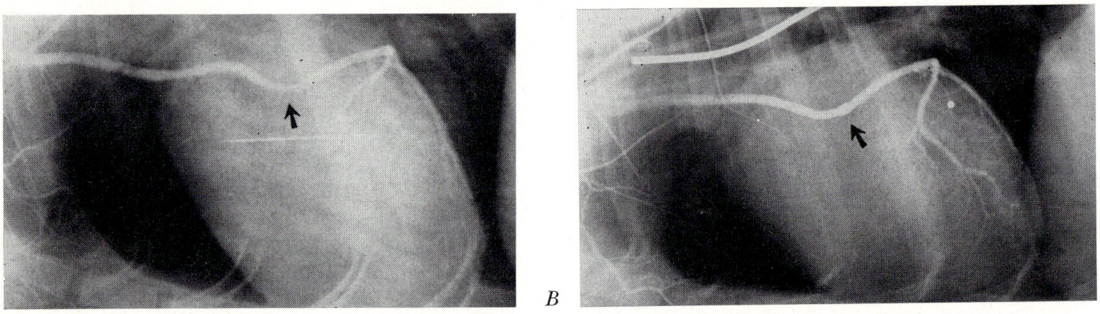

*A* *B*

**Fig. 3.** Arteriogram taken 2 weeks after anastomosis with a nylon prosthesis *(A)*, and 7 weeks after anastomosis with a stainless steel prosthesis *(B)*.

sacrifice. In vivo coronary flow studies were conducted in 14 dogs by the placement of a Kolin-type noncannulating electromagnetic flowmeter probe[7] proximal to the anastomosis on the left internal mammary artery. In 10 dogs, prior to sacrifice for anatomic studies and 13 to 17 months after construction of the anastomosis, coronary flow and central aortic pressure were recorded under Nembutal anesthesia with the chest open. Zero flow reference was repeatedly obtained by briefly clamping just beyond the probe. In the remaining 4 dogs, flow was measured daily over 2 to 4 weeks with the chest closed and the dogs in an unanesthetized state. In one of these the probe was placed about the internal mammary artery at the time of anastomosis and in the remaining 3 at the time of repeat thoracotomy 17 to 24 months after construction of the original anastomosis. Zero flow reference was secured by use of a special circumferential, nylon encapsulated, inflatable, rubber balloon placed around the internal mammary artery just distal to the flowmeter probe. This could be inflated with a known volume of fluid through a tube led externally with the flowmeter wires through a posterolateral stab wound. Postmortem studies were carried out on all dogs after death or sacrifice. The anastomoses were opened longitudinally with sharp scissors; the prosthetic cuffs were easily cut and could be flattened and slipped out of the encapsulated plane. Longitudinal sections were taken through the anastomosis for hematoxylin and eosin and elastica stains.

## RESULTS

**Occlusion time.** Construction of the anastomosis, timed from the moment of ligation of the proximal circumflex artery until flow was restored, required from 54 to 183 seconds (average 94 seconds) in 28 dogs. Ventricular fibrillation was not encountered in this group. In 5 dogs the occlusion time was 151 to 480 seconds (average 261 seconds) and in each ventricular fibrillation occurred. Ventricular fibrillation was the direct result of technical difficulties which interfered with the prompt performance of the anastomosis in 4 dogs, and occurred after onset of perfusion after 151 seconds in 1 dog. Successful defibrillation was performed in 2 animals and 1 survived with a widely patent anastomosis for 13 months.

**Electrocardiogram.** Continuous recording of lead $aV_F$ during the period of circumflex coronary arterial occlusion demonstrated various degrees of S-T and T changes consistent with acute myocardial hypoxia. These changes reverted promptly to preoperative patterns upon restoration of coronary circulation. Postoperative records of the dogs with patent anastomoses did not vary significantly from the preoperative tracings (Fig. 2).

**Arteriography.** Opacification of the internal mammary and circumflex arteries was accomplished in 8 animals. In 6, in which a radiolucent nylon cuff had been used, an excellent lumen diameter was visualized at the site of the anastomosis. Good filling of the distal circumflex artery was visualized in all 8 dogs (Fig. 3).

**Survivals.** Three dogs died at operation because of technical problems and unsuccessful anastomoses. Three died 3 to 36 hours postoperatively, 1 from separation of the anastomosis, 1 from buckling of a thin nylon cuff with thrombosis of the lumen, and 1 secondary to extensive subepicardial infarction due to repeated defibrillation. Twenty-seven dogs survived operation and the immediate postoperative period. Three of these died, 2, 3, and 13 days postoperatively from thrombosis at the anastomotic site (Table I).

Twenty-four dogs were long-term survivors with widely patent anastomoses. Three died of noncardiac causes, 7 and 10 weeks and 13 months postoperatively. Two were sacrificed in flowmeter studies 1 and 8 months postoperatively; the remaining 19 animals were sacrificed 12 to 24 months, average 15½ months, postoperatively.

**Postmortem studies.** The longitudinally opened anastomoses disclosed no thrombi or compromise of the lumen in the 24 long-term survivors (Fig. 4). The anastomoses were widely patent with occasional mild wrinkling of the intima within the prosthetic cuff which did not materially alter the lumen size. The distal coronary bed was patent in all. Small patchy areas of myo-

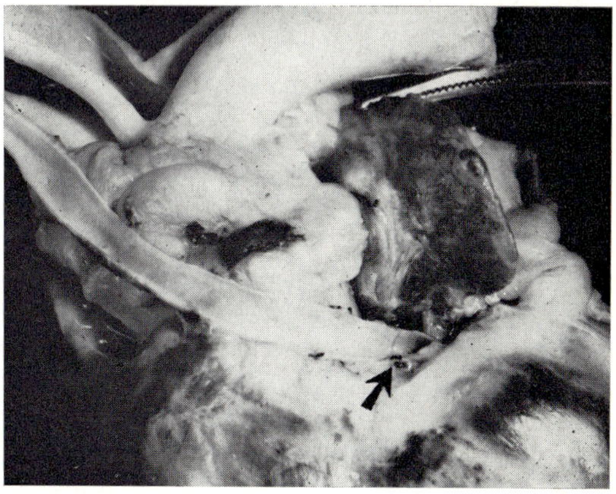

**Fig. 4.** Gross specimen from greyhound which demonstrates wide patency of anastomosis after 14 months. The left atrial appendage is retracted off the anastomosis site. The internal mammary artery has been opened longitudinally through the anastomosis into the circumflex artery.

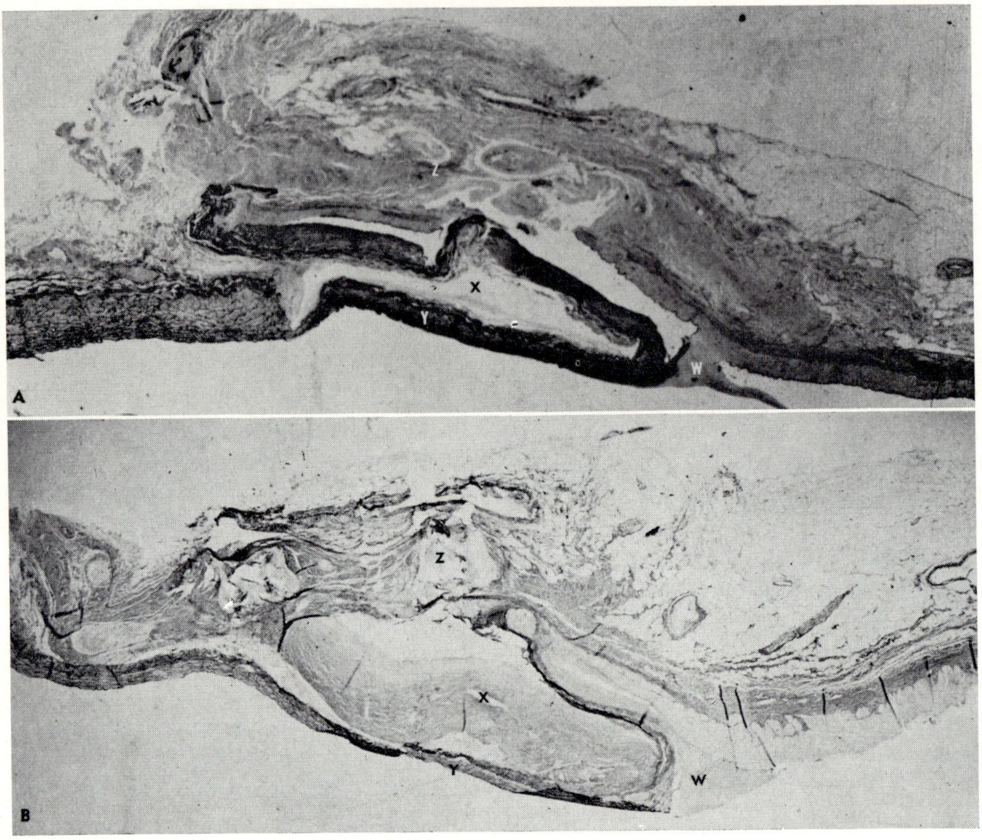


**Fig. 5.** Longitudinal sections through the internal mammary (left)–circumflex coronary (right) anastomosis. *A,* Nylon prostheses 13 months postoperatively. *B,* Stainless steel prosthesis 13½ months postoperatively. The vessel lumen is at the bottom. The fibrocollagenous wedge at the juncture of the 2 vessels is noted (*W*). Heavy fibrous reaction is seen at the site of the prosthesis (*X*) when stainless steel is used. There is thinning and compression of the elastic lamellae beneath the prosthesis (*Y*), and perivascular foreign-body reaction (*Z*) due to the circumferential ligatures. (Elastic stain; ×23; reduced 4/9.)

cardial fibrosis were seen in a few dogs in the area of distribution of the small coronary branches sacrificed in the circumflex artery dissection.

**Histologic studies.** The intima was well preserved in all chronic survivors, although in some, thinning and compression of the elastic lamellae of the internal mammary artery due to compression of an expansile vessel against the prosthesis was noted. Varying degrees of proliferative fibrous reaction were present about the prosthesis and were more intense in animals in which a steel cuff had been used. At the junction of the internal mammary and circumflex arteries, a small fibrocollagenous wedge was noted, probably secondary to organization of localized fibrin deposits at the site of juncture of the 2 vessels. This did not project into the lumen, but apparently served to smooth out the lumen at the anastomosis. This location appeared to be the site of intravascular thrombosis in the 3 animals which died of occlusion of the anastomosis in the first 2 weeks postoperatively. In one of these, a distinct circumferential thrombus formation which occluded the lumen, with origin at this junction, could be noted. Sections of the myocardium disclosed no abnormalities (Fig. 5).

**Table I.** *Survival and patency data (33 dogs)*

| | |
|---|---|
| Technical errors | |
| Died at operation (ventricular fibrillation) | 3 |
| Died 3 to 36 hr. postoperatively | 3 |
| Survived operation and immediate postoperative period | 27 |
| Died of thrombosis at anastomosis 2, 3, and 13 days postoperatively | 3 |
| Long-term survivors with patent anastomoses | 24 |
| Died of other causes 7 and 10 wk. and 13 mo. postoperatively | 3 |
| Sacrificed in flowmeter studies, 1 and 8 mo. postoperatively | 2 |
| Sacrificed 12 to 24 mo. postoperatively (average 15½ mo.) | 19 |
| Anastomoses patent by | |
| Gross observation | 24 |
| Angiography | 8 |
| Electromagnetic flowmeter data | 14 |

**Coronary flow studies.** Measurements of blood flow through the anastomosis were obtained in 14 dogs (Fig. 6). Flows of 31 to 118 ml. per minute (average 68 ml. per minute) were recorded at mean aortic pressures of 100 to 150 mm. Hg. Blood flow was again measured during the period of reactive hyperemia which immediately followed brief (8 to 15 seconds) total occlusion of the internal mammary artery. During this period peak flows of 69 to 259 ml. per minute (average 154 ml. per minute) were recorded at essentially unchanged aortic blood pressures. This represented a 1.9- to 5-fold (average 2.3-fold) increase over the control measurements. Long-term flow measurements, carried out in 4 unanesthetized animals with the chest closed were terminated in 2 to 4 weeks because of a gradual decrease to cessation of measured coronary flow. Autopsy showed a thickening of the vessel wall and thrombosis under the occlusive rubber cuff which resulted in vessel closure. Flow determination in the short- and long-term observations are tabulated in Table II.

## DISCUSSION

For a number of years surgical efforts have been directed at improving small-vessel anastomoses, especially in the coronary system, where other methods of myocardial revascularization are indirect. Systemic-to-coronary artery suture anastomoses have met with restricted success because of the significant surgical mortality rate and the high incidence of thrombotic occlusion secondary to intimal trauma. Current microsuture techniques may circumvent some of these difficulties by making possible more exacting anastomoses and consequent reduction of intimal trauma. Nonetheless, such methods remain tedious and time-consuming and, hence, continue to require a concomitant supply of oxygen-

**Table II.** *Circumflex coronary artery flow data*

| Dog. No. | Flow control | Hyperemia, peak (ml./min.) | Mean blood pressure | Heart weight (Gm.) |
|---|---|---|---|---|
| *Short-term, chest open, dog anesthetized* | | | | |
| 4 | 105 | – | 100 | 369 |
| 16 | 34 | 105 | 110 | 230 |
| 21 | 87 | 259 | 125 | 290 |
| 22 | 57 | 133 | – | – |
| 23 | 84 | 258 | 125 | 232 |
| 24 | 35 | 129 | 100 | 200 |
| 25 | 118 | 256 | 135 | 250 |
| 26 | 100 | 191 | 125 | 217 |
| 28 | 31 | 160 | 150 | 281 |
| 30 | 55 | 136 | 120 | 328 |
| *Long-term, chest closed, dog unanesthetized* | | | | |
| 1 | 42-62 | 92-124 | – | – |
| 13 | 69 | 150 | – | 285 |
| 31 | 30-41 | 69-97 | – | – |
| 33 | 52-76 | 200-232 | – | – |

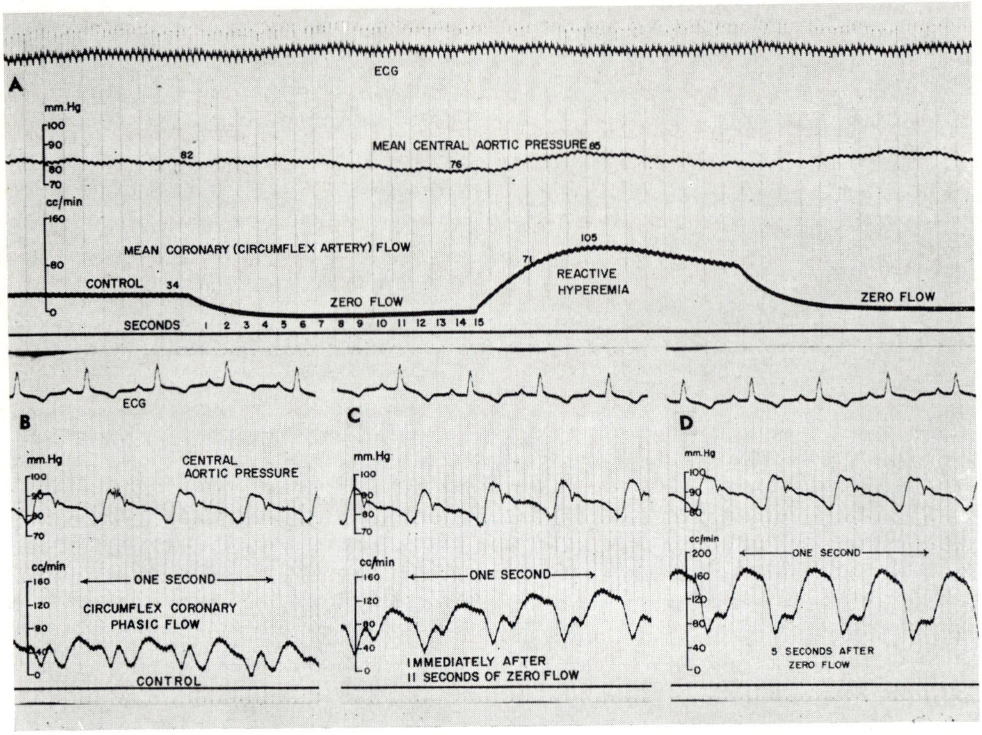


**Fig. 6.** Open-chest coronary flow measurements with an electromagnetic flowmeter 13 months after anastomosis. The perfused myocardium (Evans blue dye) weighed 55 grams. In *A*, marked reactive hyperemia is seen after brief total occlusion (mean flow). *B*, *C*, and *D* demonstrate phasic coronary flow before, immediately after, and 5 seconds after brief occlusion. *D* is during peak reactive hyperemia. The time lines are at 0.04 second intervals. Note the major flow increase during both systole and diastole. The phasic coronary flow curve is delayed slightly because of the considerably lengthened blood flow path through the internal mammary anastomosis.

ated blood to the myocardium or depression of myocardial function. A nonsuture technique is reported which combines ease and rapidity of performance and thus eliminates the need for myocardial perfusion. This, together with minimal vascular handling and intimal trauma, greatly reduces the incidence of intraluminal thrombosis. The presence of an inert prosthesis for up to a 2-year period, with surrounding mild proliferative changes, has not appeared to compromise the lumen orifice or flow through the anastomosis. In this series thrombotic occlusions at the site of the anastomosis have not occurred after the first 13 postoperative days. Widely patent anastomoses were demonstrated grossly in all long-term survivors, and electromagnetic flow studies supported the functional patency in 14 unselected animals prior to sacrifice up to 2 years after operation. Since compensatory dilatation of the coronary arteriolar bed is the first response to proximal occlusive changes in the major coronary system, the observation of striking augmentation of flow through the anastomosis during the period of reactive hyperemia is interpreted as further evidence of persistence of peripheral arteriolar tone and of wide functional patency at the anastomoses.

## SUMMARY

Nonsuture anastomosis of the internal mammary and circumflex coronary arteries is reported with observations for up to 2 years postoperatively. Twenty-four dogs, 90 per cent of those surviving operation and the immediate postoperative period, had widely patent anastomoses. Patency was confirmed by direct measurement of flow through the anastomosis by means of an electromagnetic flowmeter, by observation of significant flow augmentation during the period of reactive hyperemia after brief total occlusion, and by gross and histologic studies.

## ADDENDUM

Since preparation of this manuscript, Goetz and associates (Internal mammary–coronary anastomosis. A non-suture method employing tantalum rings, J. Thoracic Surg. 41: 378, 1961) have reported success with a similar technique. They report patency in 8 of 9 anastomoses performed in 7 dogs. Of these 7 animals, 3 were sacrificed after 6 months and the remaining 4 were alive 7 to 20 months after operation.

### REFERENCES

1. Absolon, K. B., Aust, J. B., Varco, R. L., and Lillehei, C. W.: Surgical treatment of occlusive coronary artery disease by endarterectomy or anastomotic replacement, Surg. Gynec. & Obst. **103:** 108, 1956.
2. Baker, N. H., and Grindley, J. H.: Technic of experimental systemic-to-coronary artery anastomosis, Proc. Staff Meet. Mayo Clin. **34:** 497, 1959.
3. Blakemore, A. H., and Lord, J. W.: A nonsuture method of blood vessel anastomosis: experimental and clinical study, J. A. M. A. **127:** 685, 748, 1945.
4. Carter, E. L., and Roth, E. J.: Direct nonsuture coronary artery anastomosis in the dog, U.S. Nav. Med. Res. Inst. Res. Rep. **15:** 535, 1957.
5. Egdahl, R. H., and Hume, D. M.: Nonsuture blood vessel anastomosis, A. M. A. Arch. Surg. **72:** 232, 1956.
6. Julian, O. C., Lopez-Belio, M., and Moorehead, D.: Direct surgical procedures on the coronary arteries: experimental studies, J. Thoracic Surg. **34:** 654, 1957.
7. Kolin, A., Assali, N., Herrold, G., and Jensen, R.: Electromagnetic determination of regional blood flow in unanesthetized animals, Proc. Nat. Acad. Sc. **43:** 527, 1957.
8. Moore, T. C., and Riberi, A.: Maintenance of coronary circulation during systemic-to-coronary artery anastomosis, SURGERY **43:** 245, 1958.
9. Thal, A., Perry, J. F., Miller, F. A., and Wangensteen, O. H.: Direct suture anastomosis of the coronary arteries in the dog, SURGERY **40:** 1023, 1956.
10. Weiss, E. W., and Lam, C. R.: Tantalum tubes in the nonsuture method of blood vessel anastomosis, Am. J. Surg. **80:** 452, 1950.

# Cancer risk in ulcerative colitis: formidability per patient-year of late disease

CLARENCE DENNIS, M.D.
KARL E. KARLSON, M.D.
BROOKLYN, N. Y.
*From the Department of Surgery, State University of New York Downstate Medical Center*

In 1952 we reported a series of 267 patients with idiopathic ulcerative colitis studied at the University of Minnesota Hospitals and at the Minneapolis General Hospital.[4] In this series of patients, there were 16 who up to that time had developed cancer in the large bowel, a patient incidence of 6 per cent. Four of these patients had been found to have a segmental area of colitis proximal to an obstructing carcinoma. A fifth had developed carcinoma in the stalk of one of several large polyps in the colon 3 years after the onset of colitis. The presence of colitis was regarded as incidental in these 5 cases. With the elimination of these 5 cancers, the incidence of carcinoma was 4.2 per cent. In view of the rather widely divergent opinions to be found in the literature concerning the risk of cancer development in colitis, and since we have found no other reports of an over-all incidence as high as ours is at present, an additional report on this group of patients appears appropriate.

We have endeavored to bring the follow-up on this group of patients up to date by interviews and examinations during the summer of 1957 and by correspondence since that time. Addition of 3 patients overlooked in the original study brings the total to 270. One of these, however, we have omitted from the present study because follow-up was inadequate, and we believed she would not have been found had she not died of carcinoma of the colon while under the care of a physician who knew of our interest in the problem.

Our over-all data concerning cancer development in these 269 patients are presented in Table I. The over-all patient incidence of cancer in this study was 7.4 per cent. One patient developed rectal cancer late after colectomy for colic cancer; the cancer incidence is therefore slightly higher than the patient incidence—7.8 per cent. If one excludes the 5 cases in which the tumors are considered not to be secondary to colitis, these figures are 5.7 per cent and 6.0 per cent.

Two factors had led us to re-evaluate our data rather than simply to present the figures of Table I. The first was the possibility of inaccuracy of the estimate of incidence of cancer in this group secondary to inclusion of patients who first came for attention because of appearance of cancer of the large bowel, rather than because of the presence of idiopathic ulcerative colitis without such complication. Our second reason was our failure to find in the literature any data concerning the annual cancer risk of the patient with late colitis who continues to carry all or part of the large intestine.

Four patients in this review had already developed cancer as a complication of colitis at the time they were first seen by us. These 4 patients had histories of colitis for 22 years, 15 years, 12 years, and 30 years, respectively, before they were seen. How to

Received for publication Feb. 10, 1961.

correct our figures for this distortion is not entirely clear.

It appeared more useful to determine the time of earliest appearance of cancer in this group of patients, and the annual incidence of this complication after that time. In regard to time of onset of cancer, the series contains no instance of carcinoma secondary to colitis which appeared within 10 years of the onset of colitis.

In the determination of the actual cancer incidence in patients who carried the large intestine or part of it for longer than 10 years after the onset of colitis, 2 criteria for inclusion of cases were observed. We confined our attention (1) to patients who were under observation at the University of Minnesota Hospitals or Minneapolis General Hospital at the time of the tenth anniversary of the onset of colitis, but who had no evidence of cancer of the large bowel at that time, and (2) to patients who first came to one of these clinics after the tenth anniversary of the onset of colitis without evidence of cancer at that first visit. The period of observation might be terminated by (1) death of the patient, (2) loss of the patient to follow-up, (3) development of cancer in the large bowel, or (4) removal of the colon or rectum, or both, as the case might be.

Findings are shown in Tables II and III.

## COMMENT

The figure of greatest note is the development of some 4 cancers per 100 patient-years of observation in colitis in which the whole large bowel was retained after the tenth anniversary of the onset of disease. This figure (4 per cent per year) is higher than the risk of proctocolectomy and ileostomy in the present series (under 2 per cent).[4] The risk of rectal cancer appears to be smaller than that of colon cancer, but even so it is consequential, especially in view of absence of death in the proctectomies performed after colectomy had been performed[4] and in view of retention of sexual function in 100 per cent of patients in whom the conservative proctectomy indicated in the absence of carcinoma was performed.

In our previous paper, we indicated that the risk of ileoproctostomy after colectomy is greater than the risk of proctocolectomy with ileostomy, and that the likelihood of satisfactory function after such anastomoses is less than 50 per cent. The fact that 4 of the 5 rectal cancers which we observed to develop led rapidly to the death of the patient suggests to us that the 1 per cent per annum incidence and the high fatality of cancer when it does develop in the rectum in ulcerative colitis should indicate removal of the rectum in the first place.

The decision as to what duration of chronic idiopathic ulcerative colitis should dictate proctocolectomy is difficult to make.

**Table I.** *Cancers associated with idiopathic ulcerative colitis*

| | *No.* |
|---|---|
| Ulcerative colitis cases observed | 270 |
| Patients with associated large bowel cancer | 21 |
| Case omitted for failure of follow-up | 1 |
| Cancer of rectum over 1 year after colectomy for colitis with obstructing cancer of cecum | 1 |
| Total primary cancers considered | 21 |
| Cancers primary in colon | 16 |
| Cancers primary in rectum | |
| Precolectomy | 2 |
| Postcolectomy | 3 |
| Cancers present upon first examination of patient | 4 |
| Cancers not secondary to colitis (?) | 5 |
| Surviving cancer patients* | 2 |

*Both survivors refused proctocolectomy which had been advised years before the diagnosis of cancer as a complication had been established. One had an obstructing cancer of the cecum treated by emergency colectomy, and then refused proctectomy until symptoms of a cancer there had appeared. She is well more than 5 years after proctectomy. The other has survived more than 2 years after removal of colon in which cancer was found.

**Table II.** *Cancers seen to develop in patients under observation for idiopathic ulcerative colitis*

| | |
|---|---|
| Under 10 years of ulcerative colitis | 0 cases |
| Over 10 years of ulcerative colitis | 12 cases |
| Average duration of colitis | 16 yr. |
| Average patient age at diagnosis of cancer | 35 yr. |

**Table III.** *Large bowel carcinomas which appeared in patients under observation for idiopathic ulcerative colitis*

| | *Colon or rectum without colectomy or proctectomy* | *Colon alone* | *Rectum, combined (pre- and post-colectomy)* | *Rectum after colectomy* |
|---|---|---|---|---|
| No. of patients followed | 60 | 60 | 97 | 54 |
| No. of cancers to appear | 9 | 7 | 5 | 3* |
| Patient incidence of cancer | 15% | 11.7% | 5.2% | 5.6% |
| Patient-years of observation | 218 | 216 | 443 | 229 |
| Mean duration of observation | 3.6 yr. | 3.6 yr. | 4.6 yr. | 4.2 yr. |
| Cancers per patient-year | 4.1% | 3.2% | 1.1% | 1.3% |

*Two of the rectal cancers to appear after colectomy were diagnosed in patients who had undergone ileoproctostomy (out of a total of 42 ileoproctostomies).

Several authors have presented reports of cases in which carcinomatous degeneration secondary to ulcerative colitis developed 3 to 4 years after onset of the colitis.[1, 2, 8] The rarity of such reports suggests that the risk of this complication this early in the course of idiopathic ulcerative colitis is much less than after the 10 years. As in 1952, our present data suggest that the rate of cancer occurrence rises as the years pass after the tenth anniversary of the onset of colitis. The numbers are too small for conclusive decision on this point, however. Certainly, at 10 years after onset of colitis, the risk of cancer development is already very high.[3, 5-7] It has been our policy to recommend proctocolectomy in unsatisfactorily controlled idiopathic ulcerative colitis of 3 or 4 years' duration or in the presence of advancing fibrosis which might mask the diagnosis of carcinoma by roentgen study.

A most dangerous pitfall is to judge the status of the colitis by the general apparent well-being of the patient. A healthy-looking patient all too often harbors a colon and rectum in which advanced proctocolitis or perhaps even cancer is present. Critical proctosigmoidoscopy and barium enema roentgen examination at regular intervals (no more than 6 months) are essential to conscientious care of colitic patients who retain the colon and rectum or the rectum alone. Seventeen years ago, one of the present series, a robust girl of 19 years, asked and was permitted to attend a high school dance within 6 weeks of her death from unsuspected carcinomatosis arising in the colon. Known colitis had been present for 14 years. In the light of present knowledge, this sort of tragedy is clearly avoidable.

The deplorable survival rates after vigorous therapy for cancers developing in patients under observation for idiopathic ulcerative colitis, in addition to the high incidence of cancer in colitis, dictate that our only effective therapy of this common complication is prophylactic removal of the large bowel in all cases in which colitic deformity persists beyond 3 to 4 years.

## CONCLUSIONS

1. The group of 267 patients with idiopathic ulcerative colitis reported in 1952 to have 16 large bowel cancers has been followed further. Four more cancers have been found. A fifth is omitted for statistical reasons. The over-all patient incidence of cancer complicating colitis is 7.4 per cent in this series.

2. Prolonged observation is reported in a series of 98 patients with idiopathic ulcerative colitis beyond the tenth anniversary of onset of the disease in whom there was no evidence of cancer at the start of the observation period.

3. In 60 of these patients with colons and rectums in situ and followed for a total of 218 patient-years, the incidence of cancer development was 4 per cent per year.

4. In 54 of these patients, colectomies had been performed, but the rectums had been retained. In a total of 229 patient-years of

observation, the incidence of cancer development in these rectums was 1 per cent per year.

5. We can report only 1 long-term and 1 short-term survival in the 15 patients with large bowel cancer secondary to ulcerative colitis.

6. After the tenth anniversary of the onset of disease, the patient with idiopathic ulcerative colitis bears an annual risk of cancer development of a magnitude approximately equal to that of proctocolectomy in good hands, quite apart from the other hazards of the late disease.[4] After this procedure, his outlook for survival is equivalent to that of persons of similar age without history of colitis.[4]

7. Competent care of the patient with idiopathic ulcerative colitis requires examination of the large intestine at least every 6 months. The risk of cancer is so high that removal of the colon, and preferably of the rectum also, should be performed if the bowel fails to revert to virtually normal flexibility and mucosal appearance within 3 to 4 years of onset of colitis.

The authors wish to express their thanks to Dr. O. H. Wangensteen, Surgeon-in-Chief, to Mr. Ray Amberg, Superintendent, of the University of Minnesota Hospitals, and to Dr. Claude Hitchcock, Chief of Surgery, Minneapolis General Hospital, for permission and facilities to follow and to re-examine these patients.

## REFERENCES

1. Bacon, H. E., and Trimpi, H. D.: Surgical management of ulcerative colitis, J. A. M. A. **153:** 1249, 1953.
2. Bargen, J. A., Sauer, W. G., Sloan, W. P., and Gage, R. P.: The development of cancer in chronic ulcerative colitis, Gastroenterology **26:** 32, 1954.
3. Counsell, P. B., and Dukes, C. E.: The association of chronic ulcerative colitis and carcinoma of the rectum and colon, Brit. J. Surg. **39:** 485, 1952.
4. Dennis, C., and Karlson, K. E.: Surgical measures as supplements to the management of idiopathic ulcerative colitis; cancer, cirrhosis, and arthritis as frequent complications, SURGERY **32:** 892, 1952.
5. Lyons, A. S., and Garlock, J. H.: Relationship of chronic ulcerative colitis to carcinoma, Gastroenterology **18:** 170, 1951.
6. MacDougall, I. P. M.: Ulcerative colitis and carcinoma of the intestine, Brit. M. J. **1:** 852, 1954.
7. Shands, W. C., Dockerty, M. B., and Bargen, J. A.: Adenocarcinoma of the large intestine associated with chronic ulcerative colitis, Surg. Gynec. & Obst. **94:** 302, 1952.
8. Weckesser, E. C., and Chinn, A. B.: Carcinoma of the colon complicating chronic ulcerative colitis, J. A. M. A. **152:** 905, 1953.

# Surgical history

*Conducted by* JOHN R. PAINE, M.D.

# Antyllus, the elusive surgical genius of antiquity: an analysis of his writings

RICHARD L. GRANT, M.D.
PARK FOREST, ILL.

In the study of historical figures there is occasionally encountered an enigma—an author who is afforded a great reputation, but about whom, personally, nothing is known. Just such a phantom is Antyllus, a physician and surgeon of the Graeco-Roman period whose medical and surgical writings have been known and acclaimed in almost every age. The presentation of his surgical writings will be the primary purpose of this paper. However, in spite of his wide popularity in the medical world, few facts have been uncovered concerning his life. Even the exact time in which he lived has been a subject of controversy among medical historians, although most authorities believe it to have been the early part of the second century.

Despite the dearth of information about his life, some insight into his personality can be gleaned from his writings. Although these are far from autobiographic, they do convey a considered judgment and boldness tempered with caution—principles which surely guided his life as well as his practice of medicine. Additional light may be shed on this evasive shade, Antyllus, by a consideration of the wealth of information available on the study and practice of medicine in his day. It is hoped that the speculations made from a study of this material may coincide with the unrevealed career of Antyllus.

Supported by a grant from the United States Public Health Service, National Institute of Mental Health.

## ANTYLLUS AND THE PRACTICE OF MEDICINE DURING THE ROMAN EMPIRE

The first physicians in Rome were Greek slaves, and medicine was held by the Romans to be an ignoble profession to which no free man would devote himself. Gradually, however, a change occurred principally as a result of the increased respectability and intelligence of the more recent immigrant Greek physicians. In 46 B.C. Caesar granted citizenship to physicians, and by the time of the Roman emperors Trajan (A.D. 98 to 117) and Hadrian (A.D. 117 to 138), when Antyllus probably lived, the physicians had achieved considerable social stature. They were well paid and enjoyed all the privileges and prerogatives of the Roman citizenry. They were a class unto themselves, protected by law, and accorded special guarantees by the state. If Antyllus had been as successful a physician as the character of his works leads us to assume, he undoubtedly would also have been a recipient of these special privileges and thus his life would probably have been a comfortable one.

To understand the character and knowledge of the physicians of Antyllus' day, it must be understood that long before the separation of medicine into the many specialties with which we are acquainted, good medicine was usually practiced by men with broad interests and a liberal education in the art of healing. Medicine, surgery, dietetics, pharmacy, and hygiene were indispensable parts of the whole of the practice of medicine. Men trained in all these fields abounded in the early Christian Era and are typified by the famous Galen (A.D. 133 to 200) and many others whose works are preserved in the comprehensive compilations of Oribasius (A.D. 325 to 403) and Paulus of Aegina (seventh century), 2 Byzantine physicians whose main contribution to medicine was the preservation of previous medical thought.

If the methods of treatment of these Graeco-Roman physicians sometimes seem strange and their theories of disease sometimes fallacious, it must not be ascribed to lack of intelligence or ability. Their capacity to practice medicine, so meagerly equipped with the scientific tools that appear indispensable today, is a tribute to their ability. Indeed, when one considers the lack of technical knowledge and the general level of scientific advancement of their time, these men stand out as amazingly resourceful and intelligent.

How most of these renowned physicians of antiquity obtained their training is well known, but so far as Antyllus is concerned, we can only speculate. Because of the considerable influence of previous thought discernible in his writings and because of the impact of his works on subsequent authors, it is possible that he resided in Rome, or at least lived part of his life there. He probably attended one of the many medical schools on the shores of the Mediterranean, such as Alexandria, Smyrna, Rome, Athens, or Marseilles, although definitive proof of this has yet to be discovered. Perhaps he obtained his wide experience during a tenure in one of the larger cities as public physician—an appointment which would have been earned by him for his unusual ability and great resourcefulness—or perhaps as a court physician. He may have obtained his surgical training while serving as an army physician or even as doctor for the gladiators at a gymnasium or at the arena. The latter position offered some of the best opportunities for the practice of surgical techniques and the observation of human anatomy during a time when human dissection was not practiced.

Another subject for speculation is Antyllus' nationality. It is assumed that he was a Greek, for his writings are composed in that language. Almost all of the physicians of the Roman period, including Galen, were Greek and, indeed, in the history of medicine, this period is more rightly called the Graeco-Roman period because all of medicine had its roots in Greek medical thought. Despite Rome's many contributions in other fields such as architecture, warfare, law, and politics, its medicine consisted almost exclusively of the amplification and promulgation of previous Greek thought by foreigners, mainly Greeks.

During the Graeco-Roman period there were several schools of medical philosophy, each of which held to a different idea of the causation of disease. This accounts for the diversity of treatments for the same disease which were recommended by the adherents of the several schools. By Antyllus' time there had developed an eclectic medical philosophy which drew from the other schools only principles and ideas which seemed effective and useful. Most of the unpractical theory was discarded. From the available evidence it can be concluded that Antyllus almost certainly belonged to this Eclectic School and sagaciously blended the theories of the other schools into a reasonable and practical whole. All of the theories and principles which were then so heatedly debated have long since been discarded because science has answered the questions upon which the ancients were forced to theorize. In the context of the times, however, physicians who practiced medicine in an eclectic fashion were the most progressive and contributed the most to the evolution of medical thought.

Because of the intelligence and insight of Antyllus and men like him, it was in surgery, rather than in other fields, that great progress was made during the Graeco-Roman period. Beyond this early surgical art, major improvements and innovations were not made until the advent of anesthesia and antisepsis. In fact, for more than a thousand years after the decline of Graeco-Roman medicine, much of the practice of surgery fell into disuse and ill-repute and was far below the level at which it was practiced by the physicians of the Roman Empire. One of the chief reasons for this high level of surgical practice in antiquity, with its more rational approach to treatment, is that in surgery, in contrast to medicine, the theories which contributed so much to deflecting medicine from paths of progress, did not play so large a part. The more purely technical nature of surgery with its clearly obvious results created a situation in which the usefulness and practicality of a procedure were highly prized and more easily obtained. Antyllus and the other physicians of the times, who adhered to a similar philosophy, were free to a greater extent to depend upon and learn from observation and study. They had to contend less with rigorously formal thought while attempting to analyze and categorize their ideas and findings and put them into use. It is this freedom of thought, as well as a large measure of skill, which made Antyllus' surgical works of such value to later physicians and created for him a reputation as a resourceful and experienced surgeon.

## THOUGHTS ON THE SURGICAL WRITINGS OF ANTYLLUS

Almost as elusive as Antyllus, the man, is Antyllus, the surgical author. So far as is known, none of his original writings has survived. It is fairly certain that the Byzantine encyclopedists, Oribasius (fourth century) and Paulus of Aegina (seventh century), and perhaps even the Arabian physicians, Rhazes (tenth century) and Avicenna (eleventh century), had direct access to his writings. After this time, however, no author quotes directly from any of Antyllus' works. All subsequent commentators were forced to use the writings of these four as the main sources for the study of Antyllus' thought.

The most inclusive source is the compilation by Oribasius. The translation by Bussemaker and Daremberg[3] of the Greek text of Oribasius was used for this paper, supplemented by selected parts of the writings of Antyllus found in Paulus of Aegina, as translated by Francis Adams.[5]

From the fragments available it seems that Antyllus wrote at least 2 major treatises, the first mainly concerned with medicine and the second with surgery; and although Antyllus is best known for his surgical works, his writing on other aspects of medicine show the same careful approach based on wide experience that is apparent from the surgical chapters. It is hoped that a brief outline of some of his chapters on surgery will be sufficient to demonstrate the ability and intelligence of this sage clinician. The medical works of Antyllus have been discussed in a previous paper[2] and with the exception of several methods of treatment which are actually surgical in nature, such as venesection, they will not be mentioned. Unfortunately, it would require a full reproduction of Antyllus' surgical works to do complete justice to the thoroughness and remarkable clarity with which he treats his subjects. Every page manifests the wide experience and cautious but sure judgment which served as the basis for Sir William Osler's designation of Antyllus as one of the most daring and accomplished surgeons of all time.

Most of the physicians of Antyllus' time were not specialists; they wrote on all medical subjects. Antyllus' writings, by the standards of the time, however, do not appear to be complete and by comparing them with works of other physicians of his time which have come down to us in more complete and perhaps original form, one notes wide gaps in Antyllus' subject matter. There are no specific sections on gynecology or obstetrics, dermatology, fevers, trauma, anatomy, pathology, physiology, or mental or nervous diseases, although some of these subjects are mentioned in the chapters which treat of other matters. The most likely explanation for this hiatus may be that these works were lost very early and were not included in the fragments which were available to the compilers. In view of the thoroughness with which Antyllus treats his various subjects in the chapters to which we have access, it is unlikely that he neglected to write on the topics mentioned.

## ANTYLLUS' SURGERY

For nearly 2 millennia, venesection was one of the most frequent surgical procedures. It is interesting, therefore, to note the extent of thought given and caution exercised in this important operation. Antyllus begins his section on bleeding by venesection with a detailed description of the proper vessels to be opened in different parts of the body. He cautions against thrombosis of a vessel and against incising blindly for a vessel when one is not apparent. He knowingly advises the use of a tourniquet above the site of incision on an extremity because he recognized that "never, on any part, will the band (tourniquet) cause the swelling (distention) of a vessel when it is placed below it."

One entire chapter is devoted to instructions for the actual cutting of the vein. In this he says:

> Bleeding is done, sometimes by thrusting the instrument, sometimes by raising it; by thrusting it, when the vessels are not apparent and raising it when they are very near the surface. It is not necessary to divide the vessel completely, for, in that case, the two ends retract and the blood does not jet out. . . .

Antyllus' knowledge of wound healing, in relation to the type of incision, is demonstrated in the chapters discussing the proper time for the incision and its proper size and form.

> We use the transverse incision, when we have no intention of repeating the bleeding, because once the arm is bent, the wound adheres quickly. The oblique incision is suitable when it is desired to repeat the bleeding, for during the flexion of the arm, the lips of the wound do not touch each other exactly. The straight incision (longitudinal) is also suitable when recourse will be had again to bleeding, not only the same day, but also on the third and fourth, for by flexing the arm, the lips of the wound remain notably separated from one another.

Completing the discussion on the subject of bleeding, Antyllus outlines the maneuvers which were to be resorted to if the flow of blood slowed or halted prematurely. One of the most interesting parts of this chapter is his recommendation that bands be applied to the extremities in the case of fainting due to bleeding. This corresponds to the present-day application of tourniquets to the limbs in cases of peripheral vascular collapse.

Antyllus' treatment of fistulas and abscesses constitutes a fairly complete accounting of these conditions in their various locations and degrees of complication. In fact, little improvement has been made upon his treatment of anal fistulas in the ensuing 18 centuries. His exceedingly bold, though careful, surgical approach to these conditions was mainly that of incision or extirpation in the particular manner required for the various locations. His description of the physical diagnosis and treatment of osteomyelitis is cogent and completely rational in terms of present-day knowledge. He recommends that particular attention be paid to the placement of incisions, following, if possible, the natural skin creases. His boldness was tempered with concern for the esthetic, but he did not lose sight of his real goal:

> . . . in general, it must be known that we teach the shape of the incisions by first taking into account the safety of treatment and the beauty of the form; in fact, when, with our incisions, we imitate the natural lines, we have in view, beauty; but, when we cut perpendicularly, as on the limbs and the posterior region of the neck, we are concerning ourselves with security, standing in dread of being obliged to divide some nerve or some vessel by cutting transversely. It must be recognized that we ought not to attach equal importance to security and beauty, for in all cases, I regard the consideration of the safety to be of particular concern to men.

Antyllus was not completely free of the prejudices and false theorizing of the day, despite the evidence in his works of remarkably acute powers of observation and vast experience. He was still enough of a child of his time to perpetuate the fallacious concept that:

> . . . if it is, on the other hand, an artery which has been eroded (by an abscess), there

will leak out thin, bright red blood, together with whistling and the emergence of a great deal of air.

In another chapter, he advises the surgical removal of steatomas and ganglia. An example of his experience is his caution that one should "always endeavor to remove the capsule (of a steatoma) in its entirety; for, if a part is left, this part is cause of recurrence." Although our understanding of the word steatoma may differ from his, it is obvious that he was dealing with a tumor of the skin, prone to recurrence, in which the only effective cure was complete removal.

Antyllus' best known chapter is his treatment of aneurysms, which was widely used at least until the time of John Hunter (1728 to 1793), the eminent Scottish anatomist and surgeon, who practiced and taught in London. Indeed, James Syme (1799 to 1870), the outstanding surgeon of Edinburgh and father-in-law of Lord Lister, also appears to have followed Antyllus' method. In discussing this famous chapter on aneurysm, Sir William Osler[4] says of Antyllus:

No other ancient author has anything like the same accuracy of pathologic description, and you may search the surgical literature for centuries before there is found such a gem as the account of his method, still in use, and by which his name has been permanently enshrined.

Antyllus described 2 varieties of aneurysm, those arising from a dilatation of an artery and those arising from escape of blood into surrounding tissues from a traumatized artery—perhaps leading to an ateriovenous fistula. He treated the latter type with percutaneous ligation of the area. His treatment of the former consisted of the placement of ligatures above and below the aneurysm after careful surgical exposure of the vessel, incision, and removal of the contents of the aneurysm with the ligatures left in place and without excision of the aneurysmal section. The caution expressed in his admonition not to remove the dilated section of the vessel demonstrates his experience with the occasional occurrence of loosening and accidental displacement of a ligature from the severed end of an artery, particularly one of good size, subsequent to movement and the arterial pulsations.

On the matter of hydrocephalus, Antyllus seemed to be somewhat less certain. He appears to have confused it with both cephalhematoma and caput succedaneum, for he called them all by the same name. In his description of each, he clearly differentiates them, however. He did recognize that hydrocephalus caused separation of the sutures of the skull.

One of the most daring procedures recommended by Antyllus was laryngotomy or tracheotomy:

In cases of cynanche we entirely disapprove of this operation, because the incision is utterly unavailing when the whole trachea and the lungs are affected; but in inflammations about the mouth and palate, and in cases of indurated tonsils which obstruct the mouth of the windpipe with the trachea unaffected, it will be proper to have recourse to pharyngotomy (tracheotomy), in order to avoid the risk of suffocation. When, therefore, we engage in the operation, we slit open a part of the arteria aspera (for it is dangerous to divide the whole) below the top of the windpipe, about the third or fourth ring. This is a convenient location, as being free of flesh, and because the vessels are placed at a distance from the part which is divided. Wherefore, bending the patient's head backwards, so as to bring the windpipe better into view, we are to make a transverse incision between two of the rings, so that it may not be the cartilage which is divided, but the membrane connecting the cartilages. If one be more timid in operating, one may first stretch the skin with a hook and divide it, and then, moving the vessels aside, if they come in the way, make the incision.

It is difficult to imagine that such a detailed description of a procedure as this could have been written by a person who had never performed it, but there is, currently, some question as to whether it had ever actually been performed in the Graeco-Roman period. Even Fabricius of Acquapendente (1533 to 1619), the famous Italian surgeon and anatomist and teacher of Harvey, gives an unusually lucid account of the operation, taken in part from Antyllus, but prefaced his description with the remark that he, himself, had never performed it.

Abdominal paracentesis, like tracheotomy, was performed, or at least recommended, before Antyllus' time, but ever mindful of possible difficulties, he contributed several cautions to be kept in mind during the performance of the operation. He suggested that the incision be made on the right side if there is disease of the spleen and on the left if the liver is diseased. He advised that the opening through the peritoneum should be made higher up than that of the skin in order to close more effectively the tract after withdrawal of the trochar. Another recommendation, an excellent example of Antyllus' ability to relate cause and effect, was that the discharge of water should be halted if the pulse should sink during the operation.

Antyllus included urology among his many other interests. He prescribed catheterization for urinary retention, incised for vesical calculi, and attempted correction of hypospadias. One of his omnipresent cautions was that a catheter ought not to be introduced when the retention arose from inflammation at the neck of the bladder. Unfortunately, Antyllus does not mention what should be done.

The other subjects on which Antyllus wrote were colobomas, ectropion, dropsy, hydatids, indurated tonsils, cynanche, gynecomastia, hernia (which he recognized as "a dilatation of the passage which leads from the cavity of the abdomen to the testicle"), and pterygia about the nails. In all of these is reflected the wide experience, interest, and skill of their author. We may assume that the one obvious gap in the wide variety of diseases and problems on which Antyllus touched in his surgical chapters was an intentional one. Knowing full well the penalties in his day which accompanied the performance of such a procedure, Antyllus prudently eschewed entering any of the large body cavities.

In general, most of Antyllus' surgical writings deal with procedures which could be accomplished within the limits imposed by the lack of knowledge of effective anesthetic agents and poor antiseptic technique. These procedures would be either not particularly painful, such as venesection and paracentesis, or would be carried out under conditions of dire necessity when temporizing or refusal might have led to the death of the patient, as in tracheotomy. One facet of the surgical art, which does not seem to fit into this general statement, is plastic surgery. It was usually elective, fairly time-consuming, and designed not for the saving of life or as medical treatment, but specifically for the cosmetic effect or perhaps to increase the usefulness of a part. Yet Antyllus, in the second century, did write on this subject. In fact, Castiglioni,[1] a prominent medical historian of the twentieth century, says that Antyllus'

> . . . indications relative to plastic surgery for defects of the skin and especially the eyelids, forehead, nose, and cheeks are accurate and show that the author was certainly a surgeon of wide experience and unusual ability.

Antyllus also recommended surgical correction of contractures due to scars either from burns or suppuration and had extensive experience with plastic operations on the prepuce and penis.

## CONCLUSION

From a brief sampling of his works, it is apparent that Antyllus was a life-long student of his art. Equipped with unusual perspicacity and consummate skill, he approached disease with an open mind and the sole desire to do his best for the patient. His success can be measured by his renown, and his knowledge by the few fragments of his works extant. It is hoped that this résumé of his works, in addition to presenting the thought of this truly skilled physician and surgeon, also provides some insight into the elusive personality of this enigmatic spirit of antiquity.

I wish to express my appreciation to Dr. Ilza Veith for her aid and encouragement in the preparation of this paper. I also wish to thank Dorothy H. Grant for her technical assistance.

REFERENCES

1. Castiglioni, A.: A history of medicine, New York, 1958, Alfred A. Knopf, ed. 2, p. 247.
2. Grant, R. L.: Antyllus and his medical works, Bull. Hist. Med. **24:** 154, 1960.
3. Oribasius: Oeuvres d'oribase. Translated by Bussemaker and Daremberg, Paris, 1851-1874, Imprimerie Nationale.
4. Osler, W.: Remarks on arterio-venous aneurysm, Lancet **1:** 949, 1915.
5. Paulus of Aegina: The seven books of Paulus of Aegina. Translated from the Greek with commentary by Francis Adams, London, 1844-1847, Sydenham Society.

## ERRATUM

In the paper "Myocardial Response to Prolonged Acute Oligemic Hypotension," by M. G. Weidner, Jr., M.D., Loren Roth, and F. A. Simeone, M.D., in the July, 1961, issue of SURGERY, Figs. 3 and 4 were reversed. The legend appearing under Fig. 3 belongs with Fig. 4 and vice versa.

Volume 50 Number 4

SURGERY

OCTOBER, 1961

## Clinical surgery

# Pulmonary resection for metastatic tumors of the lungs

RICHARD N. MOERSCH, M.D.*
O. THERON CLAGETT, M.D.
ROCHESTER, MINN.
*From the Mayo Clinic and Mayo Foundation*

The proper management of a patient with previously treated malignant disease in whom discrete localized lesions appear in the lungs in the absence of other evidence of recurrence is a relatively common problem. Surgical excision or resection of these apparently isolated zones of malignant spread has been carried out with increasing frequency in recent years. Gliedman and associates,[6] in an excellent review, collected reports of 289 cases from the literature in 1957, including 29 of their own. Ehrenhaft and co-workers[2] reported 28 cases the following year; additional reports[8, 12, 17, 18 22] since then have raised the total to more than 400 documented cases. Most authors have stressed the low mortality rate of the operation and the rather surprising long-term survivals that occasionally have occurred. It has been difficult to obtain survival statistics on any large number of cases, however, because of the somewhat short follow-up periods consequent to this relatively new procedure. Most series have been reported in terms of "over-all survivors" and "interval survivals."

Received for publication Nov. 18, 1960.
*Fellow in Surgery, Mayo Foundation.

Since 1941, pulmonary resection for metastatic malignant tumors has been performed on 165 patients at the Mayo Clinic. Seventy-three of these procedures were carried out more than 5 years ago. All of them were definitive operations for the treatment and attempted cure of metastatic tumors of the lung. Biopsy of the lung or deliberately incomplete resections are not included in this total. A number of cases from the earlier years of this study have been reported previously in papers from the clinic.[9, 10, 20] This communication represents a further extension of those reports.

## CLINICAL DATA

A total of 169 resections for metastatic tumors in the lungs were performed on the 165 patients. The operations were carried out from 1941 through 1959. Eighty-six of the patients were females and 79 were males; the absence of any preponderance of the male sex similar to that seen with primary pulmonary tumors has been noted before.[9, 10] The patients varied in age from 4 to 75 years, with an average age of 50 years. The median age was predictably somewhat higher, however. More than half (54 per

**Table I.** *Primary source of metastatic pulmonary tumors: 134 carcinomas*

| *Primary site of tumor* | *No. of cases* | %* |
|---|---|---|
| Rectosigmoid | 36 | 21.3 |
| Breast | 21 | 12.5 |
| Colon | 16 | 9.7 |
| Kidney | 12 | 7.3 |
| Cervix | 11 | 6.7 |
| Melanoma | 9 | 5.4 |
| Testes | 7 | 4.3 |
| Cylindroma | 6 | 3.6 |
| Squamous-cell epithelioma (skin) | 3 | 1.8 |
| Uterus | 3 | 1.8 |
| Ovary | 3 | 1.8 |
| Thyroid | 2 | 1.2 |
| Bladder | 2 | 1.2 |
| Jejunum | 1 | 0.7 |
| Jaw | 1 | 0.7 |
| Vagina | 1 | 0.7 |
| Totals | 134 | 81.0 |

*Based on the total of 165 cases.

**Table II.** *Primary source of metastatic pulmonary tumors: 31 sarcomas*

| *Type of sarcoma* | *No. of cases* |
|---|---|
| Fibrosarcoma | 8 |
| Chondrosarcoma | 4 |
| Osteogenic sarcoma | 5 |
| Synovial-cell sarcoma | 2 |
| Liposarcoma | 2 |
| Ewing's tumor | 2 |
| Undifferentiated sarcoma | 1 |
| Alveolar-cell sarcoma | 1 |
| Leiomyosarcoma | 2 |
| Rhabdomyosarcoma | 1 |
| Mesenchymoma | 1 |
| Hemangiopericytoma | 2 |
| Total | 31 (19% of all cases) |

cent) of the patients were in the sixth or seventh decade of life. Patients who had metastatic sarcomatous lesions were younger than the series as a whole, averaging 37 years at the time of pulmonary operation.

The source of the 134 primary carcinomas in this series is shown in Table I. The commonest sites of origin of the carcinomas were rectum, breast, and colon; 39 per cent of the carcinomatous lesions arose in the lower part of the intestine. This is distinctly higher than the rate in the literature as a whole.[2, 6] The kidneys, cervix, and testes were also frequent sources of such metastasis. One-fifth of the lesions were sarcomatous in nature (Table II).

Thirty-seven of the patients (22 per cent of the entire group) had multiple metastatic tumors in the lungs. In 18 of these, roentgenologic evidence of multicentricity was present prior to thoracotomy. Multiple metastatic lesions commonly were removed as part of a single inclusive resection, but multiple resections were necessary in 9 instances. On 4 occasions, second operations were performed for resection of additional or subsequent lesions.

## RECOGNITION AND DIAGNOSIS

Symptoms and clinical signs related to the thorax and lungs did not provide the primary incentive to diagnosis in this series because the majority of the patients were being seen and examined at regular intervals subsequent to previous operations for the primary malignant tumors.

A total of 88 patients, slightly more than half of the entire series, did not experience any symptoms related to the intrathoracic lesions. The recorded signs and symptoms in the remainder are shown in Table III. The commonest warning complaint was a chronic cough. This generally was mild and was attributed by the patient to smoking, a cold, or the weather. Thoracic pain was a distinct entity, most commonly encountered in patients who otherwise were free of symptoms. Little if any relationship apparently existed between the nature and duration of the symptoms and the extent and prognosis of the metastatic pulmonary lesion.

Cytologic studies of sputum or bronchial washings were performed in 65 cases in this series. Malignant cells were found in only 23 of these. Cytologic and bronchoscopic results are seen in Table IV. Results of this sort might well be expected in view of the generally peripheral nature of the lesion. Bronchoscopic examination and cytologic studies on sputum have been employed with decreasing frequency in recent years.

The lesions were visible roentgenographically in all of these cases. Roentgenologic studies of the thorax generally provided the original diagnosis. The lesion typically gave a nodular or mass shadow of a localized nature. Tomographic studies for the presence or absence of calcium were not performed routinely. As mentioned previously, the lesions in 18 cases were recognized roentgenologically as multiple. This was half of the total number reported to be multicentric by the pathologist.

## SURGICAL TREATMENT

A total of 169 operations were performed in the 165 patients (Table V). The 4 "secondary resections," which included a local excision, a segmental resection, and 2 lobectomies, were performed 1, 2, 3, and 4 years, respectively, after the initial metastatic resection. The indications were the same as those preceding the first resection.

Nearly two-thirds of the patients underwent some sort of lobectomy, and four-fifths required less than pneumonectomy. Only 4 patients required resection of the thoracic wall or diaphragm as part of the definitive operation.

All of the operations for metastatic tumors were considered to be definitive in that complete removal of all discernible malignant tissue was attempted. As noted previously, incomplete resections and simple biopsies were not included.

## RESULTS

Follow-up data were obtained as of December, 1959, on all but 4 of the 165 patients. Two of the 4 were known to have survived for 8 years after pulmonary operation, but they were lost to long-term follow-up. The third and fourth patients were last seen 6 and 4 years, respectively, after pulmonary operation. A total of 62 (38 per cent) of the patients were living at the time of this report. Forty per cent of those with metastatic carcinoma were survivors as compared to 29 per cent of those with sarcoma. The intervals of time from the pulmonary operation to the last follow-up or to death ranged from less than 1 month to more than 15 years. No relationship was apparent between this time and the source of the primary tumor. Isolated long-term survivals of 7 years or more occurred with each of the types of carcinoma, and the 3- and 5-year survival rates were comparable. However, such gross figures have little meaning by themselves. Data of more pertinence are revealed by separation of the patients into telescoping groups based on absolute survival (Table VI).

Seventy-three of the patients in this series were operated on for metastatic tumors prior to 1955; 22 (30 per cent) of these were alive 5 years or more after resection. The

**Table III.** *Signs and symptoms in metastatic pulmonary tumors**

| *Complaint* | *No. of cases* | *%†* |
|---|---|---|
| Persistent cough | 61 | 37 |
| Sputum production | 34 | 21 |
| Hemoptysis | 29 | 18 |
| Thoracic pain | 23 | 13 |
| Dyspnea | 10 | 6 |
| Wheeze | 8 | 5 |

*In 77 patients. A number of patients had more than 1 symptom or sign.

†Per cent of the total of 165 patients.

**Table IV.** *Cytologic and bronchoscopic studies in metastatic pulmonary tumors: 165 cases*

| *Procedure* | *No. of cases* | *Results* *Positive* | *Negative* | *% positive* |
|---|---|---|---|---|
| Cytology (sputum) | 52 | 19 | 33 | 37 |
| Cytology (washings) | 13 | 4 | 9 | 31 |
| Bronchoscopy | 48 | 22 | 26 | 46 |
| Bronchoscopic biopsy | 5 | 2 | 3 | 40 |

**Table V.** *Surgical procedures in metastatic pulmonary tumors: 169 operations on 165 patients*

| *Type of operation* | *No.* | *%* | |
|---|---|---|---|
| Lobectomy | 92 | 54 | 63 |
| Multiple lobectomy | 12 | 7 | |
| Lobectomy extended* | 4 | 2 | |
| Pneumonectomy | 35 | 21 | |
| Segmental resection | 15 | 9 | |
| Local excision | 11 | 7 | |

*Plus thoracic wall or diaphragm.

**Table VI.** *Survival rate in metastatic pulmonary tumors*

| Period (yr.) | Patients | | Lived beyond indicated period | |
|---|---|---|---|---|
| | Total | Traced | No. | %* |
| 1 | 131 | 131 | 93 | 71.0 |
| 2 | 113 | 113 | 55 | 48.7 |
| 3 | 99 | 99 | 35 | 35.4 |
| 5 | 73 | 71 | 22 | 31.0 |
| 7 | 51 | 51 | 12 | 23.5 |

*Based on traced patients. Inquiry as of Jan. 1, 1960. Included in the 1-year group are only patients operated on in 1958 or earlier; the 2-year group includes patients operated on in 1957 or earlier, and so forth.

survival rates decreased rather sharply during the first 3 years after operation and then leveled off. Thus, the patient who survives for the first 3 years has reasonably good prospects for the future, which is a situation analogous to that in primary carcinoma of the lung.

Survival rates in the groups with metastatic sarcomatous and carcinomatous disease are shown separately in Table VII. Gross survival statistics for the group with sarcomatous disease parallel those for the group with carcinoma but at a lower level. However, some of the long-term subgroups are rather small.

The over-all 5-year survival rate in patients who had undergone lobectomy for metastatic disease was 33 per cent. Patients requiring pneumonectomy had a 28 per cent 5-year survival rate, whereas 50 per cent of those who had undergone lesser procedures were alive after 5 years. This was related to the potentialities of the metastatic lesion and not to the surgical procedure as such.

The prognostic significance of the interval of time between the primary and the secondary operation has been considered by a number of authors[2, 6, 20] to be of less significance than the nature of the lesion itself. It has been thought, however, that patients in whom the pulmonary lesion was discovered within 1 year of the primary operation had a poorer prognosis.[1] Table VIII shows the effect of this duration on the 3-year absolute survival rate.

The size of the area of pulmonary involvement bore no discernible relationship to the prognosis in the individual case. This was true for any critical size as measured by the mean diameter. Extension to extrapulmonary structures, as pointed out previously, was significant in decreasing the survival rate.

Multicentricity of metastatic nodules, even when easily resectable, led to decreased survival rates; 79 per cent of patients with single nodules were alive 1 year after operation, whereas only 56 per cent of those who had multiple nodules of metastatic tumor survived for 1 year. Multiplicity in this sense was based on study of the pathologic material rather than on the clinical or roentgenologic appearance. The 3-year survival rates for patients with single or multicentric nodules were 50 and 19 per cent, respectively.

Only 2 of the patients in this series died during the immediate postoperative period. One of these had acute myocardial infarction on the seventh postoperative day. The second died 1 month after having undergone the pulmonary operation and before his primary jejunal carcinoma had been removed. The over-all hospital mortality rate associated with secondary pulmonary resection was 1.2 per cent in these 169 operations.

**Table VII.** *Survival rates in metastatic pulmonary tumors by type of lesion*

| Period (yr.) | Patients | | Lived beyond indicated period | |
|---|---|---|---|---|
| | Total | Traced | No. | %* |
| *Carcinoma* | | | | |
| 1 | 103 | 103 | 75 | 72.8 |
| 2 | 86 | 86 | 44 | 51.2 |
| 3 | 78 | 77 | 28 | 36.4 |
| 5 | 56 | 55 | 19 | 34.5 |
| 7 | 39 | 39 | 10 | 25.6 |
| *Sarcoma* | | | | |
| 1 | 28 | 28 | 18 | 64.3 |
| 2 | 27 | 27 | 11 | 40.7 |
| 3 | 21 | 21 | 7 | 33.3 |
| 5 | 17 | 16 | 3 | 18.8 |
| 7 | 12 | 12 | 2 | 16.7 |

*Based on traced patients. Inquiry as of Jan. 1, 1960. The 1-year group includes only patients operated on in 1958 or earlier; the 2-year group includes patients operated on in 1957 or earlier, and so forth.

**Table VIII.** *Three-year survival rates by interval between primary and secondary operations in metastatic pulmonary tumors*

| Interval (primary to secondary, yr.) | Patients | | Lived 3 or more years after pulmonary operation | |
|---|---|---|---|---|
| | Total | Traced | No. | %* |
| <1 | 22 | 22 | 3 | 13.6 |
| 1-4 | 59 | 59 | 24 | 40.7 |
| 5+ | 18 | 18 | 8 | 44.4 |
| Totals | 99 | 99 | 35 | 35.4 |

*Based on traced patients. Inquiry as of Jan. 1, 1960. Included here are only patients operated on in 1956 or earlier.

## COMMENT

The lungs have long been known to be a fertile field for the deposit and growth of metastatic tumors.[15] The incidence of pulmonary metastasis among all fatal malignant tumors was reported by Willis[23] to be 30 per cent. This rate was second only to that of metastasis to the liver. The mode of spread of metastatic tumors to the lungs is chiefly via the pulmonary and bronchial vessels. Other available routes are the thoracic duct and the hepatic veins. In approximately 15 per cent of such fatal cases, according to Farrell,[4] the lungs alone are involved by such metastatic spread. These secondary tumors may have their origin in any of the organ systems of the body.[21]

Only a small percentage of carcinomatous emboli survive on reaching the lung,[16] possibly as a result of the formation and organization of hyaline thrombi about such embolic sites, as postulated by Saphir.[19] Emboli which do survive tend to remain in a subepithelial location. King and Castleman[14] reported that the lesions in only 20 of 109 cases had infiltrated the bronchial wall or mucosa. Thus, symptoms of bronchial involvement are late and infrequent, and cytologic techniques are of less value in such cases than they are in primary bronchogenic carcinoma.[3]

Isolated reports[11, 13] have been made of the spontaneous regression of pulmonary metastatic tumors, but the prognosis when pulmonary metastasis is untreated or not palliated by physicochemical means is uniformly poor.[7, 15] Treatment of such lesions by resection was performed as early as 1898,[5] but the operation remained a surgical rarity until recent years.[1] Occasional instances of long-term survival after such procedures have been reported in detail, but the value of this treatment and its effect on prognosis in larger groups have remained uncertain.

The results of this study indicate that in properly selected cases the outlook is hopeful and certainly equal to that in many well-established operations for primary carcinoma or sarcoma.

Criteria for the selection of cases in which pulmonary resection is merited have been broadened in recent years. Multicentricity alone cannot be equated with inoperability. More than 10 per cent of the lesions in this series were known to be multiple prior to thoracotomy, and an equal additional number were found to be so by the pathologist after resection. The survival rate in patients with multiple lesions was less than in those with solitary lesions, but resection clearly is justified for multiple lesions. It is obvious that widespread dissemination of pulmonary metastatic tumors is not included in this statement. The duration of time since the discovery and treatment of the primary tumor is not a determining factor in judging operability. While careful observation for a period of weeks to months still may be advised when metastasis accompanies a primary growth, survivals may be expected after any interval of time in the absence of metastasis elsewhere. Conversely, a prolonged period between the primary operation and the appearance of pulmonary metastasis does not guarantee success. The nature and origin of the primary lesion are of little prognostic import in the individual case. All types of lesions have been associated with long-term survival. The presence or absence of clinical signs of pulmonary involvement and the results of cytologic or bronchoscopic studies are indeterminate factors in evaluation of a case.

In essence, there are 3 factors of importance to be considered in the surgical management of such patients: (1) the over-all condition of the patient and his ability to tolerate surgical intervention, (2) adequate definitive treatment of the primary lesion, and (3) the absence of local recurrent lesions or metastasis beyond the scope of the projected resection.

Secondary pulmonary growths tend to lie in a peripheral location, and the smallest resection compatible with the adequate surgical treatment of malignant tumors is indicated. Only 21 per cent of the 165 patients underwent pneumonectomy. The possibility of further contralateral resection at a future date emphasizes the importance of a limited operation. It has been suggested[6] that more extensive resection might give a better prognosis. In this series, patients who underwent the less extensive operations fared better after operation.

The inherent risk of resection of this nature is small. The hospital mortality rate in this study was 1.2 per cent, which must be balanced against the discouraging prognosis when the condition is untreated. It is undoubtedly true[6, 7, 15] that survival is related directly to the basic growth potential of the tumor. However, with no reliable method of estimating or grading this, resection in all suitable cases is justified.

## SUMMARY AND CONCLUSIONS

A total of 169 operations were carried out at the Mayo Clinic on 165 patients for removal of localized pulmonary metastatic tumors in a 19-year period. The absolute 1-year survival rate was 71 per cent, and 31 per cent of 71 traced patients eligible for 5-year studies were alive 5 years or more after resection. Patients surviving for 3 years after such operations have a greatly improved prognosis thereafter.

These figures held true for the metastatic tumors arising from a wide variety of primary carcinomas. Sarcomatous metastasis had a somewhat lower percentage of survivals. Multiple pulmonary metastatic tumors similarly carried a poorer prognosis. The duration of time since the treatment of the primary tumor and the presence or absence of clinical stigmas of pulmonary involvement did not have an appreciable effect on survival.

Thoracotomy and resection of pulmonary metastatic malignant tumors constitute a highly worthwhile and rewarding course in properly selected patients.

### REFERENCES

1. Alexander, J. and Haight, C.: Pulmonary resection for solitary metastatic sarcomas and carcinomas, Surg. Gynec. & Obst. **85:** 129, 1947.
2. Ehrenhaft, J. L., Lawrence, M. S., and Sensenig, D. M.: Pulmonary resections for metastatic lesions, A. M. A. Arch. Surg. **77:** 606, 1958.
3. Ellis, F. H., Jr., Woolner, L. B., and Schmidt, H. W.: Metastatic pulmonary malignancy: a study of factors involved in exfoliation of malignant cells, J. Thoracic Surg. **20:** 125, 1950.
4. Farrell, J. T.: Pulmonary metastasis: a pathologic, clinical and roentgenologic study based on 78 cases seen at necropsy, Radiology **24:** 444, 1935.
5. Gerulanos, M.: Eine Studie über den operativen Pneumothorax im Anschluss an einem Fall von Lungenresection wegen Brustwandsarcom, Deutsche Ztschr. Chir. **49:** 497, 1898.
6. Gliedman, M. L., Horowitz, S. and Lewis, F. J.: Lung resection for metastatic cancer; SURGERY **42:** 521, 1957.
7. Greenberg, B. E., and Young, J. M.: Pulmonary metastasis from occult primary sites resembling bronchogenic carcinoma, Dis. Chest. **33:** 496, 1958.
8. Groves, L. K., and Effler, D. B.: Surgery for metastatic neoplastic disease in the lung, Cleveland Clin. Quart. **23:** 16, 1956.
9. Habein, H. C., Clagett, O. T., and McDonald, J. R.: Pulmonary resection for metastatic tumors, A. M. A. Arch. Surg. **78:** 716, 1959.
10. Hood, R. T., Jr., McBurney, R. P., and Clagett, O. T.: Metastatic malignant lesions of the lungs treated by pulmonary resection, J. Thoracic Surg. **30:** 81, 1955.
11. Jenkins, G. D.: Regression of pulmonary metastasis following nephrectomy for hypernephroma: Eight year followup, J. Urol. **82:** 37, 1959.
12. Kelly, C. R., and Langston, H. T.: The treatment of metastatic pulmonary malignancy, J. Thoracic Surg. **31:** 298, 1956.
13. Kessel, L.: Spontaneous disappearance of bilateral pulmonary metastases, J. A. M. A. **169:** 1737, 1959.
14. King, D. S., and Castleman, B.: Bronchial

involvement in metastatic pulmonary malignancy, J. Thoracic Surg. **12:** 305, 1943.

15. Mandeville, F. B.: Roentgen and clinical problems in so-called solitary metastatic tumors in the chest, Am. J. Surg. **71:** 669, 1946.
16. Moore, G. E.: The significance of cancer cells in the blood, Surg. Gynec. & Obst. **110:** 360, 1960.
17. Parker, R. G.: The treatment of apparently solitary pulmonary metastases, J. Thoracic Surg. **36:** 81, 1958.
18. Rowlandson, R.: The surgical treatment of pulmonary metastases, Brit. J. Tuberc. **52:** 190, 1958.
19. Saphir, O.: The fate of carcinoma emboli in the lung, Am. J. Path. **23:** 245, 1947.
20. Seiler, H. H., Clagett, O. T., and McDonald, J. R.: Pulmonary resection for metastatic malignant lesions, J. Thoracic Surg. **19:** 655, 1950.
21. Turner, J. W., and Jaffe, H. L.: Metastatic neoplasms: a clinical and roentgenological study of involvement of skeleton and lungs, Am. J. Roentgenol. **43:** 479, 1940.
22. Virkkula, L.: Metastatic pulmonary lesions, Ann. chir. et gynaec. Fenniae. **48:** 37, 1959.
23. Willis, R. A.: Secondary tumours of the lungs. *In* The spread of tumours in the human body, London, 1952, Butterworth & Co., Ltd., pp. 169-177.

# Primary tumors of the small intestine

DONALD B. ROCHLIN, M.D.
WILLIAM P. LONGMIRE, JR., M.D.
LOS ANGELES, CALIF.
*From the University of California Medical Center, Department of Surgery, and Wadsworth Veterans Administration Hospital*

Because primary malignant tumors of the small intestine are relatively infrequent, knowledge of their pathologic characteristics, of the signs and symptoms, that they produce, and of their prognosis is necessarily limited. In spite of better diagnostic methods and the increased number of postmortem examinations which have been performed over the past 30 years, these lesions remain somewhat a curiosity. Although many individual case reports or studies of a specific tumor or tumor site have been published, comprehensive reviews have usually been derived, either partially or completely, from autopsy material. The relative paucity of information led us to study the literature concerning these lesions and review the pertinent case records from the University of California Medical Center and the Wadsworth General Veterans Administration Center Hospital, Los Angeles, for the period 1940 to 1959.

## REVIEW OF THE LITERATURE

The first report of a primary carcinoma of the jejunum was made by Sorlin[27] in 1824. Morgagni[20] reported lesions that descriptively seemed similar to carcinomas of the small intestine, but he failed to recognize their significance. However, in 1876, Leichtenstern[16] reported and completely described the first autopsy series of these malignant lesions. Since that time, reports of the incidence of these tumors have varied from 0.095 per cent of all malignant lesions of the gastrointestinal tract[16] to 2.3 per cent, as stated by Likely[17] in 1948. Maydl[19] reported an autopsy series in 1883 which had an incidence of 0.927 per cent. In 1903, Northnagel[21] found an incidence of 0.051 per cent, and in 1930, Rankin[25] reported an incidence of 0.62 per cent from the autopsy records of the Mayo Clinic. In reviewing the literature on the incidence of these tumors, we noted that for every case of malignancy of the small intestine, there were approximately 40 to 60 cases of malignant neoplastic disease of the colon.

In most series, approximately one-third to one-half of patients with primary malignancy of the small intestine died of intercurrent disease rather than the direct effects of the malignancy. For this reason, the majority of tumors described in the literature were found as autopsy specimens rather than primary symptomatic tumors. In the remaining 50 to 65 per cent of the patients, sufficient difficulties developed due to the primary tumor that an exploratory laparotomy was warranted to establish the etiology of symptoms. It is for this group of patients that a better understanding of the clinical manifestations, therapy, and prognosis is necessary.

In reviewing the reported series of primary malignant lesions of the small intestine from 1920 to 1960[1-3, 5-9, 11, 13-15, 18, 23, 24, 28] we found 650 cases. In individual series, depending upon the status of the patients and the number of cases reported, there was a marked variability in the relative frequency of sarcomas, carcinomas, and

Received for publication Nov. 21, 1960.

carcinoid tumors, as well as in the frequency of appearance of these lesions in various areas of the small intestine. Since many of the series included only a small number of patients, no statistical significance can be attached to the numerical values quoted in these studies.

Table I shows the relative incidence of primary malignant neoplasms of the small intestine taken from the literature. There were 136 primary tumors of the duodenum, 184 of the jejunum, and 308 of the ileum. In another 22 cases, a malignant neoplasm was found to be present in at least one other site in the small intestine. In these instances, it was not possible to decide whether 2 primary growths had arisen or whether 1 area was occupied by a metastasis from a single primary lesion. In at least 2 cases[9] a Peutz-Jegher[12, 22] syndrome was noted. The greatest number of individual malignancies was found in the ileum, but the incidence of primary carcinomas in the duodenum, jejunum, and ileum was practically identical.

Two hundred eight sarcomas, 321 carcinomas, and 121 carcinoids are included. Both the carcinoid tumors and the sarcomas were found to originate most frequently in the ileum. A progressively greater incidence of these tumors was found distally through the small intestine. The distribution of carcinomas, however, did not follow this pattern, and an almost equal incidence was noted in each of the 3 sectors. Considering all malignancies of the small intestine, however, there is a progressively greater incidence distalward in the bowel.

## CASE MATERIAL

Forty-one cases of malignancies of the small intestine were found in the records of the University of California at Los Angeles Medical Center and the Wadsworth Veterans Hospital during the years 1940 to 1959 (Table II). Five cases of sarcoma, 18 of carcinoma, and 18 of carcinoid tumor compose the series. Ten primary malignancies of the duodenum, 12 of the jejunum, and 18 of the ileum were found, as well as what appeared to be 2 primary lesions in 1 patient. The relatively small number of cases in this report precludes any statistical comparison with the larger number of cases from the literature in Table I, although the tendency for greater distalward involvement can be seen.

In 27 patients, the lesions produced sufficiently severe symptoms to require surgical intervention. In 14 cases, the lesion was an incidental finding at autopsy or at operation for other causes. Twelve of the lesions found in the latter instance were small carcinoid tumors. The series includes 38 men and 3 women. This imbalance is due to the fact that the majority of cases were taken from the records of the Veterans Administration hospital. Thirty-four Caucasians, 6 Negroes, and 1 Oriental are included. The average age of the patients in the carcinoma series was 56.4 years at the time of the initial diagnosis of malignancy;

**Table I.** *Review of the literature, 1920 to 1960, on malignant tumors of the small intestine*

| Location | No. |
|---|---|
| *Total cases* | |
| Duodenum | 136 |
| Jejunum | 184 |
| Ileum | 308 |
| Multiple | 22 |
| Total | 650 |
| *Sarcomas* | |
| Duodenum | 12 |
| Jejunum | 61 |
| Ileum | 118 |
| Multiple | 17 |
| Total | 208 |
| *Carcinomas* | |
| Duodenum | 113 |
| Jejunum | 108 |
| Ileum | 98 |
| Multiple | 2 |
| Total | 321 |
| *Carcinoid tumors* | |
| Duodenum | 11 |
| Jejunum | 15 |
| Ileum | 92 |
| Multiple | 3 |
| Total | 121 |

**Table II.** *Malignant tumors of the small intestine at University of California Medical Center and Wadsworth General Hospital, Veterans Administration Center, Los Angeles, 1940 to 1960*

| *Tumor* | *Duodenum* | *Jejunum* | *Ileum* | *Multiple* |
|---|---|---|---|---|
| Sarcoma | 1 | 2 | 2 | 0 |
| Carcinoma | 5 | 9 | 4 | 0 |
| Carcinoid tumors | 4 | 1 | 12 | 1 |
| Totals | 10 | 12 | 18 | 1 |

the oldest patient was 70 years old and the youngest 32 years old. In the series of carcinoid tumors, the average age of the patients was 51.5 years; the oldest patient was 89 years old and the youngest 50 years old. In the sarcoma series, the average age was 44.2 years, with the oldest patient 81 years old and the youngest 22 years old.

**Pathology.** The most common type of tumor found in the small intestine is the carcinoma, of which the adenocarcinoma is by far the most frequent. Various degrees of differentiation are found in pathologic sections of these lesions, but generally, well-differentiated glandular patterns are present. In carcinoma of the duodenum, as pointed out by Resnick and Cooper,[26] approximately 40 per cent of the lesions arise in the suprapapillary area, 40 per cent below the papillary area, and only 20 per cent are located in the peripapillary region. Carcinomas of the jejunum and ileum, usually present as annular constricting tumors with an ulcerating mucosal surface involving a short segment of the intestine, are very similar in appearance to carcinomas of the sigmoid area. Lymph node metastases are frequently found at the time of operation for the primary malignancy. In some cases, malignant degeneration of adenomatous polyps of the small intestine can occur as reported by Fraser,[8] and in those instances, as the polyp becomes larger, intussusception may cause acute intestinal obstruction. In our series, all tumors were pathologically shown to be adenocarcinomas with varying degrees of differentiation. No instance of the malignant degeneration of the polyp associated with Peutz-Jegher syndrome was found.

Lymphoid tumors are the most frequent type of sarcoma found in the small intestine. Lymphosarcomas, Hodgkin's disease, leiomyosarcomas, fibrosarcomas, and reticulum-cell sarcomas have all been found as primary lesions in this location. Lymphoid sarcomas may arise from follicles located within the wall of the bowel, while other sarcomas arise from other mesenchymal tissues in the same area. These lesions tend to grow outward from the serosa and muscularis. Therefore, stenosis of the lumen is a rare and late complication. The first sign produced by these lesions is displacement of the bowel on roentgenographic examination. Since encroachment on the lumen of the intestine occurs only late in the disease, sarcomas more often form palpable masses than do the small intestinal malignancies. Fraser[8] has estimated that approximately 65 per cent of sarcomas and only 29 per cent of carcinomas eventually become palpable.

In our series, an abdominal mass eventually became palpable in 17, or 62.9 per cent, of 27 patients with symptomatic tumors. In 4 cases, this was the first definitive sign that a surgical lesion was present. On pathologic examination of the sarcomas presented in this series, 3 were identified as lymphosarcomas, 1 as Hodgkin's disease, and 1 as a leiomyosarcoma.

Carcinoid tumors of the bowel arise from the Kultschitzky or argentaffin cells deep within the mucosal glands of the bowel. They are usually found in the small intestine as small, firm, yellowish, circumscribed nodules in the submucosal area. The larger tumors invade locally and may metastasize to regional lymph nodes, and occasionally to the liver. Carcinoid tumors of the gastrointestinal tract have been reported[10] to be associated with a syndrome caused by the secretion of serotonin. This clinical and pathologic picture was not found in any case of this series. All patients included in the series showed evidence of invasion of the bowel wall and this pathologic confirmation was taken as the criterion of malignancy. In 12 of the cases included, the carcinoid tumors were incidental findings at operation and in 6 patients were symptomatic lesions. Metastases to regional lymph nodes were present in 4 patients at the time of exploration. This percentage agrees closely with that reported by Dockerty[4] in which 75 per cent of all symptomatic small intestinal carcinoid tumors were found to have metastasized at the time of operation.

**Clinical signs and symptoms.** Malignant tumors of the small intestine initially manifest themselves insidiously and may mimic less serious gastrointestinal disorders for long periods of time. An index of suspicion should always be present when puzzling gastrointestinal symptoms such as unexplained bleeding or partial intestinal obstruction occur.

In our series, the symptoms appear to be divided into 3 complexes, (1) symptoms of diarrhea with large amounts of mucus present, and tenesmus; (2) obstructive symptoms producing nausea, vomiting, and cramping abdominal pain; (3) a syndrome produced by chronic blood loss into the gastrointestinal tract producing weakness, anemia, asthenia, and, on some relatively infrequent occasions, melena. In no instance in this series was there a perforation of the small intestine as was frequently noted in the report of Pridgen.[23]

The first symptom complex involves a change of bowel habit evidenced by a more frequent and diarrheal stool with a considerable quantity of mucus. This symptom complex was noted in 5 patients. In 1 case diarrhea was at times severe enough to cause as many as 10 to 12 loose, watery stools a day. These symptoms led to erroneous diagnoses of inflammatory processes, such as ulcerative colitis or regional enteritis, in 4 patients prior to the discovery of the malignancy. At times, bright blood was mixed with the choleric stool. In some instances, conservative therapy had intermittently caused symptomatic relief of difficulties, but exacerbations always followed the temporary remissions. Location rather than the type of tumor is apparently responsible for these difficulties, since 4 of the 5 patients were found to have malignant lesions of the distal jejunum and ileum.

The second symptom complex is one of partial intestinal obstruction gradually progressing to complete obstruction. In general, patients were prone to minimize the early symptoms of partial obstruction and consider them as evidence of enteritis or other similar difficulty. A history of vague, long-standing, intermittent abdominal discomfort and fullness was elicited from some patients. Because of the abdominal stress which followed every meal, the patient developed a reluctance to eat and a marked weight loss occurred. There was frequently a history of several radiologic and laboratory examinations of the gastrointestinal tract which resulted in negative reports. In some instances, small defects in the intestine were diagnosed as deformities of the small intestine due to adhesions or inflammatory processes. In the more proximal lesions, serious symptoms were manifested earlier and roentgenographic signs were more easily recognized. Diagnosis was prolonged in patients with sarcomas since these lesions, by reason of their extrinsic position, initially displaced the bowel, and it was not until ulceration of the mucosa occurred or the expanding tumor encroached on the lumen that indications for operation became apparent. This obstructive symptom complex was present in 17 of the 27 patients included in this series.

The third symptom complex is one caused by the chronic loss of blood into the gastrointestinal tract. Asthenia, anemia, and occasionally melena developed. Frequently, the only evidence of neoplasm in the bowel was revealed by laboratory studies showing anemia and the presence of occult blood in the stool. It is noteworthy that these symptoms are similar to those of cecal carcinoma.

While these symptom complexes are not always as clearly defined as presented, a combination of the symptoms may occur

**Table III.** *Duration of symptoms prior to operation*

| *Months* | *No.* |
|---|---|
| 0- 1 | 2 |
| 2- 3 | 6 |
| 4- 6 | 5 |
| 7- 9 | 3 |
| 10-12 | 5 |
| 12 | 6 |

**Table IV.** *Type of therapy*

| | *Resection* | *Bypass anastomosis* | *Inoperable* | *Radiation therapy* |
|---|---|---|---|---|
| Duodenum | 2 | 3 | 1 | 1 |
| Jejunum | 6 | 4 | 1 | 0 |
| Ileum | 3 | 3 | 2 | 2 |

with one clinical picture which is predominant.

Table III refers to the duration of symptoms of patients included in this series, prior to the time that the diagnosis of a surgical lesion was made.

Eleven patients, or 40 per cent, had initial symptoms 10 or more months prior to diagnosis. The fact emphasizes again the insidious nature of small bowel lesions.

The therapy of malignancies of the small intestine is often complicated by the fact that during operation it is found that the tumor has already invaded the regional lymphatics, foreshortened the mesentery of the bowel, and spread so extensively through it that complete irradication is impossible. Palpable nodes may be found at the root of the mesentery in the region of the superior mesenteric artery and at its origin, so that a complete removal of the tumor is not possible. While earlier diagnosis is frequently possible in tumors of the duodenum, the lesion may be unresectable because of the involvement of the retroperitoneal area as well as the presence of metastatic disease at the time of operation.

Table IV is a tabulation of therapeutic modalities used. One patient with a sarcoma of the ileum was treated by irradiation therapy with only a biopsy performed at operation. Two patients with carcinoma of the duodenum were treated with pancreaticoduodenectomy.

Curative or palliative resection was possible in 11, or 40 per cent, of patients who underwent laparotomy. In 10 patients, or 37 per cent, a palliative bypass procedure was performed and in 4 patients no attempt at palliation was possible. The operative mortality rate for apparently curative resections was 18.6 per cent.

In the entire series, 15 patients were not included in the survival data because they died of intercurrent disease of their malignancies were classified as incidental findings at the time of operation for other causes. In the sarcoma series, 1 patient is alive and apparently free of disease 11 years after operation. Three patients died of widespread metastases within 6 months of operation, and 1 operative death is listed.

Table V refers to the period of survival after resection of the carcinomas. In the group of 18 patients diagnosed as having primary adenocarcinoma of the small intestine, 5 are alive and well with no evidence of recurrence of malignant disease at the present time. Two patients are 4 months, 1 patient 3 years, 1 patient 8 years, and 1 patient 11 years postoperative. Of the patients who could be included in the series, there was a 5-year survival rate of 20 per cent.

In the series of patients with carcinoid tumors, these lesions were incidental findings in 12 patients at the time of exploratory laparotomy for other lesions in the abdomen. Six patients were primarily operated upon for symptomatic carcinoid disease. Table VI shows the postresection survival rate for these patients. One patient is alive and well 14 months postoperatively, and another is alive and well 6 years after operation.

In reviewing the case histories of patients with malignant disease of the small intestine, a large number showed other primary malignancies. In Table VII the primary tumors of the other areas are listed that had been diagnosed prior to the occurrence of malignancy of the small intestine or had developed subsequent to the operation for that disease. This high incidence of other malignancies may be due to the fact that the greatest number of cases were collected from the Veterans Administration Hospital, where elderly male patients live in the domicile associated with this institution. Because of this fact, the significance of the data in Table VII is open to question. However, it does present an interesting fact which might be corroborated in a series not as heavily weighted with elderly men.

While the prognosis of malignant neoplasms of the small intestine is relatively poor, it is probable that the 5-year survival rate could be increased by earlier diagnostic efforts and the maintenance of a high index of suspicion for the presence of these lesions. Repeated roentgenologic studies may often be indicated, and when a tumor of the small intestine is strongly suspected but not found after repeated radiologic examination, exploratory laparotomy should be performed. The therapy of choice in the treatment of these lesions is a wide resection with removal of regional lymph nodes, if this proves feasible at the time of laparotomy. If resection is impossible, a palliative short-circuiting procedure is of value. In some sarcomas, particularly those of the lymphoid series, irradiation therapy may be of value, but this modality is usually of no avail in other lesions. Chemotherapy has so far proved unsuccessful with these lesions.

Pancreaticoduodenectomy is the procedure of choice for operable duodenal carcinoma. It is interesting to note that Hallenbeck[10] quotes a 5-year survival rate of 38.5 per cent with pancreaticoduodenectomy for operable carcinoma of ampulla of Vater, while the 5-year survival rate for operable carcinoma of the jejunum and ileum was 23.9 per cent from the same institution. This is probably due to the fact that the ampullary and duodenal carcinomas produce earlier symptoms than do lesions of the jejunum and ileum. For this reason, patients with the former lesions are operated upon at an earlier date.

The importance of the recognition of any of the 3 symptom complexes cannot be overstressed, nor can the necessity for correlating the radiologic studies of the small intestine with the clinical picture that the patient presents. As earlier diagnosis of malignancies of the small intestine is made, the prognosis of surgical therapy should also become better.

## SUMMARY

A group of cases of primary malignancies of the small intestine from the University of California Medical Center, Los Angeles, and Wadsworth General Hospital, Veterans Administration Center, is presented. A total of 41 new cases of primary small bowel malignancy have been added to the literature. Of this series, 5 sarcomas, 18 carcinomas, and 18 carcinoid tumors were found.

Of this group, 27 patients had symptomatic tumors, and 14 were incidental findings at postmortem examination or at laparotomy for other reasons.

**Table V.** *Postresection survival of patients with primary carcinoma of small intestine*

| *6 mo.* | *6 mo.-1 yr.* | *1-3 yr.* | *5 yr. or more* |
|---|---|---|---|
| 5 | 4 | 4 | 2 |

**Table VI.** *Postresection survival of patients with primary carcinoid tumors of small intestine*

| *6 mo.* | *6 mo.-1 yr.* | *1-3 yr.* | *5 yr. or more* |
|---|---|---|---|
| 2 | 2 | 1 | 1 |

**Table VII.** *Primary malignancies occurring in other areas of the body in the same patients of this series*

| *Area* | *No.* |
|---|---|
| Colon | 3 |
| Prostate | 4 |
| Oral cavity | 1 |
| Pancreas | 1 |
| Lung | 2 |
| Liposarcoma | 1 |

Three symptom complexes are defined for the diagnosis of malignancies of the small intestine.

It was found that in 12 of the patients, primary malignancies of other areas occurred. The significance of this is doubtful, as it may represent the advanced age of the population included in the study.

## REFERENCES


1. Botsford, T. W., and Seibel, R. F.: Benign and malignant tumors of the small intestine, New England J. Med. **236:** 683, 1947.
2. Burman, S. O., and Van Wyk, F. Y. K.: Lymphomas of the small intestine and cecum, Ann. Surg. **143:** 349, 1955.
3. Darling, R. C., and Welch, C. E.: Tumors of the small intestine, New England J. Med. **260:** 397, 1959.
4. Dockerty, M. B.: Carcinoids of gastrointestinal tract, Am. J. Clin. Path. **25:** 794, 1955.
5. Duncan, J. A., and Ricker, W. A.: Malignant tumors of the small intestine, West. J. Surg. **58:** 401, 1950.
6. Dundon, C. C.: Primary tumors of the small intestine, Am. J. Roentgenol. **59:** 429, 1948.
7. Elias, W. S., Lund, C. C., and Yamamoto, R.: Neoplasms of the small intestine, Am. J. Surg. **88:** 384, 1954.
8. Fraser, K.: Summary of malignant tumors of small intestine, Brit. J. Surg. **82:** 479, 1945.
9. Goergenson, E. J., and Werpel, E. A.: A study of small bowel tumors with special emphasis on clinical aspects, California Med. **75:** 395, 1951.
10. Hallenbeck, G. A., Walter, W., Gray, H. K., Preslley, J. T., and Waugh, J. M.: Report on surgery of the biliary system and pancreas for 1954, Proc. Staff Meet. Mayo Clin. **30:** 640, 1955.
11. Hunt, W. H., III., Broders, A. C., Jr., and Hightower, N. C., Jr.: Primary neoplasms of the small bowel, South. M. J. **51:** 482, 1958.
12. Jegher, H., McKusick, V. A., and Katz, K. H.: Generalized intestinal polyposis and malanin spots of oral mucosa, lips, and digits, New England J. Med. **241:** 993, 1949.
13. Jenkinson, E. L., Pfisterer, W. H., and Seitz, E. R.: Primary tumors of the small intestine, Radiology **55:** 12, 1950.
14. Kleinerman, J., Yardumiun, K., and Tamaki, H. T.: Primary carcinoma of the duodenum, Ann. Int. Med. **32:** 451, 1950.
15. Kock, W.: Primary sarcomas of the small intestine; clinical study of surgically treated cases in Stockholm during 1900 to 1941, Acta chir. scandinav. **89:** 37, 1943.
16. Leichtenstern, O.: Handbuch des speciellen Pathologie und Therapie, Leipzig, 1876, F. C. W. Vogel, pp. 523-524.
17. Likely, D. S., Lesa, J. R., Stitch, M. N., and Stein, H. D.: Primary tumors of the small intestine, Arch. Int. Med. **82:** 206, 1948.
18. Maxwell, E. A., Crile, C., Jr., and Dinsmore, R. S.: Malignant tumors of the small intestine, S. Clin. North America **28:** 1149, 1948.
19. Maydl, C.: Über den Darmkrebs, Vienna, 1883, Bramisellen, p. 7.
20. Morgagni, J. B.: In which the internal preternatural tumors of the belly that remain are spoken of. *In* translation by Benjamin, A., of Miller, A., and Caldwell, T.: The seats and causes of disease, London, 1769, pp. 262-413.
21. Northnagel, H.: In Specialle Pathologie und Therapie, Vienna, 1903, Alfred Hoelder, p. 316.
22. Peutz, J. L. A.: Very remarkable case of familial polyposis of mucous membrane of the intestinal tract and nasal pharynx accompanied by peculiar pigmentation of skin and mucous membrane, Nederl. M. Aandschr. geneesk. **10:** 134, 1921.
23. Pridgen, J. E., Mayo, C. W., and Dockerty, M. B.: Carcinoma of the jejunum and ileum exclusive of carcinoid tumors, Surg. Gynec. & Obst. **90:** 513, 1950.
24. Rabinovitch, J., Grayzel, D. M., and Sawyer, A. S.: Malignant tumors of the small intestine, Am. J. Surg. **30:** 69, 1933.
25. Rankin, F. W., and Mayo, C.: Carcinoma of the small bowel, Surg. Gynec. & Obst. **50:** 939, 1930.
26. Resnick, H. L. P., and Cooper, D. R.: Carcinoma of the duodenum; review of literature from 1948 to 1956, Am. J. Surg. **9:** 946, 1958.
27. Sorlin, M.: Observation d'un squirre d'une portion de jejunum chez un sujet de quarante-neuf ans; morte a la suite de nombreux vomissements, J. gen. med. chir. et pharm. **87:** 189, 1824.
28. Strohl, E. L., Diffenbaugh, W. G., and Sarver, F. E.: The surgical significance of small bowel tumors, Surg. Gynec. & Obst. **93:** 209, 1951.
29. Thorson, A., Biorck, G., Bjorkman, G., and Waldenstrorn, J.: Malignant carcinoids of the small intestine with metastases of liver, valvular disease of right side of heart (pulmonary stenosis and tricuspid regurgitation without septal defects), peripheral vasomotor symptoms, broncho-constriction, and unusual type of cyanosis, Am. Heart J. **47:** 795, 1954.

# Chylous cysts of the abdomen

STEPHEN ENGEL, M.D.*
O. THERON CLAGETT, M.D.
EDGAR G. HARRISON, JR., M.D.
ROCHESTER, MINN.
*From the Mayo Clinic and Mayo Foundation*

Chylous cysts of the abdomen are a group of loculations of varied etiology which contain a grossly milky fluid resembling chyle.

Historically, Benevieni, a Florentine anatomist, was the first to observe a mesenteric cyst in 1507 while performing a necropsy. Rokitansky, in 1842, published the first accurate description of a chylous cyst found at necropsy.[12] The first reported successful treatment of a mesenteric cyst is credited to Tillaux. Pean, 3 years later, was the first surgeon to report the recovery of a patient with a chylous cyst treated by marsupialization.[2]

Although mesenteric cysts in general have been reported in the literature fairly frequently since then, chylous cysts seldom have been described. Beahrs and associates[1] reviewed the literature and found reports on approximately 600 abdominal cysts of mesenteric, retroperitoneal, and omental types. They reported an additional 174 cysts, including 9 of the chylous variety, encountered at the Mayo Clinic between 1911 and 1950. Since 1950, 142 similar cysts have been seen at the clinic, and among them were 14 chylous cysts. Coursley and co-workers[5] reported on 2 of the 14 in 1956. The purpose of our study is to report the 12 additional cases encountered at the clinic between 1950 and 1959 (Table I), as well as to report on the follow-up of the original cases reported by Beahrs and Coursley and their associates.

Review of the literature subsequent to 1950 showed 15 cases of chylous cysts. Burnett and associates[3] reviewed the literature and added 3 cases of mesenteric cysts, 1 of which was of the chylous variety. Simon and Williamson[11] described 3 retroperitoneal chylous cysts, and Corrao and Loyudice[4] in Argentina reported 1 case in 1958. Pack and associates[8] and Walker and Cooper[13] each reported 1 case. Raszkowski and associates[9] reported 2 cases. In addition, 6 cases of chylous retroperitoneal lymphangiomas and 79 cases of postoperative lymphocysts have been reported recently.[7, 10]

Received for publication Nov. 22, 1960.
*Fellow in Surgery, Mayo Foundation.

## CASE REPORTS

**Case 1.** A 5-year-old girl was brought to the clinic because her mother had noted that for 3 or 4 weeks her dresses had fitted more tightly than usual. The child had been seen by her local physician, and after a few days' observation it became apparent that the abdomen was indeed enlarging. Paracentesis was performed with the patient under general anesthesia. The results of all laboratory studies prior to paracentesis, including excretory urograms, were reported to be normal. A moderate amount of milky fluid was removed, and on examination this showed a trace of protein and 5,450 mg. of lipid per 100 ml. A diagnosis of chylous ascites was made and the patient was referred to the clinic. Examination showed slight drainage from the paracentesis wound and a cystic mass in the upper and middle parts of the abdomen (Fig. 1). The patient was observed for several days, during which time the size of the abdomen increased. At operation a cyst 15 by 10 by 10 cm. was found in the mesentery of the first part of the jejunum. Excision was accomplished by resection of a segment of the jejunum which formed a part of the cyst wall (Fig. 2). Microscopic examination of the specimen showed 1 large loculus with smooth muscle in the wall and with an endothelial lining and a few smaller spaces of cystic lymphangioma (Fig. 3). The patient has not had further difficulty.

**Table I.** *Summary of 12 cases encountered at Mayo Clinic between 1950 and 1959*

| *Case* | *Age (yr.)* | *Sex* | *Symptoms* | *Lesion* |
|---|---|---|---|---|
| 1 | 5 | F | Abdominal enlargement | Cystic lymphangioma (15 by 10 by 10 cm.) |
| 2 | 45 | F | Incidental | Cystic lymphangioma (15 cm. in diameter) |
| 3 | 55 | F | Abdominal mass | Cystic lymphangioma (6 cm.) |
| 4 | 52 | M | Incidental | Cystic lymphangioma |
| 5 | 8 mo. | M | Abdominal pain and mass | Multilocular cystic lymphangioma |
| 6 | 11 | M | Abdominal enlargement | Multilocular cystic lymphangioma |
| 7 | 32 | F | Abdominal mass | Cystic lymphangioma (11 cm.) |
| 8 | 4½ | F | Abdominal pain | Cystic lymphangioma (9 by 6 by 2.5 cm.) |
| 9 | 58 | M | Incidental | Cystic lymphangioma (12 by 10 by 10) |
| 10 | 33 | F | Left iliac mass after Wertheim hysterectomy | Chylous cyst (5 by 5 by 3 cm.) |
| 11 | 30 | F | Left iliac mass after Wertheim hysterectomy | Chylous cyst (35 ml. chyle aspirated) |
| 12 | 39 | F | Left iliac mass | Chylous cyst (5 cm. in diameter) |

**Case 8.** A 4½-year-old girl was seen at the clinic in 1957 with a history of pain in the right lower quadrant of 2 days' duration, for which she had undergone appendectomy elsewhere. At operation the appendix had been found to be normal, but a large retroperitoneal mass was present. Excision of this mass had not been attempted because of the operative impression that it originated from the kidney and that excretory urograms should be made prior to excision. Excretory urograms, however, were reported to be normal, and the patient was referred to the clinic. Examination did not show any gross abnormality and excretory urograms were normal. At operation a chylous cystic mass, 9 by 6 by 2.5 cm., was excised from the mesentery of the small bowel (Fig. 4). It was multilocular, and microscopic examination showed an endothelial lining and irregular bands of smooth muscle typical of cystic lymphangioma (Fig. 5). The patient had an uneventful recovery.

## DISCUSSION

In a comparison of the present series with the cases reported by Beahrs and associates[1] it is interesting to note that although more cases of mesenteric, retroperitoneal, and omental cysts have more recently been seen at the same institution in a relatively shorter time, the incidence of chylous cysts among them has increased, probably because of the greater attention paid to the character of their content since their report. In Beahrs' series there were 9 cases among 174 abdominal cysts; the percentage was 5.1. Chylous cysts have made up 9.9 per cent of the abdominal cysts since that time. The over-all incidence of chylous cysts seen at the Mayo Clinic is 7.3 per cent.

The ages of the patients varied from 24 to 62 years in Beahrs' series, and from 8 months to 58 years in the present series. Both patients in Coursley's[5] report were girls less than 15 years of age. The ages of 4 patients in our group fell in this pediatric range; 4 were in the fourth decade, 1 in the fifth decade, and 3 in the sixth decade of life. Seven patients in the present series were females and 5 were males; in Beahrs' series 5 were females and 4 were males.

Table II shows the location and symptoms of chylous cysts in both series from the Mayo Clinic and in the series from the literature.

In 5 cases a chylous cyst was found incidentally while an operative procedure was being carried out for some other reason. In 1 case a mass was not noted until routine examination. In 6 cases the primary com-

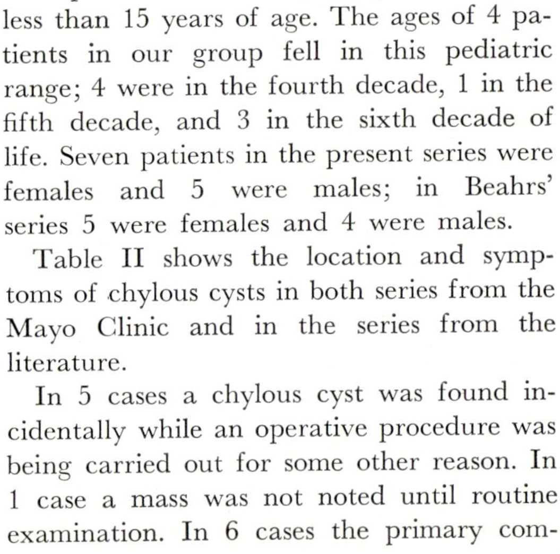

**Fig. 1.** Case 1. Prominent enlargement in upper and middle parts of abdomen is evident with patient in supine position.

plaint was increase in the size of the abdomen or the presence of an abdominal mass (Table II). Abdominal pain was reported in 3 cases. In Beahrs' series a chylous cyst was found incidentally in 1 case, while the primary complaint in 4 patients was an abdominal mass. Accompanying symptoms in all series included varying degrees of flatulence, constipation, dyspnea, and nausea. Chylous cysts developed subsequent to operation in 3 patients; pain was a symptom in 1 patient and a mass was noted on examination in the other 2 cases. Symptoms were similar in the cases of chylous cysts including those of the postoperative type reported in the literature.

Excision was the treatment of choice in 10 cases in the present series, marsupialization in 1 case, and percutaneous aspiration in 1 case (Table III). Treatment in Beahrs' series consisted of excision in 7 cases, marsupialization in 1 case, and drainage in 1 case. None of the patients were treated by marsupialization or drainage alone after 1950. The 1 patient treated by aspiration had undergone a Wertheim hysterectomy and pelvic lymphadenectomy 6 months previously. This was followed by the formation of a chylous cyst.

Further follow-up was available in 2 cases reported previously by Beahrs and associates.[1] One patient, a 37-year-old woman treated by marsupialization and drainage on 2 occasions, had not had a recurrence for 8 years and died of hypertensive cardiovascular disease and uremia. The other patient, a 58-year-old man treated by excision, lived for 8 years and died of bronchogenic carcinoma.

Two patients in the present series had recurrences which required additional operation (Cases 5 and 10); there were no deaths. Apparent recurrence and spontaneous rupture of a cyst occurred in a patient treated by marsupialization (Case 6). Seven years after operation he complained of a mass; treatment was conservative because the mass had disappeared by the time of his arrival at the clinic. Presumably the cyst had ruptured. The treatment of choice is

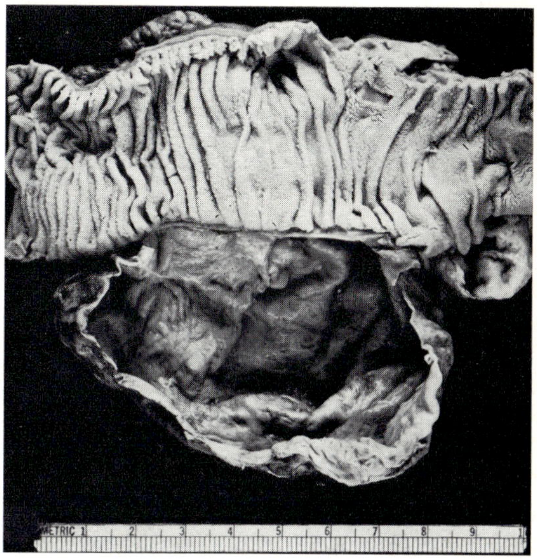


**Fig. 2.** Gross specimen of the segment of ileum which was surgically excised from a 5-year-old girl. Note the large loculus which overshadows the smaller spaces present in this cystic mesenteric chylangioma.

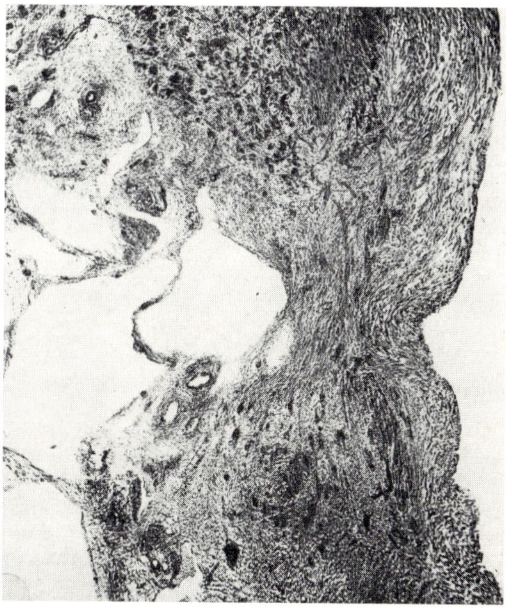

**Fig. 3.** Wall of the cystic chylangioma which was surgically excised. Only a portion of the large loculus is seen on the right; a few spaces of cystic lymphangioma, which are also lined with endothelium, are seen on the left. Smooth muscle fibers were found in the wall. (Hematoxylin and eosin; ×30.)

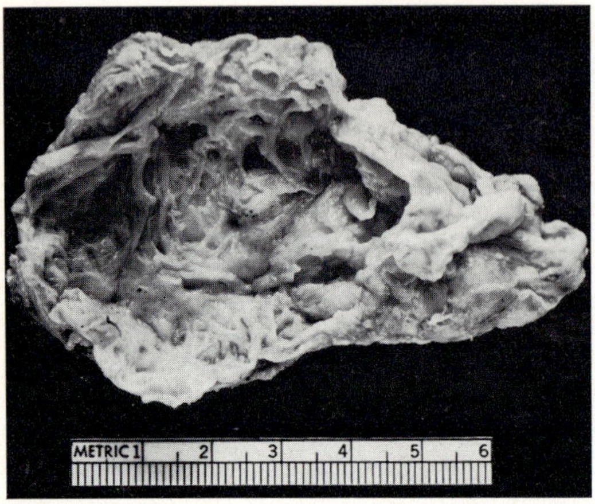


**Fig. 4.** Case 2. Gross surgical specimen shows opened large loculus of cystic lymphangioma. Note trabeculated wall.

**Table II.** *Location and symptoms of chylous cysts*

| | *Mayo Clinic series* | | *Series from literature* |
|---|---|---|---|
| | *Present series* | *Previous series** | |
| *Location* | | | |
| Mesentery of small intestine | 4 | 5 | 2 |
| Retroperitoneum | 4 | 2 | 10 |
| Mesentery of colon | 1 | 0 | 1 |
| Iliac region | 3 | 0 | 79 |
| Pancreas | 0 | 0 | 1 |
| Omentum | 0 | 2 | 0 |
| Not stated | 0 | 2 | 1 |
| *Symptoms†* | | | |
| Mass | 6 | 6 | 9 |
| Pain | 3 | 4 | 5 |
| Diarrhea | 0 | 1 | 0 |
| Nausea and vomiting | 0 | 1 | 0 |
| Constipation | 1 | 1 | 0 |
| Incidental finding | 5 | 1 | 3 |

*Beahrs and associates, 9 cases; Coursley and associates, 2 cases.

†These symptoms do not include those in the 79 cases of postoperative lymphocysts.

excision, either intact or after decompression, if the former method is not technically feasible. There were no instances of any difficulty ensuing because of rupture of cysts and spillage of chyle into the peritoneal cavity, nor did chylous ascites occur after excision. The recurrence rate was not increased in cases in which rupture of the cyst occurred during excision. Usually drains are not necessary.

There may be difficulty in determining the etiology and, therefore, in defining a classification for certain cystic lesions of the abdomen, particularly chylous cysts, partly because of the lack of any large series available for review. In considering the etiology, Beahrs and associates[1] pointed out that all cystic lesions which contain chylous fluid are not of single origin. Some are preformed or developmental anomalies, some have a traumatic origin, others may result from infection, and some may arise from neoplasia. The size of the cysts may vary from several centimeters to those so large that they fill the entire abdominal cavity or retroperitoneal space. They may be unilocular or multilocular and the lining will depend on the etiology. The content of the cyst is not a reliable means of ascertaining the origin of a chylous cyst because various circumstances may alter the content. Admittedly, there has been little if any attempt to characterize the contents of chylous cysts. Hemorrhage and inflammation in the cyst are common. Cholesterol clefts, fatty degeneration, and foam cells are seen occasionally.

The chylous cysts in 4 cases reported by Beahrs and co-workers[1] were classified as congenital or developmental. In addition, 2 were acquired, 1 was a lymphangioma, and 2 were malignant lymphangioendotheliomas. Of the 2 cysts reported by Coursley and associates,[5] 1 was a lymphangioma and the other was an acquired cyst.

In the 12 cases in the present series, 9 lesions were considered to be cystic lymphangiomas and 3 were acquired cysts which developed after Wertheim hysterectomies.

In the cases reported in the literature there were 24 retroperitoneal lymphangiomas of which 10 were chylous, 2 were lymphangiomas of the abdominal cavity, 81 were acquired chylous cysts, and 1 was a lymphangioma of the pancreas. The location of 1 cyst was not stated.

In the present series, the predominant

**Table III.** *Chylous cysts: treatment and results*

| Treatment | Present series | Previous series* | Recurrence |
|---|---|---|---|
| Excision | 10 | 7 | 0 |
| Marsupialization | 1 | 1 | 1 |
| Enucleation | 0 | 2 | 0 |
| Drainage | 0 | 1 | 1 |
| Percutaneous aspiration | 1 | 0 | 0 |

*Beahrs and associates, 9 cases; Coursley and associates, 2 cases.

pathologic finding of chylangioma is of interest. According to Ewing,[6] a chylangioma is a cavernous lymphangioma which contains a milky fluid. The chylangiomas found closely resembled cystic lymphangiomas (hygromas) seen in other parts of the body, such as those in the cervicomediastinum, but differed from them in the character of their contents. However, the etiology and pathogenesis of chylangioma are apparently similar to those of other cystic lymphangiomas and these lesions may arise from congenital sequestrations of the lymphatic system which may undergo cyst formation even in later life.

Rauch[10] recently reviewed the literature on retroperitoneal lymphangioma and found 20 cases reported to which he added 2 of his own. Eight of the lesions were chylous. These are also usually seen as unilocular or multilocular masses and are thought to be derived from congenitally misplaced lymphatic tissues rather than from obstruction of existing lymphatic channels. Raszkowski and associates[9] pointed out that there are 2 types of intra-abdominal lymphangiomas; the majority are unilocular or dumbbell in shape and the treatment of choice is simple excision. The other, less frequent, type is a multicystic lesion which is thought to invade by endothelial sprouting and has a high rate of recurrence.

Of the 9 cystic chylangiomas in the present study, 4 occurred in children and were grossly multilocular. Two of the 4 patients

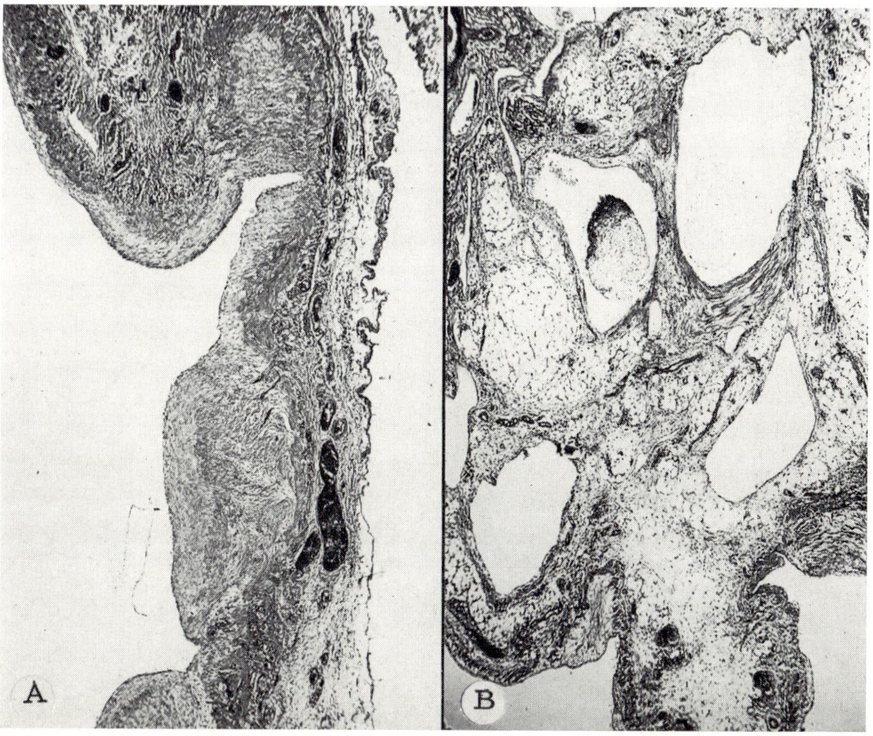


**Fig. 5.** *A*, Section of a large chylous loculus which was lined by endothelium and contained smooth muscle in its wall. *B*, Smaller loculi of typical cystic lymphangioma in same specimen as in Fig. 4. (Hematoxylin and eosin; ×30.)

had recurrent formation of cysts after operation. Only 1 required an additional surgical procedure and the cyst in the other apparently ruptured spontaneously.

The 5 cystic chylangiomas in adults were grossly unilocular, although careful microscopic examination of the wall usually revealed a few additional intramural lymphangiomatous spaces. None of the patients had an apparent postoperative recurrence. In all cystic chylangiomas an endothelial lining could be demonstrated. Smooth muscle in the cyst walls was seen as irregular, incomplete, thin bands and was similar to that found in cystic lymphangiomas in other locations in the body. Occasionally a small focal deposition of lymphocytes was noted in the wall of a cyst. The cysts had variable amounts of fibroadipose tissue from the retroperitoneum or mesentery in their walls.

The manner in which chyle accumulates in some intra-abdominal cystic lymphangiomas remains unclear. Whether this chylous fluid is derived through the return of chyle from the intestine and deposition within obstructive lymphangiomatous spaces, whether it accumulates predominantly as a transudate, or whether it results from a change in the composition of contained lymph cannot be categorically stated. Lymphangiography may prove of value in demonstrating any intestinal lymphatic or other communications with cystic chylangiomas.

All 3 chylous cysts which developed after Wertheim hysterectomy apparently were unilocular and arose in the region of the left iliac lymphadenectomy. Removal was followed by recurrence in only 1 case. The fibrous wall was available for examination in 2 cases. These cysts lacked an endothelial lining in addition to the bands of smooth muscle noted in the cystic chylangiomas. Occasionally, however, traumatic cysts may be partially lined by endothelium. Such cysts appear to arise from accumulations of lymph from lymphatics which are interrupted surgically in the course of radical dissection of pelvic lymph nodes or they may result from degenerative change in liquefying hematomas. Again, the nature of their content has not been accurately specified. Nelson and Houston[7] recently reviewed the literature and found a total of 77 similar cases, to which they added 2. They quoted Gray's series of 9 cases, which followed postoperative roentgen treatment, and Mori's series of 68 cases. The incidence of postoperative recurrence in these 2 series of cases was cited as 16.3 per cent and 48.5 per cent. Spontaneous regression was thought to occur in the majority of these cysts, and this may account for the low incidence in the present series.

## SUMMARY

In 316 cases of abdominal cysts seen at the Mayo Clinic between 1911 and 1959 there were 23 cases of chylous cysts, an incidence of 7.3 per cent, 11 of which were reported previously.

In the 12 new cases which are reported, 9 patients were considered to have chylous cystic lymphangiomas (chylangiomas) and 3 had acquired chylous cysts which developed subsequent to Wertheim hysterectomy.

Abdominal masses, noted in 8 cases, or pain and discomfort of some type were the most frequently encountered findings in these patients. Five patients were completely asymptomatic.

Chylous cysts may occur at any age and in either sex.

The results obtained predominantly favor excision as the treatment of choice. Of the 9 patients with cystic chylangiomas, 4 were children and 5 were adults. In the children the lesions were grossly multilocular; 2 were symptomatically recurrent, although only 1 required additional surgical attention because the other cyst apparently ruptured spontaneously. In the 5 adults all of the cysts were grossly essentially unilocular and did not recur postoperatively.

All 3 acquired chylous cysts developed after the patients had undergone Wertheim hysterectomy and all were located in the region of the previous left iliac lymphadenectomy. Temporization may be indicated in cases in which a chylous cyst develops after pelvic lymphadenectomy, since spontaneous regression may occur, although in persistent cases excision is the treatment of choice.

## REFERENCES

1. Beahrs, O. H., Judd, E. S., Jr., and Dockerty, M. B.: Chylous cysts of the abdomen, S. Clin. North America 1081, 1950.
2. Braquehaye, J.: Des kystes du Mésentère, Arch. gén. de méd. **170:** 291, 1892.
3. Burnett, W. E., Rosemond, G. P., and Bucher, R. M.: Mesenteric cysts: report of three cases, in one of which a calcified cyst was present, Arch. Surg. **60:** 699, 1950.
4. Corrao, F. H., and Loyudice, F.: Quiste quilifero de mesenterio, Prensa méd. argent. **45:** 2299, 1958.
5. Coursley, G., Hallenbeck, G. A., and Bernatz, P. E.: Clinically significant primary omental cysts: report of two cases, Proc. Staff Meet. Mayo Clin. **31:** 373, 1956.
6. Ewing, J.: Neoplastic diseases: a treatise on tumors, Philadelphia, 1928, W. B. Saunders Company, ed. 3, p. 254.
7. Nelson, J. H., Jr., and Houston, J. W.: Lymphocyst formation following pelvic lymphadenectomy, Am. J. Obst. & Gynec. **78:** 1298, 1959.
8. Pack, G. T., Trinidad, S. S., and Lisa, J. R.: Rare primary somatic tumors of the pancreas, A. M. A. Arch. Surg. **77:** 1000, 1958.
9. Raszkowski, H. J., Rehbock, D. J., and Cooper, F. G.: Mesenteric and retroperitoneal lymphangioma, Am. J. Surg. **97:** 363, 1959.
10. Rauch, R. F.: Retroperitoneal lymphangioma, A. M. A. Arch. Surg. **78:** 45, 1959.
11. Simon, H. E., and Williamson, B.: Retroperitoneal chylous cysts, Am. J. Surg. **91:** 372, 1956.
12. Slocum, M. A.: Surgical treatment of chylous mesenteric cyst by marsupialization, Am. J. Surg. **41:** 464, 1938.
13. Walker, J. C., and Cooper, J. A.: Lymphangioma of the mesentery of the ileum, Brit. J. Surg. **47:** 104, 1959.

# A procedure to prevent reflux after esophagogastric resection: experience with 17 patients

J. L. LORTAT-JACOB, M.D.
J. N. MAILLARD, M.D.
F. FEKETE, M.D.
PARIS, FRANCE
*From the Department of Surgery, Tenon Hospital, and Faculty of Medicine, University of Paris*

Operative techniques currently in use for reconstruction after esophagogastrectomy often prove unsatisfactory because they are complicated in the postoperative period by severe peptic esophagitis. This report describes a new procedure designed to produce a competent esophagogastric anastomosis which prevents reflux. The aim of this operative procedure is to create a valve mechanism by the implantation of esophagus into the stomach in such manner that intragastric pressure mechanically closes the esophageal lumen. A perfect apposition of the mucosa of the esophagus to that of the stomach eliminates secondary stricture. For this reason, the anastomosis, which is buried, must be very wide. To insure this, the esophagus is anastomosed to the stomach at the site of gastric transection; it is not merely implanted as in Sweet's operation.

## OPERATIVE TECHNIQUE

The operative procedure is carried out by means of a left thoracotomy through the bed of the seventh or eighth rib. After excision of the lower esophagus and the fundus of the stomach, the anastomosis is constructed at the left half of the open end of the stomach at the site of gastric transsection. Three successive rows of seromuscular sutures are placed between esophagus and stomach. Abrasion of the serosa to be apposed is carried out in order to obtain better adhesion of esophagus to stomach (Fig. 1). The first row of sutures is placed 4 to 5 cm. proximal to the clamp on the esophagus and at the same distance from the posterior edge of the site of gastric transsection. Four sutures are necessary on an average for each of these rows. After the 3 suture rows are placed, the muscular wall of the esophagus is incised, and an additional line of sutures between the muscular coat of esophagus and stomach is made. Finally, the mucosa of the esophagus is sectioned and the mucosae of stomach and esophagus are approximated edge-to-edge with the final row of sutures. It is now apparent that the posterior lip of the anastomosis protrudes well into the gastric lumen (Fig. 2). The anterior layer of the anastomosis is constructed in similar but reverse fashion (Fig. 3). A mucosal suture line is followed by a second row of sutures between the muscularis of stomach and esophagus, which is followed in turn by 3 inverting rows of sutures. The greater curvature of the stomach inverts with ease anteriorly. The gastric wall is less abundant, however, and 2 inverting rows and sometimes only 1 are possible here.

The right portion of the opened end of the stomach is now closed in 2 layers and the inversion is continued between the left side of the esophagus and the gastric wall. All layers are sutured with No. 1-0 nylon by means of a curved needle. When completed, the anastomosis resembles the protrusion of the cervix into the vagina, having the aspect of a "fish mouth." It is surrounded by a cul-de-sac of stomach wall 4

Received for publication Nov. 18, 1960.

to 5 cm. deep posteriorly and 1 to 2 cm. anteriorly.

The stomach is then sutured to mediastinal pleura in order to prevent tension on the anastomosis during the period of healing. The diaphragm is closed around the stomach and the thoracotomy closed after catheter drainage. It is essential that a long extramucosal pyloromyotomy be carried out before construction of the anastomosis is begun.

## EXPERIMENTAL OBSERVATIONS

These experiments were carried out with human autopsy material. The esophagus, stomach, and first portion of the duodenum from 10 fresh autopsy specimens were utilized. A short gastroesophageal resection was carried out, and reconstruction performed as described. A "control" preparation was made according to the procedure described by Sweet. The patency and continence of the anastomosis were then stud-

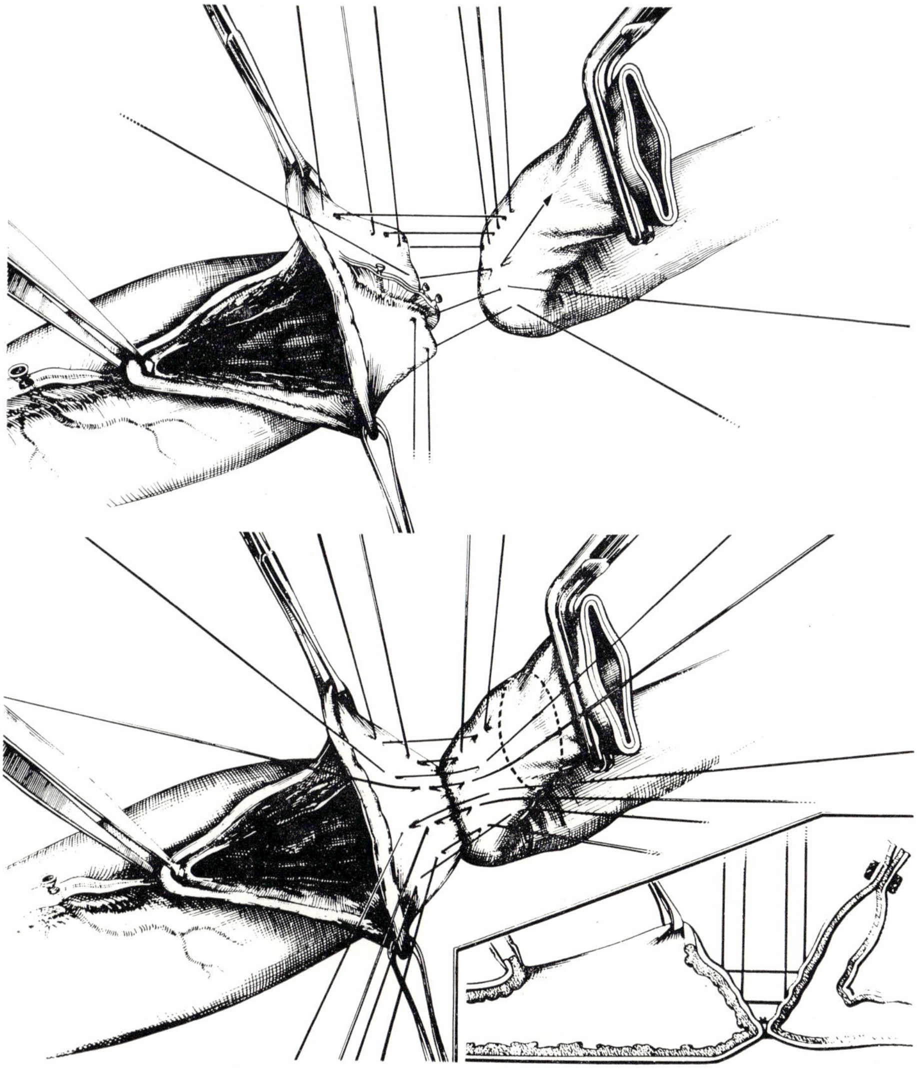

*A*

*B*

**Fig. 1.** *A,* Three posterior muscular rows of sutures. *B,* The first row is knotted. The section of the esophagus is shown by the dotted lines.

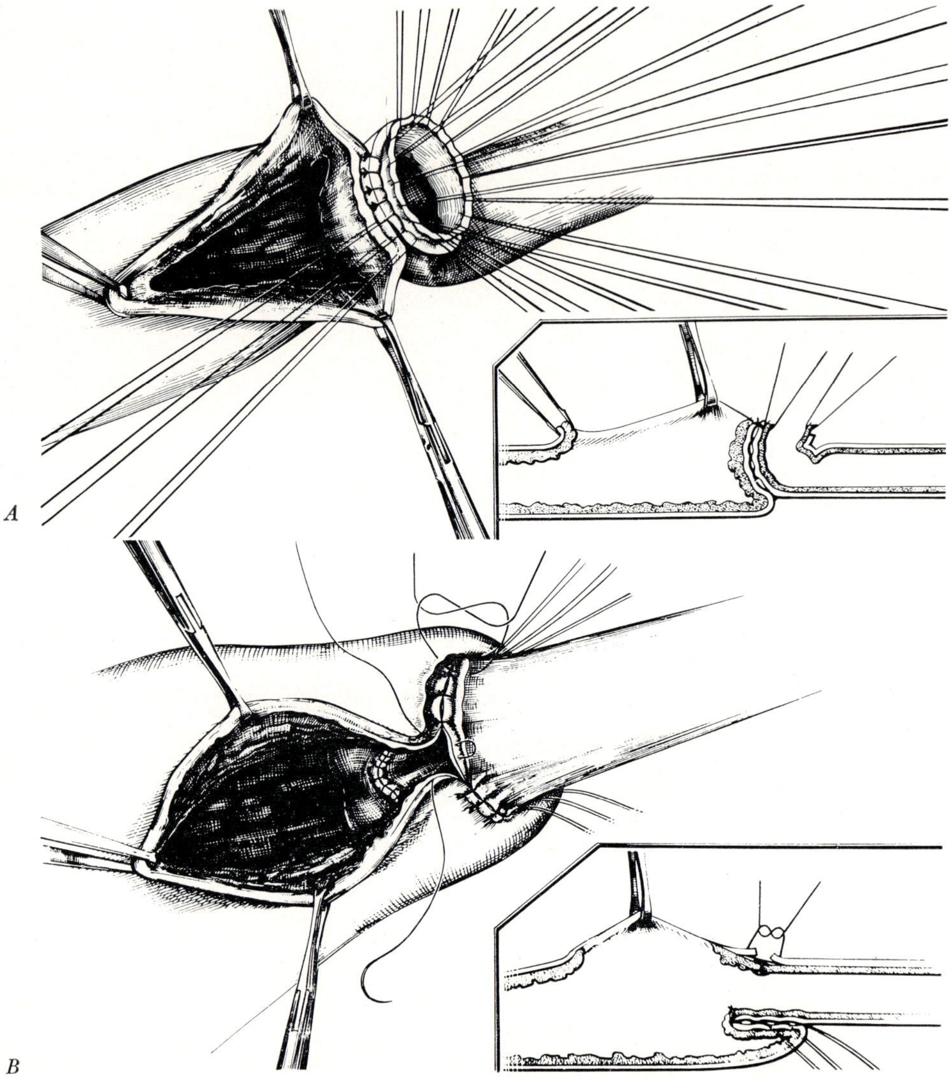

**Fig. 2.** *A,* Musculomuscular posterior layer. All the stitches are already threaded. *B,* The end of the mucomucous anterior layer, with the U point. One can see the bulging of the posterior lip of the anastomosis.

ied. The anastomosis proved to be widely patent. A large proctoscope could be introduced easily by manipulation from the esophagus into the stomach. Barium passed easily also.

The anastomosis proved to be competent, in most cases immediately after its completion, whereas a preparation made according to Sweet's description showed spontaneous reflux into the esophagus when water was introduced into the stomach. When slight manual pressure was applied, the reflux became massive. In the first 3 preparations constructed as we described, the inverting surfaces representing a papilla about 5 to 6 cm. in length, competence was found to be complete with regard to both liquid and gas even when strong manual pressure was applied to the stomach.

An attempt was made to determine just how much inversion was necessary to give the correct degree of competence. A preparation with an inversion of 1 cm. proved to be incompetent; another with an inversion of 2 cm. proved to be imperfectly competent for liquids. Two preparations with inversions of 2.5 and 3 cm. proved to be perfectly competent for liquids, but gas passed readily through under slight pressure. Two preparations with inversions of 3.5 and 4 cm. were found to be perfectly competent with regard to both liquid and gas, even under pressure (Fig. 4). We therefore believed that papillary implantation of the esophagus into the stomach with creation of a cul-de-sac around the anastomosis 3 to 4 cm. deep posteriorly and 1 to 2 cm. in front was satisfactory to prevent reflux. Any gastric pressure greater than the esophageal pressure would serve to close the valve. Thus encouraged, we have utilized this procedure during the past 2 years for 17 patients.[6, 11]

## CLINICAL OBSERVATIONS AND INDICATIONS

The patients to be described were treated exclusively for histologically benign diseases of the cardioesophageal area, namely ulcers and peptic strictures of the esophagus, esophageal varices, and megaesophagus (Table I). We have deliberately not utilized this operation in patients with malignancies. The extent of excision necessary, frequent lack of gastric acidity, and frequency of short survivals of patients with malignant disease make postoperative esophagitis less common in patients who have been operated upon for malignant tumors of gastroesophageal area. It was decided therefore, that benign lesions of the esophagus offered the best test of the operative procedure.

**Ulcers and benign strictures of the esophagus.** Some of the more limited lesions of the lower esophagus are no doubt suitable for subdiaphragmatic reposition of the cardia and local plastic operations. Out of a total of 41 patients with peptic diseases of the esophagus who have been treated surgically, 13 consecutive operations were performed, especially in older and weaker patients. The results of these operations are too frequently mediocre. Esophagogastric resection is, therefore, preferred when conditions permit it. In fact, it is often necessary for lesions which are extensive or located high, such as short esophagus or endobrachyesophagus.[10, 12] We agree with Resano that proximal gastrectomy, which in effect creates a short esophagus surgically, is not a sound procedure. Out of 10 esophagogastrectomies carried out according to the technique of Sweet, we have observed 4 patients with severe reflux esophagitis. On the contrary, higly satisfactory results have been attained with the competent anastomoses described. Out of 7 patients treated by this method, 6 made complete recoveries with no clinical or radiologic evidence of reflux esophagitis. The seventh patient died of respiratory insufficiency from atelectasis of the left lung and a right pneumothorax.

**Case 1.** P. O. U., a 62-year-old woman, had complained for a period of 1 year of thoracic pain, dysphagia, regurgitation, and hiccuping. Radiographs and esophagoscopy had shown a stricture and ulceration of the lower esophagus (Fig. 5). Radiocinematography confirmed this finding. The patient was operated upon on March

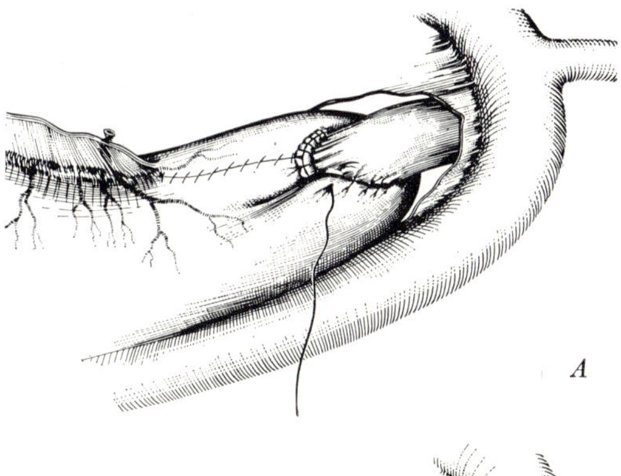

*A*

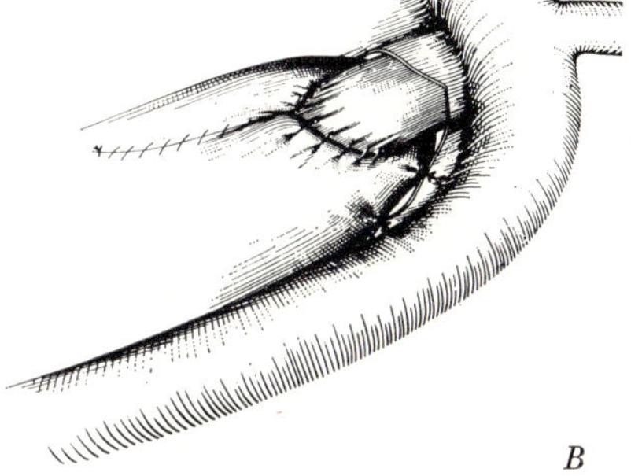

*B*

**Fig. 3.** *A*, Anterior seromuscular layer and *B*, anastomosis completed.

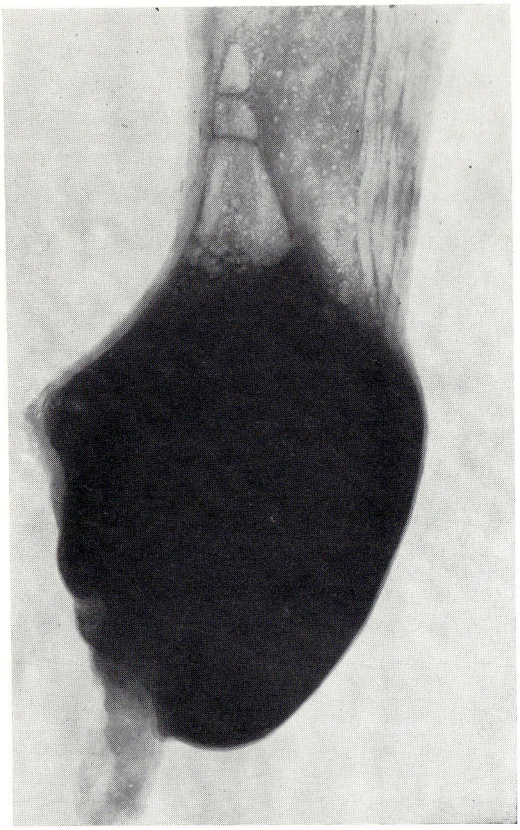

**Fig. 4.** Experimental specimen. The anastomosis is at the bottom. The stomach has been filled with barium. None of the material passes into the esophagus.

22, 1958. Thoracotomy demonstrated a brachyesophagus with stricture. It was believed that a resection of the esophagus was indicated. The specimen removed showed brachyesophagus with stenosing esophagitis. The repair was carried out according to the technique described for a competent anastomosis. The patient's postoperative course was very satisfactory. Two months after the operative procedure, the patient experienced slight dysphagia during ingestion of large pieces of solid food. This was treated symptomatically and dilatation was not necessary. It was found that the largest esophageal catheter passed easily through the anastomosis. Radiograms have confirmed the ease of passage and absence of reflux, although the patient does have frequent gaseous regurgitation. She subsequently was seen in 1959 and was asymptomatic at that time (Figs. 6 and 7).

**Megaesophagus.** Although the Heller operation remains the best possible operative treatment for spasm of the cardia, some failures are associated with its application. These are often caused by inadequate myotomy, and subsequent myotomy will be successful. Nonetheless, a certain percentage of true failures occurs after the best possible myotomy and in these patients, it is believed that esophagogastric resection is necessary.

Failure of the Heller operation can even be predicted before operation in some patients, such as those with an exaggeratedly dilated esophagus occupying the entire mediastinum or one which is bent in large sigmoid loops and is overstretched and irrecuperable. Since cardioplasty has been shown to be followed in many instances by disastrous postoperative results, we believe that a resection is indicated in these patients. If a procedure which produces a competent anastomosis can be carried out and reflux esophagitis prevented, the application of esophagogastrectomy in these instances should be feasible.

Our experience has been with 5 patients treated by esophagogastrectomy with competent anastomosis for megaesophagus. Of these patients, 4 had undergone a Heller operation previously which was followed by recurrence of the symptoms. In addition to mega esophagus, 1 of the 4 patients had a cancer. The fifth patient underwent initial proximal gastrectomy with competent anastomosis for enormous megadolichoesophagus. Because of esophageal atony, 2 of the 5 patients still complain of slight thoracic oppressiveness during meals without actual dysphagia or regurgitation. The progression of food is slowed down by the lack of peristalsis. However, one of the advantages of esophagogastric resection for megaesophagus lies in the shortening of the megadolichoesophagus, thus allowing quicker descent of the food into the stomach.

**Case 2.** Since 1940, B. A. S., a 60-year-old woman, had complained of epigastric pains, dysphagia, and regurgitation as a consequence of megaesophagus. In April, 1958, the Heller operation was carried out through an abdominal approach with resection of a longitudinal ribbon

**Table I.** *Esophagogastrectomy with competent anastomosis*

| *Indications* | *No. of cases* | *Recoveries* | *Postoperative reflux* | *Postoperative complications* | *Deaths* |
|---|---|---|---|---|---|
| Ulcer and peptic stricture of esophagus | 7 | 6 | 0 | 2 pneumothorax with recovery, 1 stricture by unfolding of invagination with recovery after reoperation | Pneumothorax and atelectasis |
| Megaesophagus | 5 | 3 | * | — | Cardiorespiratory insufficiency |
| Esophageal and gastric varices | 5 (2 extrahepatic block, 3 cirrhosis) | 4 (2 extrahepatic block, 2 cirrhosis) | 0 | 1 right pneumothorax | Hepatic coma |

*Cancer was superimposed on megaesophagus.

of the muscular layer of the esophagus over 8 to 10 cm. in length. At the end of the operation, the esophagus ruptured completely on the tape, separating from the cardia. Reanastomosis was performed in 1 layer, and the postoperative course was not remarkable. However, dysphagia persisted with dyspnea, anxiety, tachycardia, and stifling sensations when food passed. Radiograph showed the persistence of the dolichomegaesophagus without peristaltic contractions (Fig. 8). It was believed that another attempt at a Heller myotomy would be doomed to failure. The patient was operated upon again in November, 1958, at which time proximal esophagogastrectomy with competent anastomosis was carried out. Operative exploration showed that the preceding anastomosis was supple and wide, admitting the forefinger. The esophagogastric resection with excision of 3 cm. of the fundus was carried out, after which a competent anastomosis approximately 4 cm. in diameter was constructed by the technique described. At the end of the operative procedure, the stomach was inflated with air through a catheter passed through the anastomosis. Competence of the anastomosis appeared perfect. The catheter was left in situ. No pyloromyotomy was carried out. The patient was subsequently seen in March, 1959, at which time she had gained 22 pounds. This time she did not have dysphagia, showed no symptoms of reflux, and eructations were possible. Epigastric discomfort was, however, present and there was radiographic evidence of spasm of the pylorus. Subsequent to this time, we have added a pyloromyotomy as part of the operative procedure. In November, 1959, the patient had no digestive complaint and considered herself as completely recovered. Roentgenogram demonstrated a wide anastomosis (Fig. 9), and complete absence of reflux in the Trendelenburg position. Barium could be seen to outline the contours of the esophageal papilla (Fig. 10).

**Esophageal varices.** The operation is justified under these circumstances by the fact that these varicose veins are not, in reality, the spontaneous portacaval esophagocardiac anastomoses that they have been said to be. Such anastomoses do exist, but they lie below the varicosities. The varicosities themselves are submucous and the anastomoses are intramuscular. The varicose veins

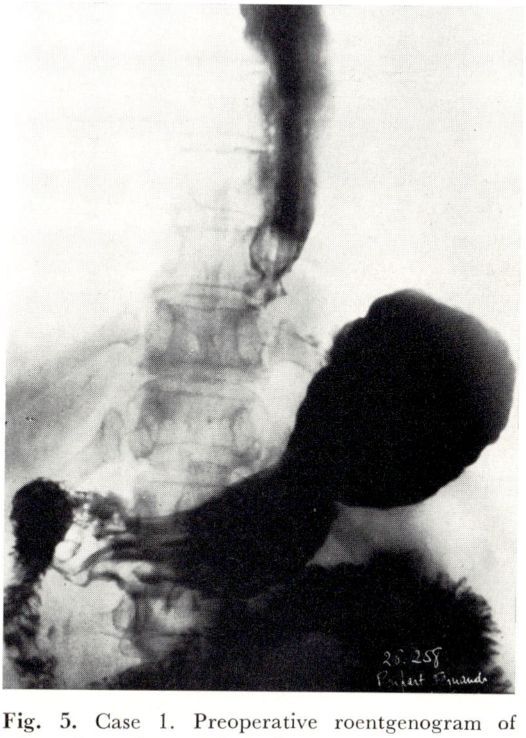

**Fig. 5.** Case 1. Preoperative roentgenogram of ulcerative stricture of esophagus.

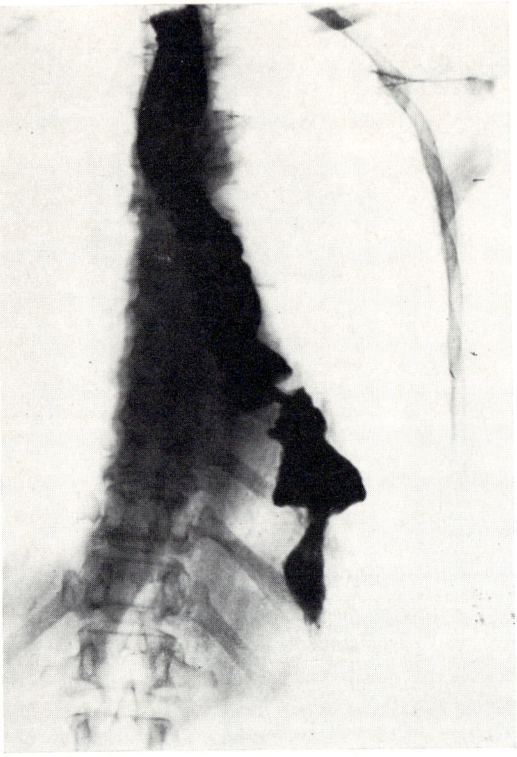

**Fig. 6.** Case 1. Roentgenogram taken 6 months after operation shows easy passage through anastomosis.

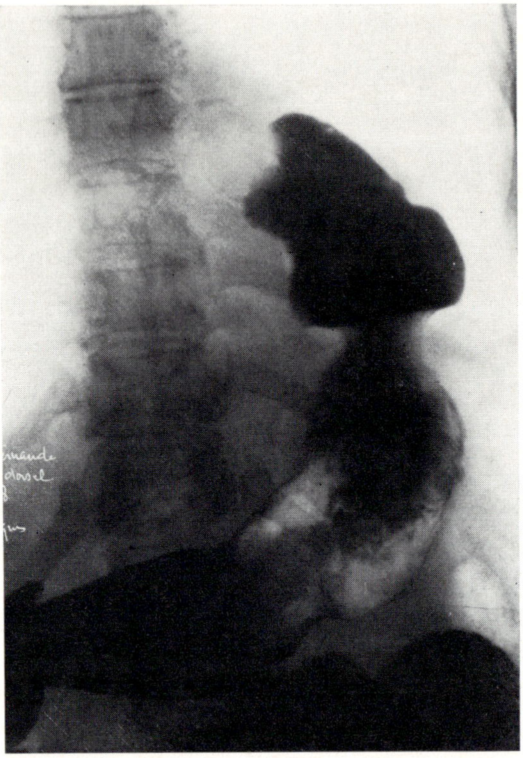

**Fig. 7.** Case 1. Six months after operation (Trendelenburg position) after esophageal lavage. There is no reflux. The bulging of the anastomosis into the stomach is clearly seen.

are actually nothing but ectasias of the finer submucous branches, truly nonfunctional venous cul-de-sacs.

The procedure of competent anastomosis described may be of value, insofar as it causes an increase in intragastric pressure which opposes the thoracic negative pressure which has been suggested to be responsible in part for the genesis of esophageal varicose veins. Reflux is also prevented and the risk of new hemorrhages by peptic ulceration of the remaining or relapsing varices is avoided without the disadvantage of total gastrectomy as proposed by Baronofsky.[3]

Proximal gastrectomy thus appears to be indicated for this disease under several conditions. Since compression by a balloon catheter usually permits a temporary cessation of hemorrhage, it is usually not applicable in instances of acute bleeding. In instances of secondary hemorrhage occurring as soon as the compressing tamponade has been released, however, the operation can be carried out. It is to be preferred to transesophageal ligation of the veins when this is carried out as the definitive operation (portacaval anastomosis impossible). The ultimate results after this operation appear to be much better, as indicated by the comparative statistics. In a collected group of 113 patients with transesophageal vein ligations (statistics of Boerema, Crile, Hamilton, Hsu, Linton, Longmire, Ludington, Marion and Desgouttes, and Roy-Cohn), there were 44 deaths and 69 survivals. Among the patients surviving, 20 experienced secondary hemorrhage and there were 28 recoveries. Twenty-three patients were secondarily treated by portacaval anastomosis. After 66 proximal gastrectomies for this condition, there were 12 deaths (18 per cent), 3 secondary deaths, and 51 recoveries (77.5 per cent). In addition to its use as described for emergency situations, proximal gastrectomy is indicated when portacaval anastomosis is impossible. For example, when there is recurrence of hemorrhage after splenectomy or splenorenal anastomosis previously performed for extrahepatic portal vein obstruction, the operation can be utilized.

**Case 3.** R. I. N., was a 17-year-old girl who developed a first hematemesis in October, 1958. Splenomegaly was discovered at this time and splenoportogram showed reflux through the gastric and esophageal veins and the absence of a portal vein trunk (Fig. 11). The patient was operated upon on March 12, 1958, at which time a splenorenal anastomosis was carried out. Postoperatively the patient did well until hematemesis occurred in June, 1959, at which time varicose veins were again demonstrated radiologically (Fig. 12). Because of succeeding hematemesis, proximal gastrectomy was decided upon. The patient was operated upon on June 11, 1959. Operation was carried out through the bed of the eighth left rib. Approximately 4 cm. of the esophagus in addition to the fundus of the stomach was resected, and competent anastomosis was carried out. The operative specimen showed numerous varicose veins under the esophageal mucous membrane. The patient was seen 6 months postoperatively and had no complaints at that time. There was no dysphagia or reflux and eructations were possible. A radiograph showed no varicose veins and continence was perfect. The patient had not had subsequent hemorrhages (Figs. 13 and 14).

In our opinion, some patients with cirrhosis seem to be benefited more by upper pole gastrectomy than by portacaval anastomosis; for example, those with associated moderate portal hypertension. Here, as with all such shunts, the portacaval anastomosis can become thrombosed and, moreover, in this circumstance a notable degree of hepatic perfusion still exists by way of the

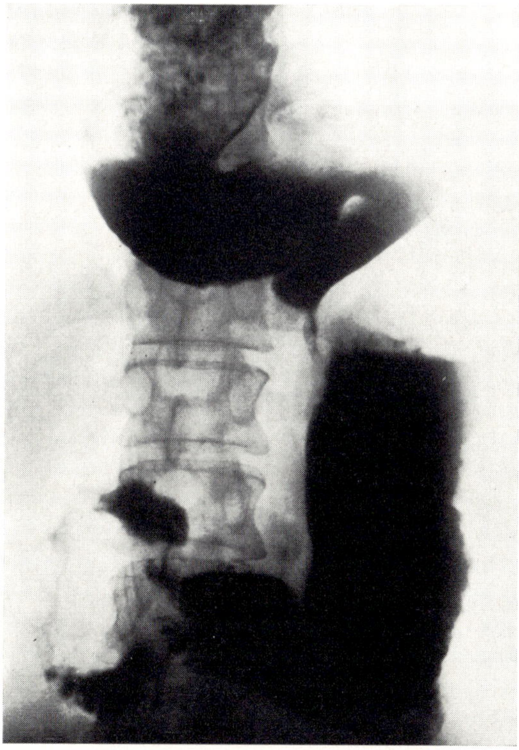

**Fig. 8.** Case 2. Preoperative roentgenogram of dolichomegaesophagus and esophageal stenosis which persisted after Heller operation.

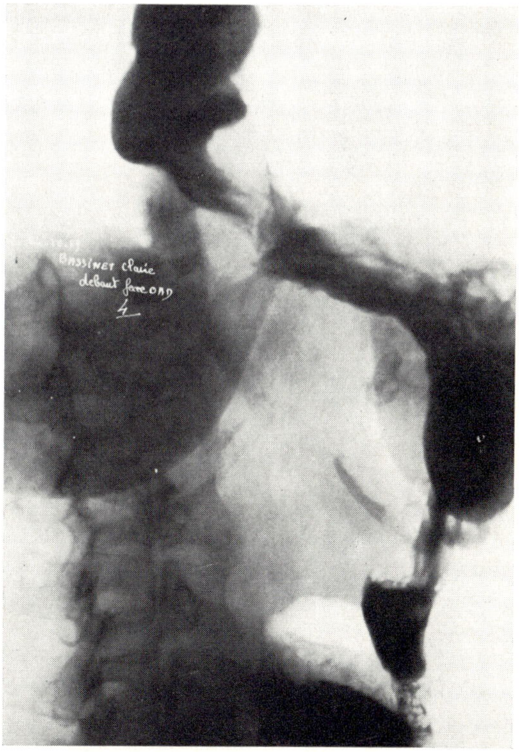

**Fig. 9.** Case 2. Roentgenogram taken 1 year after operation shows good passage through anastomosis. The esophageal caliber is quite normal.

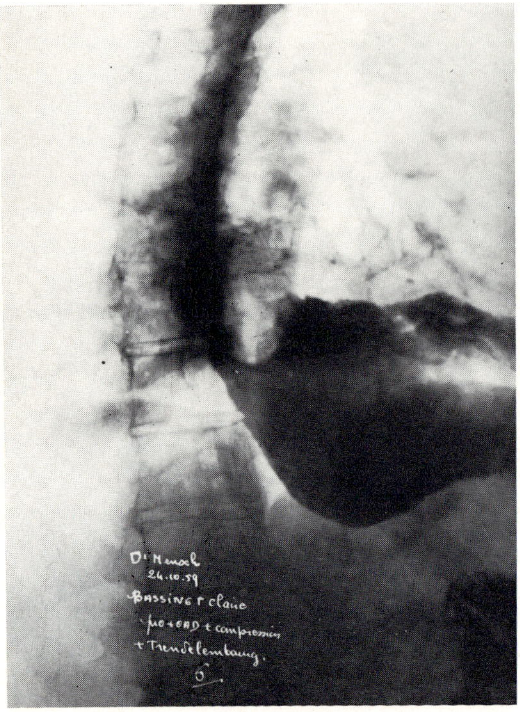

**Fig. 10.** Case 2. Roentgenogram taken 1 year after operation shows no reflux. There is neat bulging of anastomosis into gastric lumen.

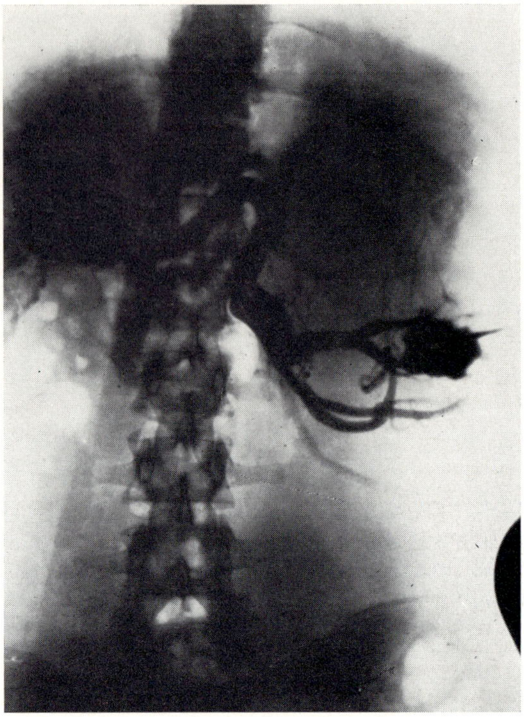

**Fig. 11.** Case 3. Cavernomatous transformation of the vena cava, with portal hypertension and esophageal varices.

portal vein and this should be retained. Also, it appears preferable in situations associated with psychiatric disorders, enabling one to see that an encephalopathy may ensue after a venous anastomosis.

Three proximal gastric resections with competent anastomoses have been carried out for this condition with 2 successes and 1 death due to hepatic coma. It must not be denied that proximal gastrectomy for varicose veins due to portal hypertension is a serious operation, a difficult one, and one often complicated by severe hemorrhage. On 2 occasions we have been obliged to abandon this operation because of a vascular periesophageal barrier which proved insurmountable.

## DISCUSSION

It is not our purpose to claim priority in research for an antireflux type of anastomosis between esophagus and stomach. Numerous techniques have been proposed for this purpose. We have given these up after trial.

Removal of gastric-acid forming zone of the stomach and esophagoantral anastomosis and pylorotomy as proposed by Wangensteen[19, 20] has long been considered to be the most successful procedure and has given excellent results. However, it is sometimes complicated by postgastrectomy problems similar to those which follow total gastrectomy, and reflux may still occur with consequent esophagitis after this operation.

Higher esophagogastric anastomosis appears theoretically to be of value. However, out of 8 patients so treated by us, 1 had disruption of anastomosis, 1 had necrosis of the fundus of the stomach, and 4 developed peptic esophagitis.

We have not been enthusiastic about the esophagojejunal anastomosis with exclusion of the stomach on a Roux Y loop (Allison). Here the problems due to gastric exclusion and the severity of the immediate postop-

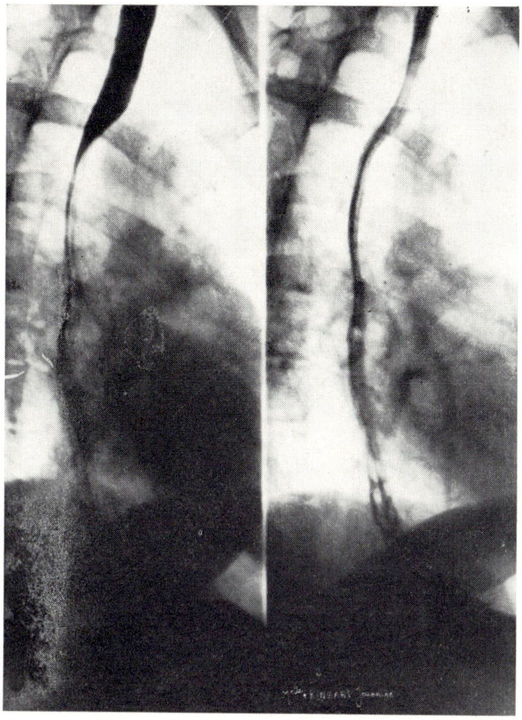

Fig. 12. Case 3. Roentgenograms which show failure of splenorenal anastomosis and reappearance of esophageal varices.

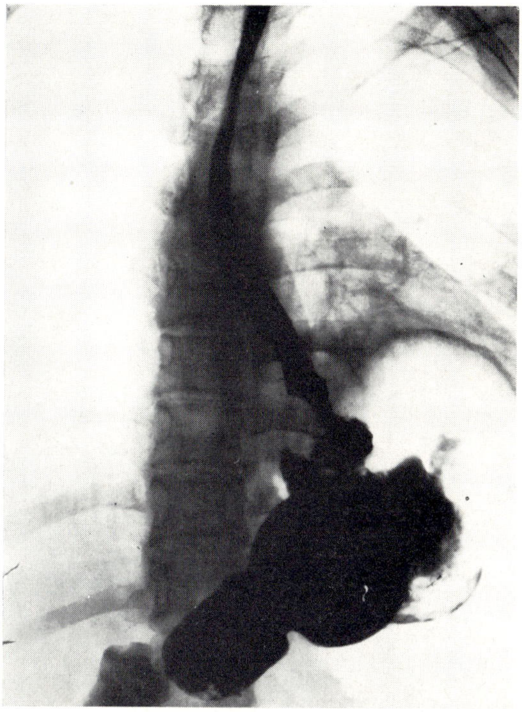

Fig. 13. Case 3. Roentgenogram taken 3 months after operation shows good passage through anastomosis. The gastric air pouch is voluminous.

erative course have led us to abandon this operation. Out of 3 patients so treated, 1 died, 1 developed esophagitis, and 1 recovered.

Interposition of an isolated loop of the small intestine between the esophagus and the stomach (Allison)[2, 4, 5, 8, 16, 18] is a serious operation and the risks of peptic jejunitis are very great. Of 3 patients so treated, 2 died and 1 developed an ulcerating hemorrhagic jejunitis in the loop. We have observed swelling and lengthening of such loops so that several reoperations were necessary to excise the extra small intestine. The use of transverse colon or ileocecum[13, 15, 17] for this purpose seems to have the same disadvantages.

Inadequacy of the various procedures led Kiriluk and Merendino[9] and Watkins[21] to suggest the building of a papilla by turning back the esophagus cut in bivalve fashion and fixing this cone into the stomach. Two clinical applications were reported by these authors, but no follow-up was given. Since 1954, no new mention of this procedure has been made to our knowledge. In any event, a cone of esophageal mucous membrane, continually bathed in gastric juice, seems to us to be inevitably doomed to peptic stenosis.

Along similar lines, Wooler[23] attempted on 3 occasions to bring the esophagus through a gastric tunnel. Adler[1] made a similar attempt and Frank[7] created a valve by invagination of a part of the fundus. The base of the invagination was closed by sutures, and the esophagogastric anastomosis was placed just in front of the gastric fold, so that the valve was applied to the opening when the intragastric pressure became higher.

Very recently, Watkins and associates[22] proposed a technique of circumferential esophagofundopexy, with the burying of the lower esophagus in the fundus, which is similar to the Witzel technique as has been

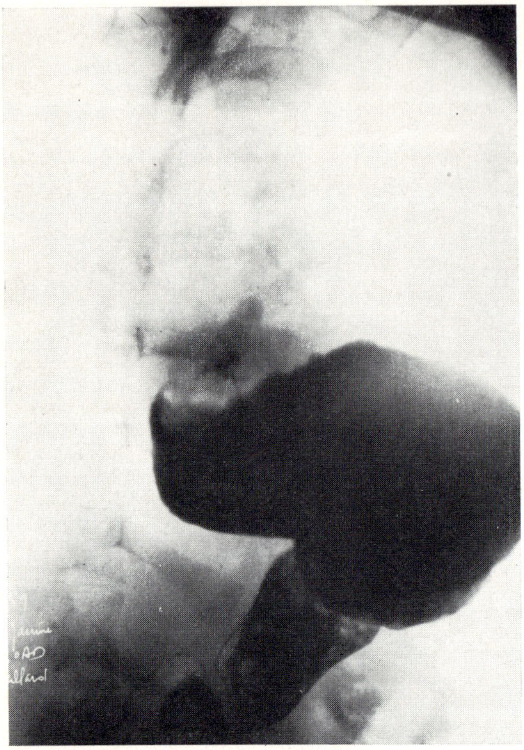

**Fig. 14.** Case 3. Roentgenogram taken 3 months after operation shows no gastroesophageal reflux.

used by Adler. No resection was carried out if the esophageal lesions were still discrete. The remainder of the operation was carried out in a manner similar to that proposed by Nissen[14] for hiatal hernia. In the case of an ulcer or esophageal stricture, Watkins and associates perform an esophageal resection, close the cardia, and reimplant the esophagus into the gastric antrum before burying it. The method, very comparable to the one we propose, seems to us to be a little more complex because of low implantation of the esophagus.

**Evaluation of the competent anastomosis.** It is necessary that there be 4 cm. of esophagus available to carry out the anastomosis correctly. The fact that the operation is utilized primarily for noncancerous lesions when resection can be reduced to a minimum limits this particular objection. The angle where the right edge of the esophagogastric implantation meets the line of gastric closure appears to be a weak point in the suture line. In actual fact, a U stitch and the esophagogastric inversion strengthen it sufficiently. It has caused no difficulty. A question may arise as to whether the mucous membrane of the esophagus thus implanted into the fundus will not be affected in the future by esophagitis and peptic stenosis. We believe that lack of clinical and radiologic evidence of reflux suggests that this will not occur. However, we have once observed stricture to occur without reflux. At a second operation, it was shown that the opening was initially too small and had been made even smaller by partial unfolding of the invagination. Abrasion of the gastric serosa at the time of placement of the sutures for inversion should make this complication avoidable.

Should excessive competence be feared? Our patients have never complained of it. Some of them have retained the capacity to eructate, and others have not noticed its disappearance. Care must be taken, however, to perform a good pylorotomy or pyloroplasty, in order to avoid gastric dilatation. This we have observed on 2 occasions because the precaution had not been taken.

**Advantages of the competent anastomosis.** The advantages can be summarized as (1) simplicity of procedure, (2) security of sutures, (3) smallness of gastric resection with remaining large reservoir essential to prevention of postoperative nutritional disorders, and (4) effectiveness in preventing reflux. Out of 17 patients operated upon, we have observed reflux only once. Although the period of follow-up is still too short to allow a definite judgment of this operative procedure, these few merits suggest the use of the competent anastomosis after all esophagogastric resections for noncancerous lesions.

## SUMMARY

An experience with 17 patients operated upon over a span of 2 years with the esophagogastric competent anastomosis is reported. This procedure, with implantation of the esophagus in the line of gastric transection, provides a valve which opposes reflux, but nevertheless allows easy passage of food through a wide anastomosis.

## REFERENCES

1. Adler, R. H.: A valve mechanism to prevent gastroesophageal reflux and esophagitis, Surgery **44:** 63, 1958.
2. Allison, P. R., Wooler, G. H., and Gunning, A. J.: Esophagojejunogastrostomy, J. Thoracic Surg. **33:** 738, 1957.
3. Baronofsky, I. D.: Portal hypertension with special reference to the acid-peptic factor in causation of hemorrhage and extensive gastric resection in its treatment, Surgery **25:** 135, 1949.
4. Dillard, D. H., and Merendino, K. A.: Experience with the interposed jejunal segment operation combined with adjunction procedures in prevention of esophagitis, S. Forum **41:** 323, 1954.
5. Ellis, F. M., Jr.: Experimental aspects of surgical treatment of reflux esophagitis and esophageal stricture, Ann. Surg. **143:** 465, 1956.
6. Fekete, F.: La gastrectomie polaire supérieure avec anastomose continente, Thèse, Paris, 1960.
7. Franke, H.: Sobre o problema da esofagite de refluxo apos ressecao do cardia, Rev. brasil. cir. **33:** 523, 1957.
8. Girvin, G. W., and Merendino, F. A.: Cardiac sphincter substitution by interposed jejunum, A. M. A. Arch. Surg. **72:** 241, 1956.
9. Kiriluk, F. B., and Merendino, K. A.: An experimental evaluation in the dog of esophagogastrectomy for the highlying gastric ulcer, Ann. Surg. **134:** 918, 1951.
10. Lortat-Jacob, J. L.: L'endo-brachy-oesophage, Semaine hôp. Ann. chir. **11:** 17, 1247, 1957.
11. Lortat-Jacob, J. L., Maillard, J. N., and Fekete, F.: La prévention du reflux après résection oesophago-gastrique par un procédé d'anastomose continente, Mém. Acad. chir. **13:** 19, 1157, 1959.
12. Lortat-Jacob, J. L., Robert, F. W., and Frentz, F.: Affections peptiques de l'oesophage, Semaine hôp. Ann. chir. **32:** 517, 1956.
13. Moroney, J.: Colonic replacement and restoration of the human stomach, Ann. Roy. Coll. Surgeons England **12:** 328, 1953.
14. Nissen, R., and Rosetti, G.: Die Behandlung von Hiatus-hernien und Refluxoesophagitis mit Gastropexie und Fundoplicatio (Indikation, Techik und Ergebnisse), Stuttgart, 1959, Georg Thieme.
15. Sirak, M. D., Clatworthy, H. W., and Elliott, D. W.: An evaluation of jejunal and colic transplants in experimental esophagitis, Surgery **36:** 399, 1954.
16. Skinner, H. H., and Merendino, K. A.: An experimental evaluation of an interposed jejunal segment between the esophagus and the stomach, combined with upper gastrectomy in prevention of esophagitis and jejunitis, Ann. Surg. **141:** 201, 1955.
17. Thomas, G., and Merendino, K. A.: An evaluation in the dog of cardiac sphincter substitution by interposed colon in presence of vagotomy and Finney pyloroplasty, Surgery **41:** 993, 1957.
18. Thomas, G., and Merendino, K. A.: Jejunal interposition operation. Analysis of thirty-three clinical cases, J. A. M. A. **168:** 1759, 1958.
19. Wangensteen, O. H.: A physiologic operation for mega-esophagus, Ann. Surg. **134:** 301, 1951.
20. Wangensteen, O. H., and Leven, W. L.: Gastric resection for esophagitis and strictures of acid-peptic origin, Surg. Gynec. & Obst. **88:** 560, 1949.
21. Watkins, D. H., Prevedel, A., and Harper, F. R.: A method of preventing esophagitis following esophago-gastrostomy, J. Thoracic Surg. **28:** 367, 1954.
22. Watkins, D. H., Rundles, W. R., and Tatom, L.: Utility of a new procedure of valvular esophagogastrostomy in cases of brachyesophagus and stricture: clinical and experimental studies of circumferential esophagofundopexy, J. Thoracic Surg. **38:** 814, 1959.
23. Wooler, G.: Reconstruction of the cardia and fundus of the stomach, Thorax **24:** 275, 1956.

# Successful inferior vena cava–superior mesenteric vein shunt in an unusual case of portal hypertension

J. MANNY SHORE, M.D.
E. CRAIG HERINGMAN, M.D.
LOS ANGELES, CALIF.
*From the Department of Surgery, Cedars of Lebanon Hospital*

The protective effect of an adequate portacaval shunt against recurrent varical hemorrhage in patients with portal hypertension has been well established by the pioneering efforts of Blakemore,[1] Child,[2] Linton,[12] Rousselot,[14, 15] and others. In cases in which the obstruction is limited to the portal vein, such as in thrombosis and cavernous transformation, and when the splenic vein is of adequate caliber, the therapeutic procedure of choice is splenectomy with splenorenal shunt. Nevertheless, there are occasions when such a procedure is not feasible and therefore some other method of control must be instituted to prevent further hemorrhage. These situations have been noted by Clatworthy,[4, 5] Koop,[11] and others[10] and may be outlined as (1) portal venous block in infants and young children (up to the age of 11) when the splenic vein is too small for an adequate splenorenal shunt, (2) concomitant thrombosis of the portal and splenic veins, (3) portal vein block, either primary or secondary to cirrhosis, treated unsuccessfully by previous splenectomy, (4) persistent portal hypertension after inadequate or thrombosed splenorenal or portacaval shunt, and (5) extreme technical difficulty resulting in inability to dissect out the portal or splenic veins.

Various approaches to these difficult situations have been proposed. In infants and young children, Clatworthy[4, 5] and Shumacker[10] advocate attempts to control the hemorrhage by medical measures, tamponade, and transesophageal ligation until the child is old enough to have a splenic vein of acceptable size for shunting. In adults, Crile[6] suggests that transesophageal ligation of the varices may be adequate definitive therapy. Habif[8] has recently advocated esophagogastric resection with jejunal interposition for cases of persistent, bleeding esophageal varices after failure of other methods of treatment. Tanner advocates "porta-azygos disconnection" by gastric resection and reanastomosis.[13] Others, such as Blakemore,[1] Child,[2] Rousselot,[14, 15] Hallenbeck,[9] and Reynolds,[16] have attempted to decompress the portal venous bed by constructing some type of shunt between a tributary or collateral of the portal system and the caval system. Recently, Julian[7] has reported his experience with portacaval anastomosis after thrombectomy of the portal vein.

In 1955 Clatworthy[5] reported the successful use of a new type of shunt which appeared promising in the treatment of children with block of the extrahepatic portal bed. In this procedure, the inferior vena cava was ligated and divided just above the bifurcation and the end of the cephalic portion swung around for anastomosis to the side of the superior mesenteric vein. Excellent results were obtained in 2 cases in which an adequate superior mesenteric vein was present. These cases all occurred in infants or children without peripheral venous disease, and there were no untoward sequelae from the vena caval ligation.[3]

Recently, a case of intrahepatic portal hypertension was encountered which was un-

Received for publication Nov. 17, 1960.

usual because it was complicated by thrombosis of both portal and splenic veins. In the control of recurrent varical hemorrhage resulting from this complex pathologic situation, a modification of the procedure used by Clatworthy has thus far proved to be satisfactory. Because this operation provides a relatively simple surgical technique in comparison to esophagogastric resection, it was believed that its use in this case merited careful evaluation and discussion.

## CASE REPORT

A 32-year-old Caucasian man was first admitted to an outside hospital on May 18, 1958, after the sudden onset of massive hematemesis and syncope. Bleeding continued for an additional 48 hours and necessitated a 4,000 ml. blood replacement. Upper gastrointestinal roentgen examination showed massive esophageal varices and the patient was transferred to the Cedars of Lebanon Hospital on May 28, 1958, for definitive therapy.

Past history showed that the patient had been in a concentration camp between the ages of 13 and 18 and had developed severe malnutrition. The physical examination on admission showed him to be normal except for an enlarged spleen which was palpable 8 cm. below the left costal margin. Results of laboratory studies were hematocrit, 38 per cent; white blood cells, 4,100; platelet count, 116,000; serum bilirubin, 1.8 mg. per cent; prothrombin time, 58 per cent; Bromsulphalein, 12 per cent (45 minutes, 22 per cent); thymol turbidity, 2.8 U.; alkaline phosphatase, 1.7 B-L units; cephalin flocculation, 3+; and serum proteins, 6.5 Gm. per cent (albumin/globulin ratio 3.5/3.0 Gm. per cent).

The preoperative diagnosis was cirrhosis of the liver with portal hypertension, esophageal varices, and splenomegaly.

Operation was performed on June 9, 1958. Immediately prior to operation a percutaneous splenoportogram (multiple exposure technique) showed obstruction of the splenic vein with filling of varices in the region of the gastric fundus (Fig. 1). At celiotomy through an upper transverse abdominal incision, the liver was found to be normal in size with a fine granular surface. Results of a frozen section examination of a liver biopsy specimen were interpreted as normal and subsequently confirmed in the permanent section. The spleen was moderately enlarged. Portal pressure taken directly from the portal vein was 36 cm. of saline solution. Since the liver appeared normal and the splenoportogram showed a splenic vein occlusion, splenectomy was performed. The splenic vein occlusion was confirmed by the inability to pass a No. 12 Fr. catheter through it toward the liver. The patient had an uneventful postoperative course.

The patient remained asymptomatic and a follow-up esophogram made 5 months after splenectomy showed moderate regression of the varices.

On Feb. 2, 1960, the patient was readmitted after the sudden onset of recurrent hematemesis. On physical examination at the time of admission, the pulse rate was 116 (minutes) and blood pressure 92/60 mm. Hg. There were tarry stools in the rectum. Bleeding ceased spontaneously within 16 hours and did not require esophageal tamponade for control. Blood volume was restored during the first 24 hours by transfusion of 2,000 units of whole blood. Results of laboratory studies were hematocrit, 36 per cent; white blood cells, 9,000; serum bilirubin, 1.4 mg. per cent; prothrombin time, 46 per cent (after vitamin K, 82 per cent); Bromsulphalein, 7 per cent (45 minutes, 14.5 per cent); thymol turbidity, 1 U.; alkaline phosphatase, 1.3 B-L units; cephalin flocculation, 2+; and serum proteins, 6.5 Gm. per cent (albumin/globulin ratio, 3.0/3.5 Gm. per cent).

An esophogram showed the presence of large varices involving the distal two-thirds of the esophagus (Fig. 2, *A*).

Operation was performed on Feb. 25, 1960. The peritoneal cavity was entered through the previous transverse upper abdominal incision. The first loop of the jejunum was identified and a jejunal vein isolated in its mesentery and cannulated with a No. 18 polyethylene catheter through which a pressure of 28 cm. of saline was recorded. A portal venogram was then made by injection of 70 per cent Hypaque through the catheter. This showed a thrombosed, recanalized

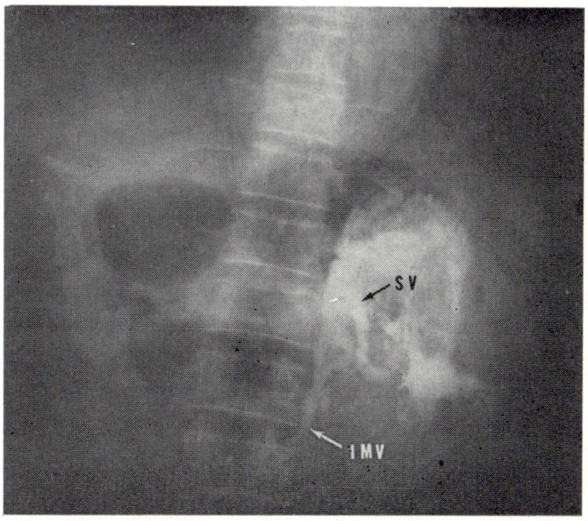


**Fig. 1.** Preoperative splenoportogram demonstrates splenic vein block. Note small size of splenic vein and filling of gastric varices from the splenic bed.

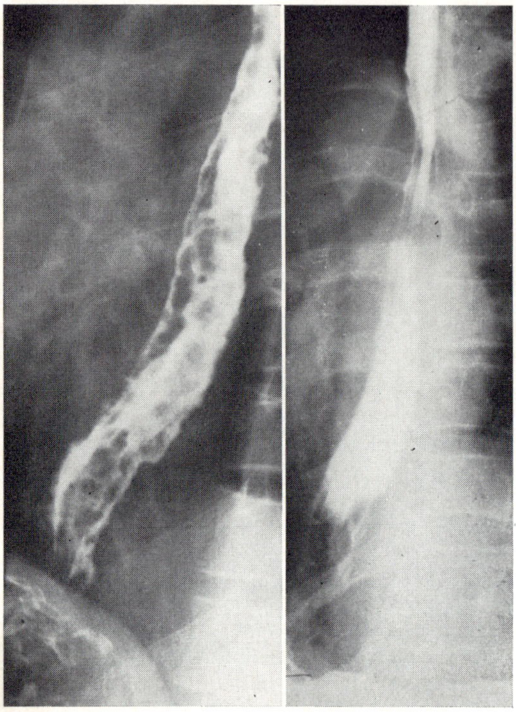

*A* *B*

**Fig. 2.** *A,* Esophogram taken before caval-mesenteric shunt demonstrates large varices which involve the distal two-thirds of the esophagus. *B,* Esophogram taken 10 months after caval-mesenteric shunt demonstrates marked regression of varices.

portal vein and a wide, patent, superior mesenteric vein (Fig. 3). At this point a decision had to be made betwen attempting a portacaval shunt, using some vessel other than the portal vein, or performing an esophagogastrectomy. Since the superior mesenteric vein appeared suitable for shunting, an anastomosis between this vessel and the inferior vena cava was elected.

Extension into a right thoracoabdominal incision was carried out. The liver appeared normal in size with a smooth, firm surface. The superior mesenteric vein was then mobilized as it crossed the third portion of the duodenum and as far as possible behind the neck of the pancreas. The portal vein thrombosis was confirmed by direct inspection and palpation. The inferior vena cava was mobilized from the renal veins to the bifurcation. It was doubly ligated with No. 2-0 silk just above the bifurcation and divided cephalad to the ligation after application of an occluding clamp just below the renal veins. Since the vena cava was not long enough to reach the superior mesenteric vein in front of the duodenum and pancreas, a tunnel was developed betwen the upper border of the third portion of the duodenum and adjoining pancreas through which the divided vena cava was brought to the superior mesenteric vein (Fig. 4). With a partially occluding vascular clamp on the superior mesenteric vein, an end-to-side anastomosis 2.5 cm. in length was created between the divided end of the inferior vena cava and the right side of the superior mesenteric vein. A continuous over-and-over suture of No. 5-0 arterial silk was used. There was an excellent flow of blood through the stoma with an immediate drop in the portal pressure to 16 cm. of saline solution.

The postoperative course was complicated by transient edema and cyanosis of both lower extremities which began on the seventh postoperative day with ambulation. This subsided completely after 1 week of bed rest, elevation of the lower extremities, and transfusion of 75 Gm. of albumin. Thereafter progressive ambulation with firm elastic support from the toes to the knees was well tolerated without edema or pain and the patient was discharged on the twenty-third postoperative day.

During the next 10 months the patient continued to improve and gained in weight and strength. There has been no recurrent hemorrhage. An esophogram taken 10 months postoperatively showed marked regression of the varices (Fig. 2, *B*). The serum bilirubin, serum protein, and hemoglobin levels have remained within normal limits. With constant elastic support during ambulation and elevation of the lower extremities when supine, the patient gradually improved his tolerance for walking and by the second postoperative month he was able to walk as much as he desired without pain or edema.

## DISCUSSION

The preoperative impression during the first admission was that of an intrahepatic type of obstruction, but the finding of a grossly and microscopically normal liver and of a splenic vein occlusion on serial splenoportography indicated that the liver was not the site of obstruction. A portal venogram taken at this time would have been of value in the interpretation of this unusual combination of findings. Although most cases of portal hypertension are either due to intrahepatic obstruction (usually portal cirrhosis) or to extrahepatic obstruction (usually thrombosis of the portal vein), one will occasionally encounter cases of intrahepatic portal hypertension in which the liver appears normal at the time of surgical exploration. It may well be that rare cases such as these are examples of what Banti originally described. The finding of an occlusion of the splenic vein in addition further complicated the present case.

The presence of a thrombosed, recanalized portal vein during the second operative procedure precluded the performance of a standard portacaval shunt. Since the splenic vein was also unavailable, there remained a choice between performance of some other type of portacaval shunt or a direct attack upon the varices themselves. The inferior vena cava–superior mesenteric vein shunt was selected because the expected mortality and morbidity rates were far lower than those of esophagogastrectomy. In addition, portal decompression could be accomplished. The rapid drop in portal pressure, the marked regression of the varices, and the clinical course of the patient to date all favor the choice of this procedure.

The inadequate length of the vena cava in this patient precluded the construction of a shunt in front of the duodenum as described by Clatworthy.[4, 5] Accordingly, a shorter route was improvised by creation of a tunnel between the superior margin of the third portion of the duodenum and the inferior border of the head of the pancreas. This proved to be an extremely helpful maneuver without which the shunt could not have been accomplished.

Although it is impossible to draw any general conclusions from a single experience, we were extremely impressed by the usefulness of the vena cava–superior mesenteric vein shunt in a case of portal hypertension in which both the portal and splenic veins were unavailable for portasystemic anastomosis. Other types of communication between the portal and systemic systems have been considered or attempted, but usually with little success. They avoid interruption of the inferior vena cava, which is the only undesirable feature of this procedure. Since the distance between the inferior vena cava and the superior mesenteric vein is too great to allow a side-to-side anastomosis, it has been bridged by a communicating venous autograft.[2, 10, 15, 16] The need for 2 anastomoses and the limited size of veins available for autograft are obvious disadvantages of this procedure. The use of collateral vessels in the portal system for anastomosis to the vena cava has usually met with failure because these vessels are often small, fragile, and thin-walled. As a result, the flow is inadequate for decompression and the shunts frequently thrombose. Poor results have been reported after the utilization of other tributaries of the portal and caval systems, such as the spermatic, ovarian, iliolumbar, renal, inferior mesenteric, and coronary veins for shunting purposes.[1, 2, 8] Occasionally, as indicated by Hallenbeck,[9] a solitary large vessel of adequate quality may be found in the porta hepatis and may be successfully utilized. The use of a double-barreled anastomosis between the divided superior mesenteric vein and the inferior vena cava carries with it the risk of thrombosis of the mesenteric vein, in addition to the need for 2 anastomoses. Anastomosis of the left renal

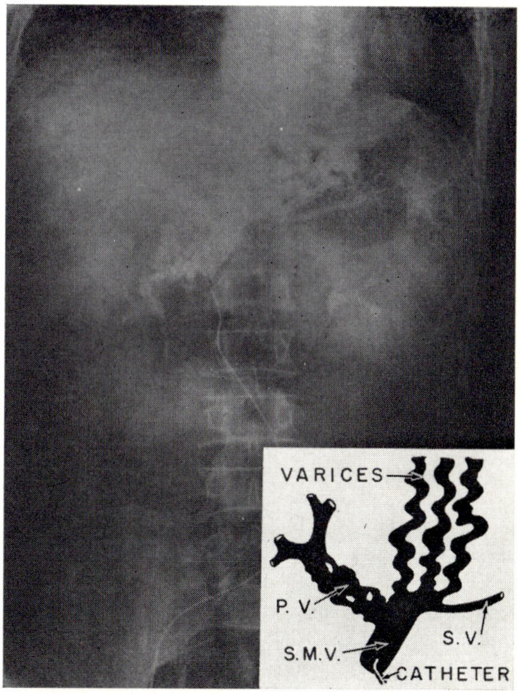


**Fig. 3.** Operative portal venogram taken at time of second operation demonstrates thrombosed, recanalized portal vein, patent superior mesenteric vein, and extensive varices and collateral vessels.

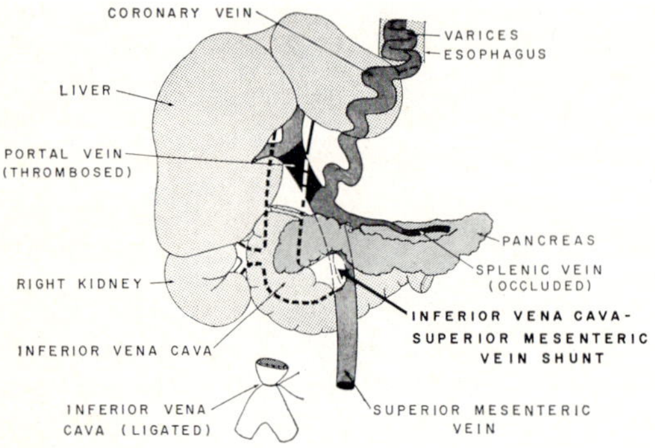


**Fig. 4.** Diagrammatic representation of surgical technique utilized in the performance of end-to-side vena cava–superior mesenteric vein shunt through a tunnel between the duodenum and the pancreas.

vein to the side of the superior mesenteric vein is another possibility which would, however, necessitate a left nephrectomy.

The inferior vena cava–superior mesenteric vein end-to-side shunt appears to be the most feasible type of shunting procedure because of its large size, single anastomosis, use of normal venous channels, and relative technical simplicity. Its main disadvantage is the necessity for ligation of the inferior vena cava. This, in itself, does not appear to be a major contraindication in view of the seriousness of the prognosis in the untreated patient and the high mortality, morbidity, and failure rates associated with other types of shunts or with esophagogastrectomy. Reluctance to ligate and divide the inferior vena cava probably stems from the unfavorable sequelae frequently encountered after this procedure is performed in the treatment of thromboembolic disease. However, in the management of these unusual cases of portal hypertension in which the veins of the lower extremities and pelvis are healthy, such fears are probably unwarranted. The reports to date of the relatively low morbidity rate encountered when this procedure has been carried out appear to support this contention.

## SUMMARY AND CONCLUSIONS

1. An unusual case of portal hypertension due to intrahepatic obstruction in the absence of demonstrable cirrhosis and complicated by obstruction of the portal and splenic veins, with bleeding esophageal varices, is presented.

2. The use of the end-to-side inferior vena cava–superior mesenteric vein shunt for the definitive control of the recurrent bleeding esophageal varices after splenectomy is described.

3. The employment of a short route through a tunnel between the duodenum and the pancreas for passage of a short vena cava is presented as a modification of the procedure.

4. The indications for, and relative merits of, the end-to-side vena cava–superior mesenteric vein shunt over other procedures in the surgeon's armamentarium for therapy of portal hypertension are described and discussed.

## REFERENCES

1. Blakemore, A. H.: Portacaval shunting for portal hypertension, Surg. Gynec. & Obst. **94:** 443, 1952.
2. Child, C. G., III: The hepatic circulation and portal hypertension, Philadelphia, 1954, W. B. Saunders Company.
3. Clatworthy, H. W., Jr.: Personal communication.
4. Clatworthy, H. W., Jr., and Boles, E. T.: Extrahepatic portal bed block in children: pathogenesis and treatment, Ann. Surg. **150:** 371, 1959.
5. Clatworthy, H. W., Jr., Wall, T., and Watman, R. T.: A new type of portal to systemic venous shunt for portal hypertension, A. M. A. Arch. Surg. **71:** 588, 1955.
6. Crile, C. J., Jr.: Transesophageal ligation of bleeding esophageal varices, Surgery **42:** 583, 1957.
7. Dye, W. S., David, D., and Julian, O. C.: Successful treatment of portal vein thrombosis associated with intrahepatic obstruction, A. M. A. Arch. Surg. **80:** 876, 1960.
8. Habif, D. V.: Treatment of esophageal varices by partial esophagogastrectomy and interposed jejunal segment, Surgery **46:** 212, 1959.
9. Hallenbeck, G. A., and Shockett, E.: Treatment of bleeding esophageal varices after splenectomy, A. M. A. Arch. Surg. **71:** 581, 1955.
10. King, H., and Shumacker, H. B., Jr.: Venous shunt procedures for portal hypertension in children, Surgery **43:** 680, 1958.

11. Koop, C. E., and Roddy, S. R.: Colonic replacement of distal esophagus and proximal stomach in the management of bleeding varices in children, Ann. Surg. **147:** 17, 1958.
12. Linton, R. R.: Surgery of Portal cirrhosis of liver, Am. J. Med. **24:** 941, 1958.
13. Mikkelson, W. P., and Pattison, A. C.: Upper gastric transection (Tanner operation), Surgery **46:** 501, 1959.
14. Rousselot, L. M.: Autogenous vein graft in splenorenal anastomosis, Surgery **31:** 403, 1952.
15. Rousselot, L. M., Ruzicka, F. F., Jr., and Doehner, G. A.: Portography in portal hypertension, S. Clin. North America **36:** 361, 1956.
16. Reynolds, J. T., and Southwick, H. W.: Portal hypertension: use of venous grafts when side-to-side anastomosis is impossible, A. M. A. Arch. Surg. **62:** 789, 1951.

# "Fore and aft" split pancreaticojejunostomy for chronic pancreatitis

RALPH P. CAMPANALE, COLONEL, USAF(MC)
BERNARD GARDNER, CAPTAIN, USAF(MC)
TRAVIS AIR FORCE BASE, CALIF.

The etiology, and therefore the rational therapy, of chronic pancreatitis has remained an enigma to most surgeons in spite of the many fine papers which have championed particular ideas on the subject. The variety of surgical procedures available, each purporting to offer the best chance of cure, testifies to our lack of knowledge concerning the true pathophysiologic nature of this perplexing disease. Experimental procedures designed to demonstrate the etiology have not produced the uniform results necessary to outline clearly the mechanisms involved. The implication of different mechanisms suggests that variable factors operating at different times and in different sites may be the logical cause of this confusing picture.

Obstruction of the main pancreatic duct alone will not produce the disease unless associated with an actively secreting gland,[5, 21, 24] and even in some of these cases, only atrophy and mild histologic evidence of inflammation occur.[14, 18] Retrojection of bile into the pancreatic duct alone will not produce the disease unless the character of the bile is drastically changed or it is under such pressure that the pancreatic acini are ruptured.[1, 2, 6] Difficulty has arisen in explaining the rise in biliary-tract pressure necessary to produce retrojection of bile into the main pancreatic duct under enough force to cause rupture of the acini.[11] Cases of pancreatitis without the presence of a common channel cannot be explained by this theory; in addition, the existence of the safety-valve action of the duct of Santorini is difficult to ignore if obstruction at the sphincter alone represents the primary etiologic condition.

Ischemia of the gland[8, 19] and tryptic activity[6, 11, 15] are 2 other factors which have been investigated experimentally and which may be involved in the pathophysiology of this disease; however, little clinical evidence is at present available to implicate these factors. Large doses of d, l-ethionine have produced pancreatitis in the experimental animal,[14] but once again the clinical significance of this is undemonstrated, although obstruction of enzyme output at the cellular membrane level has been implicated.[12]

Several factors have become clearly established. Obstruction to the main pancreatic ducts occurs sometime during the course of the disease.[3, 22, 23] Whether this is present as the primary mechanism or is secondary to the pathologic changes in the gland is unclear at the present time. Evidence for sphincter spasm has been adequately presented in the past and proximal obstruction of the duct with or without retrojection of bile is a natural consequence of this. Pathologic studies as well as studies of operative pancreaticograms have confirmed the presence of ductal obstruction in a large number of cases. Obstruction of the ducts with proximal dilatation is the mechanism of pain, at least in chronic pancreatitis when pathologic sections have shown marked fibrosis of the

Presented at the Eighth Annual Convention of the Society of Air Force Clinical Surgeons, April 14, 1960, United States Air Force Hospital Travis.
Received for publication Nov. 8, 1960.

gland and little active inflammation. Obstruction may occur not only in the head, but also in the body and tail[22]; or there may be multiple sites of obstruction, each capable of producing inadequate drainage from the particular area of the gland involved.[3, 17] Surgical therapy directed at drainage of the tail of the pancreas alone may not alleviate obstruction in the head or body of the gland. Similarly, sphincterotomy alone may only aid drainage from a small portion of the head if obstruction is present in the neck of the gland.

These factors point to the need for investigative study at the time of operation to determine the site or sites of obstruction. Finally, a combined approach to produce a completely open pancreatic drainage system throughout its length and including the sphincter, a so-called "fore and aft" procedure, seems to be a rational approach to this problem with our present state of knowledge.

## OPERATIVE PROCEDURE[17]

A routine exploration of the peritoneal cavity was carried out as the first step. With the confirmation of the clinical diagnosis of a chronic pancreatitis at operation, the next step was a routine cholecystectomy and performance of an operative cholangiogram through the cystic duct remnant in an attempt to outline both the biliary tree and the pancreatic ducts, if possible. Changes noted in the biliary tree were recorded, and if stones were present, common duct exploration was carried out. A transduodenal sphincterotomy was then performed, and a pancreaticogram is attempted via a polyethylene catheter placed in the pancreatic duct. If obstruction to the passage of dye was demonstrated, a splenectomy was carried out and the tail of the gland then amputated. The duct in the area of the tail was intubated with a fine polyethylene catheter and an anterograde pancreaticogram accomplished. The pancreaticograms usually delineated the ductal pathologic process involved. The pancreatic duct was split and laid open as far medially as practicable (Fig. 1). A Roux Y loop of jejunum was brought over the tail of the pancreas as a sheath and sutured in 2 layers to the pancreatic capsule. A catheter was left in place in the common bile duct, and Morison's pouch drained. The operation was then terminated. The common duct catheter was left in place for 2 to 4 weeks postoperatively but otherwise the postoperative care was routine.

The case reports of 2 patients illustrate some of the problems involved in the management of this disease.

## CASE REPORTS

**Case 1.** J. P., 37-year-old white male major and command pilot, was admitted to the USAF Hospital Travis on May 4, 1959, for evaluation of

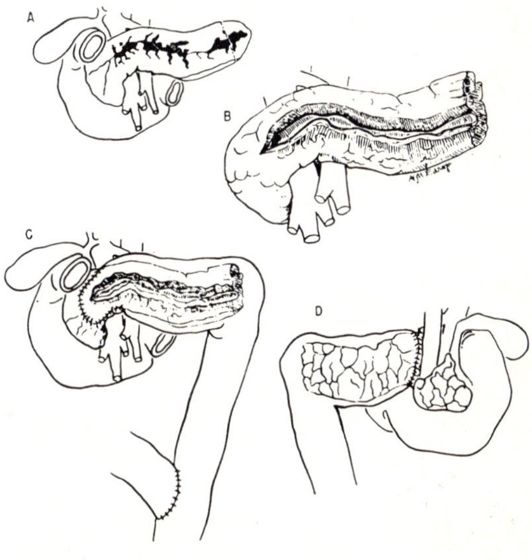


**Fig. 1.** *A,* Appearance of pancreatic ducts, as seen in some pancreaticograms. Note the alternate dilatations and stenoses that are commonly present. *B,* Pancreatic duct which is split open to show alternate stenotic and dilated areas. Catarrhal inflammation is frequently found at the stenotic narrowing, and calcification may be present at these spots. *C,* Anterior view of pancreaticojejunostomy with jejunum sutured to the right of the opened pancreas. Roux Y enteroanastomosis has been performed below the mesocolon. *D,* Posterior view of pancreaticojejunostomy with jejunum sutured to the peripancreatic tissue to the left of the superior mesenteric vessels. (From Puestow, C. B., and Gillesby, W. J.: Retrograde surgical drainage for chronic relapsing pancreatitis, A. M. A. Arch. Surg. **76:** 898, 1958.)

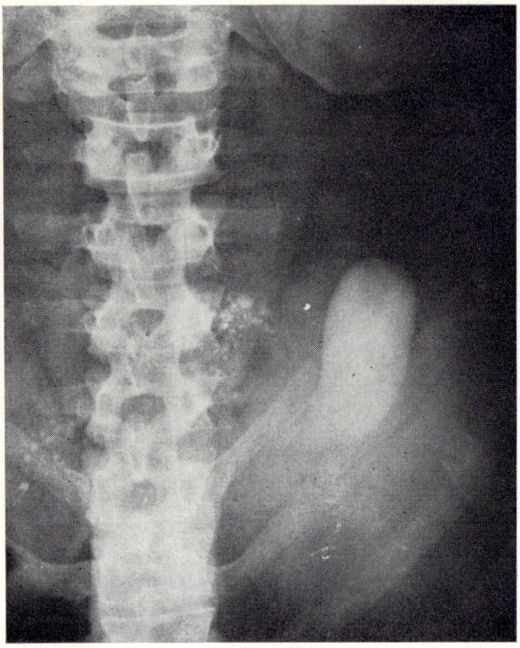

**Fig. 2.** Case 1. Note diffuse calcification in area of pancreas.

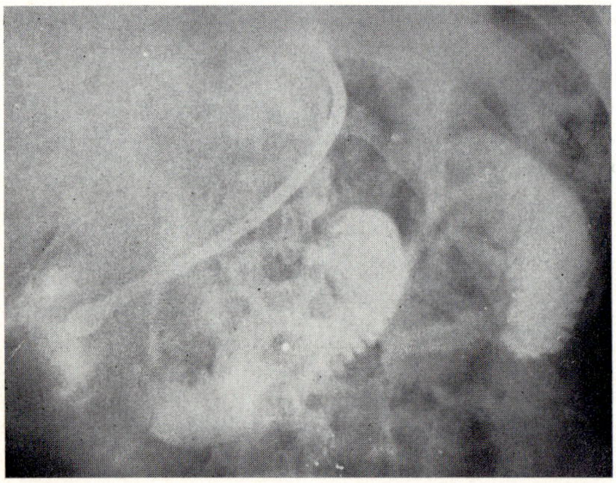

**Fig. 3.** Case 1. Operative cholangiogram. Note narrowing of intrapancreatic portion of common bile duct with proximal dilatation.

severe recurrent abdominal pain. His first hospitalization for acute pancreatitis in August, 1956, had followed consumption of a large quantity of alcohol at a party. His high alcoholic intake had remained undiminished during the subsequent 2 years while the patient continued to have intermittent abdominal pain, nausea, and vomiting which lasted for 2 to 3 days and recurred at 3 month intervals. He was again hospitalized in January, 1958, and treated conservatively, but the attacks became more frequent. In November, 1958, he was placed on a strict medical regimen, but his attacks continued unabated at weekly intervals. At the time of admission the patient weighed 125 pounds, had lost 30 pounds in the preceding 6 months, and was suffering from almost constant epigastric and back pain, nausea, and vomiting. He had occasional diarrhea of bulky stools which floated.

Physical examination showed him to be a thin, underweight, young man with abdominal and back pain. The thyroid gland was palpable, but the remainder of the physical examination was unremarkable.

The white blood cell count was 11,500 with a normal differential. Hemoglobin was 15.1 Gm. per cent and erythrocyte sedimentation rate 7 mm. Results of urinalysis were within normal limits. Prothrombin time was 100 per cent of normal. Blood calcium was 10.2 mg. per cent and serum carotene was 40 mcg. per 100 mg. Results of a glucose tolerance test were normal. Serum amylase was 266 Somogyi units.

Roentgenograms of the abdomen showed diffuse calcifications outlining the entire pancreas. A gall-bladder series was negative except for the calcifications mentioned (Fig. 2). Gastrointestinal series and chest roentgenograms were unremarkable.

On Aug. 13, 1959, an exploratory laparotomy was performed. The entire pancreas was extremely firm, almost stony in texture. The biliary tract was grossly within normal limits. A cholecystectomy was performed and a cholangiogram performed through the cystic duct remnant showed narrowing of the intrapancreatic portion of the common bile duct and proximal dilatation (Fig. 3). A transduodenal sphincterotomy was performed, and a polyethylene catheter was threaded into the pancreatic duct. A calcareous obstruction was met 2 cm. proximal to the sphincter. Amputation of the tail of the pancreas was performed after a splenectomy, a polyethylene catheter was threaded into the main duct, and a pancreaticogram was accomplished. These roentgenograms showed obstruction in the head of the gland with proximal dilatation of the main duct of Wirsung and secondary ducts (Fig. 4). A split pancreaticojejunostomy was carried out.

The patient's postoperative course was uneventful, and he was discharged on Sept. 23, 1959, to full active duty.

The patient was re-examined in April, 1960, at which time he reported that he was completely free of abdominal pain, nausea, and vomiting. His weight was 141 pounds, a gain of 16 pounds, and he was having normal bowel movements which were no longer bulky or floated. He was performing full duty and had in fact been returned to flying status. Results of a gastrointestinal series and glucose tolerance test were normal and stool specimens stained for fat were negative.

Re-examination of the patient in July, 1961, approximately 2 years postoperatively, showed that he had remained completely asymptomatic, without the loss of any time from duty. His weight was 147 pounds, a total gain of 23 pounds.

**Case 2.** K. G., a 43-year-old white male master sergeant, was admitted to the USAF Hospital Travis on July 20, 1959, for evaluation of recurrent abdominal pain. The patient habitually imbibed large quantities of alcoholic beverages and had suffered recurrent epigastric pain radiating straight through to his back for 6 years prior to admission. He had experienced 3 hospitalizations during the year prior to admission, and had suffered a 25 pound weight loss.

Physical examination showed him to be a thin, chronically ill white man, weighing 103 pounds, with marked tenderness to palpation over the mid-epigastrium. No masses were palpable. The remainder of the physical examination was unremarkable.

White blood cell count was 8,700 with a normal differential. Hemoglobin was 12.6 Gm. per cent. Results of studies of the liver function and glucose tolerance tests were within normal limits. Results of 3 serum amylase determinations performed within the first 4 days of hospitalization were 229, 320, and 400 Somogyi units, respectively.

An intravenous pyelogram, gall-bladder series, and a gastrointestinal series were unremarkable except for a slight widening of the duodenal loop and calcifications in the area of the pancreas.

On Aug. 18, 1959, an exploratory laparotomy was performed. A firm, indurated pancreas was noted with areas of calcification. The biliary tree was essentially normal. Cholecystectomy was performed and a cholangiogram accomplished through the cystic duct remnant showed slight narrowing of the intrapancreatic portion of the common bile duct (Fig. 5). A transduodenal sphincterotomy was carried out and a polyethylene catheter threaded into the pancreatic duct met obstruction 3 cm. proximal to the sphincter (Fig. 6). Splenectomy was performed, the tail of the pancreas was amputated, a polyethylene catheter was threaded anterograde through the main pancreatic duct, and a pancreaticogram was taken. These films demonstrated a dilatation of the main duct and complete obstruction in the head of the gland (Fig. 7). A split pancreaticojejunostomy was subsequently performed. A catheter was left in the common bile duct and the operation was terminated.

The patient's postoperative course was complicated by an intestinal obstruction, and on Aug. 24, 1959, a re-exploration showed an adhesive band obstructing a segment of ileum. The obstruction was relieved and the abdomen closed. Convalescence was further complicated by a wound infection which required drainage with delayed healing. The patient was discharged to full duty on Dec. 17, 1959.

Re-examination of the patient in April, 1960, showed that his abdominal pain was greatly diminished, occurring once every 3 to 4 weeks and lasting for a half day. The back pain had been completely relieved. The patient weighed 117 pounds, a gain of 14 pounds, and was able to perform full active duty. A gastrointestinal series showed a decrease in the amount of calcification

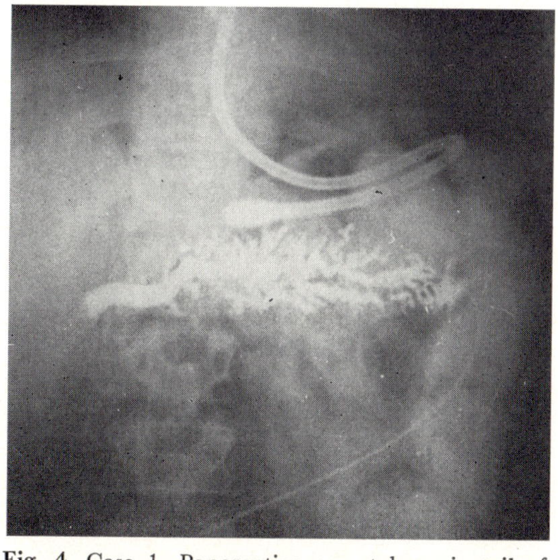

**Fig. 4.** Case 1. Pancreaticogram taken via tail of gland. Note obstruction in head of gland with proximal dilatation and tortuosity of ductal system.

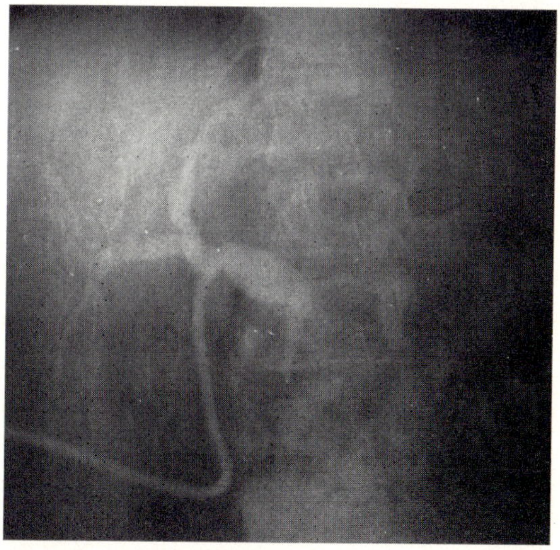

**Fig. 5.** Case 2. Operative cholangiogram. Note narrowing of intrapancreatic portion of common bile duct with proximal dilatation.

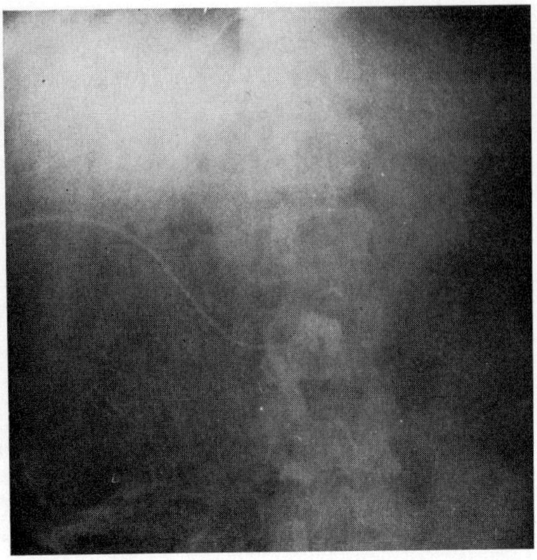

**Fig. 6.** Case 2. Operative pancreaticogram taken via sphincter which shows obstruction to passage of dye 3 cm. proximal to sphincter.

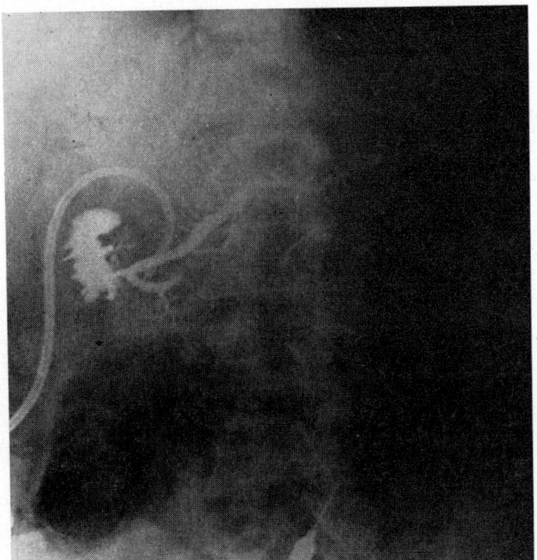

**Fig. 7.** Case 2. Operative pancreaticogram via tail of gland which shows narrowing at sphincter with proximal dilatation of major and minor ducts.

of the pancreas, and results of a glucose tolerance test were normal. The patient's stools were of normal caliber and consistency and were negative on stain for fecal fat.

In January, 1961, the patient was hospitalized because of jaundice, which followed an acute episode of pancreatitis. Exploratory laparotomy in February, 1961, showed that the head of the pancreas was enlarged to the size of an orange and was stony hard in consistency. However, the body and tail of the pancreas were essentially normal. It was considered inadvisable to attempt a choledochoduodenostomy because of technical difficulties and the operation was terminated. After recovery from the operation, the patient continued to experience attacks of moderate abdominal discomfort, which occurred once every 10 days to 2 weeks, and lasted several hours. The performance of celiac block with 1 per cent Xylocaine during an acute attack produced complete relief of pain. When these results were consistently reproduced by Xylocaine injection and injection of a saline solution failed to mitigate the pain, 7 per cent phenol was injected into the celiac plexus with excellent results. For the remainder of a 4-week hospital stay, the patient did not experience another acute exacerbation of pain. However, after his discharge from the hospital, the patient continued to experience recurring abdominal discomfort at intervals of 10 days to 2 weeks, which required the administration of analgesics for relief. It is of interest, however, that his stools continued to be of normal character, and that they failed to show any evidence of pancreatic insufficiency.

## DISCUSSION

Although the follow-up in the 2 cases reported is short, they represent fairly satisfactory results to us inasmuch as both patients, debilitated and completely incapacitated at the time we first saw them, are now returned to full active duty with the Air Force.

Split pancreaticojejunostomy has been performed successfully by Puestow[16, 17] with excellent results, and sphincterotomy has been reintroduced and performed in a large number of cases by Doubilet and Mulholland.[7] However, as far as we know, this is the first time both methods have been utilized together as a planned attack on this disease. The rationale is based upon the observed incidence of multiple sites of obstruction in the pancreatic duct as well as localized obstructions in various other parts of the gland. Although obstruction may not be the primary etiologic agent of this disease, evidence is available that it is of considerable importance in the perpetuation of the disease process, and probably for the clinical sign of abdominal pain. A review of the sections from our patients (Figs. 8 and 9) illustrates the basis for this concept. In the chronic form of the disease inflammation is not prominent and almost complete fibrosis of the gland may occur. These patients, however, complain of constant abdominal and back pain which is related, in our opinion, to the finding in pathologic specimens of ductal dilatation.

The earliest surgical attempts at treatment were designed to promote more efficient drainage,[13] and recent surgical attempts have continued this trend. Experimental work in dogs has shown regeneration of pancreatic tissue with adequate drainage.[4]

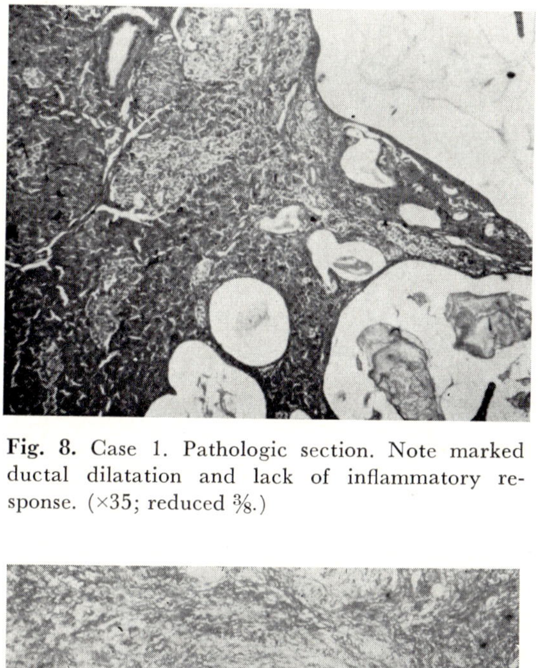

**Fig. 8.** Case 1. Pathologic section. Note marked ductal dilatation and lack of inflammatory response. (×35; reduced ⅜.)

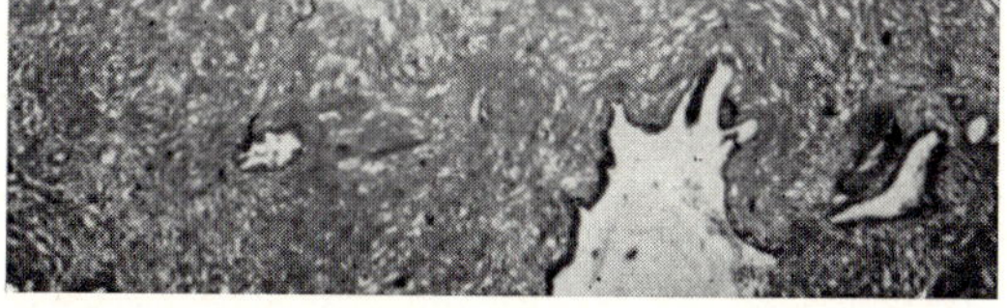

**Fig. 9.** Case 2. Pathologic section. Note almost complete fibrosis, lack of inflammatory response, and ductal dilatation. (×35; reduced ⅖.)

Sphincterotomy alone has not produced the anticipated results in the hands of several investigators[9, 20, 23] However, some of the successful results after the operation certainly indicate that sphincter spasm plays a part in the disease in some patients. The rate of recurrence after most drainage procedures may be explained by the coexistence of several factors, or by the fact that not all the involved areas of the gland are successfully drained. Success with caudal pancreaticojejunostomy is understandable on the basis of a careful selection of patients.[9, 10] When obstruction is demonstrated solely in the head of the gland and no proximal obstruction exists, caudal drainage may be successful. Marked dilatation of the pancreatic duct facilitates the mucosa-to-mucosa anastomosis and probably accounts for the continued drainage of the anastomosed gland. Often at operation, however, one can feel nodules in the fibrotic head of the gland which are indicative of disease for which drainage by this procedure is ineffective, since it exists distal to the area of obstruction. Sphincterotomy alone would not provide adequate drainage to the area of gland proximal to the obstruction. The problem of what to do for patients whose condition does not fulfill the criteria set down for performance of a caudal pancreaticojejunostomy must also be answered by the responsible surgeon. The operation that we have outlined would satisfy most of the objections. Regeneration of pancreatic tissue occurs, and there are 2 factors which would guide surgical therapy for this disease,[17] (1) adequate drainage of the pancreatic ductal system, and (2) the leaving of adequate pancreatic tissue to fulfill its secretory function satisfactorily. The operation outlined fulfills both criteria.

## SUMMARY

1. Obstruction of the pancreatic ductal system plays an important part in the pathophysiology and symptomatology of chronic pancreatitis.

2. An operation has been outlined which presents a planned attack for the produc-

tion of complete drainage of the pancreatic ductal system.

3. Two case reports are presented which illustrate clinical manifestations of the disease and the surgical results of the operative procedure.

## REFERENCES


1. Archibald, E.: The experimental production of pancreatitis in animals as the result of the resistance of the common duct sphincter, Surg. Gynec. & Obst. **28:** 529, 1919.
2. Archibald, E.: Further data concerning the experimental production of pancreatitis, Ann. Surg. **74:** 426, 1921.
3. Berrens, J. J., Baffentoss, A. H., and Gray, H. K.: Ductal changes in chronic pancreatitis, A. M. A. Arch. Surg. **68:** 723. 1954.
4. Carnevali, J. F., ReMine, W. H., Dockerty, M. B., Bollman, J. L., and Grindlay, J. H.: Experimental study of side-to-side pancreaticojejunostomy after ductal obstruction. Proc. Staff Meet. Mayo Clin. **35:** 584, 1960.
5. Coffey, R. M.: Diseases of the pancreas, M. Ann. District of Columbia **11:** 131, 1942.
6. Collins, E. N., and Owens, F. L.: Chronic pancreatitis, M. Clin. North America **40:** 465, 1956.
7. Doubilet, H., and Mullholland, J. H.: Eight year study of pancreatitis and sphincterotomy, J. A. M. A. **160:** 521, 1956.
8. Dunphy, J. E., Brooks, J. R., and Achroyd, F.: Acute postoperative pancreatitis, New England J. Med. **248:** 445, 1953.
9. Duval, M. K., Jr.: Caudal pancreatico-jejunostomy for chronic relapsing pancreatitis, Ann. Surg. **140:** 775, 1954.
10. Duval, M. K., Jr.: Pancreaticojejunostomy for chronic pancreatitis, SURGERY **41:** 1019, 1957.
11. Jones, R., Jr.: Etiology and pathogenesis of acute hemorrhagic pancreatitis, Am. J. M. Sc. **205:** 277, 1943.
12. Kahn, D. R., and Carlson, A. B.: On the mechanism of experimentally induced ethionine pancreatitis, Ann. Surg. **150:** 42, 1959.
13. Link, G.: Treatment of chronic pancreatitis by pancreatostomy: new operation, Ann. Surg. **53:** 768, 1911.
14. Noer, R. J.: Surgical considerations in the treatment of pancreatitis, Am. Surgeon **23:** 50, 1957.
15. Powers, S. R., Jr., Brown, H. H., and Stein, A.: The pathogenesis of acute and chronic pancreatitis, Ann. Surg. **142:** 690, 1955.
16. Puestow, C. B.: Personal communication.
17. Puestow, C. B., and Gillesby, W. J.: Retrograde surgical drainage of pancreas for chronic relapsing pancreatitis, Tr. West. S. A. **65:** 238, 1958.
18. Radakovich, M., Pearse, H. E., and Strain, W. H.: Study of the etiology of acute pancreatitis, Surg. Gynec. & Obst. **94:** 749, 1952.
19. Smyth, C. J.: Etiology of acute hemorrhagic pancreatitis with special reference to the vascular factors, Arch. Path. **30:** 651, 1948.
20. Thompson, J. A., and Derrick, J. R.: The diagnosis and management of acute pancreatitis, Am. J. Surg. **94:** 558, 1957.
21. Wagensteen, O. H., Leven, N. L., and Manson, M. H.: Acute pancreatitis (pancreatic necrosis), A. M. A. Arch. Surg. **23:** 47, 1931.
22. Warren, K. W.: Diagnosis and treatment of pancreatic disorders, Postgrad. Med. **21:** 548, 1957.
23. Warren, K. W.: Surgical considerations in the management of chronic relapsing pancreatitis, S. Clin. North America **35:** 785, 1955.
24. Zollinger, R. M.: Pancreatitis, Postgrad. Med. **15:** 323, 1954.

# Benign tumors of the major salivary glands

THEODOR B. GRAGE, M.D.
PAUL H. LOBER, M.D.
DONALD B. SHAHON, M.D.
MINNEAPOLIS, MINN.
*From the Departments of Surgery and Pathology, University of Minnesota Medical School*

Although a great variety of tumors take origin from the salivary glands, they are seen clinically with relative infrequency. Only a few studies have been published which have been based on a sufficiently large number of cases to permit an estimate of the clinical course, the ultimate outcome, and the best form of therapy in the management of patients with these tumors. The intimate relationship of the facial nerve to the parotid gland, by far the most common site of salivary neoplasms, disposes the surgeon to be very conservative and all too frequently leads to incomplete excision of the tumor and subsequent recurrence.

This review concerns 142 benign tumors of the major salivary glands observed and treated at the University of Minnesota Hospitals from 1932 through 1956. Particular emphasis will be placed upon the results of superficial lobectomy and of total parotidectomy with preservation of the facial nerve in the treatment of parotid tumors. Since the introduction of the latter operative technique in this hospital in 1946 by State,[8] sufficient time has elapsed to permit an evaluation of this procedure and to compare its effectiveness to that of procedures in use prior to 1946.

## MATERIAL AND METHODS

The hospital records of all patients treated at the University of Minnesota Hospitals for tumors of the major salivary glands during the time interval stated were carefully studied. Follow-up data were obtained by examination of the clinical record of periodic examinations of the patients at the Tumor Clinic and by correspondence.

Histologic sections from every tumor were reviewed and additional blocks were cut when necessary for diagnostic clarification. Special staining techniques other than the hematoxylin and eosin method were used in some of the tumors. Table I represents a histologic classification of these neoplasms and their distribution within the major salivary glands. During the time interval covered in this study, 69 malignant tumors of the major salivary glands were encountered which are not included in this report.

## MIXED TUMORS

The mixed tumors or pleomorphic adenomas (117 cases) constituted 55.4 per cent of all the salivary gland tumors seen and 82.3 per cent of the benign tumors.

**Age, sex, and location.** Mixed tumors were more common in the female. In this series, 72 tumors occurred in females and 45 in males. The ages of the patients ranged from 9 to 80 years on admission, with 7 patients being less than 16 years old (Fig. 1). The average age of the patient at the time the tumor was first noticed was 40.1 years. The site of the tumor was the parotid gland in 101 cases and the submaxillary gland in 16 instances. The tumors were equally distributed between the right and left sides.

Received for publication Jan. 15, 1961.

**Table I.** *Histologic classification of 142 benign tumors of the major salivary glands observed at the University of Minnesota Hospitals (1932 to 1956)*

| *Tumor type* | *Parotid* | *Submaxillary* | *Total* No. | *Total* % |
|---|---|---|---|---|
| Mixed tumor | 101 | 16 | 117 | 82.3 |
| Papillary cystadenoma lymphomatosum | 11 | – | 11 | 7.7 |
| Hemangioma | 7 | – | 7 | 4.9 |
| Benign lymphoepithelial lesion | 4 | – | 4 | 2.8 |
| Lipoma | 1 | – | 1 | 0.7 |
| Neurofibroma | 1 | – | 1 | 0.7 |
| Granular-cell myoblastoma | – | 1 | 1 | 0.7 |
| Totals | 125 | 17 | 142 | |

**Duration of symptoms.** In 98 of the 117 patients the duration of the tumor could be ascertained fairly accurately. The interval from onset of symptoms to the time of admission varied from 3 weeks to 70 (?) years, with an average of 5.9 years. Although the duration of symptoms varied over such a wide range, 53 per cent of the patients had noted the tumor for 3 years or less and 70 per cent of the patients were treated within 5 years after onset of symptoms.

**Signs and symptoms.** The most common complaint was of a slowly growing, nontender, palpable mass. Occasionally the tumor seemed to grow in spurts, followed by periods of quiescence. A few patients complained of numbness over the area of the tumor, although severe pain was not reported by any of the patients. In 2 patients with mixed tumors of the parotid gland, a mild facial paralysis was present prior to institution of any therapy. In both of these patients the tumor was over 6 cm. in diameter and located deep to the facial nerve.

On physical examination the tumor usually was found to be a rather firm, occasionally hard, smooth mass. Preoperative estimation of the size of the tumor, particularly the ones more deeply located, was rarely accurate. The great majority of the tumors for which the location was described in sufficient detail were located within the superficial lobe of the parotid gland.

**Gross and microscopic pathologic findings.** Grossly the tumors varied in size from 3 mm. to 11 cm., with most of them measuring from 2 to 6 cm. in diameter. They frequently appeared lobulated and invested with a capsule, which usually was quite thin and delicate and in many instances incomplete. The capsule appeared to consist of connective tissue remnants of compressed salivary gland tissue and in some of the very small tumors was entirely absent. Except for occasional secondary cyst formation, the tumors were solid and on section presented a moist and glistening surface of a gray-white color. All of the primary tumors were solitary, whereas the recurrent tumors nearly always were multiple.

The microscopic appearance of benign mixed tumors of the salivary glands has been the subject of several excellent reports and will be discussed only briefly. A wide range of histologic patterns was encountered, not only within this group but also within

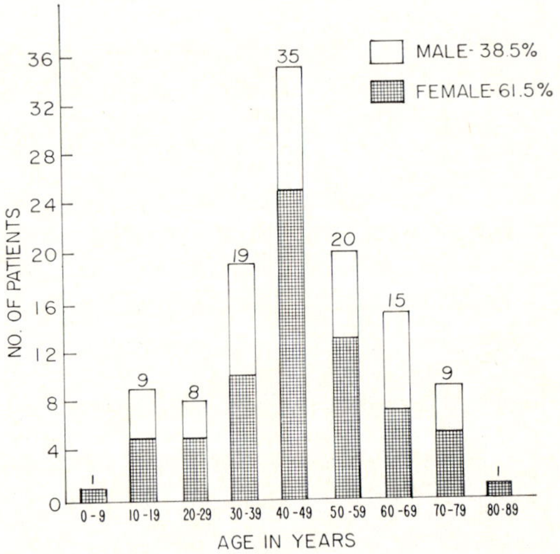


**Fig. 1.** Incidence of benign mixed tumors in various age groups (117 patients).

an individual tumor. Even though myxoid, chondromyxoid, and chondromatous patterns predominated, a few tumors were made up almost entirely of epithelial cells. In others the epithelial cells proliferated in interlacing strands and trabeculae, at times forming distinct tubular structures. Squamous metaplasia was not infrequent. Various degrees of hyalinization were present in many tumors and an occasional tumor contained areas of calcification. Formation of true cartilage and bone was not observed in this group. In several tumors epithelial nests and duct-like structures composed of large, deeply eosinophilic cells similar to those seen in papillary cystadenoma lymphomatosum were seen.

Two patients in the present group had recurrent mixed tumors that invaded the surrounding tissues, including the bone of the skull and the mandible, and therefore could not be completely removed. In both of these instances the histologic appearance of the removed tumor tissue did not differ from that seen in the other cases. Both patients ultimately died from extensive local disease. Since the term "mixed tumor" seems unlikely to be discarded, it would be well for the sake of clarity to reserve it for the pleomorphic adenomas of the salivary glands, keeping in mind that occasionally they may exhibit a more aggressive behavior and that in rare reported instances they have even given rise to metastases without histologic evidence of frank carcinomatous change.[2] The somewhat unfortunate term "malignant mixed tumor" has already been used to designate tumors which have the structural features of both mixed tumor and frank carcinoma. We have preferred to classify these as adenocarcinomas.

**Result of treatment of mixed tumors.** Of the 117 patients with mixed tumors, 113 have been followed for from 3 to 28 years. Two patients have been lost to follow-up and 2 patients have died from unrelated causes within 2 years after treatment. The results of treatment in the remaining patients are summarized in Table II. Each group will be discussed separately.

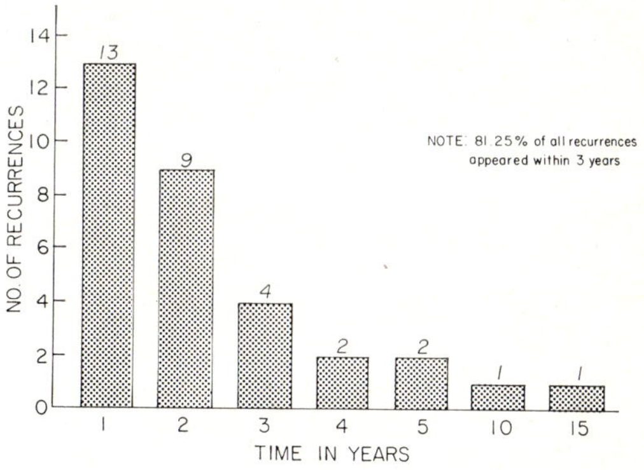


**Fig. 2.** Interval between operation and recurrence of mixed tumors (32 recurrences in 22 patients).

**Group I. Primary mixed tumors of the parotid gland treated by excision or enucleation.** Of 50 patients in this group, 48 have had a follow-up period of at least 3 years. Forty-four patients have been followed for more than 5 years and 29 of these have been followed for at least 10 years, with 10 patients having a follow-up period of over 20 years. Follow-up for the entire group averaged 14.3 years. Although the operative technique varied somewhat from patient to patient because the operations were performed by various members of the surgical staff, in all cases a direct attack upon the tumor only was made after exposure of the parotid gland. The operations were described as simple excision or enucleation, and in an occasional case the tumor was removed in piecemeal fashion. In addition to surgical removal, radiation therapy was employed for 15 patients. This consisted of deep roentgen therapy of from 1,500 to 4,500 r in 13 patients, 4 of whom also received implantation of radon seeds at the time of operation. Two other patients were treated with radium needles postoperatively.

In 5 of these 48 patients the tumor subsequently recurred. Two of the recurrences were treated by total parotidectomy and the other 3 by simple excision. All 5 patients have been free of tumor now for more than 5 years.

That spillage of tumor may be responsible for the recurrences is suggested by the fact that in 4 of the 5 patients with recurrence,

**Table II.** *Result of treatment of 113 mixed tumors of the major salivary glands*

| *Type and treatment* | *No.* | *Recurrences* | *%* | *Follow-up (yr.)* |
|---|---|---|---|---|
| Group I. Primary tumor of parotid gland treated by excision and enucleation | 48 | 5 | 10 | 14.3 (3 – 28) |
| Group II. Primary tumor of parotid gland treated by lobectomy or total parotidectomy | 29 | 0 | 0 | 8.5 (3 – 15) |
| Group III. Recurrent tumor of parotid gland treated by excision or total parotidectomy | 21 | 5 and 1* | 29 | 11.3 excision (3 – 27) 7.2 parotidectomy (4 – 11) |
| Group IV. Mixed tumor of submaxillary gland | 15 | 1* | 7 | 13.0 (3 – 26) |

*Clinically malignant, but histologically benign tumor.

the tumor had been broken into at the time of operation. However, spillage was also reported in 11 other patients without subsequent recurrence.

From these few cases it does not appear that radiation therapy offers a significant protection against recurrence. Two of the patients with recurrence had received a full course of radiation therapy at the time of the initial operation.

**Group II. Primary mixed tumors of the parotid gland treated by superficial lobectomy or total parotidectomy with preservation of the facial nerve.** Of 30 patients in this group, 16 were treated by superficial lobectomy and 14 by total parotidectomy. One patient died from unrelated causes 2 years after operation. The remaining patients have been followed for from 3 to 15 years, with an average follow-up of 8.5 years. Twenty-three patients have been followed for more than 5 years.

In addition to parotidectomy, 3 patients underwent a full course of radiation therapy for spillage of tumor in one, biopsy of the tumor 2 days prior to definitive operation in another, and the false impression that the tumor was an adenoid cystic carcinoma in the third.

There has not been a single recurrence in patients with primary mixed tumor of the parotid gland treated by superficial lobectomy or total parotidectomy as described by State.

**Group III. Recurrent mixed tumors of the parotid gland treated by excision or total parotidectomy.** This group consists of 21 patients who had 36 recurrences prior to treatment at the University of Minnesota Hospitals. An attempt was made to determine as accurately as possible the exact interval between operation and the time the recurrence made its first appearance as noted by the patient. Including the 5 patients in whom tumor recurred after treatment in this institution, this interval could be ascertained in 22 patients with a total of 32 recurrences (Fig. 2). Although in 1 patient the tumor did not recur until 15 years had elapsed, it is important to note that approximately 81 per cent of the recurrences were evident within 3 years and 94 per cent within 5 years after operation.

Of the 21 patients with recurrent tumors, 11 were treated by simple excision and 10 were treated by total parotidectomy. Nine of the patients had been treated at one time with radiation therapy elsewhere before admission.

Of the 11 patients treated by simple excision, 3 had a subsequent recurrence 2, 3, and 4 years after operation, respectively. One of these 3 patients was treated by re-excision and has been well for 26 years. Another was subsequently treated by total parotidectomy and has been free of recurrence for 9 years. The 8 remaining patients have been followed without further recurrence for an average of 11.3 years.

Total parotidectomy for recurrent mixed

tumor of the parotid gland in 10 patients was also followed by further recurrence in 3. Two of these 3 recurrences were located in the operative scar and recurred again after local excision. Since re-excision 1 patient has been followed for 4 years and the other for only 1 year. The third patient, in whom the tumor had been excised twice previously, had a hard, fixed tumor mass which had infiltrated deeply into the retromandibular space and into the skull. Despite a total radical parotidectomy the tumor could be only incompletely removed. Implantation of radon seeds and a course of roentgen therapy of 4,500 r failed to influence the course of the tumor and the patient died 8 months after operation from extensive local disease. The remaining 7 patients have been free of recurrence for an average of 7.2 years.

**Group IV. Mixed tumor of the submaxillary gland.** In this group of 16 patients, 4 had been treated initially elsewhere and had recurrent tumors when first seen at the University of Minnesota Hospitals. Each of the 16 patients was treated by complete excision of the submaxillary gland and in 2 patients an en bloc removal of the contents of the submaxillary triangle was also performed.

One patient died from an associated carcinoma of the lower lip 1 year after operation. In 1 patient, wide excision of a twice recurrent mixed tumor was followed by a recurrence which invaded the mandible and produced a pathologic fracture of the mandible. The patient refused further treatment and died 14 months later from extensive local spread. The remaining 14 patients have been followed for an average of 13 years without further recurrence.

**Incidence of facial paralysis.** Of 101 patients with mixed tumors of the parotid gland 31 sustained some loss of function of the facial nerve after operation (Table III).

In 25 of these patients the facial paralysis was partial. In the majority the resultant facial weakness was mild and usually involved the cervical or buccal division of the facial nerve. Probably because of the remarkable capacity of the facial nerve to regenerate and the existence of abundant anastomoses between its peripheral branches, most of the patients regained considerable control over the facial musculature within 2 years postoperatively. In none of the patients was it necessary to employ a plastic reconstruction or a nerve graft for the repair of the facial nerve.

In 6 patients the facial nerve was completely severed. In only 2 of them was the nerve unintentionally divided. One instance occurred during the course of an excision of a mixed tumor and in the other the nerve was cut during a superficial lobectomy. In both patients primary anastomosis of the severed nerve was rewarded with good return of function within 1 year. In 4 patients the facial nerve was intentionally sacrificed during the course of an operation for what was thought to be a malignant tumor of the parotid gland.

One patient developed a postoperative salivary fistula which closed shortly after

**Table III.** *Incidence of facial nerve injury in 101 patients treated for mixed tumor of the parotid gland*

| *Treatment* | *No.* | | *Facial nerve injury* | |
|---|---|---|---|---|
| | | | *Partial* | *Complete* |
| Group I. Primary tumor treated by excision or enucleation | 50 | | 10 | 2 |
| Group II. Primary tumor treated by superficial lobectomy or total parotidectomy | 30 | | 4 | 2 |
| Group III. Recurrent tumor | 21 | | | |
| Previous injury | | | 4 | – |
| Treated by excision | | 11 | 3 | – |
| Treated by total parotidectomy | | 10 | 4 | 2 |
| Totals | 101 | | 25 | 6* |

*In 4 of the 6 patients the facial nerve was intentionally sacrificed during the course of operation for what was thought to be a malignant tumor of the parotid gland.

1,500 r of roentgen therapy. Two patients developed gustatory sweating after operation over the area of the parotid gland.

## PAPILLARY CYSTADENOMA LYMPHOMATOSUM (WARTHIN'S TUMOR)

The symptoms in patients with papillary cystadenoma lymphomatosum are very similar to those in patients with mixed tumors. However, there are some minor differences. Warthin's tumor occurs predominantly in males and in an older age group and occasionally is bilateral. No well-documented cases of this tumor occurring in the submaxillary or sublingual glands have been reported.[6]

Of 11 patients in this group, 8 were males and 3 were females. Their ages ranged from 44 to 71 years, with an average of 61 years. The longest duration of symptoms was 4 years and in 7 patients the tumor had been noticed for less than 1 year. In 2 patients the tumor was bilateral.

The usual complaint was of a slowly growing, nontender mass. On palpation the tumor was movable and ranged in consistency from firm to soft; at times it felt fluctuant.

**Pathology.** Grossly the tumors were round or ovoid in shape, had a smooth surface, and rarely exceeded 4 cm. in diameter. The tumors were encapsulated and on cut section appeared as a partly cystic mass containing a stringy mucoid material, characteristically with a brownish tinge.

Microscopically the tumors were made up of flattened glands and slender papillary projections formed by tall columnar epithelial cells with granular acidophilic cytoplasm, in a prominent lymphoid stroma with many germinal centers.

**Treatment.** Seven patients were treated by simple excision of the tumor. A subsequent recurrence appeared in only 1 patient, in whom spillage of the tumor had occurred at the time of operation. In 1 patient the tumor was incidentally discovered during the course of a radical neck dissection for a malignant melanoma of the neck from which he died 6 weeks after operation. Three patients were treated by superficial lobectomy. One patient died 1 year after operation in a car accident. The remaining 8 patients have been followed for from 3 to 10 years with an average follow-up of 8 years without recurrence.

## HEMANGIOMAS

Hemangiomas of the salivary glands are not very common and usually occur in children. Five of 7 hemangiomas treated at the University of Minnesota Hospitals occurred in children under 5 years of age. Three of these patients were less than 1 year old. In 1 child the lesion had been present since birth and represented only 1 part of an hemangiomatous lesion involving the lower half of the ear and the cutaneous area over the parotid gland and the mandible. Beneath this skin lesion a discrete, spongy 4.5 cm. mass could be felt. In the other 6 patients the outstanding complaint was a palpable tumor with no visible characteristics of a hemangioma. The tumors had been present for from 1 month to 3 years. Two of the patients were adults, 22 and 41 years old, respectively. Three of the patients were males and 4 of them were females.

**Pathology.** All 7 hemangiomas were located within the parotid gland and varied from 2 to 7 cm. in diameter. Histologically, 5 were of the cavernous type and 2 of them, both in children, were of the capillary variety and demonstrated a high degree of cellularity.

**Treatment.** Five patients were treated by simple excision and 1 patient by a superficial lobectomy. In 1 patient a total parotidectomy was performed for a cavernous hemangioma which had diffusely involved the entire parotid area. The patients have been followed for from 3 to 21 years with an average follow-up period of 8.4 years. There have been no recurrences since treatment. Only 1 patient received roentgen therapy in 3 doses of 200 r each for a postoperative salivary fistula which promptly closed.

## BENIGN LYMPHOEPITHELIAL LESION

The diagnosis of benign lymphoepithelial lesion was made in 4 patients, 2 men and 2 women, ranging in age from 35 to 75 years. In each case the disease had a prolonged course with symptoms lasting for from 2 to 10 years before treatment. Two patients complained of mild pain over the parotid area and a painless swelling was the sole symptom in the other 2 patients.

**Pathology.** The disease may involve the entire gland diffusely or may present as scattered foci or as a localized tumor.[3] In our cases the disease involved the parotid gland diffusely in 3 patients and presented as a well-circumscribed tumor in 1 patient.

Histologically the lesions were made up of lymphoid tissue through which were scattered small and large epithelial islands. In many instances strands of epithelial cells could be traced into ductal structures. In 1 of the patients a diffusely involved gland also contained multiple cysts with contained calculi measuring up to 1 cm. in diameter. An almost identical picture was found in the opposite parotid gland of the same patient several years later. In 3 of our 4 patients the process was bilateral and in each case the parotid gland was the only site of disease.

**Treatment.** In 1 patient treatment consisted only of a biopsy of a diffuse bilateral swelling of the parotid gland which persisted until the time of his death 4 years later from unrelated cause.

In 1 patient a swelling of the parotid gland had been present for 8 years when it suddenly began to enlarge very rapidly. A total parotidectomy was performed for a diffuse process which had infiltrated into the masseter muscle and deeply into the pterygoid fossa and was believed to be a lymphosarcoma. Since postoperative irradiation with 3,600 r of deep roentgen therapy, the patient has been well for 8 years. Review of the pathologic specimen showed it to be a benign lymphoepithelial lesion.

In the third patient a well-circumscribed tumor of the left parotid gland was removed by total parotidectomy. The patient returned 8 years later with a tumor of the right parotid gland, which after excision also proved to be a benign lymphoepithelial lesion. The patient has remained well for 4 years.

The fourth patient was treated by superficial lobectomy for a diffuse involvement of the left parotid gland and 4 years later was treated by the same operation for a more localized process on the right side.

From our own experience and the reports in the literature the disease has thus far shown a benign course, notwithstanding the diffuse infiltration into the surrounding tissue seen in 1 of our patients. Because of the presence of a tumor which is usually indistinguishable clinically from other tumors of the parotid gland, most patients are treated surgically. Irradiation has given good results for others. At present too few cases have been reported for one to judge which form of treatment is more satisfactory.

## OTHER BENIGN TUMORS OF THE MAJOR SALIVARY GLANDS

**Lipoma.** One patient with a lipoma in the left parotid gland was treated by superficial lobectomy at the age of 22.

**Neurofibroma.** A 49-year-old man was treated by superficial lobectomy for a 5 cm. neurofibroma in the left parotid gland. The patient has been well for 16 years.

**Granular-cell myoblastoma.** A 48-year-old man was treated by wide excision of the right submaxillary gland for a granular-cell myoblastoma which apparently originated in or near the gland and had infiltrated the myohyoid and stylohyoid muscles. It had been excised 3 times previously. The patient has been well and without recurrence for 7 years.

## DISCUSSION

It appears from this study that superficial lobectomy and total parotidectomy with preservation of the facial nerve are well suited for the management of benign tumors of the parotid gland. In patients with primary mixed tumors of the parotid gland treated by this method and observed for from 3 to 15 years, not a single recurrence has been noted. This is in contrast to a 10 per cent recurrence rate in this institution prior to the introduction of this operation. Reports in the literature indicate an even higher recurrence rate after simple excision of mixed tumors of the parotid gland. McFarland[5] reported a recurrence rate of 48 per cent in 5 years after operation. In Rawson's[7] series 31 per cent of mixed tumors recurred within 10 years, although the majority of the recurrences took place within 4 years. Winsten and Ward[9] reported a 32 per cent recurrence rate after enucleation and a 28 per cent recurrence rate after excision of mixed tumors of the parotid gland.

Kirklin and associates[4] reviewed the experience of the Mayo Clinic up to 1945 and found a recurrence rate of 10 per cent. More recently Beahrs[1] from the same clinic reported the results of treating primary mixed tumors of the parotid gland by conservative parotidectomy. Of 47 patients so treated since 1951 none has developed a recurrence. The latter surgical technique consists of superficial lobectomy for lesions above the facial nerve and conservative total parotidectomy for lesions deep to the facial nerve. In principle at least, this appears to be very similar to the operation described by State. This striking improvement in results in both institutions is indeed encouraging and offers additional evidence that enucleation or simple excision are inadequate for benign tumors of the parotid gland.

Total parotidectomy for recurrent mixed tumors has seemingly not improved the recurrence rate. However, the number of patients so treated is too small to permit final evaluation.

We do not favor the use of a biopsy prior to removal of the tumor. The scarring and inflammation incident to a biopsy prior to definitive operation tend to make the subsequent operation more difficult and may even invite a recurrence due to spillage of tumor cells. In cases in which there is considerable doubt as to the benign nature of the tumor, a frozen section at the time of operation will usually establish the diagnosis and allow the surgeon to proceed accordingly.

## SUMMARY

A series of 142 benign tumors of the major salivary glands treated surgically at the University of Minnesota Hospitals from 1932 through 1956 has been reviewed.

The recurrence rate in 48 primary mixed tumors of the parotid gland treated by excision or enucleation was 10 per cent.

No recurrences have been observed in 28 patients with primary mixed tumors of the parotid gland treated by superficial lobectomy or total parotidectomy with preservation of the facial nerve during a 3- to 15-year follow-up period.

The recurrence rate in patients treated for recurrent mixed tumors of the parotid gland was 29 per cent, with no apparent improvement after the use of total parotidectomy.

Superficial lobectomy and total parotidectomy with preservation of the facial nerve have proved to be most effective procedures in the management of benign tumors of the parotid gland.

### REFERENCES

1. Beahrs, O. H., Woolner, L. B., Carveth, S. W., and Devine, K. D.: Surgical management of parotid lesions, A. M. A. Arch. Surg. **80:** 890, 1960.
2. Foote, F. W., and Frazell, E. L.: Tumors of the major salivary glands, Washington, D. C., 1954, Armed Forces Institute of Pathology.
3. Godwin, J. T.: Benign lymphoepithelial lesion of the parotid gland (adenolymphoma, chronic inflammation, lymphoepithelioma, lymphocytic tumor, Mikulicz's disease), Cancer **5:** 1089, 1952.
4. Kirklin, J. W., McDonald, J. R., Harrington, S. W., and New, G. B.: Parotid tumors; histopathology, clinical behavior, and end results, Surg. Gynec. & Obst. **92:** 721, 1951.
5. McFarland, J.: The histopathologic prognosis of salivary gland mixed tumors, Am. J. M. Sc. **203:** 502, 1942.
6. Orloff, M. J.: Benign epitheliolymphoid lesions of the parotid gland, papillary cystadenoma

lymphomatosum and Mikulicz's disease, Surg. Gynec. & Obst. **103:** 521, 1956.

7. Rawson, A. J., Howard, J. M., Royster, H. P., and Horn, R. C.: Tumors of the salivary glands. A clinicopathological study of 160 cases, Cancer **3:** 445, 1950.
8. State, D.: Superficial lobectomy and total parotidectomy with preservation of the facial nerve in the treatment of parotid tumors, Surg. Gynec. & Obst. **89:** 237, 1949.
9. Winsten, J., and Ward, G. E.: Mixed tumors of the parotid gland, SURGERY **42:** 1029, 1957.

# Periductal mastitis associated with reticulum-cell sarcoma in the breast

BURTON C. DYSON, M.D.
PHILADELPHIA, PA.
*From the Laboratory of the Episcopal Hospital*

A benign lesion labeled plasma-cell mastitis,[1, 4, 5, 7, 12, 17] fat necrosis,[16, 22, 23] periductal mastitis,[9, 13] comedomastitis,[32] and mammary duct ectasia[15] grossly may simulate carcinoma of the breast. Rapid frozen section study identifies it as a non-neoplastic inflammatory lesion, and unnecessary mastectomy is avoided. Periductal mastitis has been reported as an isolated lesion by most writers, but a few[9, 12, 17, 32] have described it as a minor incidental finding in association with and secondary to carcinoma. Less commonly, recognition of the typical inflammatory lesion on biopsy was followed by subsequent discovery of malignant disease elsewhere in the excised tissue.[17] There is a small but definite risk of missing a coexistent malignant lesion when incisional biopsy diagnosis is made of inflammatory reaction in tissue removed from a breast mass. For this reason, excisional biopsy of the allegedly benign mass is desirable, although in the absence of coexistent malignancy no harm results from allowing the inflammatory lesion to subside spontaneously, as it will do after simple incisional biopsy.[15]

In the case to be reported, a malignant tumor appeared in the incisional biopsy scar after an inflammatory tumor caused by periductal fibrosis had disappeared spontaneously. The rarity in the breast of the associated reticulum-cell sarcoma adds interest to the case.

## CASE REPORT

A 73-year-old white woman noted the spontaneous appearance and daily increase in size of a tender ovoid mass extending laterally from the areola in a pendulous right breast. No discharge and no retraction of the nipple were present, but skin overlying the movable mass was red and slightly edematous. After 5 days the woman sought medical advice.

Preoperative studies showed no significant physical findings other than the breast mass. Hemoglobin concentration was 10.4 Gm. per 100 ml., hematocrit 32 per cent, and white blood cell count 6,200. Urinalysis showed a specific gravity of 1.004, a faint trace of protein, no sugar, 0 to 2 white blood cells, and 0 to 2 red blood cells per high power field. On chest roentgenogram the heart and lungs were seen to be normal except for pulmonary emphysema, but osteoporotic and degenerative changes in the thoracic spine were accompanied by wedging with loss of stature of the eleventh vertebral body. Biopsy of the breast disclosed a sausage-shaped mass lying at 9 o'clock in the right breast with its medial extremity beneath the circumference of the areola, extending laterally a distance of about 4 cm. This lesion, exposed by an incision 3 cm. long, proved to be a gray, firm, solid mass which cut like a gritty pear. The cut surface was streaked with yellow and had several ducts from which soft material emerged on pressure, leading to a gross diagnosis of comedocarcinoma. No gross evidence of inflammation was seen. Upon frozen section diagnosis of "no cancer," the incision was closed without further manipulation.

In paraffin sections (Fig. 1) marked periductal inflammatory cell infiltration and fibrosis accompanied irregular dilatation of ducts within which were found innumerable foamy macrophages. Duct epithelium exhibited changes ascribed to the extensive inflammatory process. No evidence of malignancy was present. The diagnosis made was mammary duct ectasia.

The wound healed without incident, the postoperative course was afebrile, and the mass slowly decreased in size without treatment and disappeared after 10 weeks. After 4 months the patient complained of back pain of 1 week's duration, and stated that a new freely movable, nontender mass beneath the skin at the medial end

Received for publication Nov. 14, 1960.

of the biopsy scar had appeared 1 month earlier. The surgical scar was well healed. No other masses were present in either of the breasts or axillary regions. Complete physical examination again was negative except that the patient had stooped posture, tenderness over the lumbar spinous processes, and a 1 cm. subcutaneous mass at the margin of the right areola. This was removed under local anesthesia, was firm, white, and appeared grossly well demarcated from the surrounding breast tissue. On microscopic examination (Fig. 2) sheets of malignant cells with scant cytoplasm were seen extending from the main lesion irregularly into the surrounding normal mature fat. Although most of the cells could best be interpreted as forming a reticulum-cell sarcoma, plasma cells in scattered areas suggested the possibility of transition to plasmacytoma.

Chest roentgenogram again showed no evidence of disease in the heart or lungs except emphysema, and there was no change evident in the collapsed eleventh vertebral body. However, minimal compression deformity of the twelfth vertebral body was present now with mottling suggestive of malignant disease which had not been present in the films taken 4 months earlier. An upper gastrointestinal series of radioscopic studies was negative. The blood urea level was 15 mg. per 100 ml., the blood sugar level 100 mg. per 100 ml., alkaline phosphatase level 3.3 B.U., the phosphorous level 3.6 mg. per 100 ml., and albumin-globulin ratios were 3.8/5.2 and 3.1/4.4 Gm. per 100 ml. Urinalysis showed specific gravity of 1.004, faint trace of protein, no sugar, 3 to 4 hyaline casts, 6 to 8 white blood cells, and no red blood cells per high power field. Bence-Jones proteinuria was not identified. The hemoglobin concentration was 11.4 Gm. per 100 ml., hematocrit 34 per cent, and white blood cell count 4,000. With general anesthesia, right simple mastectomy with removal in continuity of attached pectoralis major fascia and fat about the axillary vein was carried out without incident. In the excised tissue no residual tumor was identified, and no metastatic tumor was found in 22 lymph nodes recovered from the axillary fat. Postoperative healing was uneventful. Irradiation of the region of the eleventh and twelfth thoracic vertebrae was begun, and 1,200 r was delivered in 8 days with temporary relief of pain. However, back pain returned and roentgenographic study 2 months after mastectomy (6 months after the initial breast mass had appeared) showed a new lesion in the body of the first lumbar vertebra.

The patient became bedfast, suffered tenderness over the right scapula and right seventh to tenth ribs posteriorly which was considered clinically to be due to metastatic disease, and 8 months after the initial breast biopsy was found to have 2 poorly defined masses, each several centimeters in diameter, in the left breast. At this time the hemoglobin concentration was 8.3 Gm. per 100 ml., hematocrit 26 per cent, reticulocyte count 1.4 per cent, and white blood cell count 5,200. Free acid was present on gastric analysis. On urinalysis the specific gravity was found to be

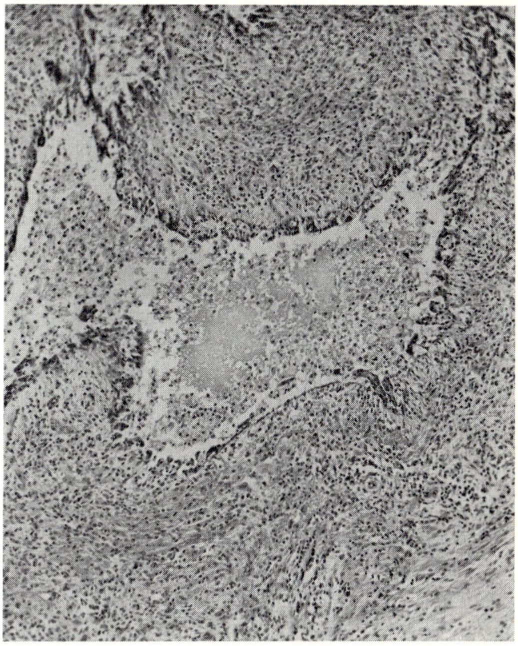

**Fig. 1.** Breast. Marked periductal inflammatory cell infiltration and fibrosis with dilatation of duct. (Hematoxylin and eosin; ×50; reduced ⅖.)

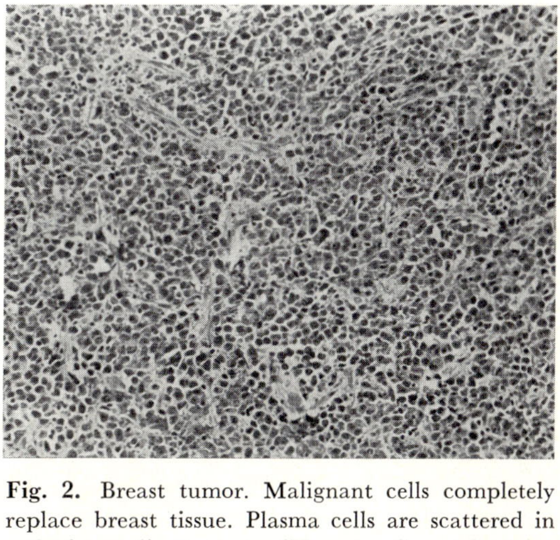

**Fig. 2.** Breast tumor. Malignant cells completely replace breast tissue. Plasma cells are scattered in reticulum-cell sarcoma. (Hematoxylin and eosin; ×230; reduced ½.)

**Table I.** *Summary of previous cases of lymphosarcoma and reticulum-cell sarcoma primary in the*

| Case No. | Author | Age | Size of lesion | Diagnosis |
|---|---|---|---|---|
| *Lesions in the lactating breast* | | | | |
| 1 | Geschickter[13] | 29 | —— | Lymphosarcoma |
| 2 | Geschickter[13] | 32 | —— | Lymphosarcoma |
| 3 | Kay[20] | 28 | —— | Lymphosarcoma |
| *Rapidly fatal cases* | | | | |
| 4 | Schreiner and Thibaudeau[28] | 69 | —— | Lymphosarcoma |
| 5 | Fox[10] | 15 | —— | Lymphosarcoma |
| 6 | Fox[10] | 63 | —— | Lymphosarcoma |
| 7 | Harrington and Miller[18] | 28 | Large, multiple | Lymphosarcoma |
| 8-12 | Geschickter[13] | 15-63 | —— | Lymphosarcoma |
| 13 | Pohl[25] | 30 | —— | Lymphosarcoma |
| 14 | Piacentini[24] | 63 | —— | Reticulum-cell sarcoma |
| 15 | Grampa[14] | 24 | "Egg" | Reticulum-cell sarcoma |
| 16 | Schottenfeld[27] | 30 | 3 cm. | Reticulum-cell sarcoma |
| 17 | Schottenfeld[27] | 75 | 10 cm. | Lymphosarcoma |
| 18 | Schottenfeld[27] | 59 | "Medium" | Lymphosarcoma |
| 19 | Raffo del Campo[26] | 12 | 4 cm. | Reticulum-cell sarcoma |
| 20 | DuRoy and Sawyer[8] | 55 | "Large" | Reticulum-cell sarcoma |
| *Small lesions cured* | | | | |
| 21 | Stringer[29] | 53 | —— | Reticulum-cell sarcoma |
| 22 | Thur[31] | 52 | —— | Lymphosarcoma |
| 23 | Harrington and Miller[18] | 38 | 3 cm. | Lymphosarcoma |
| 24 | Adair and Hermann[2] | 53 | 4 cm. | Reticulum-cell sarcoma |
| 25 | Adair and Hermann[2] | 47 | 2 cm. | Reticulum-cell sarcoma |
| 26 | Adair and Hermann[2] | 41 | —— | Lymphosarcoma |
| 27 | Geschickter[13] | — | "Small" | Lymphosarcoma |
| 28 | Schottenfeld[27] | 68 | 3 cm. | Reticulum-cell sarcoma |
| 29 | Bellini[3] | 61 | "Hazelnut" | Lymphosarcoma |
| 30 | Latteri and Santora[21] | 34 | —— | Reticulum-cell sarcoma |

1.022, and there was 1+ proteinuria, no sugar, and 15 to 20 hyaline casts per high power field. Test for Bence-Jones proteinuria again was negative. The blood urea level was 7 mg. per 100 ml. The patient refused additional studies and died at home 8 months after reticulum-cell sarcoma had been recognized in the breast. Autopsy was not permitted.

In summary, an acute, spontaneously arising, slightly tender breast mass in a 73-year-old woman was diagnosed on biopsy as mammary duct ectasia and disappeared completely after 10 weeks' observation without treatment. Shortly thereafter a new mass appeared at the medial end of the biopsy scar beneath the areola, and on biopsy proved to be a reticulum-cell sarcoma. Death occurred 8 months after removal of the reticulum sarcoma, preceded by clinical evidence of widespread metastasis.

## DISCUSSION

The typical tumor of periductal mastitis occurs in women of postmenopausal age and is located near the center of the breast not far from the areola. Retraction of the nipple occurs in 50 per cent of cases. Usually the preoperative diagnosis is cancer,[15] although the characteristic history is that of sudden onset with inflammatory signs, followed by slow regression perhaps with persistence of some induration.[13] In approximately 10 per cent of all cases reported to date, periductal mastitis has existed in conjunction with a recognized malignant lesion.[6, 7, 9, 12, 15-17, 32]

Reticulum-cell sarcoma and lymphosar-

*breast*

| *Treatment* | *Course* | *Remarks* |
|---|---|---|
| —— | Died, 4 mo. | Both breasts diffusely enlarged in all 3 cases |
| —— | Died, 4 mo. | |
| None | Died, 3 wk. | |
| Radical mastectomy and radiation | Early recurrence | Terminal when lost to follow-up at 4 yr., 9 mo. |
| Radical mastectomy | Died, 5 mo. | Cervical and axillary nodes involved at start |
| Radical mastectomy | Died, 2 mo. | Metastasis to brain |
| Radical mastectomy and radiation | Died, 7 wk. | Bilateral breast and axillary masses at start |
| —— | Died before 20 mo. | All had widespread metastases |
| Radical mastectomy and radiation | Died "soon after Rx" | Widespread metastases |
| Radical mastectomy | Died, 1 yr. | Cerebral metastasis |
| Radical mastectomy | Died, 10 mo. | Abdominal metastases |
| Local excision | Died, 5 mo. | |
| Radiation | Terminal, 3 mo. | |
| Local excision | —— | After 6 mo. vaginal bleeding from lymphosarcoma of cervix |
| Local excision and radiation | Died, 11 mo. | Recurrence at 3 mo. |
| Radical mastectomy and radiation | Died, 11 mo. | Widespread metastases |
| Simple mastectomy and radiation | Living and well, 3½ yr. | Appeared in biopsy scar 6 mo. after excision of mass labeled "chronic mastitis"; after 2½ yr. invaded entire breast and metastasized to temporal region with regression after radiation; general health excellent |
| Local excision and radiation | Living and well, 18 mo. | |
| Radical mastectomy and radiation | Living and well, 6 yr. | |
| Radical mastectomy | Living and well, 7 yr. | |
| Radical mastectomy | Living and well, 3 yr. | |
| Local excision and radiation | Living and well, 10 mo. | |
| Local excision and radiation | Living and well, 2 yr. | |
| Local excision and radiation | Died, 11 mo. | No recurrence, died of heart disease |
| Radical mastectomy and radiation | Living and well, 20 mo. | |
| Radical mastectomy and radiation | Living and well, 4 yr. | |

coma primary in the breast is a rare curiosity.[11, 19, 31] Only 30 detailed case reports with follow-up study have been recorded, all in the female breast (Table I). The tumor characteristically remains movable for a time, although microscopic infiltration of surrounding tissue already may be evident.[13] In over half of the cases reported,[6, 8, 10, 13, 14, 18, 20, 21, 25-30] death from lymphoma followed within a few weeks or months of initial diagnosis and treatment. Of 9 patients[2, 3, 13, 18, 21, 27, 31] apparently cured, 7 had been treated by irradiation. In 3 of the cases radical mastectomy had preceded irradiation, while in 4 others only local excision of the breast mass was used.

## SUMMARY

A breast mass grossly simulating carcinoma in a 73-year-old woman was diagnosed on incisional biopsy as benign periductal mastitis and subsided completely without further treatment. Four months later a reticulum-cell sarcoma was removed from the medial end of the biopsy scar beneath the areola. Widespread metastasis was followed by death 8 months later.

Excisional biopsy is advised for apparently benign periductal mastitis which simulates breast cancer.

I am grateful to Drs. John W. Klopp and Charles S. Kambe for permission to use their case report.

## REFERENCES

1. Adair, F. E.: Plasma cell mastitis, Arch. Path. **26:** 735, 1933.
2. Adair, F. E., and Hermann, J. B.: Lymphosarcoma of breast, SURGERY **16:** 836, 1944.
3. Bellini, F.: Linfosarcoma e reticulosarcoma della mammella; contributo casisto, Tumori **42:** 737, 1956.
4. Cheatle, G. L., and Cutler, M.: Tumors of the breast, Philadelphia, 1931, J. B. Lippincott Company, pp. 298-304.
5. Cromar, C. D. L., and Dockerty, M. B.: Plasma cell mastitis, Proc. Staff Meet. Mayo Clin. **16:** 775, 1941.
6. Cutler, C. W., Jr.: Plasma cell tumor of the breast with metastases, Ann. Surg. **100:** 392, 1934.
7. Cutler, M.: Plasma cell mastitis, report of a case with bilateral involvement, Brit. M. J. **1:** 94, 1949.
8. DuRoy, R. M., and Sawyer, K. C.: Lymphosarcoma of the breast; discussion and presentation of a case, Am. Surgeon **25:** 489, 1959.
9. Foote, F. W., and Stewart, F. W.: Comparative studies of cancerous versus non-cancerous breasts, Ann. Surg. **121:** 197, 1945.
10. Fox, S. L.: Sarcoma of the breast, Ann. Surg. **100:** 401, 1934.
11. Fruhling, L., and LeGal, Y.: Les sarcomes vrais primitifs de la mamella, Bull. Assoc. franç étude cancer **38:** 447, 1951.
12. Gaston, E. A.: Plasma cell mastitis, SURGERY **21:** 208, 1947.
13. Geschickter, G. F.: Diseases of the breast, Philadelphia, 1945, J. B. Lippincott Company, ed. 2.
14. Grampa, A.: Rassegna e contributo allo studio del reticolosarcoma a sede mammaria, Chirurgia **7:** 129, 1952.
15. Haagensen, C. D.: Mammary duct ectasia. A disease that may simulate carcinoma, Cancer **4:** 749, 1951.
16. Hadfield, G.: Fat necrosis of the breast, Brit. J. Surg. **17:** 673, 1930.
17. Halpert, B., Parker, J. M., and Thuringer, J. M.: Plasma cell mastitis, Arch. Path. **46:** 313, 1948.
18. Harrington, S. W., and Miller, J. M.: Lymphosarcoma of the mammary gland, Am. J. Surg. **48:** 346, 1940.
19. Hill, R. P., and Stout, A. P.: Sarcoma of the breast, A. M. A. Arch. Surg. **44:** 723, 1952.
20. Kay, S.: Lymphosarcoma of the female mammary gland, A. M. A. Arch. Path. **60:** 575, 1955.
21. Latteri, S., Jr., and Santoro, A.: Reticulosarcoma della mammella, Gior. ital. chir. **13:** 1025, 1957.
22. Lee, B. J., and Adair, F. E.: Traumatic fat necrosis of the female breast and its differentiation from carcinoma, Ann. Surg. **72:** 188, 1920.
23. Lee, B. J., and Adair, F. E.: Traumatic fat necrosis in the female breast, Ann. Surg. **80:** 670, 1924.
24. Piacentini, L.: Il reticolosarcoma sincinzioplasmodiale a sede mammaria, Arch. ital. anat. Inst. Path. **24:** 254, 1951.
25. Pohl, W.: Bosartiger Verlauf einer zunachst gutartigen Geschwulst (Lymphocymatosa mammae), Wien. klin. Wchnschr. **60:** 444, 1948.
26. Raffo del Campo, M. A., and Alperovich, A.: Reticuloblastoma de la glanula mamaria, Rev. Assoc. méd. argent. **72:** 351, 1958.
27. Schottenfeld, L. E.: Sarcoma of the breast, review of the literature with report of fourteen cases, Am. J. Surg. **88:** 229, 1954.
28. Schreiner, B. F., and Thibaudeau, A. A.: Sarcoma of the breast: report of seven cases, Ann. Surg. **95:** 433, 1932.
29. Stringer, P.: Reticulosarcoma of both breasts, Brit. J. Surg. **47:** 51, 1959.
30. Stringer, P.: Personal communication, May, 1960.
31. Thur, W.: Zur Kenntnis seltener Geschwulstformen der weiblichen Brustdruse (Lymphosarcom, Spindelzellensarkom), Arch. path. Anat. **265:** 96, 1927.
32. Tice, G. E., Dockerty, M. B., and Harrington, S. W.: Comedomastitis: a clinical and pathological study of data in 172 cases, Surg. Gynec. and Obst. **87:** 525, 1948.

# Intravisceral (topical) use of chemotherapeutic (radiomimetic) agents

LOUIS M. ROUSSELOT, M.D.
DONALD R. COLE, M.D.
NEW YORK, N. Y.
*From the Departments of Surgery, St. Vincent's Hospital and New York University School of Medicine*

Local (intravisceral) cancer chemotherapy may be defined as the regional placement of chemotherapeutic agents in a viscus by physical means. Its purpose is to minimize the effect on organs outside of the tumor zone and to permit the delivery of a higher dose to the tumor cells. Local chemotherapy in the form of topical application was the first effective form of cancer therapy. Hippocrates reported results which would be called encouraging according to current cancer reports. Many fascinating articles on the local use of chemical agents may be found in the medical literature written before the turn of the century.[6-8] Adair and Bagg[1] used mustard gas in solution for surface and interstitial tumor applications in 1931, more than 10 years before the nitrogen mustards were tried for systemic cancer chemotherapy. Reports on topical applications of modern chemotherapeutic agents indicate that while initial tumor regression was usually observed, the results in general have been unpredictable. The present situation appears to us to be similar to that of cancer therapy with roentgen rays and radium in its first decade. Good results were rare and side reactions frequent as they are today with local chemotherapy. Only after distribution and doses had been adequately controlled did radiation therapy give consistently worthwhile results. We therefore anticipate that intravisceral chemotherapy may also become a valuable tool in cancer management with improved techniques. This paper is written in the hope of stimulating interest in a new technique, which we believe may increase the survival rate without effecting morbidity or death.

Received for publication Nov. 21, 1960.

Chemotherapeutic agents may be applied to skin, to mucous surfaces, to surfaces of natural cavities, such as pleura and peritoneum, and surfaces of artificially created spaces, such as wounds. The purpose may be cure or palliation of gross tumors or prevention of local recurrence if all gross cancer is surgically removed. The use of chemical agents for the treatment of superficial tumors has been recorded as early as the fifth century by Hippocrates. Today, caustic agents are still widely used. The initiative for the first trial of modern chemotherapeutic agents for surface applications in cancer must be credited to Dr. James Ewing. While at the Army Institute of Pathology during World War I, he was impressed by the peculiar histologic reactions produced by mustard gas. In 1927, Ewing, Adair, and Bagg began animal experiments with mustard gas. They reported their clinical observations on 19 patients in 1931. Twelve of the patients were treated by superficial applications of mustard gas dissolved in water. The thirteenth patient was given an interstitial injection. They state that they saw no recurrence within 2 years, and that the skins were pliable, well healed, and painless.

In our review of the literature, we encountered 4 reports which described the use of surface applications for cancers in locations other than the skin, pleura, or peritoneal cavity. The first is by Bateman,[4] who mentions 1 patient with bladder cancer in whom intravesical instillation of triethylenethiophosphoramide (TSPA) was used. This was followed by disappearance of cancer cells from the urine. The second report is that of Schultze[27] on the treatment of 2 patients with rectal cancer who could not be operated upon. Daily enemas of Tetramine were given in addition to oral Tetramine therapy. Schultze reports "apparent cure" in one and good regression in the other. The third and fourth reports are those of Whiteside and associates[33] and Murphy[24] on the intrathecal use of Methotrexate. Much higher doses could be administered in this way than by systemic application and better results were achieved in central nervous system involvement by leukemia and lymphoma than with intravenous injections. These reports indicate to us that the intravisceral use of chemotherapeutic agents should be explored. This technique offers unique possibilities by localization to the tumor area and precise dosimetry.

Local recurrences are the cause of failure in many cancer operations; their development from implanted cancer cells was recognized by some medical pioneers. Moore,[21] in 1867, commented specifically on the danger of "seeding." To prevent it, Lack,[17] in 1876, recommended carbolic acid spray, and Babler,[3] in 1909, was using alcohol and other chemicals in operative wounds. Mayo[18] suggested the local use of phenol or cautery if complete extirpation was not possible. Ewing[11] recommended that a biopsy wound for mammary cancer be closed over a 10 per cent formalin sponge to prevent spillage of viable tumor cells during subsequent dissection.

It has now been demonstrated conclusively that cells of a malignant neoplasm are constantly being cast off.[10, 22, 25, 30, 31] Combining the first 4 reports for a total of 342 patients, we see that malignant cells were found in the wound or the abdominal cavity during cancer operations in 23 per cent. Cells which looked suspicious, but could not be classified definitely as malignant, were found in an additional 11 per cent.

The percentage of positive washes for malignant cells in the cavity depends upon the stage of the tumor as shown by the study of Moore and his group.[22] In 251 patients with abdominal cancer, positive washings were observed in noncurable cancer in 66 per cent (stomach), 58 per cent (colon), and 43 per cent (rectum); while in curable cancer positive washings were found in 33 per cent (stomach), 32 per cent (colon), and 16 per cent (rectum).

Many investigators have demonstrated that the shedding of cells is accentuated by manipulation.[2, 14, 19, 26, 30]

Chemotherapeutic agents, radiocolloids, or external roentgen therapy have been recommended for the prevention of local recurrences and metastases. The use of chemotherapeutic agents appears attractive to us because it is more economical, easier to perform, and avoids all the safety, supply, and licensing problems of radiation. Ship and colleagues[29] demonstrated the possible effectiveness of a 0.05 per cent formaldehyde solution. This material applied at times varying from 5 minutes before to 24 hours after tumor inoculation prevented growth of tumor in 80 to 85 per cent of the mice. In the untreated controls, tumor growth occurred in 100 per cent. Treated mice which developed tumor demonstrated a significant delay in time of appearance of tumor. The same concentration of formaldehyde placed in the wound 1 to 24 hours prior to tumor inoculation resulted in enhanced growth of tumor. Seal[28] compared chemotherapeutic agents with radiocolloids in transplantable ascites rat tumor. These agents were introduced into the peritoneal cavity at the same time as the tumor cells. All animals in which only the ascites tumor was injected developed cancer and died. When HN2 was injected at the same time as the implant, 80 per cent of the animals survived. Kramer and associates[15] studied the prevention of S-91 melanoma and Sarcoma 37 in mice by the use of TSPA. When TSPA was given in the tumor inoculation site at or shortly after the time of inoculation, the tumors were smaller than those in the control group. This effect was greater when tumor and TSPA were given intraperitoneally than when they were given intramuscularly. Krementz and his group[16] also investigated the effectiveness of TSPA in preventing tumor growth. They instilled Brown-Pearce tumor cells in the subcutaneous abdominal incision of 94 rabbits. In the control group, 79 per cent of the animals had growth in the wound. In the group treated with TSPA intraperitoneally, 81 per cent had tumor growth. The group in which the wound was irrigated with saline solution showed tumor growth in 74 per cent. In the group treated with TSPA instilled locally in the wound, only 40 per cent had tumor growth.

Whitehead and colleagues[34] experimented with nitrogen mustard combined with radiogold to inhibit the growth of Ehrlich ascites carcinoma in mice. The inoculations were given intraperitoneally and treatment was begun on the following day. The effectiveness was judged by the number of cells in the ascitic fluid. The authors believed that HN2-radiogold combination caused more tumor inhibition than would be anticipated if the effect of the 2 agents were merely an additive one.

On the basis of their own animal experiments, Cole and co-workers started a program of prophylactic and adjuvant injection of HN2 immediately after curative resection of carcinoma in the hope of reducing local recurrences and distant metastases.[23] This was expanded under the auspices of the Cooperative Clinical Research Program of the Cancer Chemotherapy National Service Center into a large cooperative study. Twenty-five per cent of the full dose of HN2 or TSPA was given, in this program, into the pleural or peritoneal cavity during operation, and the other 5 per cent was given intravenously. In the part of the study conducted at Veterans Administration Hospitals, the 30-day mortality rate was significantly higher in the treated than in the control group (22 versus 7 per cent for lung cancer, 23 versus 10 per cent for gastric cancer, and 12 versus 2 per cent for colorectal cancer, 1959). Since most of the agents were given intravenously, the effects of the intravisceral or intracavitary applications of chemotherapeutic agents cannot be evaluated from this study.

Hatiboglu and colleagues[12] studied the effects of various chemotherapeutic agents on tumor cells inoculated into experimental wounds in vitro and into 2 systems in vivo. The local toxicity of the agents was measured by their effects on wound healing. The ratio of the destruction of tumor cells to the impairment of wound healing was computed for each of 8 chemotherapeutic agents and was found to decrease in the following order: HN2, sodium hypochlorite, acriflavine, Clorpactin XCB, Atabrine, actinomycin D, TSPA, and Rivanol.

## SCOPE OF STUDY AND DESCRIPTION OF NEW METHOD

Under the stimulus of the need for a more effective treatment of cells shed during surgical manipulation and in the hope of thus diminishing local recurrence and metastasis from the operation itself, we have developed a technique of intravisceral topical localization of the chemotherapeutic agents during the surgical procedure. The direct intraluminal instillation of the drug assures high concentration of the agent at the tumor site with relatively prolonged action. During the development of our project in human beings, we became aware of this same suggestion by Cohn and Atik[9] in their experimental studies in rabbits. Regional leak of the agent occurs and appears to us desirable for the treatment of cells within the lymphatic and venous systems. It is possible that metastatic disease may be desirably affected by our technique. When the abdominal cavity is entered, the tumor-bearing area of intestine is immediately isolated after the technique of Cole by placement of proximal and distal umbilical tapes at the limits of conventional resection. These are tied snugly. Currently HN2 is used since our work and that of others indicates that it is still superior to other alkylating agents locally. We used 0.4 mg. per kilogram mixed so as to produce a 50 ml. solution in sterile saline solution. A purse-string suture is placed in the seromuscular coat, on the antimesenteric wall of the segment to be resected. The site selected should be some distance from the primary tumor. With a Luer-Lok syringe and attached 15 gauge needle, the chemotherapeutic solution is then slowly introduced into the lumen. After the introduction of the material, the needle is withdrawn and the suture tied. The operation is then continued in the usual fashion. The patient is followed by frequent complete blood and platelet counts and liver and kidney function tests. The specimen is examined grossly and microscopically. During the procedure, intermittent samplings of local and systemic venous blood are taken. These aliquots and the material remaining in the intestine after the removal of the specimen are analyzed for nitrogen mustard by the technique of Klatt[13] and indicate epithelial transfer and venous pickup.

To date, we have performed this procedure on 10 patients; 1 with a carcinoma of the cecum, 1 with a carcinoma of the right colon, 1 with a carcinoma of the transverse colon, 1 with a carcinoma of the splenic flexure, 3 with carcinoma of the sigmoid colon, 3 with carcinoma of the rectum, and 1 patients with chronic diverticulitis which looked grossly like carcinoma. There have been no demonstrable adverse effects locally or systemically. Wound healing has apparently been uneventful and distribution of the cytotoxic agent throughout the specimen and its vascular supply has been as predicted.

In summary, chemotherapeutic agents show promise in local attenuation of tumor growth and in the prevention of local recurrences and metastases from surgical manipulation. A new technique is described which permits a more concentrated action on the primary tumor and free tumor cells within the bowel lumen. Regional leak, via venous and lymphatic routes, appears desirable for the treatment of lymphatic and venous metastases.

## REFERENCES

1. Adair, F. E., and Bagg, H. J.: Experimental and clinical studies on the treatment of cancer by dichlorethylsulphide (mustard gas), Ann. Surg. **93:** 190, 1931.
2. Ackerman, L. V., and Wheat, M. W.: The implantation of cancer—an avoidable surgical risk? SURGERY **37:** 341, 1955.
3. Babler, E. A.: The prevention of cancer cell implantation, J. A. M. A. **52:** 182, 1909.
4. Bateman, J. C.: Chemotherapy of solid tumors with triethylene thiophosphoramide. New England J. Med. **252:** 879, 1955.
5. Bateman, J. C., and McCable, M.: Palliation of far-advanced cancer with triethylene thiophosphoramide, Acta Unio internat. contra cancrum **11:** 111, 1955.
6. Biggs, R.: Chian turpentine in cancer, Lancet **2:** 233, 1880.
7. Bulkley, L. D.: On the use of caustics in malignant disease, J. A. M. A. **22,** 982, 1894.
8. Carpenter, G. W.: Chromic acid on cancroid growths, Peoria M. Month. **1:** 34, 1880-1881.
9. Cohn, I., Jr., and Atik, M.: The influence of antibiotics on the spread of tumors of the colon, Ann. Surg. **151:** 917, 1960.
10. Dahle, T.: Transtubal spread of tumor cells in carcinoma of body of uterus, Surg. Gynec. & Obstet. **103:** 332, 1956.
11. Ewing, J.: Biopsy in mammary cancer, Illinois M. J. **63:** 482, 1933.
12. Hatiboglu, I., Moore, G., Wilkens, H., and Hoffmeister, F.: Effects of chemotherapeutic agents on wounds contaminated with tumor cells, Ann. Surg. **152:** 559, 1960.
13. Klatt, O., Griffin, A. C., and Stehlin, J. S.: Method for determination of phenylalanine mustard and related alkylating agents in blood, Proc. Soc. Exper. Biol. & Med. **104:** 629, 1960.
14. Knox, L. D.: The relationship of massage to metastasis in malignant tumors, Ann. Surg. **75:** 129, 1922.
15. Kramer, W. M., Eck, R. V., and Smith, R. R.: Inhibition of local tumor implantation with triethylenethiophosphoramide (TSPA), Cancer **11:** 999, 1958.
16. Krementz, E. T., Kerlin, M. L., and Leonard, G. L.: The effect of triethylene-thiophosphoramide on the growth of Brown-Pearce rabbit tumor in surgical wounds, S. Forum **10:** 52, 1959.
17. Lack, L.: Contribution to operative treatment of malignant disease of the larynx with special references to the danger of cancerous wound infection, Lancet **1:** 1638, 1896.

18. Mayo, W. J.: Grafting and traumatic dissemination of carcinoma in the course of operations for maligant disease, J. A. M. A. **60:** 512, 1913.
19. McGrew, E. A., Laws, J. F., and Cole, W. H.: Free malignant cells in relation to recurrence of carcinoma of the colon, J. A. M. A. **154:** 1251, 1954.
20. McPherson, C.: Dissemination of cancer cells at operation, Am. J. Proct. **11:** 414, 1960.
21. Moore, C. H.: On the influence of inadequate operations on the theory of cancer, Med.-Chir. Tr. **50:** 245, 1867.
22. Moore, G. E., Burke, E. M., Skjorten, F., Kondo, T., and Badillo, J.: Appraisal of tumor cell spread into the abdominal cavity, S. Forum **10:** 17, 1960.
23. Mrazek, R., Economou, S., McDonald, G. O., Slaughter, D. P., and Cole, W. H.: Prophylactic and adjuvant use of nitrogen mustard in the surgical treatment of cancer, Ann. Surg. **150:** 745, 1959.
24. Murphy, M. L.: Leukemia and lymphoma in children, Pediat. Clin. North America **6:** 611, 1959.
25. Quan, S. H. Q.: Cul-de-sac smears for cancer cells, SURGERY **45:** 258, 1959.
26. Saphir, O.: The transfer of tumor cells by the surgical knife, Surg. Gynec. & Obst. **63:** 775, 1936.
27. Schultze, W.: Erste Erfahrungen mit der Tetramin-Behandlung maligner Tumoren; Klinische und morphologische Beobachtungen, Deutsche med. Wchnschr. **82:** 1465, 1957.
28. Seal, S. H.: Comparison of chemotherapeutic agents with radiocolloids in transplantable ascites rate tumor. Presented at James Ewing Society Meeting, Memorial Center, New York, 1958.
29. Ship, A. G., Eck, R. V., and Smith, R. R.: Local chemotherapy of experimentally tumor-seeded wounds, Cancer **11:** 687, 1958.
30. Smith, R., and Hilberg, A. W.: Cancer-cell seeding of operative wounds, J. Nat. Cancer Inst. **16:** 645, 1955.
31. Spjut, H. J., Hendrix, V. J., Ramirez, G. A., and Roper, C. L.: Carcinoma cells in pleural cavity washings, Cancer **11:** 1222, 1958.
32. Stone, W. S.: A review of the history of chemical therapy in cancer, M. Rec. **90:** 628, 1916.
33. Whiteside, J. A., Philips, F. S., Dargeon, H. W., and Burchenal, J. H.: Intrathecal amethopterin in neurological manifestations of leukemia, A. M. A. Arch. Int. Med. **101:** 279, 1958.
34. Whitehead, R. W., Lanier, R. R., and Thompson, J. B.: The combined effect of radiogold and nitrogen mustard and radiogold and certain other compounds in the Ehrlich ascites carcinoma, Cancer **11:** 929, 1958.

# Investigative surgery

## Studies on fibrinolytic activity with venous occlusion: treatment of thrombophlebitis

E. E. CLIFFTON, M.D.
R. L. CLARKE, M.D*
J. MURPHY, M.D.
NEW YORK, N. Y.
*From the Second Surgical (Cornell) Division, Bellevue Hospital*

Thrombi can be dissolved in vivo by fibrinolytic activity and this mechanism is apparently effective in the treatment of many thromboembolic disorders.[12] Effective fibrinolytic agents have been developed for clinical use but they are still expensive and side reactions still occur, though with decreasing frequency. To increase our understanding of the mechanism of fibrinolysis we have continued to investigate methods for the induction of fibrinolytic activity by more natural means. Fibrinolytic activity has been shown to occur with many types of stress.[4]

During our studies of induced fibrinolytic activity it was noted that spontaneous fibrinolytic activity was frequently found in patients from whom it was difficult to obtain blood specimens. It occurred to us that this might be due to the prolonged venous blockage by the tourniquet. Kwaan and McFadzean[8, 9] had studied this phenomenon and Sherry and associates[11] have since reported their observations. We observed that venous occlusion by a sphygmomanometer cuff maintained at diastolic pressure resulted in significant fibrinolytic activity in a number of human subjects.[3] Increasing the duration of occlusion from 5 to 20 minutes resulted in a marked increase in the ratio of subjects demonstrating fibrinolysis—from 20 per cent with 5 minutes to 44 per cent with 20 minutes occlusion. Kwaan and McFadzean and Sherry limited their studies to short periods of occlusion and did not note the high percentage of individuals showing activity.

The present study is an extension of our previous report[3] and includes reports concerning patients with thrombophlebitis treated by this method.

### MATERIALS AND METHODS

Control blood samples were obtained either from an unobstructed vein in the antecubital fossa or over the medial malleolus. Experimental samples of venous blood were obtained distal to the sphygmomanometer cuff while it was still inflated. Blood was also obtained from a nonoccluded vein of another extremity 10 to 20 minutes after the release of pressure. The blood samples were placed on ice immediately and kept refrigerated until tested. The euglobulin method was used and fibrinolytic activity was determined by lysis of a bovine fibrin clot.[5, 10] Proteolytic activity was determined by the digestion of casein and measurement of the amount of tyrosine liberated.[6] The antiplasmin activity was determined as previously described,[2] and the prothrombin time by the one-stage method of Quick.[1] Whole-clot lysis was measured by placing a 3 ml. specimen of clotted blood in a water bath at 37° C. and measuring the time of complete lysis of the sample.

Supported by Grant H-4211, National Heart Institute, Bethesda, Md.

Received for publication Dec. 1, 1960.

*Research Fellow, National Heart Institute, Bethesda, Md.

The individuals tested were essentially healthy and none had known carcinoma or debilitating chronic illness.

## INTERMITTENT VENOUS OCCLUSION

Nine volunteer patients were used in these investigations. Two variations were employed; (1) a 20-minute period of venous occlusion followed by a 10-minute "rest" period (this cycle was then repeated), and (2) a 20-minute occlusion followed by a 20-minute "rest" period before the cycle was repeated.

A control blood sample was first obtained without obstruction from a vein in an upper extremity. An ordinary sphygmomanometer cuff was then applied to the thigh and the pressure raised to the patient's diastolic pressure in that extremity. At the end of the 20-minute occlusion period, a blood sample was obtained from an occluded vein as described.

After the 10- or 20-minute rest period, a blood sample without occlusion was obtained from an upper extremity. The entire cycle was then repeated with blood samples drawn at the end of the second occlusion period and at the end of the second rest period.

## RESULTS

Significant activity was found in the blood from the occluded vein during one or both periods of venous occlusion in 6 of 10 patients, or 60 per cent (Table I, Nos. 1, 2, 3, 5, 6, and 7). In 3 of these patients (Nos. 2, 3, and 7), the activity was poor during the first cycle, but increased significantly during the second cycle.

Four of the patients (Nos. 4, 8, 9, and 10) failed to manifest any significant increase in euglobulin fibrinolytic activity.

It is noteworthy that there was also an increase in systemic activity in 4 patients (Nos. 1, 2, 5, and 6), either after both cycles or only after the second one. In 2 of the patients (Nos. 3 and 7) in whom there was significant local activity without systemic activity, the greatest local activity occurred during the second cycle.

## PERSISTENCE OF FIBRINOLYTIC ACTIVITY

If thrombi are to be lysed in vivo it is necessary to maintain fibrinolytic activity for some time. It was important to know (1) how long the activity persists after occlusion is released and (2) whether or not the response is repeatable with subsequent courses of occlusion. To answer the first question we studied 5 patients (Nos. 11 through 15). A control sample was drawn and the occlusion was maintained for 20 minutes at diastolic pressure, a local blood sample was drawn, and the sphygmomanometer cuff removed. Samples of venous blood were then obtained from the same antecubital fossa every 20 minutes for the next hour. The local fibrinolytic activity produced by venous occlusion disappeared within 20 minutes after the release of the cuff (Fig. 1). To answer the second question we investigated 6 patients (Nos. 16 through 21) over a 6-hour period. Using periods of 20 minutes of venous occlusion separated by 20 minutes of rest (cuff

**Table I.** *Fibrinolytic activity measured in 2 successive cycles of venous occlusion at the thigh*

| *Patient* | *Occlusion/rest (min.)* | *Euglobulin fibrinolytic activity (lysis time, hr.)* *Cycle* | *Control* | *Local (lower extremity)* | *Systemic (upper extremity)* |
|---|---|---|---|---|---|
| 1 | 20:20 | 1st | 10-18 | 2 | 3-5 |
| | | 2nd | | 2 | 3-5 |
| 2 | 20:10 | 1st | 20 | 18½ | 11½ |
| | | 2nd | | 1-2 | 6 |
| 3 | 20:10 | 1st | 24 | 12½ | 24 |
| | | 2nd | | 1½-2 | 24 |
| 4 | 20:10 | 1st | 7-8 | 6-7 | 7-8 |
| | | 2nd | | 5½ | 9-10 |
| 5 | 20:10 | 1st | 24 | 5½ | 21 |
| | | 2nd | | 6-7 | 8 |
| 6 | 20:20 | 1st | 9-20 | 3 | 4 |
| | | 2nd | | 3 | 3 |
| 7 | 20:20 | 1st | ? | 24 | 24 |
| | | 2nd | | 1¼ | 24 |
| 8 | 20:20 | 1st | 7-8 | 4 | 7-8 |
| | | 2nd | | 10½ | 24 |
| 9 | 20:20 | 1st | 24 | 24 | 24 |
| | | 2nd | | 24 | 24 |
| 10 | 20:20 | 1st | 24 | 24 | 24 |
| | | 2nd | | 24 | 24 |

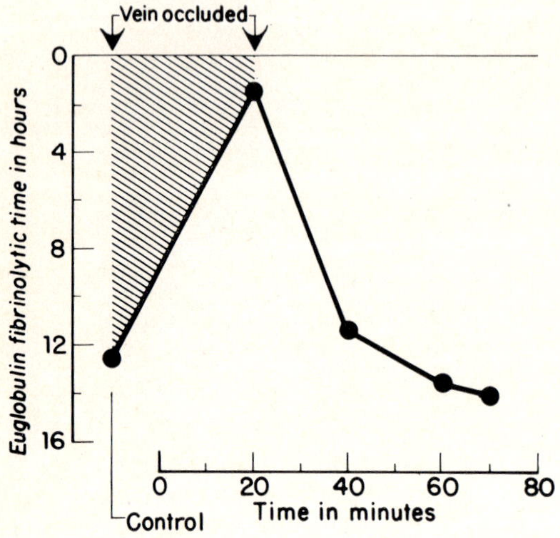


**Fig. 1.** Composite graph which shows average euglobulin fibrinolytic times of patients during and after 1 period of venous occlusion.

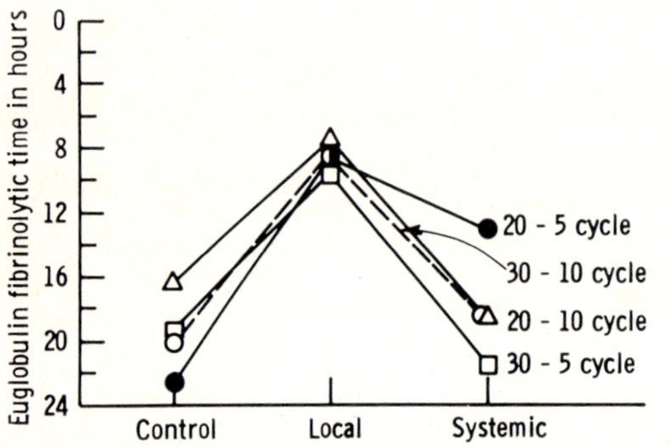


**Fig. 2.** Composite graph which shows average euglobulin fibrinolytic response to 4 different cycles of occlusion and rest; 16 experiments.

off), we obtained samples of blood from the occluded extremity each hour during the 6 hours of the test. The results indicate that this phenomenon is repeatable without any lessening of activity. That is, if the euglobulin activity increased from a control sample of greater than 24 hours to a euglobulin fibrinolytic time of 1 hour, then the activity would persist at this level throughout the test period.

## COMPARISON OF VARIOUS CYCLES

Having established the fact that significant levels of euglobulin fibrinolytic activity could be produced by successive intermittent periods of venous occlusion, we undertook to determine which of several cycles was the most effective in producing fibrinolytic activity locally and systemically. In this series the arm was used instead of the leg.

Four patients (Nos. 22 through 25) were chosen from the convalescent group on our wards. Four different cycles of occlusion are shown in Table II.

For 4 successive days each patient was subjected to a different cycle. The cycles were used in a different order for each patient.

As in our other experiments, the cuff was inflated to diastolic pressure. The local sample was obtained from the antecubital fossa prior to release of the cuff. The systemic samples were drawn from the opposite arm without occlusion. In this particular group the samples recorded are from the second cycle. Just prior to the end of the second occlusion period the local sample was obtained. At the end of the second rest period the systemic sample was drawn from the opposite arm. The same procedure was used in all the cycles. The results of these cycles on local and systemic fibrinolytic activity gave results which were similar for all the cycles tested. No one cycle was better than the others on the basis of euglobulin activity (Fig. 2). However, from a clinical viewpoint, 30 minutes of venous obstruction led to discomfort while 20 minutes did not. A rest period of 10 minutes between the cycles seemed to be more comfortable for the patients than 5 minutes of rest.

There were no significant changes in proteolytic activity, prothrombin time (Quick), or fibrinogen concentration. The whole-clot lysis time was shortened from over 48 hours to less than 6 hours in 2 local samples which showed marked fibrinolytic activity.

## EFFECT ON IN VIVO SODIUM MORRHUATE CLOTS

In view of the results described we wished to ascertain whether or not fibrinolytic activity produced by this means would dissolve recent thrombi in vivo.

According to our plan of investigation,

0.5 to 1.0 ml. of 5 per cent sodium morrhuate was injected into an occluded peripheral vein. The subjects were examined the next morning. They were accepted for investigation if the injected area showed a firm, hard cord which did not fill with blood and from which we could not draw blood. Thirteen subjects were studied. Satisfactory clots were formed in 11. Clots were formed in both legs in 3, in both forearms in 4, and in 1 forearm only in the remaining 4 subjects. In 2 we were unsuccessful in establishing a clearly demonstrated sodium morrhuate clot.

Treatment was started approximately 24 hours after formation of the clot. One of the extremities containing a thrombus was then subjected to intermittent venous occlusion for 6 hours. The other acted as a control and was subjected to the systemic effect only. The cycle used was 20 minutes of venous occlusion at diastolic pressure and 20 minutes of rest. At the end of treatment and each morning for several days thereafter the areas of the clots were closely inspected. The clot was considered dissolved only if the vein was soft and easily distensible, and if blood could be drawn from the area of the previous thrombosis.

On the side of the cuff, 8 of 11 clots (73 per cent) were dissolved during the period of intermittent venous occlusion (Table III). In one subject (No. 29) the vein failed to open during the first 6 hours of the procedure and was treated again the next day. The vein opened on the second day after 6 hours (total 12 hours) of intermittent venous occlusion. Three subjects showed persistence of the clot. Two of these underwent only 1 course, 6 hours (Nos. 31 and 32) and 1 underwent 12 hours, 2 courses (No. 35), of treatment. Of the 7 clots present in the opposite (nonoccluded) extremity, 3, or 42 per cent, dissolved (Nos. 26, 27, and 28).

All of the lysed clots recurred within 24 hours. This is to be expected because the intimal damage caused by the sodium morrhuate certainly is not healed in the period during which the subjects received their treatment. Evidence of this persistent damage is seen in the venogram (Figs. 3 and 4). Specific patients were not used as controls during this study. However, experience shows that sodium morrhuate—induced clots, once formed, will persist for at least some weeks. The coincidental lysis and rethrombosis noted during the period of observation in these experiments would be most unlikely. The phenomenon of rethrombosis in the 8 of 11 local and 3 of 7 systemic vessels that demonstrated lysis during treatment is evidence that these clots did not lyse spontaneously.

## SPONTANEOUS THROMBOSIS

This method of intermittent venous occlusion has been used on 6 patients with early superficial and deep thrombophlebitis. Because of the extreme variability of the natural history of thrombophlebitis, we wish to avoid premature opinions. All in this group have had excellent response to the treatment

**Table II.** *Cycles of occlusion*

| | *Cuff on (min.)* | *Cuff off (min.)* |
|---|---|---|
| Cycle 1 | 20 | 5 |
| Cycle 2 | 20 | 10 |
| Cycle 3 | 30 | 5 |
| Cycle 4 | 30 | 10 |

**Table III.** *Results of effect of intermittent venous occlusion for 6 hours on in vivo sodium morrhuate clots in 11 patients*

| *Patients* | *Site* | *Extremity with cuff* | *Extremity without cuff* |
|---|---|---|---|
| 26 | Legs | Open | Open |
| 27 | Legs | Open | Open |
| 28 | Arms | Open | Open |
| 29 | Arms | (1) closed, (2) open | (1) closed, (2) closed |
| 30 | Arms | Open | Closed |
| 31 | Arms | Closed | Closed |
| 32 | Legs | Closed | Closed |
| 33 | Arm | Open | * |
| 34 | Arm | Open | * |
| 35 | Arm | (1) closed, (2) closed | * * |
| 36 | Arm | Open | * |

Open means clot was lysed.

Closed means vein remained thrombosed.

*No induced clot.

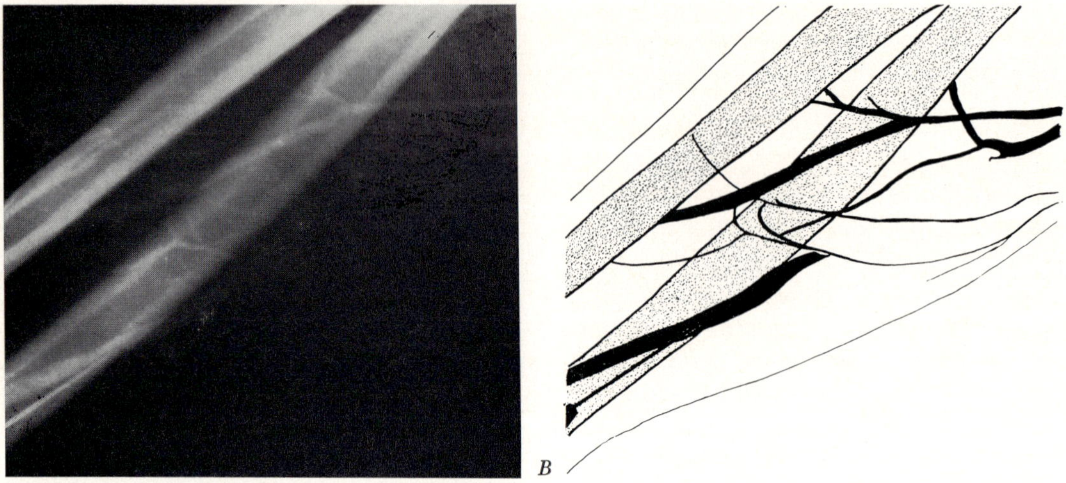

A B

**Fig. 3.** *A,* Venogram which demonstrates a forearm vein occluded by a sodium morrhuate—induced clot. *B,* Artist's illustration of original roentgenogram.

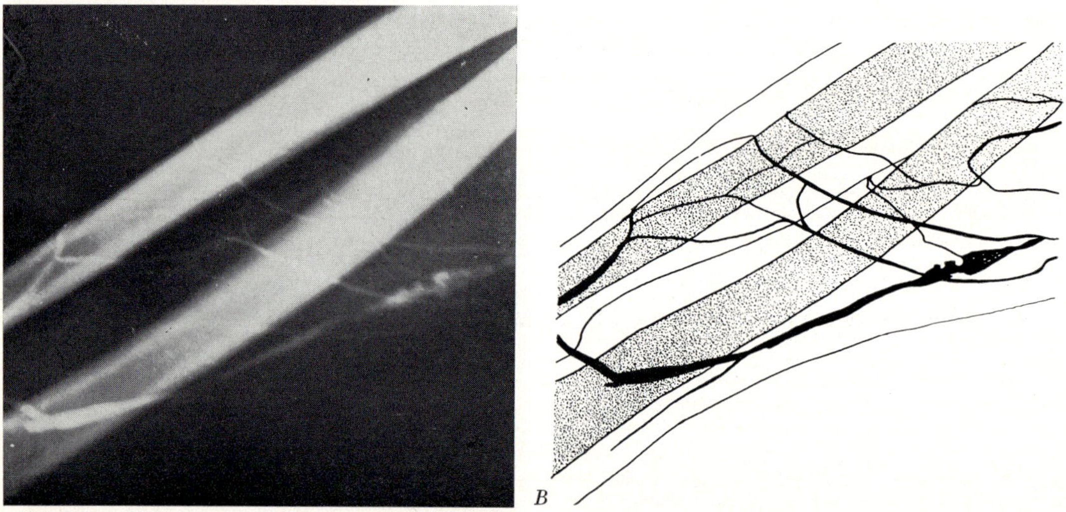

A B

**Fig. 4.** *A,* Venogram which demonstrates the open but badly damaged vein after treatment by intermittent venous occlusion. *B,* Artist's illustration of roentgenogram after treatment.

and these results warrant a more active trial. We have developed a device* which would automatically inflate and deflate a sphygmomanometer cuff at desired pressures and time intervals in order to expedite prolonged treatment periods. Patients with acute thrombophlebitis noted some discomfort with inflation of the sphygmomanometer cuff in the first hours of treatment. This was mitigated by lowering the pressure at the beginning to less than diastolic pressure and then gradually increasing it to the diastolic pressure. The following case report is typical of the results in these 6 cases.

*A prototype was designed and completed for us by W. A. Baum Co., Inc., Copiaque, L. I., N. Y.

## CASE REPORT

N. M. was a 61-year-old white textile salesman who was admitted to Doctors Hospital on March 29, 1960. His left leg was swollen with edema fluid and measured 17½ inches about the calf. The right calf measured 15 inches. There was a markedly positive Homans' sign and tenderness along the lesser and greater saphenous veins of the left leg. The symptoms had been present for 3 days. The man had been treated by bed rest, penicillin, and elevation of the left leg on 2 pillows. On admission intermittent venous occlusion with a "20-20" cycle was begun and lasted 6 hours. At the end of that time the left leg was normal in regard to swelling and pain. The circumference was 15½ inches and there was no tenderness along the saphenous veins of the leg. The next day the treatment was repeated. Since that time the patient has had no medications, was never treated with anticoagulants, and has had no symptoms while working a full day as a textile salesman. He has been advised to wear a below-knee stocking to help prevent recurrence.

## DISCUSSION

In this and a previous paper[3] we have attempted to evaluate the effect of venous occlusion on fibrinolytic activity in human beings. It has been noted that after 5 minutes of venous occlusion significant activity appears distal to the tourniquet in 20 per cent of the patients, but with more prolonged occlusion (up to 20 minutes) a higher percentage (60 per cent) is obtained. In an effort to determine whether or not this phenomenon was transitory, the system of intermittent cycles of occlusion was evolved. From a practical point of view, the 20-minute period of venous occlusion with a 10- or 20-minute rest period was found to be most effective. We also were able to demonstrate that high levels of activity could be maintained for long periods. Our study with successive cycles seems to indicate that activity produced by this means is cumulative and that if activity does not appear with the first cycle it may appear later.

The experimentally produced sodium morrhuate clots served as a means of determining the thrombolytic effectiveness of the fibrinolytic activity produced. Eight of the 11 thrombi (72 per cent) on the treated side were dissolved by the local fibrinolytic activity. This is as effective as systemic therapy with use of fibrinolytic agents for 4 to 6 hours. The relative effectiveness of the systemic activity produced was demonstrated by the lysis of 3 of 7 (43 per cent) of the clots in the opposite extremity (systemic effect) as compared with the 8 of 11 (73 per cent) lysed on the side of the occlusion (local effect).

The relationship between this type of activity and that seen in the classical examples of "spontaneous" fibrinolytic activity is not known at present. However, we hope to be able to contribute to this knowledge with additional studies of the plasminogen—activator—plasmin relationship in occluded venous blood. Studies on the complicated metabolic changes with occlusion are also in order, since changes in pH, oxygen, carbon dioxide, and tissue breakdown products may be of importance in the production of the lytic activity. It is hoped that additional study will furnish methods to increase the percentage of good results. Studies of the effects of a combination of small amounts of fibrinolytic agents and intermittent venous occlusion are being undertaken. It will also be necessary to evaluate combinations of occlusion with other drugs, such as pyrogens and nicotinic acid, and particularly local paravascular injections of drugs such as adrenalin. A thorough clinical trial with a large number of patients will be undertaken as soon as the preliminary studies are completed. This principle of treatment of thrombotic disease was suggested in the past, but was discontinued because of the unreliability of the results.[7] The reasons for the unsatisfactory results seem to be clear at this point. The method was used on patients with old thrombi and arteriosclerosis, which would respond very poorly, if at all. The cycle used, venous occlusion for 3 to 5 minutes, would not be expected to be satisfactory on the basis of our present studies. With the cycles shown to be effective by these studies, it is conceivable that effective treatment of recent thrombi may be accomplished.

## SUMMARY

1. It has been shown that significant fibrinolytic activity may be produced by venous occlusion alone.

2. Periods of occlusion separated by periods of rest produce continued levels of fibrinolytic activity in the majority of patients.

3. The cycle with 20 minutes of occlusion followed by 10 to 20 minutes of rest was found to give the most satisfactory results in this study.

4. The fibrinolytic activity so produced will dissolve sodium morrhuate clots both locally (8 of 11) and systemically (3 of 7).

5. This mechanism is an effective, nontoxic, method of producing therapeutic levels of fibrinolysin in a significant percentage of patients.

## REFERENCES

1. Biggs, R., and Macfarlane, R.: Human blood coagulation and its disorders, Oxford, 1957, Blackwell Scientific Publications, ed. 2, p. 402.
2. Burchell, A. R., and Cliffton, E. E.: Inhibition of fibrinolysis by hyperlipemia. Thromb. et Diath. Haem. **5:** 463, 1961.
3. Clarke, R. L., Orandi, A., and Cliffton, E. E.: Tourniquet induction of fibrinolysis, Angiology **11:** 367, 1960.
4. Cliffton, E. E.: Variations in the proteolytic reactions of serum: effect of disease, trauma, x-ray, anaphylactic shock, ACTH and cortisone, J. Lab. & Clin. Med. **39:** 105, 1952.
5. Cliffton, E. E., and Cannamela, D.: Fibrinolytic and proteolytic activity of a human plasminogen prepared from fraction III of human plasma, J. Appl. Physiol. **6:** 42, 1953.
6. Cliffton, E. E., and Cannamela, D.: Variations in the proteolytic activity of serum of animals including man, Proc. Soc. Exper. Biol. & Med. **77:** 305, 1951.
7. Collens, W. S., and Wilensky, N. D.: Use of intermittent venous compression in treatment of peripheral vascular diseases, Am. Heart J. **11:** 705, 1936.
8. Kwaan, H. C., and McFadzean, A. J. S.: On plasma fibrinolytic activity induced by ischemia, Clin. Sc. **15:** 245, 1956.
9. Kwaan, H. C., and McFadzean, A. J. S.: On the production of plasma fibrinolytic activity within veins, Clin. Sc. **16:** 241, 1957.
10. Remmert, L. F., and Cohen, P. P.: Partial purification and properties of proteolytic enzymes of human serum, J. Biol. Chem. **181:** 431, 1949.
11. Sherry, S., Lindemeyer, R. I., Fletcher, A. P., and Alkjaersig, N.: Studies on enhanced fibrinolytic activities in man, J. Clin. Invest. **381:** 810, 1959.
12. Symposium on fibrinolysis sponsored by the Sloan-Kettering Institute, New York, March 25-26, 1960, Am. J. Cardiol. **6:** 367, 1960.

# Physiologic effects of gastric hypothermia. I. The effect on estimated hepatic blood flow in the normal anesthetized dog

STEPHEN L. WANGENSTEEN, M.D.*
RICHARD C. ORAHOOD, B.A.**
WALLACE K. LUKE, B. A.
WILLIAM V. HEALEY, M.D.
NEW YORK, N. Y.
*From the Department of Surgery, Columbia University College of Physicians and Surgeons, and the Surgical Service of the Presbyterian Hospital*

Since the recent introduction of gastric hypothermia as a method to control massive upper gastrointestinal hemorrhage, encouraging and often dramatic results have stimulated increasing interest in and use of this technique.[9] Of all causes of massive upper gastrointestinal hemorrhage, probably the most difficult to manage has been bleeding esophageal varices. Experience to date at The Presbyterian Hospital indicates that esophagogastric hypothermia is effective in the temporary control of massive hemorrhage from bleeding esophageal varices.

O. H. Wangensteen and associates[10] have amply demonstrated several changes in gastric physiology that attend local gastric cooling. One of the alterations noted was depression in gastric blood flow amounting to approximately 66 per cent. Since the arterial supply to the stomach and the liver stem from the same source, it suggested that gastric cooling might result in a reduction of hepatic blood flow as well. If hepatic blood flow were reduced as significantly as gastric blood flow, serious consequences could follow the use of gastric cooling in patients with marked liver damage. The present study was performed to determine the effect of gastric hypothermia upon estimated hepatic blood flow in the normal normothermic anesthetized dog.

Supported by Research Grant H-5372 from the National Institutes of Health, United States Public Health Service.
Received for publication June 15, 1961.

*Special Research Fellow, National Heart Institute.
**Post Sophomore Research Fellow, National Institutes of Health.

## METHODS

Total estimated hepatic blood flow was measured by the Bromsulphalein (BSP) removal method described by Bradley.[1] Ample evidence has accumulated that supports the assumptions on which the BSP method depends.

Twenty adult mongrel dogs of both sexes which weighed between 14 and 27 kilograms were used in the experiments. Two experimental designs were employed.

**Plan I.** Three dogs were subjected to measurements of hepatic blood flow (1) with an empty intragastric balloon, and (2) after inflation of the gastric balloon with 500 ml. of fluid at body temperature. These measurements were obtained to determine whether or not there was reduction in hepatic blood flow from the inflated, noncooled gastric balloon.

**Plan II.** Fourteen dogs were subjected to measurements of hepatic blood flow (1) with an intragastric balloon filled with 500 ml. of fluid at body temperature (same procedure as the second step in Plan I), and (2) during gastric hypothermia with 500 ml. of circulating fluid in the gastric balloon and maintenance of body temperature.

Three dogs were subjected to all of the procedures and are included in both plans. Thus, there are 6 dogs in Plan I and 17 dogs in Plan II.

Pentobarbital sodium was given intravenously to maintain light anesthesia. In 4 animals which received gastric cooling, arterial pH, carbon dioxide tension, carbon dioxide content, and $HCO_3$ were determined to be certain ventilation was constant. A polyethylene catheter was surgically placed in the left common hepatic vein under sterile conditions according to the method of Shoemaker[8] several days prior to the blood flow studies. Peripheral arterial samples were obtained from a catheter inserted in the femoral artery. A solution of BSP in isotonic saline solution was infused at a constant rate into a peripheral vein after a priming dose of 50 mg. of BSP. The rate of BSP infusion was kept at 1 mg. per minute in most instances because this rate was found to maintain the most nearly constant peripheral plasma concentration. The infusion was allowed to run at least one-half hour before any determinations were performed so that BSP equilibration could occur. When gastric cooling was employed, at least 1 hour was allowed to elapse before determinations were performed. Duplicate serum concentrations of BSP were determined on an Evelyn colorimeter by the method described by Gaebler.[3] Peripheral mean arterial blood pressure was recorded on a mercury manometer from a catheter inserted in the femoral artery. Rectal temperature was monitored by a thermistor probe inserted in the rectum.

Gastric hypothermia was employed with a machine, plastic coaxial tube assembly, and balloon previously described.[12] The inflow temperature of the circulating fluid was routinely 0 to 2° C. Body temperature was maintained by external heating with electric heating pads.

## RESULTS

The calculation of estimated hepatic blood flow was obtained by multiplying the estimated hepatic plasma flow by the factor $\frac{1}{1-Hct}$. In these experiments hematocrit determinations were not performed during the stage of gastric cooling. Subsequently it was noted that gastric cooling produced an increase in the large vessel hematocrit, although a normal body temperature was maintained. Mere inflation of the gastric balloon with fluid at body temperature induced no significant change in the hematocrit, however. In order to obtain a reasonable value for hepatic blood flow during gastric hypothermia, we used the average hematocrit increase noted in another study from this laboratory[7] for the calculation of average hepatic blood flow results. In these studies, gastric cooling was performed for the same period and the general protocol of the experiment was identical except that parameters of renal hemodynamics were studied. In 9 dogs the average increase in the large vessel arterial hematocrit after 1 hour of gastric cooling was 17 per cent. A similar result has been obtained during studies on the effect of gastric cooling on total circulating blood volume.[11] These studies afford reasonable assurance that in response to 1 hour of gastric cooling the average hematocrit increase is approximately 17 per cent. In the present study the average precooling hematocrit of the dogs in Plan II was 37 per cent. After 1 hour of gastric cooling, we assume the average hematocrit to be 43 per cent, an increase of 17 per cent. Since the hematocrit increases with gastric cooling, the reduction in hepatic blood flow is less marked than the reduction in hepatic plasma flow.

In Plan I, 6 dogs underwent measurements of hepatic blood flow with an empty intragastric balloon (Table I). The mean hepatic plasma flow was 335 ml. per minute or 17.0 ml. per kilogram per minute. The mean hepatic blood flow was 605 ml. per minute (31.2 ml. per kilogram per minute).

With the introduction of noncooled fluid into the gastric balloon (Plan I, second step) the mean hepatic plasma flow was reduced to 288 ml. per minute (14.6 ml. per kilogram per minute). The mean hepatic blood flow was reduced to 522 ml. per minute (27.2 ml. per kilogram per minute). In 2 of the dogs there was no depression in flow after inflation of the gastric balloon. Statistical analysis of these results shows that these changes are not significant ($p < 0.4$).

In Plan II (first step), 17 dogs were subjected to measurements of hepatic blood flow with an inflated noncooled intragastric balloon (Table II). The average hepatic plasma flow was 340 ml. per minute (18.8 ml. per kilogram per minute and the average hepatic blood flow was 557 ml. per minute (30.9 ml. per kilogram per minute).

**Table I.** *The effect of gastric hypothermia on estimated hepatic blood flow in Plan I*

| Dog No. | Wt. (Kg.) | P* | | Ex%† | | Hepatic plasma flow‡ (ml./min.) | | Hepatic plasma flow‡ (ml./Kg./min.) | | Hepatic blood flow‡ (ml./min.) | | Hepatic blood flow‡ (ml./Kg./min.) | |
|---|---|---|---|---|---|---|---|---|---|---|---|---|---|
| | | 1 | 2 | 1 | 2 | 1 | 2 | 1 | 2 | 1 | 2 | 1 | 2 |
| 330 | 19 | 0.00014 | 0.00014 | 13 | 25 | 516 | 280 | 27.1 | 14.7 | 920 | 500 | 48.4 | 26.3 |
| 335 | 20 | 0.00001 | 0.00019 | 20 | 17 | 454 | 489 | 22.7 | 24.4 | 928 | 998 | 46.4 | 49.9 |
| 340 | 16 | 0.00009 | 0.00000 | 41 | 22 | 234 | 337 | 14.6 | 21.0 | 403 | 580 | 25.2 | 36.2 |
| 350 | 19 | 0.00004 | 0.00018 | 41 | 26 | 258 | 220 | 13.5 | 11.5 | 392 | 332 | 20.6 | 17.5 |
| 396 | 27 | 0.00004 | 0.00006 | 35 | 38 | 263 | 212 | 9.7 | 7.8 | 516 | 416 | 19.1 | 15.4 |
| 392 | 17 | 0.00001 | 0.00016 | 13 | 10 | 290 | 188 | 17.0 | 11.0 | 476 | 309 | 28.0 | 18.1 |
| Mean<br>S.D. | 19.7 | — | — | 27 | 23 | 335<br>±118 | 288<br>±112 | 17.0<br>±6.4 | 14.6<br>±6.4 | 605<br>±251 | 522<br>±254 | 31.2<br>±12.9 | 27.2<br>±13.5 |

*P = change in arterial BSP concentration (milligrams per milliliter of plasma per minute).

$$†Ex\% = \frac{\text{arterial–heptatic BSP difference (mg.\%)}}{\text{arterial BSP (mg.\%)}} \times 100$$

‡Estimated.

**Table II.** *The effect of gastric hypothermia on estimated hepatic blood flow in Plan II*

| Dog No. | Wt. (Kg.) | P* | | Ex%† | | Hepatic plasma flow‡ (ml./min.) | | Hepatic plasma flow‡ (ml./Kg. min.) | | Hepatic blood flow‡ (ml./min.) | | Hepatic blood flow‡ (ml./Kg./min.) | |
|---|---|---|---|---|---|---|---|---|---|---|---|---|---|
| | | 1 | 2 | 1 | 2 | 1 | 2 | 1 | 2 | 1 | 2 | 1 | 2 |
| 209 | 15 | 0.00009 | 0.00000 | 54 | 54 | 151 | 152 | 10.0 | 10.0 | 231 | | 15.4 | |
| 217 | 17 | 0.00010 | 0.00006 | 38 | 33 | 331 | 249 | 19.4 | 14.6 | 473 | | 31.5 | |
| 218 | 17 | 0.00006 | 0.00014 | 47 | 48 | 400 | 155 | 23.5 | 9.1 | 648 | | 38.1 | |
| 230 | 19 | 0.00000 | 0.00016 | 58 | 86 | 217 | 118 | 11.4 | 6.2 | 360 | | 19.0 | |
| 232 | 19 | 0.00005 | 0.00000 | 29 | 19 | 612 | 251 | 32.2 | 13.2 | 1090 | | 57.3 | |
| 239 | 17 | 0.00000 | 0.00052 | 28 | 15 | 328 | 408 | 19.3 | 24.0 | 544 | | 32.0 | |
| 240 | 18 | 0.00000 | 0.00004 | 27 | 25 | 421 | 421 | 23.3 | 23.3 | 560 | | 31.1 | |
| 245 | 14 | 0.00004 | 0.00032 | 18 | 9 | 212 | 130 | 15.1 | 9.3 | 341 | | 24.4 | |
| 248 | 17 | 0.00058 | 0.00008 | 28 | 14 | 281 | 55 | 16.5 | 3.2 | 530 | | 31.2 | |
| 256 | 19 | 0.00000 | 0.00038 | 41 | 33 | 450 | 372 | 23.7 | 19.5 | 725 | | 40.2 | |
| 262 | 21 | 0.00004 | 0.00028 | 53 | 39 | 247 | 166 | 11.7 | 7.9 | 418 | | 20.0 | |
| 263 | 24 | 0.00008 | 0.00028 | 21 | 35 | 580 | 285 | 24.1 | 11.9 | 998 | | 41.6 | |
| 270 | 23 | 0.00018 | 0.00040 | 27 | 10 | 365 | 326 | 15.8 | 14.2 | 403 | | 21.0 | |
| 273 | 14 | 0.00044 | 0.00040 | 37 | 13 | 254 | 155 | 18.1 | 11.1 | 374 | | 26.7 | |
| 335 | 20 | 0.00019 | 0.00016 | 17 | 17 | 489 | 111 | 24.4 | 5.5 | 998 | | 49.9 | |
| 340 | 16 | 0.00000 | 0.00023 | 22 | 19 | 337 | 217 | 21.0 | 13.5 | 580 | | 36.2 | |
| 392 | 17 | 0.00016 | 0.00044 | 11 | 26 | 113 | 129 | 6.6 | 7.6 | 188 | | 11.0 | |
| Mean<br>S.D. | 18.0 | — | — | 33 | 29 | 340<br>±140 | 218<br>±111 | 18.8<br>±6.5 | 12.1<br>±5.9 | 557<br>±265 | 381 | 31.0<br>±12.2 | 21.2 |

*P = change in arterial BSP concentration (milligrams per millileter of plasma per minute).

$$†Ex\% = \frac{\text{arterial–heptatic BSP difference (mg.\%)}}{\text{arterial BSP (mg.\%)}} \times 100$$

‡Estimated.

It is noted that these average results, when they are considered on a per kilogram basis, are as high as those of either step in Plan I.

With the employment of gastric hypothermia (Plan II, second step), the hepatic plasma flow fell to an average of 218 ml. per minute (12.1 ml. per kilogram per minute), a reduction in plasma flow of 35 per cent ($p < 0.005$) from the first step. In this step of the experiment it is necessary to employ the increased hematocrit value in the calculation of hepatic blood flow. This gives an estimated hepatic blood flow of 381 ml. per minute (21.2 ml. per kilogram per minute), which is a 31 per cent reduction in blood flow rather than 35 per cent. In 4 dogs no depression in blood flow occurred during gastric cooling.

The arterial pH, carbon dioxide tension, carbon dioxide content, and $^{-}HCO_3$ were determined in 4 of the animals. In 1 dog there was a rise in carbon dioxide tension during gastric hypothermia. No significant changes were noted in the pH measurements or in carbon dioxide content. In all of the dogs there was a depression in hepatic flow during intragastric cooling.

No changes were noted in the mean arterial blood pressure during inflation of the intragastric balloon or gastric cooling.

## DISCUSSION

It has previously been reported that gastric blood flow is unchanged upon inflation of an intragastric balloon without cooling.[10] The data in the present study suggest that on occasion the position and weight of the filled noncooled balloon within the stomach may reduce hepatic blood flow, perhaps by resting on the portal vein. If the left lobes of the liver are encroached upon during inflation of the balloon, we may see an artificial reduction in flow since the hepatic venous sampling catheter was placed in the left common hepatic vein. On the other hand, the per kilogram flow results obtained with a filled gastric balloon in Plan II are similar to the results obtained with an empty intragastric balloon in Plan I, although the values are quite similar. This suggests that as more animals are measured the occasional reduction in hepatic flow seen in an animal will not be significantly reflected in the mean results, and that, in general, the hepatic blood flow is not influenced by inflation of the balloon alone.

Under the conditions of this study there was a definite decrease in estimated hepatic blood flow in most animals when gastric hypothermia was employed, in addition to any "tamponade" effect that may have been present from the inflation of the balloon.

Hallet,[4] using the BSP removal method, has described the depression in hepatic blood flow that occurs in systemic hypothermia. The fall in hepatic blood flow parallels the reduction in cardiac output. A depression in hepatic blood flow of similar magnitude to that noted in the present study was reached at 30° to 32° C.

Heimburger and colleagues[5] found no reduction in portal venous flow or portal venous oxygen saturation at the end of one-half hour of gastric cooling when the stomach wall temperature was maintained at 20° C. At the end of 2 hours portal flow was significantly reduced, but this reduction appeared to be the result of the experimental preparation rather than gastric cooling. Nicoloff,[6] on the other hand, reports that portal flow is reduced approximately 25 per cent during gastric cooling as measured by an electromagnetic flowmeter. He found relatively little change in hepatic arterial flow. Our data give no indication which component of hepatic inflow is affected since only total estimated hepatic blood flow was measured.

In the patient with cirrhosis and intrahepatic block, portal inflow to the liver is reduced and hepatic arterial inflow is believed to convey most of the circulation to the damaged, distorted parenchyma. If gastric hypothermia does reduce hepatic arterial flow significantly, it could further impair the already limited blood supply to the liver in the cirrhotic patient with bleeding esophageal varices.

In 16 patients bleeding from esophageal

varices treated with gastric hypothermia, clinical deterioration has not been observed during cooling. In fact, the reverse has been true. Clinical improvement noted during cooling may have been related to the arrest of hemorrhage, which was effected in every instance. We have reduced the circulating volume used clinically in patients with liver disease from the originally recommended 800 to 1,000 ml. to 200 to 400 ml. without sacrificing control of hemorrhage. The use of a small circulating volume with concentration on the placement of a single-lumened, gourd-shaped balloon in the esophagus and upper stomach has been satisfactory and appears worthwhile.

## CONCLUSIONS

1. Measurements of estimated hepatic blood flow by the BSP removal method were performed in 20 anesthetized dogs.
2. In general, inflation of the intragastric balloon without cooling does not produce a reduction in hepatic blood flow.
3. Gastric hypothermia significantly reduced hepatic blood flow under the conditions of the experiment.
4. The clinical significance of a reduction in hepatic blood flow during gastric cooling has not been determined.

### REFERENCES

1. Bradley, S. E., Inglefinger, F. J., Bradley, G. P., and Curry, J. J.: Estimation of hepatic blood flow in man, J. Clin. Invest. **24:** 890, 1945.
2. Burton-Opitz, R.: The vascularity of the liver. II. Influence of portal blood flow upon the hepatic artery, Quart J. Exper. Physiol. **24:** 390, 1945.
3. Gaebler, O. H.: Determination of Bromsulphalein in normal, turbid, hemolyzed, or icteric serums, Am. J. Clin. Path. **15:** 452, 1945.
4. Hallet, E. B.: The effect of lowered body temperature on estimated hepatic blood flow, S. Forum **6:** 332, 1955.
5. Heimburger, I., Teramoto, S., and Schumacher, H. B.: Influence of general hypothermia and local gastric cooling on portal blood flow, SURGERY **47:** 534, 1960.
6. Nicoloff, D.: Personal communication, 1961.
7. Orahood, R. C., Wangensteen, S. L., and Luke, W. K.: Physiologic effects of gastric hypothermia. II. The effect on renal blood flow, renal plasma flow, and glomerular filtration rate in the normal anesthetized dog, SURGERY **50:** 656, 1961.
8. Shoemaker, W. C., Walker, W. F., Van Ittalie, T. B., and Moore, F. D.: A method for simultaneous catheterization of major hepatic vessels in a chronic canine preparation, Am. J. Physiol. **196:** 311, 1959.
9. Wangensteen, O. H., Root, H. D., Jenson, C. D., Imamoglu, K., and Salmon, P. A.: Depression of gastric secretion and digestion by gastric hypothermia: its clinical use in massive hematemesis, SURGERY **44:** 265, 1958.
10. Wangensteen, O. H., Salmon, P. A., Griffen, W. O., Paterson, J. R. S., and Fattah, F.: Studies of local gastric cooling as related to peptic ulcer, Ann. Surg. **150:** 346, 1959.
11. Wangensteen, S. L., Orahood, R. C., and Luke, W. K.: Physiologic effects of gastric hypothermia. III. The effect on circulating blood volume and large vessel hematocrit. In preparation.
12. Wangensteen, S. L., and Smith, W. H.: A gastric hypothermia machine, SURGERY **47:** 924, 1960.

# Physiologic effects of gastric hypothermia. II. The effect on renal blood flow, renal plasma flow, and glomerular filtration rate in the normal anesthetized dog

RICHARD C. ORAHOOD, B.A.*
STEPHEN L. WANGENSTEEN, M.D.**
WALLACE K. LUKE, B.A.
NEW YORK, N. Y.
*From the Department of Surgery, Columbia University College of Physicians and Surgeons, and the Surgical Service of the Presbyterian Hospital*

In a few patients who have received gastric hypothermia for the control of massive upper gastrointestinal hemorrhage, a depression in urine output has been noted. In our series of patients treated for massive bleeding by gastric cooling, 70 per cent have been in shock prior to the initiation of gastric hypothermia. In addition to hemorrhage, myocardial infarctions and other cardiovascular accidents have contributed to the hypotensive episode. In view of depressions noted in gastric and hepatic blood flows, the question has been raised whether or not gastric hypothermia itself is a contributing factor in renal ischemia.

Ample evidence has accumulated that gastric hypothermia markedly alters gastric function.[14] Recent findings indicate that the physiologic changes induced by this form of cooling are not limited to the stomach. Data from this laboratory and elsewhere have shown that gastric cooling affects hepatic blood flow,[15] circulating blood volume,[16] and pancreatic function.[9]

The purpose of the present study was to ascertain the effects of gastric hypothermia on renal hemodynamics in normal anesthetized dogs.

## METHODS

The experiment was designed to determine changes, if any, in effective renal plasma flow, effective renal blood flow, and glomerular filtration rate rendered by (1) the weight of a fluid-filled balloon in the stomach and (2) chilling of the fluid to near freezing while maintaining body temperature. The experiment consisted of 3 stages. In Stage I the animal was lightly anesthetized and considered to be in a basal state. These values represent the base line. Since each dog served as its own control, results obtained in the later stages were compared to these figures. In Stage II a gastric balloon was positioned in the stomach and filled with noncooled fluid to the volume used during the gastric hypothermia stage (250 to 400 ml., depending on the animal's weight). This stage demonstrates the effect of the fluid-filled noncooled gastric balloon. In Stage III the fluid in the balloon was cooled while body temperature was maintained. One hour of intragastric cooling was employed before any determinations were obtained. Electric heating pads were utilized to maintain body temperature. In this stage, the effect of gastric

Supported by Grant H-5372 (C1) from the National Institutes of Health, United States Public Health Service.
Received for publication June 15, 1961.

*Post Sophomore Research Fellow, National Institutes of Health.

**Special Research Fellow, National Heart Institute.

hypothermia is added to the effect of the filled balloon.

Mongrel dogs which weighed from 10.3 to 19.0 kilograms and had been fasted for 24 hours but given water ad libitum were anesthetized with 30 mg. per kilogram of pentobarbital sodium administered intravenously. Anesthesia was supplemented throughout the experiment with small doses to maintain light anesthesia. Catheters were placed proximally into the aorta via the femoral artery and into the urinary bladder. Priming doses of sodium para-aminohippurate (PAH) (8 mg. per kilogram) and inulin (50 mg. per kilogram) were administered intravenously to achieve the desired plasma levels of 0.02 and 0.25 mg. per milliliter, respectively. These were followed by a sustaining dose in isotonic saline solution infused intravenously by a constant infusion pump to maintain the desired plasma levels. Except for the infusion containing PAH and inulin (1.0 to 2.0 ml. per minute), no infusions were given at any time during the experiment.

After a 30-minute wait for equilibration, the bladder was emptied and timed urine collection periods were begun which lasted 15 to 30 minutes, depending on urine output. If urine output was below 1.0 ml. per minute the experiment was discontinued at this point, since accurate determinations are difficult to achieve with highly concentrated urine. Midway in the urine collection period an arterial blood sample was drawn and hematocrits were determined on a portion of these samples by the microhematocrit method. The remainder was used for plasma determinations of PAH and inulin concentrations. Two urine collections were obtained for each of the 3 stages of the experiment. Renal plasma flow and glomerular filtration rate were measured by the renal clearance of PAH and inulin, respectively.[4, 12] Renal blood flow for each stage of the experiment was calculated from the PAH clearance and the stimultaneous arterial hematocrit.

Gastric hypothermia was obtained by the circulation of fluid at 0° to 2° C. through a latex gastric balloon attached to a plastic coaxial tube assembly with the gastric hypothermia machine which was previously described.[17]

Rectal temperature was monitored by a thermistor probe inserted into the rectum. Any animal in which the body temperature fell more than 5° C. during the experiment was eliminated.

Mean arterial blood pressure was monitored by a mercury manometer via the femoral arterial catheter.

## RESULTS

Nine mongrel dogs of 14.8 kilograms mean body weight were used in the present study. The large-vessel arterial hematocrit, PAH clearance results (effective renal plasma flow), and calculated renal blood flow for the 3 stages of the experiment are shown in Table I. The mean arterial hematocrit for Stage I was 43.1 per cent. In 5 animals arterial hematocrits were determined in Stage II and the average was 45 per cent. After 1 hour of gastric cooling the mean arterial hematocrit rose to 50.4 per cent, an increase of 17 per cent ($p < 0.01$).

In Stage I the mean effective renal plasma flow was 191 ml. per minute or 12.9 ml. per minute per kilogram. In all experiments the renal plasma flow decreased in the final 2 stages; the average was 146 ml. per minute (9.9 ml. per minute per kilogram) in Stage II and 116 ml. per minute (7.8 ml. per minute per kilogram) in Stage III, a 23.5 per cent ($p < 0.001$) reduction in Stage II and a 39 per cent ($p < 0.001$) decrease in Stage III from base-line levels.

The mean control effective renal blood flow (Stage I) was 335 ml. per minute or 22.6 ml. per minute per kilogram. The calculation of the renal blood flow depends upon the renal plasma flow and the simultaneous arterial hematocrit. Only 5 hematocrit determinations were obtained during the second stage. It was assumed that these 5 experiments typified the change in hematocrit for all the experiments. On this assumption the mean effective renal blood flow for Stage II was determined from the mean renal plasma flow of all the experiments and the average hematocrit of these 5 experiments.

**Table I.** *The effect of gastric hypothermia on renal hemodynamics*

| Dog No. | Weight (Kg.) | Hematocrit | | | Effective renal plasma flow (ml./min./Kg.) | | | Effective renal blood flow (ml./min./Kg.) | | |
|---|---|---|---|---|---|---|---|---|---|---|
| | | I | II | III | I | II | III | I | II | III |
| 474 | 13.3 | 42 | — | 54 | 15.9 | 11.5 | 8.5 | 27.5 | — | 18.5 |
| 488 | 18.6 | 38 | — | 46 | 14.6 | 9.1 | 8.1 | 23.6 | — | 14.9 |
| 505 | 19.0 | 47 | — | 54 | 10.8 | 7.9 | 6.8 | 20.4 | — | 14.7 |
| 516 | 13.3 | 41.5 | — | 60.5 | 12.3 | 10.4 | 6.9 | 21.2 | — | 17.5 |
| 540 | 14.0 | 44 | 42.5 | 44 | 12.9 | 11.1 | 10.2 | 22.9 | 19.4 | 18.2 |
| 100 | 15.9 | 40.5 | 41.5 | 44 | 12.1 | 8.9 | 5.9 | 20.3 | 15.3 | 10.6 |
| 104 | 14.0 | 45 | 46.5 | 52 | 11.6 | 10.6 | 9.6 | 20.9 | 18.4 | 20.1 |
| 110 | 10.3 | 48 | 48 | 49 | 11.9 | 10.5 | 7.8 | 23.0 | 20.2 | 15.2 |
| 112 | 15.0 | 42 | 46 | 50 | 14.1 | 10.3 | 7.3 | 24.4 | 19.2 | 14.5 |
| Mean | 14.8 | 43.1 | — | 50.4 | 12.9 | 9.9 | 7.8 | 22.6 | 17.6 | 15.9 |
| S.D. | | | | | ±1.6 | ±1.1 | ±1.4 | ±2.34 | | ±2.8 |

**Table II.** *The effect of gastric hypothermia on renal hemodynamics*

| Dog No. | Glomerular filtration rate (ml./min./Kg.) | | | Filtration fraction | | | Urine volume (ml./min./Kg.) | | |
|---|---|---|---|---|---|---|---|---|---|
| | I | II | III | I | II | III | I | II | III |
| 474 | 5.8 | 4.1 | 4.4 | 0.3632 | 0.3529 | 0.5133 | 2.22 | 2.44 | 2.67 |
| 488 | 3.5 | 3.5 | 2.7 | 0.2426 | 0.3882 | 0.3333 | 5.56 | 3.33 | 2.62 |
| 505 | 3.3 | 2.9 | 2.1 | 0.3024 | 0.3733 | 0.3101 | 1.90 | 1.81 | 1.38 |
| 516 | 4.7 | 4.7 | 3.9 | 0.3841 | 0.4532 | 0.5652 | 1.60 | 3.02 | 0.44 |
| 540 | 3.9 | 4.1 | 4.1 | 0.3000 | 0.3654 | 0.3986 | 1.77 | 1.76 | 4.30 |
| 100 | 3.8 | 3.4 | 2.7 | 0.3125 | 0.3803 | 0.4574 | 1.93 | 1.82 | 1.70 |
| 104 | 3.1 | 3.3 | 3.4 | 0.2716 | 0.3333 | 0.3556 | 2.80 | 2.55 | 3.20 |
| 110 | 4.4 | 4.4 | 3.4 | 0.3658 | 0.4167 | 0.4375 | 1.37 | 1.52 | 1.46 |
| 112 | 3.2 | 3.1 | 3.2 | 0.2264 | 0.3052 | 0.4404 | 1.16 | 1.60 | 1.22 |
| Mean | 3.9 | 3.6 | 3.2 | 0.3074 | 0.3743 | 0.4235 | 2.26 | 2.19 | 2.11 |
| S.D. | ±0.9 | ±0.6 | ±0.7 | ±0.0554 | ±0.0482 | ±0.0837 | | | |

The resulting figure was 260 ml. per minute (17.6 ml. per minute per kilogram), a reduction of 22.5 per cent ($p < 0.001$) from Stage I. In Stage III the renal blood flow was 235 ml. per minute (15.9 ml. per minute per kilogram). This value represents a 30 per cent ($p < 0.001$) decrease from base line.

The change in glomerular filtration rate during the experiment was much less marked than that of the renal blood or plasma flows (Table II). The mean base-line value (Stage I) was 58 ml. per minute or 3.9 ml. per minute per kilogram. In Stage II 4 animals failed to exhibit any change and in 2 animals the filtration rates increased. The mean value of 54 ml. per minute (3.6 ml. per minute per kilogram) showed an over-all reduction of 7.0 per cent ($p < 0.3$) from Stage I. A more marked change occurred in Stage III when the mean value of 48 ml. per minute (3.2 ml. per minute per kilogram) was a reduction of 17 per cent ($p < 0.02$) from the value in Stage I.

As one would expect from the PAH and inulin clearances, the filtration fraction increased from a control mean value of 0.3074 to 0.3743 in Stage II and further to 0.4235 in Stage III. The Stage II result is an increase of 22 per cent ($p < 0.002$) from Stage I and Stage III is 38 per cent ($p < 0.001$) above the base-line level.

The urine volumes remained relatively constant throughout the experiment, showing only a slight mean decrease in amount as the experiment progressed. Indeed, in 3 experiments the urinary output increased slightly. Prior to 1 experiment an animal was supplemented by a 400 ml. infusion of 5 per cent dextrose in water and the urine volume increased markedly in Stage III.

The mean arterial blood pressure was not affected by either the filled intragastric balloon or gastric hypothermia.

## DISCUSSION

The base-line renal plasma flow, renal blood flow, and glomerular filtration rate obtained in this study were slightly lower than the mean normal values determined in 75 dogs by Houck.[5] Anesthesia is known to significantly affect renal hemodynamics and his values were obtained from trained, unanesthetized dogs. The mean renal blood flow in the present study approximates the value of 21.3 ml. per minute per kilogram in anesthetized dogs which was reported by Smythe and his associates.[13]

In Stage II the inflated intragastric balloon significantly affected renal hemodynamics. Fig. 1 graphically illustrates the "tamponade" effect on renal blood and plasma flows. The decreases in renal plasma flow and renal blood flow were essentially equal, accompanied by an insignificant increase in large-vessel hematocrit. A less significant decrease in glomerular filtration rate was associated with this marked decrease in renal blood and plasma flow resulting in an increase in filtration fraction.

The mechanism or mechanisms responsible for the effect of Stage II are not clearly understood. The possibility of partial occlusion of the renal veins or inferior vena cava from the overlying weight of the intragastric balloon must be reasonably discarded, since Blake and associates[2] reported that fivefold elevations of venous pressure must be obtained before alterations in renal blood flow or glomerular filtration rate are observed. However, partial occlusion of the aorta or renal arteries due to "tamponade" may be involved. Also, inflation of the gastric balloon may initiate a reflex mechanism mediated by the splanchnic nerves and thereby cause the effects seen. However, at present, no evidence is available to substantiate either of the latter 2 possibilities. Whatever the mechanism involved, intrinsic renal regulation maintains the glomerular filtration rate at nearly normal levels.

To demonstrate the effect of gastric hypothermia alone, the results from Stage II (inflated balloon) and Stage III (gastric cooling) were compared. The differences showed that renal plasma flow was decreased 16 per cent ($p < 0.001$), renal blood flow was decreased 7.5 per cent, and glomerular filtration rate was decreased 10 per cent ($p < 0.05$). In view of the depression in renal plasma flow, a decrease in glomerular filtration rate might be expected since less plasma was presented to the glomeruli for filtration.

In Fig. 1 the effects of gastric hypothermia on renal blood flow, renal plasma flow, and hematocrit are illustrated. A significant increase in large-vessel arterial hematocrit was noted after 1 hour of gastric cooling. The red blood cell volume perfusing the kidneys per minute in Stage III has remained unchanged from Stage II, yet the plasma flow is further depressed. Renal blood flow is the product of renal plasma flow and the arterial hematocrit. Because of the rise in arterial hematocrit, renal blood flow was decreased less markedly than renal plasma flow.

An investigation of the effect of gastric hypothermia on circulating blood volume, in

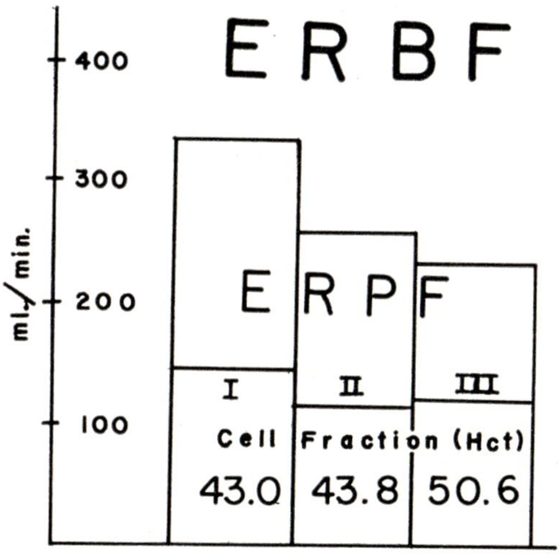


Fig. 1. The effect of a filled intragastric balloon and gastric hypothermia on effective renal blood flow *(ERBF)*, effective renal plasma flow *(ERPF)*, and large-vessel arterial hematocrit *(Hct)*.

which both plasma and red blood cells were tagged by radioactive materials, showed a marked depression in circulating plasma volume and a reduction in total blood volume.[16] These results suggest that the effects of gastric cooling observed in the present study may be a manifestation of the more general circulatory effects of this form of cooling, and not alterations in intrinsic renal hemodynamics.

The effects of generalized hypothermia on renal hemodynamics have been reported by several investigators.[1, 3, 6-8, 10, 11] These studies show that there is a 50 to 60 per cent reduction in renal blood flow and glomerular filtration rate in the temperature range of 25° to 30° C.

Thus it appears that the principal effect of intragastric cooling on renal hemodynamics is due to the inflated noncooled gastric balloon. This finding is in contrast to the investigations of gastric and hepatic blood flows in which the inflated balloon caused little or no effect and intragastric cooling resulted in a marked depression of blood flow.[14, 15]

Clinically, from the findings of the present study it seems unlikely that renal ischemia could result from gastric hypothermia. Considering the depression in renal plasma flow and glomerular filtration rate effected by this technique, accumulation of plasma-carried substances might result from decreased clearance by the kidneys.

## CONCLUSIONS

1. Renal plasma flow, renal blood flow, and glomerular filtration rate were measured in normal anesthetized dogs under conditions of gastric hypothermia with maintenance of body temperature.

2. Renal blood flow was decreased significantly by a fluid-filled, noncooled gastric balloon.

3. Gastric hypothermia causes a significant increase in large-vessel arterial hematocrit.

4. Gastric hypothermia reduces significantly renal plasma flow, but decreases renal blood flow to a lesser extent.

5. Glomerular filtration rate remains relatively unaffected by a fluid-filled noncooled gastric balloon.

6. Gastric cooling causes a depression in glomerular filtration rate.

## REFERENCES

1. Bergstrand, A., and Sterky, G.: Renal function in hypothermia, Acta physiol. scandinav. **31:** 13, 1954.
2. Blake, W. D., Wegria, R., Keating, R. P., and Ward, H. P.: Effect of increased renal venous pressure on renal function, Am. J. Physiol. **157:** 1, 1949.
3. Blatteis, C. M., and Horvath, S. M.: Renal, cardiovascular and respiratory responses and their interrelation during hypothermia, Am. J. Physiol. **192:** 357, 1958.
4. Goldring, W., and Chasis, H.: Hypertension and hypertensive disease, New York, 1944, The Commonwealth Fund.
5. Houck, C. R.: Statistical analysis of filtration rate and effective renal plasma flow related to weight and surface area in dogs, Am. J. Physiol. **153:** 169, 1948.
6. Miles, B. E., and Churchill-Davidson, H. C.: The effect of hypothermia on the renal circulation of the dog, Anesthesiology **16:** 230, 1955.
7. Morris, G. C., Moyer, J. H., Cooley, D. A., and Brockman, H. L.: The renal hemodynamic response to hypothermia and to clamping of the thoracic aorta with and without hypothermia, S. Forum **5:** 219, 1954.
8. Moyer, J. H., Morris, G., and De Bakey, M.: Hypothermia. I. Effect on renal hemodynamics and on excretion of water and electrolytes in dog and man, Ann. Surg. **145:** 26, 1957.
9. Nabseth, D. C., Goodale, R. I., and Reif, A. E.: Studies on the effect of intragastric cooling on acute experimental pancreatitis, Surgery **47:** 542, 1960.
10. Onnis, M., Bounous, G., and Shumacker, H. B., Jr.: Renal blood flow in moderate hypothermia, A. M. A. Arch. Surg. **80:** 593, 1960.
11. Page, L. B.: Effects of hypothermia on renal function, Am. J. Physiol. **181:** 171, 1955.
12. Smith, H. W.: Principles of renal physiology, New York, 1957, Oxford University Press.
13. Smythe, C., Heinemann, H. O., and Bradley, S. E.: Estimated hepatic blood flow in the dog; effect of ethyl alcohol on it, renal blood flow, cardiac output and arterial pressure, Am. J. Physiol. **172:** 737, 1953.
14. Wangensteen, O. H., Salmon, P. A., Griffen, W. O., Jr., Paterson, S., and Fattah, F.: Studies of local gastric cooling as related to peptic ulcer, Ann. Surg. **150:** 346, 1959.

15. Wangensteen, S. L., Orahood, R. C., and Luke, W. K.: Physiolgoic effects of gastric hypothermia. I. The effect on estimated hepatic blood flow in the normal anesthetized dog, SURGERY **50:** 651, 1961.
16. Wangensteen, S. L., Orahood, R. C., and Luke, W. K.: Physiologic effects of gastric hypothermia. III. The effect on circulating blood volume and large-vessel hematocrit, In preparation.
Wangensteen, S. L., and Smith, W. H.: A gastric hypothermia machine, SURGERY **47:** 924, 1960.

# Role of pancreatic and biliary juices in regulation of gastric secretion: pathogenesis of the Mann-Williamson ulcer

RENÉ MENGUY, M.D., PH.D.*
HAROLD MINGS, M.D.
OKLAHOMA CITY, OKLA.
*From the Department of Surgery, University of Oklahoma Medical Center and Oklahoma City Veterans Administration Hospital*

The Mann-Williamson operation or duodenal drainage procedure remains one of the more reliable methods of producing an experimental peptic ulcer in dogs.[4] The ulcer, which appears on the jejunal side of the gastrojejunostomy within several weeks to several months after the duodenum has been transplanted to the terminal ileum, is generally attributed to unopposed action of acid gastric juice because of diversion of alkaline duodenal contents from the gastric outlet zone. To explain the Mann-Williamson ulcer by a change in the equilibrium of the pH of the gastric outlet zone seems plausible. However, there is some evidence which suggests that a more complex physiologic disturbance in the gastrointestinal tract may be responsible. Several groups of investigators have observed an increase in gastric secretion from Heidenhain pouches after a Mann-Williamson operation.[2, 3, 8] Removal of the duodenal mechanism of acid inhibition has been considered responsible for this increase in gastric secretory activity.[1] One dissenting opinion has been raised by Okinaka and associates[7] who, working with a modified Mann-Williamson preparation, did not observe an increase in gastric secretion after duodenal drainage to the ileum.

Supported in part by Public Health Service Grant A3934, National Institute of Arthritis and Metabolic Diseases, and by American Cancer Society Grant E-186.

Received for publication Nov. 28, 1960.

*Markle Scholar in Medical Sciences. Present address: Department of Surgery, University of Kentucky Medical Center, Lexington, Ky.

Studies previously reported from this laboratory have shown that inhibition of gastric secretion normally produced by fat in the intestine fails to occur in the absence of pancreatic and biliary secretions from the proximal small intestine.[5] Obviously, in dogs which have undergone a Mann-Williamson operation the proximal small intestine is devoid of pancreatic and biliary juices and inhibition of gastric secretion by fat can no longer be expected to occur. Failure of this inhibitory mechanism could presumably cause an increase in gastric secretory activity.

Our purpose in these studies was to determine whether or not an increase in gastric secretion occurs in dogs after diversion of biliary and pancreatic juices from the duodenum without interfering with the duodenal acid inhibition mechanism.

## MATERIALS AND METHODS

Denervated fundic (Heidenhain) pouches were constructed in 4 adult mongrel dogs. Strict asepsis was observed. Pouch secretions were drained via a metal-sheathed plastic cannula into a rubber bag changed every 24 hours prior to feeding. The animals were fed a mixture of horse meat (450 Gm.) and dog meal (450 Gm.) at the same hour every day, including Sundays. Salt was added to the diet in the amount of 5 Gm. per 100 ml. of gastric juice secreted during the preceding 24 hours. Daily collections of pouch secretions were started 3 weeks after the operation. The 24-hour output of gastric juice was measured, titrated for free hydrochloric acid concentration with Töpfer's reagent, and the amount of free hydrochloric acid secreted per 24 hours was calculated. Also, the pouch output of free hydrochloric acid in response to a standard meal was measured at hourly intervals for a period of 5 hours after the meal. The hourly collections were then included in the total 24-hour output. Three such experiments were performed in 3 dogs. After a 15-day control period the animals were again operated upon and a short (4 cm.) cuff of duodenum which incorporated both pancreatic and biliary ducts was resected and transplanted to the terminal ileum at a point 50 cm. proximal to the cecum (Fig. 1). Duodenal continuity was re-established by an end-to-end anastomosis. For the first 3 postoperative days the dogs were maintained on parenteral fluids. Thereafter, they were fed as before and pouch collections were resumed for another 15-day period. In addition to measurements of 24-hour pouch secretion, the hourly output of free hydrochloric acid in response to the standard meal was studied over a 5-hour period in 3 animals as described. After completion of the second 15-day collection period the dogs were again operated upon. Pancreatic and biliary secretions were shunted back to the duodenum by mobilization of the duodenal cuff which had been previously transplanted to the ileum and anastomosis of it to the side of the duodenum after closure of its proximal end. Ileal continuity was re-established by an end-to-end anastomosis. Pouch collections were then resumed in the same manner as described in the 2 dogs that survived the third operation.

## RESULTS

All 4 dogs exhibited an increase in the daily output of hydrochloric acid from the Heidenhain pouches after diversion of pancreatic and biliary juices to the ileum. Increases in the average daily output after the shunt ranged from 80 to 566 per cent. After pancreatic and biliary juices were shunted back to the duodenum, the secretory rate of the pouches immediately returned to control levels in the 2 dogs which survived the third operation (Table I, Fig. 2). In the 3 animals in which the hourly response of the Heidenhain pouch to the standard meal was studied, the pattern of the response was considerably altered by the diversion of pancreatic and biliary secretions to the

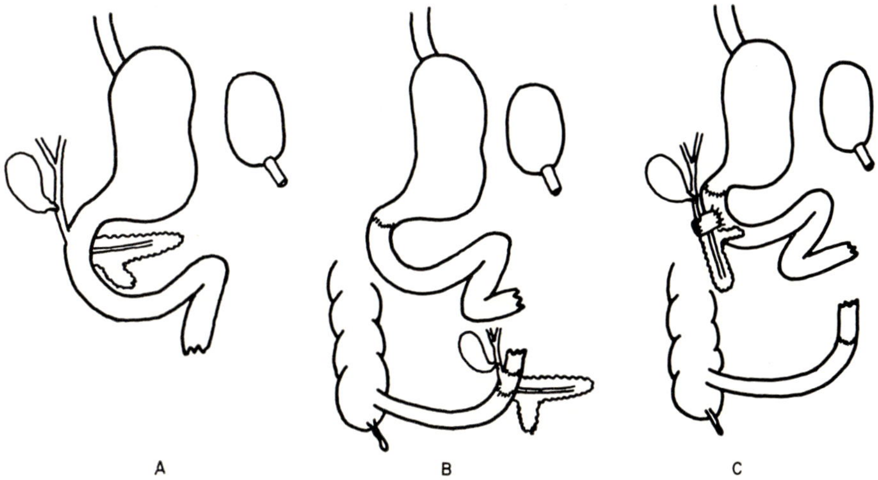

**Fig. 1.** Schematic representation of experimental preparation used in this study. *A,* Construction of Heidenhain pouch. *B,* Diversion of pancreatic and biliary juices to ileum by transplantation of a short cuff of duodenum which incorporates pancreatic and biliary ducts to terminal ileum. *C,* Pancreatic and biliary juices returned to duodenum.

**Table I.** *Twenty-four hour output of free hydrochloric acid from Heidenhain pouches*

| | Control period | | Biliary and pancreatic secretions shunted to terminal ileum | | | | Biliary and pancreatic secretions shunted back to duodenum | | |
|---|---|---|---|---|---|---|---|---|---|
| Dog No. | No. 24 hr. collections | Av. 24 hr. output of free HCl ($x_1$)* | No. 24 hr. collections | Av. 24 hr. output of free HCl ($x_2$)* | Significance of $x_2$-$x_1$ | % deviation from controls | No. 24 hr. collections | Av. 24 hr. output of free HCl ($x_3$)* | Significance of $x_2$-$x_3$ |
| 1† | 15 | 5.5 ± 2.4 | 15 | 21.3 ± 4.0 | $p < 0.001$ | +287 | — | — | — |
| 2† | 15 | 9.1 ± 1.7 | 15 | 16.4 ± 5.0 | $p < 0.001$ | + 80 | — | — | — |
| 3 | 15 | 1.5 ± 1.2 | 15 | 10.0 ± 5.2 | $p < 0.001$ | +566 | 15 | 3.5 ± 2.0 | $p < 0.001$ |
| 4 | 15 | 0.7 ± 0.5 | 15 | 3.5 ± 1.4 | $p < 0.001$ | +400 | 15 | 0.4 ± 0.4 | $p < 0.001$ |

*Milliequivalents ± standard deviation.
†Dog did not survive third operation.

**Table II.** *Hourly output of free hydrochloric acid from Heidenhain pouches in response to a standard meal*

| | Control period (mEq.) | | | | | Pancreatic and biliary secretions shunted to terminal ileum (mEq.) | | | | | Pancreatic and biliary secretions reshunted to duodenum (mEq.) | | | | |
|---|---|---|---|---|---|---|---|---|---|---|---|---|---|---|---|
| Dog No. | 0*-1 hr. | 1-2 hr. | 2-3 hr. | 3-4 hr. | 4-5 hr. | 0*-1 hr. | 1-2 hr. | 2-3 hr. | 3-4 hr. | 4-5 hr. | 0*-1 hr. | 1-2 hr. | 2-3 hr. | 3-4 hr. | 4-5 hr. |
| 1† | 0.00 | 0.04 | 1.02 | 0.39 | 0.50 | 0.15 | 1.30 | 1.97 | 1.68 | 2.41 | — | — | — | — | — |
| | 0.00 | 0.5 | 0.08 | 0.33 | 1.08 | 0.17 | 0.80 | 1.71 | 1.29 | 1.18 | — | — | — | — | — |
| | 0.00 | 0.8 | 0.75 | — | 0.47 | 0.42 | 1.33 | 1.87 | 1.49 | 1.05 | — | — | — | — | — |
| 3 | 0.00 | 0.14 | 0.1 | 0.07 | 0.06 | 0.57 | 0.81 | 0.67 | 0.57 | 0.00 | 0.00 | 0.02 | 0.07 | 0.20 | 0.30 |
| | 0.00 | 0.00 | 0.02 | 0.01 | 0.03 | 0.50 | 0.69 | 0.35 | 0.34 | 0.24 | 0.02 | 0.19 | 0.15 | 0.20 | 0.23 |
| | 0.00 | 0.00 | 0.07 | 0.04 | 0.03 | 1.04 | 1.51 | 0.87 | 0.60 | 0.73 | 0.00 | 0.10 | 0.16 | 0.13 | 0.36 |
| 4 | 0.00 | 0.00 | 0.00 | 0.00 | 0.01 | 0.03 | 0.10 | 0.12 | 0.27 | 0.13 | 0.00 | 0.00 | 0.00 | 0.00 | 0.00 |
| | 0.00 | 0.00 | 0.00 | 0.00 | 0.00 | 0.01 | 0.10 | 0.20 | 0.50 | 0.30 | 0.00 | 0.00 | 0.00 | 0.00 | 0.00 |
| | | | | | | 0.00 | 0.07 | 0.36 | 0.50 | 0.46 | 0.00 | 0.00 | 0.00 | 0.00 | 0.00 |

*Meal given at hour 0.
†Dog did not survive third operation.

ileum. In all 9 experiments the 3 dogs showed a more active and more sustained secretory rate than during the control period. After the third operation the secretory response of the pouches to the same meal returned to control levels in the 2 surviving animals (Table II, Fig. 3).

## DISCUSSION

It can be concluded from these data that gastric secretory activity is increased when pancreatic and biliary secretions are absent from the proximal small intestine. Our results confirm those of other workers who have observed an increase in gastric secretion in dogs after a Mann-Williamson operation.[2, 3, 8] In the classic Mann-Williamson operation, the entire duodenum is removed from its normal intestinal continuity and anastomosed to the terminal ileum.[4] With this preparation 2 important physiologic changes take place in the gastrointestinal tract. Duodenal juices are absent from the proximal small intestine. Also, the duodenum, being removed from the acid stream, becomes predominantly alkaline and would no longer be capable of exerting on the stomach the inhibitory influence initiated by a low duodenal pH (duodenal acid inhibition phenomenon). The former change is an obvious one, the latter is more theoretical in nature. Dragstedt and associates,[1] who have observed an increase in acid output from Heidenhain pouches after a Mann-

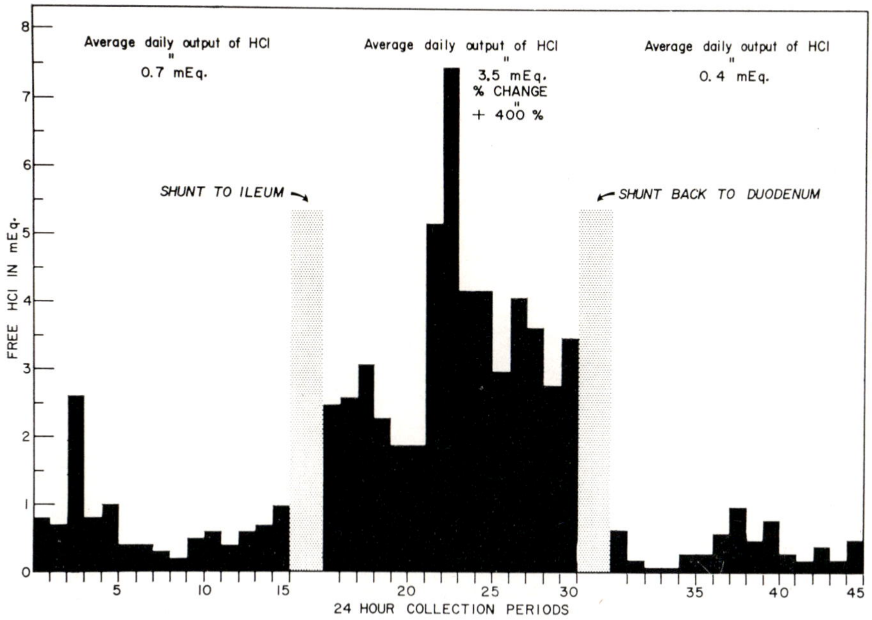


**Fig. 2.** Graphic representation of daily output of free hydrochloric acid from Heidenhain pouch in Dog 4 shows increase in gastric secretory activity after diversion of pancreatic and biliary juices to the ileum and disappearance of gastric hypersecretion after these juices were returned to duodenum.

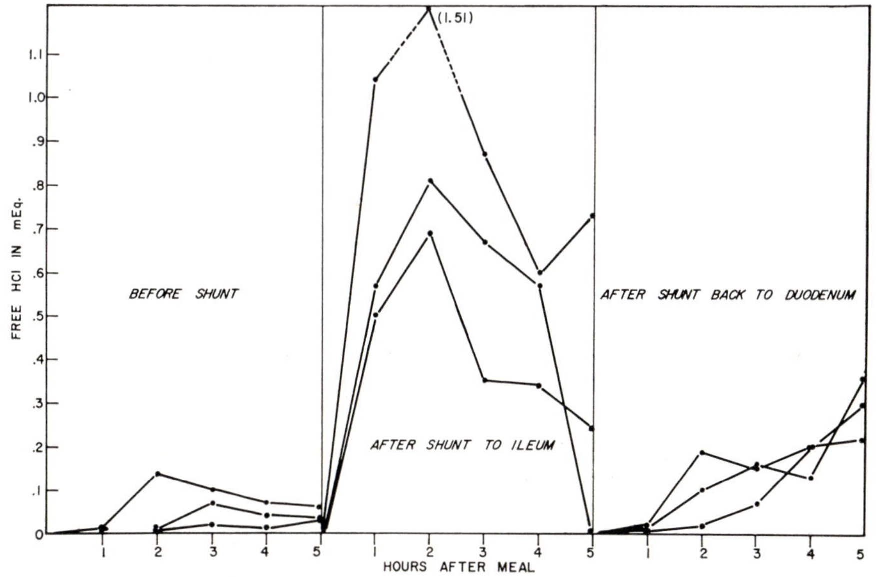


**Fig. 3.** Graphic representation of secretory response of Heidenhain pouch to a standard meal (Dog 3) shows pronounced increase in secretory response to the meal after diversion of pancreatic and biliary juices to the ileum and reversion to control values of the secretory response after these juices were shunted back to the duodenum.

Williamson operation, believe that this gastric hypersecretion is due to the absence of gastric inhibition which occurs under normal conditions when gastric acid comes in contact with duodenal mucosa. In our preparation, the anatomic continuity of the duodenum was disturbed only by a short duodenal cuff which incorporated both pancreatic and biliary ducts. Under these experimental conditions, the major physiologic change in the intestinal tract was diversion of pancreatic and biliary secretions from the proximal small intestine. The resulting augmentation of secretion exhibited by the Heidenhain pouches was of the same order of magnitude as observed by Dragstedt and his associates after a classic Mann-Williamson operation.[8] Therefore, our results suggest that gastric hypersecretion present in Mann-Williamson dogs is not due merely to removal of the duodenal acid inhibition mechanism (if indeed such a mechanism is operative within the physiologic range of duodenal pH). The logical inference is to consider the absence of pancreatic and biliary juices from the small intestine responsible for the gastric hypersecretion by some as yet unexplained mechanism. The increase in the hourly output of acid after a standard meal which was observed in the absence of pancreatic and biliary juices from the proximal small intestine suggests that the pouch mucosa was responding to a greater humoral stimulus or that some humoral inhibitory mechanism was impaired.

The antrum would be one obvious source of increased humoral stimulus. However, recent experiments from Dragstedt's laboratory showed that gastric hypersecretion produced by classic Mann-Williamson operation was not prevented by antrectomy.[1] A humoral secretagogue of intestinal origin could also be invoked. This does not seem likely in view of the rather small amount of gastric secretion of intestinal origin even under conditions of normal digestion.

Therefore, one must consider the possibility that this hypersecretion was due to normal antral function unopposed by the inhibitory mechanisms which operate under physiologic conditions. As mentioned in our introductory statements, we have found in working with rats that fat in the intestine failed to inhibit gastric secretion when pancreatic and/or biliary secretions were absent from the small intestine.[5] Extending this work to dogs, we observed that fat, carbohydrate, and protein in the form of olive oil, starch, and albumin were capable of decreasing histamine-stimulated Heidenhain pouch secretion when introduced into the duodenum. This inhibition failed to occur after pancreatic and biliary secretions had been diverted to the ileum.[6] These data suggest the existence of an intestinal inhibitory mechanism related to and dependent upon proper digestion of food substances. Impairment of digestion due to absence of pancreatic and biliary secretions from the small intestine, as in our experimental preparation, or as in the classic Mann-Williamson operation, would result in the loss of this intestinal inhibitory mechanism. The stomach would then lose a braking mechanism and, like a machine with a broken governor, would hypersecrete excessively with each meal. We suspect that the absence of this intestinal inhibitory mechanism which is dependent upon food digestion is responsible for the gastric hypersecretion characteristic of the Mann-Williamson operation. In all probability this hypersecretion, unopposed by alkaline juices at the gastric outlet zone is, in turn, responsible for the Mann-Williamson ulcer.

## SUMMARY

Denervated fundic (Heidenhain) pouches were constructed in 4 dogs. Twenty-four hour collections of pouch output were made over a 15-day control period. After this control period pancreatic and biliary juices were diverted to the terminal ileum by transplantation of a short duodenal cuff which incorporated both pancreatic and biliary ducts to the ileum at a point 50 cm. proximal to the ileocecal valve. After this procedure, all dogs exhibited a substantial increase in the 24-hour output of free hydrochloric acid from the Heidenhain pouches.

This gastric hypersecretion disappeared after pancreatic and biliary juices were returned to the duodenum. In this preparation the major portion of the duodenum was left in its normal continuity. Therefore, it is concluded that gastric hypersecretion characteristic of the Mann-Williamson animal is not due solely to removal of the duodenal acid inhibition mechanism. Etiology of this hypersecretion may be the loss of intestinal inhibitory mechanisms which are dependent upon proper digestion of food substances.

## REFERENCES

1. Baugh, C. M., Bravo, J., Dragstedt, L. R., and Dragstedt, L. R., II: The pathogenesis of the Exalto-Mann-Williamson ulcer. II. Relation of the antrum to the hypersecretion of gastric juice in Mann-Williamson animals, Gastroenterology **39:** 330, 1960.
2. Brackney, E. L., Thal, A. P., and Wangensteen, O. H.: Role of duodenum in control of gastric secretion, Proc. Soc. Exper. Biol. & Med. **88:** 302, 1955.
3. Ivy, A. C., and Bachrach, W. H.: An abnormal mechanism for the excitation of gastric secretion in the dog, Am. J. Digest. Dis. **7:** 76, 1940.
4. Mann, F. C., and Williamson, C. S.: The experimental production of peptic ulcer, Ann. Surg. **77:** 409, 1923.
5. Menguy, R.: Studies on the role of pancreatic and biliary secretions in the mechanism of gastric inhibition by fat, SURGERY **48:** 195, 1960.
6. Menguy, R.: Unpublished data.
7. Okinaka, A., Moody, F., Gineen, J., Beal, M. J., and Martin, K. A.: Experimental production of peptic ulcers without increased secretion of acid, SURGERY **46:** 70, 1959.
8. Storer, E. H., Oberhelman, H. A., Woodward, E. R., Smith, C. A., and Dragstedt, L. R.: Effect of the Exalto-Mann-Williamson procedure on gastric secretion, A. M. A. Arch. Surg. **64:** 192, 1952.

# Portacaval shunt in the rat

S. H. LEE, M.D.
BERNARD FISHER, M.D.
PITTSBURGH, PA.
*From the Department of Surgery, Laboratory of Surgical Research, University of Pittsburgh, School of Medicine*

Certain precise physiologic and metabolic studies related to portacaval shunting have been hampered by the necessity of resorting to the use of the dog and other large test animals in which the creation of controlled experimental conditions is at best difficult. It would be advantageous, particularly in investigations related to liver regeneration, if the Eck fistula could be performed on the laboratory rat. In fact, the stimulus to perfect such a technique arose from our interest in (1) evaluating in animals with shunts the humoral factor which has been reported to be associated with liver regeneration,[2, 6, 7, 10] and (2) evaluating the experiments of Weinbren[12] which suggest that, contrary to the reports of numerous prior investigators,[3, 9, 11] liver deprived of its portal blood supply is capable of regeneration.

The purpose of this report is (1) to describe a technique for portacaval shunt in the rat which has been performed over 100 times during the past year and a half (by S. H. L.) with an operative mortality rate of less than 5 per cent and by which shunts have remained patent indefinitely, and (2) to present certain observations made on animals with such shunts.

## METHOD

**Surgical techniques.** End-to-side and side-to-side portacaval shunts were performed on Sprague-Dawley rats which weighed more than 140 Gm. Clean, but not sterile, surgical technique was used in animals anesthetized with ether. The abdomen was opened and the intestines retracted laterally to expose the portal vein and vena cava, the anatomic relationships of which are shown in Fig. 1, *A*. After mobilization of the portal vein with ligation of its coronary venous tributary and partial freeing of the vena cava at and above the entrance of the renal vein, these vessels were occluded (Fig. 1, *B*). A small hemostat, curved to resemble a Satinsky blood vessel clamp, was used on the vena cava, and a mosquito hemostat was placed across the portal vein. The blades of both clamps were ground and polished to reduce their thickness, and they were rubber shod. An elliptical opening was made in the vena cava, the portal vein was severed after ligation of the end proximal to the liver, and an anastomosis was performed with No. 7-0 braided silk attached to 2 three-eighths circle taper needles.* Over-and-over stitches were employed. After removal of the clamps oozing was readily controlled by a few moments of slight pressure with a gauze sponge. The portal vein was completely occluded for from 10 to 12 minutes.

The technique for side-to-side shunt was identical to that for end-to-side anastomosis, except that an elliptical opening was made in the portal vein and this vessel was easily approximated to the vena cava in longi-

Supported by United States Public Health Grant A-369.
Received for publication Nov. 29, 1960.

*David and Geck (American Cyanamid).

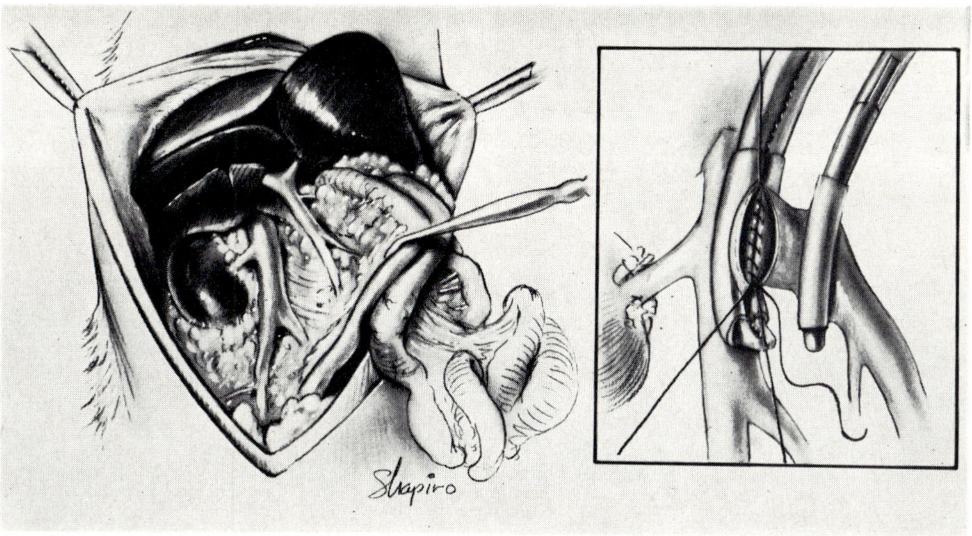


*A* *B*

**Fig. 1.** Technique of portacaval shunt in the rat. *A,* Anatomic relationships of portal vein and vena cava. *B,* Microsuture technique.

tudinal fashion. For visual aid a binocular magnifier with a 2.25 diameter magnification and a 10 inch focal length was worn by the operator.

After shunting, animals were maintained on an ad libitum chow checker diet, except those for which food consumption was recorded. These received measured amounts of ground chow. All animals were housed in separate cages and permitted water as desired. At intervals splenoportograms or mesenteric portograms were performed to determine patency of the shunts. These were accomplished by insertion of a 21 gauge needle into either the splenic pulp or a tributary of the mesenteric vein. Attached to the needle was a length of polyethylene tubing through which 1.25 ml. of radiopaque material (70 per cent Urokon) was injected. Roentgenograms were taken with exposure factors of 50 kv., 50 Ma., one-twentieth second, and a target film distance of 29 inches.

Blood ammonia determinations were made in duplicate on 0.5 ml. of blood drawn from the femoral vein. Submicrodiffusion units were used, and ammonia level was determined by the technique described by Conway.[4]

Liver analyses were carried out in the conventional fashion already described from this laboratory[5] and by Gurd and associates[8] in their work on liver regeneration. Sections of liver were examined by use of routine histologic techniques.

## RESULTS

None of the animals in which technically satisfactory end-to-side portacaval shunts had

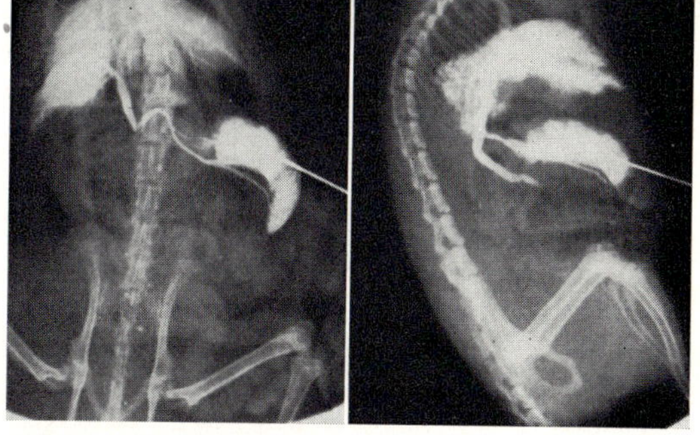

**Fig. 2.** Splenoportograms in normal rats.

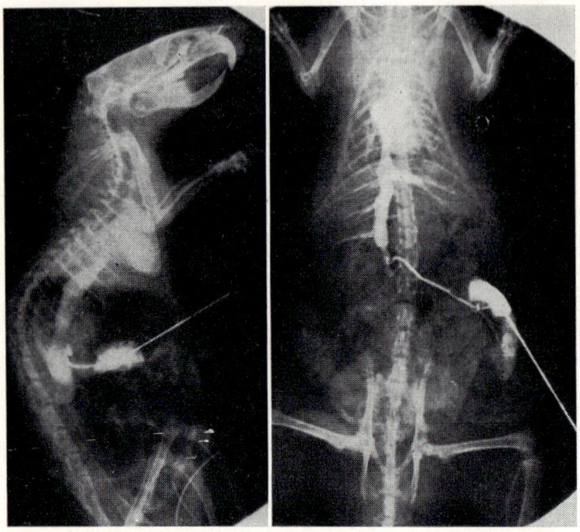

**Fig. 3.** Splenoportograms taken 4 months after shunt.

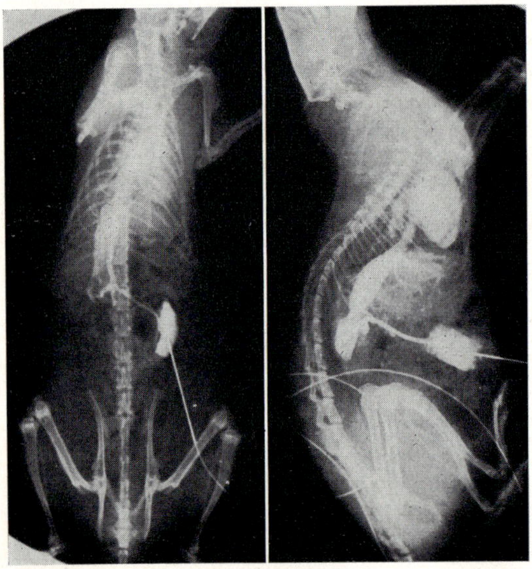

*A* *B*

**Fig. 4.** Splenoportograms taken *A,* 5 months after shunt, and *B,* 7 months after shunt (note retrograde filling of hepatic veins).

been performed demonstrated closure of the shunts when followed for as long as 7 months. Representative splenoportograms from normal rats and those with shunts observed from 4 to 7 months (Figs. 2 through 4) demonstrate patency of the shunts, and no evidence of portal collaterals was observed in such animals.

While animals with shunts appeared well and healthy, weight curves demonstrated a striking difference from that observed in control rats. By 1 week all 6 animals with sham operation which had been fed ad libitum exceeded their preoperative weights and continued to gain, so that by 3 months they had almost doubled their body weights (Fig. 5, *A*). Those subjected to end-to-side shunt lost weight postoperatively—some precipitously (Fig. 5, *D* and *E*), some gradually (Fig. 5, *B*)—and did not return to their preoperative weights for from 2 to 3 months. An occasional animal (Fig. 5, *F*) did not lose weight, but did fail to gain for the first few months. With return to the preoperative level, body weights tended to plateau so that no additional substantial weight gains were observed in animals followed for as long as 5 months.

In several animals food consumption was recorded at intervals after shunting. Sham control rats consumed from 17 to 22 Gm. of food per day while continuing to gain approximately 2 Gm. of weight per day. Three to 4 months after shunting these animals ate an average of 18 Gm. of food each day with no appreciable weight increase.

Seventeen normal rats were found to have a blood ammonia level of 2.2 ± 0.6 $\gamma$ per milliliter. By 60 to 90 days after shunting (end-to-side) this valve had increased to 6.1 ± 1.6 $\gamma$ per milliliter, where it remained in subsequent determinations.

Composition of the liver 5 to 144 days after portacaval shunt was little different from that of normal control animals (Table I). Aside from the fact that the size of the liver, when expressed in terms of per cent of body weight, was smaller in animals with shunts than in control rats, no marked difference in fat, protein, glycogen, or water was apparent. Microscopic examination of livers from such animals with long-term shunts showed a slight increase of fat in some but no increased alteration from normal (Fig. 6).

## DISCUSSION

To our knowledge this is the first report of the successful creation of Eck fistulas, which remained indefinitely patent, in rats by a technique similar to that used in human

**Table I.** *Composition of liver after end-to-side portacaval shunt in the rat*

| | No. of rats | Days after shunt | % body weight | Composition of liver (% wet weight) | | | |
|---|---|---|---|---|---|---|---|
| | | | | Water | Protein | Fat | Glycogen |
| Controls | 25 | — | 3.2 | 70.1 | 20.3 | 3.5 | 3.6 |
| Rats with shunts | 5 | 134 | 2.3 | 69.9 | 21.6 | 2.8 | 3.1 |

beings. In 1946, Whitaker[13] reported the creation of such fistulas by piercing the lumina of the inferior vena cava and superior mesenteric vein with a curved needle and attached suture. The latter, which had been passed through both veins, was firmly ligated. Several days later, the proximal portal vein was tied off. This technique, however, prove unreliable[12] and its use has not been productive.

Recently Bono and his group[1] demonstrated that cirrhotic rats develop portal hypertension and a hemodynamic response which is practically indistinguishable from that seen in human beings with this condition. Certainly only through such an experimental model can it be expected that further progress in our understanding of the pathologic physiologic aspects of portal hypertension will be made. It is anticipated that studies now being conducted in this laboratory in which end-to-side and side-to-side portacaval shunts are performed on such cirrhotic animals as described by Bono and his colleagues will contribute to a better understanding of the value of such operations for portal hypertension.

In this laboratory past experience in maintaining dogs with portacaval shunts for prolonged periods has been similar to that of others. Animals lose or do not gain weight, present nutritional problems, and readily become debilitated. Of interest and worthy of further investigation is our observation that, after shunting, rats maintained under ideal circumstances failed to gain weight, in spite of the fact that food consumption was not dissimilar to that of control animals. The possibility of impaired intestinal absorption after Eck fistula construction is to be considered.

Thus, with the availability of this tech-

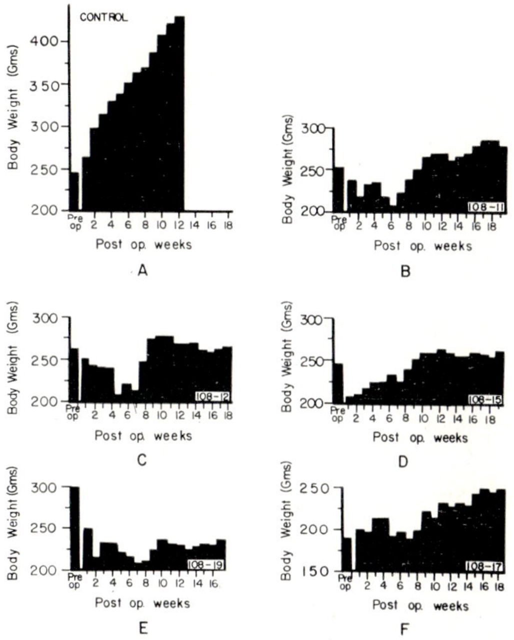


**Fig. 5.** Weekly weight charts from control rats *(A)* and those with portacaval shunts (*B* through *F*).

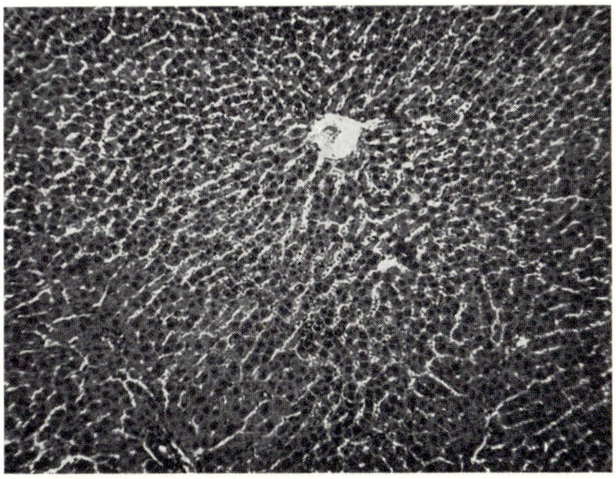

**Fig. 6.** Microscopic section of liver which was taken from rat 7 months after portocaval shunt. (×150; reduced 3/7.)

nique for portacaval shunt in the rat, it is anticipated that more precise data regarding nutrition, hepatic regeneration, and metabolic and physiologic parameters consequent to Eck fistula construction will be forthcoming.

## SUMMARY

Portacaval shunt, carried out by a technique similar to that employed in the human being, has been performed with a minimum of deaths. Animals observed for as long as 7 months demonstrated patency of the Eck fistulas. While maintaining the appearance of good health, these animals failed to gain weight in a fashion comparable to that observed in control rats. Data concerning food consumption, liver composition, blood ammonia levels, and histologic study are presented. It is anticipated that more precise information on liver regeneration and certain metabolic and physiologic parameters subsequent to Eck fistula formation in both normal and cirrhotic animals will be obtained in a controlled fashion which was previously most difficult in larger animals.

### REFERENCES

1. Bono, R. F., Moreno, A. H., Rousselot, L. M., and Panke, W. F.: Studies on portal hypertension. V. A comparison between the experimentally induced state of portal hypertension and that observed in human beings, Surgery **48:** 119, 1960.
2. Bucher, N. L. R., Scott, J. F., and Aub, J. C.: Regeneration of the liver in parabiotic rats, Cancer Res. **11:** 457, 1951.
3. Child, C. G., Barr, D., Holswade, G. R., and Harrison, C. S.: Liver regeneration following portacaval transposition in dogs, Ann. Surg. **138:** 600, 1953.
4. Conway, E. J.: Microdiffusion analysis and volumetric error, London, 1957, Crosby Lockwood and Son, Ltd.
5. Fisher, B., Russ, C., and Bluestone, C.: Composition of the regenerated dog liver following partial hepatectomy and total arterialization, Am. J. Physiol. **181:** 203, 1955.
6. Friedrich-Freksa, Von H., and Zaki, F. G.: Spezifische Mitose-Auslosung in normaler Rattenleber durch Serum von partiell hepatektomierten Ratten, Ztschr. Naturf. **9:** 394, 1954.
7. Glinos, A. D., and Gey, G. O.: Humoral factors involved in the induction of liver regeneration in the rat, Proc. Soc. Exper. Biol. & Med. **80:** 421, 1952.
8. Gurd, F. N., Vars, H. M., and Ravdin, I. S.: Composition of the regenerated liver after partial hepatectomy in normal and protein depleted rats, Am. J. Physiol. **152:** 11, 1948.
9. Mann, F. C., and Magath, J. B.: The production of chronic liver insufficiency, Am. J. Physiol. **59:** 485, 1922.
10. Smythe, R. L., and Moore, R. O.: A study of possible humoral factors in liver regeneration in the rat, Surgery **44:** 561, 1958.
11. Stephenson, G. W.: Experimental pathology of the liver. IX. Restoration of the liver after partial hepatectomy and partial ligation of the portal vein, Arch. Path. **14:** 484, 1932.
12. Weinbren, K.: The portal blood supply and regeneration of the rat liver, Brit. J. Exper. Path. **36:** 583, 1955.
13. Whitaker, W. L.: Portal vein ligation and Eck fistula in the rat, Proc. Soc. Exper. Biol. & Med. **161:** 420, 1946.

# The investigation of renal complications of aortic clamping

JOSEPH E. WHITLEY, M.D.*
RICHARD L. WITCOFSKI, M.S.
JOHN H. FELTS, M.D.
I. MESCHAN, M.D.
WINSTON-SALEM, N. C.
*From The Bowman Gray School of Medicine and the North Carolina Baptist Hospital*

Acute renal insufficiency is one of the major complications of aortic operations, particularly in elderly patients who undergo aneurysmectomy and replacement grafting.[1] Serious renal complications have been encountered after this procedure on our surgical service and have focused attention on this problem. We chose to investigate it with radioactive compounds selectively secreted by the kidney[11] in acute dog experiments.

## EQUIPMENT

Measuring equipment consisted of matched collimated probes (1½ by 1 inch sodium iodide [T1] crystals), matched rate meters, and a dual rectilinear chart recorder. The crystals were recessed 7.0 cm. from the face of the cone, which had an aperture of 8.4 cm.

## METHODS

Our initial approach to the problem was to investigate this syndrome in dogs anesthetized intravenously with pentobarbital sodium. A midline laparotomy was performed. The kidneys were located and marked externally for ease in positioning the scintillation detectors. An umbilical tape ligature was placed about the aorta below the origin of the renal arteries. Ureteral catheters were then passed up the ureters via a cystotomy wound, and minute-to-minute urine collections made before, during, and after each experimental procedure.

The external scintillation probes were positioned over the kidneys, 1 $\mu$c. per kilogram of orthoiodohippuric acid $I^{131}$ injected intravenously, and an external "renogram" performed. The renogram was continued until an excretory plateau was reached (about 20 minutes). Interpretation of the curves was performed by a previously described method.[12]

The umbilical tape was tightened to occlude the aorta and the renogram repeated 1 or more times during the occlusion. The ligature was then removed from the aorta and the renogram repeated 2 or more times.

This experiment was performed in 9 dogs with clamping intervals of from 20 minutes to 1 hour. A typical result is shown in the upper sequence of curves of Fig. 1 (control).

In an effort to prevent the deterioration of the renogram pattern, 4 methods were utilized just prior to aortic clamping; (1) administration of a ganglionic blocking agent (phenoxybenzamine*) intravenously (0.1 mg. per kilogram) in 3 dogs; (2) administration of 2 per cent Procaine infiltrated into the tissues of 1 renal pedicle (1.0 to 1.5 ml.) in 2 dogs (with the other kidney as a control); (3) administration of small amounts of normal saline solution infiltrated into the tissues of 1 renal pedicle (1.0 to

Supported by National Institutes of Health Grants H.T.S.-5392 and H5418, The North Carolina Heart Association, and The James Picker Foundation.

Received for publication Dec. 9, 1960.

*Fellow in Radiological Research, James Picker Foundation, Department of Radiology.

*Provided as Dibenzylene by Smith Kline & French Laboratories.

1.5 ml.) in 2 dogs; and (4) administration of large volumes of normal saline solution infiltrated into the tissues of 1 renal pedicle (4 to 6 ml.) in 2 dogs.

## RESULTS AND ANALYSIS

In the control experiments, consistent results were obtained bilaterally in all 9 dogs. Immediately after ligation of the aorta, there was a significant increase in the height and apparent function as measured by the renogram. This transient change in the renogram was soon superseded (in 10 to 20 minutes) by a gradual deterioration of the renogram pattern first evidenced in the excretory phase with a so-called "obstructive pattern." With continued clamping, the over-all height was diminished and the secretory and the excretory phases markedly prolonged, indicating diminished renal function. After the removal of the clamps, there was a gradual return toward normal function over a period of the next several hours. The rapidity of this return to the normal was not directly related to length of clamping time in our limited experience.

Administration of phenoxybenzamine intravenously did not prevent the transient "increase in function" as seen by the renogram. The increase in height of the complex was followed by a return to normal conditions bilaterally.

Administration of Procaine into 1 renal pedicle resulted in the curves shown in Fig. 1. As is evident from the illustration, the unprotected kidney (left) went through the control cycle. The protected side (right) followed the same course that the phenoxybenzamine protection produced.

The dogs which received infiltration of small amounts of normal saline solution in the renal pedicle showed no alteration from the course observed in the control side. However, distention of the renal pedicle with larger doses of normal saline produced results similar to those seen with Procaine.

## DISCUSSION

In response to clamping of the aorta below the origin of the renal arteries, there is a transient increase in vascular distending pressure and in renal blood flow. These changes are evidenced on the renogram by an increase in the height of the complex with an unchanged time relationship of the component parts of the curve. During the next phase there is a decreased renal blood flow and decreased urine output, with no change in the concentrating ability of the tubules. This is evidenced in the renogram by return of the height of the complex to control or below control height without change in the time intervals of the vascular or secretory phases, but with prolongation of the excretory phase. This reflex increase in renal resistance has been believed to be of etiologic significance in the development of acute tubular necrosis.[6]

The results of the attempts to alter the deterioration of the pattern of the renogram demonstrated that these changes were preventable with phenoxybenzamine or by the injection of a local anesthetic into the renal pedicle. Distention of the renal pedicle with a large volume of saline solution apparently produces the same result (this may be due to either mechanical compression of nerve conduction or alteration of transmural pressure). These studies confirm the previous observations[5, 7] that the diminution in renal function which follows acute aortic occlusion is probably partially mediated by the renal nerves. Haddy's group[3] is at variance with these findings in that renal nerve section did not alter the initial decrease and subsequent increase in renal resistance. The local renal vascular receptor and the autoregulatory mechanism of the kidney may resolve this apparent variance.[8-10]

Ganglionic blocking agents have the possible disadvantage of producing systemic hypotension.[4] Infusion directly into the renal artery is a means by which this hazard could possibly be lessened.[2]

Because all patients subjected to aortic clamping do not develop renal damage, it is difficult to assess the prophylactic effects of anesthetic agents or inert materials infiltrated into the renal pedicle. Serial renograms taken during such procedures might

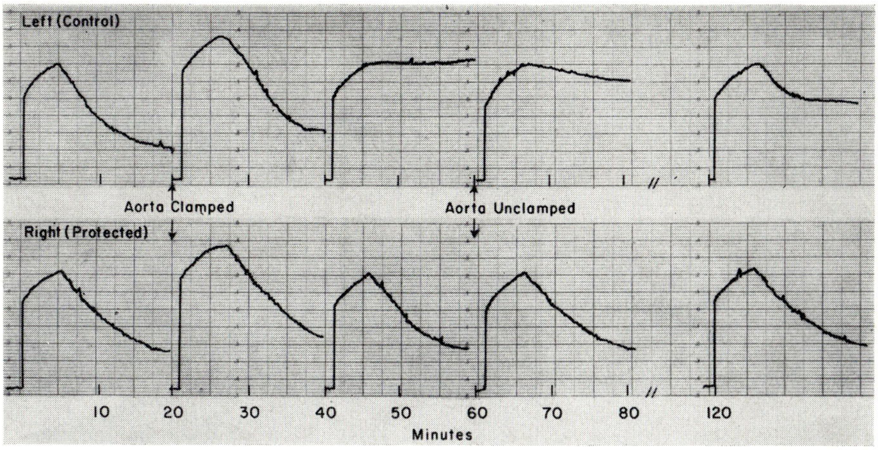


**Fig. 1.** Serial renograms obtained with the right renal pedicle injected with Procaine before, during, and after aortic occlusion below the level of the renal arteries.

clarify the problem and permit further assessment of renal function during aortic operations.

## SUMMARY AND CONCLUSIONS

1. Clamping the aorta below the level of the origin of the renal arteries causes initially "improved" renal function, as judged by the renogram.

2. In 10 to 20 minutes, there occurs a progressive deterioration of the renogram pattern and diminished urine flow.

3. This secondary response may be abolished by the intravascular administration of phenoxybenzamine, or by the injection of the renal pedicle with a local anesthetic or a large volume of saline solution.

4. We believe this syndrome of transient renal failure may be similar to that encountered in the human being under similar situations and may be preventable by the same measures.

We are grateful for the technical assistance of Claudius D. Walker, B.S.

### REFERENCES

1. Doolan, P. D., Wiggins, R. A., Thiel, G. B., Lee, K. J., and Martinez, E.: Acute renal insufficiency after aortic surgery, Am. J. Med. **28:** 895, 1960.
2. Ginsburg, J., and Duff, R. S.: Inhibition of levarterenal by intra-arterial phenoxybenzamine in man, Circulation Res. **6:** 751, 1958.
3. Haddy, F. J., Scott, J., Fleishman, M., and Emanuel, D.: Effect of changes in flow rate upon renal vascular resistance, Am. J. Physiol. **195:** 111, 1958.
4. Moyer, J. H., and Handley, C. A.: Renal hemodynamic and blood pressure response to N-phenoxyisopropyl-N-benzyl-B-chlorethylamine (SKF 688A), J. Pharmacol. & Exper. Therap. **104:** 329, 1952.
5. Nanson, E. M., Noble, J. G., and Ernson, H.: The effect on the kidneys of cross clamping the aorta distal to the renal arteries, S. Forum **9:** 347, 1959.
6. Oliver, J., MacDowell, M., and Tracy, A.: The pathogenesis of acute renal failure associated with traumatic and toxic injury. Renal ischemia, nephrotoxic damage and ischemuric episode, J. Clin. Invest. **30:** 1307, 1951.
7. Powers, S. R., Boba, A., and Stein, A.: The mechanism and prevention of distal tubular necrosis following aneurysmectomy, SURGERY **42:** 156, 1957.
8. Semple, S. J. G., and DeWardener, H. E.: Effect of increased renal venous pressure on circulatory "autoregulation" of isolated dog kidneys, Circulation Res. **7:** 643, 1959.
9. Tobian, L.: Physiology of the juxtaglomerular cells, Ann. Int. Med. **52:** 395, 1960.
10. Waugh, W. H.: Myogenic nature of autoregulation of renal flow in absence of blood corpuscles, Circulation Res. **6:** 363, 1958.
11. Whitley, J. E., Witcofski, R. L., Meschan, I., and Felts, J. H.: Experimental comparison of orthoiodohippuric acid and iodopyracet in renal function evaluation, Radiology **76:** 464, 1961.
12. Witcofski, R. L., Whitley, J. E., Meschan, I., Painter, Wm. E., and Felts, J. H.: A method and parameters for the analysis of renal function by external scintillation detector techniques. Radiology **76:** 621, 1961.

# Surgical fact or fancy. I. Fate of cholecystojejunostomy in the absence of common bile duct obstruction

SCOTT J. BOLEY, M.D.
WILLIAM M. P. McKINNON, M.D.
ARTHUR R. WRIGHT, M.D.
QUEENS, N. Y.
*From the Departments of Surgery, Kew Gardens General Hospital and Queens General Hospital*

Education of a surgeon through the years, and to a large degree even today, has been based upon the passing of knowledge from master to pupil. Often principles which determine basic procedures have come through several generations and are accepted without question. The purpose of our series of experiments was to separate surgical fact from fancy. Re-evaluation of accepted maxims which are being questioned by a new generation of surgeons is worth while, regardless of the results.

The performance of a cholecystojejunostomy in the absence of biliary tract obstruction has its place in the management of neoplastic and inflammatory diseases which are eventually expected to obstruct the common bile duct. Nonresectable pancreatic and gastrointestinal neoplasms are the most common indications. Surgical preceptors and the surgical literature criticize this procedure "because the anastomosis will close in the absence of obstruction." Is the latter maxim surgical fact, or fancy?

## METHOD OF STUDY

With Nembutal anesthesia, side-to-side cholecystojejunostomies were performed on 6 healthy dogs. The anastomoses varied in diameter from 2 to 5 cm., depending upon the size of the gall bladder. Two-layer anastomoses were performed with the inner layer of either continuous or interrupted No. 4-0 chromic catgut sutures and the outer layer interrupted No. 5-0 silk sutures. The site of anastomosis was from 6 to 12 inches from the ligament of Treitz.

All of the animals recovered well from the operation with the exception of 1 dog that ate poorly for several days. They were fed the usual laboratory diet.

Re-exploration was performed at 5 to 9 months after creation of the anastomosis. Patency of the anastomoses was first estab-

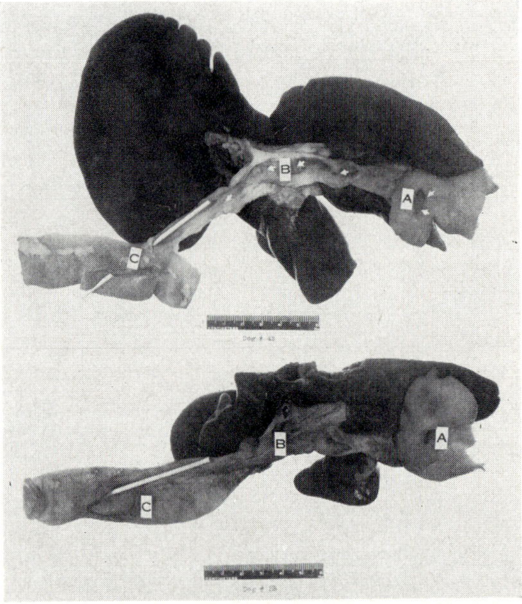


**Fig. 1.** Specimens from Dogs 4B and 5B which show patent cholecystojejunostomies *(A)* and absence of obstruction in common bile duct *(B)* and at the ampulla of Vater *(C)*.

Received for publication Dec. 5, 1960.

**Table I.** *Data on 6 dogs with cholecystojejunostomies*

| Dog No. | Diameter of anastomoses (cm.) At original operation | Time of sacrifice | Interval between operation and sacrifice (mo.) | Comments |
|---|---|---|---|---|
| 1B | 3.5 | 2 | 8½ | Debris in gall bladder |
| 2B | 3.5 | 1.5 | 7 | Debris in gall bladder and common bile duct; common bile duct appeared dilated but was thin-walled |
| 3B | 2.5 | 1.0 | 7¼ | Some foreign material in gall gladder |
| 4B | 4.5 | 3 | 5 | Gall bladder filled with debris |
| 5B | 2.5 | 1.5 | 6 | Debris present in gall bladder |
| 6B | 3 | 2.0 | 6¾ | Mucosal bridge across anastomoses; suture incorporating anterior and posterior walls clearly demonstrated |

lished by injection of saline solution into the jejunum while the intestine above and below the cholecystojejunostomy was occluded. The anastomosis and the biliary tract were then dissected after the animal had been sacrificed.

## RESULTS

The cholecystojejunostomy stoma was patent in all 6 animals. Saline solution passed easily from jejunum into the gall bladder. Table I lists the diameter of the anastomoses at postmortem examination and at the original procedure. In Dog 6B a bridge was found across the center of the patent stoma. It could be demonstrated that the posterior wall had been incorporated during placement of the anterior inner layer of sutures. In spite of this, stomas 0.5 cm. in diameter were present on both sides of the mucosal bridge.

Dissection of the biliary tracts showed the absence of any obstruction (Fig. 1). Probes were easily passed from the gall bladder into the duodenum.

In all of the dogs except Dog 6B, partially digested debris was present in the gall bladder. There was no evidence of any gross inflammation of the gall bladders or extrahepatic ducts. Grossly the livers appeared to be normal. Microscopically there was minimal infiltration of the periportal spaces by chronic inflammatory cells in Dogs 2, 5, and 6.

## DISCUSSION

Based upon this experiment it appears that a cholecystojejunostomy performed in the absence of common duct obstruction will remain patent for at least 6 to 9 months in dogs. Certainly most inoperable neoplasms in man for which the procedure might be indicated would have involved the common duct or caused death within this period. The diameters of the anastomoses suggest that the stomas would have remained patent much longer, if not indefinitely. The presence of food debris within the gall bladder supports the use of the Roux Y type anastomosis or an enteroenterostomy with the side-to-side cholecystojejunostomy. The minimal evidence of ascending cholangitis is probably not applicable to man because of differences in bacterial content of the portal blood and liver.

## SUMMARY

1. The statement that a cholecystojejunostomy will not remain patent in the absence of biliary obstruction has been questioned.

2. Cholecystojejunostomies were created in 6 dogs and were patent 5 to 9 months later. Absence of any biliary obstruction was proved at re-exploration.

3. Experimental observations show definitely that a cholecystojejunostomy performed in anticipation of common bile duct obstruction can be expected to remain patent.

# Pediatric surgery

*Conducted by* MARK M. RAVITCH, M.D.

# Idiopathic muscular hypertrophy of the gastrointestinal tract in a child

ROWENA SPENCER, M.D.
THOMAS L. HUDSON, M.D.
NEW ORLEANS, LA.
*From the Department of Surgery, Louisiana State University School of Medicine, and Charity Hospital of Louisiana at New Orleans*

Idiopathic muscular hypertrophy of any portion of the gastrointestinal tract except the pylorus is rare, and most reported instances have occurred in elderly adults with only a short segment involved. After finding extensive and massive hypertrophy of the muscularis of the gastrointestinal tract in a small child, we searched the literature and found only 1 previously recorded similar case. Review of the medical records of the Charity Hospital of Louisiana at New Orleans revealed no previous case of muscular hypertrophy of the bowel except of the pylorus.

Hypertrophy of the muscularis may be classified as primary (idiopathic) or secondary. Manifestations of primary hypertrophy vary with the location of the lesion. In hypertrophic pyloric stenosis of infants or adults, the hypertrophy causes obstruction; in other portions of the gastrointestinal tract, however, primary lesions apparently neither cause nor result from obstruction, as the hypertrophy was an incidental finding at autopsy in most of the reported cases.

Secondary hypertrophy is seen in the dilated segment of bowel immediately proximal to an acquired chronic partial obstruction or a congenital partial or complete obstruction. This compensatory hypertrophy results from the obstruction.

Received for publication Jan. 12, 1961.

The present case is exceptional in that the condition was found at laparotomy in a child with protracted vomiting. Extensive idiopathic hypertrophy in this patient was most prominent in the muscularis of the duodenum and jejunum.

## CASE REPORT

B. R., a 4-month-old white pseudohermaphrodite who was later found to be a male, was admitted on Sept. 13, 1955, because of vomiting, weight loss, and constipation. The constipation had been present since birth and the vomiting had begun 2 weeks later. Both had become progressively more severe until, at the time of admission, no stool was passed spontaneously and no food was retained.

Prenatal history was not remarkable. Birth weight was 7½ pounds. One older sibling was normal.

Physical examination showed the infant to be poorly nourished, poorly developed, and moderately dehydrated. He weighed 6 pounds, 14 ounces. The uvula was bifid and the second and third toes webbed bilaterally. Heart and lungs were normal. There were marked peristaltic waves across the epigastrium, a palpable pyloric tumor, and "a firm, cordlike structure palpated from the umbilicus to the suprapubic region." Bilateral inguinal masses were thought to be gonads. The clitoris was hypertrophied and the fused labia fleshy and saclike. The urethral (vaginal?) meatus was just below the phallus. No uterus could be palpated on rectal examination.

Results of a routine blood count, urine analysis, and serum electrolyte determinations were not remarkable except for a low potassium level (3.7

mEq. per liter). Excretory urogram and cystogram were normal, and a gastrointestinal series showed gastric retention.

Because 24-hour urinary excretion of 17-ketosteroids (1.4 mg.) and corticoids (0.13 mg.) was considered suggestive of adrenal hyperplasia, cortisone was given before, during, and after operation.

After appropriate intravenous therapy, operation was performed under local anesthesia on Sept. 23, 1955. The pyloric tumor was said to be much larger than it had felt through the abdominal wall, and a Ramstedt pyloromyotomy was carried out. Since no other viscera were mentioned in the operative note, it is assumed that the abdomen was not explored and that the nature of the "cordlike structure" was not determined.

The infant did well postoperatively in spite of the fact that the serum potassium level remained low. The parents refused further investigation and removed the patient from the hospital on Oct. 8, 1955.

The patient was next admitted on July 1, 1957, at the age of 2 years because of vomiting for 6 months, weight loss, and febrile convulsions.

The child was microcephalic and retarded both mentally and physically. The chest was normal. The abdomen was not distended but the "spleen" was felt 2 or 3 cm. below the costal margin.

Blood count and urine examination were normal. Results of blood chemistry studies were within normal range except that the potassium level was 4.1 mEq. per liter. Gastrointestinal series was strongly suggestive of continued pyloric obstruction. Urinary 17-ketosteroids were 1.6 mg. in 24 hours (upper limit of normal for age). Skin biopsy failed to show any female chromatin in the nuclei.

Vomiting was controlled with tincture of belladonna and the patient was discharged on Aug. 7, 1957.

On the third admission, on July 7, 1958, the child had been vomiting for 2 weeks. The infant was found to be moderately dehydrated, but the abdomen was said to be normal. However, a note dated 2 days after admission described a "rubbery, hoselike mass in the upper abdomen that moves easily and is not indentable like feces."

Blood count and urine analysis were again normal. Electrolyte studies showed a chloride level of 62.5 mEq. per liter, sodium level of 127 mEq. per liter, and potassium level of 2.4 mEq. per liter. Lumbar puncture yielded no abnormal findings.

Fluids and cortisone were given intravenously. After remaining semicomatose for several days, the child improved slowly and was discharged on Aug. 13, 1958.

On Sept. 24, 1958, the child, now 3 years, 4 months old, was again admitted because of continued vomiting. The mother, a poor historian, now stated that the patient had never really stopped vomiting after the operation for pyloric stenosis.

Past history on this occasion showed that 1 sibling had been operated upon for pyloric stenosis and that another (aged 2 years) also had microcephaly, retardation, and pseudohermaphrodism. Two other siblings, 1 older and 1 younger than the patient, were normal.

The child was pale, weak, and listless and weighed only 17 pounds. Microcephaly and pseudohermaphrodism were again noted. The abdomen was not distended, but a freely movable abdominal mass measuring 7 or 8 by 2 cm. was easily palpable.

The only abnormality found after blood count, urine examination, and blood chemistry determinations was a potassium level of 3.5 mEq. per liter.

The patient was hydrated and operation undertaken on Sept. 26, 1958. After a smooth induction of anesthesia without respiratory difficulty, cardiac arrest occurred the instant an endotracheal tube was inserted. When the chest was opened, the heart was found to have resumed normal function.

The abdomen was opened through a right paramedian incision and a few thin, fibrous adhesions divided. The palpable abdominal mass was found to be the proximal jejunum. Exploration showed that the pyloric hypertrophy was still present, but that the pyloric obstruction had been definitely relieved by the clearly visible pyloromyotomy. The stomach and first portion of the duodenum were rather thick and edematous, but the remainder of the duodenum and the proximal half of the jejunum were uniformly involved in a process grossly identical to hypertrophic pyloric stenosis. This 30 to 35 cm. segment of bowel was 2 to 3 cm. in diameter, pale, thick and rubbery, and relatively inflexible. The thickening gradually decreased in the distal jejunum, and the ileum and colon appeared normal.

Biopsy of the proximal jejunum showed that most of the thickness of the bowel wall consisted of pale, gristly muscle, and the pathologist reported that the microscopic findings on frozen section were identical to those of hypertrophic pyloric stenosis. The biopsy site was closed in 2 layers, the serosal surface being simply approximated because the inflexible muscularis prevented inversion. A 2-layer gastrojejunostomy was performed, bringing the relatively normal distal jejunum anterior to the colon, and the abdomen was closed in layers.

The patient recovered promptly from anesthesia. Urinary output remained relatively depressed, and an increase in intravenous fluids was accompanied by an increase in drainage from the

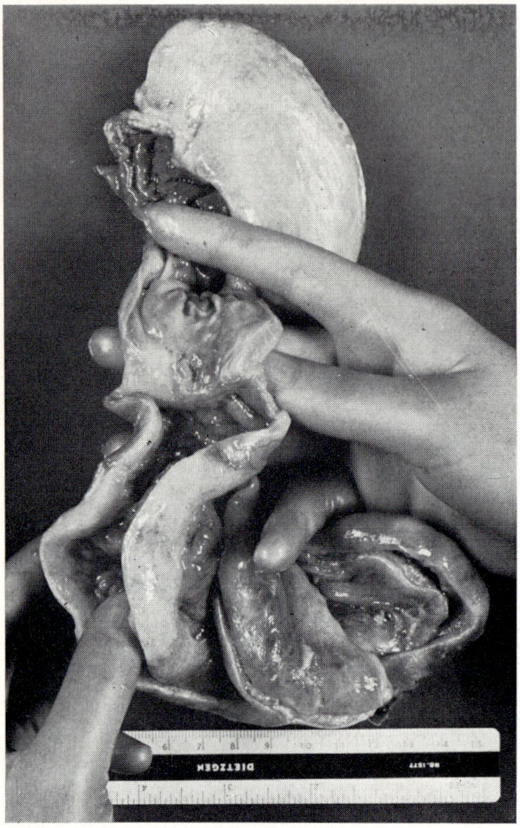

**Fig. 1.** The autopsy specimen shows the thickness of the pylorus and the duodenum.

nasogastric tube. There was no indication that the gastrojejunostomy was functioning. On the fifth postoperative day cortisone was instituted, and urinary volume improved. However, the next day the patient became grossly edematous and a right inguinal hernia was noted. During the night the abdomen became massively distended and roentgenograms showed pneumoperitoneum.

At operation performed on Oct. 3, 1958, with local anesthesia, the biopsy site in the jejunum was seen to be completely disrupted. The jejunal incision was again closed in layers and reinforced with an omental graft, but the child failed to respond after operation and died 4 hours later.

Autopsy findings included microcephaly with gyral abnormalities, stenosis of the aqueduct of Sylvius with mild ventricular dilatation, and hypoplasia of the medullary pyramids; pulmonary edema, pneumonitis, and atelectasis; and pseudohermaphrodism with histologically normal undescended testes and a right indirect inguinal hernia.

Most interesting was the gastrointestinal tract (Fig. 1). There was gross hypertrophy of the muscularis of the esophagus, stomach, pylorus, duodenum, jejunum, and ileum. The process was most marked in the esophagus, the pylorus, the distal three-fourths of the duodenum, and the proximal half of the jejunum (Fig. 2). Serosal surfaces reflected the inflammatory changes of recent peritonitis, and the mucosa of the involved bowel was thicker than normal. Most of the thickness of the bowel wall, however, consisted of massively hypertrophied muscularis, the inner circular layer being most prominently involved (Fig. 3).

There was no intra- or extraluminal obstruction of any portion of the gastrointestinal tract, nor was there any dilatation. The gastroenterostomy was healed and anatomically patent. The entire mesentery appeared normal. An incidental finding was a diverticulum of the second portion of the duodenum extending into the head of the pancreas.

Microscopic examination of the gastrointestinal tract showed small aggregations of lymphocytes in the wall of the esophagus, severe esophagitis attributed to the indwelling nasogastric tube, and acute peritonitis of the abdominal viscera. There was moderate hypertrophy of the muscular wall of the stomach, first portion of the duodenum, and proximal ileum, and massive hypertrophy of the muscularis of the esophagus, pylorus, distal duodenum, and proximal jejunum. In all involved bowel, the circular muscle was approximately twice as thick as the longitudinal. The mucosa and muscularis mucosae of the involved bowel were also thicker than normal. Myenteric plexuses and ganglion cells were large, easily identified, and seemed more prominent than normal.

**Comment.** Two questions immediately arise. Were (1) the "cordlike structure" present at the age of 4 months, (2) the "spleen" palpated at the age of 2 years, and (3) the "rubbery, hoselike mass" found at the age of 3 years all the same mass that was found at operation? Would that the first surgeon had explored the abdomen when he performed the pyloromyotomy!

**Table I.** *Normal and hypertrophied segments of the gastrointestinal tract (mm.)*

| | *Age 3⅓ yr.* | | *Age 11 yr.* | |
|---|---|---|---|---|
| *Segment* | *Normal** | *Patient B. R.* | *Normal* | *Guthrie's patient* |
| Esophagus | 1.0 | 2.5 | 2.0 | 8.0 |
| Stomach | 1.3 | 2.25 | — | — |
| Pylorus | 1.7 | 6.0 | 3.0 | 10.0 |
| Duodenum (first part) | 0.28 | 2.5 | — | — |
| Duodenum (distal) | 0.25 | 5.25 | 2.0 | 5.0 |
| Jejunum | 0.25 | 5.0 | 2.0 | 5.0 |
| Ileum | 0.25 | 1.0 | 2.0 | 3.0 |

*The "normal" child, who had died of burns, was exactly the same age as Patient B. R. but weighed twice as much.

The second question concerns the etiology of the vomiting. Was it due to congenital defects of the central nervous system or to muscular hypertrophy of the duodenum and jejunum? It was determined at operation (and confirmed at autopsy) that the pyloromyotomy had relieved the pyloric obstruction. It is tempting to assume that the muscular hypertrophy of the duodenum and jejunum had continued to cause obstruction.

## REVIEW OF THE LITERATURE

Review of the literature yielded only 2 cases of idiopathic muscular hypertrophy of the gastrointestinal tract in children. Pritchart and Hiller[13] reported simply that a 3-month-old male who died of hypostatic pneumonia was found to have muscular hypertrophy of the esophagus, pylorus, and ileocecal sphincter. A case reported by Guthrie,[8] however, is of particular interest because it was remarkably similar to ours.

Guthrie's patient was an 11-year-old girl who was admitted after a brief illness consisting of vomiting, diarrhea, and abdominal pain followed by a convulsion. The parents, questioned later, denied any history of gastrointestinal symptoms other than an occasional "bilious attack." Death shortly after admission was found at autopsy to have been due to acute nephritis.

> The lower two-thirds [of the esophagus] where the muscle is non-striated had assumed the form of thick-walled tube of a rubber-like consistency as a result of muscular hypertrophy of the wall, fairly uniform throughout although tending to increase slightly towards the lower end, and ceasing abruptly at the cardia where there was no sign of obstruction. The gullet was not dilated, the condition being one of pure hypertrophy.
>
> The distended stomach had a rather thin wall, except in the pyloric canal which showed massive muscular hypertrophy. The caliber of the duodenum and jejunum was greatly increased and the wall so thick that on palpation it felt like heavy rubber tubing. The small bowel gradually decreased in size from above down and reached normal dimensions in the terminal ileum. There was no abnormality of the ileo-caecal valve or of the colon.

The mucosa in the hypertrophied area was "considerably thickened with unusually prominent rugae." Histologic examination showed massive hypertrophy of the circular muscle and moderate hypertrophy of the

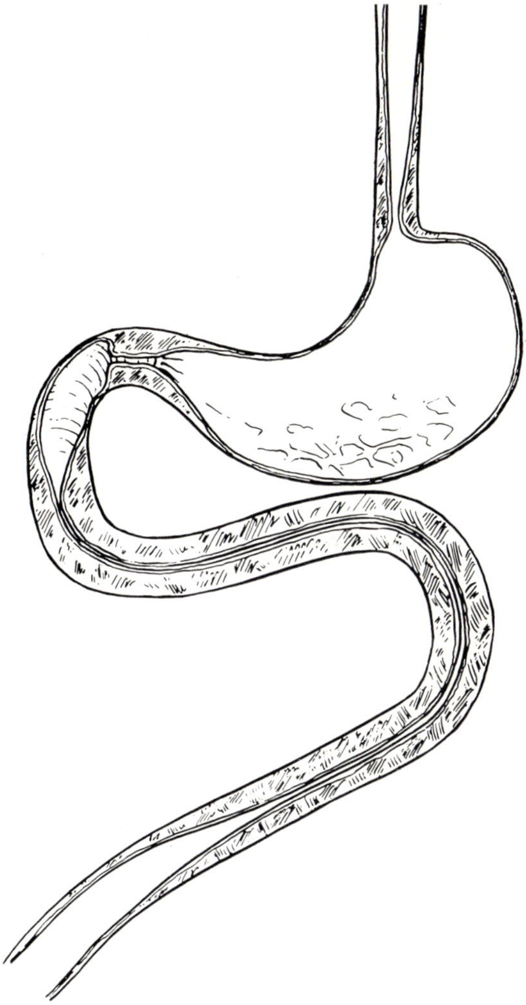

**Fig. 2.** Diagram of the upper gastrointestinal tract (in longitudinal section) shows the relative thickness of the muscular wall of the involved bowel.

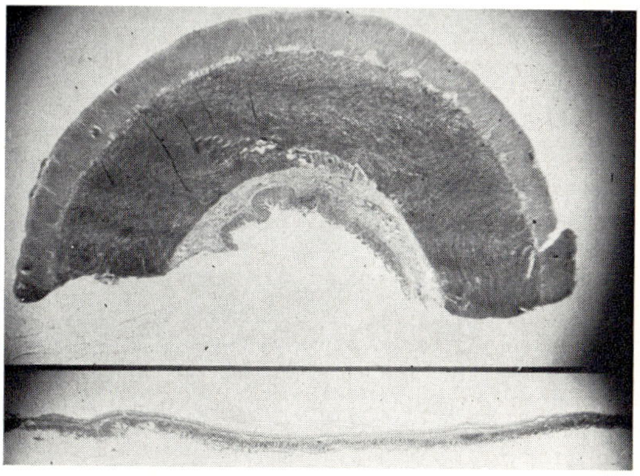

**Fig. 3.** Photomicrograph shows the duodenum of 2 patients 3⅓ years old, 1 normal and 1 with idiopathic muscular hypertrophy.

**Table II.** *Collected series of 23 cases of idiopathic muscular hypertrophy*

| *Case* | *Author and year* | *Age (yr.)* | *Sex* | *Location* | *Symptoms* |
|---|---|---|---|---|---|
| 1 | Reher, 1885 | 60 | M | Esophagus | Yes |
| 2 | Pitt, 1888 | 68 | F | Esophagus | ? |
| 3 | Rolleston, 1899 | 59 | M | Esophagus | No |
| 4 | Elliesen, 1903 | 39 | M | Esophagus | "Careful" |
| 5 | Ehlers, 1907 | 56 | M | Esophagus, pylorus | No |
| 6 | Mollison, 1919 | 62 | ? | Esophagus | ? |
| 7 | Pritchart, 1920 | 3 mo. | M | Esophagus, pylorus, ileocecal sphincter | ? |
| 8 | Rake, 1926 | 67 | M | Esophagus | No |
| 9 | von Brücke, 1928 | 67 | M | Esophagus | Yes |
| 10 | | 63 | M | Esophagus | No |
| 11 | Goedel, 1929 | 39 | M | Esophagus | No |
| 12 | Wood, 1932 | 69 | M | Esophagus | No |
| 13 | Rössle, 1935 | 67 | M | Pylorus, jejunum | ? |
| 14 | | 27 | F | Antrum, ileum | Yes |
| 15 | | ? | M | Esophagus, pylorus | ? |
| 16 | | 57 | M | Esophagus | ? |
| 17 | Helmke, 1939 | 41 | M | Esophagus | No |
| 18 | | 57 | M | Esophagus | No |
| 19 | | 64 | M | Esophagus | No |
| 20 | | 59 | M | Esophagus, pylorus | No |
| 21 | Guthrie, 1945 | 11 | F | Esophagus, pylorus, duodenum, jejunum | No |
| 22 | Schroeder, 1949 | 74 | M | Stomach | Yes |
| 23 | Spencer, 1961 | 3 | M | Esophagus, pylorus, duodenum, jejunum | Yes |

*Autopsy findings included pyelonephritis and nephrosclerosis, pulmonary emphysema and pneumonia, rheumatic valvular disease

longitudinal muscle. The walls contained small collections of leukocytes but there was no trace of chronic inflammatory change. "The myenteric nerve plexuses with their ganglion cells remained in a state of good preservation, free from atrophy or fibrosis."

This case is almost identical to ours. The involvement in both was most marked in the esophagus, pylorus, distal duodenum, and proximal jejunum, and only moderate in the first portion of the duodenum and distal small bowel (Table I).

## IDIOPATHIC MUSCULAR HYPERTROPHY IN ADULTS

In contrast to the extensive lesions in children, muscular hypertrophy of the gastrointestinal tract in the adult is usually limited to the esophagus of elderly men. The conditions are apparently related, however, as the gross and microscopic appearances are similar in the two age groups.

Baillie,[2] in 1799, included an example of thickening of the esophagus in a series of engravings, but according to Albers[1] the tumefaction was in the submucosa, and "the muscle layer itself is atrophic." Förster,[6] Niemeyer,[11] and Zenker and Ziemssen[22] postulated that this condition might occur and Birch-Hirschfeld[3] seems to have described the lesion, but none of these authors cites a specific case.

The earliest documented record of idiopathic muscular hypertrophy (in the esophagus) was reported in 1885 by Reher[15] (Table II). Including that case, 17 instances of esophageal involvement in adult patients have been recorded to date. In 3 of these, the pylorus also showed hypertrophied muscularis. In 3 additional reports, hypertrophy

| *Associated pathologic process* | *Cardiac enlargement* | *Renal disease* | *Remarks* |
|---|---|---|---|
| — | No | No | Died, carcinoma of rectum |
| — | Yes | Yes | Cerebral hemorrhage |
| Pylorus small, no thickening of wall | Yes | No | Fracture of ribs, bronchitis, erysipelas |
| — | No | No | Tuberculous meningitis |
| — | Yes | Yes | Emphysema, pneumonia, dilatation of stomach |
| Sessile papillomas in esophageal mucosa | Yes | Yes | — |
| "Pea-sized" polyp in cardia | ? | ? | Hypostatic pneumonia |
| Inflammation of ganglia and nerves | No | No | ? Carcinoma of tongue, pneumonitis, heart atrophied |
| Small myoma | No | No | Died after operation of pneumonia |
| Small myoma | Yes | No | Hemiplegia |
| — | ? | ? | — |
| — | No | No | Acute colitis, fatty liver, heart ¾ normal size |
| Polypoid gastritis and duodenitis | ? | Yes | — |
| Tuberculosis of lung, intestine, peritoneum | No | No | Adhesions |
| — | ? | ? | — |
| — | ? | ? | Hernias and adhesions |
| Small myoma | Yes | Yes | — |
| Small myoma | Yes | No | Emphysema |
| Myomas | Yes | No | — |
| Myomas | Yes | No | — |
| — | No | Yes | — |
| Peach pit in stomach | ? | ? | Died 6 years later* |
| — | No | No | Microcephaly, pseudohermaphrodism |

myocardial infarction, and aneurysm of ascending aorta. No additional hypertrophy of the gastrointestinal tract was found.[19]

of the gastric or intestinal musculature was found without involvement of the esophagus.

Idiopathic muscular hypertrophy occurs most often in the esophagus of elderly white men. Only 2 cases have been reported in women. Ages of the patients ranged from 27 to 74, and 15 of the 18 whose ages were stated were over 56 years (Table II).

As far as can be determined, this condition has not been seen in a Negro. It is assumed, perhaps erroneously, that all patients from England and Germany were white. Of the 2 patients from the United States, Schroeder said his was white, and Wood described his as "an American grocer."

## SYMPTOMS

In view of the extent of involvement found at autopsy, it is amazing that idiopathic muscular hypertrophy is usually an asymptomatic lesion. In most patients it was stated specifically that there was no history of dysphagia or gastrointestinal disturbance, but in a few, some symptoms were described.

The patient with esophageal hypertrophy reported by Reher died with carcinoma of the rectum but had complained of a feeling of obstruction in the esophagus in addition to constipation. Elliesen's[5] patient with esophageal involvement had been "careful" with his food since the age of 15, but his wife did not know why. In von Brücke's[20] first case, difficulty in swallowing had been diagnosed fluoroscopically as "spasm," but an operation was necessary 9 years later because of persistent and increasing dysphagia. Operative findings and procedure were not recorded, but the patient died after the operation and at autopsy was found to have hypertrophy in the esophageal muscularis.

Rössle's[17] female patient had had abdominal "colic," but this is not surprising in the light of autopsy findings of tuberculous enteritis and peritonitis with adhesions. It is possible that the hypertrophy of the ileum in this patient was secondary to chronic partial obstruction (dilatation was not mentioned), but this would hardly explain the associated hypertrophy of the muscularis of the antrum. One patient who did have symptoms was the one described by Schroeder,[18] but the obstruction was due to a peach pit impacted above the muscular hypertrophy in the midportion of the stomach; similar symptoms 6 years previously had subsided when the patient was restricted to a bland diet.

## PATHOLOGY

In the typical case, idiopathic muscular hypertrophy is an unexpected, unexplained finding at autopsy. By definition, all hypertrophy associated with proximal dilatation or distal obstruction is excluded from this report.

Of the 23 patients in this series, 3 (all adults) had involvement of the stomach, of the pylorus and jejunum, and of the antrum and ileum, and 20 had hypertrophy in the esophagus. In 14 adults the esophagus alone was involved, and in 3 others, esophagus and pylorus. All of the 3 children had hypertrophy of the esophageal and pyloric muscularis, but one also had involvement of the ileocecal sphincter and the other 2 had additional involvement of the duodenum and jejunum.

In instances in which a detailed description of the lesion was reported, the segment of muscular hypertrophy showed fusiform involvement, with a gradual onset and termination. In cases of esophageal involvement in which the hypertrophy continued to the cardia, the termination was more abrupt than in those in which the marked hypertrophy ended a few centimeters above the cardia.

The circular muscle was more markedly hypertrophied than the longitudinal. Minimal increase in the connective tissue between muscle bundles in some cases and small groups of lymphocytes in others were not interpreted as indicative of significant inflammatory reaction. Autonomic ganglia were reported as entirely normal except in Rake's[14] patient with marked inflammatory infiltration of the ganglion cells and nerves.

Associated lesions of the involved segment were occasionally seen. One of Rössle's[17] patients, with hypertrophy of the pyloric and jejunal musculature, had polypoid gastritis and duodenitis, and another, a female with involvement of the antrum and ileum, also had tuberculous peritonitis and enteritis.

Ehlers[4] noted that his patient had a small diverticulum of mucosa into the muscle of the esophagus, but gives the impression that this was due to overgrowth of the muscularis and was not a true diverticulum. Mollison[10] reported his patient to have small sessile papillomas of the esophageal mucosa associated with hypertrophy of the muscle, but these lesions apparently did not represent cause and effect because there was no proximal dilatation. Pritchart's[13] 3-month-old patient had a "pea-sized" polyp at the cardia in addition to hypertrophy of the esophagus, pylorus, and ileocecal sphincter.

Each of von Brücke's[20] 2 patients had a myoma of the esophagus in association with muscularis hypertrophy, and the occurrence of 1 to many myomas of the esophagus of all 4 of Helmke's[9] patients caused him to consider the possibility that muscular hypertrophy was a form of myomatous hyperplasia.

## ETIOLOGY

The etiology of "idiopathic" muscular hypertrophy is unknown, but various factors have been considered. A congenital predisposition seems unlikely in view of the predominance of the lesion in elderly patients. In the earlier literature the role of the adrenal gland was discussed.[13]

Wood,[21] among others, considered the possibility that this lesion in the esophagus might represent compensated achalasia. He stated, "Hypertrophy occurs as long as compensation is maintained, then dilatation.

This is analogous to what happens with the heart in hypertension, and with the urinary bladder in obstruction, and in fact, is true of any tubular-muscular organ." However, compensated achalasia should be found in young patients since the decompensation would presumably occur with increasing age, yet muscular hypertrophy is usually found in elderly patients.

Helmke[9] attributed the hypertrophy of the esophageal musculature to smooth muscle spasm resulting from the irritation of the contracting heart, because all of his patients had cardiac hypertrophy and/or dilatation. His interesting study of the dry weight of the esophageal muscle in patients with normal and enlarged hearts lends some support to his theory, as cardiac enlargement was found to be associated with increased weight of the esophageal muscle. However, some patients with muscular hypertrophy of the esophagus were reported to have a small heart, and involvement of other portions of the gastrointestinal tract could hardly be explained on the basis of cardiac disease.

Lesions in the heart (in 9 patients), kidneys (in 7), and lungs (in 6) probably represented the unrelated cause of death in patients with asymptomatic muscular hypertrophy.

## DIAGNOSIS AND TREATMENT

Roentgenographic features of muscular hypertrophy of the gastrointestinal tract are unknown. Von Brücke's first patient was diagnosed fluoroscopically as having "spasm" of the esophagus 9 years before the lesion was found at autopsy, and roentgenologic examination of Schroeder's patient showed an hourglass stomach presumed to be due to carcinoma. The child in the present report had gastrointestinal series at 4 months and at 2 years of age, but on neither occasion did the radiologist describe any abnormality of the esophagus or upper small bowel, nor can any obstruction in these areas be recognized with certainty on any of the films. However, the marked narrowing of the lumen, inflexibility of the wall, and thickening of the mucosa seen at postmortem examination might be recognized fluoroscopically if symptoms direct the attention of the radiologist to the involved segment.

It would be difficult to recommend treatment for a condition which is usually an incidental finding at autopsy. However, as operation was performed on 3 patients in this series, it is possible that on rare occasions the surgeon will be called upon to make a decision regarding therapy. Isolated lesions of the stomach or short segments of involved intestine will probably be resected, for diagnosis if not for treatment. In extensive involvement, as in Guthrie's patient and the one in the present report, a short circuit procedure may be performed, but it is not certain that this will be indicated if the gastrointestinal series fails to show obstruction. Biopsy incisions should be closed with care and reinforced with an omental graft, as the inflexible muscularis will prevent inversion of the bowel wall.

## SUMMARY

The case is reported of a 3-year-old child with idiopathic muscular hypertrophy of the esophagus, stomach, pylorus, duodenum, jejunum, and ileum, with particularly massive hypertrophy of the esophagus, pylorus, distal duodenum, and proximal jejunum. Vomiting was the principal symptom, and the hypertrophied bowel was palpable through the abdominal wall. There have been 2 previous reports of this condition in children. There have been 20 reports of a similar condition in adults, usually limited to the esophagus. The etiology is unknown. In adults the condition appears to have been almost asymptomatic.

### REFERENCES

1. Albers: Erläuterungen zu dem Atlasse der pathologischen Anatomie. II. Abteilung, Bonn, 1839.
2. Baillie, M.: Series of engravings, accompanied with explanations, to illustrate the morbid anatomy of the human body, fasc. 1, 1799.
3. Birch-Hirschfeld, F. V.: Lehrubuch der pathologischen Anatomie, Leipzig, 1887, F. C. W. Vogel.
4. Ehlers, H. W. E.: Ein Fall von wahrscheinlich kongenitaler Hypertrophie der Ösoph-

agusmuskulatur bei gleichzeitig bestehender kongenitaler hypertrophischer Pylorusstenose, Virchows Arch. path. Anat. **189:** 512, 1907.
5. Elliesen: Über idiopathische Hypertrophie der Oesophagusmuskulatur, Virchows Arch. path. Anat. **172:** 501, 1903.
6. Förster, A. J. T.: Handbuch der speziellen pathologischen Anatomie, Leipzig, 1863, Leopold Voss.
7. Goedel, A.: Idiopathische diffuse Oesophagushypertrophie, Wien. med. Wchnschr. **79:** 967, 1929.
8. Guthrie, Katherine J.: Idiopathic muscular hypertrophy of oesophagus, pylorus, duodenum, and jejunum in a young girl, Arch. Dis. Child. **20:** 176, 1945.
9. Helmke, K.: Über Oesophagushypertrophie, Virchows Arch. path. Anat. **304:** 79, 1939.
10. Mollison: Case presentation, Proc. Roy. Soc. Med. **12:** 73, 1919.
11. Niemeyer, F.: Lehrbuch der speziellen Pathologie und Therapie, Berlin, 1865, A. Hirschwald.
12. Pitt, G. N.: Hypertrophy of the circular muscular coat of the esophagus associated with an hypertrophied heart, Tr. Path. Soc. Lond. **39:** 107, 1888.
13. Pritchart, Eric, and Hillier, W. T.: Specimens of a case of hypertrophic pyloric stenosis with associated hypertrophies, Proc. Roy. Soc. Med. **13:** 33, 1920.
14. Rake, G. W.: A case of annular hypertrophy of the oesophagus: achalasia of the cardia without oesophageal dilatation, Guy's Hosp. Rep. **76:** 145, 1926.
15. Reher, H.: Beiträge zur Casuistik der Oesophaguserkrankungen, Deutsches Arch. klin. Med. **36:** 454, 1885.
16. Rolleston, H. D.: Idiopathic hypertrophy of the oesophagus, Tr. Path. Soc. Lond. **1:** 69, 1899.
17. Rössle, R.: Die Pylorushypertrophie des Erwachsenen, Schweiz. med. Wchnschr. **65:** 174, 1935.
18. Schroeder, C. M.: Hourglass stomach caused by annular muscular hypertrophy: report of a case, Ann. Surg. **130:** 1085, 1949.
19. Schroeder, C. M.: Personal communication.
20. von Brücke, H.: Über idiopathische Hypertrophie der Spieseröhre, Virchows Arch. path. Anat. **270:** 880, 1928.
21. Wood, D. A.: Primary idiopathic muscular hypertrophy of the esophagus with narrowing of the lumen, Arch. Path. **14:** 766, 1932.
22. Zenker, F. A., and Ziemssen, H.: Handbuch der speziellen Pathologie und Therapie, Leipzig, 1878, F. C. W. Vogel.

# Hydronephrosis associated with aberrant renal vessels in infants and children

N. O. ERICSSON, M.D.
ULF RUDHE, M.D.
ALEX LIVADITIS, M.D.
STOCKHOLM, SWEDEN
*From the Surgical Department of the Pediatric Clinic, Karolinska Sjukhuset*

The association of aberrant renal vessels with hydronephrosis was first described by Boogard[3] in 1857. There is much controversy concerning the exact role played by the aberrant renal vessels in the production of hydronephrosis. There is also a lack of unanimity in regard to the proper surgical management of this condition. Many authors consider the presence of aberrant renal vessels to have a secondary causative significance. There are, however, cases in which correction of the vascular anomaly alone results in complete cure or marked improvement of the condition. In these cases, it would be reasonable to accept the primary etiologic importance of the aberrant renal vessels. This is true especially for patients in the pediatric age group, in whom secondary obstructive lesions are less likely to develop.

Urinary obstruction may be produced either by direct vascular compression of the ureter[5, 16, 17] or by interference with its peristaltic activity.[7, 14] Some authors suggest that aberrant renal vessels act only as a subsidiary factor aggravating the hydronephrosis initiated by other lesions, such as ureteropelvic fixation or ureteral stricture.

The frequency of supernumerary renal vessels is estimated to be 26 per cent. The incidence of aberrant renal vessels in patients with hydronephrosis varies from 4 to 90 per cent (Table I). The variety of criteria used in the classification of hydronephrosis on an etiologic basis probably accounts for this discrepancy.

Hydronephrosis may be asymptomatic; however, hydronephrosis of vascular origin often is associated with painful acute episodes. Aortography may provide specific diagnostic information. One form of treatment is division of the aberrant renal vessels. This, however, may lead to necrosis of a major renal segment if the vessel is sizeable. For this reason, vessels preferably should not be divided, but rather transposed as recommended by Hellstrom.[8, 9]

Our observations are derived from a study of 12 patients with vascular hydronephrosis seen at Karolinska Sjukhuset within a 7-year period (1952 to 1959).

## MATERIAL

Among 70 children with hydronephrosis operated upon between the years 1952 and 1959, 12 had aberrant renal vessels. These were of such size and in such close relation to the ureter that they undoubtedly were the definite cause of obstruction. Only large vessels which cross the ureter transversely and anteriorly and producing evident compression were considered. Smaller aberrant renal vessels of horizontal or vertical course are not considered in this study. With these criteria, the incidence of vascular hydronephrosis was 17 per cent (Table I). The age at onset of symptoms was from 1 to 15 years. The left side was involved in 8 patients and the right in 3. Bilateral aberrant renal vessels

Received for publication March 9, 1961.

**Table I.** *Incidence of hydronephrosis associated with aberrant renal vessels*

| *Author* | *%* |
|---|---|
| Campbell[4] | 4 |
| Lowsley and Kirwin[11] | 11 |
| Helstrom[8] | 24 |
| Soley[15] | 30 |
| Nixon[12] | 32 |
| Henline[10] | 41 |
| White and Wyatt[17] | 90 |
| Authors | 17 |

**Table II.** *Treatment and results in 12 cases of hydronephrosis due to aberrant renal vessels*

| *No. of cases* | *Surgical procedure* | *Results* |
|---|---|---|
| 4 | Transposition of aberrant renal vessels | All free of symptoms, all free of infection, all regression of dilatation |
| 5 | Transposition of aberrant renal vessels plus resection of the renal pelvis | All free of symptoms, 4 free of infection, 4 regression of dilatation |
| 3 | Primary nephrectomy | All free of symptoms, all free of infection |

were found in 1 case. Periodic pain was the most common clinical feature in this series. This symptom proved to be helpful in the differentiation of the nature of obstruction preoperatively. Pyuria was noted in 3 cases. The hydronephrosis was asymptomatic in 2 additional cases and the condition was discovered during an emergency operation for a flank injury with rupture of the kidney. Intravenous pyelograms were obtained in all cases. The ureteropelvic junction could not be clearly demonstrated in any of these studies. Since a short defect at the upper part of the ureter is common in other types of hydronephrosis, this finding was not considered pathognomonic of vascular obstruction. Retrograde pyelography was not used because of the danger of infection. The diagnosis was established at operation in each case. All patients showed a marked degree of hydronephrosis (Figs. 1 and 2). Surgical judgment was always conservative, in an effort to preserve the kidney and its vascular supply intact. Division of the aberrant renal vessels was avoided. They were merely displaced and fixed at a higher level on the renal pelvis. In this way, the ureteropelvic junction was relieved from the vascular compression. The fixation was performed with interrupted catgut stitches. The adventitia of the vessel was sutured to the superficial layer of the renal pelvis.

In 4 cases, only transposition of the aberrant renal vessels was performed. In 5 cases, the transposition was combined with resection of the renal pelvis. In 3 cases, the renal parenchyma was so badly destroyed that nephrectomy was indicated. The surgical treatment and results are shown in Table II. Postoperatively, all patients are asymptomatic. However, 1 patient has persisting asymptomatic urinary tract infection as evidenced by pyuria and bacilluria. All patients subjected solely to transposition of the aberrant renal vessels show satisfactory regression of hydronephrosis (Figs. 1 and 2). The follow-up time varies from 2 months to 3 years.

## DISCUSSION

Pediatric patients seem most suitable for the study of the primary cause of hydronephrosis. During the relatively short period of illness, secondary changes have less chance to develop and to complicate the clinical picture. The vascular hydronephrosis may be associated with other obstructive factors, the most common being ureteral fixation of the renal pelvis, kinking of the ureter by adhesions, and ureteropelvic stenosis. Adhesions can be congenital in origin[18] or secondary to hydronephrosis with or without infection. There is no unanimity of opinion concerning the significance of adhesions in the causation of hydronephrosis. It is a common experience that mere lysis of these adhesions has not brought about improvement as would be expected if these were the direct cause of obstruction. Actual strictures at the ureteropelvic junction are less often associated with aberrant renal vessels.[12] Such strictures may appear secondary to the vascular compression of the ureter. It is therefore advisable in all patients with aberrant renal vessels to open the pelvis and calibrate the pelvic outlet. If a stricture is found, it should be corrected at the same time.

A prerequisitive for regression of hydronephrosis after surgical relief of the obstruction is the maintenance of the elasticity and contractility of the renal pelvis. For this reason, it is advisable to correct the obstruction early before secondary fibrotic changes develop. In hydronephrosis of undetermined origin, the decision in favor of conservative or surgical treatment is not always easy. In doubtful cases and particularly when aberrant renal vessels or other type of ureteropelvic obstruction is suspected, early operation is indicated. Concerning operative technique, we favor the transposition of the aberrant renal vessels as advocated by Hellstrom.[8, 9] Although division of the aberrant renal vessels may not have clinical sequelae,[1] necrosis of the renal parenchyma can result.[6, 13] This is not surprising since recent studies have demonstrated that in 51 per cent of patients, the lower pole vessels supply the 2 lower pyramids, but in 11 per cent they supply 5 or 6 pyramids corresponding to one-fourth to one-half of the kidney substance.[2]

We have had no personal experience with the Hamilton-Stewart operation; this requires more complicated operative steps than a simple transposition. In cases in which ureteropelvic resection is performed, the aberrant renal vessels can be displaced behind the reconstructed junction.

The results of this series seem to justify our opinion regarding the true causative significance of the aberrant renal vessels. Among 100 adult patients with hydronephrosis, Hellstrom and associates[9] found 24 in which aberrant renal vessels were considered the primary or secondary cause of obstruction. Four of them were operated upon with only transposition of the aberrant renal vessels. The results were good in 2. The remaining 2 were recently operated upon. Nixon[12] made a comprehensive analysis of 78 cases of hydronephrosis in children. Twenty-five had obstruction of vascular origin, although 16 of them presented some additional anomaly in the form of adhesions with ureteropelvic fixation or kinking of the upper part of the ureter. Nixon considers vascular obstruction a complication of the hydronephrosis rather than its cause. In his series, operations were successful in 89 per cent of the cases of vascular obstruction. For ureteropelvic stricture, they were successful in 60 per cent, and for ureteropelvic fixation, in only 33 per cent. A possible explanation of this difference might be the earlier detection of the vascular hydro-

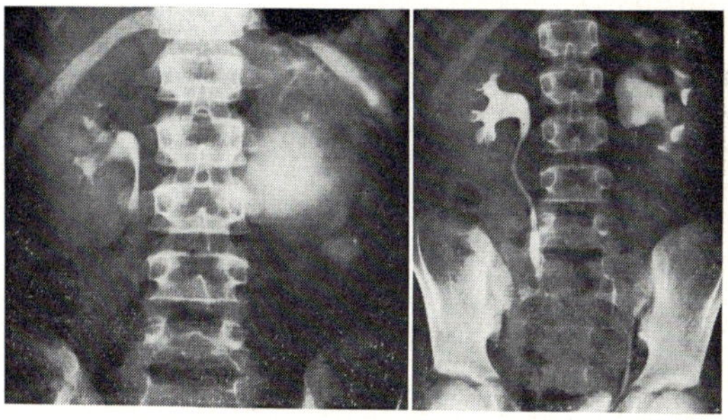

*A* *B*

**Fig. 1.** Boy, 10 years of age. There had been pain in the left flank for some years. *A,* Preoperative marked hydronephrosis on left side, obstructed outflow from renal pelvis. Operation consisted of only transposition of aberrant vessel. *B,* Two months after operation there was slight dilatation of pelvis and no obstruction of outflow.

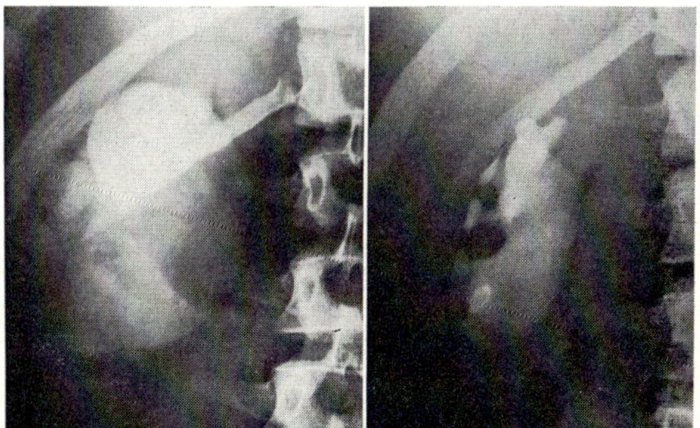

*A* *B*

**Fig. 2.** Boy, 15 years of age. There had been 1 year of severe pain in the right flank and 2 weeks of urinary tract infection with fever. *A,* marked hydronephrosis on right side and obstructed outflow from renal pelvis. Operation consisted of only transposition of aberrant vessel. *B,* 6 months after operation there is regression of hydronephrosis and no obstruction of outflow.

nephrosis. In our experience, however, there is nothing to indicate that vascular hydronephrosis is recognized earlier than other types of ureteropelvic obstruction. The fact that the results with vascular obstruction, even when combined with adhesions, are better than results with adhesions only may indicate the etiologic importance of the vessel.

## SUMMARY

1. Twelve cases of hydronephrosis in children caused by aberrant renal vessels are presented. Five of the patients were male and 7 female; their ages varied from 1 to 15 years. The right side was involved in 3 cases, the left in 8 cases, and there was bilateral involvement in 1.

2. In 9 patients, transposition of the aberrant renal vessels, alone or combined with resection of the renal pelvis, was performed. In 3 additional patients, nephrectomy was indicated.

3. Good function and marked regression of the anatomic changes were observed.

4. Early operation before the establishment of irreversible kidney damage is recommended.

5. Transposition of the aberrant renal vessels is considered the operation of choice.

### REFERENCES

1. Bergendahl, S.: Zur Frage der Hydronephrose bei Nierengefasservarianten unter besonderer Berucksichtigung ihrer Behandlung durch Gefassresektion, Acta chir. scandinav., suppl. 54, 1936.
2. Boijsen, E.: Angiographic studies of the anatomy of single and multiple renal arteries, Acta radiol., suppl. 183, 1959.
3. Boogard, J. A.: Wearneming eener Uitzetting van Hetregter Nierhekken met. Doodelijken Afloop, Nederl. tijdschr. geneesk. **1:** 145, 1857.
4. Campbell, M. F.: Vascular obstruction of the ureter in children, J. Urol. **65:** 734, 1951.
5. Cecil, A. B.: Aberrant renal vessels a cause of kidney disease, S. Clin. North America **10:** 983, 1930.
6. Deming, C. L.: Ureteropelvic obstruction due to extrinsic lesions of the ureter as a clinical entity and its treatment, J. Urol. **50:** 420, 1943.
7. Fey, M.: Role prepondérant des artères anormales dans la pathogénie des hydronéphroses, Bull. mém. Soc. nat. chir. **54:** 383, 1928.
8. Hellstrom, J.: A contribution to the knowledge of the relation of abnormally running vessels to hydronephrosis and an investigation of the arterial condition in 50 kidneys, Acta chir. scandinav. **61:** 289, 1927.
9. Hellstrom, J., Giertz, G., and Lindblom, K.: Pathogenesis and treatment of hydronephrosis, VIII Congress of International Urological Society, Barcelona, 1949, p. 163.
10. Henline, R. B.: The case and treatment of non-calculous ureteropelvic obstructions, J. Urol. **34:** 584, 1935.
11. Lowsley, O. S., and Kirwin, T. J.: Clinical urology, Baltimore, 1944, The Williams & Wilkins Co.
12. Nixon, H. H.: Hydronephrosis in children. A clinical study of seventy-eight cases with special reference to the role of aberrant renal vessels and the results of conservative operations, Brit. J. Surg. **60:** 601, 1953.
13. O'Conner, V. J.: Conservative surgery of hydronephrosis, J. Urol. **46:** 1051, 1942.
14. Quinby, W. C.: Factors influencing the operative procedure in hydronephrosis, J. A. M. A. **93:** 1709, 1929.
15. Soley, P. J.: Ureteropelvic obstruction in children. Incidence and etiology, J. Urol. **55:** 46, 1946.
16. Walters, W.: Resection of the renal pelvis for hydronephrosis, its complication and results, Surg. Gynec. & Obst. **51:** 811, 1930.
17. White, R. R., and Wyatt, G. M.: Surgical importance of the aberrant renal vessel in infants and children, Am. J. Surg. **58:** 48, 1942.
18. Ostling, K.: The genesis of hydronephrosis, Acta chir. scandinav., suppl. 72, 1942.

# The management of familial gastrointestinal polyposis involving stomach and colon

SCOTT J. BOLEY, M.D.
WILLIAM M. P. McKINNON, M.D.
VINCENT F. MARZULLI, M.D.
BROOKLYN, N. Y.
*From the Department of Surgery, Queens Hospital Center, and the Pediatric Surgical Service, Jewish Hospital of Brooklyn*

Familial polyposis may occur in any or all segments of the gastrointestinal tract.[23] When the entire tract is involved it is impossible to eradicate the disease and therapy is limited to the complications, such as intussusception or hemorrhage, as they occur. With polyposis of the large bowel alone, complete extirpation is possible and the well-recognized high incidence of carcinoma in this condition has made total colectomy with ileostomy, or subtotal colectomy with ileoproctostomy, the accepted therapy. Polyposis involving the entire stomach would necessitate total gastrectomy to eliminate the disease. The complications and sequelae of this operation are generally considered as arguments against its use in the absence of a malignancy. Fortunately, total excision by limited gastric resection is possible in over one-half of the cases of gastric polyposis because of the localized distribution of the disease.[12, 15, 21, 26]

Combined polyposis of the colon and stomach falls somewhere between the other types and poses a most difficult therapeutic problem. While complete extirpation is possible, it may leave the individual with a "cure worse than the disease." Restricting intervention to treatment of complications, on the other hand, exposes the patient to the risk of development of malignancies. This is clearly established in colonic polyposis and less certainly in gastric polyposis. Thus, the place of operation in the treatment of this form of the disease cannot be stated with assurance. In the cases to be reported, the problem was further complicated by the diagnosis of the disease in 2 sisters at 11 and 16 years of age.

In deciding upon the course of treatment for a child with established polyposis of both the colon and stomach, we attempted to answer 4 pertinent questions.

**Is any operation indicated?** The almost certain development of carcinoma in familial polyposis of the colon is an absolute indication for colectomy if at all feasible. We believe that the presence of polyposis in the large and small bowel contraindicates extirpative operation. However, if it can be established that the small bowel is completely free of polyps, then colectomy at the least can be performed without the fear of subsequent crippling loss of small bowel by resection necessitated by intussusception, hemorrhage, or malignant degeneration. The presence of concomitant gastric polyposis should not influence the decision for colectomy, and may be an indication for partial gastrectomy.

**At what age should operation be performed?** The prevention of the development of carcinoma of the colon is the primary indication for operation. This complication has been described in children 12 to 15 years of age[11, 18, 27] and thus temporization is not justified in relation to colectomy.[19] The effects of colectomy on nutrition and growth have not been adequately studied but in many instances (as in Case 1) weight gain

Received for publication April 5, 1961.

and development have improved after resection of the involved intestine.[10] Since most pediatric surgeons[7, 16, 22, 25] perform some sort of ileoproctostomy rather than total colectomy and ileostomy, the psychological damage of the latter procedure is not a consideration and is not a reason for delaying operation.

The question as to when any attack should be made on the gastric lesions is more difficult to answer because the dangers inherent in their presence are not firmly established. Normal development of children after partial gastrectomy and, in 1 case, total gastrectomy[9] is well documented,[4, 24, 27] but the effect of combined gastric and colon resections in children has never been assessed. It is possible that removal of the diseased stomach may actually have a beneficial effect on nutrition.

**What type of procedure upon the colon?** Subtotal colectomy with ileoproctostomy remains the procedure of choice in children,[7, 16, 22, 25] although retention of the rectum carries the risk of subsequent malignancy regardless of the attention given to postoperative fulguration of new polyps. Everson and Allen[8] reported an incidence of carcinoma of the colon developing after this method of treatment of 5.2 per cent in 115 patients of all ages. Hubbard[14] found that 1 of 17 children (5.7 per cent) subsequently had a rectal carcinoma, but most of these patients were followed less than 10 years. Ravitch[25] devised and recommends subtotal colectomy and anal ileostomy with removal of all of the rectal mucosa.

Recognizing the danger inherent in retaining the rectum, we believe that the risk is worth while in order to preserve a continent anal sphincter. In children the psychological effect of ileostomy is an additional reason for subtotal rather than total colectomy.

**What type of procedure upon the stomach?** Whether or not any operative attack on the gastric polyposis should be made is the first question. Gastric polyposis by itself has been reported to be associated with carcinoma of the stomach in 10 to 40 per cent of cases,[2, 13, 20, 26] but this figure might be higher if only cases of familial gastrointestinal polyposis were studied. Although no definite statement can be made concerning the malignancy potential of gastric polyposis, there is presumptive evidence that the pathologic changes in the stomach and colon follow a similar pattern. Obviously, removal of this lesion is desirable.

The effects of total or radical subtotal gastrectomy are such that these procedures in children might result in the production of "gastrointestinal cripples," especially if the procedures are superimposed on a subtotal colectomy. Surgical approach to the gastric lesions is therefore necessarily limited. Fortunately, as stated, total excision by limited gastric resection is possible in over one-half of the cases of gastric polyposis because of the localized distribution of the disease. Luckily this localized distribution of the gastric polyps obtains in approximately the same percentage when the colon is also involved.[12, 15, 21]

Our approach to the question of what to do with the stomach was based upon the probable, though unproved, malignancy potential of gastric polyposis and the frequency with which these lesions are amenable to limited local resection. Halsted and associates,[12] in the only other recent report of such cases (in 4 adults), chose to observe the gastric lesions and recommended colectomy alone. Two of their patients and another member of the family with gastric polyposis alone have been followed for 10 years, and have not to Bartlett's[1] knowledge developed any gastric malignancy.

## PLAN OF THERAPY

We referred to all of the literature available on this subject in our attempts to answer the foregoing questions. From this information a plan evolved and was undertaken in the treatment of the patient in Case 1.

Initial laparotomy is used to determine the extent of the disease. Since the stomach and colon are known to be involved, the small bowel is examined first by endoscopy through 2 or 3 enterostomies. If polyposis of the jejunum or ileum is found, eradication of the disease is obviously impossible. The procedure is terminated and further treatment limited to the correction of complications. In the absence of small bowel involvement, the stomach is examined through a gastrotomy. If the disease is localized, partial gastrectomy is performed, preferably with reconstruction of gastroduodenal continuity. If the gastric involvement is diffuse, as many of the polyps as possible should be removed locally through the gastrotomy. The first procedure is then terminated.

Having determined the absence of small bowel polyposis, and having determined the extent of, and treated, the gastric polyposis, we then begin treatment of the colon. Multiple fulgurations of the rectum are performed until the rectal mucosa is clear up to the point where resection is to be performed. In children and adolescents this is best performed under general anesthesia.

After preparation of the rectum subtotal colectomy and ileoproctostomy are performed. Postoperatively sigmoidoscopic examinations and fulguration of any new polyps should be carried out every 3 months.

Even in patients in the pediatric age group we believe that this plan should be instituted as soon as the diagnosis is made.

## CASE REPORTS

**Case 1.** An 11-year-old white girl was referred to the Queens Hospital Center because of marked pallor. She had suffered fatigue, dizziness, and fainting intermittently for 8 months and occasional vomiting, but no observed hematemesis or melena. She had always eaten poorly and had gained weight slowly. While she usually had 3 to 4 bowel movements a day, she had no diarrhea.

A younger brother had died at 5 years of age from massive intestinal bleeding per rectum. Investigation of the parents and 2 older sisters disclosed polyposis in 1 of the sisters.

The child weighed only 59 pounds, the hemoglobin was 4 Gm. with a hematocrit of 22 per cent and a red blood cell count of 2.9 million. The stools showed ova of *Hymenolepis nana* and 1 specimen was positive for occult blood. Sigmoidoscopy showed numerous large and small polyps in the rectum and rectosigmoid, and the barium enema showed multiple colonic polyps. A gastrointestinal series showed numerous gastric polyps.

At laparotomy multiple polyps were palpated in the large bowel. None were felt in the small intestine. A sigmoidoscope was threaded through the small bowel, through 2 separate enterotomies, but no polyps were disclosed. Through a gastrotomy the gastric polyps were seen to be limited to the lower third of the stomach, and a subtotal gastrectomy and Billroth I gastroduodenostomy were performed. The gastric polyps were histologically benign and ranged in size from 0.5 to 3 cm. in diameter (Fig. 1).

The rectal polyps were fulgurated sigmoidoscopically on repeated occasions after operation until, after approximately 2 months, no additional polyps were visible. An abdominal colectomy with ileorectostomy was then performed. At the time of operation no polyps were palpable in the stomach. The polyps were distributed throughout the colon (Fig. 2), and those examined histologically showed no evidence of malignancy.

The child has been examined regularly at 3-month intervals since the operation, and the polyps which have reappeared (with decreasing frequency) have been fulgurated upon each occasion. Thirty months after colectomy and gastrectomy the child is in good health, having grown in weight and height to levels normal for her age. She has 2 to 3 bowel movements with formed stools a day on a full diet and without medication.

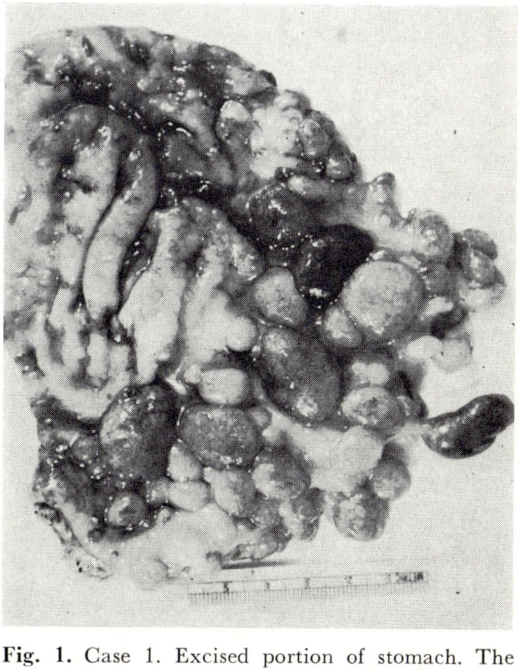

**Fig. 1.** Case 1. Excised portion of stomach. The polyps were localized to the distal one-third of the stomach.

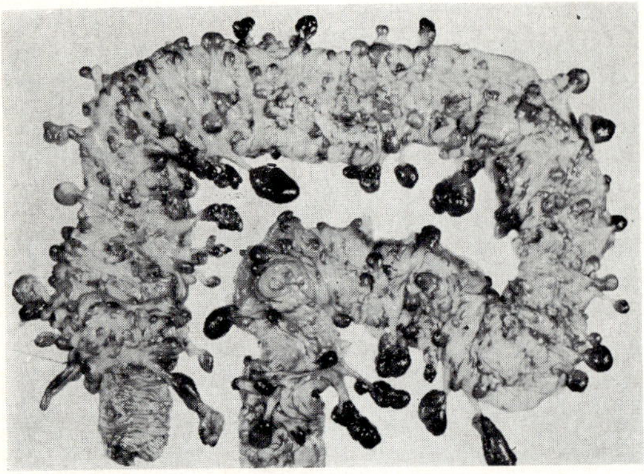

**Fig. 2.** Case 1. The tremendous involvement of the entire colon shows the extent of the disease when the child was 11 years old.

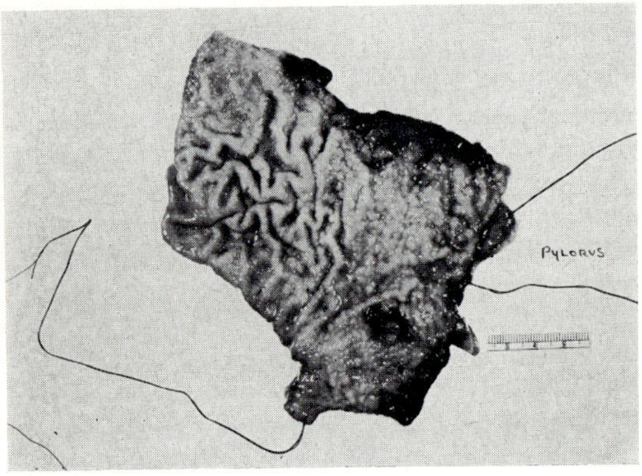


**Fig. 3.** Case 2. Excised segment of stomach. The early cobblestone changes that were present in the residual stomach can be seen at the left. The marked polypoid changes were limited to the prepyloric region.

*Comment.* The localization of the gastric polyps to the distal portion of the stomach and the absence of polyps in the small intestine made operative therapy feasible. It appears that in this instance the condition is familial since 1 brother died with intestinal bleeding and 1 sister has been found to have colonic polyposis.

**Case 2.** The 16-year-old sister of the patient in Case 1 was asymptomatic and had been found to have colonic polyps as a result of investigation of the family. The hemoglobin was 10.5 Gm. and the stools positive for occult blood. Sigmoidoscopy showed numerous polyps of the rectum and sigmoid, some as large as 1.5 cm. in diameter, and barium enema showed polyps throughout the colon. No polyps were seen in the stomach or small bowel on radiographic examination.

After repeated fulgurations of the rectal polyps over a period of 3 months, laparotomy was performed. Although the gastrointestinal series had failed to show gastric polyps, the stomach in this patient was found to be involved, as in the younger sister. There were numerous polyps in the prepyloric area and, in addition, the remaining gastric mucosa had a cobblestone appearance (Fig. 3). A distal gastrectomy and Billroth I gastroduodenostomy were well tolerated. The polyps were histologically benign. Three months later, after further fulguration of the rectal polyps, a subtotal colectomy with ileosigmoidostomy was performed. There were innumerable benign polyps in the portion of the colon removed. In the 26 months since operation the patient has undergone repeated fulgurations for recurrent rectal polyps which seem to show a tendency to decrease in numbers. A bout of mechanical intestinal obstruction due to adhesions has required operative relief. The patient is in good health, has 2 to 3 formed stools a day, and maintains her preoperative weight.

*Comment.* The distribution of the gastric and colonic polyps in this patient is like that in her sister, and obviously suggests a familial pattern. In this patient, perhaps unwisely, the colon was resected to a level above the peritoneal reflection.

## DISCUSSION

The incidence of familial polyposis involving both the stomach and colon has never been determined, but isolated case reports have appeared in the literature since 1896.[21] Mayo[17] is of the opinion that 5 per cent of patients with polyposis of the colon have gastric involvement, but has presented no statistics to support this. Dukes[5] writes that none of the patients at St. Mark's Hospital have had known stomach lesions, but no effort was made to determine their presence. Halsted and colleagues[12] made the only other prior report of familial cases. The occurrence of the gastric and colonic combination is much more common than involvement of the entire gastrointestinal tract.[15, 17, 29]

Radiographic demonstration of polyposis of the colon is relatively simple. The diagnosis of gastric polyposis, however, can often be made only by gastroscopy or at laparotomy, as in Case 2. In Halsted's[12] series, gastroscopic examination was necessary in all 5 cases, although the roentgenographic study was suggestive in 1. Preoperative determination of small bowel polyps is completely unreliable by present means. Operative enteroscopies proved successful in our 2 patients and only 2 enterostomies were required for visualization of the entire small bowel.

The removal of gastric polyps in the absence of complications is in opposition to the approach of Halsted and his group. We believe that when possible, local resection is advisable, although the early cobblestone appearance of the residual gastric mucosa in Case 2 may be preliminary to new polyps. It must be acknowledged, however, that no instance has been reported in which carcinoma of the stomach has developed in a patient who has undergone subtotal colectomy for colonic polyposis.

The postoperative courses of both girls appear to demonstrate that subtotal colectomy combined with partial gastrectomy is compatible with normal development. The marked improvement in nutrition and growth of the younger child may be due to removal of the gastric or of the colonic disease or both. Diarrhea has not been a problem and both girls have had a normal life.

Although spontaneous disappearance of residual rectal polyps after subtotal colectomy has been reported,[3, 6, 14, 28] it did not occur in our patients and repeated fulgurations have been necessary at 3-month intervals.

As Ravitch[23] has said, the occurrence of these potentially malignant lesions at both ends of the gastrointestinal tract poses a difficult surgical problem. The occurrence in 2 children was an additional source of concern. Because the correct treatment of familial polyposis of the stomach and colon is as yet undetermined, our approach to the problem was based upon the desire to eradicate as much of the malignancy potential as possible without interfering with normal nutrition and growth.

## SUMMARY

1. The problems inherent in the treatment of children with familial polyposis involving both the stomach and colon have been presented.

2. The authors base their therapeutic approach upon 6 premises and facts expressed in the literature. First, polyposis involving the stomach and colon is more common than diffuse involvement of the gastrointestinal tract. Second, polyposis of the colon has a malignancy potential approaching 100 per cent. Third, polyposis of the stomach has a malignancy potential, but of an undetermined degree. Fourth, polyposis of the stomach is often localized enough to permit extirpation by partial gastrectomy. Fifth, carcinoma in polyposis of the colon has occurred in patients as young as 12 years of age. Sixth, growth and development of children after subtotal gastrectomy or colectomy have been good.

3. The course described is recommended when the presence of polyposis in the colon and stomach is established. Definitive operation is suggested in children at whatever age the diagnosis is made. Exploratory laparotomy is performed and the small bowel explored endoscopically through multiple enterotomies. If polyps are found eradication of disease is impossible and no resection is indicated. If no polyps are found in the small bowel, a gastrotomy is performed to evaluate the involvement of the stomach. Extirpation of the polyps by partial gastrectomy is performed if feasible, and if not, simple excision of as many polyps as possible is carried out. Four to 6 weeks later, after preliminary fulguration of the rectal polyps, subtotal colectomy and ileoproctostomy are performed. The retained rectum is examined every 3 months and new polyps fulgurated.

4. Two cases of polyposis of the stomach and colon in which the suggested course of therapy was employed are presented.

The authors express their appreciation to the many members of the surgical and pediatric services of the Queens Hospital Center whose cooperation and care made possible completion of the therapeutic program undertaken in the cases reported.

## REFERENCES

1. Bartlett, M. K.: Personal communication.
2. Berg, J. W.: Histologic aspects of the relation between gastric adenomatous polyps and gastric cancer, Cancer **11:** 1149, 1961.

3. Cole, J. W., and Holden, W. D.: Postcolectomy regression of adenomatous polyps of rectum, A. M. A. Arch. Surg. **79:** 385, 1959.
4. Craver, W. L., and Glenn, F.: Peptic ulceration in childhood, A. M. A. Arch. Surg. **77:** 833, 1958.
5. Dukes, C. E.: Personal communication.
6. Dunphy, J. E., Patterson, W. B., and Legg, M. A.: Etiologic factors in polyposis and carcinoma of colon, Ann. Surg. **150:** 488, 1959.
7. Eckert, C.: Intestinal polyposis, *in* Ariel and Pack: Cancer and allied diseases of infancy and childhood, Boston, 1960, Little, Brown & Company.
8. Everson, T. C., and Allen, M. J.: Subtotal colectomy with ileosigmoidostomy and fulguration of polyps in retained colon, A. M. A. Arch. Surg. **69:** 806, 1954.
9. Finney, D. C. W., Schnauffer, L., and Stafford, E. S.: Total gastrectomy in an infant made necessary by ingestion of tinning paint, Ann. Surg. **151:** 891, 1960.
10. Gordon, D. L., Hallenbeck, G. A., Dockerty, M. B., Kennedy, R. L., and Jackman, R. J.: Polyps of the colon in children, A. M. A. Arch. Surg. **75:** 90, 1957.
11. Gross, R. E.: The surgery of infancy and childhood, Philadelphia, 1953, W. B. Saunders Company.
12. Halsted, J. A., Harris, E. J., and Bartlett, M. K.: Involvement of the stomach in familial polyposis of the gastrointestinal tract, Gastroenterology **15:** 763, 1950.
13. Hay, L. J.: Surgical management of gastric polyps and adenomas, Surgery **39:** 114, 1956.
14. Hubbard, T. B., Jr.: Familial polyposis of the colon: the fate of the retained rectum after colectomy in children, Ann. Surg. **23:** 577, 1957.
15. Lazar, H. P., and Bendix, R. M.: Familial polyposis with external manifestations, Gastroenterology **36:** 841, 1959.
16. Longino, L. A., and Holder, T. M.: Rectal bleeding in children, Pediat. Clin. North America **6:** 1153, 1959.
17. Mayo, C. W.: Discussion of Estes, W. L. Ann. Surg. **127:** 1055, 1948.
18. McKenny, D. C.: Multiple polyposis, Am. J. Surg. **46:** 204, 1939.
19. Mellish, R. W. P.: Timing in pediatric surgery, Pediat. Clin. North America **6:** 987, 1959.
20. Pearl, F. L., and Brunn, H.: Multiple gastric polyposis, Surg. Gynec. & Obst. **76:** 257, 1943.
21. Port, K.: Multiple polypenbildung im tractus intestinalis, Deutsche Ztschr. Chir. **42:** 181, 1896.
22. Potts, W. J.: The surgeon and the child, Philadelphia, 1959, W. B. Saunders Company.
23. Ravitch, M. M.: Polypoid adenomatosis of the entire gastrointestinal tract, Ann. Surg. **128:** 283, 1948.
24. Ravitch, M. M., and McGoon, D. C.: Teratoid tumors and dermoid cysts, *in* Ariel and Pack: Cancer and allied diseases of infancy and childhood, Boston, 1960, Little, Brown & Company.
25. Ravitch, M. M., and Sabiston, D. C.: Anal ileostomy with preservation of the sphincter, Surg. Gynec. & Obst. **84:** 1095, 1947.
26. Spriggs, E. I., and Marxer, O. A.: Polyps of the stomach and polypoid gastritis, Quart. J. Med. **12:** 1, 1943.
27. Swenson, O.: Pediatric surgery, New York, 1958, Appleton-Century-Crofts, Inc.
28. Turell, R.: Colonic and anorectal function and disease, Internat. Abstr. Surg. **107:** 417, 1958.
29. Wechselman, L.: Polyp u carcinom in magen darm kanal, Beitr. klin. Chir. **70:** 855, 1910.

# The surgical school of Theodor Billroth

KAREL B. ABSOLON, M.D.*
MINNEAPOLIS, MINN.
*From the Department of Surgery, University of Minnesota Medical School*

> He who combines the knowledge of physiology and surgery, in addition to the artistic side of his subject, reaches the highest ideal in medicine.
>
> Billroth, 1885

The metamorphosis from barber surgeon to modern surgeon had been completed by the time Theodor Billroth appeared on the scene. The technical aspects of surgery had made this discipline stand apart from internal medicine until the early 1800's. Historically, one may trace the nature and origin of the separate lines which had become very definite in the seventeenth century. Gradually the schism lessened. During the nineteenth century, the dividing lines between medicine and surgery were recognized as unnecessary; oftentimes they proved to be an obstacle and consequently were removed. Billroth represented the pinnacle of this development and at the same time laid the foundations on which present-day surgery was to be built, foundations which were to be completed by his pupils. Billroth's energy, artistry, and scientific fervor illuminated their paths. Billroth became the greatest of surgeons, but at the same time he assumed an important place in the cultural and historical development of his time.[4, 43, 47, 64, 83]

Supported by the Institutional Grant, University of Minnesota Medical School, United States Public Health Service Grant No. H5433, and the Minnesota Heart Association.

Presented at the quarterly Seminar of History of Medicine, University of Minnesota Medical School, Dec. 12, 1960.

*Part of this study was carried out during the tenure of a United States Public Health Service Fellowship.

Through conquest of the unknown, Billroth and his pupils were dedicated to improve the fate of people suffering of hitherto incurable diseases. This was accomplished by free quest, clinical and experimental, into the technical, mechanical, and scientific aspects of surgical disease.

The impact that Billroth's school had on the surgical development of this century forces our surgical generation to make repeated inquiries into the period in which these men lived and labored and review the circumstances under which they searched and the procedures by which they obtained results.

This experience was to the author one of serene satisfaction and fulfillment. Are not all of us related to this school of surgery by identification and acceptance of its basic principles?

Only rarely is a surgical school crowned with as many pioneering accomplishments as Billroth's. Stimulating his pupils and by active transfer of his principles to them, Billroth built up a movement which is comparable only to his own achievements. The master continued to live through those who followed him; his pupils searched out the flaws in technique or reasoning of both their teacher and themselves. With his help, they advanced to even greater heights (Fig. 1).

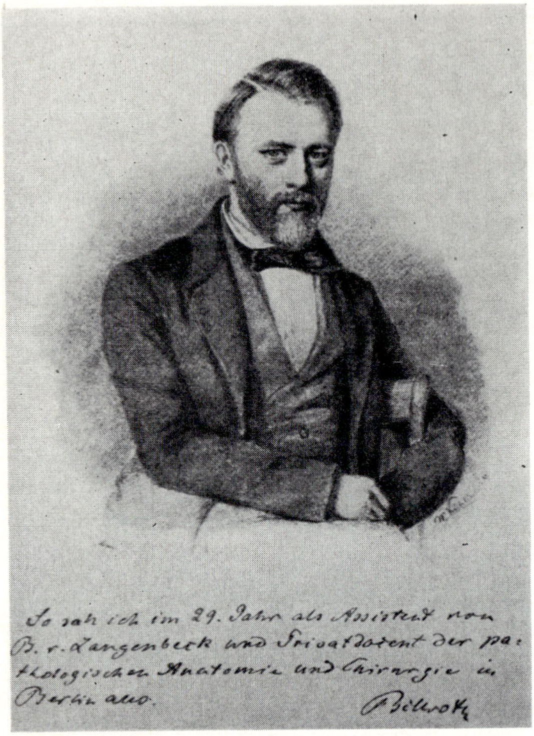


**Fig. 1.** Billroth at the age of 29 years when he became assistant to B. v. Langenbeck and Docent of Pathological Anatomy and Surgery in Berlin.

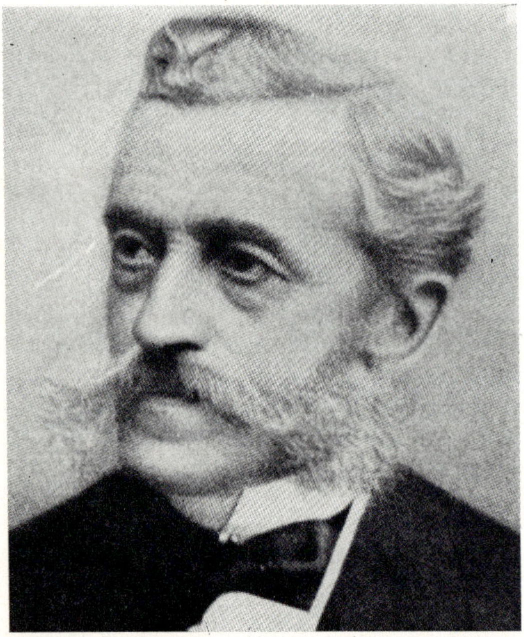

**Fig. 2.** Bernhard v. Langenbeck, Professor of Surgery, Berlin (1848 to 1882).

> The greatest happiness of my life was founding a school that carries on my aims of scientific and humanitarian accomplishments.
>
> Billroth to His, 1893

## BILLROTH (1829 TO 1894)

From the day he entered the medical arena of the Austrian capital in 1867 until he was forced into limited activity by congestive heart failure 25 years later, Billroth's aim was to build a school of new surgical thought.[86] He had already shown his capabilities when in 1860, at the age of 31, he was appointed Director of the Surgical Clinic in Zurich.

The influence of Bernhard v. Langenbeck (Fig. 2), his teacher in Berlin, was conspicuous. Langenbeck had transferred from the study of physiology (Professor of Physiology, Göttingen) to the practice of surgery (Professor of Surgery in Kiel and Berlin). The same path was followed by Billroth. His dissertation thesis, suggested to him by Schönlein's former assistant, Ludwig Traube, was entitled *Nature and Cause of Pulmonary Affections Produced by Bilateral Vagal Section.*[6] For this work, Billroth obtained his degree in medicine at the age of 23 years.

Billroth admired his authoritarian teacher greatly, commonly recalling to his students the "resonance of the 'viva vox' (lively, loud, and energetic voice) of old Langenbeck." The following excerpt from Langenbeck's letter to Billroth, dated May 24, 1882, proves the esteem the teacher held for his pupil. At the same time, it presents a valuable cultural and historical document on the relationship between Berlin and Vienna.

> Yesterday evening the faculty considered my successor. I suggested that you be the only candidate proposed to the Minister and this suggestion was accepted without discussion. That, I believe, has never happened at the Berlin faculty; it must make you happy that this unanimity was not produced by my influence in the faculty, for I have never possessed any, but was due to your scientific importance.
>
> I came home happy and here I find your negative answer; that was a cold shower for me. I consider your letter as never having been written. . . . I don't have to ask you to reconsider. The points to be adjudged are that the Fatherland, which would greet you with enthusiasm upon your

return, is increasing in its importance. It also possesses better student material. . . . I recognize the anti-German tendencies in Austria. Even with the great reputation which you are known to enjoy in Vienna, they never will cease to consider you as an intruder.

The departure from my dear Berlin will be unusually hard, and it would be made easier if you should be holding my position. I, also would put the Surgical Congress in your hands. My advice and my desire is that you will mention this letter to no one and that you will accept the call. I am asking you insistently to attend the Congress, and I am inviting you for dinner on June 2 at 6:00 P.M.

Billroth did not heed the advice. He was culturally and spiritually part of the Austrian life and loved by the Austrian people.[50] He appreciated the atmosphere of Johannes Brahms' artistic Vienna and respected the scientific development accomplished by freedom-loving men. Brahms was originally a northern German himself and benefited by the cultural atmosphere of Vienna in his musical development. Billroth had divorced himself completely from the polished Prussian mustache and uniform.

The Berlin surgical chair fortunately came to be occupied by Ernst v. Bergmann, who, among other important accomplishments, pioneered in aseptic surgery.

Upon becoming head of the Second Surgical Department in Vienna on Oct. 11, 1867, Billroth proclaimed in his inaugural lecture, "The future of a school is based on the work of the pupils, as is the future of a country on the work of its citizens." Billroth outlined to his pupils epigrammatically, "He who cannot quote his therapeutic experiences in numbers is a charlatan; be truthful for clarity's sake, do not hesitate to admit failures, as they must show the mode and places of improvement." And again in 1876 he redefined the ideal of a university of learning when he stated, "If one considers the heights of the medical schools in Vienna, Prague, Würzburg, Göttingen, Berlin, Freiburg, and Leipzig which persist even today, one can see that it is not the men of formal medical pedagogy that attract students; contrariwise, scientists are the magnets for these schools. A school's purpose is not to unify a group of people and spread their identical thought. Controversy in investigation will never disappear. The principle, method and the goal of investigations is recognition of truth, even though the truth may be in conflict with our social, ethical and political circumstances. This is the binding force of a modern university."

To anticipate development, to judge collaborators correctly, to stimulate his coworkers in the proper direction is the prerogative of only the greatest of men. Billroth's influence on scientists in their fields was boundless. The importance of his discovery of the Streptococcus[15] on the development of bacteriology was credited by Robert Koch in a letter to Billroth dated April 29, 1890. "As I started my first investigations, I was entirely under the influence of your studies on Coccobacteria Septica that were published at that time, and this impression did not fade to this day. . . ." Billroth's vision of the development of chemotherapy was expressed in the studies on the relationship of living animal and vegetable cells (1890). "The malarial and syphilis organisms can be killed with quinine, arsenic, and mercury or iodine respectively," he stated. "The duty of generations to come is to find similar agents for the tuberculosis bacillus and the cancer microbes."[9]

Billroth's views on surgical training were unique for the time in which he lived. It was his opinion that the student would be ready to start his surgical training only after he had absorbed his medical studies and enlarged his points of view in hospitals. Performing operations on cadavers and experimental animals, 2 or 3 years' assistantship in a surgical department, studies of surgical monographs, writing of patient histories, and acquiring practical experience in the hospital were necessary to prepare the surgeon for independent work. Anything that concerned the patient, including nursing duties, had to be experienced by the surgeon. Billroth knew that all this could be accomplished with perserverance and diligence; he demonstrated that there is no short road to knowledge that can be accomplished in any prescribed period of time while moulding pupils. The physician's role was always to find the cause of the pathologic process, to predict its course, and to bring it successfully to an end. Billroth documented by example that empiric knowledge clarified by scientific investigation is the procedure by which satisfactory solutions of mysterious medical problems are reached.[17]

Billroth's pupils were called enthusiastically as professors to other universities. It was common knowledge that they were selected, trained, and screened through Billroth's hands. Billroth insisted that they be well founded in anatomy, pathology, physiology, and experimental research—all necessary prerequisites for the academic surgeon today as well. His pupils were to supply the answers to his current interest; they supplied many answers that surgery had been waiting for. Billroth helped secure publication of the works of his pupils in prominent scientific journals and brought their names before the scientific world (Fig. 3).

## BILLROTH'S PUPILS

From his many pupils, a number became professors of surgery and heads of surgical clinics. They made important contributions to the medical sciences and especially surgery. The most important representatives (Fig. 4) were R. Gersuny (Vienna), V. Czerny (Freiburg, Heidelberg), C. Gussenbauer (Prague, Vienna), V. Hacker (Innsbruck, Graz), A. Wölfler (Graz, Prague), J. Mikulicz-Radecki (Krakow, Breslau), A. Eiselsberg (Utrecht, Königsberg, Vienna), A. Winiwarter (Liege), and A. Fränkel (Vienna).

**Czerny (1842 to 1916).** Vincenz Czerny, the son of a pharmacist, was born in 1842 in Trautenau, Bohemia. After obtaining his first teaching appointment in Vienna in 1871 as Docent, he was called to Heidelberg in 1877 as Professor of Surgery. His major contributions pertained to cancer research and abdominal surgery.[45] In 160 surgical papers, he discussed technical aspects and therapeutic results of procedures such as gastric and intestinal resections, gall-bladder operations, esophagectomy, and operations on the thyroid and larynx.[19-21]

In 1878, Czerny performed the first vaginal panhysterectomy with modern technique. In May, 1877, he was the first to extirpate successfully a napkin-ring cancer of the cervical esophagus in a 51-year-old woman. By means of an incision along the left anterior border of the sternocleidomastoid muscle, the esophagus was exposed, the tumor freed from the surrounding tissues, and a segment 6 cm. long removed after proximal transection at the pharynx. The 2 esophageal apertures were brought to the skin and the distal one used for feeding purposes. The patient survived the operation and 5 months later was able to work, but died of recurrent cancer. In 1884 another Billroth pupil, Mikulicz, performed a similar operation, establishing esophageal continuity with 2 wing-shaped skin flaps.[70] The edges of the inverted flaps were sewed together with catgut and the outside skin was closed with silver wire sutures. Ten days after operation the patient was able to take solid foods, but 10 months later died of recurrent cancer. In 1908, Hacker, a later assistant to Billroth, reported a successful simultaneous resection of both the cervical esophagus and larynx.[57]

It is clearly evident that Billroth exerted great influence on his students. In 1872 he wrote on experimental esophageal resections and the therapeutic potential of this procedure.[10] From 1878 Billroth popularized partial laryngectomy, a procedure first performed by Maas of Breslau in 1876. Even though the first total laryngectomy had been performed by Watson of Edinburgh in 1866 for syphilis, Czerny together with Billroth performed the first total laryngectomy for cancer on Dec. 31, 1873. Czerny developed this procedure on dogs and demonstrated experimentally its practical feasibility as early as 1870. The final and equally important step, namely rehabilitation of the laryngectomized patient, was accomplished by Gussenbauer's construction of an artificial larynx for one of Billroth's patients operated on in 1874. In 1879, Billroth removed the entire larynx except the epiglottis, a large part of the pharynx, the esophagus up to the manubrium, and the entire thyroid gland for an invasive carcinoma of the larynx. The patient withstood the procedure well but died of a mediastinal suppuration and suppurative pericarditis 6 weeks after the operation. This complication was a consequence of a false passage produced by esophageal dilatation. Billroth remarked that even though a human being could endure so extensive a procedure remarkably well, such an operation had no future.[8]

Czerny was an excellent teacher. In addition to the practical aspects of surgery, he emphasized the historical development of surgical methods and the place for improvement that lay ahead. His monograph, *Relationship of Surgery to Natural Sciences,* and his study, *The Development of Surgery During the Nineteenth Century and Its Relationship to Teaching* (Heidelberg, 1904), reveal this aspect of his interests.

Prior to Czerny's appointment as Professor in Heidelberg, he held the chair of surgery in Freiburg. There he married Kussmaul's daughter.

Because of limited hospital bed space he found time for his favorite preoccupation, the study of experimental surgery and pathologic histology. Stimulated by his associations with Langhans, Nothnagel, and Kussmaul, Czerny contributed in this period to various aspects of bone tuberculosis, osteitis deformans, fat embolism, colonic absorption, and intestinal suturing.[45]

His major research in the cancer field was yet to come. Retiring as Professor of Surgery (replaced by another pupil of Billroth, Albert Narath), he worked toward the development of a cancer institute, the first of its kind in Germany.[18] Stimulated by his visit to the State Institute for the Study of Malignant Disease in Buffalo, New York, he built the new institute and became its director in 1906. Czerny published some 40 studies on cancer; the technique of tumor transplantation into the anterior chamber was one of his discoveries.

The many accomplishments of Czerny were honored by presidencies of the Deutsche Gesellschaft für Chirurgie in 1901, of the International Surgical Congress in 1908, and of the International Association for Cancer

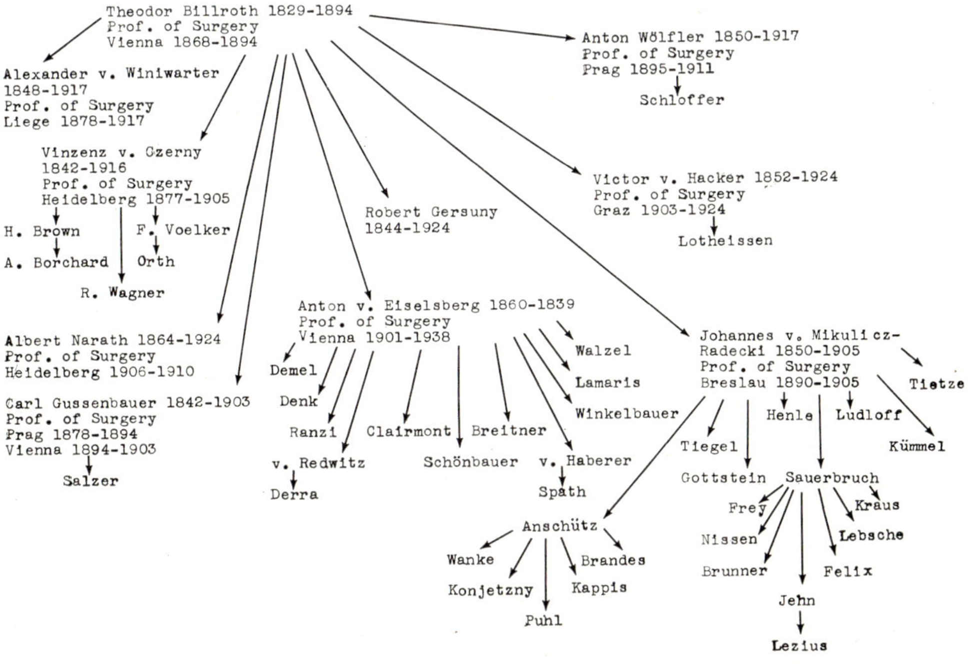


**Fig. 3.** The Billroth surgical school.

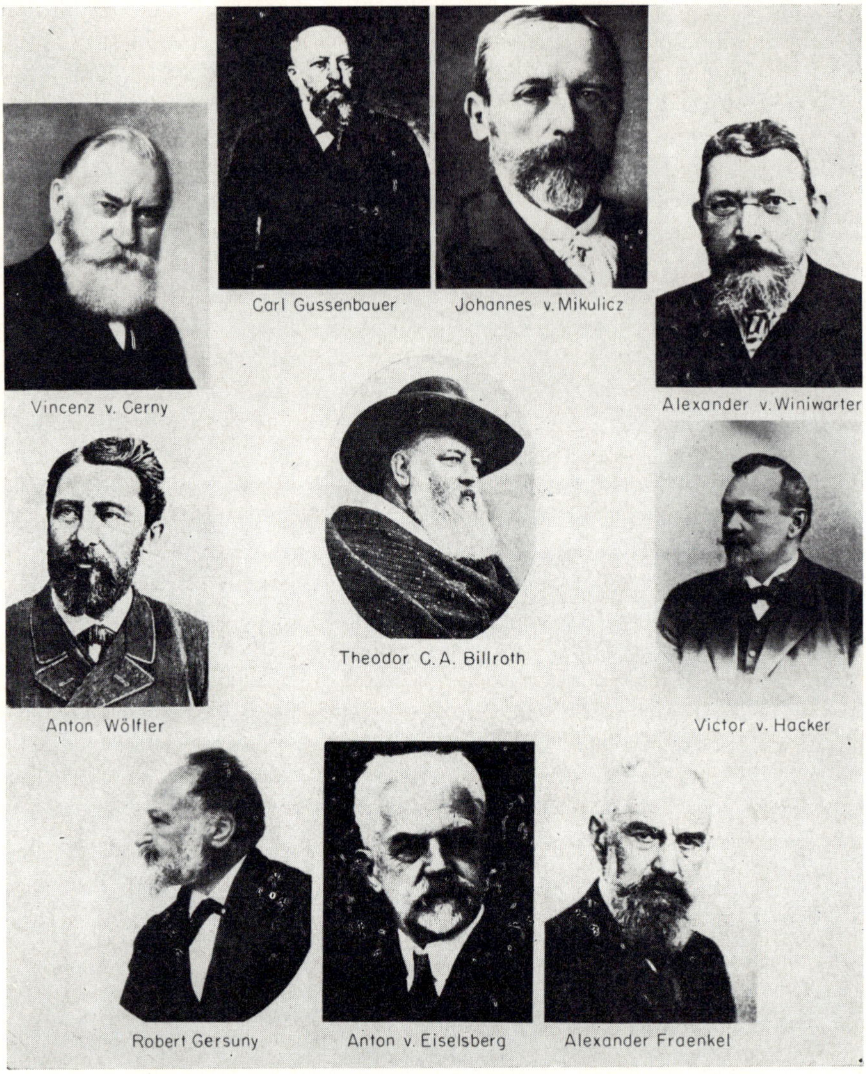


**Fig. 4.** Billroth and his pupils.

Research in 1910. In 1885, Czerny was made an Honorary Fellow of the American Surgical Association.

**Gussenbauer (1812 to 1903).** Billroth's surgical chair came to be occupied by Carl G. Gussenbauer, then Professor of Surgery in Prague. Gussenbauer, the son of a physician in Obervallach, Austria, was born in 1842. It was logical that a pupil of Billroth should become the new head of the now famous Second Surgical Clinic.[28] Gussenbauer entered into apprenticeship under Billroth shortly after obtaining his medical degree in 1866. His first works were anatomic and concerned the musculature of the atrioventricular valves in the human being, healing of wounds, and the trauma of skeletal muscle (1871). His interest in cancer is evident from his study of lymphatic spread of malignant tumors (1872). Gussenbauer's contributions to clinical surgery include the description of Billroth's techniques of laryngectomy (1874) and studies on partial gastrectomy in dogs (1876), subtotal colectomy of the descending colon (1879), and extirpation of pharyngeal tumors by the oral route (1879). He was the first to treat a pancreatic cyst surgically by marsupialization.[48]

Billroth's interest in bone surgery and fracture treatment was sporadic. This was perhaps due to the fact that the prominent Viennese surgical figure of the 1880's, Eduard Albert, Chairman of the First Surgical Clinic, considered bone and joint pathology and surgery one of his major interests. This activity had great impact on the development of the Viennese School of Orthopedics by Albert's pupil, Heinrich Lorenz, and influenced Billroth as well as some of his pupils. Gussenbauer discussed the methods of surgical osteolysis in 1875. This study again may have presented the background for the first hemipelvectomy performed by Billroth in 1891, who himself contributed to joint resection in his early years.[13, 14]

Gussenbauer made inroads into brain surgery by his works on the extirpation of "myelogenic" cranial tumors and the surgical therapy of deep traumatic brain abscesses.[46, 49] One of the great honors conferred upon Gussenbauer was his election as the first foreigner to the presidency of the German Surgical Society in 1894.

**Gersuny (1844 to 1924).** Robert Gersuny, son of a physician, was born in Bohemia. After finishing his medical course in Prague, he became private assistant to Billroth and later chairman of the surgical pediatric department.[29]

Just as Billroth, most of his students were broadly oriented. Gersuny, for example, introduced the bow-shaped osteotomy, performed the first cholecystogastrostomy, and recognized the surgical significance of peritoneal adhesions and the clinical picture these may produce. The colporrhaphy procedure which he developed for treatment of uterine prolapse gained wide use[41]; his technique of twisting the female urethra and rectum for incontinence showed ingenuity.[39, 42] The introduction of a lampwick as a drain provided a useful implement in surgical therapy. He demonstrated before Kocher that Dupuytren's contracture could be cured by careful excision of the palmar fascia and emphasized early esophageal dilatation in chemical burns of the esophagus.[37, 40] Some of his more popular writings were translated into English.[38]

Gersuny was highly regarded as diagnostician and teacher.[36, 44]

**Winiwarter (1848 to 1917).** The multifaceted personality of Alexander v. Winiwarter reflects Billroth's spirit. It was he who inherited the job of revising the ninth through the sixteenth editions of Billroth's famous *Allgemeine Chirurgische Pathologie und Therapie.* The first edition of this classic work, which later was translated into 10 foreign languages, was published in 1860 at the time when Billroth obtained the Professorship of Surgery in Zurich.

Billroth, recognizing his own limitations, relinquished a work closer to his heart than any other. "When some time ago the editors asked me to prepare the new printing of this book," he stated, "I realized that I could not do it as thoroughly as I was able to years ago. My surgical work, teaching and

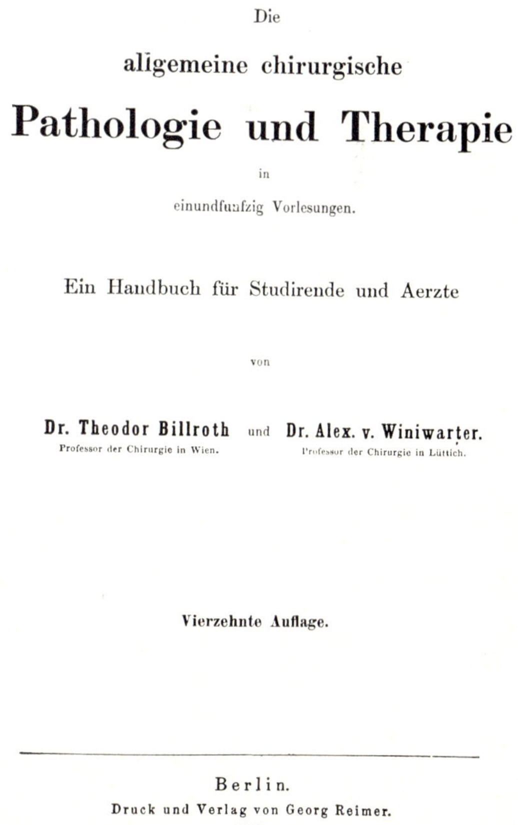
Die

allgemeine chirurgische

Pathologie und Therapie

in

einundfunfzig Vorlesungen.

Ein Handbuch für Studirende und Aerzte

von

Dr. Theodor Billroth — Professor der Chirurgie in Wien.
und
Dr. Alex. v. Winiwarter. — Professor der Chirurgie in Lüttich.

Vierzehnte Auflage.

Berlin.
Druck und Verlag von Georg Reimer.
1889.

**Fig. 5.** Title page of Billroth's classic textbook.

public activities absorbed my energy to such a degree that it was made impossible for me to follow the theoretical sciences, the backbone of medicine. . . . Along these lines, I am saying goodbye as a surgical writer to the readers who gave me so much friendship. I wish to state with pride that my efforts to stimulate the students for this beautiful art and science of surgery were brilliantly rewarded." He complimented Winiwarter on having revised his book with competence with regard to the views of the modern and future surgeon, while simultaneously keeping with piety the spirit of the original author (Fig. 5).

Alexander v. Winiwarter was born in 1848. He obtained his medical degree in 1870 in Vienna and after 6 years as assistant to Billroth, became Docent in 1876. While working under Billroth, he wrote on the pathologic anatomy of the liver (1872), lymphomas (1874), and plexiform neuromas of the peripheral nerves (1876). In 1878, promoted to the surgical professorship in Liege, he made additional contributions to surgical pathology and therapy, writing on surgical diseases of the skin (1892), the male genitals (1906), and operations on the biliary tree,[85] as well as developing cholecystoenterostomy, perineorrhaphy according to Lawson Tait, and the use of arsenicals in the treatment of lymphomas. Once he had settled in Belgium, it was a logical decision for Winiwarter and his family to become Belgian patriots. Although not a Belgian by birth, he enthusiastically adopted his new country despite the reproaches and enmity of his Viennese friends during World War I.[2, 84]

In 1867, Billroth had pointed out the importance of examining one's conscience in evaluating the results of surgical therapy. Winiwarter, probably on Billroth's prompting, published in 1878 a statistical evaluation of breast cancer cures accomplished in Billroth's clinic. This was 3 years after v. Volkman had published the first statistics on cancer in the history of medicine. Winiwarter showed that 4.7 per cent of 170 patients were alive and well 3 or more years after mastectomy. The public was impressed by these figures, however meager. The clinic in Billroth's and his assistants' hands no longer was a place for only the poor to come and die. The eloquence of facts and numbers replaced the therapeutic nihilism aggressively associated with scientific diagnostic investigations or interpretations of the earlier days of Joseph Skoda and Carl Rokitansky. As Winiwarter proved on the basis of rational statistical analyses, surgical diseases, including cancer, were curable.[87]

Alexander Winiwarter's younger brother, Felix, while under the tutorship of Billroth from 1876 to 1878, described as an entity thromboangitis obliterans—Winiwarter's disease.[88]

In 1877, Billroth stated "that no unsurmountable obstacles to partial excision of the stomach existed, either on anatomical, physiological or operative grounds." His indications and justification for surgical procedures, even so new and drastic for that time, were defined strictly but humanely. "One may perform surgical procedures only if there is a little chance of success. To operate without having a chance means to prostitute the beautiful art and science of surgery. Surgery would otherwise become suspicious to our lay public and to our colleagues."

Billroth's pupils Gussenbauer, Winiwarter, and Czerny (1874) developed the technique of gastric resection in dogs. The first partial gastrectomy in dogs had been successfully accomplished by D. Merrem in 1810, who proposed this operation for treatment of gastric cancer in human beings. It was appropriate that Billroth's clinic, after re-evaluation of the experimental subtotal gastrectomy, should play the pioneering role in the development of gastric surgery for cancer.

**Wölfler (1850 to 1917).** Anton Wölfler, son of a physician, came from Kopecany in Bohemia, obtained his medical degree in 1874 in Vienna, and worked subsequently under Billroth. In the letters of Billroth one may see the satisfaction he found in Wölfler's accomplishments which he foresaw. Wölfler recognized that surgery did not consist of operations viewed as theatrical performances by individuals, but that only with the aid of new investigative advances could surgery grow into a real science. Scientifically disciplined, his energy grew with the magnitude of problems on hand.[82]

In 1881, 2 major milestones in surgery of the stomach were accomplished. Wölfler performed the first successful gastroenterostomy (antecolic), following the suggestion of Nicoladoni.[62, 89] It was Billroth himself, of course, who performed the first successful subtotal gastrectomy for cancer of the stomach (Billroth I type) on Jan. 29, 1881.[5, 12, 62, 89] Two previous gastrectomies for cancer by Pean on April 9, 1879, and Rydygier on Nov. 16, 1880, had not been successful. Rydygier stated that Billroth did not know about the 2 previous gastrectomy attempts in human beings.

Wölfler wrote more than 20 papers on the pathology and therapy of the thyroid gland. He described the "fetal adenoma" of the thyroid gland and his detailed pathologic studies of the thyroid gland expanded on the previous works of Virchow.[91] "Wölfler's sign" for clinical diagnosis of the hourglass stomach was helpful prior to diagnostic roentgenography. His classical publications, *The Resection of the Carcinomatous Pylorus Carried out by Billroth* (1881), *Amputations in Professor Billroth's Clinic* (1880), and *The Surgical Treatment of Goiter* (1891), and his writings on carcinoma of the tongue and kidney (1881) and foreign bodies in the human gastrointestinal tract (1909) established Wölfler's place in the history of modern surgery. Wölfler's technique of intestinal suture from inside the lumen out, which he described in his report on gastrectomies, must be considered as one of his major technical accomplishments. We scarcely realize today that intestinal suture ever presented a problem of sorts.

Antisepsis, surprisingly enough, was accepted by Billroth with some misgivings. It appeared scientifically insecure to this early student of bacteriology. Carbolic acid as a disinfectant perhaps was repulsive to Billroth's fine senses. He was not allergic to

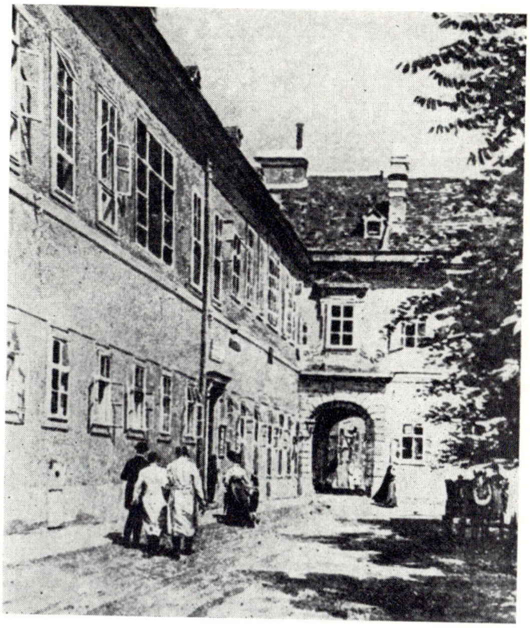

**Fig. 6.** Billroth's clinic in the 1880's.

carbolic acid as suspected by some of his students. Allergy to carbolic acid was a common drawback to its use. Lorenz, for example, was forced into orthopedics just because of this.

It was reported that Billroth encountered Lister while the latter was traveling through Germany demonstrating his "spray" and caught him rather off balance by asking why many surgical wounds heal "per primam" without pus formation, while deep-seated abscesses in the knee joint form without evidence of injury. Despite the antagonism to the carbolic acid spray, Billroth sent Wölfler to Volkmann's clinic in Halle and to Lister's clinic in Edinburgh to investigate the antiseptic techniques. Upon his return, the open-minded Billroth gave Wölfler an operating room to test the carbolic acid spray's effectiveness. The results supported Lister's contentions. Gersuny reported Billroth's remarks, "I have seen such results with other methods." Replied Wölfler, "Not as constantly." Wölfler succeeded in persuading his chief to adopt the Edinburgh technique in Vienna.

Asepsis was soon to replace antisepsis. "All surgeons wear antiseptic uniforms and individuality recedes into the background," muttered Billroth in 1889. But 2 years later, observing the successes of his pupils, he remarked happily, "With clean hands and conscience the least experienced surgeons accomplish better results than the most famous professors of surgery in yesteryear." Wölfler was appointed Professor of Surgery in Graz (1886) and reorganized the somewhat stagnant surgical department of his predecessor, Rzehaczek. In 1895, he moved to the same position in Prague. This new professorship of greater stature gained him popularity and a following of students. Wölfler's other works included development of a technique of herniorrhaphy with transplantation of the cord, experimental studies on the transplantation of the mucosa, and the parasacral approach to proctectomy.[90, 92, 93]

**Mikulicz (1850 to 1905).** Discoveries in scientific and practical surgery were the goal of Johann v. Mikulicz-Radecki. He was Billroth's most brilliant pupil, judged from his many original contributions.[81] Born in Czernowitz in the eastern Austrian province of Bukowina, he obtained his medical degree in Vienna in 1875. He was a short, mercurial young man with small thin hands, an accomplished pianist. Through Billroth's chamber music group, he set forth toward the successful accomplishment of his great ambitions. Working under Billroth until 1882, he became Professor of Surgery in Krakow in 1883 and held this appointment for 4 years. Rydygier became his successor. Mikulicz left for a new appointment in Königsberg in 1887 and finally settled in Breslau in 1890.

Improvements in antisepsis, disinfection, and anesthesia were some of his early successes,[75] and continued to interest him throughout his life.[71, 80] After introducing the surgical mask and cotton gloves into surgery in 1896, he eventually adopted Halsted's use of rubber gloves.[74]

Mikulicz's invention and development of the esophagoscope and gastroscope in 1881 gained him the title of Father of Gastroscopy and Esophagoscopy.[77] Laryngoscopy had been presented at the Hunterian Society of London in 1829 by Benjamin Babington. Waldenburg, in 1870, had constructed a tubular scope with which he was able to visualize an esophageal diverticulum. Desormaux, in 1865, had observed the interior of the bladder as well as the esophagus. But only Kussmaul, elongating Desormaux's scope to 73 cm., was able to perform true esophagoscopy. In 1868 he visualized the cardia of the stomach and diagnosed a cancer of the esophagus.[61] Mikulicz established that although the pharynx and esophagus are not in a straight line, the 2 organs could be channeled, permitting use of straight rigid tubes for direct inspection by means of reflected light. For gastroscopy, he recommended an angulated apparatus. Equally great merit goes to Mikulicz's technical collaborator, Leiter, who developed the illuminating system for the gastroscope and esophagoscope.

Mikulicz introduced new techniques of thyroidectomy, pyloroplasty, and developed original methods for treatment of torticollis and scoliosis. Mikulicz acknowledged Heineke's independent development of pyloroplasty.[73] A novel technique of the Billroth II type gastrectomy was introduced by him in 1889. Mikulicz fashioned a retrocolic side-to-side gastrojejunostomy with isoperistaltic alignment of the jejunum.[67, 68] A type of foot amputation for diseases of the talus and calcaneus is known as the Mikulicz-Wladimirowsky operation.[72] His pathologic studies included descriptions of the characteristics of rhinoscleroma in 1876 (Mikulicz cells) and of that peculiar pathologic entity of the salivary glands, called Mikulicz's disease and Mikulicz's syndrome 12 years later.[76, 79]

Billroth's interest in the parotid gland must be recalled[7] as he described tumors of this region in great detail and coined the term "cylindroma." In 1884, Mikulicz successfully operated on a perforated typhoid ulcer, a pioneering achievement by itself. The monograph on diseases of the mouth (1898) is a classic treatise.

Mikulicz found that the abdominal esophagus could be operated upon without an ensuing tension pneumothorax, and he was the first to successfully perform a gastric cardiectomy (1898).

A pioneer accomplishment evolved from his collaborations with Sauerbruch, namely, the experimental and clinical demonstration of the feasibility of transpleural thoracotomy under differential pressure (1904). Mikulicz thus coauthored the opening stages of an entirely new surgical era, the surgical penetration of the thoracic cage.[78]

Two generations were to pass from Billroth's time before Sauerbruch's pupil, Rudolph Nissen, accomplished the first total pneumonectomy for bronchiectasis in 1931. Nissen employed mass ligation of the hilum and allowed the lung to slough. Two years later Evarts Graham performed the first successful one-stage pneumonectomy for cancer of the lung (1933).

In 1903 Mikulicz described the treatment of colon cancer by exteriorization.[69] This was essentially the procedure utilized by Bryant (1882), Bloch (1892), and Paul (1895).

Just as the immortal Evarts Graham became a victim of cancer of the lung, which he had been the first to cure surgically, Mikulicz's life was cut short by an inoperable stomach cancer. He, himself, made the diagnosis by palpating the abdominal mass, which proved to be a carcinomatous extension from the posterior wall of the stomach invading the pancreas.[24] Von Eiselsberg established its inoperability on exploration. Mikulicz spent the final days prior to his death holding meetings in his home, encouraging and advising his pupils in what directions to carry their life's work. So close a parallel existed between the life and spirit of Billroth and Mikulicz that Billroth's letter in 1894 to Gersuny, written while looking across the sea in Abbazia and speculating beyond his worldly enclosure, could well have been written by Mikulicz: "My life was overly rich. I have received a lot and I was glad to give as much as I was able. Now, at the end of my life, in beauty and harmonious form it fades noiselessly from me. I hope the same for my good wife, my dear children, and my good faithful friends."

Mikulicz's letter to v. Eiselsberg a few days before his death said, "I am saying goodbye without reproach. I am satisfied with my life. I worked as hard as I was able to, I have been accorded considerable recognition, and I have been happy." Mikulicz died at the height of his activity and fame. The pupil of a master surgeon, Mikulicz had become an acknowledged leader in his profession.

Mikulicz's trip in 1903 to England and the United States where he lectured and demonstrated his surgical procedures which were new on our continent, was a triumph. Honorary degrees were conferred on him in Edinburgh, Glasgow, and Philadelphia; he was elected to the membership of the American Surgical Association, the College of Physicians, and the New York Academy of Medicine.

The monthly, *Mitteilungen aus den Grenzgebieten der Medizin und Chirurgie,* which Mikulicz founded with Naunyn in 1896, was carried on in the hands of Anton v. Eiselsberg.

**Hacker (1852 to 1933).** Viktor v. Hacker was a product of Vienna. Born in 1852, he received his medical degree in 1878. After his assistantship under Billroth, he became director of the Sophien-Spital in Vienna.[66] He was appointed Professor of Surgery first in Innsbruck (1895) and later in Graz (1903). The experience with antiseptic treatment of wounds by the Billroth Clinic was summarized by Hacker in 1883. The translation of this book into the English language attests to its great importance in that day.[52] In 1886, he summarized the experience of the Billroth Clinic with gastrectomies,[53] and coauthored another study, *Gastric Operations in Cicatrical Stenoses* (1895), with G. Lotheissen. Hacker's works on chemical esophageal stenoses (1889), congenital anomalies and injuries of the esophagus (1905), replacement of the esophagus with the transverse colon (1914), and surgery of the esophagus (1926), approached the most difficult field in the surgical treatment of the digestive system.[59] In his other studies he contributed to plastic surgery,[55, 58] treatment of tracheal strictures,[56] mediastinitis,[54] and neurosurgery.[51]

**Fränkel (1857 to 1929).** Billroth's interest in surgical therapy of war injuries stemmed from his experiences in the field hospitals in Weissenburg and Mannheim (1870). Alexander Fränkel continued these endeavors. Born in Jassy, Rumania, he obtained his medical doctor's degree in 1880 in Vienna. After 3 years as Demonstrator in Pathology, he was assistant in the Billroth Clinic from 1884 to 1890.

In the Balkan campaign and in World War I he brought military surgery to a higher level.[30] From 1895 to 1929, as Chief of Surgery of the Wiener Allgemeine Polyklinik, he published studies on thrombosis, embolism, peritoneal sepsis, coverage of cranial defects, treatment of umbilical hernia, traumatic epilepsy, wound healing, surgical therapy of tuberculosis, cancer, and so forth.[31-35] Fränkel was editor of the *Wiener Klinische Wochenschrift* for 25 years.

**Eiselsberg (1860 to 1939).** All of Billroth's assistants acquired some characteristics of their friend and teacher, Theodor Billroth. He again was well aware of the qualities and potential of his pupils. He had called Eiselsberg, then in the early stages of his professional development, "an eminent surgeon of the first order." Eiselsberg surpassed Billroth in one respect, namely, 19 of his assistants succeeded to chairmanships of departments of surgery or as heads of surgical specialties.[22, 83] In the history of surgical education, only our great Halsted has been able to equal this record.[17]

Anton Eiselsberg was born in 1860 in Steinhaus, Austria. After studies in Würzburg, Zurich, Paris, and Vienna, he obtained his medical degree in 1884. Assistant to Billroth since 1887, he was appointed 6 years later as Chairman of the Surgical Clinic in Utrecht succeeding Salzer.

The fame of Billroth was such that his assistants were called to foreign lands as surgeons-educators, even though they hardly spoke a word of the country's tongue. The fact that Winiwarter, when called to Liege, had to learn French in 3 months in order to deliver his lecture course, was impressive. Eiselsberg learned Dutch in as short a period of time. In 1896, he accepted the chair of surgery in Königsberg, having been offered the professorship in Prague the same year.

A distinguished career for Eiselsberg was assured by his appointment in 1901 as Albert's successor. For Eiselsberg to replace Albert was not a small task. Albert was the greatest speaker and teacher since Josef Hyrtl. His lecture course was more popular with the students than Billroth's, a fact that Billroth reluctantly accepted in one of his writings.[16] His precise evaluation of a disease process as a pathologic entity was exemplary.[65] Albert's *Diagnosis of Surgical Diseases,* which reached 9 editions, demonstrated the diagnostic excellence for which he was famous and its clarity was hailed as an example of medical writing. The honor of being the only Austrian up to that time to be elected to the membership of the Royal College of Surgeons in England proved his international reputation.

Eiselsberg's monograph on fracture treatment continued the traditions of his predecessor, but he looked into new fields. He made contributions in the experimental laboratory as well as in clinical investigations. He was the first to transplant a sarcoma to a rat and thus stimulated the field of experimental oncology.[26]

To improve his bacteriologic knowledge, Billroth sent young Eiselsberg to Robert Koch's laboratory in Berlin. Studies on detection of cocci in the blood and sweat, on the bacterial content of soaps and dressings, and on tetanus were stimulated by this association. The demonstration of pyogenic organisms in blood smears from patients suffering from infections with a septic clinical course was of practical significance.[25]

The early clinical works of Eiselsberg concerning surgery of the thyroid gland and its relationship to the development of tetany after total thyroidectomy for a functional thyroid carcinoma are classical. Temporary postoperative hypothyroidism was relieved spontaneously when metastases appeared in the skull and recurred upon excision of the secondary deposits. In 1892, Eiselsberg successfully transplanted autologous thyroid glands into the abdominal wall of thyroidectomized cats.[27] Upon excision of the grafts, the animals developed tetany; the parathyroid glands were at that time, of course, unknown.

Surgery of the gastrointestinal tract was Eiselsberg's major preoccupation during his lifetime. In 1895, he reported on 38 operations for gastric cancer that included 28 gastroenterostomies with a mortality rate of 25 per cent and 10 gastrectomies with a mortality rate of 50 per cent. The anastomoses were performed in 3 layers. As early as 1897, he could report on 40 major anastomotic surgical procedures by his hand with a mortality rate of 17.5 per cent. None of the patients had died of a leak in the suture line, an unusual achievement for this period.

Eiselsberg brought gastrointestinal surgery as practiced in his day to a high level of performance. These accomplishments, which Billroth foresaw, must have been a great satisfaction to him. Billroth often reminisced about his own early surgical days. Trying to gain experience, he had performed laparotomies mostly in hopeless cases but without concern for complications. Billroth admitted that the number of patients lost was great. Some were saved, however, and experience was gained for the future.

Hypophyseal surgery was developed in Vienna under Eiselsberg's leadership.[23] One of his pupils, Bernard Aschner, was able in 1909 to obtain survivals in puppies after hypophysectomy and demonstrate, thus, the growth function of the pituitary gland.[1] Eiselsberg was one of the first to treat acromegaly by surgical intervention, reporting in 1912 on 16 hypophyseal operations. Eiselsberg's studies on the vertebral column and brain gave impetus to the growth of neurosurgery. It remained for Harvey Cushing, however, to develop this discipline into an entirely independent specialty. In 1907, Eiselsberg performed his first successful removal of a spinal tumor and as early as 1913 was able to report with Ranzi on 208 brain and spinal tumor operations.

Eiselsberg, just as Billroth, chose his students with great care. Everyone had to prove himself in another medical discipline, be it anatomy, pathology, bacteriology, chemistry, or internal medicine, prior to entering his clinic. The only subject of no importance in this selection was surgical "know-how"; that he was able to supply himself.[83]

Billroth was of the same opinion. "The art of operating," he stated, "has as any other art, a certain basic technique which can be taught and learned. The operative technique is based on knowledge of anatomy and individual ability. Technical talent can be replaced by constant exercise, as long as other attributes pertaining to a physician are available."

The admiration and love of his pupils was expressed in the *Lehrbuch der Chirurgie A. von Eiselsberg* (Berlin, 1930). Anton v. Eiselsberg received many honors and became the second surgeon to be awarded the coveted Lister gold medal. He was awarded honorary doctors' degrees from the Universities of Athens, Budapest, Debreczin, Edinburgh, Geneva, Leiden, Vienna and the Sorbonne. Such distinctions as the presidencies of the German and International Surgical Societies did not spoil a humble man. When Eiselsberg reached 75 years of age, he declined the holding of any official public ceremonies in his honor.

## THE VIENNA SURGICAL SCHOOL, BILLROTH, AND THE SELECTION OF HIS SUCCESSORS

Founding of the Allgemeine Krankenhaus (Fig. 7) in 1784 was the first essential step in the development of the Viennese Surgical School. Ferdinand Joseph v. Leber, Vinzenz v. Kern, and Joseph v. Wattman were its early members. The two most important surgical figures of the pre-Billroth era were Johann v. Dumreicher and Franz Schuh (Figs. 8 and 9).

Dumreicher, who was famous for the unitarian concept of medicine and surgery which he had developed in his thesis *De Unione Medicinae et Chirurgiae,* was in-

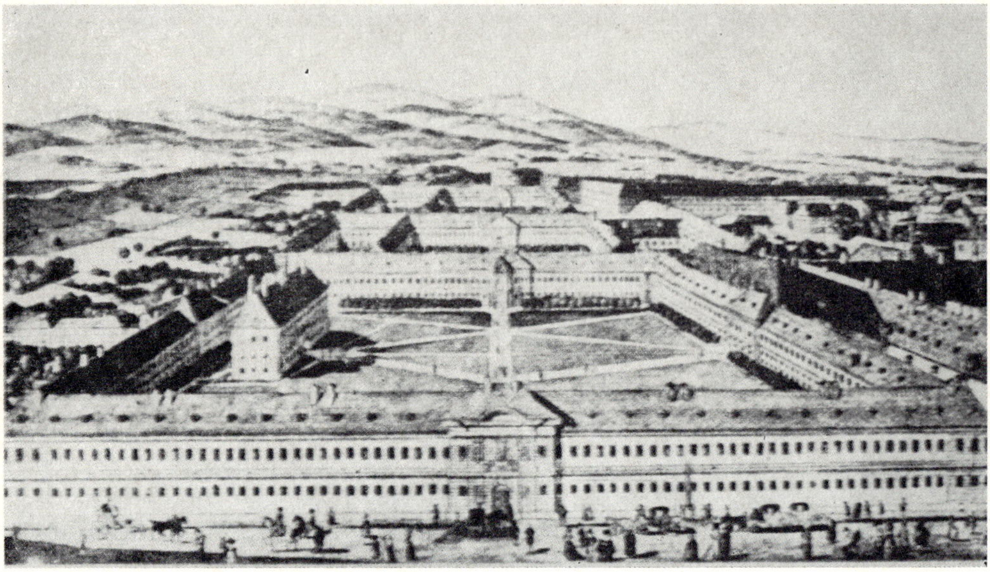

**Fig. 7.** Das Allgemeine Krankenhaus at time of foundation by Joseph II in 1784.

FOUNDING OF DAS ALLGEMEINE KRANKENHAUS - 1784

Ferdinand Joseph v. Leber
1729-1808
Prof. of Surgery 1762-1805

Conrad M. Langenbeck
1776-1851
Prof. of Surgery
Göttingen 1814-1848

B.V. Langenbeck
1810-1887
Prof. of Surgery
Berlin 1848-1882

Vinzenz v. Kern
1760-1829
Prof. of Surgery 1805-1823

Joseph v. Wattmann
1789-1866
Prof. of Surgery 1830-1847

1842
Surgical
Service Split
Into

1st Surgical Division

Johann v. Dumreicher
1815-1880
Prof. of Surgery 1848-1880

Eduard Albert
1841-1900
Prof. of Surgery 1881-1900

Anton v. Eiselsberg
1860-1939
Prof. of Surgery 1901-1938

Egon Ranzi
1875-1939
Prof. of Surgery 1938-1939

L. Schönbauer
1888-
Prof. of Surgery 1939-
Presently Emeritus

2nd Surgical Division

Franz Schuh
1805-1867
Prof. of Surgery 1842-1867

Christian Albert Theodor Billroth
1829-1894
Prof. of Surgery 1868-1894

Karl Gussenbauer
1842-1903
Prof. of Surgery 1894-1903

Julius v. Hochenegg
1859-1940
Prof. of Surgery 1904-1930

Wolfgang Denk
1882-
Prof. of Surgery 1931-
Presently Emeritus

**Fig. 8.** The genealogy of the Vienna surgical school.

strumental in splitting the growing surgical university service in 1841.

Schuh, the first head of the newly built Second Surgical Clinic, adopted and expanded Joseph Skoda's clinical diagnostic techniques for the surgical patient. He was the first to aspirate successfully a pericardial effusion by means of a trocar and cannula in 1841.

It is odd that Billroth, who must have been familiar with his predecessor Schuh's successes concerning pericardial paracenthesis, vehemently opposed this procedure. His statement as late as 1882 that "paracenthesis of the dropsical pericardium is an operation which, in my opinion, is very near what some surgeons call prostitution of the art of surgery and others call surgical frivolity" was whimsical but retarded progress in this field. There is no evidence that Billroth ever opposed Schuh in any other way. A keen student of history, Billroth must have been familiar with the original suggestion to aspirate pericardial fluid by Riolanus (1649) and Morgagni's demonstration that pressure upon the heart by effusion in the pericardial sac could cause cardiac arrest. Two years after Billroth's pronouncement, we find Gussenbauer (1884) draining a pericardial effusion through the thorax with complete recovery of the patient. He resected the left fifth rib anteriorly with the intention of draining a thoracic empyema. In 1895, Eiselsberg successfully drained a purulent pericardial accumulation.

Surgery of the thoracic cavity and the heart presented to Billroth a psychological barrier. He was not able to foresee the development of cardiac surgery when he wrote in 1883, "The surgeon who would attempt suture of a cardiac wound should lose the respect of his colleagues." Tempora mutant!

Dumreicher, head of the First Surgical Clinic, and highly influential in the reigning circles, after rebuilding Austrian military medicine, urged Albert's appointment as his successor. Albert also had the support of Joseph Skoda, as acknowledged in his speech at the occasion of his twenty-fifth jubileum (1899).

Billroth and Albert together accomplished the reorganization of medical studies at Austrian universities (1878). Billroth's analysis of the Austrian and German university systems was translated into English which attested to its world-wide importance.[11] These attempts at reforms were of similar importance, even though not executed on as large a scale as the reforms of v. Swieten in Vienna 50 years before, or those of our own great medical educator, Simon Flexner, son of an immigrant coal miner from Bohemia, 30 years later.

By the time Albert took over Dumreicher's department, he was a seasoned surgeon, having held the professorship in Innsbruck from 1873 to 1881. Whereas Billroth was the more aggressive, adventurous, experimental surgeon, Albert was inclined to contemplative theorizing. His special fortes were diagnosing in the old tradition and precise performance of established surgical procedures. Albert's mastery of philosophy, mathematics, and descriptive geometry, which was acknowledged by his contemporaries in those specialties, helped in investigations on mechanisms of joint function, skeletal architecture, and heat economy of the heart and lungs. He published over 160 clinical and physiologic experimental studies, some of purely theoretical nature. His *History of Surgery* and several volumes of poetry are

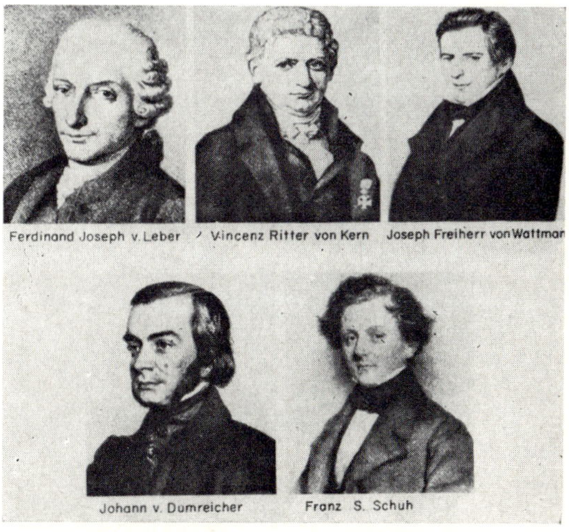


**Fig. 9.** Members of the Vienna surgical school, 1762 to 1880.

examples of his broad interests. Albert's appointment as Professor of Surgery despite Billroth's support of his own assistant, Czerny, was a great personal victory.

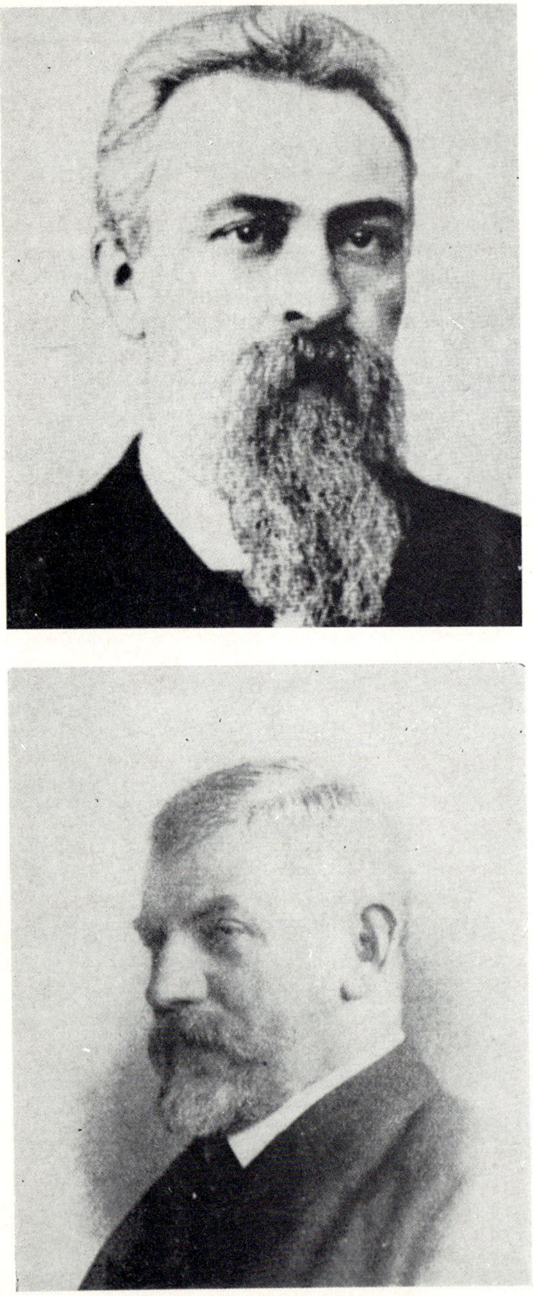

*A*

*B*

**Fig. 10.** *A,* Eduard Albert, Professor of Surgery, University of Vienna (First Surgical Division), 1848 to 1880, and *B,* his pupil, Julius Hochenegg, Professor of Surgery, University of Vienna (Second Surgical Division), 1904 to 1930.

Czerny's vindication must have been the offer extended to him in 1894 to succeed Billroth in Vienna. This was perhaps the greatest honor anyone could bestow on him. Despite Albert's urging, Czerny abruptly declined the appointment.[62] He was involved in planning his major accomplishment of building the cancer institute. In addition, it is likely that already at this time he was suffering from chronic leukemia.

The Second Surgical Service of Billroth was occupied by Gussenbauer until 1904, upon whose death Julius Hochenegg, the able pupil of Albert, was appointed Professor[60] (Fig. 10).

Eiselsberg's appointment to Albert's surgical professorship historically completes the circle. Justice was thereby done to both rival branches of the Vienna surgical school.

Billroth's musical talents favorably compare with Albert's poetic inclinations. Science and art imbibe from the same fountain! Billroth wrote to Brahms in 1886 saying that he had never known a scientist, or read about one, who in principle was not an artist with a rich and childish phantasy.

One may speculate why so many pupils of Billroth and, in general, many professors at the University in Vienna, such as Skoda, Rokitansky, Hebra, and Albert, came from provincial areas (Bohemia, Moravia, and Transylvania). The Austro-Hungarian empire was a multilingual conglomeration of German, Czech, Hungarian, Polish, Slovak, Ukranian, Rumanian, Croatian, and Italian speaking peoples. A strong element of centralization in Vienna, due to the fact that this city was the seat of the Emperor and the central government, brought greater support to its institutions of learning. This fact induced many ambitious individuals from the provinces to seek employment and advance their cause under more favorable circumstances. Greater competition produced better men and these men were able to build a university unequalled on the continent of Europe in the second half of the nineteenth century.

Surgeons always have built concepts, many of which disappeared and were forgotten as time passed by. It is of more than passing significance how many concepts introduced in Vienna by Billroth and his school still remain with us.

Billroth and his pupils probed in the laboratory, observed on the wards, and achieved in the operating theater!

The search for truth, the look into the future, with knowledge of what was accomplished in the past, was the credo of Billroth's surgical school.

I am grateful to Dr. Owen H. Wangensteen, Chief, Department of Surgery, University of Minnesota, for stimulating this study and for helpful assistance; to Dr. H. Schoenbauer, Professor of History of Medicine, University of Vienna; to Dr. A. S. Leonard, Department of Surgery, University of Minnesota; and to Mr. J. G. Ziegler, Greenwich, Connecticut, for corrections and advice. The assistance of Mrs. S. Matsuyama-Kobe, B.A., in the search for the pertinent references was greatly appreciated. I am also grateful for the materials used in the illustrations which were obtained from many sources, including L. Schoenbauer, *Das Medizinische Wien;* A. Hurwitz and G. A. Rogenshein, *Milestones in Modern Surgery;* the United States Public Health Service, Bethesda, Maryland; *Wiener Klinische Wochenschrift; Bulletin de l'Académie royale de médicine de Belgique;* and the Archives of History of Medicine, Department of Surgery, University of Minnesota.

## REFERENCES

1. Absolon, K. B.: Bernhard Aschner: surgeon, scientist, and scholar, SURGERY **48:** 979, 1960.
2. Anonymous: Alex. v. Winiwarter, Wien med. Wchnschr. **67:** 2166, 1917.
3. Billroth, T.: Die Allgemeine Chirurgische Pathologie und Therapie, Berlin, 1880, G. Reimer.
4. Billroth, T.: Aphorismen zu Lehren und Lernen der Medizinischen Wissenschaften, Wien, 1886, C. Gerold's So.
5. Billroth, T.: Magenresection, Wien. med. Presse **22:** 205, 1881.
6. Billroth, T.: De natura et causa affectionis, quae nervo vago utroque dissecto exoritur, Berolinum, 1852, thesis.
7. Billroth, T.: Speicheldrüsengeschwülste, Arch. path. Anat. **17:** 357, 1859.
8. Billroth, T.: Totalextirpation des ganzen Esophagus von Pharynx bis zum Sternum; eine Totalextirpation des ganzen Larynx mit der ganzen Schilddrüse, Verhandl. deutsch. Gesellsch. Chir. **8:** 7, 1879.
9. Billroth, T.: Über die Einewirkung lebender Pflanzen und Tierzellen aufienander. Eine biologische Studie, Wien, 1890, A. Hölder.
10. Billroth, T.: Über Esophagus—resection, Arch. klin. Chir. **13:** 65, 1872.
11. Billroth, T.: Über das Lehren und Lernen der Medizinischen Wissenschaften an den Universitäten der deutschen Nation, nebst allgemeinen Bemerkungen uber Universitäten, Wien, 1876, C. Gerold's So.
12. Billroth, T.: Über einen neuen Fall von gelungener Resection des Carcinomatösen Pylorus, Wien. med. Wchnschr. **31:** 1427, 1881.
13. Billroth, T.: Über die Resection des Kniegelenkes, Deutsche Klinik **33:** 1859.
14. Billroth, T.: Über die Resection des Oberschenkelkopfes, Deutsche Klinik **28,** 1859.
15. Billroth, T.: Untersuchungen über die Vegetationsformen von Coccobacteria Septica und deren Anteil welchen sie an die Entstehung und Verbreitung der accidentellen Wundkrankheiten haben, Berlin, 1874, G. Reimer.
16. Billroth, T.: Wie Sollen die Unterrichtsräume einer Chirurg. Klinik in Wien Beschaffen sein und wie könnten die in Ansicht genommenen Kliniken in dem Rahmen der k. und k. Allgemeinen Krankenhauses eingefügt werden? Eine Klinisch-tektonische Studie, Wien. klin. Wchnschr. **2:** 2, 1889.
17. Carter, B. N.: The fruition of Halsted's concept of surgical training, SURGERY **32:** 518, 1952.
18. Czerny, V.: Das Heidelberger Institute für Experimentelle Krebsforschung, Tübingen, 1912, H. Laupp.
19. Czerny, V.: Neue Operationen. Resection d. Esophagus, Zentralbl. chir. **4:** 433, 1877.
20. Czerny, V., and Rindfleisch, W.: Darmnähte und Darmresectionen, Beitr. klin. Chir. Festschr. T. Billroth, 1892.
21. Czerny, V., and Rindfleisch, W.: Über die an der Heidelberger Chirurg. Klinik ausgeführten Operationen an Magen und Darm, Beitr. klin. Chir. **9:** 661, 1892.
22. Denk, W.: Anton v. Eiselsberg, Sein Lernen u. Wirken, Wien. klin. Wchnschr. **53:** 55, 1940.
23. Eiselsberg, A.: Hypophysenoperation bei Degen. Adiposogenitalis, Wien. klin. Wchnschr. **21:** 1115, 1908.
24. Eiselsberg, A.: Johann v. Mikulicz-Radecki, Wien. klin. Wchnschr. **18:** 671, 1905.
25. Eiselsberg, A.: Nachweis von Eiterkokken im Blut als diagnostisches Hilfsmittel, Wien. klin. Wchnschr. **3:** 731, 1890.
26. Eiselsberg, A.: Transplantation eines Fibrosarkoms bei Ratten, Wien. klin. Wchnschr. **3:** 927, 1890.
27. Eiselsberg, A.: Transplantat der Katzen-

schilddrüse und Auftreten von Tetanie nach Entfernung des engeheilten Transplantats, Wien. klin. Wchnschr. **5**, 1892.
28. Fränkel, A.: Carl C. Gussenbauer, Wien. klin. Wchnschr. **16:** 757, 1903.
29. Fränkel, A.: R. Gersuny, Wien. klin. Wchnschr. **37:** 1197, 1924.
30. Fränkel, A.: Kriegschirurgische Mitteilungen aus dem Deutschen Ordenspitale in Belgrad, Wien. med. Wchnschr. **36:** 381, 1886.
31. Fränkel, A.: Zur Lehre von der Krebskrankheit, Wien. med. Wchnschr. **72:** 229, 1922.
32. Fränkel, A.: Nabelhernien, Wien. klin. Wchnschr. **21:** 1558, 1908.
33. Fränkel, A.: Schädeldefect und Epilepsie, Wien. klin. Wchnschr. **18:** 982, 1905.
34. Fränkel, A.: Über peritoneale Infection, Wien. klin. Wchnschr. **4:** 291, 1891.
35. Fränkel, A.: Über postoperative Thromboembolie, Arch. klin. Chir. **86:** 531, 1908.
36. Gersuny, R.: Aphoristisches und Darmchirurgie, Int. klin. Rundschau **8:** 73, 1894.
37. Gersuny, R.: Eine Dauersonde für die Speiseröhre, Wien. med. Wchnschr. **37:** 1645, 1887.
38. Gersuny, R.: Doctor and patient: hints to both, London, 1898, J. Wright & Co.
39. Gersuny, R.: Eine neue Operation zur Heilung der Incontinentia Urinae, Zentralbl. Chir. **16:** 433, 1889.
40. Gersuny, R.: Operation bei Kontraktur der Palmaraponeurose, Wien. med. Wchnschr. **34:** 969, 1884.
41. Gersuny, R.: Die Septumnaht bei Prolapsoperationen, Wien. klin. Wchnschr. **16:** 1105, 1893.
42. Gersuny, R.: Eine Sphincteroplastik am Darm, Zentralbl. Chir. **20:** 553, 1893.
43. Gersuny, R.: Theodor Billroth, Meister d. Heilkunde, Rikola Ed., 1929.
44. Gersuny, R.: Über Falsche Diagnosen, Wien. med. Wchnschr. **37:** 1645, 1887.
45. Gersuny, R.: Vinzenz Czerny, Wien. klin. Wchnschr. **29:** 1375, 1916.
46. Gussenbauer, C.: Ein Beitrag zur Kenntniss und Extirpation der Schädelgeschwülste, Ztschr. f. Heilk. **5:** 139, 1884.
47. Gussenbauer, C.: In memoriam. T. Billroth, Wien. klin. Wchnschr. **10:** 982, 1897.
48. Gussenbauer, C.: Zur Operativen Behandlung der Pankreascysten, Arch. klin. Chir. **29:** 358, 1883.
49. Gussenbauer, C.: Zur Operativen Behandlung der tiefliegenden traumatischen Hirnabcesse, Prag. med. Wchnschr. **10:** 1, 1885.
50. Gussenbauer, C.: Theodor Billroth, Prag. med. Wchnschr. **19:** 89, 1894.
51. Hacker, V.: Ersatz von Schädeldefecten durch unter die Kopfschwarte verschobene oder umgeklappte Periostknochenlappen beziehungsweise Periostlappen, Beitr. klin. Chir. **38:** 499, 1903.
52. Hacker, V.: Introduction to the antiseptic treatment of wounds according to the method in use at Prof. Billroth's clinic in Vienna, London, 1891, Parcival & Co.
53. Hacker, V.: Die Magenoperationen an Prof. Billroth's Klinik, 1880 bis März 1885, Wien, 1886, Toeplitz-Deuticke.
54. Hacker, V.: Zur operativen Behandlung der periesophagealen und mediastinalen Phlegmone nebst Bemerkungen zur Technik der Mediastinotomie, Arch. klin. Chir. **44:** 478, 1901.
55. Hacker, V.: Über den autoplastischen Ersatz der Streck und der Beugesehnen der Finger durch entbehrliche Sehnen des Handrückens, Beitr. klin. Chir. **66:** 259, 1910.
56. Hacker, V.: Über die Behandlung der Narbenstricturen des Luftrohres und die Mangoldt'sche Laryngo-Tracheoplastic, Beitr. klin. Chir. **44:** 762, 1904.
57. Hacker, V.: Über Resection und Plastik am Halsabschnitt bei Carcinom, Verhandl. deutsch. Gesellsch. Chir. **37:** 359, 1908.
58. Hacker, V.: Wangenplastik mit am Sternalrand gestielten, gegen die Schulter verlaufenden Brusthautlappen, Wien. klin. Wchnschr. **23:** 48, 1910.
59. Hacker, V., and Lotheissen, G.: Chirurgie der Speiseröhre, Stuttgart, 1926, G. Enke.
60. Heyrowsky, H.: V. v. Hochenegg, Wien. klin. Wchnschr. **53:** 499, 1940.
61. Hochberg, L. A.: Thoracic surgery before the 20th century, New York, 1960, Vantage Press.
62. Hurwitz, A., and Regensheim, G. A.: Milestones in modern surgery, New York, 1958, Paul B. Hoeber, Inc.
63. Jirásek, A.: Eduard Albert, Prague, 1946, Cěskoslov. Chir. Spol.
64. Leonardo, R. A.: Lives of master surgeons, New York, 1948, Froben Press, Inc.
65. Lorenz, A.: Eduard Albert, Wien. klin. Wchnschr. **13:** 895, 1900.
66. Lotheissen, G.: Victor v. Hacker, Wien. med. Wchnschr. **83:** 775, 1933.
67. Mikulicz-Radecki, J.: Beiträge zur Technik der Operation des Magencarcinoms, Arch. klin. Chir. **57:** 524, 1898.
68. Mikulicz-Radecki, J.: Bericht über 103 Operationen am Magen, Arch. klin. Chir. **51:** 9, 1896.
69. Mikulicz-Radecki, J.: Chirurgische Erfahrumgen über den Darmcarcinom, Arch. klin. Chir. **69:** 28, 1903.
70. Mikulicz-Radecki, J.: Ein Fall Von Resection des carcinomatosen Esophagus mit plastischen Ersatz des excidierten Stückes, Prag. med. Wchnschr. **11:** 10, 1886.

71. Mikulicz-Radecki, J.: Die Methoden der Schmerzbetäubung und Ihre gegenseitige Abgrenzung, Arch. klin. Chir. **64:** 209, 1901.
72. Mikulicz-Radecki, J.: Eine neue Osteoplastische Resectionsmethode am Fusse, Arch. klin. Chir. **26:** 494, 1881.
73. Mikulicz-Radecki, J.: Zur operativen Behandlung des stenosierenden Magengeschwüres, Arch. klin. Chir. **37:** 80, 1888.
74. Mikulicz-Radecki, J.: Das Operieren in sterilisierten Zwirnhandschuhen und mit Mundbinde: ein Beitrag zur Sicherung des aseptischen Verlaufs von Operationswunden, Zentralbl. Chir. **24:** 713, 1897.
75. Mikulicz-Radecki, J.: Über die Anwendung der Antisepsis bei Laparatomien mit besonderer Rücksicht auf die Drainage der Peritonealhöhle, Arch. klin. Chir. **26:** 111, 1881.
76. Mikulicz-Radecki, J.: Über eine eigenartige Erkrankung der Tränen und Mundspeicheldrüsen, Beitr. klin. Chir. Festschr. T. Billroth, 1892.
77. Mikulicz-Radecki, J.: Über Gastroscopie und Oesophagoscopie, Zentralbl. Chir. **8:** 673, 1881.
78. Mikulicz-Radecki, J.: Über Operationen in der Brusthöhle mit Hilfe der Sauerbruchschen Kammer, Deutsch. med. Wchnschr. **30:** 530, 1904.
79. Mikulicz-Radecki, J.: Über das Rhinoslerom (Hebra), Arch. klin. Chir. **20:** 458, 1876.
80. Mikulicz-Radecki, J.: Versuche über Resistenzvermehrung des Peritoneums gegen Infection bei Magen und Darmoperationen, Arch. klin. Chir. **73:** 347, 1904.
81. Sauerbruch, E. F.: Johann v. Mikulcz-Radecki, München. med. Wchnschr. **52:** 1297, 1905.
82. Schloffer, H.: Anton Wölfler, Wien. med. Wchnschr. **67:** 47, 1917.
83. Schönbauer, L.: Das Medizinische Wien, Wien, 1944, Urban u. Schwarzenberg.
84. Willems, M.: A. Winiwarter, Bull. Acad. roy. méd. Bélg. **5:** 541, 1925.
85. Winiwarter, A.: Ein Fall von Gallenretention bedingt durch Impermeabilität des Ductus Choledochus. Anlegung einer Gallenblasen-Darmfistel, Heilung, Prag. med. Wchnschr. **7:** 201, 1882.
86. Winiwarter, A.: Vor sechsundreissig Jahren. Errinerungen an T. Billroth, Wien. klin. Wchnschr. **20:** 309, 1907.
87. Winiwarter, A.: Synopsis of the statistics of carcinoma mammae, from the clinic of Prof. Billroth at Vienna (translated by G. Wieber from Beitr. Statistik der Carcinome), Ann. Anat. & S. Soc. Brooklyn **1:** 23, 1879.
88. Winiwarter, F.: Über eine Eigentümliche Form von Endarteritis und Endophlebitis mit Gangrän des Fusses, Arch. klin. Chir. **23:** 202, 1879.
89. Wölfler, A.: Gastroenterostomie, Zentralbl. Chir. **8:** 705, 1881.
90. Wölfler, A.: Die Radikaloperation des freien Leistenbruches, Beitr. klin. Chir. Festschr. T. Billroth, 1892.
91. Wölfler, A.: Über die Entwicklung und den Bau des Kropfes, Arch. klin. Chir. **29:** 754, 1883.
92. Wölfler, A.: Über den Parasacralen und Pararectalen Schnitt für Blosslegung des Rectum, des Uterus und der Vagina, Wien. klin. Wchnschr. **2:** 296, 1889.
93. Wölfler, A.: Über die Technik und Wert von Schleimhautübertragungen, Arch. klin. Chir. **37:** 709, 1888.

# An intimate view of the Letheon controversy

GEORGE A. DEGENSHEIN, M.D.
ALFRED HURWITZ, M.D.
BROOKLYN, N. Y.
*From the Department of Surgery, Maimonides Hospital*

The discovery of anesthetics was like the opening of the door to an endless corridor flanked on either side with countless other doors, all slightly ajar and waiting for someone to push them open and reveal their secrets. The importance of this milestone is self-evident, but the tremendous impact it had on the development not only of surgery, but also of related fields, was immeasurable. It marked the end of the era of stop-watch surgery, and provided the "open sesame" to a surgical attack on all organs of the body. In contradistinction to the rapid and crude operations that had to be practiced in the preanesthetic era, surgical procedures could now be refined to embrace careful hemostasis, painstaking exposure, and meticulous handling of tissues.

In 1824 Hickman attempted to relieve pain by inhalation of gas. This work was negated by the Royal Society when Davy, who had also reported the analgesic properties of nitrous oxide, was president. Jackson, who first familiarized Crawford Long with the properties of ether, failed to recognize its value and its eventual impact on mankind. The ill-fated Horace Wells, who failed in his attempt to introduce nitrous oxide as an anesthetic, committed suicide. Pope actually performed the first dental extraction under ether administered by Clarke, but he also was unaware of its potentialities. Crawford Long removed a tumor from the neck of a patient under ether anesthesia in 1842, but did not report the incident until 1846. His discovery was based on the observation of insensibility to pain induced during "ether frolics" which were in vogue in Georgia at that time.

It remained for Morton (Fig. 1) to convince Dr. John C. Warren, a senior surgeon at the Massachusetts General Hospital in Boston, of the efficacy of ether as an anesthetic agent. The success of the experiment (Fig. 2) received immediate acclaim and initiated the impetus to its widespread use. Morton, who had given up a lucrative dental practice, then tried to patent ether under the name of Letheon. He actually received a patent, but it was rescinded. Wells, Jackson, and Long all filed claims to priority and the fight was carried to the United States Senate. A patent was refused after several attempts, and even the President of the United States became involved. In 1862 Morton, broken and humiliated, returned to his farm, where he lived in poverty until 1868. Goaded on by a new pamphlet written by Jackson, he journeyed to New York to file suit against him and died there of a stroke a few days later. It is a paradox that a discovery which was to relieve more suffering than any other should have brought so much misery to the principals who were responsible for it. The Letheon controversy received considerable publicity and the good name of medicine suffered.

In our researches for *Milestones in Modern Surgery* we came across an article written by Mrs. William T. G. Morton (Fig. 3) on the fiftieth anniversary of her husband's demonstration of his discovery. We have not been able to identify the magazine since the pages carried no name in the heading.

Although volumes have been written on the subject, this article gives such a heart-rending personal account of Morton's fate, that we considered it worthy of reproduction.

## THE DISCOVERY OF ANESTHESIA*

### Dr. W. T. G. Morton and his heroic battle for a new idea. How painless surgery began fifty years ago.

**By Elizabeth Whitman Morton**

My husband, whose full name was William Thomas Green Morton, was born in Charlton, Massachusetts, August 19, 1819. The family house stood on a farm of about one hundred acres, and was an old-fashioned wooden structure with an immense stone chimney in the centre. It was shaded by old trees, and covered by creepers and climbing plants. It was a typical New England farm-house, and the boy grew up among wholesome surroundings, gaining a strength of body that served him in the severe strain of later years. Curiously enough, even at an early age his mind turned naturally toward medicine, and he was nicknamed "doctor" by his playmates, for whose imaginary ills he used to prescribe learnedly from an outfit of elder-tree vials and bread pills. On one occasion he nearly caused the death of his little sister by pouring down her throat some extraordinary concoction of his own, while she lay asleep in her cradle.

The instruction he received was imparted in the schools of his native town and at the neighboring academies of Leicester and Northfield, where he studied hard for three years, leaving at the age of seventeen, when he went to Boston to begin earning his living. Here he gained employment in the publishing house of the editor of the "Christian Witness," James B. Dow, whose beautiful wife took a great interest in him and arranged that he should live with them. Both Mr. and Mrs. Dow showed themselves staunch friends to the young man, and recognized his unusual talents. The friendship was maintained to the end of Dr. Morton's life. Kind as they were to him, however, he soon became dissatisfied, his duties allowing him little time for study, which was his great ambition. So devoted was the boy to books that all his leisure moments were spent in reading. A few months of this busy life convinced him that he could never be happy in that way of existence, and, uncertain what to do and homesick, he went back to his father's house in Charlton. He then concluded to study dentistry, which at that time had attained the dignity of a respected profession.

His success was rapid. In 1844, two years after his graduation at the Baltimore College of Dental Surgery (the first dental college established in America), he was earning from his profession an income of about ten thousand dollars, being already recognized as one of the most skilful dental surgeons in Boston. He had established himself in Boston a little before our marriage, I being a young girl of seventeen, just out of Miss Porter's school at Farmington, Connecticut, where my father lived. For a year before, Dr. Morton had paid me attentions, which were not well received by my family, he being regarded as a poor young man with an undesirable profession. I thought him very handsome, however, and he

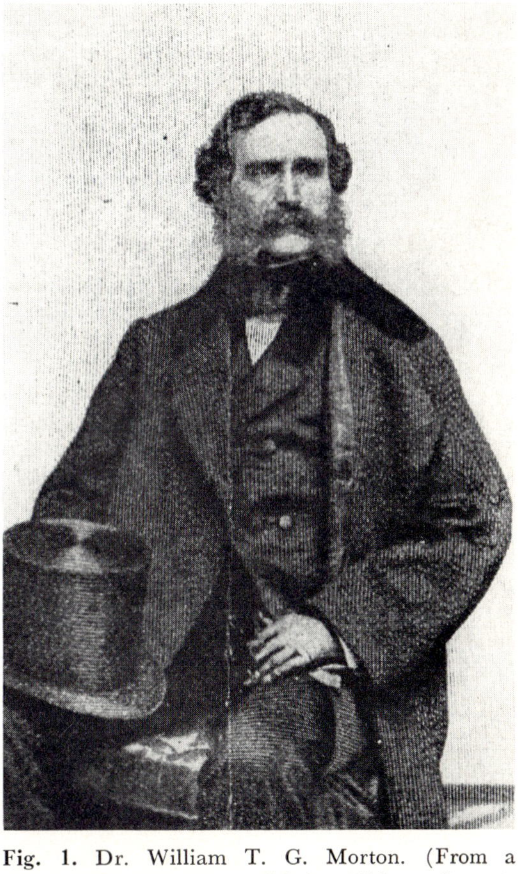

**Fig. 1.** Dr. William T. G. Morton. (From a photograph taken in 1854 by Silsbee, Case & Co., Boston, Mass.)

*It will be fifty years on the 16th of next October since Dr. Morton publicly proved his priceless discovery, and the jubilee of the events is to be celebrated in Boston.

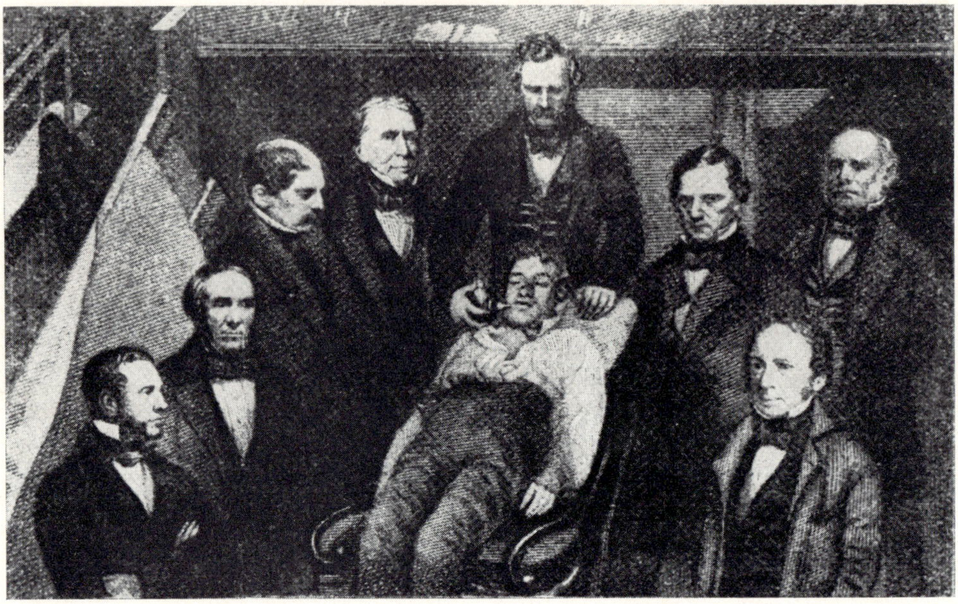

**Fig. 2.** Dr. Morton making the first public demonstration of etherization at the Massachusetts General Hospital, Boston, Oct. 16, 1846. (After a steel engraving published in *Trials of a Public Benefactor,* by Nathan P. Rice, M.D., New York, 1859, Pudney and Russell, Publishers.)

was much in love with me, coming regularly from Boston to visit me. I learned later on that from the first day he saw me he had determined to marry me if he could, and after his death I found in an old diary of that year an entry written just after my first meeting with him, where he expressed his intention of making me his wife, and even noted the gown and hood I wore. In my eighteenth year he took me from the fine old homestead we lived in—quite an historic mansion it was, where John C. Calhoun had often visited my father's family—and brought me to Boston. My uncle Lemuel was then a classmate of Calhoun's in Yale, and later on a member of Congress from Connecticut. Two others of my Whitman ancestors, father and son, were graduated at Harvard, one in 1668, and the other in 1696. The son settled in Farmington as one of the earliest ministers.

Dr. Morton was one of those tremendously earnest men who believe they have a high destiny to fulfil. How may times he said to me in the months preceding his great discovery: "I have a work to do in this world, Lizzie!" Or, again: "The time will come when I will do away with pain!" During our early married life, while he was making himself known as one of the most skilful dentists in Boston and carrying on an enormous business, he found time in addition to pursue his medical studies at the Harvard Medical School, in order to take a medical degree, for he had promised my mother to give up dentistry. Every morning he used to rise between four and five o'clock to get time for what he called his serious work; and never shall I forget my sensation as a young bride at sleeping in a room where a tall, gaunt skeleton stood in a big box near the head of the bed. After the first successful use of the sulphuric ether, the immense responsibilities that came upon him, and the unceasing anxiety and annoyances, compelled him to give up the study of medicine and devote himself to anesthesia. This was a great grief to him, because he was at that time within a few months of taking his degree.

At the time of our marriage Dr. Morton was twenty-four years old, and, as I have said, his mind was already occupied with thoughts destined to lead to his discovery. Every spare hour he could get was spent in experiment. At Wellesley, Massachusetts, where was our summer home, there was a spring which contained a number of gold-fish, and I noticed that my husband would often go to it, and I would see him catching the fish and looking at them intently as if studying them as he held them wriggling in his hand. Then he used to make experiments nearly every day on "Nig," a black water-spaniel, a good-sized dog that had belonged to his father. I was only a girl of eighteen at this time, and had not the least idea of what he was trying to do; nor would I have understood the importance of his experiments had he told me. I only knew that his clothes seemed always saturated with the smell of ether, and I did not like it. One day he came running into the house in great distress (for he was always tender-hearted), leading the dog, which walked rather queerly, and said:

"Poor Nig; I've had him asleep a long time. I was afraid I had killed him."

"Do you put the fish asleep, too?" I asked, laughing.

"I try to," he said quite seriously, "but have not succeeded yet."

I laughed again, thinking it was all a joke, but my husband became very grave, and said:

"The time will come, my dear, when I will banish pain from the world."

It was at this time also that he used to bottle-up all sorts of queer bugs and insects, until the house was full of crawling things. He would administer ether to all these little creatures, and especially to the big green worms he found on grapevines.

I remember how Dr. Morton's friends laughed at these queer experiments, and I am afraid I joined with them sometimes. But he continued on his way undaunted, frequently saying: "I shall succeed; there must be some way of deadening pain."

As he began to near success I became alarmed, for, not satisfied with trying the ether on bugs and animals, my husband began experimenting upon himself. He sent out his assistants offering a reward of five dollars to any person who would have a tooth drawn while under the influence of his pain-annulling agency. There were many people suffering from aching teeth which needed to be extracted, and the five dollars was an object; but no one could be induced to take the risk. Finally his two assistants allowed him to experiment upon them, but the result was not satisfactory, because of impurities in the ether. Having detected this, my husband, with characteristic persistence, at once procured a supply of pure ether, and, unwilling to wait longer for a subject, shut himself up in his office, and tested it upon himself with such successs that for several minutes he lay there unconscious. That night he came home late, in a great state of excitement, but so happy that he could scarcely calm himself to tell me what had occurred; and I, too, became so excited that I could scarcely wait to hear. At last he told me of the experiment upon himself, and I grew sick at heart as the thought came to me that he might have died there alone. He went on to say that he was resolved not to sleep that night until he had repeated the experiment, and declared that, late as it was, he must still find a patient. Returning to his office, he could find no one who could be induced to have a tooth drawn by the "painless method," which was what the doctor was now so eager to demonstrate. Discouraged, he was on the point of etherizing himself once more, and having one of his assistants extract a tooth from his own head, when there came a faint ring at the bell.

It was long past the hour for patients, but there stood a man with his face all bandaged, and evidently suffering acute pain. And strangest of all were his words.

"Doctor," he said, "I have the most frightful toothache and my mouth is so sore I am afraid to have the tooth drawn. Can't you mesmerize me?"

The doctor could almost have shouted with delight, but, preserving his self-possession, he brought the man into his office and told him he could do something better than mesmerize him. Then he explained the purpose of administering the sulphuric ether, and the man eagerly consented. Without delay my husband saturated a handkerchief with ether, and held it over the man's face, for him to inhale the fumes. The assistant, Dr. Hayden, who held the lamp, trembled visibly when Dr. Morton introduced the forceps into the mouth of the man and prepared to pull the tooth. Then came the strain, the wrench, and the tooth was out, but the patient made neither sign nor sound; he was quite unconscious.

Dr. Morton was overjoyed at the result. Then,

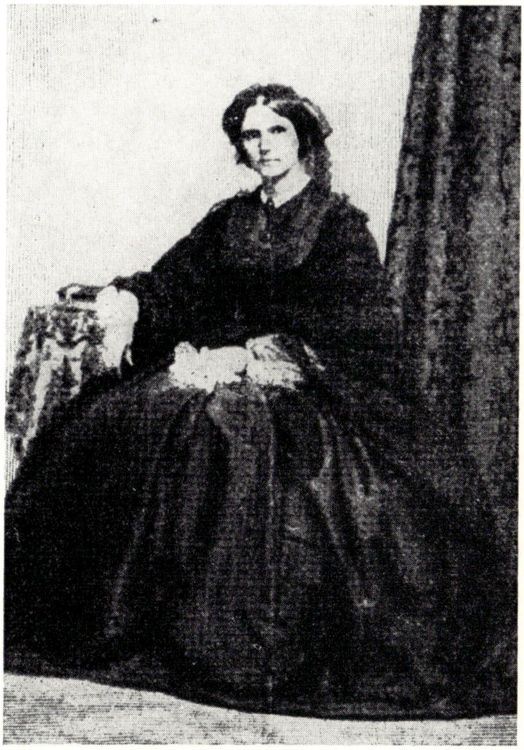

**Fig. 3.** Elizabeth W. Morton, wife of Dr. Morton. (From a photograph taken in Washington in 1862.)

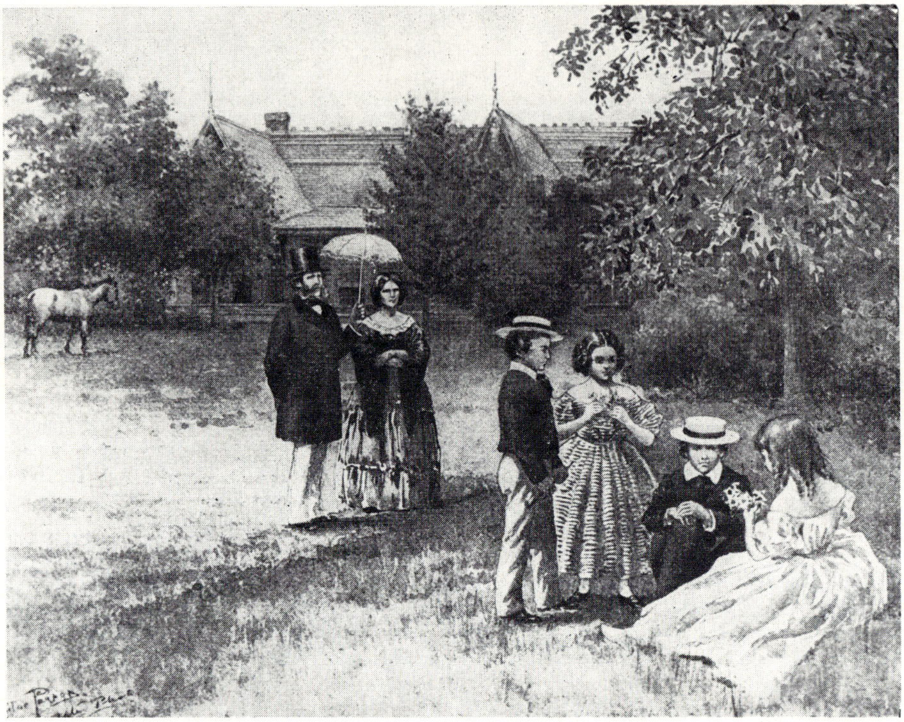

Dr. and Mrs. Morton and their children at their summer home at Wellesley. (Drawn by Victor Perard from a photograph taken in 1856.)

as the man continued to make no movement, he grew alarmed, and it flashed through his mind that perhaps he had killed his patient. Snatching up a glass of water, he emptied it full into the face of the unconscious man, who presently opened his eyes and looked about him in a bewildered way.

"Are you ready now to have the tooth out?" asked the doctor.

"I am ready," said the man.

"Well, it is out now," said the doctor, pointing to the tooth lying on the floor.

"No!" cried the man in greatest amazement, springing from the chair, and being a good Methodist, shouting, "Glory! Hallelujah."

From that moment Dr. Morton felt that the success of sulphuric ether was assured. Thenceforward he was unceasing in his efforts to bring his discovery before the medical world, and, after many discouragements, he succeeded in inducing Dr. John C. Warren, senior surgeon in the Massachusetts General Hospital, to allow him to visit the hospital and try his discovery upon a patient who was about to be operated upon.

The night before the operation, my husband worked until one or two o'clock in the morning upon an inhaler he had devised, and then regarded as essential to the operation, although it has since been discarded. I assisted him, nearly beside myself with anxiety, for the strongest influences had been brought to bear upon me to dissuade him from making this attempt. I had been told that one of two things was sure to happen; either the test would fail and my husband would be ruined by the world's ridicule, or he would kill the patient and be tried for manslaughter. Thus I was drawn in two ways; for while I had unbounded confidence in my husband, it did not seem possible that so young a man (he was only twenty-seven years old at this time) could be wiser than the learned and scientific men before whom he proposed to make his demonstration.

After resting a few hours, Dr. Morton was off early in the morning to see the instrument-maker, for there were still changes necessary in the inhaler. From that moment I saw nothing of him for twelve hours, which were hours of mortal anxiety. How they dragged along as I sat at the window, expecting every moment some messenger to tell me that the patient had died under the ether and the doctor would be held responsible! Two o'clock came, three o'clock, and it was not until nearly four that Dr. Morton walked in, with his usually genial face so sad that I felt failure must have come. He took me in his arms, almost fainting as I was, and said tenderly: "Well, dear, I succeeded."

In spite of these words, his gloom of manner and evident depression made it impossible for me to believe the good news. It seemed as if he should have been so highly elated at having accomplished one of the most splendid achievements of the century, and yet there he was, sick at heart, crushed down, one would have said, by a load of discouragement. This was due not only to bodily fatigue and the reaction after his great efforts, but to an intuitive perception of the troubles in store for him. It is literally true that Dr. Morton never was the same man after that day; his whole life after was embittered through this priceless boon he had conferred upon the human race.

Of the three men now living who saw this first operation upon a patient under the influence of ether, one is Dr. Robert Davis of Fall River. He was then a medical student in Boston, and he has given me the description of what happened on this memorable occasion. The amphitheater of the operating-room was crowded with members of the medical profession, doctors and students, all curious, and all skeptical, as to the outcome of the experiment to be made. All the greatest surgeons of Boston were present, including the celebrated Dr. Jacob Bigelow, whose son, Dr. Henry J. Bigelow, a young and enthusiastic surgeon of about Dr. Morton's age, was a warm friend of Dr. Morton's and perhaps the only man present who had faith in him. It must be said, however, that he had more grounds for this belief than the others, since he had been privileged to witness some of my husband's previous tests with ether in private.

The hour for the operation arrived and Dr. Morton was not on hand. Five minutes passed, ten minutes, and then Dr. Warren, the eminent surgeon, looking around with a smile on his face, slightly sarcastic, suggested that, as Dr. Morton was not present, it might be well to let the operation go on in the usual way. The patient had meantime been brought in, and was lying on the operating-table deathly white, doubly apprehensive of what was to come. At that moment Dr. Morton came in, breathless from haste, carrying the inhaler, which had just been delivered to him by the maker and had nearly been the cause of the failure of the test.

Without any delay, and with a coolness and self-possession in strong contrast with the general nervous tension of the assembly, Dr. Morton proceeded to administer sulphuric ether to a human being, for the purpose of destroying pain by forced anesthesia in a surgical operation, for the first time in the world's history. Pouring the liquid into the inhaler, he lifted the latter to the patient's nostrils, and held it there for some minutes, allowing the man to breathe the fumes. Then, looking into his face intently, and feeling the pulse, he turned to Dr. Warren, who stood near with his surgeon's knife behind him, and said in a quiet tone that sounded plainly through the silence:

"Your patient is ready, doctor."

Then in all parts of the amphitheatre there came a quick catching of the breath, followed by a silence almost deathlike, as Dr. Warren stepped forward and prepared to operate. The sheet was thrown back, exposing the portion of the body from which a tumor was to be removed, an operation exceedingly painful under ordinary conditions, although neither very difficult nor very dangerous. The patient lay silent, with eyes closed as if in sleep; but everyone present fully expected to hear a shriek of agony ring out as the knife struck down into the sensitive nerves. But the stroke came with no accompanying cry. Then another and another, and still the patient lay silent, sleeping, while the blood from severed arteries spurted forth. The surgeon was doing his work, and the patient was free from pain, so it seemed at least; and all in wonder strained their eyes and bent forward, following eagerly every step in the operation. Those in the front rows leaned far over or knelt on the floor, so that those behind might see better. The operation advanced quickly and easily to its finish. The tumor was taken away, the arteries fastened with ligatures, the gaping wound sewed up, then dressed and bandaged. Half an hour covered the whole of it. During that time no cry or groan escaped the patient, no indication of suffering.

Dr. Morton aroused the patient after the operation was completed, and said, "Did you feel any pain?" The patient replied, "No." Then Dr. Warren, turning to the company, said in his impressive manner, "Gentlemen, this is no humbug." All pressed about Dr. Morton and congratulated him upon his success.

Many successful operations, followed quickly. The hospital authorities, though, refused to make further use of the discovery, on the ground that they did not know the nature of the drug employed in inducing unconsciousness. My husband at once offered to give them full information on this point; but opposition had been aroused, and for several weeks operations at the hospital were performed by the old method of making the patient bear the torture.

Partly with a view to keeping this discovery out of the hands of persons who might use it unwisely, and acting upon the advice of Rufus Chate and Caleb Cushing, lawyers of national reputation, Dr. Morton patented his application of sulphuric ether; but he never enforced the patent, for his humanity was too great to keep back from suffering millions so precious an agency of relief. Yet he was criticized on all sides for taking out the patent, and cruel attacks were made upon him that cut him to the heart. At this time, it seemed to us who had to bear the brunt of these attacks that the value of this greatest of blessings, brought so suddenly and unexpectedly to the suffering, was lost sight of in the attempt to traduce the discoverer's character and motive. Abuse and ridicule were showered upon him by the public press, from the pulpit, and also by prominent medical journals, for presuming or daring to claim that he could prevent the pain of surgical operations. In those days I feared to look into a newspaper, for what wife does not feel more keenly unjust aspersions on her husband than he for himself? Then, too, the world's way—jealousy, malice, and envy—was new to me. Soon there sprang up contestants to Dr. Morton's title of discovery; men who claimed as theirs the work which he had accomplished with such infinite labor and for which he had hazarded life and reputation.

After the successful use of the sulphuric ether at the hospital, it became necessary to find a name for the new agent, and much discussion ensued. A meeting of physicians was called at the house of Dr. A. A. Gould, among those present being Dr. Oliver Wendell Holmes, Professor Agassiz, and Dr. Henry J. Bigelow, one of Boston's most eminent surgeons, who had encouraged Dr. Morton in his experiments at a time when many were in doubt or against him. Dr. Gould read a list of names that had been suggested, and on hearing the word "Letheon," my husband exclaimed: "That is the name; I want the discovery christened 'Letheon.' " Others were of the same opinion, but finally the suggestion of Dr. Holmes was accepted, and the word, "anesthesia" was chosen.

In spite of the various efforts that were made during subsequent years to obtain recognition from the United States government of Dr. Morton's services to the country and to the world, nothing was ever done. This was, perhaps, the greatest sorrow of my husband's later years, a sorrow rendered all the more keen from the fact that other governments hastened to bestow upon him orders and decorations. Russia gave him the "Cross of the Order of St. Vladimir"; Norway and Sweden gave him the "Cross of the Order of Vasa"; and the French Academy of Arts and Sciences sent him a gold medal, the Montyon prize. What he regarded as his greatest treasure was a small silver casket containing one thousand dollars in money, and presented by the trustees of the Massachusetts General Hospital. This was given "in honor of the ether discovery, September 30, 1846." The casket, medal, and decorations are now in the Historical Rooms in Boston, as well as many original documents relating to the discovery, the medals and the orders. In 1852, Dr. Morton received the honorary degree of Doctor of Medicine from his original alma mater, the Washington University of Medicine, afterwards merged into the College of Physicians and Surgeons, of Baltimore, Maryland.

During the war my husband served with Grant in the battle of the Wilderness, and with General Burnside at Fredericksburg, and had abundant opportunity to demonstrate the value of his discovery in the treatment of surgical cases on the battlefield. The following is an extract from one of his letters, which was written to a friend in May, 1864:

"When there is any heavy firing heard, the ambulance corps, with its attendants, stationed nearest to the scene of action starts for the wounded. The ambulances are halted near by, and the attendants go in with stretchers and bring out the wounded. The rebels do not generally fire upon those wearing ambulance badges.

"Upon the arrival of a train of ambulances at a field hospital, the wounds are hastily examined, and those who can bear the journey are sent at once to Fredericksburg. The nature of the operations to be performed upon the others is then decided upon, and noted on a bit of paper pinned to the pillow or roll of blankets under each patient's head. When this had been done, I prepared the patients for the knife, producing perfect anesthesia in an average time of three minutes, and the operators followed, performing their operations with dexterous skill, while the dressers in their turn bound up the stumps."

Dr. John H. Brinton of Philadelphia, in a valedictory address to the graduating class of Jefferson Medical College of Philadelphia in 1892, relates an interesting incident from personal reminiscence.

"In the early summer of 1864, during the fierce contest in the Virginia wilderness, I was present officially at the headquarters of Lieutenant-General Grant, on whose staff I had previously served. When in conversation with him, an aide approached, and said to him that a stranger, a civilian doctor, wished to see him for the purpose of obtaining an ambulance, for his personal use in visiting the field hospitals. The answer of the general was prompt and decided: 'The ambulances are intended only for the sick and wounded, and under no circumstances can be taken for private use.' This response was carried, as given, to the waiting applicant, a travel-stained man in brownish clothes, whom at the distance, I thought I recognized. I went to him and found that he was Dr. W. T. G. Morton. I asked him to wait a minute, and returned to the general. On repeating his request, I received the same answer. 'But, general,' I ventured to say, 'if you knew who that man is, I think you would give him what he asks for.'

" 'No, I will not,' he replied. 'I will not divert

an ambulance to-day for any one; they are all required elsewhere.'

" 'General,' I replied, 'I am sure you will give him the wagon, he has done so much for mankind, so much for the soldier—more than any soldier or civilian has ever done before; and you will say so when you know his name.'

"The general took his cigar from his mouth, looked curiously at the applicant, and asked, 'Who is he?'

" 'He is Dr. Morton, the discoverer of ether,' I answered.

"The general paused a moment; then said, 'You are right, doctor, he has done more for the soldier than any one else, soldier or civilian, for he has taught you all to banish pain. Let him have the ambulance and anything else he wants.'

"Afterward, during his stay, by order of the general commanding, he was tendered the hospitalities of the headquarters, ambulance, tent, mess, and servant."

Now I come to the last days of my husband's life. On July 6, 1868, he left Etherton Cottage for New York, to reply to an article that had recently appeared in one of the monthlies advocating Dr. Jackson's claim to be the discoverer of sulphuric ether. It was some time since anything of the sort had appeared, for medical journals the world over had admitted Dr. Morton's right to the discovery, and this article agitated him to an extent I had never seen before. The weather was very hot, and on July 11 he telegraphed me that he was ill and wished me to come to him. I went at once, and found he was suffering with rheumatism in one leg. Under the treatment of the distinguished Dr. Sayre, my husband improved, and on Wednesday, after dinner, he proposed we should drive to Washington Heights and spend the night there at the hotel, as a change from the hot city. We started out about eight o'clock in the evening, Dr. Morton himself driving.

After a little he complained of feeling sleepy, but refused to give me the reins or to turn back. Just as we were leaving the Park, without a word he sprang from the carriage, and for a few moments stood on the ground, apparently in great distress. Seeing a crowd gathering about, I took from his pocket his watch, purse, also his two decorations and the gold medal. Quickly he lost consciousness, and I was obliged to call upon a policeman and a passing druggist, Dr. Swann, who assisted me. We laid my husband upon the grass, but he was past hope of recovery. We sent at once for a double carriage, but it was an hour before one came. Then two policemen lifted him tenderly upon the seat, I being unable to do anything from the condition I was in: the horror of the situation had stunned me, finding myself alone with a dying husband, surrounded by strangers, in an open park at eleven o'clock at night.

We were driven at once to St. Luke's Hospital, where my husband was taken in on the stretcher, and immediately the chief surgeon and house physicians gathered about him. At a glance the chief surgeon recognized him, and said to me: "This is Dr. Morton?"

I simply replied, "Yes."

After a moment's silence he turned to the group of house pupils, and said: "Young gentlemen, you see lying before you a man who has done more for humanity and for the relief of suffering than any man who has ever lived."

In the bitterness of the moment, I put my hand in my pocket, and taking out the three medals, laid them beside my husband, saying: "Yes, and here is all the recompense he has ever received for it."

Dr. Morton died at the age of forty-eight. He was buried in Mt. Auburn Cemetery, near Boston, in the presence of many noted physicians of Boston. Over his grave stands a monument erected by the citizens of Boston, with this inscription, written by the late Dr. Jacob Bigelow of Boston:

"William T. G. Morton, Inventor and Revealer of Anesthetic Inhalation. By whom pain in surgery was averted and annulled. Before whom in all times surgery was agony. Since whom science has control of pain."

Dr. Morton's recreation was work on his farm at Wellesley, the town which is now the seat of Wellesley College. He was always a great lover of nature. People did not interest him very much, and he cared little for clubs. Not long after our marriage he purchased from a brother of Edward Everett a small place at Wellesley, then West Needham, where we went to live in the spring of 1846, having built a new cottage, and where several of our children were born.

My husband loved his children and made companions of them. He taught his boys to shoot as soon as they were large enough to hold a revolver, and vied with them in target practice until they became experts. My second son, Edward, possibly influenced by this early training, served through the Zulu war in South Africa, as a member of the Cape Mounted Rifles, gaining the decoration of the Victoria medal. Two sons are practising physicians, and the two daughters are married. Our home at Wellesley was sold some years ago; a public library has been erected upon the site of our cottage, and the grounds are a public park.

It has been a great pleasure to me to know that within the last two years my husband's name has been enrolled upon the base of the dome in the new chamber of the House of Representatives in the State House in Boston, among the selected fifty-three of Massachusetts's most distinguished citizens. "The names have been selected in such a way that each shall either mark an epoch, or designate a man who has turned the course of events." In the outside walls of the new Public Library in Boston are thirty arches filled with memorial tablets, inscribed with about five hundred names of writers, artists, and scientists. In this "roll of honor" also is inscribed my husband's name.

Volume 50 Number 5

SURGERY

NOVEMBER, 1961

Clinical surgery

# Elective uptake of radioiodine by cancer of the stomach

W. H. CLODE*
J. M. V. SOBRAL*
E. LIMA BASTO, F.A.C.S.
A. M. BAPTISTA*
LISBON, PORTUGAL
*From the Laboratório de Isótopos Abílio Lopes do Rego, Instituto Português de Oncologia*



It is well known that the stomach plays a part in the iodine cycle. The absorption of iodine through the gastrointestinal system happens very rapidly and the iodine concentration in the gastric juice reaches very high values as has been demonstrated with use of radioiodine as a tracer.[1]

Our attention was recently called to a patient who received a therapeutic dose of 16,000 rad of $I^{131}$ for the treatment of very severe hyperthyroidism. Two months later the patient returned to our laboratory because of his awareness of a nodule in the lower left side of the neck.

A thyroid scan was performed which showed a definite uptake of radioiodine over the supraclavicular node. Histologic examination after biopsy showed a lymph node invaded by a neoplastic glandular structure which could be interpreted as a metastatic gastric carcinoma or, inasmuch as the histologic characteristics were not perfectly typical, as a possible thyroid neoplasm, the diagnosis being supported by the radioiodine uptake.

Six months later the patient died of cancer of the stomach which had been symptomatic for only 2 months, but had been too far advanced for surgical treatment. This case called our attention to the possibility that iodine could play an important part in the metabolism of gastric neoplasms and we now present our first results of this study.

## MATERIAL AND METHODS

In 6 cases in which cancer of the stomach was diagnosed by the usual clinical and radiologic methods, we administered intravenously 1 $\mu c$ of $I^{131}$ (carrier-free sodium iodine from the Radiochemical Center, Amersham) 24 hours before surgical intervention. The tumor was removed, carefully washed in normal salt solution, and fixed for 24 hours in formol. Fragments of the tumor and of normal stomach were taken

Received for publication Dec. 20, 1960.

*Centro de Estudos de Física da Comissão de Estudos de Energia Nuclear do Instituto de Alta Cultura.

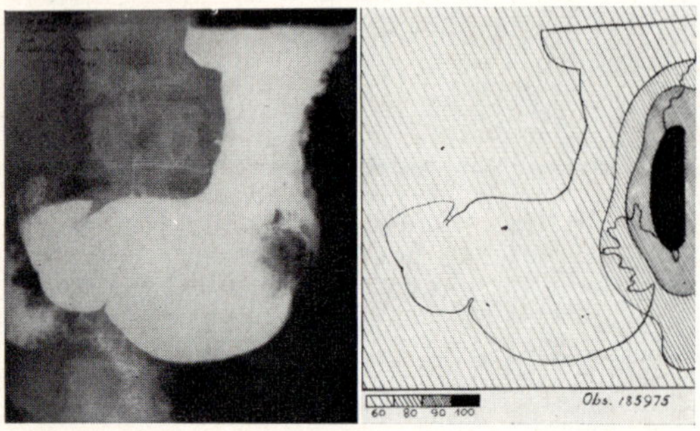

**Fig. 1.** Adenocarcinoma of stomach. Scanning of stomach after intravenous administration of 300 μc of $I^{131}$.

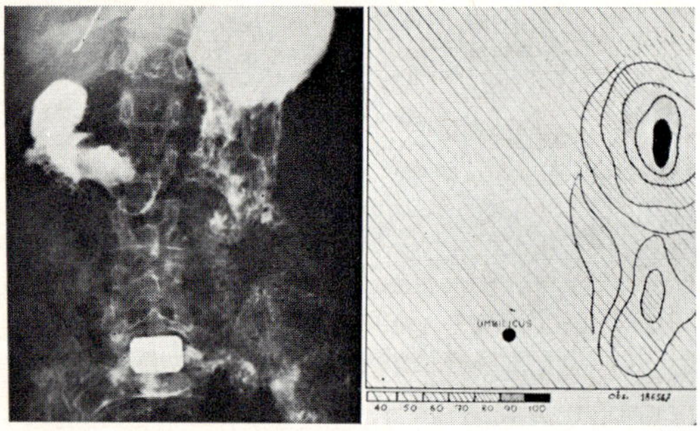

**Fig. 2.** Adenocarcinoma of stomach. Relatively increased radioactivity at the site of the cancer was shown by scanning after the administration of radioactive iodine.

and weighed and, after digestion for 24 hours in sulfuric acid, the radioactivity was measured in a well-type scintillation detector.

We studied only patients with the clinical diagnosis of cancer who were more than 50 years old, and therefore we were not particularly worried about the thyroid dose. Efforts are being directed toward making the use of much smaller amounts of radioiodine possible for the in vivo counting.

We believe from first results with a scanning apparatus which has a very much increased sensitivity and with photographic recording, that the $I^{131}$ amount can be substantially reduced. In a few patients, radioactive scanning of the stomach was performed before the operation in order to discover if an increased radioactivity was to be observed over the tumor-bearing region.

For this purpose we used a manual scanner with a scintillation (thallium activated) sodium iodide crystal, 4 by 4 cm. shielded by 5 cm. of lead. The cylindrical aperture of the collimator had a diameter of 1.5 cm. and was 12 cm. high. The patient was in a dorsal decubitus position and the counter, perpendicular to the plane of the bed, was moved laterally to cover all the abdomen. Counting in each position was from 0.5 to 1 minute.

Table I shows the results obtained from specific radioactivity measurements of the normal mucosa and of the tumor tissues.

Fig. 1 shows the results of scanning over the stomach of Patient 2 after the intravenous administration of 300 μc of sodium iodine ($I^{131}$). The scanning showed a tumor of the greater curvature. This cancer was inoperable but a lymph node removed from the greater omentum during the operation had a higher specific radioactivity than the normal tissue. The results in a few other cases up to now always revealed the presence of tumors (Fig. 2).

One case was particularly interesting (Table I, Patient 6) in which the lesion macroscopically resembled an ulcerated carcinoma. As shown in Table I, the relation of tumor radioactivity to the normal radioactivity was less than 1. A careful histologic examination showed the lesion to be a callous peptic ulcer.

In order to disprove the suggestion that the higher concentration observed was due

**Table I**

| *Patient* | *Tumor specific radioactivity* / *Normal tissue specific radioactivity* | *Observations* |
|---|---|---|
| 1. E. T. B. | 3.3 | Adenocarcinoma |
| 2. A. J. P. | 3.4 | Lymph node fragment with metastasis of inoperable adenocarcinoma |
| 3. A. J. A. | 3.5 | Adenocarcinoma |
| 4. P. P. V. | 21.8 | Adenocarcinoma |
| 5. P. M. | 30.9 | Adenocarcinoma |
| 6. M. R. C. | 0.58 | Callous peptic ulcer |

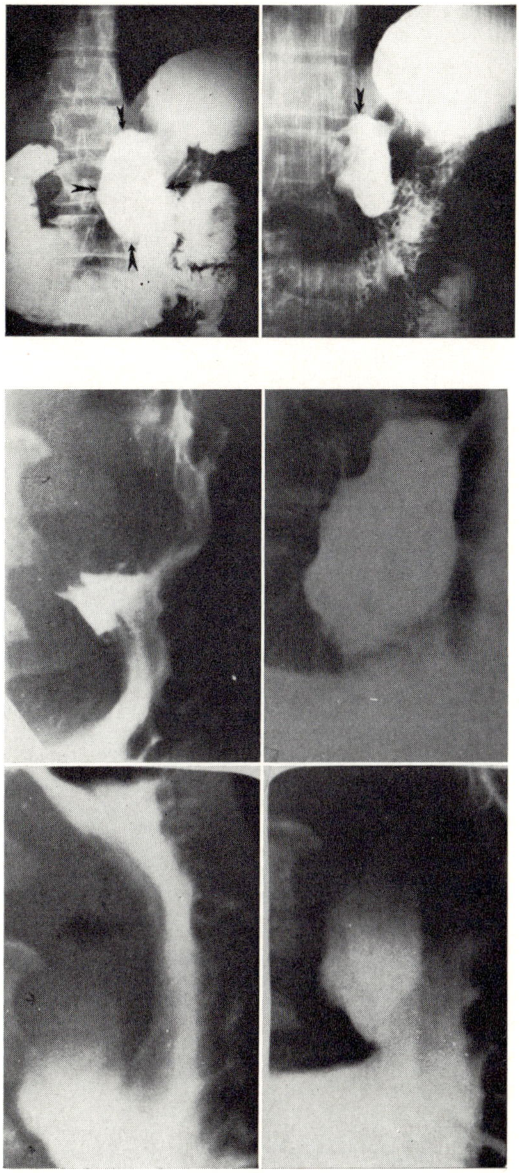

*A*

*B*

**Fig. 3.** *A,* Roentgenograms which offer a suspicion of cancer of the stomach. *B,* Scanning after the administration of radioactive iodine showed no specific concentration. Later gastrectomy showed the lesion to be a giant benign ulcer.

to an increased vascularization of the tumor without any specific concentration mechanism for iodine, a study was made in 1 case in which 300 $\mu c$ of $I^{131}$-labeled human serum albumin was injected 15 minutes before the gastrectomy. We obtained for the relative radioactivity of tumor and normal tissue the value of 0.79.

It is also interesting to see that a suspected cancer of the stomach (Fig. 3) did not give the expected result after scanning. It later proved to be a giant benign ulcer. The scanning in other ulcer cases failed to show any specific radioactivity uptake.

## SUMMARY AND CONCLUSIONS

In all of the patients studied until now, it was shown that cancer of the stomach is indeed able to pick up radioiodine and that its specific radioactivity is higher than that of the normal gastric mucosa.

Scanning over the stomach region also showed a higher concentration of the radioactivity over the tumor in accordance with the previous findings. These facts suggest a new diagnostic procedure for cancer of the stomach, because in normal patients (hyperthyroid patients who were treated with radioiodine) we have never observed similar findings.

The results are particularly interesting because until now, an increased radioiodine uptake detected over a region was related to the possible existence of a metastasis of thyroid cancer.

Work is being done to extend the number of observations and, in particular, to study the biochemical and metabolic aspects of this problem and its possible implications in the diagnosis and therapy of cancer of stomach.

## REFERENCE

1. Schiff, L., Stevens, C. D., Molle, W. E., Steinberg, H., Kumpe, C. W., and Stewart, P.: Gastric (and salivary) excretion of radioiodine in man, J. Nat. Cancer Inst. **7:** 349, 1947.

# A simple cooling device for treatment of upper gastrointestinal bleeding

MARSH H. HOLT, M.D.
CHICAGO, ILL.
*From the Department of Surgery, Northwestern University Medical School*

The use of local hypothermia in the treatment of upper gastrointestinal hemorrhage as recently introduced by Wangensteen[3-5] and his associates has gained increasing interest and trial. The rationale behind this technique stems from the studies by Wangensteen which demonstrated the effectiveness of local hypothermia in depressing peptic activity, suppressing gastric secretions, decreasing bowel motility, and diminishing local blood flow.

The routine practical use of local hypothermia for intractable hemorrhage, however, is limited to centers with the specialized equipment and personnel necessary for this type of procedure.

Utilizing our experience derived from the use of intragastric cooling in general hypothermia,[1, 2] we have developed a simple, safe, and inexpensive device which can be used in a routine hospital procedure in the treatment of uncontrolled upper gastrointestinal hemorrhage.

## MATERIALS

The device consists of a basic pump–cooling unit (Fig. 1, *A*), plastic tubing with intragastric or esophageal balloons (Fig. 1, *B* and *C*), and a physiologic cooling solution. The unit can be used with either an open or closed circulation system.

The pump–cooling unit is composed of (1) a heat exchanger, (2) a fluid reservoir, (3) an automatic leveling device, and (4) a small centrifugal pump.

Supported in part by Public Health Service Grant No. H-2879.
Received for publication Dec. 8, 1960.

The heat exchanger is composed of 18 feet of three-eighths inch Tygon plastic tubing wound in a spiral fashion around a stainless steel frame. The unit is constructed to fit within a common operating room bucket and to be covered with chipped ice. A monitoring thermometer is interposed at the inflow and outflow ends of the tubing.

The fluid reservoir is a 1 L. graduated Lucite cylinder which is attached to the steel framework above the ice level. It is used only during open-circuit perfusion. The cooling solution drains by syphon from the stomach and enters the top of the reservoir through a screen filter. The fluid is then drawn from the reservoir via a bottom outlet and pumped through the heat exchange unit and back into the stomach.

The automatic leveling device, used only with the open-circuit technique, is attached to the reservoir where it serves to maintain a constant circulating volume. The device employs an Acro snap action switch* which is mounted on the reservoir and attached by a lever to the end of a finger cot connected directly to a nipple on the reservoir. As the reservoir fluid level varies with the outflow-inflow difference, the finger cot fills or collapses, moving the attached switch lever causing an on-off regulation of the pump. The sensitivity is adjustable to within 50 ml. by alteration of the position of the switch. During closed-system use the leveling device is bypassed and constant circulation is maintained. A 3-way master switch provides an on-off or automatic setting.

*Acro Switch Company, Columbus, Ohio.

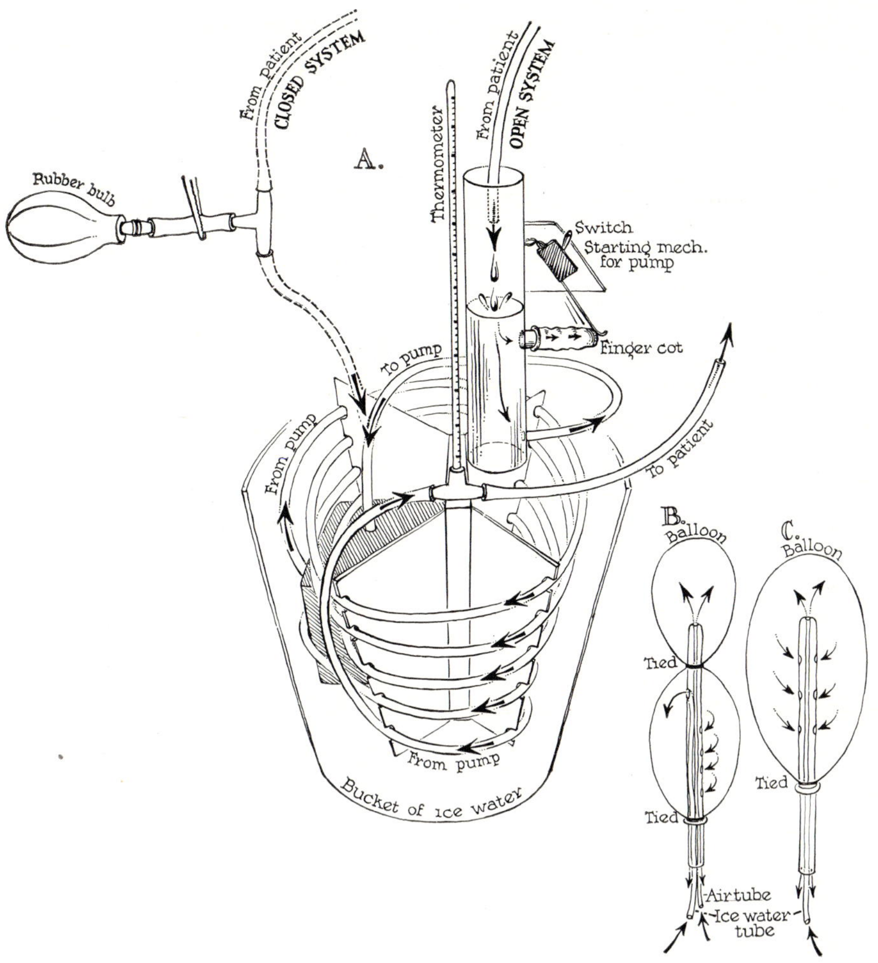


**Fig. 1.** *A,* Schematic drawing of the cooling unit assembled and in use which shows both open system (solid-line tube from patient) and closed system (broken-line tube from patient). *B,* Balloon used for cooling and compressing bleeding esophageal varices. *C,* Balloon used for closed-system cooling of the stomach.

The pump used is a small, submersible centrifugal sump pump ($25.00) with a removable brass head (Little Giant*). The pump is attached to the steel frame and submerged in ice to maintain a safe operating temperature.

The tubing with intragastric and esophageal balloons is shown in Fig. 1, *B* and *C.* This can be easily made from an 18 Fr. K-55 Pharmaseal urinary drainage tube as an outer shell and an inner tube of polyethylene (PE320). A condom is attached to the outer shell with thread to form a sealed circulation chamber. The esophageal unit contains a small additional tube leading to a separate intragastric compartment which can be filled with air or water. The appropriate intraesophageal pressure, according to the Sengstaken principle, is determined with a single mercury manometer connected to the closed circulation system.

During open circulation, a Levin tube for inflow is placed in the stomach via one nostril, while an 18 Fr. K-55 Pharmaseal multiperforated outflow tube also lies within the stomach after being passed through the other nostril.

The fluid used for open intragastric perfusion is that recommended by Wangensteen

*Little Giant Vaporizer Company, Oklahoma City, Okla.

**Table I.** *Open-system cooling solution*

| | |
|---|---|
| Glucose | 50 Gm. |
| $NH_4Cl$ | 2 Gm. |
| KCl | 0.75 Gm. |
| $NaHCO_3$ | add to adjust pH to 7.4 |
| Distilled water | 1 L. |

From Wangensteen.[3]

(Table I). We have used this solution on 4 occasions in the induction of general hypothermia and have perfused the stomach for 4 hours in each instance. Evaluations of pH and potassium, sodium, and chloride levels in the solution before and after perfusion showed only an average decrease in pH from 7.4 to 5.2 and no significant electrolyte alterations.

## METHOD OF OPERATION

The patient is examined to determine the site of hemorrhage as nearly as possible (esophageal varices or gastric or duodenal lesion). An attempt is then made to relieve the stomach of clotted blood by an orally inserted Ewald or colon tube.

After passage of a nasogastric Levin tube, the appropriate cooling tube is inserted by way of the other nostril. Cooling in the closed system is started after distention of the balloon with 300 ml. of water by way of a T connector or in the open system after filling of the stomach with the same amount of cooling solution.

During closed-system perfusion, constant gastric lavage with cold saline solution is performed through the Levin tube until there is no evidence of further hemorrhage. Constant low suction is maintained thereafter.

During open perfusion, the stomach is evacuated every hour and the fluid lost through the pyloric canal replaced. The average loss was 100 ml. per hour.

When the fluid is circulated at 600 ml. per minute, the temperature of the cooling fluid is from 5 to 10° C. and that of the returning fluid is approximately 4° C. higher in the closed system and 7° higher in the open system.

The total fluid contents of the cooling apparatus is 1,200 ml. in the open system. The stomach contains 300 ml., the heat exchanger 400 ml., and the reservoir approximately 500 ml. In the event that the automatic leveling device should fail, only the contents of the reservoir could be pumped into the stomach. This protection against acute severe gastric distention is possible because of the limited capacity of the unit and the inherent inability of the pump to function when filled with air from the empty reservoir. The closed system contains 700 ml. of water, 300 ml. of which is in the stomach balloon.

## SUMMARY

An inexpensive, relatively simple, and safe apparatus is described which can be used by the average house officer in the primary treatment of uncontrolled upper gastrointestinal hemorrhage.

This device, in a modified form, will be available shortly from Gorman-Rupp Industries, Inc., Bellville, Ohio.

### REFERENCES

1. Holt, M. H., Benvenuto, R., and Lewis, F. J.: General hypothermia with intragastric cooling, Surg. Gynec. & Obst. **107:** 251, 1958.
2. Holt, M. H., Benvenuto, R., and Lewis, F. J.: General hypothermia with intragastric cooling: a further study, S. Forum **9:** 287, 1959.
3. Wangensteen, O. H., Salmon, P. A., Griffen, W. O., Jr., Paterson, J. R. S., and Fattah, F.: Studies of local gastric cooling as related to peptic ulcer, Ann. Surg. **150:** 346, 1959.
4. Wangensteen, O. H., Root, H. D., Jenson, C. B., Imamoglu, K., and Salmon, P. A.: Depression of gastric secretion and digestion by gastric hypothermia: its clinical use in massive hematemesis, Surgery **44:** 265, 1958.
5. Wangensteen, O. H., Root, H. D., Salmon, P. A., and Griffen, W. O., Jr.: Depressant action of local hypothermia upon gastric digestion: its use in the control of massive hematemesis, J. A. M. A. **169:** 1601, 1959.

# Treatment of cardiospasm (achalasia of the esophagus) in children

W. SPENCER PAYNE, M.D.
F. HENRY ELLIS, JR., M.D.
ARTHUR M. OLSEN, M.D.
ROCHESTER, MINN.
*From the Mayo Clinic and Mayo Foundation*

Cardiospasm, or achalasia of the esophagus, although commonly encountered in adults, is rare in children. Moersch[6] found 12 patients less than 14 years of age in a series of 691 patients treated for cardiospasm. Among adult patients in that series, less than 5 per cent had the onset of symptoms during childhood. Olsen and associates[8] noted a similar incidence in their series of 601 patients. Only a few reports concern this condition in children, and more information is needed with regard to the methods of management and results of treatment in this age group.

## MATERIAL

The present study is a review of the cases of 27 children 14 years of age and younger who were treated for cardiosapsm at the Mayo Clinic in the 25-year period from Jan. 1, 1935, through Dec. 31, 1959.

The diagnosis of cardiospasm was established in each case on the basis of characteristic symptoms and roentgenographic findings. Eight patients underwent esophagoscopic examination, in addition to the usual diagnostic studies, as part of the diagnostic investigation. Because of technical difficulties in performing esophageal motility studies in the very young,[7] complete documentation of the diagnosis of cardiospasm by this method was available in only 4 cases.

Eleven of the children were female and 16 were male. The 27 patients ranged in age from 13 months to 14 years (Table I) when first seen. The duration of symptoms ranged from 1 month to 10 years and averaged 2.6 years. The apparent age at onset of achalasia according to duration of symptoms is shown in Table II.

Regurgitation and obstruction to swallowing were the most frequent complaints, and weight loss or failure of growth and development were the second most common. Occasionally, weight loss of 30 to 40 pounds was encountered in children with severe obstructive symptoms. Less than half complained of pain referable to the esophagus. Nine had experienced recurrent episodes of pneumonitis secondary to aspiration of esophageal contents.[1] Children with cardiospasm were more severely incapacitated by their symptoms than were adult patients. However, the severity of the disease with respect to the degree of esophageal dilatation noted on initial roentgenograms of the esophagus was less in these children than we have noted in adult patients.[8, 9] In the present series, only 6 patients had severe dilatation. The rest had either mild or moderate dilatation.

Eleven of the patients had undergone some form of esophageal dilation, usually on multiple occasions, prior to examination and treatment at the clinic. It was either the recurrence of symptoms after treatment or the failure of previous dilations to relieve symptoms that caused these patients to seek additional medical aid.

## METHODS OF TREATMENT

Since there is no known means of restoring normal peristaltic activity to the esoph-

Received for publication Dec. 15, 1960.

**Table I.** *Age distribution of 27 children with achalasia of esophagus*

| Age (yr.) | 1 | 2 | 3 | 4 | 5 | 6 | 7 | 8 | 9 | 10 | 11 | 12 | 13 | 14 |
|---|---|---|---|---|---|---|---|---|---|---|---|---|---|---|
| No. of patients | 1 | 4 | 1 | – | – | 4 | – | 2 | 3 | – | 2 | 2 | 4 | 4 |

**Table II.** *Apparent age at onset of achalasia in 27 children*

| Age (yr.) | 0-¼ | ½-1 | 2 | 3 | 4 | 5 | 6 | 7 | 8 | 9 | 10 | 11 | 12 | 13 | 14 |
|---|---|---|---|---|---|---|---|---|---|---|---|---|---|---|---|
| No. of patients | 5 | 5 | – | – | 1 | 2 | 2 | 2 | – | 2 | 2 | 1 | 4 | 1 | – |

agus in patients with achalasia, treatment at present is limited to relief of the distal esophageal obstruction. In the present series this was accomplished either by mechanical dilation of the cardia or by esophagomyotomy.

The preferred method of esophageal dilation for cardiospasm at this institution is hydrostatic dilation by means of a Plummer hydrostatic dilator,[8] which is passed over a previously swallowed thread. However, in some small children and in infants hydrostatic dilation may be hazardous, and some of these patients were treated by the passage of graduated sounds or bougies only. In children, unlike in adults, general anesthesia is occasionally required for these procedures.

Surgical treatment was undertaken in some patients who had failed to respond to mechanical dilations. Esophagomyotomy by means of a modified Heller procedure[2, 9] was the only surgical treatment employed in this series.

Thus, of the 27 children in this study, 26 were treated by dilation (8 by bougienage only and 18 by hydrostatic dilation) and 5 patients were treated by esophagomyotomy, 4 of them after previous treatment by mechanical dilations. One patient had only surgical treatment.

## RESULTS OF TREATMENT

For the purpose of evaluating the results of treatment, the entire group was divided into patients who had received conservative treatment (mechanical dilation, 26 cases) and those who received surgical treatment (esophagomyotomy, 5 cases). Thus, 4 patients are included in both groups, namely, those who first received conservative treatment and, that failing, then underwent operation.

No hospital morbidity or deaths occurred in the group treated conservatively. All patients experienced symptomatic improvement immediately after the first course of treatment.

Among the 5 patients who underwent surgical treatment, all noted immediate and gratifying relief of their symptoms after operation. Only 1 patient experienced significant postoperative complications; empyema developed, necessitating decortication of the lung. No hospital deaths occurred among the group operated upon.

**Late results.** Complete follow-up information in the form of clinic examination or response to follow-up letters or both was available for review for 25 of the 26 children treated by dilation and for all 5 of those treated surgically.

Among the 25 children treated by dilation, the length of follow-up ranged from 1 to 19 years and averaged 9.6 years. The length of follow-up in the surgical group ranged from 1½ to 3 years and averaged 2.3 years.

The criteria for evaluating the effectiveness of treatment were similar to those used in previous studies.[2, 8, 9] The over-all effectiveness of treatment was judged with regard to the need for additional treatment and the status of the patient at the time of the most recent follow-up contact. Thus, the patient's condition was judged as being "improved" only if lasting symptomatic remission followed the initial trial of a given form of treatment. It was considered "poor" if additional treatment of the same or of a different type was necessary to relieve the patient of his symptoms.

Patients were classified as having excellent

results if they were completely asymptomatic, had gained weight, and had returned to full activity. They were classified as having good results if they fulfilled the aforementioned requirements but continued to notice occasional dysphagia when eating too rapidly or when nervous. Certain types of food, such as apples, raw vegetables, or peanut butter, may occasionally inconvenience these patients. Patients were judged to have fair results if they fulfilled most of the basic criteria and were definitely improved but continued to have occasional to frequent episodes of dysphagia with certain foods and occasional regurgitation. Patients were classified as having poor results if they showed no improvement or had a worsening of the condition.

The results of late follow-up of patients treated by conservative means were generally unsatisfactory (Table III). Of the 8 patients treated by simple bougienage, 3 have had persistent improvement and 5 had recurrence of symptoms within 1 year of the initial treatment. In the 3 patients who showed improvement, the results were only fair at the time of follow-up. All 5 patients who experienced recurrence of symptoms have been retreated by other means.

Of the 17 patients treated by hydrostatic dilations, 7 have had persistent improvement since the first treatment (Table III). Ten patients had recurrence of symptoms and required retreatment. Symptoms recurred in this group from 6 months to 4 years after initial treatment. The status of the 17 patients at the time of the last follow-up contact, including the results of all retreatments, was excellent in 2, good in 3, fair in 5, and poor in 7. Unfortunately, the data are incomplete with regard to the number of retreatments that were necessary to accomplish these results; many of these children have undergone subsequent dilations elsewhere. However, some are known to have improved with as few as 2 courses of treatment and others with as many as 12 at our institution. No morbidity or deaths were associated with any of the retreatments in this series.

The late results of surgical treatment have been most gratifying (Table III). All 5 patients have had persistent improvement. Four had excellent results and 1 good. None of these patients has required retreatment of any type, and none has experienced esophageal reflux or other late complications. The data in these 5 cases are considered in detail in Table IV.

## COMMENT

The present study seems to confirm previous reports that the late results of mechanical dilation of the esophagus for cardiospasm are less satisfactory in children than they are in adults.[8] On the other hand, esophagomyotomy by means of a modified Heller procedure seems to offer the best means of producing sustained symptomatic improvement in patients of all ages.[9]

The children in this study who were treated by mechanical esophageal dilation have required many courses of treatment,

**Table III.** *Late results of treatment of 26 children with achalasia*

| Type of treatment | No. of patients* | Results of treatment | | | | Average duration of follow-up (yr.) |
|---|---|---|---|---|---|---|
| | | Improved | | | Same or worse | |
| | | Excellent | Good | Fair | Poor | |
| *Conservative* | | | | | | |
| Simple bougieneage | 8 | 0 | 0 | 3 | 5 | 7.3 |
| Hydrostatic dilations | 17† | 1 | 1 | 5 | 10 | 11.2 |
| *Surgical* | | | | | | |
| Modified Heller procedure | 5 | 4 | 1 | 0 | 0 | 2.3 |

*Four of the patients included in the surgical group received conservative treatment initially and are listed also in that group.
†One patient treated by hydrostatic dilation was lost to follow-up and is not included.

**Table IV.** *Late results of Heller operation for achalasia in children**

| *Case No.* | *Age (yr.)* | *Sex* | *Duration of symptoms (yr.)* | *Duration of follow-up (yr.)* | *Result* |
|---|---|---|---|---|---|
| 1 | 3 | F | 1 | 3 | Excellent |
| 2 | 14 | F | 1 | 2½ | Excellent |
| 3 | 6 | M | 5 | 2½ | Excellent |
| 4 | 9½ | M | 1½ | 2 | Excellent |
| 5 | 11½ | M | 1 | 1½ | Good |

*All patients except 1 (case 3) had undergone previous treatment. Moderate dilatation of the esophagus was present in all 5 patients.

often over a period of years. Some have had to continue such treatment into adult life. Treatment by bougienage alone has rarely given more than temporary relief. Hydrostatic dilation, if it is to be effective, must be a drastic procedure, and often the endoscopist performing the dilations is unwilling to be as vigorous in these small patients as he might be in the adult. The necessity for general anesthesia in some of the very young patients undoubtedly increases the risk of the procedure.

In spite of the many unfavorable aspects, esophageal dilation was accomplished with little risk to the patient in this series. This procedure is capable of producing good symptomatic improvement for short periods and can be used in lieu of gastrostomy in preparing the severely malnourished child for more definitive treatment. Hydrostatic dilations seem preferable to simple bougienage, and an occasional patient may sustain a satisfactory remission of several years' duration. Unfortunately, the larger the number of dilations required, the less favorable the result. Local reaction produced by repeated dilations could lessen the surgeon's chance of obtaining a completely satisfactory result.

Experience with the surgical treatment of achalasia in infants and children has been limited. King[5] reported good results with esophagomyotomy in a 6½-month-old infant. Ferguson and Burford[3] operated on several children, the youngest of which was 9 months of age. Others have reported their experiences with the Wendel[10] and the Grøndahl[4] procedures in children with achalasia.

Esophagomyotomy by means of a modified Heller procedure is the preferable surgical treatment for cardiospasm. In the patient with symptoms whose general condition permits, we see no reason to delay operation because of age once the diagnosis has been established. Some form of definitive therapy is desirable before the esophagus has become greatly distended and decompensated. Thus, it appears that the younger the child, the greater the indication for surgical treatment as opposed to mechanical dilation. The growth factor does not appear to have any particular effect on the end result in these young patients treated by myotomy.

The diagnosis of cardiospasm may be difficult to establish in infants and children. They are often unable to cooperate satisfactorily for the necessary diagnostic studies, particularly for studies of esophageal motility. Occasionally, surgical exploration will be indicated to rule out some other condition. Malignancy in this region is rare in children. However, 2 patients not included in this study underwent surgical exploration after a clinical diagnosis of cardiospasm and were found at operation to have lower esophageal leiomyomas, which accounted for their symptoms. Satisfactory esophageal motility studies could not be obtained in these cases because neither patient was old enough to make this possible. The need for techniques of performing such studies in infants and children is obvious.

## SUMMARY

Cardiospasm, or achalasia of the esophagus, is rare during infancy and childhood, but it should be considered in the differential diagnosis of young patients with feeding problems, regurgitation, and dysphagia. There is nothing characteristic about the patient's age at onset of symptoms. The degree of esophageal dilatation is often less than that seen in adults with this condition, although the symptoms are usually more severe. Often the diagnosis is difficult to establish in this age group.

Several forms of treatment were employed in the present series. Of 5 patients treated surgically by means of a modified Heller procedure, the results were excellent in 4 and good in 1. Patients treated by repeated hydrostatic dilations or by simple bougienage had comparatively poorer results.

It is concluded that the modified Heller procedure can be used effectively in the treatment of infants and children with achalasia; it is the treatment of choice when the diagnosis is established in the patient with symptoms. Dilation therapy can be used effectively in lieu of gastrostomy in preparing the severely malnourished patient for operation.

## REFERENCES

1. Andersen, H. A., Holman, C. B., and Olsen, A. M.: Pulmonary complications of cardiospasm, J. A. M. A. **151:** 608, 1953.
2. Ellis, F. H., Jr., Olsen, A. M., Holman, C. B., and Code, C. F.: Surgical treatment of cardiospasm (achalasia of the esophagus): considerations of aspects of esophagomyotomy, J. A. M. A. **166:** 29, 1958.
3. Ferguson, T. B., and Burford, T. H.: An evaluation of the modified Heller operation in the treatment of achalasia of the esophagus, Ann. Surg. **152:** 1, 1960.
4. Johnston, J. H., Jr., and Twente, G. E.: Esophageal achalasia (cardiospasm): report of two cases with unusual manifestations, SURGERY **29:** 196, 1951.
5. King, R.: Surgical correction of achalasia of the esophagus in infants, J. M. A. Georgia **42:** 466, 1953.
6. Moersch, H. J.: Cardiospasm in infancy and in childhood, Am. J. Dis. Child. **38:** 294, 1929.
7. Olsen, A. M., Code, C. F., and Clagett, O. T.: Role of motility patterns in the diagnosis of esophageal disease, J. A. M. A. **172:** 319, 1960.
8. Olsen, A. M., Harrington, S. W., Moersch, H. J., and Andersen, H. A.: The treatment of cardiospasm: analysis of a twelve-year experience, J. Thoracic Surg. **22:** 164, 1951.
9. Payne, W. S., Ellis, F. H., Jr., and Olsen, A. M.: Achalasia of the esophagus: a follow-up study of patients undergoing esophagomyotomy, A. M. A. Arch. Surg. **81:** 411, 1960.
10. Swenson, O., and Oeconomopoulous, C. T.: Achalasia of the esophagus in children, J. Thoracic Surg. **41:** 49, 1961.

# The 2-limb temporary gastrostomy tube

MARIO E. JASCALEVICH, M.D.
NEW YORK, N. Y.
*From the Surgical Department, New York Polyclinic, Medical School, and Hospital*

A review of the literature of the past 50 years shows several reports on the role of nasogastric intubation in the development of lesions of the upper respiratory and digestive tracts, and particularly in the production of ulcerative and later stenosing esophagitis.[2, 4-10] Because of this experience there is an increasing tendency in surgical centers across the country to resort more often to temporary gastrostomy in aged, debilitated, and poor-risk patients who will not tolerate a nasogastric tube well. Temporary gastrostomy would also be indicated in situations in which there is a history of nasopharyngolaryngeal or esophageal disease. Highly emotional and uncooperative individuals are also candidates for this procedure. In all such cases a lower incidence of pulmonary complication, a more comfortable patient, and the guarantee of a suction system that is very effective and easy to maintain are early rewards of temporary gastrostomy. Moreover, operations on the upper gastrointestinal tract in those situations can be further assisted if, in addition to the advantages of direct gastric drainage which avoids the nasal route, there could be independent suction from the stomach and/or afferent anastomotic loop and injection of feeding solutions into the efferent loop. The pioneering work of Abbott and Rawson[1] and others[9] partially accomplished this plan. Their device is a nasogastric tube with a single body and double lumen which, when used after gastroenterostomy and Billroth II gastrectomy, does not allow for suction in situ of the afferent loop that is particularly prone to obstruction and should be better kept decompressed. Mersheimer[12] in 1942 made the first attempt to do this by using dual and separate tubes for suction and feeding. He employed 2 No. 12 Levin tubes coupled with silk ligatures which were passed through the nose down to the stomach prior to operation. At this time, before performing the anterior layer of the gastroenterostomy, the surgeon places the distal ends of these tubes separately in the corresponding anastomotic limbs of the jejunum. Although in our hands the system appeared to be poorly tolerated by the patient and shares the criticism of nasogastric intubation in general when applied in the particular situations discussed, its principle stands with regard to the importance of direct and independent care of the proximal and distal anastomotic loops. This was accomplished successfully with our 2-limb temporary gastrostomy tube, an appliance which allows for jejunal feeding together with suction of the afferent loop, while at the same time provides the advantages of a gastrostomy type of drainage. As intravenous alimentation becomes replaced by enteral feeding, this device will render a particular service in postoperative recovery after upper gastrointestinal operations on patients with cardiorespiratory decompensation who otherwise would stand the double burden of an intravenous drip and the partial upper respiratory obstruction produced by the nasogastric tube. Moreover, in radical operations for carcinoma of the same area the device offers

Received for publication Dec. 8, 1960.

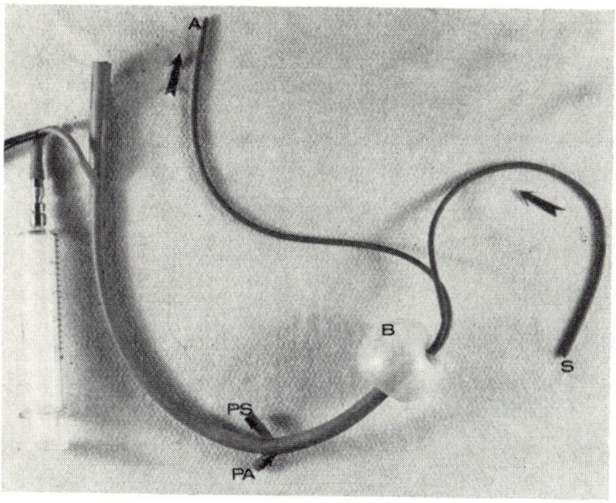


**Fig. 1.** Two-limb temporary gastrostomy tube with balloon inflated. *B,* Balloon; *A,* alimentary limb; *PA,* proximal end of limb *A*; *S,* suction limb; and *PS,* proximal end of limb *S.*

a solution to the double need for effective suction and the early administration of a complete nutritional support.

## DESCRIPTION OF THE INSTRUMENT

The 2-limb temporary gastrostomy tube (Fig. 1) has been improvised very effectively. The tip of a No. 28 Foley catheter is cut off just distal to the bag *(B)* and through its lumen the proximal ends of 2 No. 12 Fr. red tubes are passed *(S)* and *(A)* which emerge at a variable distance from the balloon, approximately 10 to 12 cm. *(P.S.* and *P.A).* For this purpose, 2 parallel orifices are made on the shaft of the Foley catheter at that level, with care not to enter

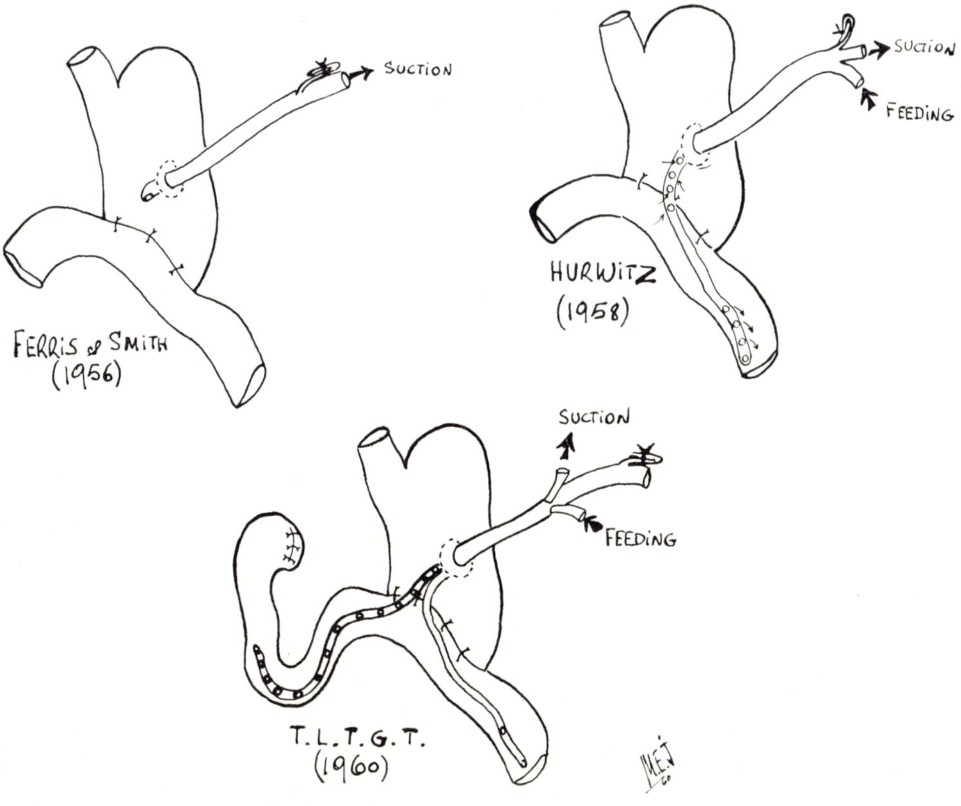


**Fig. 2.** The temporary gastrostomy tube described compared with other previously described models.

the channel that governs bag inflation. The openings permit snug passage of each French tube. These emerge from the host catheter for a distance of 2 cm. which is enough to insure connecting ends for the feeding and suction lines without undue shortening of the limbs of the instrument. Thus, the legs will measure 12 to 13 cm. long and can be prepared as necessary for their future use. The aspirating limb *(S)* will have multiple orifices cut out along the entire length at intervals of 2 cm. which are of a diameter sufficient to allow good suction without weakening the shaft of the tube itself. The feeding limb *(A)* will have only 1 orifice made at the distal end, about 2 cm. from the tip. To insure easy identification, the body and the cuff of each red tube are properly marked "suction" or "output" and "feeding" or "input." This will prevent cross misplacement of the aspirating and alimentary lines by the surgeon and misconnections by the staff in charge of the postoperatory care. When the integrity of the balloon and the patency of the channels have been tested, the 2-limb temporary gastrostomy tube is ready for use. Fig. 2 shows the type of gastrostomy tube used by Farris and Smith[6] and the model of Hurwitz[9] in comparison with the one described.

## CLINICAL APPLICATION

A gastrotomy by the usual technique for gastrostomy is performed and each limb of the tube is introduced (with the help of a director if preferred) and placed. The aspirating limb is passed to the segment where suction is needed, either the stomach, duodenum, or afferent loop of a gastroenterostomy (Fig. 3), and the feeding limb is introduced far along the duodenum or efferent loop, depending on the particular situation. The distal end of the Foley catheter is then passed inside the stomach, the

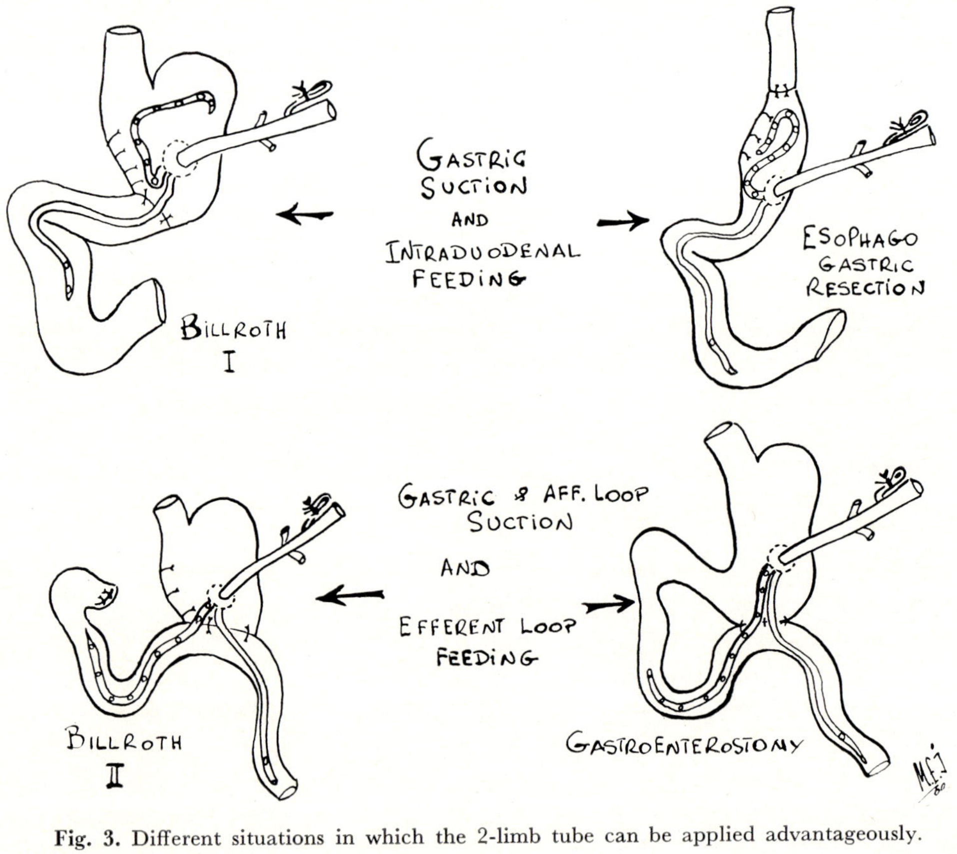


**Fig. 3.** Different situations in which the 2-limb tube can be applied advantageously.

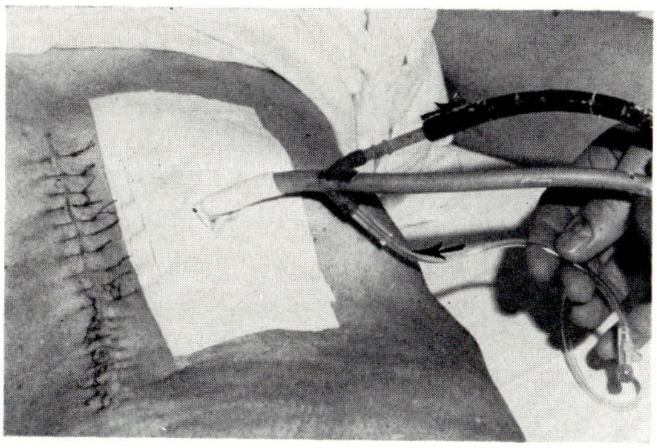

**Fig. 4.** Actual patient with tube applied. Note input and output lines *(arrows)* approaching the body of the Foley catheter through which they will reach the gastric lumen.

balloon inflated, and the gastrostomy completed with a typical Stamm technique. The proximal end with the twin French tubes is brought out of the abdomen through a stab wound. Finally, a silk stitch is placed to fix the Foley catheter to the skin edge of the stab incision.

Immediately after operation the output end of the tube is connected to a Wangensteen intermittent suction machine and the desired drip solution is attached to the input end. Twenty-four to 48 hours after the procedure a highly blended liquid feeding mixture can be passed through the input line. The aspirated fluids, if aseptically collected, could also be injected through this channel when necessary. Fig. 4 shows a typical 2-limb temporary gastrostomy tube in use.

## SUMMARY

A 2-limb tube for temporary gastrostomy which permits simultaneous and independent suction and jejunal feeding is presented and its mode of use described. Its particular value in gastroenterostomy and Billroth II gastrectomy is stressed, as well as its application after upper gastrointestinal operations on patients with cardiorespiratory decompensation and radical resections for carcinoma in the aged and debilitated individual.

Our recent favorable experience with emergency gastrostomy and insertion of a 2-limb tube in a case of severe duodenal fistula after a Billroth II gastrectomy, which allowed an effective aggressive approach of the blow-out of the stump, will be the subject of a future report.

## REFERENCES

1. Abbott, W. O., and Rawson, A. J.: A tube for use in the postoperative care of gastroenterostomy cases, J. A. M. A. **108:** 1873, 1937.
2. Bartels, E. C.: Acute ulcerative esophagitis; a pathological and clinical study of eighty-two cases observed at necropsy, Arch. Otolaryng. **23:** 550, 1936.
3. Bingham, J. A. W.: Esophageal strictures after gastric surgery and nasogastric intubation, Brit. M. J. **2:** 819, 1958.
4. Butt, H. E., and Vinson, B. P.: Esophagitis. Anatomy and physiology and a review of the literature, Arch. Otolaryng. **23:** 550, 1936.
5. Douglas, W. K.: Esophageal strictures associated with gastroduodenal intubation, Brit. J. Surg. **43:** 404, 1956.
6. Farris, J. M., and Smith, G. K.: An evaluation of temporary gastrostomy; a substitute for nasogastric intubation, Ann. Surg. **144:** 475, 1956.
7. Gilchrist, R. K.: Gastrostomy tubes, Surg. Gynec. & Obst. **106:** 631, 1958.
8. Graham, J., Barnes, N., and Rubenstein, A. S.: The nasogastric tube as a cause of esophagitis and stricture, Am. J. Surg. **98:** 116, 1959.
9. Hurwitz, A.: A new dual purpose gastrostomy tube, A. M. A. Arch. Surg. **77:** 79, 1958.
10. Iglauer, S., and Molt, W. F.: Severe injury to the larynx resulting from indwelling duodenal tubes, Ann. Otol. Rhinol. & Laryngol. **48:** 886, 1939.
11. McKeown, K. C.: Esophageal stenosis after partial gastrectomy, Brit. M. J. **2:** 819, 1958.
12. Mersheimer, W. L.: A double-tube method for drainage and feeding following gastric resection or gastroenterostomy, Surgery **12:** 563, 1942.

# Magnetic intubation

H. FRANK McCARTHY, M.D.
H. PHILIP HOVNANIAN, M.S.
TIMOTHY A. BRENNAN
PHILIP L. GAGNER, B.S.
WILMINGTON, MASS.
*From the Research and Advanced Development Division, Avco Corporation*

External magnetic forces may be used to guide a gastroduodenal tube through the pylorus into the duodenum. The system has provided successful decompression in patients with obstruction in a few minutes. This technique eliminates the delay associated with usual intubation methods and permits more rapid intestinal decompression in patients with serious distention.

A small permanent magnet is imbedded within the tip of a Cantor or Miller-Abbot tube. This tube is introduced into the stomach in the usual manner. It is then externally directed through the pylorus with the aid of the electromagnet.

## THE ELECTROMAGNET

Six different electromagnets were fabricated and tested for magnetic field intensity, heat generation, weight, and power requirements.

Figs. 1 and 2 demonstrate the final design of electromagnet in position on the right flank of the subject. A central iron core is wound with aluminum strips (instead of copper wire) in order to reduce weight to approximately 14 pounds. A thumb microswitch on the magnet handle turns the power on or off. The magnetic field configuration has been designed to diminish excessive attraction of the tube as it approaches the magnet face. This provides a gentle pull upon the tube tip at all times, regardless of the relative proximity of the magnets. The thumb-controlled microswitch provides intermittent attraction at will and minimizes magnet heating. The direct current power supply of the electromagnet operates from an alternating current line at

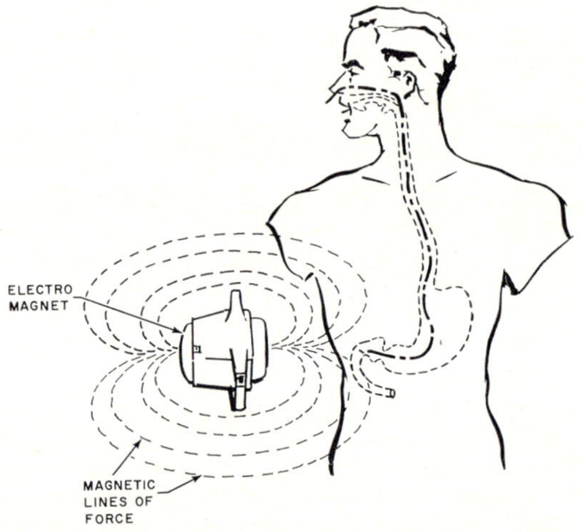


**Fig. 1.** Magnetic intubation diagram shows relative position of external magnet for transport through pyloric sphincter. Note that body does not present any insulation to magnetic lines.

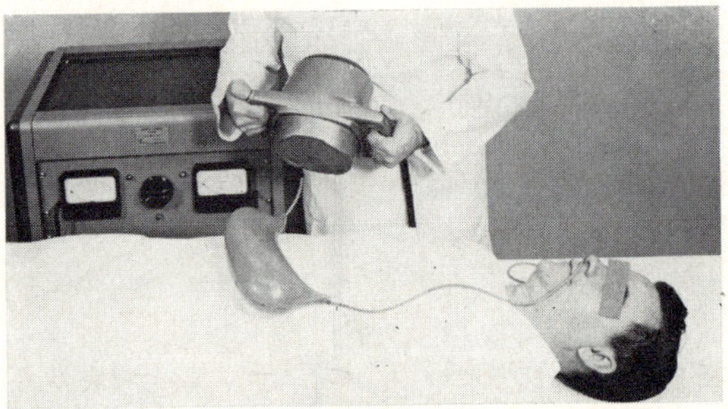

**Fig. 2.** Schematic photograph shows the relative positions of external electromagnet and the gastroduodenal tube with embedded magnet.

Received for publication Dec. 19, 1960.

115 v. and a little under 15 amp. at maximum power.

At times some manipulative procedures are concurrently needed, for example, freeing of the tip of the gastroduodenal tube from a stomachic fold caused by intestinal distention.

## CONCLUSION

Tests on patients indicate that the magnetic technique is feasible for rapidly directing the gastroduodenal tube with ease. The technique has proved to be safe.

Thanks are extended to Dr. Elton Watkins, Jr., of the Lahey Clinic, Boston, Massachusetts, Dr. Nicandro F. DeCesare of Clover Hill Hospital, Lawrence, Massachusetts, and to Dr. Samuel Klauber of the McCarthy Clinic in Lawrence, Massachusetts for their cooperation in the performance of tests on patients.

# Peritoneal tap in abdominal trauma

THEODORE DRAPANAS, M.D.
JOHN McDONALD, M.D.
BUFFALO, N. Y.
*From the Department of Surgery, University of Buffalo School of Medicine, and the Edward J. Meyer Memorial Hospital*

Along with the increasing incidence of traumatic lesions seen by physicians and emergency units of hospitals, the occurrence of multiple injuries after vehicular accidents has become a common problem.[4, 6] All too frequently, although a serious abdominal injury is present, it may be masked by concurrent head injury in a patient who may be unable to give an accurate history. In another patient, obvious injuries to the extremities and thorax may so detract from the symptomatology of abdominal trauma that serious delays in treatment may occur. Furthermore, the physician may be confronted with a patient so critically ill that complete diagnostic studies are not deemed advisable.

The control of hemorrhage from injured abdominal viscera continues to be the most common emergency measure to be necessitated by abdominal trauma. Williams and Zollinger,[8] in a recent review of 200 patients with abdominal trauma, state, "Eighty-eight per cent of deaths from nonpenetrating abdominal wounds were due to hemorrhage. . . . Of perhaps the most significance was a delay in diagnosis and treatment in half the patients who died."

It is apparent, therefore, that any attempts to decrease the mortality rate of abdominal trauma should be directed toward earlier diagnosis and treatment rather than improvement of surgical techniques which are fairly well standardized at the present time.

Received for publication Dec. 2, 1960.

One of the most valuable adjuncts in the diagnosis of suspected abdominal injury is the use of the so-called "peritoneal tap" or abdominal paracentesis. Despite numerous articles[1-3, 5, 7, 8] advocating acceptance of this valuable and simple diagnostic tool, some physicians continue to deplore its use, stating that it is a dangerous and ineffective procedure. Other physicians have not had adequate experience in performing this procedure or do not understand its merits or limitations.

In our institution, we have performed numerous peritoneal taps in the past 10 years, and the procedure has been an important tool in the differential diagnosis of abdominal trauma. It is the purpose of this report to present our experience and a brief review of the techniques of peritoneal tap in an attempt to emphasize the merits of this valuable procedure.

## TECHNIQUE

The method of recovering fluid from the peritoneal cavity has undergone few changes in the past half century.[3] Fig. 1 depicts the sterile tray for peritoneal tap which is always available in our emergency room. Frequently, however, in a critical situation, a single sterile syringe and a long 18 or 20 gauge spinal needle will suffice. The patient, shortly after voiding or after catheterization if he is unable to void, is placed in the supine position and a rapid skin preparation is performed. We have preferred to use a dilute iodine solution followed by alcohol because of ready availability of these agents.

The abdomen is carefully examined and scars or other points of fixation of bowel to the abdominal wall are avoided in order to prevent penetration with the needle.

Subcutaneous skin wheals are raised at each puncture site with a 25 gauge needle and a few milliliters of a local anesthetic agent is infiltrated into the abdominal wall. Ordinarily, infiltration only of the skin and peritoneum is necessary. A long 18 or 20 gauge, short beveled spinal needle attached to a 10 ml. syringe is inserted through the abdominal wall until the peritoneum is entered, as determined by a slight "give" to the needle. Gentle suction is intermittently applied to the syringe as the needle is advanced slowly or carefully changed in position in searching for the desired fluid. If a positive tap is obtained, the needle is withdrawn and the procedure terminated. We have usually considered a minimum of 0.1 ml. of fluid as evidence of a positive tap. On occasions, when fluid other than blood is obtained, it is immediately placed in a sterile test tube for subsequent culture and also smeared on a slide for microscopic examination. If the initial tap is negative or any question of the source of the aspirated fluid arises, taps are repeated in other sites or quadrants.

Figs. 2 and 3 show the usual sites preferred for 4-quadrant or bilateral flank taps. We believe that puncture through the rectus sheath anteriorly should be condemned for 3 reasons. First, rectus sheath hematoma may result because of the course of the inferior epigastric vessels as shown. Second, the chance of needle penetration of the bowel is higher because gas-filled loops of bowel will tend to float anteriorly in an abdomen containing fluid or blood. Finally, aspiration laterally along the peritoneal gutters will increase the chances of success of the tap if only small amounts of fluid are present. In our experience, bilateral flank taps are equally as reliable as those performed in all 4 quadrants.

We have obtained a positive tap with as little as 200 ml. of blood present in the peritoneal cavity measured at the time of laparotomy. Giacobine and Siler,[3] in an excellent experimental study with dogs, showed that a 78 per cent positive tap rate can be achieved with a volume of blood comparable to 500 ml. in the average human adult.

Table I shows the accuracy of peritoneal tap reported by other authors in recent publications. A positive tap rate approximating 80 per cent can be anticipated with correct technique, and emphasizes the accuracy of this procedure.

## COMPLICATIONS

Complications attendant to this procedure are rare. We have seen only 1 complication in our series and this was attributed to faulty technique resulting from puncture

**Table I.** *Results of peritoneal taps in recent experimental and clinical reports on abdominal trauma*

| *Report* | *No. of cases* | *% accuracy* |
|---|---|---|
| Giacobine and Siler (1960) | 101 patients | 82 |
| Williams and Zollinger (1959) | 200 patients | 79 |
| Baxter and Williams (1960) | 80 dogs | 90 |
| Economy and associates (1960) | 47 patients | 83 |
| Authors' series | 80 patients | 82 |

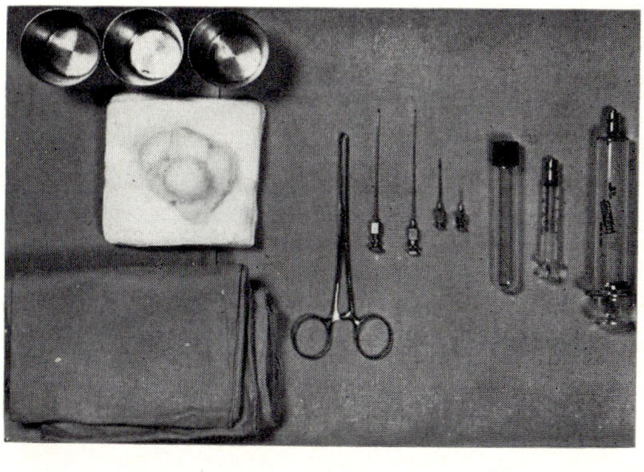

**Fig. 1.** Tray for abdominal paracentesis available in emergency room for immediate use.

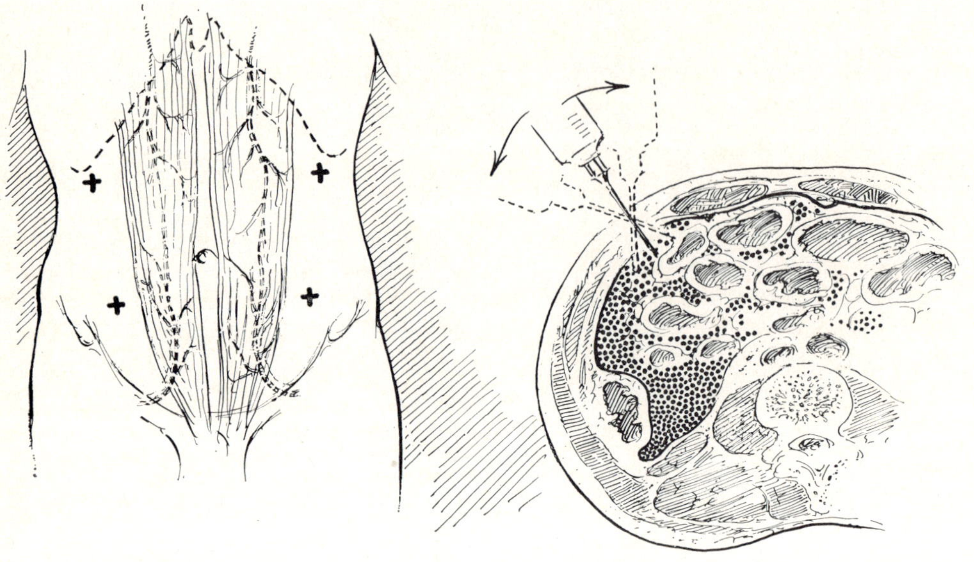

**Fig. 2.** Technique for 4-quadrant peritoneal taps. Preferred location for aspiration of each quadrant is shown. Note that puncture through the rectus sheath is avoided.

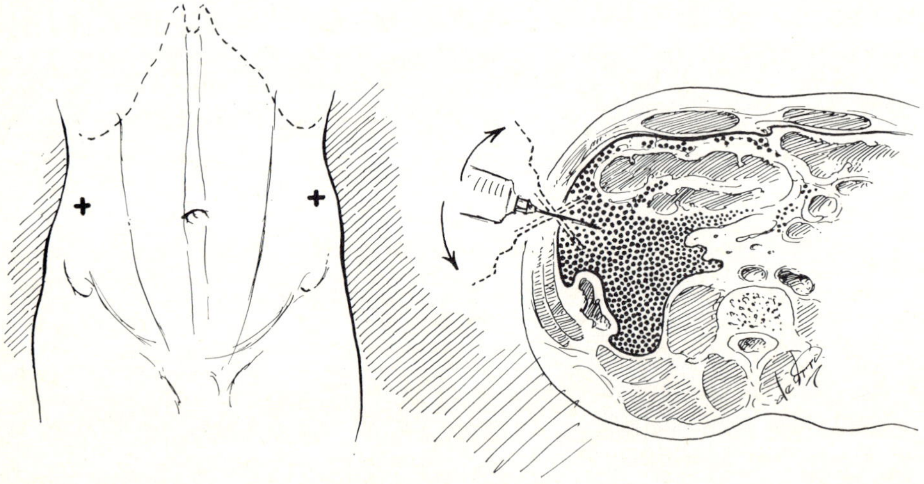

**Fig. 3.** Technique for bilateral flank taps. Aspiration is performed in each flank midway between costal margin and iliac spine. In our experience, bilateral flank taps are equally as reliable and more easily performed than 4-quadrant taps in cases of abdominal trauma.

through the rectus sheath and laceration of the inferior epigastric artery which necessitated subsequent drainage of a hematoma. Although in some instances bowel content was aspirated, no known complications have occurred. At subsequent laparotomy in most of the patients, no evidence of the puncture wound in the bowel causing continued leakage and requiring suture has been found. We have not considered this occurrence to be a serious drawback to the procedure inasmuch as direct puncture of the bowel with an 18 gauge needle performed during other surgical procedures rarely, if ever, requires suturing because of the self-sealing action of the bowel wall. Similar conclusions have been reached by most authors on this subject. Nevertheless, at least on theoretical grounds, it is believed that peritoneal tap should probably be avoided in the presence of distended bowel in which the elevated intraluminal pressure may tend to cause continued leakage, even through a small needle puncture.

A careful perusal of our experience and that reported in the literature does not show any known instances of laceration of an intraperitoneal or mesenteric vessel attributed to a peritoneal tap.

Examples of the invaluable information obtained by peritoneal tap can perhaps be emphasized by case reports.

## CASE REPORTS

**Case 1.** C. P., a 20-year-old man, was admitted 15 minutes after an accident involving an automobile which he was driving. He was unconscious and did not respond, even to painful stimuli. There was a large scalp laceration, and the pupils were unequal and responded poorly to light. The initial blood pressure was 120/75 mm. Hg, pulse rate was 120 per minute, and respirations were irregular. Breath sounds were diminished on the right and paradoxical motion of the right upper anterior chest was present. The abdomen was soft with normal peristalsis. Deep-tendon reflexes were absent in the left upper extremity, and bilateral Babinski signs were present. Chest roentgenogram showed a right pneumothorax and multiple right rib fractures. A closed-tube thoracostomy and tracheostomy were performed, resulting in marked improvement of the patient's condition. Catheterization showed a grossly bloody urine. Despite negative abdominal signs, peritoneal taps were performed in both flanks shortly after admission and these showed a free flow of blood from the right side. A transfusion was promptly started, and the patient received a total of 2,000 ml. of blood and 2,000 ml. of saline solution in the next 2 hours while the neurological status was being carefully evaluated. A laparotomy was performed, and approximately 3,000 ml. of blood found in the peritoneal cavity from a ruptured spleen and a liver laceration. Splenectomy and suture of the liver laceration were carried out. Postoperatively, the patient remained comatose for the next 4 days, then gradually regained consciousness. Lumbar puncture on the fifth day showed xanthochromic fluid. The patient's subsequent course was uncomplicated except for a residual neurological deficit in the left upper extremity related to a probable brachial plexus injury.

This case illustrates the necessity of peritoneal taps despite the absence of abdominal signs in an unconscious patient with multiple injuries. In this instance, blood replacement was rapidly instituted and operation was promptly performed to control intraperitoneal bleeding. At no time was the patient in oligemic shock. A considerable delay in diagnosis of the abdominal injury might have occurred in this patient had peritoneal taps not been so promptly performed.

**Case 2.** W. P., a 30-year-old woman, was admitted to the psychiatric service with acute alcoholic intoxication, tremors, and confusion. Studies in the hospital yielded a clinical diagnosis of chronic Laennec's cirrhosis with hepatosplenomegaly. Four months after admission, because of continued hepatomegaly, a needle liver biopsy was performed through the tenth intercostal space at the anterior axillary line without event. The next day because of anorexia, mild abdominal distention, and questionable tenderness in the epigastrium, surgical consultation was obtained. Blood pressure at that time was 110/70 mm. Hg and pulse was 116 per minute. Hemoglobin was 11.5 Gm. Four-quadrant peritoneal taps were performed, and 50 ml. of dark blood was obtained from the right lower quadrant. Transfusion of 1,000 ml. of blood and a laparotomy were performed. A 2 cm. laceration of the liver and 2,000 ml. of blood were found in the peritoneal cavity. Suture of the liver laceration was performed, additional transfusions were given, and the patient had an uneventful recovery.

This case, like the previous one, also emphasizes the value of diagnostic peritoneal taps in a patient with equivocal clinical signs in whom an earlier diagnosis was made and the necessity for blood replacement and operation was recognized before the appearance of clinical shock.

**Case 3.** J. G., a 45-year-old man, was admitted to the hospital in a disoriented state 2 hours after an automobile accident. Blood pressure was 110/80 mm. Hg and pulse was 88 per minute. Physical examination was negative except for lack of conjugate eye movement and mild upper abdominal tenderness and spasm. Hematocrit was 40 per cent. Four-quadrant peritoneal taps gave negative results. Roentgenograms of the skull and abdominal scout films were negative. Despite the negative peritoneal taps, exploratory laparotomy was performed, and a retroperitoneal laceration of the duodenum was found and repaired. No free fluid was present in the peritoneal cavity. The postoperative course was uneventful.

This case is presented to emphasize the need for abdominal exploration in a patient with abdominal signs after blunt abdominal trauma despite negative roentgenographic evidence and negative results of peritoneal taps. A negative peritoneal tap should not replace surgical judgment in this instance, for only positive taps are to be considered significant.

## SUMMARY

1. Peritoneal tap is a useful, safe, and highly accurate procedure. The indications, techniques, and evaluation of results of peritoneal tap are discussed.

2. The most significant causes of death in acute abdominal trauma continue to be a delay in diagnosis and inadequate resuscitation and control of hemorrhage. It is believed that the frequent use of peritoneal tap as a diagnostic adjunct, in addition to the established surgical principles, will prevent delay and lead to earlier surgical intervention in the patient with occult intraperitoneal injury.

### REFERENCES

1. Baxter, C. F., and Williams, R. D.: Blunt abdominal trauma. Presented to the American Association for the Surgery of Trauma, Oct. 5, 1960, Coronado, Calif. J. Trauma **1:** 241, 1961.
2. Economy, D., Koucky, C., and Novack, R. L.: Non-penetrating injuries to the spleen, Am. J. Surg. **99:** 647, 1960.
3. Giacobine, J. W., and Siler, V. E.: Evaluation of diagnostic abdominal paracentesis with experimental and clinical studies, Surg. Gynec. & Obst. **110:** 676, 1960.
4. Kennedy, R. H., Blum, L., Bryer, B. F., and Payson, B. A.: The multiple injury patient, Bull. Am. Coll. Surgeons **42:** 107, 1957.
5. Shaftan, G. W., Gliedman, M. L., and Cappelletti, R. R.: Liver injuries—a review of one hundred and eleven cases. Presented to the American Association for the Surgery of Trauma, Oct. 5, 1960, Coronado, Calif. In press.
6. Shortliffe, E. C., Hamilton, T. S., and Noroian, E. H.: The emergency room and the changing pattern of medical care, New England J. Med. **258:** 20, 1958.
7. Thompson, C. T., and Brown, D. R.: Diagnostic paracentesis in the acute abdomen, SURGERY **35:** 916, 1954.
8. Williams, R. D., and Zollinger, R. M.: Diagnostic and prognostic factors in abdominal trauma, Am. J. Surg. **97:** 575, 1959.

# Technique in resection of esophageal diverticulum

J. MURRAY BEARDSLEY, M.D.
PROVIDENCE, R. I.
*From the Department of Surgery, Rhode Island Hospital*

The one-stage operation for Zenker's diverticulum of the esophagus is now generally accepted as the operation of choice. Other techniques, such as suspension, inversion of the diverticulum, and the two-stage procedure, have little to recommend them. Although the one-stage operation has been generally accepted, certain refinements can be applied which will tend to ensure a more perfect end result.

The 2 main pitfalls that have long been recognized are, first, inadequate removal of the sac and, second, the danger of narrowing at the point of excision (Fig. 1). In order to avoid these 2 errors, we have for some years employed a method that has been extremely helpful to us and, in our opinion, allows the surgeon to accomplish the operation with a greater degree of perfection.

The operation is routinely carried out with a nasogastric tube in place, and some surgeons believe that as the diverticulum is being resected, the "open" method will guard against the aforementioned dangers. This is not always true since it may still be difficult to pinpoint the exact junction between the esophagus and the diverticulum, especially at the inferior border. If the slightest amount of diverticulum is left at this point, recurrence is likely. Furthermore, even with a Levin tube in the esophagus, it is still possible to angulate the esophagus as the dissection is being carried out.

After exposure of the esophagus, either through a vertical incision along the anterior border of the sternal mastoid or a curved transverse incision (we prefer the latter for cosmetic reasons), the diverticulum is identified and partially dissected out. At this stage, the anesthetist threads a McGill tube over the nasogastric tube and the surgeon gently assists its passage beyond the

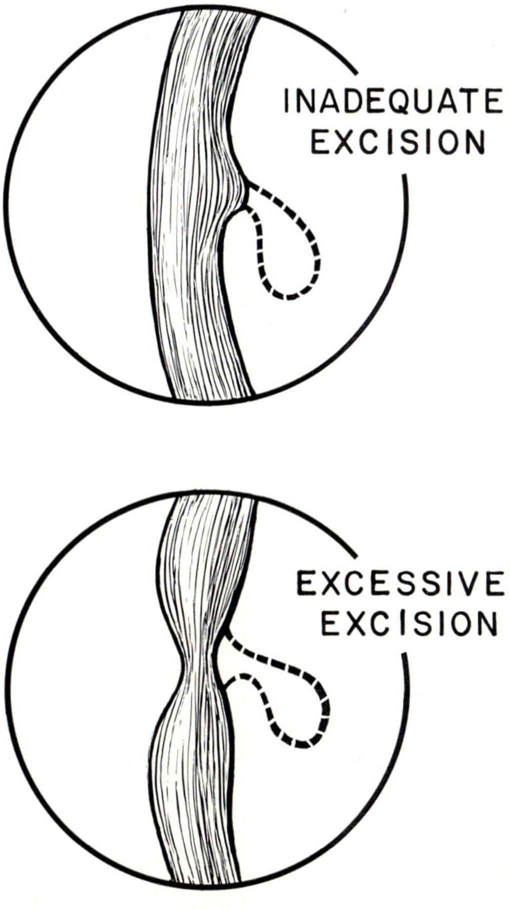


Fig. 1.

Received for publication Jan. 9, 1961.

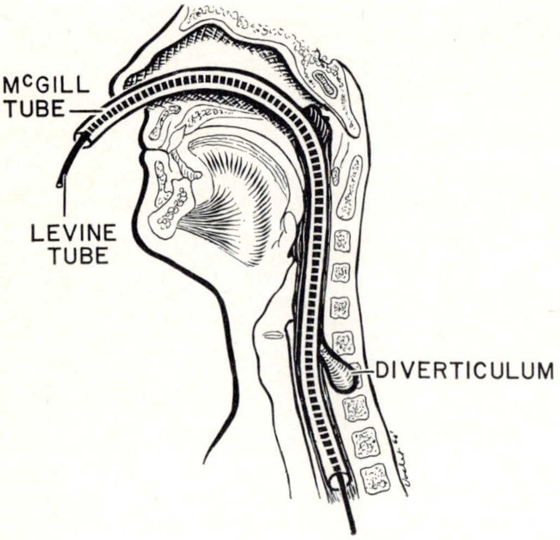


**Fig. 2.**

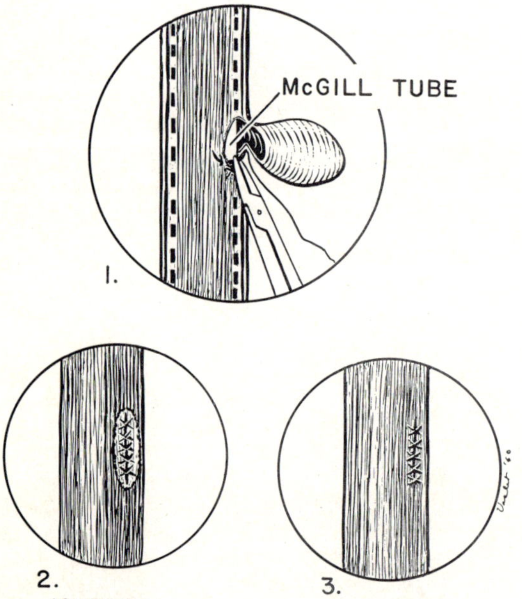


**Fig. 3.**

neck of the diverticulum (Fig. 2). With this wide-caliber rigid tube in place, the dissection is continued. It is now impossible to

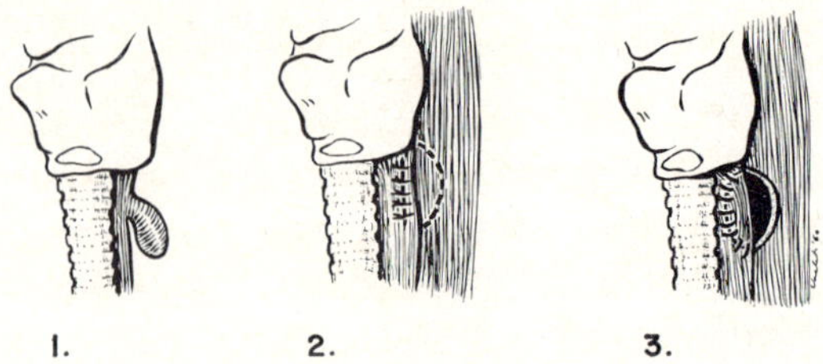


**Fig. 4.**

angulate the esophagus and thus narrowing is prevented. Furthermore, the normal diameter of the esophagus is demonstrated and preserved which allows a definitive dissection, excision, and closure of the mucosal layer.

No crushing instruments should ever be placed on the esophageal side. Sutures are placed as the untraumatized mucosa is cut and closed over the McGill tube. As the diverticulum is excised, closure is made with atraumatic interrupted sutures of No. 4-0 silk in a manner similar to that used in dividing and closing the bronchus. The McGill tube is visible as this step is being carried out. After closure of the mucosal layer, the McGill tube is withdrawn to allow for a relaxed closure of the muscular layer (Fig. 3).

Drains should never be placed in proximity to the suture line since this will encourage fistula formation. However, there is no real objection to placing a small rubber tissue drain 2 to 3 cm. distant from the line of suture. With the present technique, we have never had a fistula develop and, as a matter of fact, we employ drainage only occasionally.

We have continued to use a pedicle flap of prevertebral fascia as a buttress to the suture line, as previously reported (Fig. 4).

**REFERENCE**

1. Beardsley, J. M.: Diverticulum of esophagus, Am. J. Surg. **88:** 331, 1954.

# Metastatic malignant schwannoma with bilateral pulmonary resection

K. H. RONALD CHANG, M.D.
FAUSTINO N. NIGUIDULA, M.D.
BUFFALO, N. Y.
*From the Department of Health, State of New York; J. N. Adam Memorial Hospital; and the Department of Surgery, Buffalo General Hospital*

Although pulmonary resection for solitary pulmonary metastatic lesions after the primary lesion has been controlled is now an established procedure, resection for multiple pulmonary metastatic nodules with bilateral involvement has been very rarely performed and, in fact, is not advocated by most thoracic surgeons. Review of the English literature up to 1959 has shown that only 12 cases have been reported in which bilateral resection for metastatic lesions were performed (Table I).

Schwannoma or neurilemmoma is generally considered to be a benign, slow-growing tumor. Malignant degeneration is very rare and only 4 documented instances have been reported.[12, 16] This rarity may be actual but the confusion in the nomenclature of this tumor may indicate that the malignant forms are more frequent. Furthermore, the embryonal origin of Schwann cells from the neural crest may make it indistinguishable from other malignant tumors of similar origin, such as sympathicoblastomas.[16]

This case is presented because (1) malignant schwannoma is very rare, (2) bilateral resection for multiple metastatic pulmonary lesions is seldom performed, and (3) the patient is alive 3 years after the first lobectomy and 2½ years after the second lobectomy.

## CASE REPORT

U. D., a 64-year-old white man, had a tumor removed from the left side of the neck beneath the angle of the mandible in February, 1950. The lesion had been first discovered by the patient 3 years previously. At that time it was about the size of a pea, and by the time of excision its size had increased to that of a "small egg." The histologic picture of the resected growth was that of a neurofibrosarcoma.

In May, 1954, 4 years after the first excision, the tumor recurred, and it was removed locally. Microscopically the tissue removed showed interlacing bundles of elongated cells arranged in a plexiform manner. The nuclei were large, irregular, and hyperchromatic with an occasional mitosis. A diagnosis of malignant schwannoma was made (Fig. 1). Another local excision was performed in September, 1954, for the recurrence of a mass in the same area, but the histologic section at that time showed only granulation tissue.

Two years later, July, 1956, the patient was admitted to the Roswell Park Memorial Institute for recurrence of the growth in the left submaxillary area. The patient stated at that time that the rate of growth appeared to be faster. Excisional biopsy was carried out. The tissue removed was 3 by 2 by 1 cm. in size. The tumor mass was lobulated and encapsulated with a histologic picture similar to that present in 1954. This local excision was followed by left radical neck dissection. Although the excised lymph nodes were reported to be free of tumor, a portion of the muscle and connective tissue was found to be invaded by malignant cells. Chest roentgenograms at that time did not show any evidence of lung metastasis. The patient was followed, thereafter, at the Roswell Park Memorial Institute and no recurrence of the tumor in the neck or evidence of metastasis was noted.

The patient was next admitted to the J. N. Adam Memorial Hospital on July 8, 1957 for complaints of nonproductive cough, easy fatigue, pain in the left side of the chest, and some difficulty in swallowing. He had lost 16 pounds of weight during the preceding 6 months, and a chest roentgenogram made shortly before admission showed an abnormal shadow in the left lung field (Fig. 2). The patient had been smoking 1

**Table I.** *Reported cases of bilateral pulmonary resection for metastatic lesions*

| Year | Author | Lesion | Procedure | Interval* 1 | Interval* 2 | Remarks |
|---|---|---|---|---|---|---|
| 1940 | Churchill[4] | —— | Bilateral partial lobectomy | — | — | No details |
| 1947 | Alexander[1, 2] | Spindle-cell neurosarcoma | Bilateral lobectomy | 1 yr. | 1 yr. | Alive after 9½ yr. |
| 1951 | Ehrenhaft[6] | Leiomyosarcoma | Resection of lingula | 46 mo. | 2 mo. | Died 6 mo. after lung operation, 4½ yr. after primary operation |
| 1955 | Higginson[8] | Teratocarcinoma | (1) Multiple segment, right, (2) multiple segment, left, (3) segment, left lower lobe | 23 mo. | 2 wk.<br>6 mo. | 8 mo. after lung operation had left nephrectomy and adrenalectomy, died |
| 1955 | Higginson[8] | Adenocarcinoma of stomach | (1) Left lower lobectomy, (2) segment, right lower lobe | 45 mo. | 17 mo. | Only 3 mo. follow-up with no recurrence |
| 1955 | Jones[10] | Malignant melanoma | (1) Lower lobectomy, (2) lower lobectomy | 8 yr. | 8 mo. | Died 7 mo. after second lobectomy |
| 1955 | Weinberg[21] | Osteosarcoma of femur; had hemipelvectomy | Local excision | Few months | | No follow-up |
| 1956 | Groves and Effler[7] | Hemangiopericytoma of skin of back | (1) Local excision, (2) local excision, right lung | 13 yr. | 2 yr. | No follow-up |
| 1956 | Groves and Effler[7] | Hemangiopericytoma of femur | (1) Local excision, left upper lobe, (2) local excision, right upper lobe | 1 yr. | 14 mo. | 1½ yr., no recurrence |
| 1956 | Strieder[19] | Adenocarcinoma of colon | (1) Right upper lobectomy, (2) left lower lobectomy | 1 yr. | 7 mo. | Died 2 yr. later |
| 1956 | Strieder[19] | Adenocarcinoma of colon | (1) Segment, left upper lobe, (2) left upper lobectomy | 5 yr. | 4 yr. | Alive 71 mo. after second operation |
| 1959 | Rumel[16] | Osteogenic sarcoma | (1) Right middle lobectomy, (2) left lower lobectomy and lingulectomy | — | 3 wk. | 7-year "cure" |
| 1960 | Chang | Malignant schwannoma | (1) Right upper lobectomy, (2) right upper lobectomy | 6 yr. | 10 mo. | 3 years, alive |

*1, Interval between removal of primary lesion and first pulmonary resection. 2, Interval between the 2 pulmonary resections.

pack of cigarettes per day for the past 48 years. He had worked as a farmer and later as a buffer in a tanning factory. He had resided almost exclusively in western New York.

Physical examination on admission showed him to be a well-developed, fairly well-nourished white man in no acute respiratory distress. The temperature was normal. There was a healed incisional scar in the left submandibular area. The lungs were clear to auscultation and percussion. The results of a tuberculin test and sputum examinations for tumor cells were negative. Several 24- and 72-hour sputum specimens were negative for the presence of acid-fast bacilli when studied by the concentration and culture methods.

Chest roentgenograms showed an abnormal density located anteriorly in the left upper lobe. No cavity was demonstrated in planigraphic views. Bronchoscopy and bronchograms failed to show signs of any endobronchial disease. The planigrams showed 2 separate, fairly discrete shadows with surrounding haziness.

On Aug. 20, 1957, a left thoracotomy was performed. The palpable and visible disease was limited to the left upper lobe and consisted of a dimpling and retraction at the junction of the anterior and apicoposterior segments. A hard irregular mass, measuring 3 by 4 cm., was first removed by wedge excision but when the frozen section showed malignant schwannoma a left upper lobe lobectomy was performed (Fig. 3). The thickened area in the operative scar of the neck was likewise excised a few days later, but was found to be free of tumor on microscopic examination.

The patient was then followed in the Outpatient Department and monthly chest roentgenograms did not show any change until 8 months later when new disease was seen in the right upper lobe (Fig. 4). By this time, the patient had again developed a cough, but it was productive of 30 to 100 ml. of mucoid sputum per day. He was readmitted to the J. N. Adam Memorial Hospital on April 24, 1958. Physical examination yielded essentially negative results. Results of tuberculin and histoplasmin skin tests were negative. The sputum was negative for acid-fast bacilli and tumor cells. Pulmonary function studies showed a maximum breathing capacity of 47 L. and a vital capacity of 2,850 ml., or 74 per cent of predicted normal. On May 26, 1958, a right upper lobe lobectomy was performed. The resected lobe contained 3 large nodules, 1 in the apical segment, a smaller one in the anterior segment, and another small one at the junction of the anterior and posterior segments. Microscopic sections showed involvement of the subpleural parenchyma and also the overlying pleura. The cells were long and spindle-shaped, arranged in interlacing bundles with tendency to palisade. The nuclei varied in size and shape, and there were as many as 7 mitotic figures per high power field (Fig. 5). The postoperative course was complicated by an auricular fibrillation which responded to digitoxin and quinidine. Since discharge from the hospital on July 11, 1958, the patient has been followed in the Outpatient Department. He has maintained his weight at around 170 pounds. He complains only of moderate dyspnea on exertion which he claims prevents him from any gainful occupation. Serial chest roentgenograms have not shown significant change or evidence of a new lesion (Fig. 6).

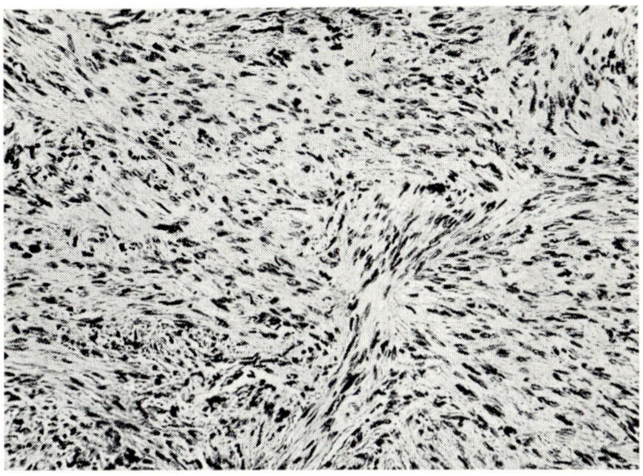

**Fig. 1.** Section from the original lesion from left side of neck shows interlacing bundles of elongated cells arranged in plexiform manner. The nuclei are large, irregular, and hyperchromatic with occasional mitosis. (Hematoxylin and eosin; ×100; reduced 4/7.)

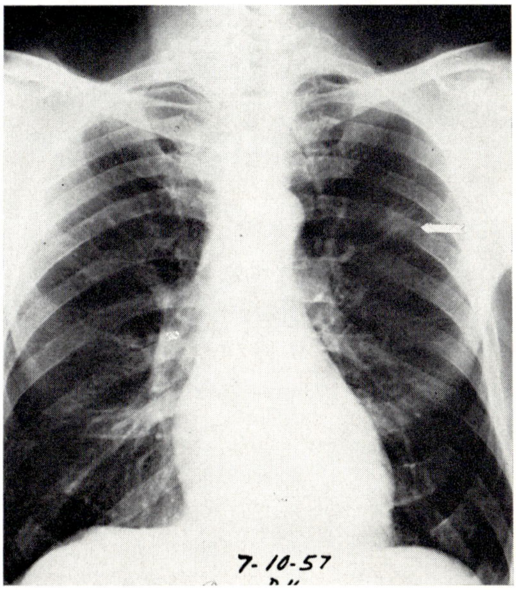


**Fig. 2.** Chest roentgenogram taken in 1957 shows the lesion in the left upper lung field.

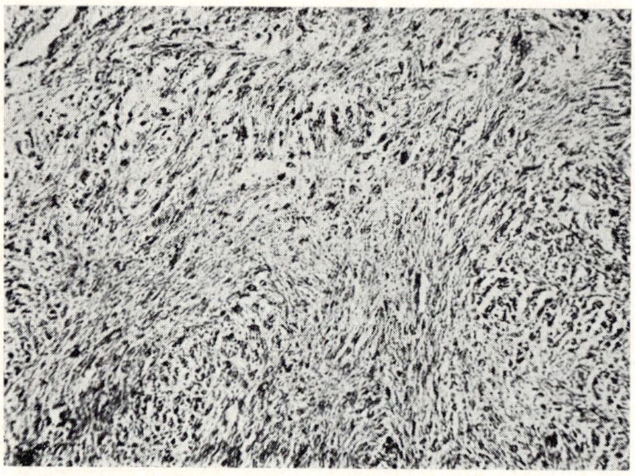

**Fig. 3.** Microscopic section of the lesion removed from the left upper lobe shows a very similar pattern to that seen in Fig. 1. (Hematoxylin and eosin; ×100; reduced 4/7.)

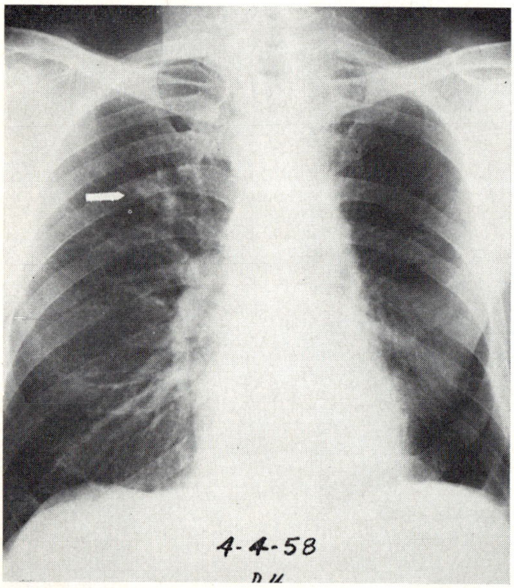


**Fig. 4.** Chest roentgenogram taken 8 months after the first film shows new disease in the right upper lung field.

## DISCUSSION

Robinson, in a recent survey of all the thoracic surgeons in the United States, found that 91.8 per cent, or a total of 279, of the responding surgeons resect solitary pulmonary metastatic lesions.[15] Although not openly admitted, resection for metastatic lesions, when the primary site has been controlled, is now widely practiced and even recommended as an advisable procedure. The extent of resection advocated is very limited and in most cases is performed in the guise of palliation.

In the majority of cases the removal of a solitary pulmonary nodule is motivated by the absence of a definite diagnosis. The appearance of a nodule in the lung sometime after removal of an extrapulmonary malignancy is no indication that it is necessarily metastatic. The chance of its being another primary lesion is from 3.2[3] to 4.1 per cent.[13] Several authors have set criteria for differentiating a metastatic nodule from a primary lesion, but even this is not helpful to the surgeon, who usually has to make the final decisions as to whether or not thoracotomy should be performed.[5-11]

The lung is the second most common site of metastatic lesions for most malignancies.[14] Pulmonary metastases result from embolization after tumor invasion of the regional veins at the primary site.[16] If the primary growth had been completely controlled, no further embolization and lung involvement need be expected. In 18.3 per cent of lung metastases, there is an invasion of the bronchial wall. It is therefore very likely that further spread in the lung from the metastatic focus can be accomplished by both hematologic and bronchogenic pathways.[14] Coexistent multiple metastatic foci need not necessarily arise from the original extrapulmonary primary focus.

In the majority of cases reported, there was a time interval between the appearance of the various lung lesions. Removal of 1 focus and subsequent appearance of another focus again raises the possibility of the latter nodule being a primary tumor. Again, thoracotomy is performed mainly for diagnosis and secondly for prevention of complications such as hemoptysis, bronchial obstruction, and suppuration. The morbidity and mortality rate for exploratory thoracotomy has now been reduced to a minimum so that even for palliative purposes, resection may be offered.

Analysis of the 12 reported cases and our case, in which bilateral resections have been performed, showed no correlation between the type of tumor and the length of survival period after pulmonary resection. Six of the 13 patients (46 per cent) survived over 1 year after the second operation, whereas the survival rate for 1 year and over after pulmonary resection for unilateral metastatic lesion is 75 per cent.[19]

## SUMMARY AND CONCLUSION

A case of a 64-year-old white man who underwent bilateral lobectomy for metastatic pulmonary lesions arising from a previously removed malignant schwannoma of the neck is presented. The patient is alive and well 2½ years after bilateral pulmonary resection. Malignant degeneration of schwannoma (neurilemmoma) is very rare. Bilateral pulmonary resection for metastatic lesions is occasionally performed and, so far, only 12 cases are reported in the English literature.

Resection for multiple metastatic lesions in the lung, when the removal is surgically feasible and will not incapacitate the patient, appears to be justified in certain selected cases not only for palliation, but also in hope of cure.

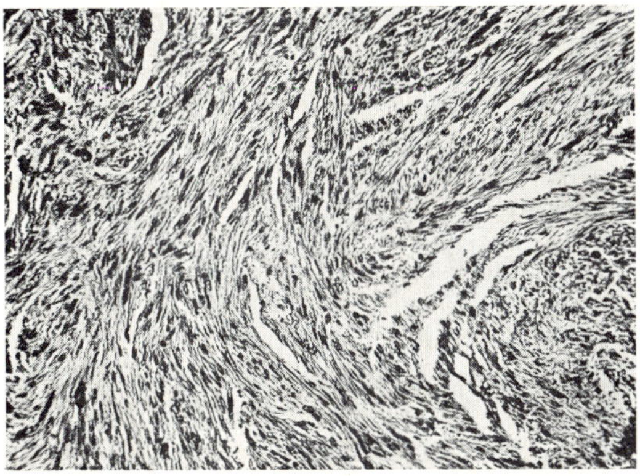

**Fig. 5.** Section from the right upper lobe. The cells are long and spindle shaped, arranged in interlacing bundles with tendency to palisades. The nuclei vary in size and shape and there are numerous mitotic figures. (Hematoxylin and eosin; ×100; reduced ⅘.)

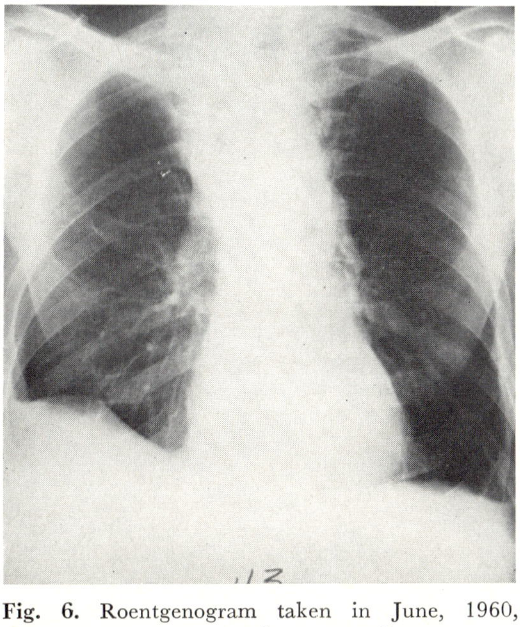

**Fig. 6.** Roentgenogram taken in June, 1960, shows no recurrence and no new disease.

### REFERENCES

1. Alexander, J.: Discussion of Alexander, J., and Haight, C.[2]
2. Alexander, J., and Haight, C.: Pulmonary resection for solitary metastasis, Surg. Gynec. & Obst. **85:** 29, 1947.
3. Cahan, W. G.: Lung cancer associated with cancer primary in other sites, Am. J. Surg. **89:** 494, 1955.
4. Churchill, E. D.: Resection of lung, SURGERY **8:** 961, 1940.
5. Cotton, B. H.: Differential diagnosis of primary and metastatic malignancy of the lung, Am. J. Surg. **54:** 173, 1940.
6. Ehrenhaft, J. L.: Pulmonary resection for metastatic lesions, Arch. Surg. **63:** 326, 1950.
7. Groves, L. K., and Effler, D. B.: Surgery for metastatic neoplastic disease of the lung, Cleveland Clin. Quart. **23:** 16, 1956.
8. Higginson, J. F.: A study of excised pulmonary metastatic malignancy, Am. J. Surg. **90:** 241, 1955.
9. Hood, R. T., McBurney, R. P., and Clagett, O. T.: Metastatic malignant lesions of the lungs treated by resection, J. Thoracic Surg. **30:** 81, 1955.
10. Jones, J. C.: Discussion of Higginson, J. F.[8]
11. Kelly, C. R., and Langstron, H. T.: Treatment of metastatic pulmonary malignancy, J. Thoracic Surg. **31:** 298, 1956.
12. Kragh, L. V., Soule, E. H., and Masson, J. K.: Benign and malignant neurilemmomas of the neck and head, Surg. Gynec. & Obst. **111:** 211, 1960.
13. Moetel, C. G., Anderson, H. A., and Baggentass, A. H.: Coexistence of primary lung cancer and other primary malignant neoplasms, Dis. Chest **35:** 343, 1959.
14. Reingold, I. M., and Konwaler, B. E.: Metastatic malignant tumors of the bronchus

found in bronchial biopsy and secretion, Dis. Chest **18:** 162, 1950.
15. Robinson, J. L., Jones, J. C., and Meyer, B. W.: Indication for lobectomy in treatment of cancer of the lung, J. Thoracic Surg. **32:** 500, 1956.
16. Rumel, W. R., Cutler, R. R., and Halliday, W. R.: Metastatic osteogenic sarcoma with bilateral pulmonary resection, Dis. Chest **35:** 106, 1959.
17. Schlumberger, H. G.: Malignant schwannoma. Tumors of mediastinum, Armed Forces Institute of Pathology, 1951.
18. Seiler, H. H., Clagett, O. T., and MacDonald, J. R.: Pulmonary resection for metastatic malignant lesions, J. Thoracic Surg. **19:** 655, 1950.
19. Strieder, J. W.: Surgical management of neoplastic pulmonary metastasis, New England J. Med. **254:** 1059, 1956.
20. Warren, S., and Gates, O.: Multiple primary malignant tumors. Survey of literature and statistics, Am. J. Cancer **16:** 1358, 1932.
21. Weinberg, J. A.: Discussion of Higginson, J. F.[8]

# Anuria after operation for abdominal aortic aneurysm treated by hemodialysis with complete recovery

JÖRGEN HINDBERG, M.D.
SATORU NAKAMOTO, M.D.
WILLEM J. KOLFF, M.D.
CLEVELAND, OHIO
*From the Department of Artificial Organs and Division of Research, The Cleveland Clinic Foundation, and The Frank E. Bunts Educational Institute*

Acute renal failure is one of the common and most severe complications of grafting of the aorta, and it is often the direct cause of death. Anuria after aortic operations may be due to any of 5 causes.

First, emboli of atheromatous material may be whirled up the clamped part of the aorta and lodged in the renal arteries.[5] This is the most frequent cause of anuria and is almost always fatal,* but it occurs less frequently in patients who are handled by experienced surgeons.

Second, ischemia due to low blood volume, shock, and temporary occlusion of renal vessels may result in acute tubular necrosis.

Third, blood transfusion accidents or overheating of cold blood may cause hemoglobinuric tubular damage.

Fourth, tubular damage occurs more often when a large number of transfusions have been given, and also when necrosis of an extremity is present. It is likely that sludging of blood may play a role in the pathogenesis of this type of tubular damage.

Fifth, anuria may result from a combination of the factors described. An excellent review of the pathogenesis of renal failure after aortic operations has recently been given by Doolan and associates.[1]

Received for publication Nov. 25, 1960.

*We saw 6 of these occurrences in 1 year, but have never seen one originate among the patients operated on at the Cleveland Clinic.[2, 3]

## CASE REPORT

A 54-year-old man who had suffered increasingly severe lumbar pain for a period of 9 months was found to have a large abdominal aortic aneurysm. A Dacron aortic graft was inserted. The aneurysm extended from the immediate subrenal level to the bifurcation of the aorta with calcification of the aortic wall and the common iliac arteries. The operation lasted over 9 hours and was difficult because of an unusual amount of adhesions and dense inflammatory connective tissue around the aneurysm. Lacerations of the right renal artery and the left renal vein occurred. The right renal artery had to be reanastomosed so that the right kidney was without a blood supply for approximately 90 minutes. The left renal vein, being obstructed for approximately 4 hours, was replaced by a venous autograft taken from the saphenous vein. After operation, there were good pulsations in both femoral and pedal arteries. During the operation 7 pints of whole blood and 1 pint of plasma were given to the patient. There was no evidence of incompatibility.

Postoperatively, the patient was given Levophed and Sol-Cortef for 2 days. He was also treated with cortisone, calcium gluconate, and Aureomycin, because of the need to maintain the blood pressure with vasopressors. Daily fluid intake was about 2 L. Immediately after the operation he developed severe oliguria with a daily urinary output of less than 150 ml. The blood urea level increased to 104 mg. per 100 ml. on the third day; serum creatinine reached 13 mg. per 100 ml.; carbon dioxide content was 22 mEq. per liter, serum potassium, 5.8 mEq. per liter; and sodium, 134 mEq. per liter.

The patient was tranferred to the Cleveland Clinic Hospital on the fourth postoperative day for evaluation and treatment with the artificial kidney.[4] Upon admission to the Clinic, he was alert

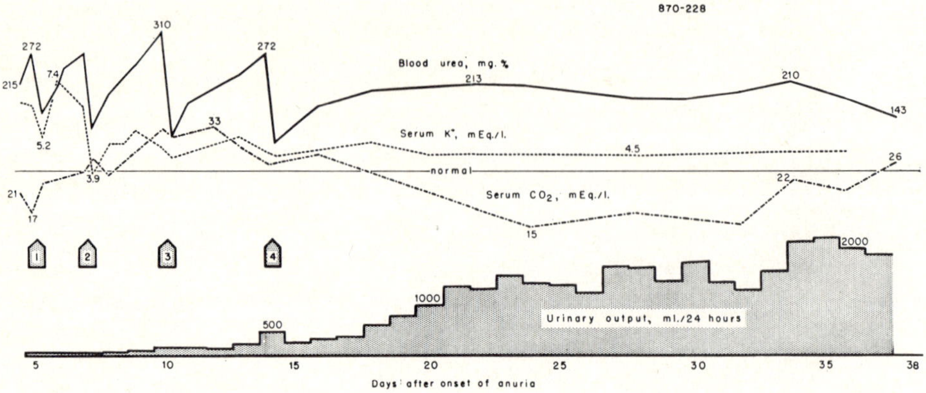


**Fig. 1.** The course of blood urea, serum potassium, and carbon dioxide content in patient with renal shutdown after aortic grafting operation. The horizontal line indicates the normal level of blood urea, serum potassium, and carbon dioxide content. Note the drop in blood urea at each of the 4 dialyses. Also note that a urine volume between 1,000 and 2,000 ml. was not sufficient to lower the blood urea level to under 200 mg. per 100 ml. Six months after discharge, blood urea level was 52 mg. per 100 ml., serum potassium level 4.8 mEq. per liter, and carbon dioxide content 23 mEq. per liter.

and cooperative. The skin was somewhat dry, but pulmonary or peripheral edema was not evident. The abdomen was rather distended but peristalsis was active. The serum electrolytes were sodium, 136; potassium, 6.6; chloride, 94; and carbon dioxide, 21 mEq. per liter. The hemoglobin count was 14.1 Gm. per 100 ml., and cell volume, 43 per cent. The blood urea level was 215 mg. per 100 ml. On the fifth postoperative day, the patient underwent treatment with the artificial twin-coil kidney* for 3 hours.[4] The blood urea level decreased from 272 to 158 mg. per 100 ml. and creatinine from 13.6 to 10.0 mg. per 100 ml.

Because the patient was oliguric until the seventeenth postoperative day, he was treated with the artificial kidney 4 times. Corrections of electrolytes and lowering of retention products were obtained each time (Fig. 1). The daily urinary output was slowly increasing, and after 34 days it was more than 2,000 ml. per 24 hours. The blood urea level was reduced to 104 mg. per 100 ml. at the end of the fourth hemodialysis, rose to 213 mg. per 100 ml., then was stabilized at around 200 mg. per 100 ml. for 2½ weeks, and finally started to decrease. On the day of discharge, the thirty-eighth postoperative day, the blood urea level was 143 mg. per 100 ml. The recovery was uneventful except for a slight fever (90° to 101° F.) from the eighth to the thirty-first postoperative day which was treated with antibiotics. A pleural effusion present from the twenty-second to the twenty-sixth postoperative day was treated with thoracentesis with removal of a total of 1,800 ml. of transudate. The patient was in excellent condition when examined 6 months after operation. He had a normal blood urea level and apparently was fully recovered.

*Travenol Laboratories, Inc., Morton Grove, Ill.

## DISCUSSION

The case report illustrates the importance of intensive treatment of acute renal failure which follows anuria after vascular operations. The patient was oliguric for 17 days and did not reach a daily urinary output of 2,000 ml. until the thirty-fourth postoperative day.

Therapy in cases of acute renal failure should include a general supportive program with a high caloric, low protein diet, large doses of vitamins, and the restriction of certain electrolytes such as sodium and potassium. Administration of fluid is based upon a daily record of body weight and fluid intake and output, and more than 700 ml. per 24 hours is rarely given during the anuric phase, although compensation can be made for both fluid and electrolyte losses. Frequent dialyses with ultrafiltration greatly facilitate fluid and electrolyte management. Administration of antibiotics is desirable in the prevention and treatment of infections. Treatment with the artificial kidney is indicated if the blood urea level is greater than 200 mg. per 100 ml., if serum potassium exceeds 7 mEq. per liter, if plasma carbon dioxide content is less than 12 mEq. per liter, or if the clinical condition of the patient deteriorates.

Our present policy is to dialyze frequently in the hope that the patient can avoid the clinical symptoms of uremia and that he can be left in optimum clinical condition so that he can eat better, his wounds can heal faster, and he can be ambulated. Recovery of renal function is thus made more comfortable.

In the diuretic phase which follows the oliguria, the fluid and electrolytes are replaced at a slower rate than that at which they are excreted. Nearly all the patients lose weight during this period, which indicates that they are actually overhydrated.

## SUMMARY

A case is presented of acute renal failure after an abdominal aortic operation. The patient required 4 treatments with the artificial twin-coil kidney.

Early and frequently repeated dialyses offer the best possible way for patients to recover from renal failure after operations on the aorta. Such treatment should continue as long as there is a chance for recovery and occlusion of the renal arteries or other irreparable renal damage has not been proved to be present.

## REFERENCES

1. Doolan, P. D., Wiggins, R. A., Thiel, G. B., Lee, K. J., and Martinez, E.: Acute renal insufficiency following aortic surgery. A discussion of the pathogenesis and a consideration of gangrene of an extremity as a complication, Am. J. Med. **28:** 895, 1960.
2. Humphries, A. W., deWolfe, V. G., and LeFevre, F. A.: Major arterial grafting in one hundred sixty-nine consecutive cases; a preliminary report on incidence of success and failure, A. M. A. Arch. Surg. **74:** 65, 1957.
3. Humphries, A. W., deWolfe, V. G., and LeFevre, F. A.: The present status of major arterial grafting, Ohio M. J. **53:** 1413, 1957.
4. Kolff, W. J., and Watschinger, B.: Further development of coil kidney: disposable artificial kidney, J. Lab. & Clin. Med. **47:** 969, 1956.
5. Thurbeck, W. M., and Castleman, B.: Atheromatous emboli to the kidneys after aortic surgery, New England J. Med. **257:** 442, 1957.

# Temperature gradients associated with extracorporeal perfusion and profound hypothermia

BERNARD FISHER, M.D.
E. J. FEDOR, PH.D.
J. W. SMITH, M.D.
PITTSBURGH, PA.
*From the Department of Surgery, Laboratory of Surgical Research, University of Pittsburgh School of Medicine*

It is now recognized that thermal gradients which exist in the body under normal conditions become more pronounced with the induction of hypothermia.[1, 6, 13, 20] Most of the available data have been obtained when surface cooling was employed. In 1948, Haterius and Mason[9] noted as much as 3° C. difference between the liver and rectum of dogs so cooled. Hegnauer and Penrod[11] reported a brain temperature higher than that of the rectum, with the heart intermediate, and other investigators[5, 22] have demonstrated that the temperature in the rectum is usually several degrees lower than that in the esophagus. Differences of several degrees have been recorded[21] between rectum, muscle, and subcutaneous tissue when animals were cooled to 25° C.

While such variations in internal body temperature have been noted to occur with the use of extracorporeal perfusion and direct blood cooling,[4, 8, 18, 22] detailed data are lacking. This study was undertaken to obtain more knowledge of these temperature differences.

## METHODS

Mongrel dogs of both sexes, averaging 14 kilograms in weight, were anesthetized with pentobarbital sodium attached to a Medtronic automatic respirator, an extracorporeal system consisting of a T. M.-2 Sigmamotor perfusion pump, a 13 inch Kay-Cross convoluted disc oxygenator, and a gas type heat exchanger.[15] The unit was primed with heparinized blood. Vascular connections were made with catheters which had been inserted via a femoral artery into the aorta at the level of the renal arteries and through the femoral and jugular veins into the venae cavae. In 1 group of dogs, prior to cooling and after laparotomy and thoracotomy, copper Constantan thermocouples* were implanted at various sites throughout the body. In other groups they were inserted at different positions within the same organ and temperatures were compared with those recorded from the esophageal thermocouple which was always placed at midesophagus. Animals were sacrificed at the conclusion of each experiment, and the precise position of the thermocouples was confirmed. A Leeds-Northrup Speedomax type G recorder, which registered automatically every 30 seconds, was used to monitor temperatures. Temperature variations as slight as 0.1° C. were detectable. A perfusion rate of approximately 50 ml. per kilogram per minute was maintained during cooling and rewarming. Rewarming was begun when the esophageal temperature registered 10° C., and perfusion was stopped when this temperature reached 25° to 30° C.

Supported by United States Public Health Service Grant H-2065, Department of Army Contract No. DA-49-007-MD-715, and Southwestern Pennsylvania Heart Association.

Received for publication Dec. 7, 1960.

*Type NN-30-DT Cu-Constantan-30 gauge BNS, nylon insulation, Thermo Electric Co., Inc., Saddle Brook, N. J.

## RESULTS

**Body thermal gradients.** Probes were placed in various locations in 10 dogs, and temperatures simultaneously recorded. To facilitate presentation, temperature curves obtained have been divided in Fig. 1, *A* and *B*. It is apparent from these illustrations (which represent mean values) that a considerable thermal gradient occurs from site to site during cooling and rewarming.

Six minutes after inception of cooling, when the esophageal temperature registered 24.3 ± 3.7° C., values ranged from 31.4 ± 2.4° C. (subcutaneous) to 24.7 ± 3.5° C. (liver). With further cooling, the spread increased. Just prior to rewarming (esophageal 9.0 ± 1.0° C.), temperatures from all locations lay between 8.2 ± 2.3° C. (liver) and 18.0 ± 2.0° C. (subcutaneous). A fairly constant thermal relationship between the various sites was observed during the cooling phase. It is evident that the liver temperature more closely approximated the esophageal temperature than did that from any other site.

The esophageal temperature fell more rapidly and to a greater extreme than any of the others recorded during cooling, and upon rewarming became the most elevated. The liver temperature continued its esophageal relationship. Aside from the latter, however, no similar correlations could be established during the rewarming phase. A remarkable temperature gradient was maintained even to the time of cessation of perfusion. At this point the esophageal temperature was 30.7 ± 1.2° C., and the spleen had failed to rise above 25.6 ± 2.4° C.

**Organ thermal gradients.**

*Brain.* That all parts of the brain do not cool and rewarm similarly may be seen in Fig. 2, *A* and *B*. For clarity of presentation, brain area temperatures which approximated each other throughout within less than 1 degree were averaged and plotted as 1 curve. In all instances, temperature differentials were accentuated as cooling progressed. In the animals studied the esophageal temperature was lower—sometimes as much as 3° C. —than that recorded from the area of the brain with the lowest temperature (usually the base of the brain). Temperature gradient between the esophagus and other areas was as much as 10° C., as exemplified in Fig. 2, *A* (occipital lobes and esophagus). No consistent temperature relationship existed between the various areas of the brain. Areas which cooled most rapidly were most readily rewarmed. Occasionally, when the esophageal temperature approximated 30° C., temperatures of certain areas of the brain remained depressed (Fig. 2, *B*).

*Heart.* Data were obtained from 14 dogs in which thermocouples were inserted into various sites in the right and left sides of the heart. A composite of the results obtained from the right and left ventricular myocardia and chambers (mean with standard deviation), (Table I) suggests that no significant gradient in temperature occurred

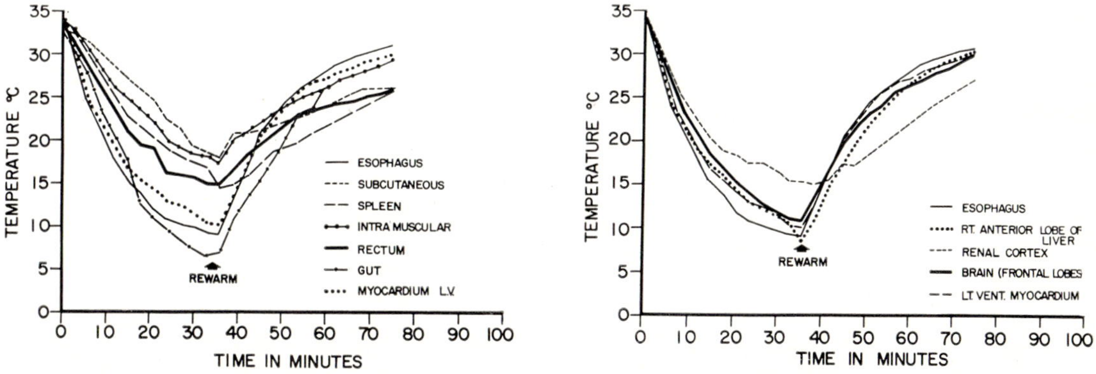


**Fig. 1.** Temperature variations in dogs subjected to extracorporeal cooling and rewarming. Each curve represents the mean of 10 animals.

**Table I.** *Mean temperatures from various parts of hearts of 14 dogs*

| *Position of thermocouple* | *Time of extracorpore[al]* | | | | |
|---|---|---|---|---|---|
| | *Cooling (C.)* | | | | |
| | *0* | *3* | *6* | *12* | *18* |
| Esophagus | 34.1 (1.2) | 29.7 (2.5) | 24.1 (3.7) | 18.6 (3.0) | 14.0 (2.6) |
| Right ventricle (chamber) | 34.2 (0.9) | 30.2 (1.7) | 23.6 (3.6) | 18.2 (4.7) | 14.9 (4.1) |
| Right ventricle (myocardium) | 33.3 (0.4) | 31.0 (1.4) | 25.0 (2.6) | 18.7 (4.3) | 14.6 (4.4) |
| Left ventricle (chamber) | 34.3 (0.7) | 30.8 (1.8) | 24.7 (4.1) | 18.4 (5.1) | 14.9 (5.2) |
| Left ventricle (myocardium) | 34.5 (0.8) | 30.4 (1.8) | 24.6 (3.3) | 19.1 (4.4) | 15.4 (4.4) |

Numbers in parentheses indicate standard deviation.

from one region to another and between heart and esophagus. From Fig. 3, *A, B,* and *C* it may be seen that such data are misleading. Actually, cardiac gradients—in some instances quite marked—were present in every dog studied. Temperature differences were more apparent as the body temperature was lowered. Similar gradations persisted during the entire rewarming phase. No constant temperature relationship was found to exist between the esophagus and the various parts of the heart. As the temperature was reduced the gradient between the two became more pronounced, so that, for example, in some animals at 10° C. the esophageal temperature was as markedly different as ± 5° C.

*Liver.* In some animals there was a marked temperature gradient between different lobes of the liver which, as in the other organs, became more pronounced as cooling progressed (Fig. 4, *A*). In others (Fig. 4, *B*), less of a differential was observed. But in no animal was cooling and rewarming uniform throughout the liver.

*Kidney.* In 6 animals thermocouples were placed in the renal cortex, medulla, pelvis, artery and vein, and beneath the capsule. Temperature gradients at once became apparent upon cooling (Fig. 5), the greatest differences being observed just prior to rewarming when the esophageal temperature was 9.2 ± 1.3° C. At that time the renal cortex was 15.2 ± 1.5° C., the medulla 11.5 ± 2.0° C., the subcapsular area 11.9 ± 2.4° C., and the renal pelvis 8.6 ± 1.3° C. The renal artery temperature, which was similar to that of the blood entering the aorta, was 3.6° C. lower than that noted in the renal vein. A marked lag in rewarming of the kidney was apparent, but the gradients between capsule, cortex, and medulla observed during cooling diminished. At cessation of perfusion, when the esophageal temperature (30.2° C.) approximated that of the renal artery (31.4° C.), the renal cortical and medullary temperatures were still depressed (27.0° C.).

## DISCUSSION

It is readily apparent from this study that with the use of extracorporeal perfusion in the production of hypothermia uniform body cooling does not occur. Marked differences in temperature exist not only from one area of the body to the other, but also within each organ. With progressive reduction of body temperature to more profound levels (10° C.) such variances become further accentuated. The more rapid the cooling and rewarming (that is, with use of increased flow rates), the greater these differentials become. While it is generally accepted[20] that in hypothermia use of the rectal temperature as an index of temperature throughout the rest of the body may be inaccurate, it seems that the same is true for temperature recorded from the esophagus.

Temperature differences from various parts of the heart during cooling and rewarming were interesting. Aside from spec-

| *erfusion (min.)* | | | | | | | | |
|---|---|---|---|---|---|---|---|---|
| | | | *Rewarming (C.)* | | | | | |
| *24* | *30* | *36* | *3* | *6* | *12* | *18* | *30* | *39* |
| 11.9 | 10.5 | 9.2 | 11.9 | 16.8 | 21.9 | 25.2 | 28.6 | 30.3 |
| (2.0) | (1.5) | (1.8) | (3.3) | (3.2) | (3.0) | (2.5) | (1.3) | (1.5) |
| 12.5 | 11.4 | 9.8 | 13.5 | 17.7 | 23.7 | 26.6 | 29.5 | 30.2 |
| (3.5) | (3.0) | (3.1) | (2.3) | (3.4) | (3.3) | (2.7) | (1.4) | (0.7) |
| 12.8 | 11.5 | 10.8 | 12.9 | 17.5 | 24.1 | 26.5 | 29.5 | 29.1 |
| (3.4) | (2.8) | (2.4) | (2.4) | (3.7) | (3.9) | (3.2) | (1.7) | (1.0) |
| 12.3 | 10.2 | 9.6 | 12.0 | 15.4 | 20.4 | 24.4 | 28.2 | 29.6 |
| (3.9) | (3.1) | (2.6) | (2.5) | (3.7) | (4.3) | (4.4) | (2.3) | (1.5) |
| 12.9 | 11.5 | 10.1 | 13.0 | 16.7 | 22.0 | 25.6 | 28.4 | 29.9 |
| (3.5) | (3.1) | (3.0) | (2.4) | (3.6) | (4.3) | (3.0) | (1.0) | (1.1) |

ulation that such gradients might be responsible for fibrillation in hypothermia,[3, 11] no experimental evidence had been presented to confirm or deny this. Recently it was reported by us[7] that no relationship exists between such thermal differentials and the production of ventricular fibrillation encountered in hypothermia. In some animals during cooling and rewarming temperature variations in the heart as great as 10° C. were found. While fibrillation was not usually encountered under such circumstances, it was observed when little or no temperature gradient was recorded.

The marked difference in brain and esophageal temperatures found by us and others[16, 17, 23] and the variations from one portion of the brain to another may well explain the neurological sequelae occasionally observed with circulatory arrest of a protracted period when the esophageal temperature is used as an index of depth of hypothermia. In practically all of the animals the temperature in the frontal lobes lagged the most from that of the esophagus, while the probe at the base of the brain registered temperatures closest to that of the esophagus.

Our observation that the renal cortical temperature was consistently higher than that of the medulla and kidney pelvis and that a difference existed in the temperatures of the renal arterial and venous blood suggests that total kidney perfusion does not take place, but that precortical arteriovenous shunts are in effect. Likewise, as evidenced by the differences in temperature between the various lobes, uniform perfusion of the liver does not always occur. A most likely explanation for all of the thermal gradients which vary from animal to animal rests on the premise that there is a difference

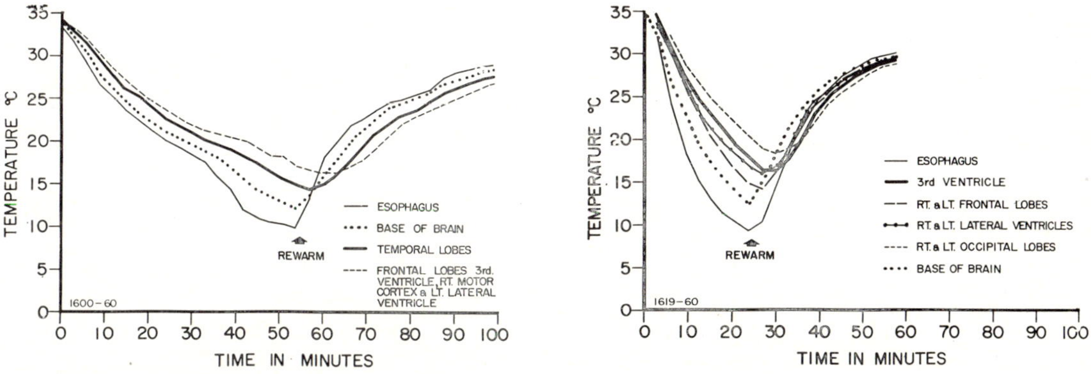


**Fig. 2.** Temperature differentials recorded from various parts of the brain.

in blood flow through various parts of the body. This in turn is probably related to catheter position, pump flow rates, and other as yet undescribed hemodynamic changes. Consequent to the blood flow and thermal variances, it is reasonable to assume that significant oxygen gradients likewise exist.

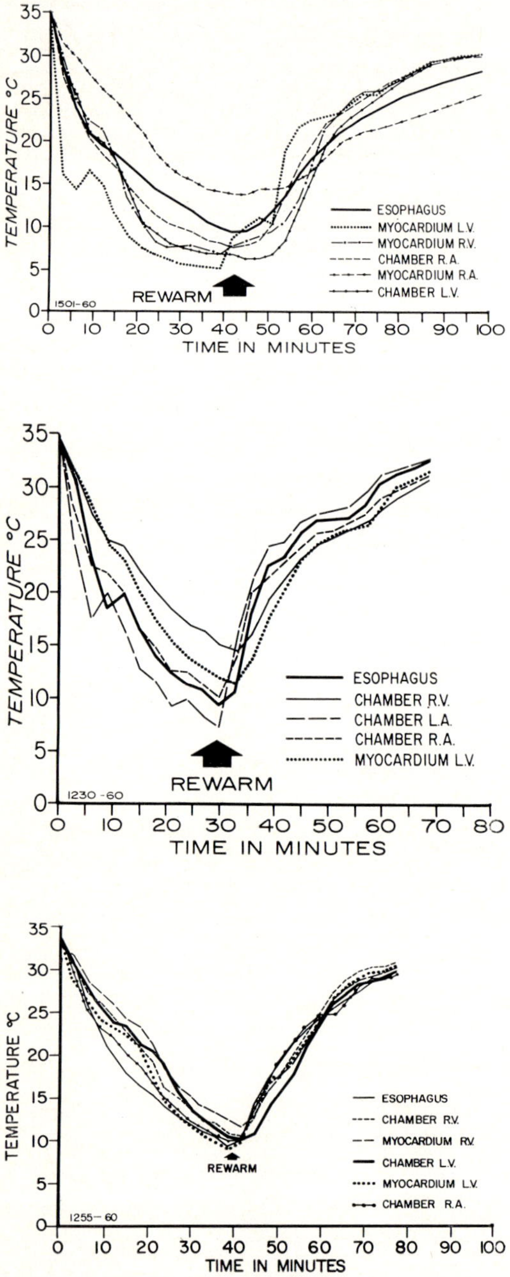


**Fig. 3.** Cardiac temperature gradients from 3 representative animals.

Certainly, one of the practical objectives of profound hypothermia is to permit prolonged circulatory arrest. This is feasible only if oxygen requirements at these low temperatures are markedly reduced and are adequately met. Bigelow and associates,[2] using surface cooling, reported an almost linear relationship between oxygen consumption and temperature to 20° C. when the former was 15 per cent of normal. By extrapolation of the curve, they concluded that at 10 to 12° C. oxygen consumption would be minimal. Results with extracorporeal cooling apparently are not similar. Heimbecker and associates[12] reported a variation of oxygen requirements of from 0.6 to 20 per cent of basal in 7 dogs with body temperatures between 8.5 and 12° C. when flow rates were about 65 ml. per kilogram per minute. In a recent study, Kameya and colleagues,[14] reported that at 10° C., with a flow rate of 60 ml. per kilogram per minute, oxygen consumption was 1.2 ml. per kilogram per minute, or about 17 per cent of that in monothermic animals at equivalent flow rates, but that with lower perfusion rates oxygen debt may occur. Sealy and his colleagues[19] found oxygen consumption at 20° C. to be 20 to 25 per cent of normal, while at 10° C. they believed it might be 10 per cent of normal. They also reported that after extracorporeal cooling to profound levels, circulatory arrest of 1 hour resulted in a 70 to 80 per cent reduction of oxygen in mixed venous blood with an oxygen debt occurring.

It may well be assumed from this evidence of continued substantial oxygen consumption at such profound levels of cooling that, due to lack of uniform cooling, oxygen debt in certain tissues may be more profound than in others, and that frank damage due to anoxia may result. If further prolongation of circulatory arrest in the profoundly cooled man or animal is contemplated, it seems that effort should be expended to obtain more uniform cooling.

## SUMMARY

The use of extracorporeal perfusion and heat exchange to produce profound hypo-

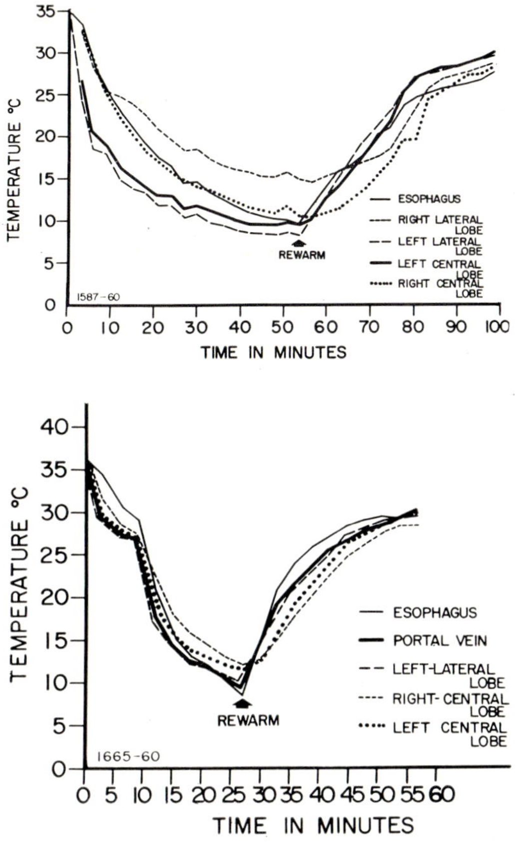


**Fig. 4.** Characteristic temperature variations in the liver after extracorporeal cooling and rewarming.

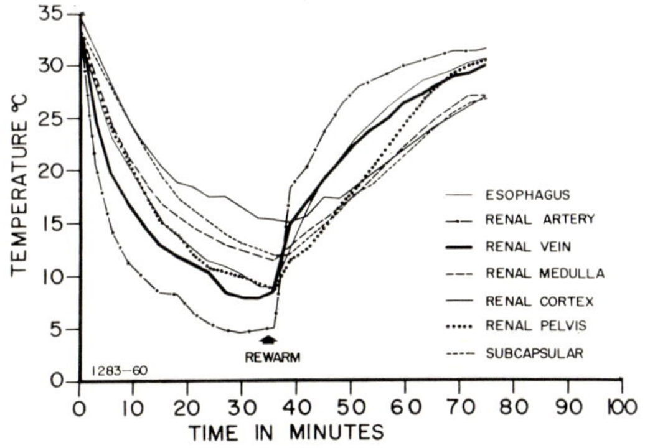


**Fig. 5.** Temperatures recorded from different parts of the kidney.

thermia results in marked temperature gradients throughout the body during the periods of both cooling and rewarming. This variation not only exists from organ to organ, but is observed when temperatures are recorded from different parts of the same structure. Simultaneously recorded temperatures from different parts of the brain, heart, kidney, and liver demonstrate evidence of markedly uneven cooling and rewarming. The lower the temperature, the more pronounced become such gradients. No correlation could be established between such thermal differentials in the heart and the onset of ventricular fibrillation encountered in hypothermia. The relation of these findings to oxygen consumption is commented upon, and it is concluded that if protracted circulatory arrest is to be contemplated with profound hypothermia, effort must be made to obtain more uniform cooling.

## REFERENCES

1. Bazett, H. C., Love, L., Newton, M., Eisenberg, L., Day, R., and Forster, R.: Temperature changes in blood flowing in arteries and veins in man, J. Appl. Physiol. **1:** 3, 1948.
2. Bigelow, W. G., Lindsay, W. K., Harrison, R. C., Gordon, R. A., and Greenwood, W. F.: Oxygen transport and utilization in dogs at low body temperature, Am. J. Physiol. **160:** 125, 1950.
3. Brooks, C. M., Hoffman, B. F., Suckling, E. E., and Orias, O.: Excitability of the heart, New York, 1955, Grune & Stratton, Inc., p. 172.
4. Brown, I. W., Jr., Smith, W. W., Young, W. G., Jr., and Sealy, W. C.: Experimental and clinical studies of controlled hypothermia rapidly produced and corrected by a blood heat exchanger during extracorporeal circulation, J. Thoracic Surg. **36:** 497, 1958.
5. Cooper, K. E., and Kenyon, J. R.: A comparison of temperatures measured in the rectum, oseophagus and/or the surface of the aorta during hypothermia in man, Brit. J. Surg. **44:** 616, 1956-57.
6. Cranston, W. I., Gerbrandy, J., and Snell, E. S.: Oral, rectal and oesophageal temperatures and some factors affecting them in man, J. Physiol. **126:** 347, 1954.
7. Fisher, B., and Fedor, E. J.: Cardiac temperature gradients during extracorporeal perfusion and profound hypothermia, Proc. Soc. Exper. Biol. & Med. **106:** 275, 1961.
8. Gollan, F., Tysinger, D. S., Grace, J. T., Kory, R. C., and Meneely, G. R.: Hypothermia of 1.5° C. in dogs followed by survival, Am. J. Physiol. **181:** 297, 1955.
9. Haterius, H. O., and Mason, G. L.: Experimental hypothermia and rewarming in the

dog. Recovery after severe reduction in body temperature, Am. J. Physiol. **152:** 225, 1948.
10. Hegnauer, A. H.: Cold injury, Transactions of Second Conference, Josiah Macy Jr. Foundation, New York, 1952, p. 181.
11. Hegnauer, A. H., and Penrod, K. E.: United States Air Force Technical Report No. 5912, 1950.
12. Heimbecker, R. O., Young, W. E., and Sanford, D. C.: Experimental studies on the production of deep hypothermia by means of a pump oxygenator and heat exchanger with a note on the clinical application, Canad. J. Surg. **3:** 79, 1959.
13. Horvath, S. M., Rubin, A., and Foltz, E. L.: Thermal gradients in the vascular system, Am. J. Physiol. **161:** 316, 1950.
14. Kameya, S., Oz, M., Neville, W. E., and Clowes, G. H. A., Jr.: A study of oxygen consumption during profound hypothermia induced by perfusion of the entire body, S. Forum **11:** 190, 1960.
15. Kaplan, A., Fisher, B., Fedor, E. J., and Carrol, F.: A gas type heat exchanger for induction of profound hypothermia and rewarming. In press.
16. Lesage, A. M., Freese, J. W., Sealy, W. C., and Young, W. G., Jr.: Study of the effects of complete circulatory arrest in the profoundly hypothermic dog, S. Forum **11:** 188, 1960.
17. Lesage, A. M., Sealy, W. C., Brown, I. W., Jr., and Young, W. G., Jr.: Hypothermia and extracorporeal circulation, A. M. A. Arch. Surg. **79:** 607, 1959.
18. Peirce, E. C., and Polley, V. B.: Differential hypothermia for intracardiac surgery, A. M. A. Arch. Surg. **67:** 521, 1953.
19. Sealy, W. C., Young, W. G., Jr., Brown, J. W., Jr., Smith, W. W., and Lesage, A. M.: Profound hypothermia combined with extracorporeal circulation for open-heart surgery, Surgery **48:** 432, 1960.
20. Severinghaus, J. W.: Temperature gradients during hypothermia, Ann. New York Acad. Sc. **80:** 515, 1959.
21. Spurr, G. B., Horvath, S. M., Hamilton, L. H., and Hutt, B. K.: Temperature gradients in the hypothermic dog, Am. J. Physiol. **186:** 47, 1956.
22. Stupfel, M., and Severinghaus, J. W.: Internal body gradients during anesthesia and hypothermia and effect of vagotomy, J. Appl. Physiol. **9:** 380, 1956.
23. Zingg, W., and Kantor, S.: Observations on the temperatures in the brain during extracorporeal differential hypothermia, S. Forum **11:** 192, 1960.

# Percutaneous iliofemoral arteriography

ROBERT A. SCHOBINGER, M.D.

BRONX, N. Y.

*From the Bronx Veterans Administration Hospital and Department of Surgery, Albert Einstein College of Medicine*

Angiography has contributed greatly to the better understanding, and thus to the therapy, of arterial and venous disease states. The accelerated interest in diagnosis and therapy of arterial insufficiency represents one typical example of the increased activity in this challenging and important field of human pathology. It is well established that adequate surgical therapy for peripheral occlusive arterial disease depends upon the objective evidence provided by properly executed arteriograms. Increasing experience has demonstrated that occlusive arterial disease in the leg may be associated with definite, yet asymptomatic, arteriosclerotic changes within the abdomen.[4, 12] These alterations may be diffuse or segmental and of variable degrees. Such changes affecting the arterial system above Poupart's ligament may sooner or later progress to complete obstruction of the arterial lumen and jeopardize the success of well-performed peripheral arterial operations. Arterial disease cephalad to the femoral canal is frequently not suspected and therefore not investigated if both femoral pulses appear to be of equal quality and if the symptomatology points only toward femoropopliteal involvement.

In the presence of unequal femoral pulsations, aortography is usually considered to be the diagnostic method of choice. By aortography is meant the direct translumbar approach and not the intravenous type of aortography, since the latter technique, in my opinion and the opinions of other workers in this field,[6, 8, 11] has yet to demonstrate a reliability similar to that of the time-honored and well-established direct method. Initially we extended the use of aortography to patients who exhibited evidence of peripheral arterial occlusive disease with rather rapid cephalad progression of the morbid process. In such patients aortography rather than femoral arteriography was performed, even if both femoral pulses were of equal quality. In so doing, we occasionally discovered unsuspected involvements of the aorto-iliac system which imposed a modification on the original surgical planning.

For the past 18 months we have made an effort to opacify the iliac arteries and distal aorta in the course of percutaneous femoral arteriography. We have found that the introduction of contrast medium at the level of the common femoral artery allowed excellent opacification of the aortoiliac system in surprisingly many cases in addition to permitting the visualization of the more peripheral arterial tree. This was considered to represent a definite advantage over aortography by which the proper evaluation of the arterial outflow tract in the calf was occasionally not possible or often was obtained only with difficulty.

Our present indications for iliofemoral arteriography include peripheral occlusive arterial disease, regardless of the slow or rapid cephalad progression of the arterial disease process. Earlier we performed iliofemoral arteriograms only in patients with bilaterally equal femoral pulses. Now we

Received for publication Dec. 12, 1960.

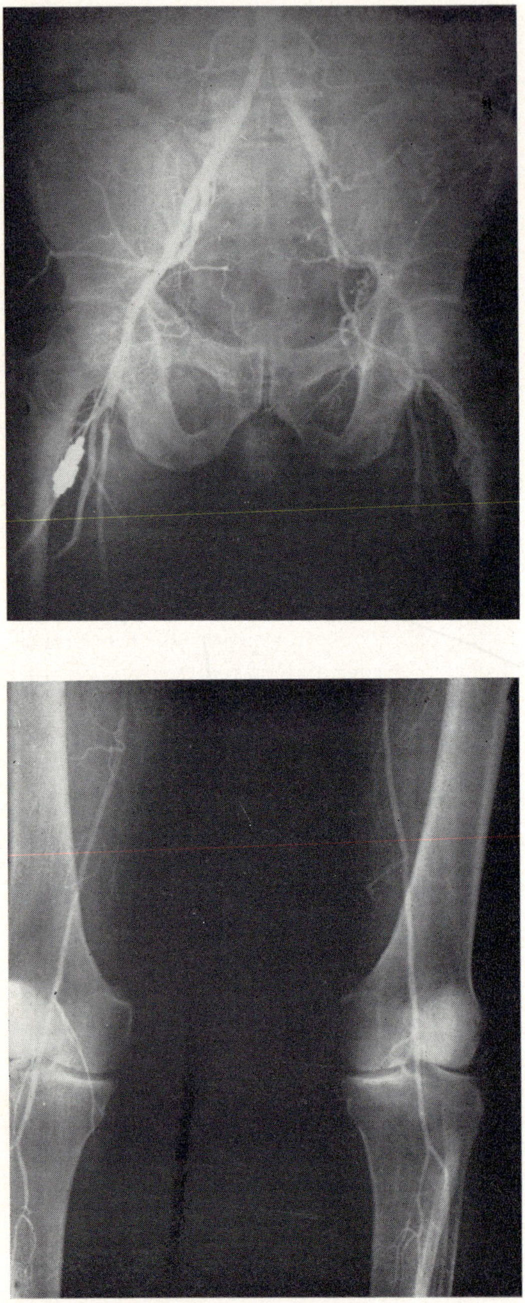

**Fig. 1.** Right percutaneous iliofemoral arteriogram performed on patient under 2 per cent procaine local anesthesia. Two sets of films. Total amount of contrast medium was 40 ml. Right pedal and left femoral pulses were clinically absent and right popliteal pulse was weak. Arteriogram shows block in right superficial femoral artery and narrowing of popliteal artery. There is absent opacification of the iliofemoral system on the left with replacement by an extensive collateral network, and faint outlining of the distal aorta.

employ this method also in subjects with bilaterally palpable, yet unequal, femoral pulses and whenever possible, even in patients with only one pulsating common femoral artery (Fig. 1). Translumbar aortography can always be resorted to, should, in this last category of patients, the aortoiliac system escape satisfactory opacification by unilateral femoral injections. From this brief exposé can be seen that we have become increasingly selective in our indications for aortography.

## RATIONALE

Symptomatic peripheral arterial occlusive disease may, as was already mentioned, coexist with asymptomatic arterial changes at a more proximal level (Figs. 2 and 3). Since the natural history of arteriosclerosis is toward progression, there sooner or later will come the moment of symptomatic proximal arterial insufficiency. From the therapeutic and prognostic points of view it seems important to recognize such latent changes prior to the institution of definitive operation on the major branches of the femoropopliteal axis. The evaluation of the arterial inflow tract may have been unduly neglected in the past in favor of a rather detailed investigation of the various outflow or "run-off" patterns. More attention should be paid to the condition of the arterial tree over some distance proximal to a peripheral arterial occlusion. This precaution may further improve the selection of patients for operation and the type of procedure could also be better adapted to an individual situation. The second point to be emphasized is that the unilaterality of symptoms of arterial occlusive disease does not necessarily correspond to the ipsilaterality of maximal arterial involvement. We have on several occasions seen patients who presented symptoms of ischemia only in 1 leg, but who on arteriography exhibited a comparatively more advanced occlusive process in the opposite asymptomatic lower extremity. Such observations were mainly made because of our insistence to routinely obtain arteriograms of both lower extremities at the same sitting, even if only 1 leg appeared involved.

## PRINCIPLE

The procedure consisted usually of simultaneous bilateral percutaneous femoral arteriography with retrograde opacification of the iliac arteries and distal aorta. Obviously, when only 1 femoral pulse is palpable, the procedure is restricted to that side. Two purposes are thus fulfilled. First, the proximal arterial system can be evaluated in conjunction with that of the leg and, second, both femoral arteries and their branches are outlined simultaneously for valuable comparative studies. In other words, an attempt is made to roentgenographically evaluate the arterial inflow and outflow tracts of both lower extremities by a rather simple and safe method, an attempt which in the vast majority of instances is successful. Similar thinking led Sammons and Mahin[9] to employ retrograde aortography and pelvic arteriography. These workers apparently resort only to a unilateral percutaneous femoral puncture and apply a tourniquet distal to the site of injection in order to favor the retrograde diffusion of contrast medium within the iliac arteries, aorta, and opposite femoropopliteal system. The principle of this technique is not new. It is in this respect worth while to recall the pioneering work of Castellanos and Pereiras[1, 2] and the stimulating contributions of Fariñas,[5] Peirce,[7] and Seldinger.[10] In contradistinction to the customary practice of applying a tourniquet distal to the site of injection in order to facilitate the countercurrent diffusion of contrast material, we prefer not to subject an already diseased artery and extremity to the additional insult of external constriction. A partial or total arterial occlusion below the common femoral artery acts as an obturator of sufficient im-

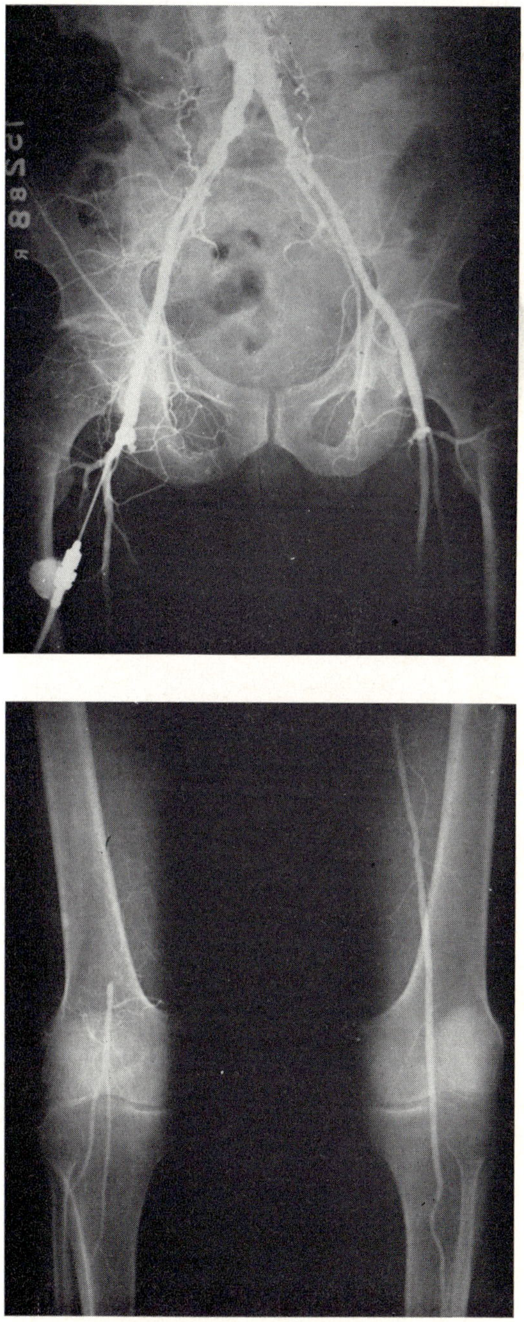

**Fig. 2.** Right percutaneous iliofemoral arteriogram. Spinal anesthesia was used. Total amount of contrast medium was 40 ml. Composite picture combines the abdominal phase of the first set of films with the femoropopliteal pattern of the second set exposed 6 seconds later. There were clinically absent pulses on the right below a strongly pulsating common femoral artery. Left lumbar sympathectomy had been performed previously. Arteriogram shows marked sclerosis of distal aorta and right common iliac artery, complete obstruction of right superficial femoral artery from its origin down, high origin of right anterior tibial artery, and diffuse sclerotic changes of left superficial femoral artery with poor popliteal outflow tract.

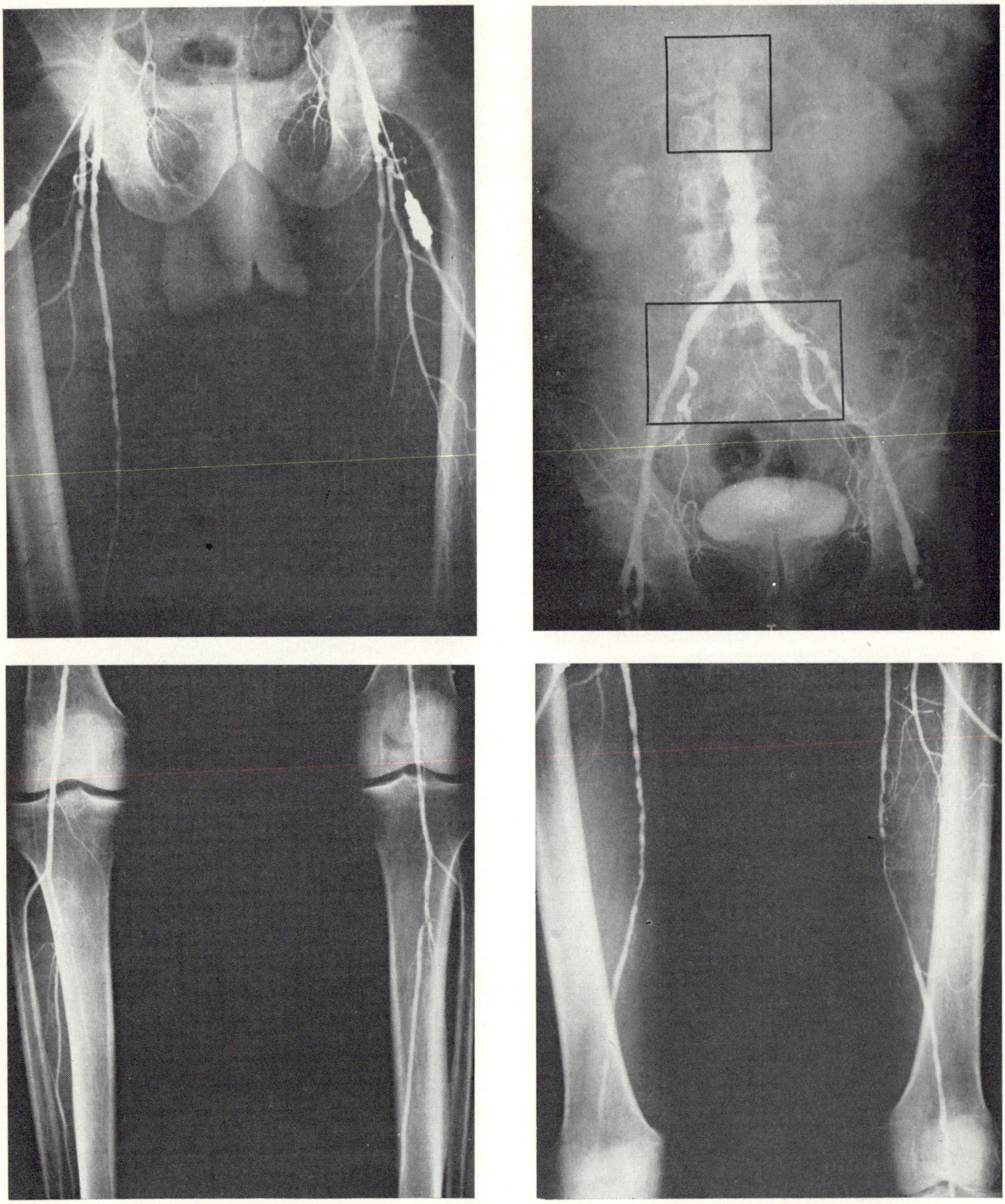

*A* *B*

**Fig. 3.** *A,* Bilateral percutaneous femoropopliteal arteriogram. Spinal anesthesia was used and 30 ml. of contrast medium was simultaneously injected into each artery. Clinically there were unequal common femoral and popliteal pulses (weaker on left), faint posterior tibial pulse on left, and absent pedal pulses on right. The picture is composite. Diffuse sclerotic changes of the superficial femoral arteries are demonstrated, particularly on the right, with bilaterally narrowed popliteal outflow tracts. *B,* Bilateral ileofemoral arteriogram of same patient. Simultaneous, forceful injection of 40 ml. of medium into each artery was used. This is the first set of films. The aorta is opacified to slightly above the renal vessels. Arteriogram shows sclerotic changes of entire visualized portion of abdominal aorta, iliac vessels, and both superficial femoral arteries. Note unsuspected sclerotic changes in aorta and right renal artery (upper box), and narrowing of right internal and left external iliac arteries (lower box).

portance to permit satisfactory retrograde opacification of the aortoiliac system without the aid of external measures.

## ANESTHESIA

Iliofemoral arteriography can satisfactorily be performed on a patient under local, spinal, or general anesthesia. We have employed all 3 modalities, but have adopted spinal anesthesia as the method of choice whenever possible since it is usually well accepted by the patient, can be carried out readily in the x-ray room, and provides maximal vasodilatation. If local anesthesia is to be used, it is important to adequately sedate the patient with Demerol (100 mg.) and Seconal (100 mg.) administered 1 hour prior to the procedure. A solution of 2 per cent procaine is employed, 3 to 4 ml. of which is injected directly into the artery 1 to 2 minutes prior to the injection of contrast medium. The introduction of procaine usually produces a sensation of warmth and occasionally of burning, the appearance of which at the various levels in the leg is a precious guide for the proper timing of the roentgenographic exposures. We did not observe any immediate or late ill effects after the intra-arterial injection of 2 per cent procaine, and the arteriographic details have, in our hands at least, been highly satisfactory (Fig. 1).

## TECHNIQUE

In view of the increased interest in peripheral vascular diseases, many institutions have developed their own type of roentgenographic device for single or multiple exposures. Seriography is almost always required for the adequate capture of the vascular pattern distal to a complete occlusion. This is frequently accomplished exposure to 2 series of films at 3 to 5 second intervals. Whatever device is employed, the large-size films should be used to make adequate aortofemoral or femoropopliteal arteriograms. In our institution we employ two 14 by 17 inch films contained in grid cassettes in lengthwise juxtaposition in a film tunnel to allow the exposure of 2 sets of films at any desired interval. This arrangement normally encompasses the entire lower extremity or the aorta from the level of the renal arteries to the trifurcation of the popliteal artery (Fig. 3, *A*).

Comfortable positioning of the patient can easily be achieved by placing a long piece of foam rubber, sandwiched between 2 folded bed sheets, on top of the roentgenographic device. This arrangement, furthermore, will allow the effortless modification of the patient's position by simply pulling in the desired direction on the lower sheet.

For femoropopliteal arteriography the patient is positioned in such a manner as to include in the proximal film both anterior superior iliac spines. This positioning allows the capture of the arterial system of the leg from slightly above Poupart's ligament to a point slightly above the ankles (Fig. 3, *B*). It is advisable to rotate the legs of the patient internally by spreading the heels and taping the overlapping toes together. This internal rotation opens the interosseous space roentgenographically and allows a much better identification of the various branches of the popliteal artery. Preliminary scout films are always obtained to verify the correct positioning of the patient and the various roentgenographic factors. The latter are, for femoropopliteal arteriography, 300 Ma., 75 to 80 KVP, one-fourth second. For aortofemoral arteriography, the factors are 300 Ma., 85 to 90 KVP, one-fourth second. The beam is filtered by 2 mm. of aluminum. In order to compensate for the difference in density between the abdomen and the thighs or the thighs and the calves, respectively, a sheet of black paper is placed over the distal film at the time of the loading of the cassette. We found that this method is more easily remembered by the x-ray technician than the change from a conventional to a tapered filter. The focus–film distance is 5 feet in both instances.

For iliofemoral arteriography the patient's position is modified to situate the upper edge of the film at the level of the xiphoid process.

Principles of strict asepsis must be followed during the entire procedure. The person performing the injection should wear cap and mask. Both inguinal areas, which should have been shaved, are widely disinfected with 3 layers of tincture of Merthiolate which is prevented from running down along the genitals by properly placed sponges. Then the groins are suitably outlined by sterile towels. A 17 gauge spinal needle with a long bevel is employed for arterial cannulation. The site of puncture is ideally situated 1 fingerbreadth below Poupart's ligament. For a right handed person standing on the right of the patient, the artery is palpated with the middle finger and index finger of the left hand, which are slightly spread. The needle, with stylet in place and at a 45 degree angle with its tip aimed cephalad, is introduced between these 2 fingers. Once the needle reaches the femoral sheath, transmitted pulsations may be felt. Further advancement of the needle will, as a rule, lead to compression of the arterial lumen. At this moment the pulsations above the needle will usually persist, though diminished in intensity, and can still be felt by the middle finger, while they are obliterated by the needle in a distal direction and escape palpation by the index finger. Further advancement of the needle will place its tip into the arterial lumen. The stylet is gently withdrawn and if the needle is properly placed a jet of arterial blood accompanied by rhythmical motions of the needle is observed. Should no arterial blood flow from the needle upon removal of the stylet, it is best to slowly withdraw the open needle with a rotary motion. Often both walls of the artery have been traversed and slight withdrawal of the needle will place its tip correctly within the lumen of the artery. The absence of a free flow of blood accompanied by a rhythmical motion of the needle in a

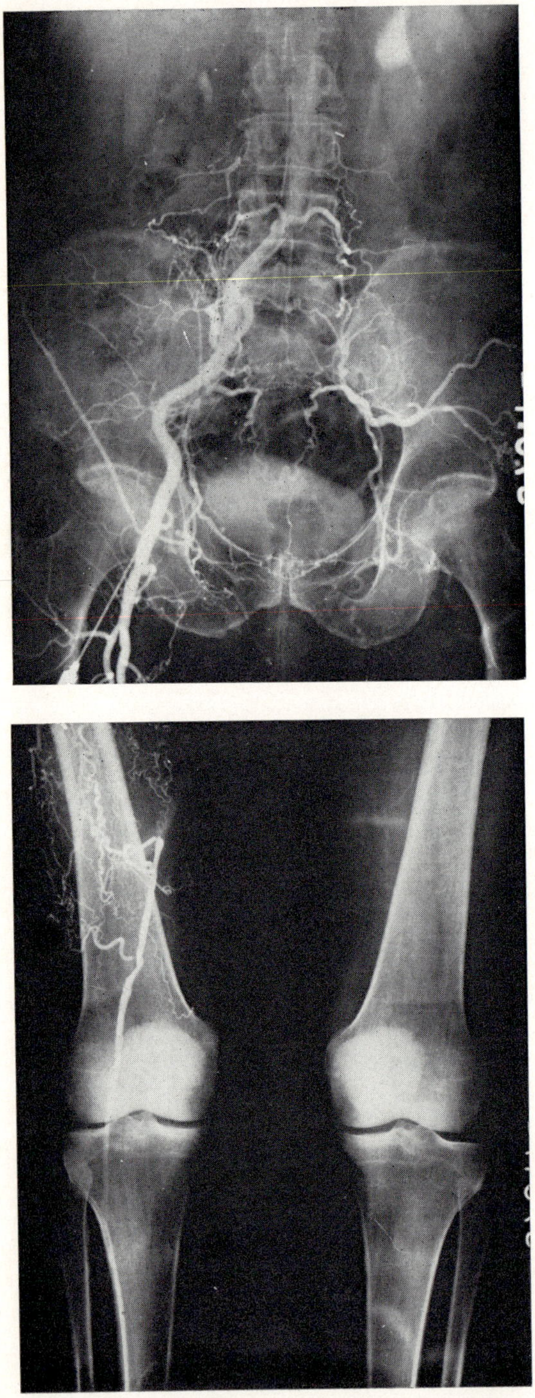

**Fig. 4.** Right percutaneous iliofemoral arteriogram. Spinal anesthesia was used. Total amount of medium was 30 ml. There were clinically absent pulses at all levels in the left lower extremity and a strongly pulsating common femoral artery with weak popliteal and pedal pulses on the right. Picture is composite, and the second set of films was exposed 8 seconds after the first. Arteriogram shows block of left external iliac artery bridged by collaterals and segmental narrowing of origin of right superficial femoral artery. Both superficial femoral and popliteal arteries are somewhat narrowed, including the outflow tracts in the calves.

horizontal plane, or a slow flow of dark blood, indicates that the needle had been placed laterally to the artery. The detail of bidigital palpation of the artery shortens the time required for arterial cannulation and eliminates blind poking or traumatic "fishing" for the vessel. The introduction of the needle with sylet in place prevents obliteration of its lumen by fragments of soft tissues or calcified material. Once the needle is properly placed it is, without stylet, gently advanced about 2 cm. in a cephalad direction so as to place its tip within the lumen of the external iliac artery. The stylet is then replaced and the opposite common femoral artery cannulated in a similar fashion if bilateral arteriograms can be performed. The plastic tubings which previously had been filled with sterile normal saline solution and to which a 2-way stopcock had been applied on the syringe side, are now connected to the needles. Each tube is immediately flushed clear of all blood with saline solution and the stopcock closed while the solution is being injected. This will replace the metallic stylet with a physiologic obturator consisting of incompressible liquid. From this moment on the needle is no longer manipulated. All the handling is done at the other end of the plastic tubing in order to minimize the danger of dislocation or contamination of the needle. Superimposition of the plastic tubing on the femoral artery can be avoided by deflection of the tubing laterally. If the examination is carried out under local anesthesia we customarily inject 3 to 4 ml. of 2 per cent procaine into each artery just prior to the connection of the tubings to the needles. This injection precedes the introduction of contrast medium by 1 to 2 minutes.

Bilateral femoropopliteal arteriograms are obtained by having 2 persons introduce simultaneously and under constant pressure 30 ml. of contrast medium into each artery. The contrast material employed in all our arteriograms consists of a 50 per cent solution of diatrizoate (Hypaque). Synchronization is important and the time required for such a manual injection amounts to approximately 4 seconds. This rate of injection is used to create an adequate bolus of contrast medium. The first set of films is exposed while the last 3 to 4 ml. of medium is injected and the second set 4 to 8 seconds later. The shorter interval is selected when only a moderate degree of ischemia of the extremity exists, when incomplete occlusions are anticipated, or when a careful clinical examination of the extremities has shown a palpable flow through collateral arteries such as the genicular vessels. A 6 to 8 second interval is chosen in the presence of advanced ischemia or of a complete block without palpable collaterial circulation. Immediately after the injection the needles and tubings are thoroughly flushed with saline solution and the stopcock closed. The needles are not withdrawn until the immediately developed films have been inspected and the arteriograms found to yield the desired information.

For iliofemoral arteriograms the patient's positioning is modified in the manner described. Either new syringes are employed or the previously used ones thoroughly flushed with saline solution to prevent clogging. These little details are purposely emphasized because it is amazing how frequently they are forgotten! Each syringe is filled with 40 ml. of contrast medium which this time is forcefully injected, again simultaneously by 2 persons. The timing of the roentgenographic exposure corresponds to that mentioned for femoropopliteal arteriography. We thus have obtained retrograde arteriograms encompassing both iliac arteries and the aorta up to and including the renal arteries (Fig. 3, *A* and *B*).

During the period ranging from Jan. 1, 1959, to June 30, 1960, inclusively, we performed bilateral femoral arteriograms on 82 patients. Excellent opacification of both femoropopliteal systems was obtained in 80 patients, while in the remaining 2 patients only the arteries in 1 leg were visualized because of unilateral extravasation of contrast medium. The iliac vessels and distal aorta were outlined to a degree satisfactory for diagnosis in 71 patients. The reasons for inadequate aortoiliac angiograms in 6 patients were unilateral extravasation (2), motion (2), and faulty timing of the roentgenographic exposure (2) Adverse reactions to the contrast medium after the first injections rendered repeat injections inadvisable in 2, and in 3 patients no attempt at retrograde opacification of the aortoiliac system was made. Unilateral femoral punctures with counter-current opacification of the iliac arteries, aortic bifurcation, and contralateral iliofemoropopliteal system was performed in 10 additional patients, bringing the total of patients included in this study to 92. The latter examination was successful in 9 instances. In the remaining patient the contralateral femoropopliteal arterial tree could not be visualized adequately because of its involvement by extensive occlusive disease.

## SUMMARY

The described technique allows the opacification of the arterial inflow and outflow tracts in arterial occlusive disease of the lower extremities as well as a simultaneous comparative angiographic study of the arterial system of each leg.

The angiographic data collected in the course of such examinations have confirmed the presence of diffuse and/or segmental arterial occlusive disease at levels usually not encompassed by conventional peripheral femoral arteriography.

It can be anticipated that such extended and well-tolerated angiographic studies will shed more light on the over-all process of arteriosclerosis. They will also invite additional improvements in the selection of patients for direct arterial operations. The more adequate evaluation of the hitherto somewhat neglected inflow tract may influence the planning of therapeusis. The discussed method of bilateral simultaneous opacification of the entire arterial system of both lower extremities provides also a unique opportunity to study the vascular status of an asymptomatic leg, the counterpart of which is affected by symptomatic occlusive arterial disease. Thus, improved diagnostic insight may lead to a better therapeutic approach and even have prognostic implications.

### REFERENCES

1. Castellanos, A., and Pereiras, R.: Counter-current aortography, Rev. cubana de cardiol. **2:** 187, 1939-40.
2. Castellanos, A., and Pereiras, R.: Retrograde or counter-current aortography, Am. J. Roentgenol. **63:** 559, 1950.
3. Crawford, E. S., Beall, A. C., Moyer, J. H., and De Bakey, M. E.: Complications of aortography, Surg. Gynec. & Obst. **104:** 129, 1957.
4. De Bakey, M. E.: Discussion of Wylie, E. J., and Goldman, L.[12]
5. Fariñas, P. L.: New technique for arteriographic examination of the abdominal aorta and its branches, Am. J. Roentgenol. **46:** 641, 1941.
6. Hodes, P. J.: Personal communication.
7. Peirce, E. C.: Percutaneous femoral artery catheterization in man with special reference to aortography, Surg. Gynec. & Obst. **93:** 56, 1951.
8. Ruzicka, F. F., Jr.: Personal communication.
9. Sammons, B. P., and Mahin, H. P.: New technique of contrast visualization of the distal aorta, pelvic and lower extremity arterial system in obliterative vascular disease, Am. J. Roentgenol. **81:** 835, 1959.
10. Seldinger, S. I.: Catheter replacement of the needle in percutaneous arteriography, Acta Radiol. **39:** 368, 1953.
11. Shapiro, J.: Personal communication.
12. Wylie, E. J., and Goldman, L.: The role of aortography in the determination of operability in arteriosclerosis of the lower extremities, Ann. Surg. **148:** 325, 1958.

# A new operation for transposition of the great vessels

HARRIS B. SHUMACKER, JR., M.D.
INDIANAPOLIS, IND.
*From the Department of Surgery and Research Center, Indiana University School of Medicine*

Up to the present time, transposition of the great vessels has been treated primarily by various palliative procedures designed to increase the admixture of venous and arterialized blood either by creation of an atrial septal defect or by partial venous retransposition.[2, 3, 5] Since Albert's[1] suggestion that complete correction might be accomplished by intra-atrial retransposition, several additional operations aimed at this end[4, 6, 7] have been proposed. This report describes another method by which this can be achieved. That it effectively shunts vena caval and coronary sinus blood into the posterior ventricle through the mitral valve and pulmonary venous return into the anterior ventricle through the tricuspid valve is evident from animal experiments and 2 clinical cases.

## OPERATIVE PROCEDURE

An incision is made in the right atrial wall close to and parallel to the interatrial groove (Fig. 1). Another longer curved incision is made toward the left side of the right atrium, beginning near the left side of the inferior vena cava and ending near the left side of the superior vena cava. Through this incision the right atrial cavity is inspected and the atrial septum is excised as completely as possible. The right side of the atrial flap is sutured to the right lateral margins of the venae cavae, the right lateral margins of the septal ring, and the left atrial wall to the left of the points of entry into the left atrium of the pulmonary veins. The left side of the flap is then sutured to the left lateral margins of the posterior caudal wall of the right atrium, beginning at the left side of the inferior vena caval orifice and extending in a cephalad direction to the left of the coronary sinus, the cut edge of the base of the septum, and across the remaining cephalad posterior aspect of the right atrial wall up to the left lateral margin of the superior vena cava. The vena caval and coronary sinus flow has now been diverted into the posterior ventricle. The procedure is completed by suturing an oval graft to the right and left edges of the free right atrial incisions and the presenting anterior surfaces of the superior and inferior venae cavae. This shunts the pulmonary venous drainage around and over the previously constructed tunnel into the anterior ventricle via the tricuspid valve.

The same objective can be gained with a modification (Fig. 2). The original incision through the right side of the right atrial wall is made a little farther to the left of the interatrial groove. After the second incision is made and a somewhat narrower double-pedicled flap created, an oval patch of Teflon felt or other suitable material is sutured to the right edge of the flap. This graft is then similarly approximated to the left atrial wall to the left of the points of entry of the pulmonary veins. The left edge of the flap is sutured in place as previously described. The remaining free edges of the

Supported by grants from the James Whitcomb Riley Memorial Association and United States Public Health Service Research Grant H-2035(C-5) from the National Heart Institute.

Received for publication Jan. 3, 1961.

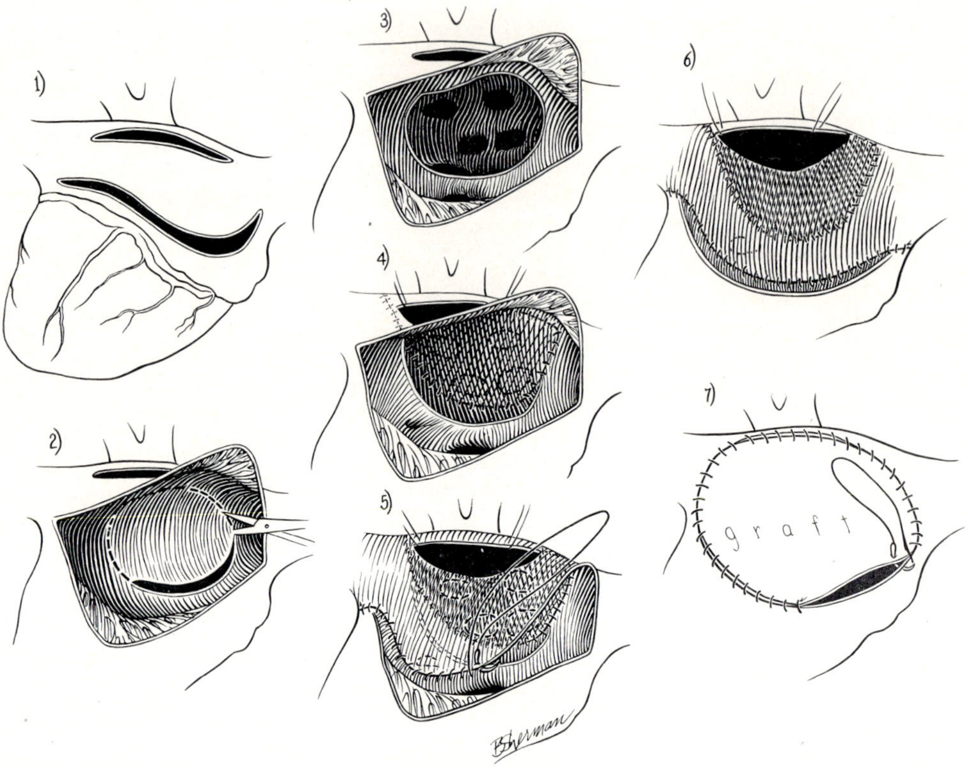


**Fig. 1.** Drawings which illustrate intra-atrial retransposition. *1,* The right atrial incisions; *2,* excision of atrial septum; *3,* view of pulmonary veins and portion of mitral orifice; and *4,* suture of right side of atrial flap to the right of the mitral orifice. For clarity of illustration, length of the line of suture is exaggerated and represents the point of attachment to the left atrial wall. Actually, since the side of the right atrial flap is shorter, the left atrial wall is "tented up" or "purse-stringed" in a fashion as the suture is accomplished. *5* and *6,* Suture of left side of right atrial flap to atrial wall. The vena cava–coronary sinus tunnel is now complete. *7,* Reconstruction of anterior atrial wall by means of a graft.

right atrium are then directly approximated and sutured above and below to the anterior walls of the superior and inferior venae cavae.

In experimental animals, the completeness of the transposition is evident from roentgenographic studies with contrast material. When contrast material is injected into a pulmonary vein, the right ventricle and the pulmonary arterial tree become opacified. When the injection is made into a vena cava, the vena caval tunnel and the coronary sinus are opacified, as well as the left ventricle, the coronary arteries, and the aorta.

## CASE REPORTS

**Case 1.** The patient was a very ill 10½-month-old male infant who had had cyanosis since birth, progressive respiratory difficulty, and poor weight gain. He weighed only 8 pounds, 13 ounces, at the time of operation. He was admitted to the hospital on Sept. 5, 1960. Catheterization and cineangiographic studies through the saphenous vein and by percutaneous ventricular puncture established the diagnosis of transposition with bidirectional shunt through an atrial septal defect. Pressures were 101/11 mm. Hg in the right ventricle, 113/64 in the aorta, 2.4 in the right atrium, and 5.4 in the left atrium. The femoral blood was 48.7 per cent saturated and rose only to 53.6 per cent saturation during oxygen inhalation. The patient was treated for diarrhea and with digitalis and diuretics for heart failure. Though the lungs remained relatively free of râles and the liver was not remarkably enlarged, peripheral edema became progressively more marked while the infant was in the hospital in spite of intensive treatment. He remained listless and cyanotic.

Operation was carried out on September 30.

The infant seemed nearly moribund at the time. Arterial pressure could not be obtained by sphygmomanometric means and as soon as the radial artery was catheterized for this purpose shortly after induction of anesthesia, the systolic pressure was only 20 mm. Hg. It improved, however, after the administration of vasopressors. The left iliac vein was catheterized through the left saphenous vein for intravenous administration of fluids. The inferior vena cava was catheterized through the right common iliac vein exposed through a right lower quadrant extraperitoneal incision. At the same time, the arterial cannula was introduced into the right iliac artery. A right anterolateral thoracotomy incision was made. The tissues at the site of each incision were markedly edematous. There was free pleural fluid and marked increase in the amount of pericardial fluid. It had been hoped that it would be possible to catheterize the superior vena cava via the azygos vein but the latter was too small to permit introduction of a catheter of adequate size. Consequently, the superior vena cava was catheterized directly through its anterior wall. Inflow and outflow catheters were connected with a rotating disc oxygenator, partial bypass was begun, and the patient was cooled to a rectal temperature of 26.7° C. The venae cavae were now occluded and ventricular fibrillation induced by electric shock. The first operative procedure described was then carried out without significant difficulty. On exploration of the atrium, a secundum type defect approximately 1 cm. in diameter was found. The septum was excised. The vena cava–coronary sinus tunnel was created with the double-pedicled right atrial flap and the anterior atrial wall was reconstructed with a patch of woven Teflon. Warming was begun. When the temperature had risen to 29° C. ventricular fibrillation ceased spontaneously with return of good ventricular contractions. The color of the patient improved remarkably. When the extracorporeal circulation was discontinued, the heart action remained quite good for a while. Unfortunately, the operative procedure was now necessarily prolonged because of difficulty in securing hemostasis, particularly from the sutured iliac vessels. There was also some lesser difficulty in securing hemostasis along the edges where the patch had been sutured to the atrial wall and venae cavae. During this period, the blood pressure dropped to approximately 60 mm. Hg systolic. The wounds were closed and the patient returned to the recovery room. The color remained good but the pressure continued at about the level of 50 or 60 mm. Hg in spite of blood replacement and the use of vasopressors. About 4:00 P.M. the child died. Postmortem examination showed no other congenital defects and the retransposition seemed to have been adequately performed.

**Case 2.** The second patient was a 2-day-old infant who was admitted on Oct. 12, 1960. He had been cyanotic and, in spite of oxygen administration, had had rapid and difficult respiration since birth. He was found to be cyanotic and had fast irregular breathing, hepatomegaly, and peripheral edema. Cardiac catheterization and cineangiography performed on Oct. 24 showed evidence of transposition of the great vessels, a ventricular septal defect with bidirectional shunt, a patent foramen ovale, and a patent ductus arteriosus. The aortic blood was only 67.5 per cent saturated while the infant was breathing oxygen. In spite of diuretics and digitalization, the peripheral edema increased.

At the time of operation on November 16, the infant weighed only 9 pounds, 6 ounces. No blood pressure could be obtained when he was brought to the operating room, though it was 50 mm. Hg systolic when the internal mammary artery was later catheterized. The inferior vena cava was cannulated via the left common iliac vein and later the superior vena cava was cannulated through the azygos vein. The arterial inflow cannula was placed in the external iliac artery. A bilateral thoracotomy incision was made. All the tissues were markedly edematous. The patent ductus arteriosus was isolated and ligated when partial bypass was begun. The patient was cooled to 25° C. rectal temperature. The heart went into standstill as this low temperature was reached. The atrial retransposition was accomplished without difficulty according to the modified procedure previously described. A small segment of Dacron graft was sutured to the right side of the atrial flap and after the vena cava–coronary sinus tunnel had been created, the anterior atrial wall was closed directly and sutured across either end to the anterior surfaces of the superior and inferior venae cavae. The ventricular septal defect was repaired through a ventriculotomy incision.

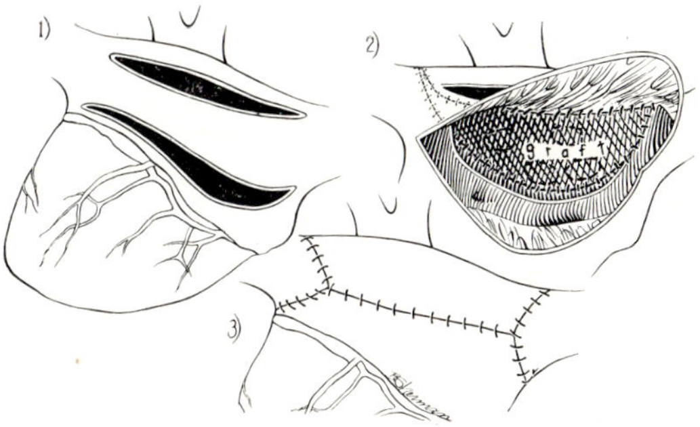


**Fig. 2.** Drawings which illustrate modified procedure. *1,* The atrial flap is created; *2,* the graft is sutured to right side of flap and to left atrial wall; and *3,* the procedure is completed.

Unfortunately, the venous outflow catheters were so small that it was impossible to use an adequate perfusion rate. Indeed, at one time the rate had to be reduced to 180 ml. per meter squared. In spite of this poor perfusion, the blood pressure ranged between 40 and 50 mm. Hg systolic throughout the procedure. It was possible to cool the infant fairly rapidly, but because of the poor flow rate it took an inordinately long time to rewarm him. Though the repair was completed within approximately 1 hour, it was nearly 3 hours before the patient was adequately rewarmed. As the patient became warm, the heart went into ventricular fibrillation. This was corrected with electric shock. Because of the poor perfusion during rewarming, cardiac massage was also carried out. A blood pressure ranging between 40 and 70 mm. Hg was thus maintained. When the extracorporeal circulation was discontinued when the infant's temperature was 35° C., the blood pressure was approximately 40/20, the heart was seemingly contracting well, and the patient's color was good. During closure of the anterior chest wall, however, cardiac arrest occurred and it was impossible to bring about resuscitation.

Operation in both cases was undertaken as a desperate measure with the realization that there was relatively little chance of success. Both infants were in very poor condition and in marked heart failure. One weighed less than 9 pounds and the other only 9 pounds, 6 ounces. Disappointing as the outcome was, there were some gratifying aspects. It was satisfying to know that the procedure could be accomplished in such tiny infants. After repair, both had a period of apparently good color and reasonably good heart action. In both cases, difficulties arose which should be averted in future attempts. In the first, the operation was unduly prolonged by difficulty in securing hemostasis, particularly from the repair of the iliac vessels. In the second, it was greatly prolonged because of the small caliber of the venous drainage tubes and the consequent poor perfusion rate.

## DISCUSSION

The operation described consists essentially in the diversion of vena caval and coronary sinus blood flow into the posterior ventricles by creation of a tunnel constructed by means of a double-pedicled right atrial flap and reconstruction of the anterior right atrial wall so as to permit pulmonary venous blood to flow through the tricuspid valve into the anterior ventricle. The first alternative method outlined works well in the dog and was accomplished without difficulty in the first clinical case. Though there is considerable disparity between the length of the right side of the atrial flap and the distance between the points of caval-atrial junction around the left atrium to the left of the points of entry of the pulmonary veins, this seems to present no real difficulty. Sutures are simply placed more closely on the flap than on the left atrial wall. It appears likely that its use in all patients except those with massive right atrial enlargement would necessitate reconstruction of the right anterior atrial wall by means of a graft rather than by direct suture. I believe that it would be better to utilize a pericardial graft covered with thin Teflon felt since this might permit an easier blood-tight closure.

The second modification was easily carried out in the second case. Adding a plastic extension of an appropriate size and shape to the right side of the atrial flap permits a narrower atrial flap, and it is likely that reconstruction of the anterior wall of the right atrium could be accomplished fairly regularly by direct-suture closure.

The first is probably the better method since one can make the anterior atrium as large as he wishes and thus can be assured of adequate room around the vena cava–coronary sinus tunnel for free flow of blood from pulmonary veins through the tricuspid valve. It appears to have certain potential advantages over previously described methods. The use of the atrial septum itself as described by Albert is unlikely to prove suitable for human beings in view of the small size of the septum and the frequency with which the amount of available septal tissue is still further decreased because of the presence of an atrial septal defect. The creation of the interatrial tunnel exclusively by means of a prosthesis, as suggested by Merendino and his associates[6] and by Creech and his colleagues,[4] appears unwise since it would not grow with increasing size of the patient and the heart. With either of the 2 procedures I have described, the grafts used constitute only a portion of the repair and viable autogenous tissue makes up the rest. Hence, there should be no difficulty with growth. The multiple-flap method of Senning[7] has to commend it the incontrovertible fact that it is, as far as I know, the only method yet successfully applied in human beings. The proposed procedures seem to be simpler in execution.

Just what approach would prove best remains to be seen. In the first clinical case, a right anterior thoracotomy incision was quite satisfactory. In this instance, there was no additional anomaly except for the atrial septal defect. In the second, in which a patent ductus arteriosus was present, a bilateral anterior thoracotomy incision worked well. If a ventricular septal defect were present and there were no patent ductus arteriosus, perhaps a sternum-splitting incision would be better. This matter could be settled by further clinical trials.

The difficulty encountered in the first case in securing hemostasis should be obviated by use of a pericardial graft, perhaps best also covered with thin Teflon felt, for reconstruction of the anterior atrial wall and use of the proximal end of the right subclavian artery for the arterial inflow catheter. I have subsequently found that the right subclavian artery can be adequately mobilized even through a sternum-splitting incision to permit introduction of the inflow catheter through its proximal end into the aorta. The subclavian artery can then be ligated at the completion of the procedure, eliminating the necessity for arteriorrhaphy on such a tiny vessel. When the iliac vein is exceedingly small as was true in this case, it could be safely ligated rather than repaired. The inadequate venous outflow in the second case presented a more difficult problem but a solution seems to be at hand. At the moment, it is my feeling that if a similar situation is encountered I should place the outflow catheters initially in the inferior vena cava via the common iliac vein and in the superior vena cava via the azygos vein. Before beginning perfusion, however, I would introduce a large catheter into the right atrium at a point where the atriotomy could subsequently be incorporated in one of the incisions made to create the atrial flap. This catheter would then be used during the cooling phase for venous outflow and should permit adequate perfusion. Once a low body temperature had been reached, the smaller catheters placed into the superior and inferior venae cavae could be used instead to maintain some extracorporeal circulation during the period of interatrial retransposition. When the corrective procedure had been accomplished, quick rewarming should be possible by draining off venous blood through a fairly large catheter placed through the posterior ventricle into the pulmonary artery.

## SUMMARY

A new method for interatrial venous retransposition has been described. It seems applicable to cases of transposition of the great vessels.

### REFERENCES

1. Albert, H. M.: Surgical correction of transposition of the great vessels, S. Forum **5:** 74, 1954.
2. Baffes, T. G.: A new method for surgical correction of transposition of the aorta and pulmonary artery, Surg. Gynec. & Obst. **102:** 227, 1956.
3. Blalock, A., and Hanlon, C. R.: The surgical treatment of complete transposition of the aorta and the pulmonary artery, Surg. Gynec. & Obst. **90:** 1, 1950.
4. Creech, O., Mahaffey, D. E., Sayegh, S. F., and Sailors, E. L.: Complete transposition of the great vessels. A technique for intracardiac correction, Surgery **43:** 349, 1958.
5. Lillehei, C. W., and Varco, R. L.: Certain physiologic, pathologic, and surgical features of complete transposition of the great vessels, Surgery **42:** 898, 1957.
6. Merendino, E. A., Jesseph, J. E., Herron, P. W., Thomas, G. I., and Vitto, R. R.: Interatrial venous transposition. A one-stage operation for the conversion of complete transposition of the aorta and pulmonary artery to corrected transposition, Surgery **42:** 898, 1957.
7. Senning, Å.: Surgical correction of transposition of the great vessels, Surgery **45:** 966, 1959.

# Resection of inferior vena cava and graft replacement (aortic homograft) for retroperitoneal sarcoma

CHARLES J. McPEAK, M.D.
NEW YORK, N. Y.
*From Memorial Hospital*

This report concerns the removal of a right retroperitoneal sarcoma with the resection of the right kidney, along with 13.5 cm. of the infrahepatic portion of the vena cava including the distal 1.5 cm. of the left renal vein. The resected portion of the vena cava was replaced by a segment of preserved homologous abdominal aorta. The divided end of the left renal vein was anastomosed to an opening made in the side of the preserved graft.

## CASE REPORT

In 1948, at the age of 50, a woman had begun to experience a dull, rather severe, deep epigastric pain. It occurred predominantly on the right side and penetrated through to the patient's back. Because of persistent pain, and after complete but nonrevealing clinical and laboratory studies, the patient underwent an exploratory laparotomy, at which time no intra-abdominal disease was found. In September, 1952, after a similar nonrevealing survey, the patient underwent a second exploratory laparotomy. At this time, there was a firm mass in the right retroperitoneal area thought to be carcinoma of the pancreas; no resection was attempted. In January, 1953, an exploratory laparotomy was performed and the previously described retroperitoneal tumor mass confirmed. An attempt to remove this retroperitoneal tumor showed that the mass could not be dissected away from the vena cava.

After this operation, the woman was given a course of radiation therapy, the factors of which are unavailable. She experienced transient relief after this treatment, but the pain soon recurred and became increasingly severe. She was admitted to Memorial Hospital where she was given a calculated tumor dose of 3,000 r to the area of the mass through a 10 by 10 cm. anterior portal by the cobalt therapy machine. For nearly 2 months after this treatment there was marked, but again transient, relief of symptoms.

The patient was readmitted to Memorial Hospital in October, 1955. She described the same severe, dull, persistent pain in the right upper abdominal quadrant with penetration straight through to the back. Examination showed her to be a pale, lean woman who evidenced chronic weight loss. In the right upper abdominal quadrant there was a poorly defined mass which did not move on respiration or on bimanual manipulation. There was no evidence of metastases by clinical or laboratory determinations. The inferior vena cava was outlined by injection of Urokon into the left femoral vein through a polyethylene catheter (Fig. 1). This study demonstrated the

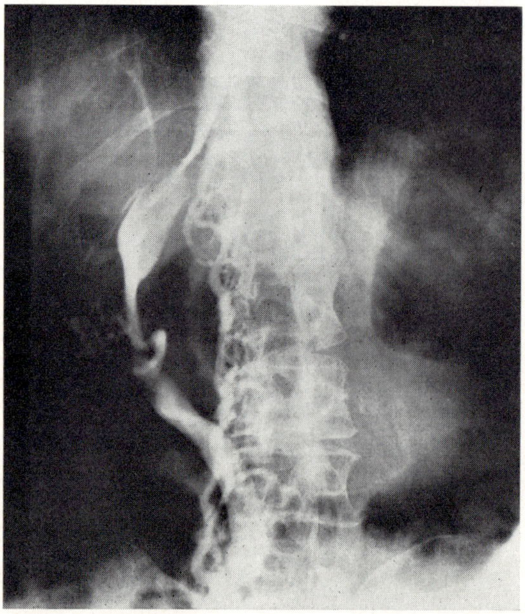

**Fig. 1.** Venogram (Urokon) which shows displacement and partial rotation of the vena cava by retroperitoneal tumor.

Received for publication Jan. 2, 1961.

vena cava to have a maximum point of displacement 2½ inches to the right of its normal course. The displacement curve began inferiorly at $L_3$ and extended up to the level of $D_{11}$. In addition to the lateral displacement, there appeared to be flattening and longitudinal rotation of the vein by the tumor mass. Intravenous pyelogram showed an indistinct mass in the right renal area, but the kidney itself could not be outlined and there was no evidence of dye excretion from the right kidney. The left kidney was normal in position, outline, and function.

After correction of a deficit in the blood volume, the patient was prepared for operation. Exposure of the operative area was obtained through a transverse epigastric incision. Later, as it became necessary to mobilize the liver superiorly, a right thoracotomy incision was made to divide the diaphragm.

There were diffuse adhesions throughout all the planes of the upper abdomen which resulted from the 4 previous operations as well as the 2 courses of radiation therapy. The pancreas, duodenum, and portal structures were identified and reflected to the left and superiorly. It was then apparent that the tumor was rather discrete and lay posteromedially to the right kidney, posteriorly and more to the left of the vena cava, but anteriorly and to the right of the aorta (Fig. 2). Although this rather firm tumor lay directly over a segment of the aorta and both renal arteries, it was possible to free them of the tumor by dissection in the subadventitial plane of these arterial structures. Such dissection was not possible with the corresponding veins, however, for the vena cava and right renal vein were inseparable from the tumor.

The removal of the tumor mass with the adjacent invaded tissues required the resection of the right kidney, right adrenal gland, and the involved segment of the vena cava. The vena cava segment measured 13.5 cm. in length. In order to provide a free cuff of vena cava superiorly, it was necessary to dissect the vessel free from the inferior 1.5 cm. of the liver. This required the division of the two lowermost hepatic veins. It was found that the left renal vein could be divided between the ovarian vein and the vena cava. A homograft of an abdominal aorta measuring 13.5 cm. in length, which had been prepared by the freeze-dry method, was sutured in place.

In order to anastomose the divided end of the remaining renal vein to the graft without tension, a left nephropexy was performed to support the kidney in a more medial and anterior position. An ellipse was excised from the wall of the homograft to correspond to the size of the left renal vein. The end of the vein was then anastomosed to the side of the homograft with the same type

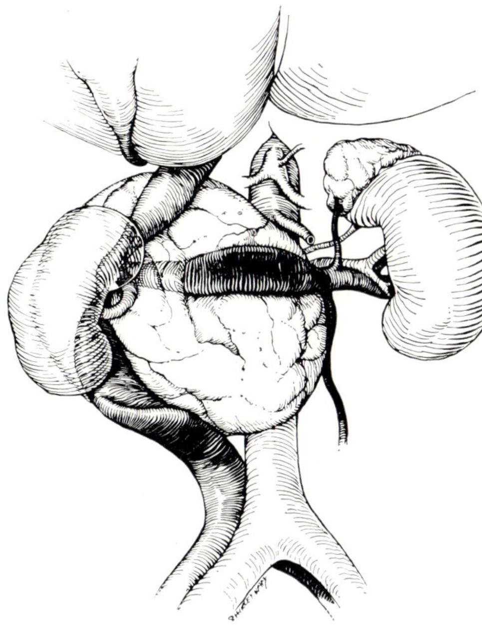

**Fig. 2.** Sketch which shows the anatomic relationship and position of the tumor.

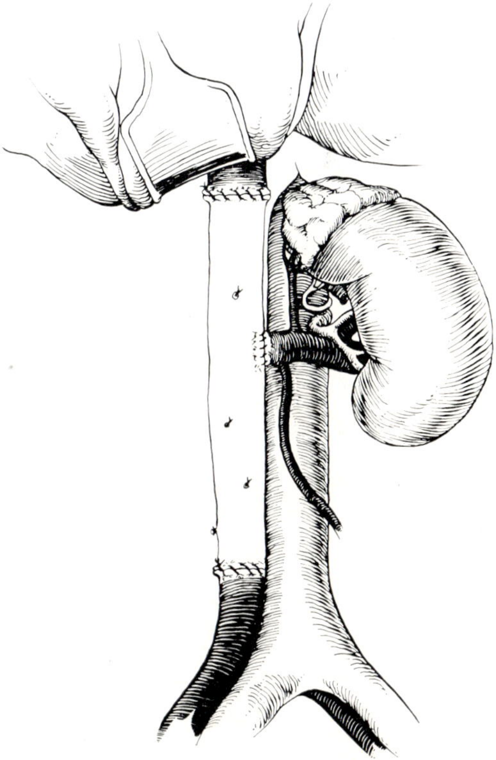

**Fig. 3.** Drawing illustrates the blood vessel anastomoses with the graft (aortic hemograft) in place.

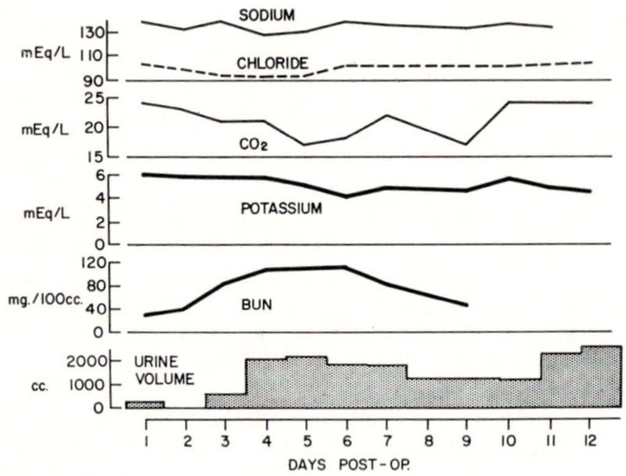


**Fig. 4.** Graph shows function of left kidney (with renal vein–vena cava anastomosis) as reflected by daily urinary output and simultaneous blood chemistry studies. The elevated potassium level started to fall almost immediately when the urinary output returned on the fourth postoperative day, whereas the fall in the blood urea nitrogen level did not begin until the sixth postoperative day. Note that the potassium level rose again for a brief period at the time of the massive thrombosis on the tenth day.

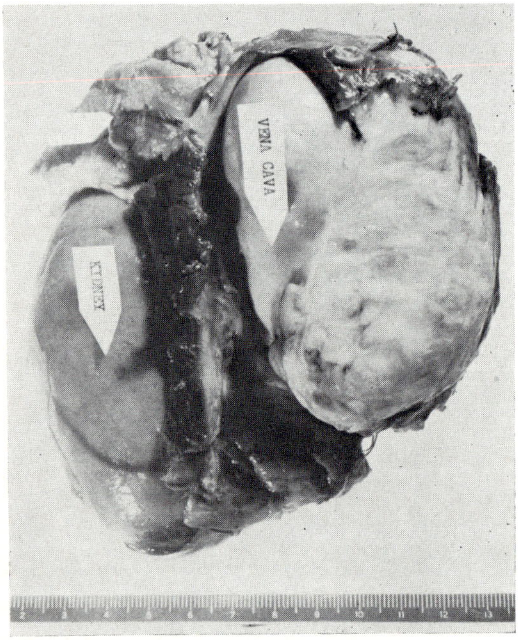


**Fig. 5.** Gross specimen which shows invasion and replacement of wall of vena cava by tumor.

of everting No. 5-0 arterial silk suture (Fig. 3). The anastomotic sites were irrigated freely with dilute heparin solution during the procedure. Air was aspirated from the open vessels and replaced with normal saline solution before blood flow was allowed to resume through the graft.

The chest was closed after an underwater drainage system was in place. Two large Penrose drains were left in the right renal space and allowed to emerge through the right lateral end of the laparotomy wound. The patient received 10 units of blood (5,000 ml.) during the operation.

While the inferior vena cava was temporarily occluded, the blood pressure in the arm dropped to 70 to 80 mm. Hg systolic for 1 hour and 20 minutes. The blood pressure rose to 100 systolic after the vena cava clamps had been removed.

Postoperatively, the patient was given heparin in the fluids which were administered intravenously by a continuous drip through a polyethylene catheter inserted into the common femoral vein by way of the saphenous vein. Approximately 200 mg. of heparin was used daily in this manner.

The patient was doing well when, on the tenth postoperative day, she rather abruptly lapsed into coma associated with a fall in blood pressure to 78/0 and an increased pulse rate to 132 per minute. She responded from this hypotensive state with the rapid administration of 600 ml. of plasma and 1,000 ml. of whole blood. At the same time, she was noted to have increased swelling and mottling of both legs and buttocks, especially on the right. The polyethylene catheter in the femoral vein was obstructed and attempts to replace it were unsuccessful, presumably because of a thrombus in both iliac veins. This thrombophlebitis developed in the presence of Ace elastic bandages on both legs from toes to upper groins, as well as a continuous drip of diluted heparin into the venous system below the anastomosis. The massive thrombophlebitis was treated by bed rest, elevation of both legs, and the application of warm wet towels to both lower extremities.

Two weeks after the onset of the thrombophlebitis, the edema of the buttocks began to subside, followed soon afterward by the edema of the thighs and legs. At the time of discharge, 42 days after operation, there was only minimal edema of both ankles after the patient had been out of bed for several hours.

Fig. 4 illustrates the marked depression in urinary output over the first 3 postoperative days. The blood chemistry levels are correspondingly shown.

**Pathology report.** The specimen as received had the over-all measurements of 14 by 12 by 6 cm. and included the right kidney, right adrenal gland, a segment of the inferior vena cava, and the retroperitoneal tumor. The portion of vena cava was tortuous, and was distorted by the tumor. The vena cava segment measured 11.0 cm. in

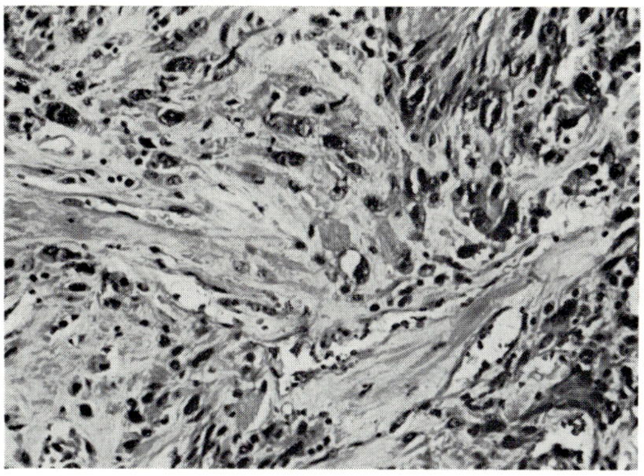

**Fig. 6.** Photomicrograph of section of tumor which shows both the marked hyalinization and the undifferentiated pleomorphic cellular component of the tumor tissue.

length and showed gross invasion of the wall by the tumor. The tumor mass measured 10.6 by 6.5 by 6.5 cm. It was very firm in consistency, and on sectioning presented a variegated tan to yellow to dark red appearance with a whorled and trabeculated pattern.

The right kidney measured 10.5 by 5 by 3.5 cm. Its capsule was thickened, but it did strip with ease to reveal a smooth cortical surface. The kidney was estimated to weigh 80 grams. On its cut surface the cortex was thin, measuring only 0.3 cm. in dimension. The medullary portion did not appear unusual. The pelvis was slightly dilated, as were the pelvic calyces, but the 2.0 cm. of ureter attached to the renal pelvis was not dilated. The right renal vein showed a normal origin from the vena cava and no obvious site of occlusion (Fig. 5).

**Microscopic description.** The bulk of the tumor was hyalinized, relatively avascular, and with only scattered, small tumor cells (Fig. 6). The next most common pattern was at the other extreme—an extremely cellular, poorly differentiated, and pleomorphic tumor with many giant cells characteristic of radiation reaction. Inflammation and necrosis were present, but not constant. A few foci were less anaplastic and better differentiated. The sections from the vein wall showed complete replacement of the wall by tumor.

The diagnosis was anaplastic fibrosarcoma with evidence of radiation reaction. The patient had lived without pain in complete comfort and with a full scope of activity for 1 year when pulmonary metastases were discovered. She died shortly thereafter.

# A technique of attaching a synthetic graft to the side of a severely arteriosclerotic aorta

JOHN R. DERRICK, M.D.
GALVESTON, TEXAS
*From the Department of Surgery, University of Texas, Medical Branch*

Currently, bypass grafts are being used with increasing frequency for severe occlusive disease of the major branches that arise from the aorta. The generalized nature of the degenerative process that is known as arteriosclerosis often results in changes in the aorta which mitigate against the successful attachment of a bypass graft. The surgical accessibility of the lower abdominal aorta makes this an ideal region for the attachment of bypass grafts for major abdominal or peripheral arteries; yet, this area is often the most severely involved by arteriosclerosis. The severe degeneration and calcification often leave only a thin layer of fibrous adventitial tissue which does not readily hold sutures, or, if it does, it is found to lack both strength and uniformity.

Received for publication Jan. 7, 1961.

A buffer graft around the area affords easy, secure attachment of grafts without the necessity of resection of the severely degenerated portion and extension of the operative procedure. Use of a sheet of woven Teflon around the site, as illustrated in Fig. 1, permits the attachment of a bypass graft. Fig. 2

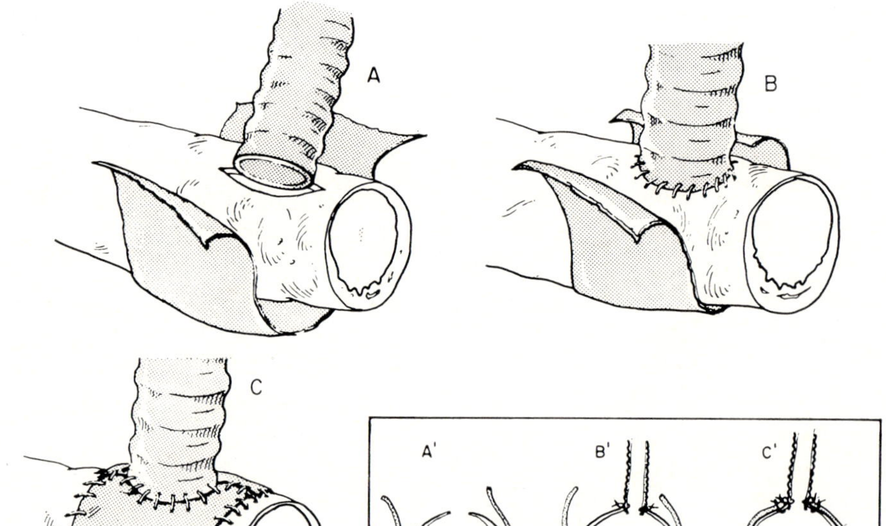


**Fig. 1.**

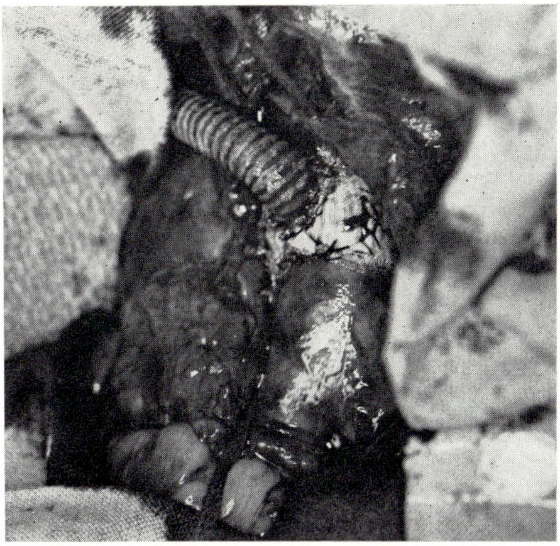

**Fig. 2.**

is a photograph taken at operation of a retrograde flow graft (De Bakey's side-arm graft) which is attached to the lower abdominal aorta and going to the right renal artery.

The graft is initially sutured to the thinned, friable edges of the aortotomy with No. 4-0 arterial silk. The Teflon sheet is then placed around the aorta and trimmed to conform to the graft and the aorta, as illustrated in Fig. 1, *C*. A second row of No. 3-0 arterial sutures, snugly approximating the Teflon sheet to the graft, adds strength and secures the anastomosis. To prevent bleeding and dissection beneath the buffer graft, a running No. 3-0 arterial suture is then made, with use of the adventitial coat of the aorta and the Teflon at a distance of 3 to 10 mm. from the graft anastomosis.

This technique may provide a simple means of graft attachment without the necessity of extensive aortic resections in instances in which the bypass graft attachment is insecure or is not feasible because of severe degenerative changes.

Investigative surgery

# Physiologic evidence of lymphatic repair after skin homotransplantation

R. C. A. WEATHERLEY-WHITE, M.D.*
RICHARD B. STARK, M.D.
MARGIE DE FOREST, A.A.
NEW YORK, N. Y.
*From the Surgical Service (Plastic), St. Luke's Hospital in the City of New York*

The immunologic nature of the homograft rejection response has been amply documented.[4, 10] Less clear, however, are the means by which this response is initiated.

Evidence at this time points to the regional lymphatic system of the host as a primary mediator of homograft rejection. Scothorne and McGregor,[7] who pointed out that the rabbit's ear is drained unilaterally to a regional node at the base of the ear, demonstrated a marked increase in weight of that node after homografting of skin distal to it, while the contralateral node was not affected. There was no gain of weight due to the operative procedure or to absorption of toxic products from a graft that was being rejected. Furthermore, Stark and associates[9] showed that the weight gain due to homografting was significantly higher than that which follows autografting. Histologic studies[6] showed the presence of "large lymphoid cells" in the ipsilateral node after homografting. These large cells were postulated to be the site of antibody formation, which, when disseminated through the blood stream, are responsible for graft rejection. Stark and Dwyer[8] carried the argument one stage further when they showed that interruption of the lymphatic pathway by resection of the regional node produced enhanced survival of homografts. They also showed that if homografts are placed on both ears, and only 1 node resected, then both grafts are lost without enhancement. This strongly suggests that a localized connection between the graft and the lymphatic system of the host is necessary for the systemic immunologic response.

Evidence based on anatomic studies indicates that lymphatic continuity is re-established within 4 to 6 days of grafting.[1, 3, 5] One could therefore postulate a mechanism whereby homograft antigen is sequestered within the graft until lymphatic connections develop between the graft and the host's bed. The antigen is then conducted to the node where the systemic homograft response is initiated.

Certain inconsistencies are immediately apparent in this hypothesis. If immunity depends on establishment of lymphatic repair, and this takes 4 to 6 days, then it is difficult to explain nodal enlargement and histologic changes characteristic of homotransplantation which occur within 2 days of the procedure. Furthermore, it is impossible to ascribe to lymphatic mediation the rapid rejection of the "second-set" homograft.

One of these premises must be wrong. Either immunity must begin independently of lymphatic repair, or current methods of identifying lymphatics (India ink or fluo-

Received for publication Dec. 17, 1960.

*Present address: University of Colorado Medical Center, Denver, Colo.

rescein dye) do not demonstrate early functioning connections.

We decided to study the development of lymphatic repair using, as a parameter, the clearance of radioactive albumin from the intradermal tissues of the graft, since it has been shown that this protein is cleared selectively by the lymphatics rather than by capillaries.[2] Therefore, this method represents a functional rather than an anatomic approach to the timing of lymphatic re-establishment.

## METHOD

For this experiment, rabbits of disparate strains (chinchillas and New Zealand whites) were used. Thirty-six animals were divided into 2 equal groups as donors and recipients, and 2 rabbits were used as controls to investigate the clearance of $I^{131}$-tagged albumin from the intact ear. One ear of each of 18 rabbits was injected intradermally with 0.25 ml. of $I^{131}$-tagged albumin containing 30 $\mu$c. The following day, with sterile technique and intravenous Nembutal anesthesia, circular full-thickness grafts measuring 2.5 cm. in diameter were taken so as to include the previously marked injection site. The grafts were transplanted immediately to the ears of 18 recipient rabbits. The purpose of the 24-hour delay was to allow intact lymphatics of the donor animal to carry away any albumin which, through faulty technique of injection, might have found its way into the subcutaneous tissue. Thus, at the time of grafting we assume that there was present only intradermally trapped albumin without contamination of the underside of the graft.

Immediately after the procedure, radioactivity was quantitated from the newly transplanted graft. A thallium-activated collimator with a 4-inch sodium iodide crystal was used, shielded with one-half inch lead through which was bored a circular aperture the size of the grafts. Each area was counted for 100 seconds. Daily readings were taken from the grafts to show clearance of albumin by the lymphatics, and from the flank of each animal to demonstrate systemic pickup of circulating $I^{131}$-tagged albumin.

The second part of the experiment concerned the role played by the regional auricular lymph node proximal to the graft. The day of grafting and each day thereafter, 2 rabbits underwent bilateral nodal resection. The nodes were weighed and the radioactivity measured in vitro with a well-type counter. By continuation of the count for 15 minutes, an accurate assessment could be obtained of the time when $I^{131}$-tagged albumin first appeared in the regional node. Furthermore, by correlation of the rate of albumin clearance from the grafts with the time of node resection, it was possible to assess the effect of nodal resection upon lymphatic clearance of protein from the grafts.

Finally, a sham operation was carried out in 2 animals, with exposure but not resection of the nodes, so as to estimate the effect that operative trauma with subsequent inflammatory reaction might have upon lymphatic clearance.

The method of graphically representing the results bears explanation. Because of the unavoidable disparity in volume of injected material, the ordinate of all grafts, representing the quantity of radioactivity present, is expressed as a percentage of initial count. The average initial raw count was between 4,000 and 6,000 counts per second. Furthermore, all counts are adjusted for radioactive decay, with a factor of 0.917 per day.

On the same graph is plotted the systemic appearance of radioactivity as measured by the same counter over the animal's flank. This, however, is presented in counts per second rather than percentage of initial count because the quantity involved is too small (up to 100 counts per second).

## RESULTS

The pattern of clearance of radioactive albumin from an injection site in the intact ear conformed with the results of previous work[2] (Fig. 1).

Measurements were taken at hourly intervals for 12 hours and daily thereafter. As may be seen, there was a rapid initial loss. Fifty per cent of the injected albumin was

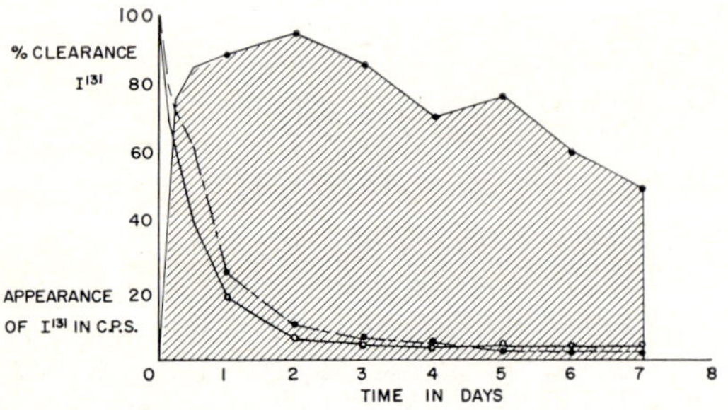


**Fig. 1.** The rapid rate of clearance of $I^{131}$-tagged albumin from the intradermal tissues of the intact ear is shown. Fifty per cent of activity is cleared within 24 hours. The solid area represents the average systemic radioactivity in counts per second.

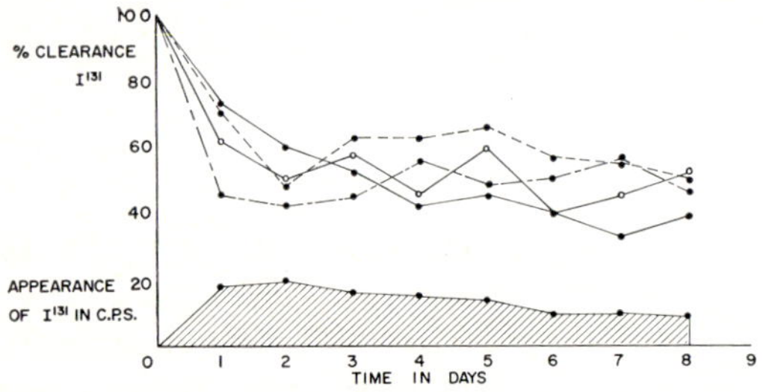


**Fig. 2.** The rate of clearance of $I^{131}$-tagged albumin from the homografts of 4 rabbits. Initial clearance takes place in the presence of an intact lymphatic system in the recipients, because they represent the late nodal resection group. Thirty-eight per cent of base-line activity is cleared within 24 hours. The solid area represents the average systemic activity in counts per second.

cleared in the first 12 hours. At the end of 8 days, only 1 to 2 per cent remained at the injection site. In counts per second this was little more than the generalized background present in the body. The level of body radiation was seen to rise correspondingly with the rapid clearance by the lymphatics, and then dwindled slowly as the protein was metabolized and excreted.

When the albumin was contained in the intradermal tissues of a graft, predictably the rate of clearance was slower. However, there was no "trapping" of albumin for several days as expected and a significant loss occurred at 24 hours. The patterns of albumin clearance from 4 animals which underwent nodal resection on the seventh and eighth posthomotransplantation days are shown in Fig. 2. Thus, the initial loss of albumin, in this series, took place in the presence of an intact lymphatic drainage system in the recipient.

As can be seen, there was an immediate loss of radioactivity from the grafts. An average of 38 per cent of base-line activity was cleared within 24 hours. The curves flattened out in 2 to 3 days. Systemic radioactivity was not elicited in the hour after the graft procedure, but was definitely present at 24 hours. The average body count at that time was 18 counts per second.

When the lymphatic drainage pathway is interrupted by surgical ablation of the regional node, the clearance of radioactive albumin is delayed significantly. Four animals underwent resection of this node either at the time of homografting or 24 hours subsequently. As can be seen (Fig. 3), the initial loss was considerably less than in the previous group. An average of 11 per cent was cleared in the first 24 hours as opposed to 38 per cent in the previous group. The curves remained shallow for 3 days, at which time they took a steeper course and then leveled off at the fifth day. Similarly, less systemic radiation was noted at first. The body count at 24 hours was only 6 counts per second and rose to a peak at 3 days. These findings—the delayed clearance of protein-bound matter after lymph node resection—provide a theoretical basis for the phenomenon of graft enhancement after regional lymph node resection.

Fig. 4 shows the superimposed mean patterns for each group, early and late node resection, which illustrate the disparity of clearance between the 2 groups. The third curve represents the pattern of clearance of 2 rabbits in which, after homotransplantation, a sham operation was carried out at the base of each ear, with exposure but not resection of the regional node. As can be seen, albumin clearance was not delayed in those animals, which demonstrates that the disparity between the groups was due to actual interference with the lymphatic system rather than to operative trauma and subsequent inflammatory reaction.

After resection of the auricular nodes from each rabbit, nodes were weighed and the amount of radioactivity determined by means of a well-type, thallium-activated sodium iodide counter. Because of the small amount of activity present, each node was counted for 15 minutes. After this, an equal time was used to measure machine and room background. The activity present is expressed in counts per second, with allowance for radioactive decay and machine background. Table I shows the results of this phase of the study.

As seen, activity was picked up by the node draining the ear which was operated upon within 2 days of grafting. That this was due to a genuine lymphatic pathway rather than to the blood stream via capillary regeneration is strongly suggested by the fact that, at that time, no activity was demonstrable in the contralateral node. In fact, throughout the experiment virtually no radiation was found on that side. The only 2 occasions were when the over-all body level was disproportionately high as seen by the irregular figures in the ipsilateral node.

Review of the nodal weights again demonstrates that the node on the homografted side increases in size more than that on the nongrafted side, confirming previous work.

## SUMMARY AND CONCLUSIONS

1. Previous experiments implicate the regional lymphatic system as a primary mediator of homograft rejection. A physiologic study has been made of the time of lymphatic repair between graft and host bed.

2. The ears of 18 rabbits were injected with $I^{131}$-tagged albumin. The next day, full-thickness grafts were taken so as to include the injection site and were transplanted homologously. Radioactivity of the graft was measured daily to show clearance of albumin by the lymphatics and was counted from the flank to show systemic pickup. Furthermore, 2 rabbits daily underwent resection of lymph nodes. The nodes were weighed and in vitro radioactivity measured.

3. Results indicate that clearance of al-

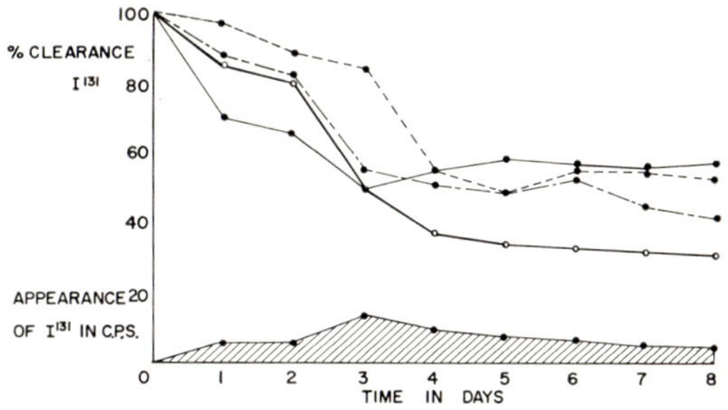


**Fig. 3.** The greatly impeded clearance of $I^{131}$-tagged albumin from the homografts of 4 rabbits which underwent lymph node resection at the time of grafting. They represent the early nodal resection group. Eleven per cent of base-line activity is cleared within 24 hours. The solid area represents the average systemic activity in counts per second and shows a slower pick-up by the body.

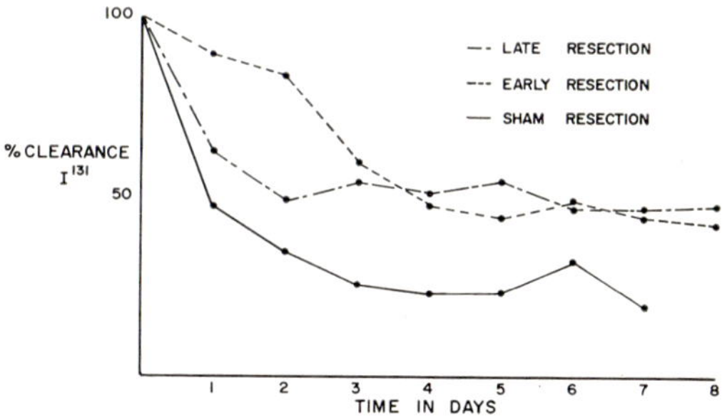


**Fig. 4.** The mean pattern of clearance of $I^{131}$-tagged albumin from both early resection and late resection groups, superimposed for comparison. The third curve shows the clearance pattern of the animals which underwent sham resection and demonstrates that clearance is not delayed by operative trauma.

**Table I.** *Weight and in vitro radioactivity of ipsilateral and contralateral auricular nodes*

| | *Grafted ear* | | *Nongrafted ear* | |
|---|---|---|---|---|
| *Day* | *Average weight of nodes (mg.)* | *Counts per sec.* | *Average weight of nodes (mg.)* | *Counts per sec.* |
| 1 | 120 | 0 | 115 | 0 |
| 2 | 135 | 2 | 140 | 0 |
| 3 | 427 | 2 | 100 | 0 |
| 4 | 925 | 13 | 203 | 2 |
| 5 | 325 | 4 | 95 | 0 |
| 6 | 500 | 4 | 170 | 0 |
| 7 | 690 | 8 | 260 | 2 |
| 8 | 392 | 3 | 240 | 0 |

bumin begins within 24 hours of grafting. By 24 hours, between 3 per cent and 67 per cent of base-line activity was lost from the grafts, and all animals showed systemic activity. Radioactivity was found in the node at the base of the ear within 24 hours and rose to a peak at 4 to 7 days. Virtually no activity was detectable in the opposite node, indicating that clearance from the homograft was via a lymphatic pathway rather than the blood stream. The rate of albumin clearance was impeded by node resection.

4. A hypothesis which implicates the regional node in graft immunity and is dependent upon the clearance of protein-bound antigen by regenerated lymphatic connections has been proposed.

We wish to thank Dr. Richard P. Keating, Chief of the Radioisotope Laboratory at St. Luke's Hospital in the City of New York, for his helpful criticism regarding radioisotope methods.

## REFERENCES

1. Egdahl, R. H., and Varco, R. L.: Intradermal fluorescein test for homograft rejection period, Transplantation Bull. **3:** 152, 1956.
2. Ju, D., and Blakemore, A. H.: A lymphatic function test, S. Forum **5:** 607, 1954.
3. McGregor, I. A., and Conway, H.: Development of lymph flow from autografts and homografts of skin, Transplantation Bull. **3:** 46, 1956.
4. Medawar, P. B.: *In* Preservation and transplantation of normal tissues, Ciba Foundation Symposium **1:** 22, 1955.
5. Scothorne, R. J.: Lymphatic repair and the genesis of homograft immunity, Ann. New York Acad. Sc. **73:** 673, 1958.
6. Scothorne, R. J.: Studies on the response of the regional lymph node to skin homografts, Ann. New York Acad. Sc. **64:** 1028, 1957.
7. Scothorne, R. J., and McGregor, I. A.: Cellular changes in lymph nodes and spleen following skin homografting, J. Anat. **89:** 283, 1955.
8. Stark, R. B., and Dwyer, E. B.: The enhancement of homografts of skin, SURGERY **46:** 277, 1959.
9. Stark, R. B., Dwyer, E. B., and de Forest, M.: Effect of surgical ablation of regional lymph nodes on survival of skin homografts, Ann. New York Acad. Sc. **87:** 104, 1960.
10. Voisin, G. A., and Maurer, P.: Studies on the role of antibodies in the failure of homografts, Ann. New York Acad. Sc. **64:** 1053, 1957.

# Experimental ascites. I. Production of ascites by gradual occlusion of the hepatic veins with an internal vena caval cannula

MARSHALL J. ORLOFF, M.D.*
GILBERT B. SNYDER, M.D.
DENVER, COLO.
*From the Department of Surgery, University of Colorado School of Medicine*

In 1728, Richard Lower[6] first described the experimental production of ascites in animals by occlusion of the thoracic inferior vena cava. In 1907, Bolton[1] confirmed Lower's studies and in recent years McKee and associates[9] have clearly established this technique as a simple and reliable method of producing ascites. Results of a number of studies indicate that the ascites arising from partial occlusion of the thoracic inferior vena cava is derived largely from the surface of the liver and is a consequence of obstruction of hepatic venous outflow.[2, 4, 8] Some evidence suggests that much of the ascitic fluid originates directly from the hepatic lymphatics.[3, 4, 10]

In human beings with cirrhosis of the liver, evidence indicates that obstruction of hepatic venous outflow is an important causative factor in the development of ascites, much as it is in the experimental animal. The studies of Madden and associates[7] and of Welch and his group[11] in human beings have clearly demonstrated an intrahepatic block involving the hepatic veins. However, the clinical and experimental conditions are not truly comparable because in the human being with liver disease the block involves the hepatic veins within the liver and the inferior vena caval pressure is not significantly elevated, while in the animal with partial occlusion of the thoracic inferior vena cava the obstruction is extrahepatic and produces a marked elevation of pressure in the vena cava as well as within the liver. Consequently, it has not been possible to evaluate experimentally the measures directed at decompressing the liver by shunting hepatic venous blood into the systemic venous system.

The present investigation was undertaken in an attempt to produce in dogs hepatic venous outflow obstruction comparable to that which occurs in human beings with liver disease, without producing an elevation of pressure in the inferior vena cava. It represents a modification of the technique first described in 1958 by Kling and Allen[5] and involves the insertion of a thin-walled polyvinyl cannula into the inferior vena cava at the level of entrance of the hepatic veins.

## PROCEDURE

**Operation.** Forty-seven healthy adult male and female mongrel dogs which varied in weight from 19 to 28 kilograms were used as subjects. Anesthesia was produced intravenously with pentobarbital sodium in a dose of 30 mg. per kilogram of body weight and positive-pressure respiration was maintained with an automatic respirator which delivered a mixture of air and oxygen through an endotracheal tube. The operations were performed with sterile technique. During the operative procedure each dog received 5 per cent dextrose in water intra-

Supported in part by United States Public Health Service Grant. No. A-3048.

Received for publication Feb. 10, 1961.

*Markle Scholar in Medical Science. Present address: Department of Surgery, University of California School of Medicine, and Harbor General Hospital, Los Angeles, Calif.

**Fig. 1.** Photograph of the vena caval cannula made of dyed polyvinyl chloride. Dimensions are 3 to 3.5 inches in length, 0.025 inches in wall thickness, and 0.375 to 0.438 inches in outer diameter.

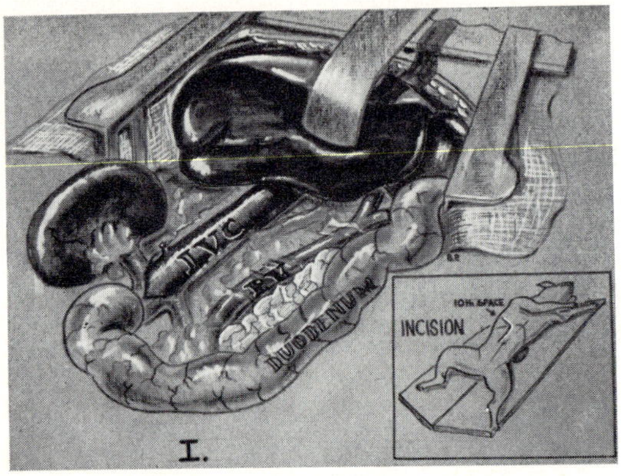


**Fig. 2.** Drawing which shows exposure of the abdominal inferior vena cava from the level of the renal veins to the level of its disappearance into the liver (I). The position of the dog and the right thoracoabdominal incision are shown in the inset.

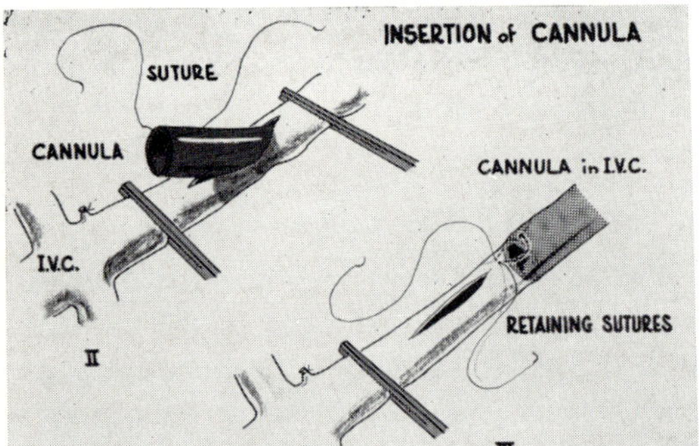


**Fig. 3.** Drawings which show introduction of the cannula into an incision in the anterior wall of the abdominal inferior vena cava (II), and completed insertion of the cannula which is being fixed to the vena cava by bringing the double-needle suture through the anterior wall of the vein (III). Note that the double-needle suture was attached to the inferior end of the prosthesis prior to insertion.

venously in a dose of 30 to 50 ml. per kilogram of body weight. Postoperatively food and water were offered ad libitum. All animals received procaine penicillin intramuscularly in a dose of 600,000 U. daily for 4 days including the day of operation. The cannula to be inserted into the vena cava was siliconized on its internal surface prior to operation in order to minimize clot formation in the lumen. The external surface was left unaltered for the purpose of obtaining reactive fibrosis around the hepatic vein orifices. Several types of cannulas made of polyethylene and polyvinyl chloride were tested before the procedure was standardized. The one selected for extensive trial was made of dyed polyvinyl chloride* and is employed commercially to cover electrical wires (Fig. 1). The cannulas measured 3 to 3.5 inches in length and had a wall thickness of 0.025 inches. Cannulas of 2 diameters were used, one with an outer diameter of 0.375 inches and the other with an outer diameter of 0.438 inches, the choice depending on the diameter of the vena cava. It is important to emphasize that the diameter of the cannula should be slightly smaller than that of the vena cava and the cannula should slide easily into the vessel. A tight-fitting cannula invariably produces acute occlusion of the hepatic veins and death.

The dog was placed in the left oblique position for a right thoracoabdominal incision. A pad was placed under the animal at the level of the costal margin. The incision extended through the right tenth intercostal space, across the costal cartilages, and onto the abdominal wall as a right rectus incision (Fig. 2). The diaphragm was incised along the lines of its fibers from the periphery to the central tendon and the wound edges were held widely apart with a self-retaining retractor. The abdominal vena cava was mobilized from the level of the renal veins to the level of its disappearance into the liver (Fig. 2).

*Natvar "400" tubing made by Natvar Corp., Woodbridge, N. J., and supplied by Electrical Specialty Co., Denver Colo.

Prior to insertion of the cannula an atraumatic swaged No. 5-0 silk suture with needles attached to both ends was placed through the distal end of the cannula for subsequent fixation of the tube to the wall of the vena cava. Before insertion of the prosthesis, heparin in a dose of 1 to 1.5 mg. per kilogram was administered intravenously. In early experiments, protamine in an intravenous dose of 2.0 mg. per kilogram was given before the wound was closed, but in later studies administration of protamine was abandoned.

The abdominal vena cava was occluded with vascular clamps at 2 levels, just inferior to the liver and just above the renal veins, and a 2 cm. longitudinal incision was made in its anterior wall between the 2 clamps. The cannula was inserted into the opening in the vena cava and the abdomen was filled with an isotonic saline solution containing heparin (20 mg. per 100 ml. of saline) until the vena cava was completely submerged (Fig. 3). The superior clamp was then removed and the cannula was pushed cephalad into the vena cava until its inferior end was just superior to the upper limit of the incision in the vena cava. The superior end of the cannula extended well into the thoracic inferior vena cava above the level at which the superior hepatic vein entered. The cannula was fixed to the vena cava by bringing the double-needle suture through the anterior wall of the vein and tying its ends (Fig. 3). Failure to suture the cannula to the wall of the vessel leads to migration of the tube into the right auricle. The opening in the vena cava was occluded with a Satinsky clamp, vena caval blood flow was restored by removal of the inferior vascular clamp, and the incision in the vein was approximated with a continuous No. 5-0 vascular silk suture (Fig. 4). The incisions in the diaphragm and in the thoracic and abdominal walls were closed in layers with chromic catgut sutures and the costal cartilages were approximated with heavy silk sutures. The skin edges were approximated with sutures of fine silk. A large rubber tube was left in the pleural cavity

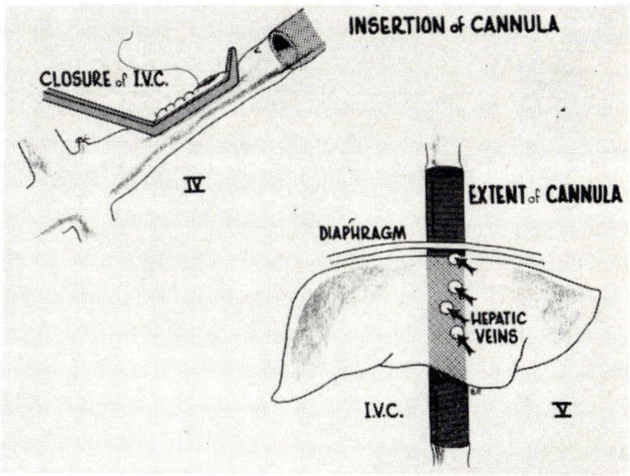


**Fig. 4.** Drawings which show closure of the vena caval incision over a Satinsky clamp after the blood flow has been restored (IV), and the completed operation with the cannula in position opposite the orifices of the hepatic veins (V).

until the closure of the wound was completed when, after aspiration of the pleural cavity, it was removed.

**Pressures.** Pressures in the abdominal inferior vena cava and portal vein were determined by needle puncture during operation and before and after insertion of the cannula. A spinal manometer filled with a heparin-saline solution was employed and the level of the vein in which pressure was being measured was used as the reference point. In 4 animals, pressure determinations were repeated 1 to 4½ months after operation.

**Angiograms.** Inferior vena caval angiograms were obtained from 3 weeks to 10 months postoperatively from most of the animals which survived for more than 2 weeks. The dogs were lightly anesthetized intravenously with pentobarbital sodium and a polyethylene catheter was inserted through a saphenous vein into the inferior vena cava to a level just superior to the entrance of the renal veins. Seventy per cent Urokon in a dose of 25 ml. was injected rapidly and 8 roentgenograms were obtained serially at 1-second intervals.

**Paracentesis.** All animals were subjected to abdominal paracentesis when ascites was apparent clinically and the amount of fluid obtained was measured. Subsequently, paracentesis was repeated intermittently. Para-

**Table I.** *Pressures in abdominal inferior vena cava and portal vein immediately before and after insertion of cannula in 47 dogs*

| | Control pressure (cm. saline) | | Pressure after cannula inserted (cm. saline) | | | | Pressure change (cm. saline) | |
|---|---|---|---|---|---|---|---|---|
| | Mean | Range | Mean | Range | % animals | | Mean | Range |
| Inferior vena cava | 7.5 | 2.0-13.0 | 3.8 | 1.0- 9.2 | Fall | 98 | 3.7 | 0.4-8.4 |
| | | | | | No change | 2 | — | — |
| | | | | | Rise | 0 | — | — |
| Portal vein | 11.5 | 6.0-15.0 | 13.5 | 8.0-21.0 | Fall | 4 | 0.6 | 0.4-0.7 |
| | | | | | No change | 15 | — | — |
| | | | | | Rise | 81 | 2.5 | 0.3-7.0 |

**Table II.** *Pressure measurements in abdominal inferior vena cava and portal vein in 4 dogs, repeated 1 to 4½ months after insertion of cannula*

| Dog No. | Cannula patency | Interval between measurements (mo.) | Pressures (cm. saline) Inferior vena cava | | | Portal vein | | |
|---|---|---|---|---|---|---|---|---|
| | | | Initial | Repeat | Change | Initial | Repeat | Change |
| 59-423 | Patent | 1 | 3.5 | 3.0 | −0.5 | 14.5 | 26.5 | +12.0 |
| 60-22 | Patent | 4½ | 2.5 | 3.0 | +0.5 | 13.5 | 23.4 | + 9.9 |
| 60-43 | Occluded | 4½ | 4.0 | 8.0 | +4.0 | 15.3 | 27.0 | +11.7 |
| 60-176 | Occluded | 2½ | 8.0 | 10.0 | +2.0 | 15.5 | 25.6 | +10.1 |

centesis was performed with a large trocar under local procaine anesthesia. The animal was placed in the prone position on a special table containing an opening through which the abdomen could be drained from a position underneath the table.

**Autopsies.** All animals died or were sacrificed and were subjected to autopsy examinations. In each dog the viscera were studied grossly and particular attention was given to the liver and to the vena cava containing the prosthesis. Sections of liver were examined microscopically.

## RESULTS

**Mortality rate.** Thirty-three animals failed to survive for sufficiently long periods of time to develop ascites. The majority of these (76 per cent) died within 48 hours of operation and at autopsy the liver was found uniformly to be enlarged and congested. It is believed that death was a consequence of acute occlusion of the hepatic veins from a tight-fitting cannula. Four animals died from wound infections or pneumonia, 1 dog was lost, and the cause of death could not be determined in 3 dogs which died during the first postoperative week.

Fourteen animals (30 per cent) lived for 3 weeks to 10½ months and were considered long-term survivors in that they were alive for a sufficient length of time to have developed ascites. Six of these died from 21 to 60 days postoperatively as a result of inanition associated with massive ascites. The remaining 8 dogs were sacrificed 5 weeks to 10½ months postoperatively.

**Pressures.** In all but 1 of the 47 dogs there was a fall in abdominal inferior vena caval pressure after insertion of the cannula (Table I). In 1 animal there was no change in pressure. The mean pressure decrease was 3.7 cm. saline and the range was 0.4 to 8.4 cm. There was no significant difference in the magnitude of the drop in pressure in the dogs which subsequently died and in those which survived. The fall in vena caval pressure is believed to have resulted from a decrease in the flow of hepatic venous blood into the vena cava as a consequence of obstruction of the hepatic vein orifices by the prosthesis.

The portal venous pressure increased after insertion of the cannula in 38 of 47 animals (81 per cent, Table I). The mean rise was 2.5 cm. saline and the range was 0.3 to 7 cm. Again, there was no significant difference between dogs which died and those which lived. In 5 dogs no change in pressure was found and in 2 dogs there was a slight pressure drop of less than 1 cm. Hepatic venous outflow obstruction with back pressure on the liver and portal venous system is believed to have been responsible for the rise in portal pressure which occurred in the majority of animals.

In 4 animals pressures in the inferior vena cava and portal vein were again determined just prior to sacrifice 1 to 4½ months after operation (Table II). Two of these animals had a patent cannula and 2 had developed thrombosis of the prosthesis. In all 4 animals the portal venous pressure had increased markedly to hypertensive levels as a result of progressive hepatic venous outflow obstruction. The rise ranged from 9.9 to 12 cm. saline above the final level obtained at the time of operation.

In the dogs with a patent cannula the inferior vena caval pressure had not changed significantly. In 1 dog there was a 0.5 cm. rise and in the other a 0.5 cm. fall in pressure. In the 2 animals with thrombosis of the cannula, the vena caval pressure was found to have increased 4 cm. in one and 2 cm. in the other. The rise was not nearly as great as might be expected, probably because of the profuse collateral circulation which had developed.

**Ascites.** Twelve of 14 long-term survivors developed massive ascites (Table III). The ascites was first detected clinically between 9 and 44 days postoperatively and varied in amount from 1.5 to 11.5 L. (Fig. 5). The

**Table III.** *Onset and magnitude of ascites and patency of cannula in long-term survivors*

| *Dog No.* | *Clinical onset ascites (postoperative day)* | *Volume of fluid (ml.)* | *Angiogram* | *Time of death and cause* | *Autopsy findings* |
|---|---|---|---|---|---|
| 59-122 | 21 | 6,000 | — | 21 days, inanition | Cannula patent |
| 59-130 | 14 | 2.300 | — | 21 days, inanition | Cannula patent |
| 59-131 | 34 | 10,000 | Cannula patent | 2 mo., inanition | Cannula patent |
| 59-261 | 13 | 1,500 | Cannula blocked | 10½ mo., sacrificed | Thrombus in cannula |
| 59-423 | 9 | 4,000 | Cannula patent | 1 mo., inanition | Cannula patent |
| 60-22 | 38 | 4,000 | Cannula patent | 4½ mo., sacrificed | Cannula patent |
| 60-43 | 31 | 3,000 | Cannula blocked | 4½ mo., sacrificed | Thrombus in cannula |
| 60-59 | 44 | 3,000 | Unsuccessful | 51 days, inanition | Cannula lost |
| 60-141 | 40 | 2,800 | — | 2 mo., inanition | Cannula patent |
| 60-143 | None | — | Cannula blocked | 3 mo., sacrificed | Low insertion of cannula, superior hepatic vein open, thrombus in cannula |
| 60-176 | 25 | 11,500 | Unsuccessful | 2½ mo., sacrificed | Thrombus in cannula |
| 60-188 | None | — | Cannula blocked | 2½ mo., sacrificed | Low insertion of cannula, superior hepatic vein open, thrombus in cannula |
| 60-246 | 30 | 1,800 | Unsuccessful | 5 weeks, sacrificed | Thrombus in cannula |
| 60-XXX | 30 | 3,000 | — | 6 mo., sacrificed | Thrombus in cannula |
| Summary | 9-44 days | 1.5-11.5 L. | 43% patent | — | 46% patent |

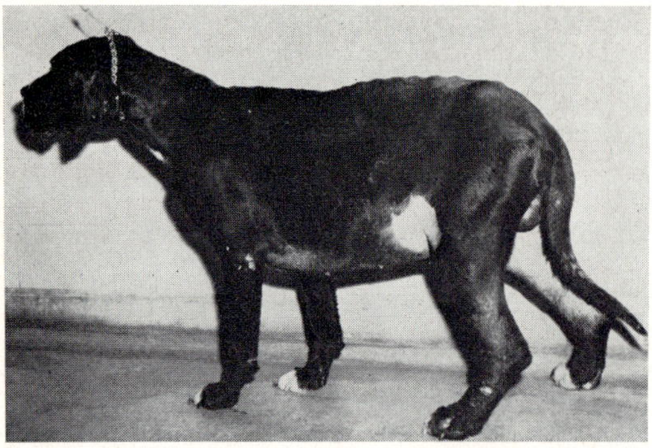

**Fig. 5.** Photograph of dog No. 59-131 taken 45 days after insertion of the internal vena caval cannula shows massive ascites. Immediately after the photograph was taken, paracentesis produced 10 L. of ascitic fluid.

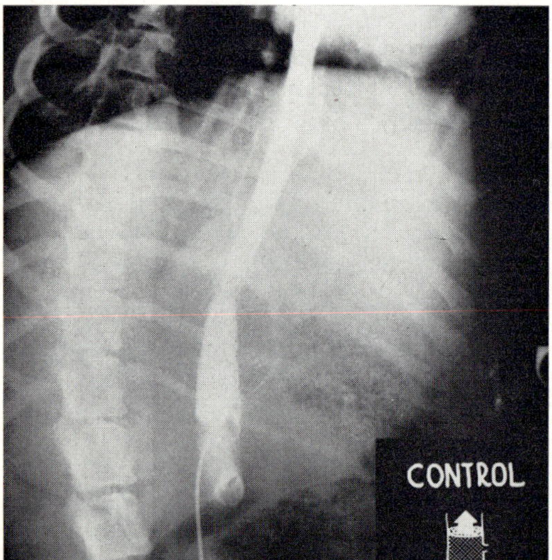


**Fig. 6.** Vena caval angiogram from dog No. 60-22 performed 4½ months after operation shows a patent cannula with rapid passage of dye into the heart. The catheter was positioned about 2 inches below the cannula. The animal had 4 L. of ascitic fluid at the time of this study.

fluid was straw colored and had the typical composition of a transudate of plasma. Once ascites developed, it persisted until the animal died or was sacrificed. Six dogs died from 21 to 60 days postoperatively as a result of inanition associated with the ascites, while the remaining 8 animals were sacrificed from 5 weeks to 10½ months after operation.

The failure to produce ascites in 2 animals was clearly explained by autopsies which in both cases showed that the cannula had not been inserted sufficiently high in the vena cava and had failed to occlude the large superior hepatic vein.

**Angiograms.** Inferior vena caval angiography was attempted in 10 animals from 3 weeks to 10 months postoperatively. In 3 dogs the procedure was unsatisfactory, while in 7 animals adequate visualization of the vena cava was obtained. The cannula was found to be patent in 3 animals (43 per cent), 3 weeks, 1 month, and 4½ months, respectively, after operation (Fig. 6), and was occluded in 4 animals. In each instance of occlusion, the block was demonstrated at the inferior end of the prosthesis and numerous large collateral vessels were seen bypassing the obstruction (Fig. 7).

**Autopsies.** Postmortem examinations were performed in all animals. In 1 of the 14 long-term survivors the cannula was lost during the autopsy and it is not known whether or not the cannula was patent. In 6 of the remaining 13 dogs (46 per cent), the cannula was found to be patent from 21 days to 4½ months postoperatively while in 7 animals studied 5 weeks to 10½ months after operation, the prosthesis was found to be completely occluded by an organized thrombus (Table III). Numerous large collateral veins attached to the vena cava below the level of the cannula were observed in animals in which thrombosis had occurred.

In each instance the cannula was surrounded by a smooth, shiny neointima of fibrous material which completely occluded the orifices of the hepatic veins. In 2 dogs which failed to develop ascites because of low insertion of the prosthesis, the orifice of the large superior hepatic vein was open.

In all animals the liver was greatly enlarged, hard, and congested and fibrinoid material was deposited on its surface. Massive ascites was present in all but the 2 dogs referred to previously. Microscopic examination of the liver showed dilatation of the entire hepatic vasculature, intense congestion of the sinusoids, dilatation of the lymphatic spaces, and focal areas of necrosis.

## DISCUSSION

The insertion of a polyvinyl cannula into the inferior vena cava at the level of entrance of the hepatic veins is a simple method of producing ascites by gradual selective occlusion of the hepatic venous outflow tract. The reactive material of which the cannula is made stimulates the formation of a fibrous neointima which surrounds the prosthesis and completely covers the orifices of the hepatic veins. The ascites which develops is massive and persistent. The hepatic venous outflow obstruction leads to progressive portal hypertension. The mechanism by which ascites is produced, therefore, is similar to that which is believed to occur in human beings with ascites due to cirrhosis of the liver. In a significant number of animals, 46 per cent in this study, the cannula remains patent for long periods and when such is the case, the pressure in the inferior vena cava is normal. In this regard, the method affords a distinct advantage compared to the technique of partial thoracic inferior vena caval occlusion which by its nature results in marked elevations of inferior vena caval pressure.

There are 2 problems associated with the internal cannula technique of producing ascites, namely, acute hepatic venous occlusion and thrombosis of the cannula. The first difficulty, acute occlusion of the hepatic veins, results from a cannula which fits too tightly in the vena cava and it is followed invariably by death within 24 to 48 hours. It is believed that acute hepatic venous outflow obstruction was responsible for most of the deaths in this study. It is desirable to use a prosthesis which slides easily into the vein but at the same time fills the lumen, since small cannulas which fit loosely in the vena cava rapidly develop thromboses. Unfortunately, it is often not possible during the operation to determine accurately when the cannula is producing too much obstruction of hepatic venous outflow.

The second problem, thrombosis of the cannula, is a consequence of the introduction of a foreign body into the low-flow, low pressure vena cava. Clot formation has been a major stumbling block associated with the use of synthetic materials in the venous system and the development of occlusion of the prosthesis in a number of the animals was not surprising. Indeed, it was surprising that so many of the cannulas (46 per cent) remained patent for long periods of time. Perhaps siliconizing the internal surface of the cannula and the use of systemic heparinization increased the incidence of success.

Although thrombosis of the cannula and

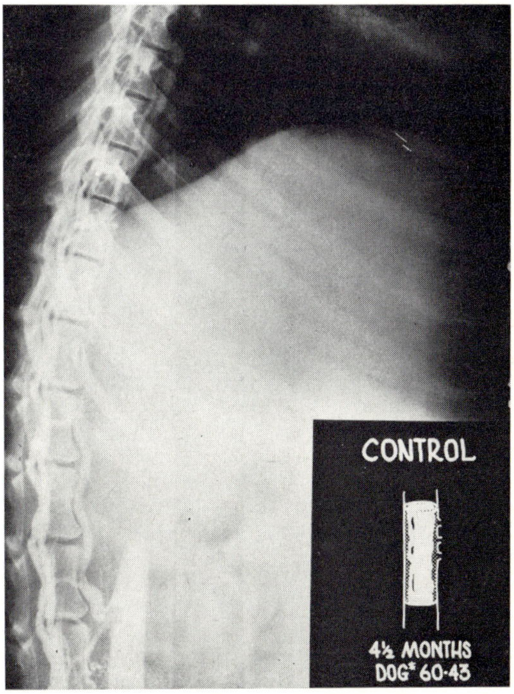


**Fig. 7.** Vena caval angiogram from dog No. 60-43 performed 4½ months postoperatively shows thrombosis of the cannula and large collateral vessels bypassing the obstruction. The collateral vertebral veins are particularly prominent. The roentgenogram shown was the first in the series. The dye had disappeared from the vena cava 3 seconds later, indicating efficient function of the collateral vessels. The animal had 3 L. of ascitic fluid.

the resultant vena caval obstruction did not seem to increase or decrease the rate of ascitic fluid formation, it would be expected to nullify the main advantage of the internal cannula technique. It is of interest, therefore, that in the 2 dogs in which pressure determinations were repeated some time after the development of thrombosis, the vena caval pressures had increased only slightly (2 and 4 cm.). Gradual development of thrombosis and development of an extensive collateral circulation are presumed to have prevented a marked increase in vena caval pressure. The most prominent collateral pathways involved the vertebral and spinal veins.

With the exception of the internal vena caval cannula technique, no simple method of producing ascites has been described by which hepatic venous outflow is selectively obstructed, inferior vena caval pressure is not elevated, and consistently massive ascites is produced. Although problems such as thrombosis of the cannula and death from acute hepatic venous occlusion often complicate the use of the internal cannula method, the results of this investigation indicate that further use of this technique is warranted, particularly as a tool for investigating the effects on ascites of various portal-systemic venous shunts.

## SUMMARY AND CONCLUSIONS

A simple method for producing ascites by gradual occlusion of the hepatic veins without obstruction of the inferior vena cava was evaluated in 47 dogs. The technique involved the introduction of a thin-walled polyvinyl cannula into the inferior vena cava at the level of entrance of the hepatic veins. The reactive polyvinyl stimulated the gradual formation of a fibrous neointima which completely covered the orifices of the hepatic veins.

After insertion of the prosthesis there was a fall in inferior vena caval pressure in 98 per cent of the animals, presumably because of obstruction of the flow of hepatic venous blood into the vena cava. At the same time, there was a rise in portal venous pressure in 83 per cent of the dogs, believed due to hepatic venous outflow obstruction with back pressure on the portal system. Determination of pressures again after long intervals of time in 4 dogs showed a progressive elevation of portal pressure in all, no change in vena caval pressure in the 2 animals with a patent cannula, and a slight rise in vena caval pressure in the 2 dogs with thrombosis of the cannula.

Fourteen animals survived the operation for significant periods. The majority of animals which failed to survive died within 48 hours, presumably from acute occlusion of the hepatic veins due to a tight-fitting cannula. Twelve of the 14 long-term survivors developed massive persistent ascites varying in amount from 1.5 to 11.5 L. within 9 to 44 days postoperatively. The 2 animals which failed to develop ascites were found to have patent superior hepatic veins as a result of insertion of the cannula too low in the vena cava.

Angiograms and autopsies showed a patent cannula in 46 per cent of the surviving animals for periods of up to 4½ months. In the remainder of the dogs, the cannula developed thrombosis.

Despite the problems of acute hepatic venous occlusion and thrombosis of the cannula, the incidence of success is sufficiently high to warrant further use of this technique, particularly as a means of studying the effects on ascites of portal-systemic shunts. No other technique is available presently for this purpose.

### REFERENCES

1. Bolton, C.: Pathology of dropsy produced by obstruction of venae cavae, Proc. Roy. Soc. London **79:** 267, 1907.
2. Freeman, S.: Recent advances in the physiology and biochemistry of the liver, M. Clin. North America **37:** 109, 1953.
3. Gray, H. K.: Clinical and experimental investigation of the circulation of the liver, Ann. Roy. Coll. Surgeons England **8:** 354, 1951.
4. Hyatt, R. E., and Smith, J. R.: The Mechanism of ascites: a physiologic appraisal, Am. J. Med. **16:** 434, 1954.

5. Kling, S., and Allen, P. B. R.: The effects of gradual complete occlusion of the hepatic veins, S. Forum **9:** 550, 1959.
6. Lower, R.: Tractatus du corde, item de motu et colore sanguinis, London, 1728, ed. 6, p. 127.
7. Madden, J. L., Lore, J. M., Jr., Gerold, F. P., and Ravid, J. M.: The pathogenesis of ascites and a consideration of its treatment, Surg. Gynec. & Obst. **99:** 385, 1954.
8. Mallet-Guy, P., Devic, G., Feroldi, J., and Desjacques, P.: Étude expérimentale des ascites; sténoses veineuses post-hépatiques et transposition du foie dans le thorax, Lyon Chir. **49:** 153, 1954.
9. McKee, F. W., Schloerb, P. R., Schilling, J. A., Tishkoff, G. H., and Whipple, G. H.: Protein metabolism and exchange as influenced by constriction of the vena cava, J. Exper. Med. **87:** 457, 1948.
10. Nix, J. T., Flock, E. V., and Bollman, J. L.: Influence of cirrhosis on proteins of cisternal lymph, Am. J. Physiol. **164:** 117, 1951.
11. Welch, C. S., Welch, H. F., and Carter, J. H.: The treatment of ascites by side to side portacaval shunt, Ann. Surg. **150:** 428, 1959.

# Coagulation studies on bleeding surgical patients

KARL E. KARLSON, M.D.
BERNARD LERNER, M.A.
BROOKLYN, N. Y.
*From the Department of Surgery, State University of New York Downstate Medical Center, and Kings County Hospital*

Studies reported here concern a group of patients admitted to the hospital with gastrointestinal hemorrhage and another group with excessive uncontrollable oozing during operation. The tests used in these studies for the various components of the coagulation mechanism are of such nature that they may be performed relatively quickly without elaborate equipment or extensive special knowledge. Therefore, they may be applicable to the evaluation of these problems on a routine basis.

It is generally accepted that most gastrointestinal hemorrhage results initially from involvement of blood vessels in the local lesion. Prolongation of the bleeding may disturb physiologic processes and alter certain components of the coagulation mechanism. In patients with excessive oozing during or immediately after operation, this bleeding from small vessels has been demonstrated in some cases to be associated with defects in the coagulation mechanism.

The coagulation tests used were chosen because they indicate the nature of many of the possible deficiencies in the clotting mechanism. A knowledge of an existing deficiency allows intelligent use of one or more of the specific therapeutic agents which have been advocated in the literature for these deficiencies. For example, vitamin K is effective for prothrombin and factor VII deficiencies in the presence of adequate liver function. Fibrinogen administration has been advocated for hypofibrinogenemia. Albumin has been suggested to supply antifibrinolysin (antiplasmin) since this enzyme is contained in the albumin fraction of the plasma. Platelet transfusions are used in cases of severe platelet deficiency. Fresh blood and fresh frozen plasma are usually effective for deficiencies in platelets (fresh blood only contains platelets), factor V, and other constituents of phase I of the coagulation mechanism. Fresh blood and fresh frozen plasma are generally helpful in bleeding due to all possible coagulation causes when the defects are severe or not definitively understood.

The coagulation abnormality most frequently reported during gastrointestinal bleeding from otherwise benign disease processes is prothrombin deficiency, and somewhat less often factor V and platelet deficiencies. Occasionally abnormal results have been observed in almost all of the other usual coagulation measurements.[1, 6, 10, 29] Some of the deficiencies have been of severity commonly implicated as dangerous, but in most of the cases reported the patients appeared to have had no serious impairment of hemostasis.

Patients with gastrointestinal bleeding and associated liver diseases show an even greater incidence of abnormality. Low prothrombin values, prolonged recalcification times, decreased factor V, prolonged thrombin times, low platelet counts, low fibrinogen levels,

Supported in part by United States Public Health Service Research Grant No. A-1811.
Received for publication Sept. 19, 1960.

and fibrinolysis have been commonly found in patients with liver disease.[1, 6, 10, 15, 21, 28, 30, 33, 38] The role of the liver in production of prothrombin, factor V, fibrinogen, and other factors determines this relationship.

Decreased blood flow to the liver with accompanying hepatic anoxia has been demonstrated during hemorrhage from the gastroduodenal artery.[23] However, a detrimental effect on coagulation from liver hypoxia during upper gastrointestinal bleeding has not been shown.

With surgical oozing, decreased numbers of platelets are frequently observed, but in most cases they are not decreased sufficiently to explain the abnormal bleeding.[13, 14, 20, 40, 43, 45] Measurements which reflect platelet decreases, such as clot retraction, bleeding time, tourniquet test, and prothrombin consumption have been noted to be correspondingly affected.[40]

Decreased fibrinogen levels are reported by several groups in some, but not all, patients with oozing. Afibrinogenemia is almost never seen in surgical patients.[8, 31, 43, 45] Fibrinolysis has been observed in patients with oozing.[7, 8, 13, 24, 31, 40, 43, 45] This is thought to have little clinical importance by some,[40, 43] whereas others consider it to be an etiological factor in the bleeding.[7, 45]

Factor V deficiency has been reported to occur more frequently in patients with oozing than in those without.[45] Abnormalities in several measurements (platelets, recalcification time, thromboplastin generation, prothrombin consumption, prothrombin activity, fibrinogen, and fibrinolysis) were shown to be similar in one study of patients with oozing and a control group of patients without, and the conclusion was drawn that unevaluated factors were involved in the former group.[43]

While oozing has been known to be closely associated with massive blood transfusions of approximately 5,000 ml. or more, it has not been demonstrated that this is a consistent relationship.[17, 20, 40, 43, 45] Transfusion reactions have been cited as the basis for the development of oozing,[12, 13, 26] while some authors have questioned the role of transfusion reactions.[45] A heparinoid substance has been related to oozing.[12] It has been demonstrated that the citrate from large infusions of bank blood will not cause oozing.[45]

It does not appear that a single coagulation abnormality can be demonstrated to be the common cause for oozing.[43, 45] It has been indicated, however, that oozing is more frequently associated with multiple coagulation abnormalities.[45]

## METHODS AND MATERIALS

Analytically, 11 tests were employed to detect vascular and coagulation defects. These tests and their general relationship to the blood and tissue coagulation mechanisms are illustrated by the form used by the laboratory to report results (Fig. 1). It is useful to note that some measurements reflect defects in both vascular integrity and coagulation mechanism, and some measurements reflect defects in more than one phase of coagulation.

**Bleeding time.** The method of Ivy was used.[27] Normal was 1 to 5 minutes. Occasionally the method of Duke was employed.[19, 32] Normal was 1 to 3 minutes. Three millimeter lancets were used.*

**Tourniquet test.** The positive pressure method for 5 minutes was used[19, 27] (normal, no petechiae).

**Clotting time.** The clotting-time test was performed by a 3-tube Lee-White method.[22] Modifications were a 2-syringe technique, a 38° C. bath, and no saline in the syringes or tubes. Normal was 5 to 10 minutes for the third tube.

**Clot retraction.** Retraction in the clotting-time tubes was judged after 1 hour at 38° C. Retraction was graded "good" when the clot occupied one-half to two-thirds of the total volume,[25] "fair" for lesser degrees of retraction, and "poor" for no retraction. "Good" retraction was normal.

**Platelet smear.** A Wright-stained smear was examined under oil immersion (×970).[19, 27] Two per high power field (about 100 red blood cells per field) was adequate.

*Medi-Point Lancets, Brooklyn, New York.

BLOOD COAGULATION REPORT

Patient's Name: ______________________________ Date: __________

Ward: __________ Age: __________ Sex: __________ Time: __________

______________________________________________

______________________________________________

VASCULAR*

Bleeding Time: ______________________________ Normal: 1-5 min. (Ivy)
1-3 min. (Duke)

Tourniquet Test: ______________________________ Normal: No petechiae

PHASE I. BLOOD OR TISSUE THROMBOPLASTIN FORMATION

Prothrombin Consumption: ______________________________ Normal: 85-99%

Clotting Time (Lee-White 38° C.): ______________________________ Normal: 5-10 min. 3rd tube

Clot Retraction (1 hr. 38° C.): ☐ GOOD ☐ FAIR ☐ POOR

Platelet Smear: ______________________________ "Adequate": 2/HPF (100 RBC/HPF)

Factor V Corrects Proth. Act. to: ____________________ % of control

Factor VII Corrects Proth. Act. to: ____________________ % of control

Deficient: Corrects prothrombin activity more than halfway to 100%

PHASE II. THROMBIN FORMATION

Prothrombin Activity: Control: __________ secs. __________

Patient: __________ secs. = __________ % of control
Normal: 65-100%

PHASE III. FIBRIN FORMATION

Fibrinogen: ______________________________ Normal: 180-390 mg.%

Fibrinolysis (24 hrs. 38° C.): ______________________________ Negative: No lysis in 24 hrs.

*Some measurements reflect vascular structure and coagulation mechanism. Some measurements reflect more than one phase of coagulation.

**Fig. 1.** Blood coagulation report form.

**Prothrombin activity.** The Quick[32] method was used, but with 8 mm. inner diameter tubes. Simplastin* was the thromboplastin source, and Protrol† served as the control plasma. The per cent of control was obtained from a dilution curve supplied with the Simplastin. Normal was 65 to 100 per cent, which corresponds to about 3 seconds over control.[9, 16]

**Factor V deficiency.**[4, 5, 39] When the prothrombin activity was less than 65 per cent, the ability of factor V to correct the abnormality was determined by dilution of the plasma with prothrombin-free plasma (P.F.P.)‡ and determination of the prothrombin activity of the dilution (80 per cent P.F.P. and later 50 per cent P.F.P. dilution was used). Factor V deficiency is considered to be present when the abnormal prothrombin activity is corrected by the addition of P.F.P. (factor V) more than halfway toward 100 per cent from the uncorrected value.

**Factor VII deficiency.**[4, 39] When factor V correction of prothrombin activity was inadequate, the ability of factor VII to correct the abnormality was determined by dilution of plasma with normal serum§ (9 to 1), and determination of prothrombin activity of the dilution. Factor VII deficiency is considered to be present when abnormal prothrombin activity is corrected by the addition of serum (factor VII) more than halfway toward 100 per cent from the uncorrected value. (Note: Adequate correction by either factors V or VII implies a normal prothrombin content and a normal content of the other factor. Inadequate correction by both factors implies a deficiency in prothrombin, prothrombin plus factors V and/or VII, or in factors V plus VII).

**Prothrombin consumption.**[32, 41] Serum prothrombin activity was determined on serum from the clotting-time tubes after 1 hour at 38° C., but 0.1 ml. P.F.P. was blown into the Simplastin just before addition of the serum. The per cent prothrombin consumption equals 100 per cent less the per cent serum prothrombin activity. Normal was 85 to 99 per cent, which corresponds to serum prothrombin time of about 25 seconds or higher (Protrol, 11 to 12 seconds).

**Fibrinogen (method I).** The method up to the formation of the Biuret color is essentially that of Ratnoff and Menzie.[34] The color was developed by the addition of 4.0 ml. of saline, followed by 5.0 ml. of dilute biuret reagent,[44] and allowing the solution to stand 30 minutes in a 38° C. bath. Absorption was measured in a Coleman 14 spectrophotometer at 550 mu., and the fibrinogen concentration calculated on the basis of a bovine albumin* calibration curve. Normal was 180 to 390 mg. per cent.

**Fibrinogen (method II).** Later determinations were performed by a serial dilution method,[35] which was calibrated by the use of saline-diluted human plasma against method I. Titers of 32, 64, and 128 consistently corresponded to values of 100, 150, and over 200 mg. per cent fibrinogen. The use of freshly dissolved thrombin (in saline) was important in this range. Normal was a titer of 128 (tube 7) equal to over 200 mg. per cent.

**Fibrinolysis.** Fibrinolysis was detected by observation of the clotting-time tubes in a 38° C. bath for 24 hours[39] (negative, no lysis).

Clot lysis was adopted as the determination of choice for clinical purposes because fibrinolytic enzymes with activity insufficient to effect clot lysis are probably insignificant clinically as the cause of bleeding.[39] Therefore, the more elaborate methods for detection of profibrinolysin, fibrinolysin, antifibrinolysin, and other proteolytic enzymes were not employed.

**Blood volume.** Blood volumes were determined by $I^{131}$ and hematocrit.[36] Lowest normal red blood cell mass (R.C.M.) was considered to be 30 ml. per kilogram.

*Simplastin, Warner-Chilcott Laboratories, Morris Plains, N. J.

†Protrol, Knickerbocker Biologicals, New York, N. Y.

‡Prothrombin-Free Beef Plasma (P.F.P.), Hyland Laboratories, Los Angeles, Calif.

§Normal serum. Blood clotted 2 hours at 38° C., and serum separated and frozen in aliquots at –20° C.

*Pro-Sol, Standard Scientific, New York, N. Y. Vendor analysis for Kjeldahl nitrogen.

**Table I.** *Diagnostic classification of 143 patients with gastrointestinal bleeding*

| *Diagnosis* | *No. of patients* |
|---|---|
| *Benign Lesions* | |
| Duodenal ulcer | 50 |
| Gastric ulcer | 26 |
| Marginal ulcer | 3 |
| Hiatus hernia | 3 |
| Gastritis | 2 |
| Enteritis | 2 |
| Duodenal adenoma | 1 |
| Cholecystitis | 1 |
| Sigmoid diverticulosis | 2 |
| Colonic polyps | 2 |
| Colonic bleeding | 3 |
| Internal hemorrhoids | 1 |
| Bleeding site unknown | 14 |
| Total | 110 |
| *Malignant lesions* | |
| Carcinoma of stomach | 6 |
| Carcinoma of colon | 6 |
| Carcinoma of rectum | 7 |
| Total | 19 |
| *Associated hepatic disease* | |
| Cirrhosis | 10 |
| Metastatic carcinoma to liver | 3 |
| Hepatomegaly (cause undetermined) | 1 |
| Total | 14 |
| Three-Group total | 143 |

**Gastrointestinal hemorrhage.** Diagnostically, the patients with gastrointestinal hemorrhage were classified into 3 groups (Table I). These groups were composed of patients with (1) benign lesions, (2) malignant lesions, and (3) associated hepatic disease.

Laboratory estimation of blood volumes on 134 of the patients showed an average red blood cell mass (R.C.M.) of 16.4 ml. per kilogram, which represents a blood loss of 45 per cent of normal[18] (Table II). Sixty-two per cent of these patients had a red blood cell mass less than 18 ml. per kilogram, equivalent to an average blood loss of 40 per cent.

Blood transfusion, except in the hepatic disease group, was infrequent before coagulation studies were performed. Only 17 per cent of all the patients had received blood before analysis. The average transfusion was 1,600 ml., a quantity which is usually not considered detrimental to the coagulation processes.

The relative amounts of blood loss indicated in Table II for the 3 groups are the result of the methods employed for patient selection and might be different under other circumstances.

**Surgical oozing.** Twenty patients who bled excessively from small vessels during operation or the postoperative period were studied for coagulation or vascular defects (Table III). The bleeding was in all cases of the small-vessel oozing type and was considered excessive for the operation being performed. Descriptions of the oozing came from the surgeons involved and from the patients' charts. Although simultaneous large vessel bleeding did occur in some of the cases, troublesome excessive small vessel oozing was present in every case. All analytical work was carried out while the patient was experiencing the excessive oozing, but not always at the most critical period of the episode.

Table III is arranged in order of increasing blood transfusion received up to the time of analysis. The average amount of blood received was 5,600 ml. Ten of the patients received less than 5,000 ml. when coagulation studies were performed. Almost all of the patients received additional blood before the oozing episode was over, so that total amounts for the episodes are somewhat higher.

Oozing was first noted during operation in 13 of the 20 patients, and in the other 7 almost immediately postoperatively. Three analyses were performed while the operation was in progress, 9 the day of operation, and 4 each the first and second days postoperatively.

The oozing was controlled in 18 of the 20 patients within 1 day of the analytical work. Two patients continued oozing up until the time they died on the day of operation. They had been given apparently adequate blood replacement throughout. Three more patients died within 3 days of operation, but the oozing had been previously controlled. Of the 5 patients who did not survive, 4 had received over 10,000 ml. blood at the time of analysis.

In addition to the bank blood, fresh blood was administered to 6 patients (Patients 8, 11, 12, 14, 15, and 19), and fresh frozen plasma to 2 others (Patients 1 and 13). Vitamin K was given whenever abnormal prothrombin activities indicated the necessity. A multivitamin preparation (containing vitamin C) was routinely given all patients postoperatively.

## RESULTS

**Gastrointestinal hemorrhage.** The frequency of abnormal results of coagulation measurements among the 3 groups of patients with gastrointestinal bleeding is shown in Table IV. The 110 patients with benign lesions suffered only 5 per cent abnormal coagulation measurements, and the 19 patients with malignant lesions only 8 per cent.

The most frequently abnormal measurements in patients with benign lesions were prothrombin consumption (abnormal in 16 per cent), and prothrombin activity (abnormal in 12 per cent). In the patients with malignant lesions, the greatest number of abnormalities occurred in the same 2 measurements, but to a slightly greater extent. Prothrombin consumption was decreased in 22 per cent of the patients and prothrombin activity in 16 per cent.

It is apparent from Table IV that the bleeding patients who had associated hepatic disease showed considerably more abnormal measurements (22 per cent) than did the others. The 2 tests most frequently abnormal were the same ones as in the other 2 groups, but in reversed order—prothrombin activity (abnormal in 71 per cent), and prothrombin consumption (abnormal in 40 per cent).

Of the 10 patients with hepatic disease, the decreased prothrombin activities in at least 3 were due to factor V deficiency and in 1 to factor VII deficiency. Two of the abnormal prothrombin consumptions were caused by factor V deficiency (cirrhosis), and the other 2 were due to defects in non-specified phase I factors, antihemophilic globulin, plasma thromboplastic component, or others (metastatic hepatic carcinoma).

Examination of the available records of 85 of these patients was made to determine the presence of clinical shock at or immediately prior to the time of coagulation studies. Of 19 patients in shock, 8 (42 per cent) had 1 or more abnormal result of coagulation tests and 3 (16 per cent) had 2 or more abnormal results. Of 66 not in shock, 17 (26 per cent) had 1 or more abnormal test result and 7 (11 per cent) had 2 or more abnormalities. Prothrombin consumption was abnormal in 3 of 10 patients without obvious liver disease in shock in whom the test was performed, and in 2 of 22 similar patients not in shock.

**Surgical oozing.** The analytical data for the 20 patients who oozed abnormally during operation are shown in Table V. Only 1 patient displayed no coagulation disturbance whatever. A total of 189 measurements were performed on these 20 patients. Sixty (32 per cent) of the 189 values were abnormal.

Sixteen per cent of the measurements were abnormal in the group of 10 patients who received less than 5,000 ml. of blood, whereas 47 per cent of the measurements

**Table II.** *Evaluation of blood loss in patients with gastrointestinal bleeding*

| *Diagnostic group* | *No. of patients* | *Average R.C.M. (ml./Kg.)* | *% patients with R.C.M. < 18 ml./Kg.** | *% of patients transfused†* |
|---|---|---|---|---|
| Benign lesions | 110 | 15.2 | 67 | 15 |
| Associated hepatic disease | 14‡ | 18.5 | 60 | 50 |
| Malignant lesions | 19 | 21.7 | 32 | 11 |
| | Average | 16.4 | 62 | 17 |

*An 18 ml. per kilogram red blood cell mass (R.C.M.) represents R.C.M. loss of approximately 40 per cent.
†Average transfusion was 1,600 ml. These are transfusions given before analyses were performed.
‡Bleeding esophageal varices in 7.

**Table III.** *Clinical description of 20 patients with surgical oozing*

| *Patient No.* | *Sex* | *Age* | *Diagnosis* | *Operation* | *Blood received before analysis (ml.)** | *Oozing first noted* | *Time of analysis* | *Oozing controlled* |
|---|---|---|---|---|---|---|---|---|
| 1 | F | 50 | Obstructive jaundice | Cholecystostomy | None | Postoperatively | Postoperatively | 1 day postoperatively |
| 2 | F | 22 | Cirrhosis | Common bile duct exploration | 500 | At operation | At operation | At operation |
| 3 | M | 24 | Carcinoma, cecum | Laparotomy | 500 | At operation | Postoperatively | Postoperatively |
| 4 | F | 23 | Tuberculosis | Lobectomy | 2,000 | At operation | At operation | Postoperatively |
| 5 | M | 42 | Appendicitis | Appendectomy | 2,000 | Postoperatively | 2 days postoperatively | 2 days postoperatively |
| 6 | F | 58 | Gastric ulcer | Subtotal gastrectomy | 2,500 | At operation | 1 day postoperatively | 1 day postoperatively |
| 7 | F | 13 | Scoliosis | Spine fusion | 2,500 | At operation | Postoperatively | Postoperatively |
| 8 | F | 43 | Tuberculosis | Thoracoplasty | 4,000 | At operation | Postoperatively | 1 day postoperatively |
| 9 | M | 75 | Mesenteric thrombosis | Small bowel resection | 4,000 | Postoperatively | 2 days postoperatively | 2 days postoperatively |
| 10 | M | 34 | Pancreatitis | Cholecystectomy | 4,500 | Postoperatively | 1 day postoperatively | 1 day postoperatively, died 2 days postoperatively |
| 11 | F | 39 | Stomal ulcer | Subtotal gastrectomy | 5,000 | At operation | 2 days postoperatively | 3 days postoperatively |
| 12 | F | 55 | Tuberculosis | Pneumonectomy | 5,500 | Postoperatively | 1 day postoperatively | 1 day postoperatively |
| 13 | F | 24 | Peptic ulcer | Gastrectomy, repair hepatic vein laceration | 6,000 | At operation | At operation | 1 day postoperatively |
| 14 | M | 32 | Tuberculosis | Pneumonectomy | 8,000 | At operation | Postoperatively | Postoperatively |
| 15 | M | 72 | Carcinoma, pancreas | Pancreatectomy | 8,500 | Postoperatively | 1 day postoperatively | 1 day postoperatively |
| 16 | M | 20 | Cirrhosis | Portacaval shunt | 9,500 | At operation | 2 days postoperatively | 2 days postoperatively |
| 17 | M | 62 | Carcinoma, rectum | Attempted resection, colostomy | 11,000 | At operation | Postoperatively | Died postoperatively, still oozing |

**Table III**—*Cont'd*

| Patient No. | Sex | Age | Diagnosis | Operation | Blood received before analysis (ml.)* | Oozing first noted | Time of analysis | Oozing controlled |
|---|---|---|---|---|---|---|---|---|
| 18 | F | 51 | Cirrhosis | Portacaval shunt | 11,500 | At operation | Postoperatively | Died 3 days postoperatively, oozing |
| 19 | F | 43 | Ruptured aortic aneurysm | Resection, aneurysm | 12,000 | At operation | Postoperatively | Postoperatively, died |
| 20 | M | 35 | Pancreatitis | Pancreatectomy | 12,000 | Postoperatively | Postoperatively | 2 days postoperatively, died 3 days postoperatively |

*Most of the patients received additional blood before the end of the oozing episode.

**Table IV.** *Abnormal coagulation measurements in patients with gastrointestinal bleeding*

| Coagulation measurements | Benign lesions | | Malignant lesions | | Associated hepatic disease | |
|---|---|---|---|---|---|---|
| | No. of tests* | % of tests abnormal | No. of tests | % of tests abnormal | No. of tests | % of tests abnormal |
| *Vascular* | | | | | | |
| Bleeding time | 103 | 3 | 17 | 6 | 11 | 18 |
| Tourniquet test | 99 | 1 | 17 | 12 | 11 | 0 |
| *Phase I* | | | | | | |
| Prothrombin consumption | 52 | 16† | 9 | 22† | 10 | 40† |
| Clotting time | 110 | 4 | 19 | 0 | 14 | 7 |
| Clot retraction | 109 | 5 | 19 | 5 | 14 | 14 |
| Platelet smear | 53 | 4 | 9 | 11 | 11 | 18 |
| Factor V | 100 | 4 | 18 | 0 | 8 | 38 |
| Factor VII | 100 | 2 | 18 | 11 | 8 | 13 |
| *Phase II* | | | | | | |
| Prothrombin activity | 107 | 12† | 19 | 16† | 14 | 71† |
| *Phase III* | | | | | | |
| Fibrinogen | 50 | 6 | 6 | 0 | 11 | 27 |
| Fibrinolysis | 108 | 1 | 19 | 5 | 14 | 14 |
| Average | | 5 | | 8 | | 22 |

*Each patient was tested once only.

†Two most frequently abnormal tests in each group.

were abnormal in the 10 patients who received more than 5,000 ml. of blood. This represents a significant increase in the number of abnormal measurements with increasing blood loss.

The distribution of the 60 abnormal values among the 11 determinations is summarized in Table VI.

Prothrombin activity, abnormal in the greatest number of patients with oozing (65 per cent), is followed by prothrombin consumption (55 per cent), bleeding time (50 per cent), and clot retraction (45 per cent). The other 7 values were abnormal in a smaller number of patients. They ranged from factor V (38 per cent) and fibrinogen (25 per cent) to tourniquet test (22 per cent), platelet smear (15 per cent), clotting time and fibrinolysis (10 per cent each), and finally factor VII (8 per cent).

**Table V.** *Occurrence of abnormal coagulation measurements in patients with surgical oozing*

| | *Vascular* | | *Phase I* | | |
|---|---|---|---|---|---|
| *Patient No.* | *Bleeding time (min.)** | *Tourniquet test†* | *Prothrombin consumption (%)* | *Clotting time, 3rd tube (min.)* | *Clot retraction* |
| 1 | — | — | 53§ | 10:00 | Good |
| 2 | — | — | 90 | 9:00 | Good |
| 3 | 3:30 | Negative | over 90 | 6:00 | Good |
| 4 | — | — | 89 | 6:00 | Good |
| 5 | over 10:00§ | Negative | over 90 | 8:00 | Good |
| 6 | 2:30 | Negative | over 90 | 5:00 | Fair§ |
| 7 | 8:00§ | Negative | 87 | 3:30 | Good |
| 8 | — | — | 89 | 6:00 | Good |
| 9 | over 15:00§ | Negative | 88 | 8:00 | Good |
| 10 | 4:00 | — | 82§ | 6:00 | Fair§ |
| 11 | 13:00§ | Positive§ | 72§ | 9:30 | Good |
| 12 | 9:00§ | Negative | 79§ | 8:30 | Fair§ |
| 13 | 4:00 | — | 64§ | 11:00§ | Poor§ |
| 14 | over 10:00§ | Negative | 80§ | 29:00§ | Poor§ |
| 15 | 3:00 | — | 37§ | 7:00 | Fair§ |
| 16 | 4:00 | — | 80§ | 6:30 | Fair§ |
| 17 | — | — | 79§ | 9:00 | Good |
| 18 | 6:00§ | — | 74§ | 6:00 | Fair§ |
| 19 | — | — | 66§ | 7:30 | Good |
| 20 | 5:00 | Positive§ | over 90 | 7:30 | Poor§ |

*Duke method for Patients 10, 13, 18.

†Ten petechiae (Patient 11), and 30 petechiae (Patient 20) in area of dime in antecubital fossa.

‡Rosenberg method for Patients 5, 7, 9, 11, 13, 14, 18, 20.

§Abnormal values. Sixty out of 189 (32 per cent).

## COMMENT

The severity of the abnormal values in the patients with gastrointestinal bleeding extended from very mild to severe, with no particular pattern obvious. There was no correlation with severity of hemorrhage or diagnosis. Values for the 2 most frequently abnormal determinations are illustrative. Abnormal prothrombin consumptions, with the exception of one 39 per cent value, ranged from 70 to 84 per cent (average 77 per cent). Abnormal prothrombin activities ranged from 10 to 64 per cent (average 43 per cent).

One-half of the decreased prothrombin consumptions in the patients with gastrointestinal bleeding were due to defects in unspecified phase I factors, and the remainder were caused in equal numbers by platelet and factor V deficiency.

The specific causes for decreased prothrombin activities in these patients cannot be evaluated precisely because of incomplete data concerning factors V and VII. However, the available measurements indicate that deficiencies in factor V or VII are at least as frequent a cause for decreased prothrombin activities as is prothrombin deficiency.

It seems justifiable to conclude that there is no representative or serious coagulation defect which aggravates bleeding in the usual patient with gastrointestinal hemorrhage without significant liver disease or obvious hemorrhagic diathesis. There is no clinical evidence that coagulation was impaired in this group of patients.

The data on the patients with hepatic disease agree with the known high incidence of abnormal coagulation in patients of this type. It is possible that many of the patients studied bled unusually severely because of the coagulation abnormality present.

Our data indicate that there are 2 measurements, prothrombin activity and prothrombin consumption, which gave abnormal

| | | | *Phase II* | *Phase III* | |
|---|---|---|---|---|---|
| *Platelet smear* | *Factor V deficiency* | *Factor VII deficiency* | *Prothrombin activity (%)* | *Fibrinogen (mg. %)‡* | *Fibrinolysis* |
| Adequate | No | No | 100 | 397 | Negative |
| Adequate | No | No | 70 | 356 | Negative |
| Adequate | Yes§ | No | 59§ | 468 | Negative |
| Adequate | No | No | 85 | 298 | Clot lysis 24 hr.§ |
| Adequate | — | — | 57§ | over 200 | Negative |
| Adequate | No | No | 78 | 498 | Negative |
| Adequate | No | No | 72 | over 200 | Negative |
| Adequate | No | Yes§ | 59§ | 274 | Negative |
| Adequate | Yes§ | No | 59§ | over 200 | Negative |
| Adequate | — | — | 53§ | 288 | Negative |
| Adequate | — | — | 55§ | over 200 | Negative |
| Adequate | Yes§ | No | 57§ | 150§ | Negative |
| Adequate | Yes§ | No | 27§ | 150§ | Negative |
| Adequate | — | — | 23§ | over 200 | Negative |
| Less than 1/h.p.f.§ | No | No | 79 | 248 | Negative |
| None on smear§ | No | No | 68 | 302 | Negative |
| Adequate | — | — | 39§ | 164§ | Clot lysis 90 min.§ |
| None on smear§ | — | — | 53§ | 150§ | Negative |
| Adequate | Yes§ | No | 35§ | 151§ | Negative |
| Adequate | — | — | 10§ | over 200 | Negative |

results more often than any other tests in the patients studied. These 2 tests appear to be the most useful ones for screening patients with gastrointestinal bleeding for possible coagulation defects.

Abnormalities in coagulation may be more frequent in patients in shock than in those who do not exhibit signs of clinical shock. Studies of hemorrhagic shock in animals suggest that early in shock (first hour) coagulation is accelerated but that as shock continues deficiencies in coagulation occur.[37, 42]

The existence of a large number of abnormal values in the patients with oozing lends strong support to the belief that coagulation difficulties are the important element in the oozing phenomenon. The severity of the abnormalities extends over a wide range, from seemingly mild to severe. The severely abnormal values could be suspected of contributing to the oozing. It is also conceivable that some of the milder aberrations may render coagulability ineffective to prevent hemorrhage in cases of extensive surgical procedures. In the case of fibrinogen it has been suggested that levels of approximately 150 mg. per cent are not adequate to control the bleeding in patients with surgical oozing.[31]

It would be useful to know if the coagulation defects seen in the oozing patients are present at the start of oozing or if they appear later as a result of increasing blood loss or transfusions. The fact that there are more abnormal measurements in the patients with the greatest amount of transfusion does not unequivocally answer this question. Only by more frequent analytical determinations on each patient could the time of onset of coagulation disturbance be determined.

Several of the values are abnormal in a large number of patients, and these can be considered as the most useful tests for patients with surgical oozing. However, it is important to ponder that even the most frequently abnormal determination, prothrombin activity, is within normal limits in 7 of 20 patients

**Table VI.** *Distribution of individual abnormal coagulation values in patients with surgical oozing*

| *Coagulation measurements (20 patients)* | *No. of tests** | *% of tests abnormal* |
|---|---|---|
| *Vascular* | | |
| Bleeding time | 14 | 50 |
| Tourniquet test | 9 | 22 |
| *Phase I* | | |
| Prothrombin consumption | 20 | 55 |
| Clotting time | 20 | 10 |
| Clot retraction | 20 | 45 |
| Platelet smear | 20 | 15 |
| Factor V deficiency | 13 | 38 |
| Factor VII deficiency | 13 | 8 |
| *Phase II* | | |
| Prothrombin activity | 20 | 65 |
| *Phase III* | | |
| Fibrinogen | 20 | 25 |
| Fibrinolysis | 20 | 10 |

*Each patient was tested once only.

**Table VII.** *The interpretation of abnormal coagulation values as specific coagulation defects in patients with surgical oozing*

| *Coagulation defects (20 patients)* | *No. of patients tested* | *% of patients with defects* |
|---|---|---|
| 1. Vascular | 14 | 50 |
| 2. Clot retraction (unknown cause) | 20 | 25 |
| 3. Antihemophilic globulin, plasma thromboplastic component, or others in phase I | 20 | 25 |
| 4. Platelets | 20 | 15 |
| 5. Factor V | 13 | 38 |
| 6. Factor VII | 13 | 8 |
| 7. Prothrombin or combined prothrombin factors | 20 | 35 |
| 8. Fibrinogen | 20 | 20 |
| 9. Fibrinolysis | 20 | 10 |

with oozing (35 per cent). Thus, there is no single abnormal measurement which is characteristic of the 20 patients with surgical oozing.

A consideration of abnormal measurements without an understanding of the causative defects has only limited value. It is a knowledge of the underlying defect which has etiological and therapeutic importance. The 60 abnormal coagulation measurements found in the patients with surgical oozing (Tables V and VI) have been interpreted in terms of 9 coagulation defects (Table VII). Interpretations are made within the limitations imposed by an analytical scheme of limited scope, and by current knowledge of the coagulation mechanism:

1. Vascular defect: Abnormal bleeding time or tourniquet test not related to platelet deficiency.
2. Clot retraction defect (unknown cause): Impaired clot retraction not due to platelet deficiency or elevated fibrinogen level.
3. Defect in antihemophilic globulin, plasma thromboplastic component, or others in phase I: Insufficient prothrombin consumption or prolonged clotting time, but adequate platelets and normal factor V.
4. Platelet defect.
5. Factor V defect.
6. Factor VII defect.
7. Prothrombin or combined prothrombin factors defect: Decreased prothrombin activity not correctable by prothrombin-free plasma or normal serum. The defect may be in prothrombin, in prothrombin plus factors V and/or VII, or in factors V plus VII.
8. Fibrinogen defect: Not due to demonstrable fibrinolysis. Elevated levels are not considered a defect.
9. Fibrinolysis defect.

Defects found in the greatest number of patients were the vascular defect, the factor V defect, and the prothrombin or combined prothrombin factors defect. Defects in the vascular component have not been cited previously as occurring in a significant number of cases of oozing during operation. This experience emphasizes the necessity of considering this factor. The other 6 defects are of less importance to the group as a whole, although in individual cases they may have been the chief cause of oozing. The inability to demonstrate rapid clot lysis in all but 1 instance should, according to Stefanini and Dameshek,[39] eliminate fibrinolysis as a major defect causing bleeding at the time of the analyses in this group of cases. However, fibrinolysis has been characterized as being rapidly transitory[45] and may have been missed in some of the patients. Four patients who were shown to have low fibrinogen levels (about 150 mg. per cent) suggest this possibility. Fibrinolysis has been considered to be significant in some previous studies, although more recently it has not been given as much emphasis.

The single most frequently occurring defect, the vascular defect, is not present in 7 out of 14 patients with oozing (50 per cent), which indicates that there is no single coagulation defect which is characteristically present in these 20 patients with surgical oozing. Lack of a characteristic defect (or measurement) emphasizes the importance of detailed coagulation study of individual patients.

Occurrence of multiple coagulation defects (2 or more defects being considered multiple) is summarized in Table VIII. A positive correlation of multiple defects with clinical oozing has been made previously.[45] However, the occurrence of multiple coagulation defects is not characteristic of these 20 patients with oozing since 9 of them (45 per cent) have single defects or no defects.

Occurrence of multiple coagulation abnormalities in these patients serves to emphasize the usefulness of fresh whole blood and fresh frozen plasma in therapy. When laboratory facilities are unavailable, fresh blood or plasma is indicated because they contain most of the necessary coagulation factors. Often the usual tests show multiple abnormalities with no single striking defect, and again fresh blood or plasma is most important.

**Table VIII.** *Occurrence of multiple* coagulation defects in patients with surgical oozing*

| *No. of defects per patient* | *No. of patients* |
|---|---|
| None | 2† |
| 1 | 7 |
| 2 | 3 |
| 3 | 6 |
| 4 | 2 |

*Two or more defects were considered multiple.

†Patients 2 and 6. The fair clot retraction in Patient 6 is considered to be a reflection of the elevated fibrinogen level.

## SUMMARY

1. The coagulation mechanism of 163 patients with surgical bleeding was studied by means of 11 tests which reflect vascular integrity and all phases of blood coagulation.

2. In 143 patients with gastrointestinal bleeding the hemorrhage had resulted in an average estimated blood loss of 45 per cent of normal red blood cell mass. Patients with benign lesions had very few coagulation abnormalities, and patients with malignant lesions had only slightly more abnormal measurements. However, hepatic disease was associated with major coagulation disturbances. Two of the 11 tests, prothrombin activity and prothrombin consumption, were most frequently abnormal. They are the most useful for screening patients with gastrointestinal bleeding for coagulation defects.

3. Twenty patients were surgical patients who oozed excessively during operation or immediately thereafter. A high percentage of the coagulation measurements (32 per cent) during these bleeding episodes were abnormal. Those most frequently abnormal were prothrombin activity (abnormal in 65 per cent of patients), prothrombin consumption (abnormal in 55 per cent), and bleeding time (abnormal in 50 per cent). These are the most useful tests for the etiological diagnosis of patients with surgical oozing.

4. When the abnormal coagulation measurements were interpreted in terms of more specific coagulation defects, those most frequently present were a vascular defect, a factor V defect, and a defect in prothrombin or combined prothrombin factors. These defects were those most likely related to the oozing in the 20 patients.

5. Despite the large number of abnormal measurements and coagulation defects found in the patients with surgical oozing, there was no single one which was characteristic. The presence of multiple defects, present in 55 per cent of the patients, was likewise not characteristic. The need for assay of coagulation factors of individual patients is therefore indicated. Therapeutic use of fresh blood or plasma, because they contain most of the necessary constituents for coagulation, is also emphasized.

**REFERENCES**


1. Aggeler, P. M., and Lucia, S. P.: Hemorrhagic disorders, Chicago, 1949, Chicago Press.
2. Austurheim, K.: Some peculiar clinical pictures in metastasizing carcinoma of the stomach, Acta med. scandinav. **155:** 185, 1956.
3. Biben, R. L., and Tynan, M. L.: Hemorrhagic diathesis in carcinoma of the stomach. A case report, Ann. Int. Med. **49:** 917, 1958.
4. Biggs, R., and MacFarlane, R. G.: Human blood coagulation, Oxford, 1957, Blackwell Scientific Publications.
5. Brinkhous, K. M.: Hemophilia and hemophilioid diseases, Chapel Hill, 1957, University of North Carolina Press, p. 81.
6. Chalmers, T. C., Bigelow, F. S., and Desforges, J. F.: The effects of massive gastrointestinal hemorrhage on hemostasis. II. Coagulation factors, J. Lab. & Clin. Med. **43:** 511, 1954.
7. Cliffton, E. E., Grossi, C., and Siegel, M.: Hemorrhage during and after operation secondary to changes in the clotting mechanism: physiology and methods of control, SURGERY **40:** 37, 1956.
8. Coon, W. W., and Hodgson, P. E.: Fibrinolysis in surgery patients. I. Possible relationship to a hemorrhagic diathesis, Surg. Gynec. & Obst. **95:** 717, 1952.
9. DeGruchy, G. C.: Clinical hematology in medical practice, Springfield, Ill., 1958, Charles C Thomas, Publisher.
10. Desforges, J. F., Bigelow, F. S., and Chalmers, T. C.: The effects of massive gastrointestinal hemorrhage on hemostasis. I. The blood platelets, J. Lab. & Clin. Med. **43:** 501, 1954.
11. Frick, P. G.: Acute hemorrhagic syndrome with hypofibrinogenemia in metastatic cancer, Acta haemat. **16:** 11, 1956.
12. Friesen, S. R., Harsha, W. N., and McCroskey, C. H.: Massive generalized wound bleeding during operation with clinical and experimental evidence of blood transfusion reactions, SURGERY **32:** 3, 1952.
13. Friesen, S. R., and Nelson, R. M.: The occurrence of massive generalized wound bleeding during operation, Am. Surgeon **17:** 609, 1951.
14. Gollub, S., Winchell, H. S., Ehrlich, E., and Ulin, A.: Thrombocytopenia in massive transfusion, SURGERY **45:** 366, 1959.
15. Harrington, W. J., Manheim, R. H., Desforges, J. F., Minkel, H. P., Crow, C. B., and Stohlman, F.: The bleeding tendency in hepato-cellular and obstructive jaundice, Bull. New England M. Center **12:** 121, 1950.
16. Howland, W. S.: Cardiovascular and clotting disturbances during massive blood replacement, Anesthesiology **19:** 140, 1958.
17. Howland, W. S., Schweizer, O., Boyan, C. P., and Dotta, A. C.: Physiologic alterations with massive blood replacement, Surg. Gynec. & Obst. **101:** 478, 1955.
18. Karlson, K. E., Enquist, I. F., Dennis, C., and Fierst, S.: Results of three methods of therapy for massive gastroduodenal hemorrhage, Ann. Surg. **148:** 594, 1958.
19. Kracke, R. R., and Parker, F. P.: Textbook of clinical pathology, Baltimore, 1940, William Wood & Company.
20. Krevans, J. R., and Jackson, D. P.: Hemorrhagic disorder following massive whole blood transfusions, J. A. M. A. **159:** 171, 1955.
21. Kwaan, H. C., McFadyean, A. C. S., and Cook, J.: Plasma fibrinolytic activity in cirrhosis of the liver, Lancet **270:** 132, 1956.
22. Lee, R. I., and White, P. D.: A clinical study of the coagulation time of blood, Am. J. M. Sc. **145:** 495, 1913.
23. LeVeen, H. H., Mulder, A. G., and Prokup, F.: The physiological mechanism for death in massively bleeding peptic ulcer, Surg. Gynec. & Obst. **94:** 433, 1952.
24. Lincoln, A. F., Moorman, J. A., and Schultz, R. L.: Fibrinolysis following thoracic surgery, Surg. Gynec. & Obst. **105:** 541, 1957.
25. MacFarlane, R. G.: A simple method for measuring clot retraction, Lancet **1:** 1199, 1939.
26. McCroskey, C. H., and Friesen, S. R.: Hemorrhagic transfusion reactions, J. Kansas M. Soc. **53:** 1, 1952.
27. Miller, S. E.: Textbook of clinical pathology, Baltimore, 1955, Williams & Wilkins Company.
28. Mindrum, G., and Glueck, H. I.: Plasma prothrombin in liver disease: its clinical and prognostic significance, Ann. Int. Med. **50:** 1370, 1959.
29. Ofstad, A. J.: Blodets protrombininnhold ved akutt gastrointestinalblødning, Nord. med. **60:** 1754, 1958.
30. Owren, P. A.: The diagnostic and prognostic significance of plasma prothrombin and factor V levels in parenchymatous hepatitis and obstructive jaundice, Scandinav. J. Clin. & Lab. Invest. **1:** 131, 1949.
31. Phillips, L. L., Rowley, P. T., and Habif, D. V.: Hypofibrinogenemia in surgical patients, Surg. Gynec. & Obst. **103:** 443, 1956.
32. Quick, A. J.: The physiology and pathology of hemostasis, Philadelphia, 1951, Lea & Febiger.
33. Rapaport, S. I., and Goodman, J. R.: Clotting factor abnormalities in chronic liver disease, Mil. Med. **121:** 251, 1957.

34. Ratnoff, O. D., and Menzie, C.: A new method for the determination of fibrinogen in small samples of plasma, J. Lab. & Clin. Med. **37:** 316, 1951.
35. Rosenberg, A. A.: Plasma fibrinogen determination. A rapid titration method, Clin. Chem. **2:** 331, 1956.
36. Senn, L. Y., and Karlson, K. E.: Methodologic and actual error of plasma volume determinations, SURGERY **44:** 1095, 1958.
37. Smith, J. J., Hartwick, J. P., and Regan, M. J.: Coagulation mechanism in hemorrhagic shock, Fed. Proc. **16:** 120, 1957.
38. Stefanini, M.: The hemorrhagic diathesis of liver dysfunction and obstructive jaundice, Intern. Soc. Hemat., 3rd Internat. Cong. Cambridge, 1950, p. 484.
39. Stefanini, M., and Dameshek, W.: The hemorrhagic disorders, New York, 1955, Grune & Stratton, Inc.
40. Stefanini, M., Mednicoff, J. B., Solomon, L., and Campbell, E. W.: Thrombocytopenia of replacement transfusion. A cause of surgical bleeding, Clin. Res. Proc. **2:** 61, 1954.
41. Sussman, L. N., Cohen, I. B., and Gittler, R.: Clinical application of simplified serum prothrombin consumption test, J. A. M. A. **156:** 702, 1954.
42. Turpini, R., and Stefanini, M.: The nature and mechanism of the hemostatic breakdown in the course of experimental hemorrhagic shock, J. Clin. Invest. **38:** 53, 1959.
43. Ulin, A. W., Gollub, S. W., Winchell, H. S., and Ehrlich, E. W.: Hemorrhage and massive transfusion, J. A. M. A. **168:** 1971, 1958.
44. Weichselbaum, T. E.: An accurate and rapid method for the determination of proteins in small amounts of blood serum and plasma, Am. J. Clin. Path. **16:** 40, 1946.
45. Zucker, M. B., Siegel, M., Cliffton, E. E., Bellville, J. W., Howland, W. S., and Grossi, C. E.: Generalized excessive oozing in patients undergoing major surgery and receiving multiple blood transfusions, J. Lab. & Clin. Med. **50:** 849, 1957.

# Evaluation of the dissolution effect of fibrinolysin (plasmin) on induced vascular microthrombi

W. H. LEE, JR., M.D.
R. R. BRADHAM, M.D.
B. THREAT, B.A.
C. DAVENPORT, B.A.
LOS ANGELES, CALIF., AND CHARLESTON, S. C.
*From the Departments of Surgery, University of California Medical Center and the Medical College of South Carolina*

The development of a relatively purified, standardized preparation of human fibrinolysin† has caused a recent flurry of investigation, notably clinical and laboratory evaluation of the efficacy of this material in dissolving clots. The results of these investigations at the time of this writing are conflicting. Some of the reasons for the conflict in data concerning the assessment of fibrinolysin are apparent upon review of the available literature.

One problem has been the variance in the experimental methods of producing a clot in vivo. Some methods produced trauma to vascular endothelium and would theoretically perpetuate the tendency for thrombosis. Examples of these methods are the injection of chemical irritants into a vein, production of thrombosis by the passage of an electrical current through the wall of a vessel, direct crushing of a vessel between hemostats, and so forth. Other methods which have been used to stimulate thrombosis did not produce obvious trauma to the endothelium. Examples of these methods include the injection of thrombin into an isolated segment of vein and the production of complete stasis in a segment of vein by temporary "atraumatic" ligatures. Methods which produce venous thrombosis without overt trauma to the vascular endothelium may be analogous to clinical studies concerning phlebothrombosis, whereas methods which do produce trauma to the vascular endothelium may be more analogous to the clinical investigation of thrombophlebitis. The difficulty of evaluating the degree of inflammatory element in clinical venous thrombosis is a possible cause of the conflict in data from clinical studies regarding the evaluation of fibrinolysin therapy.

A second factor in the conflict of available data has been the tendency for investigators to utilize an indirect approach in attempting to measure the ability of fibrinolysin to dissolve a clot in vivo. Suggestive evidence, however strong, lacks definitive demonstration of clot dissolution in the living organism.

A third factor has been a considerable variance in the dosage of drugs employed, and the apparent difference in activity of 2 different commercially available preparations of fibrinolysin.[5] A fourth variable frequently controlled inadequately (as to dosage and individual tolerance) has been the concomitant use of anticoagulants (heparin).

A previous report[1] attempted to assess the efficacy of one preparation of fibrinolysin* by a method which employed a "trau-

Supported by training grants Nos. HTS-5337 and HTS-5337 (C2), National Institutes of Health.

Received for publication Dec. 19, 1960.

†All fibrinolysin used in this study was supplied by the Ortho Research Foundation, Raritan, N. J.

*Actase, fibrinolysin supplied by Ortho Research Foundation, Raritan, N. J.

matic" but standard venous clotting technique and evaluation of the result by direct observation of the clot. However, the experimental control in this series of experiments depended upon the use of the contralateral femoral vein in the dog as the "control" to establish evidence of thrombosis. In addition, the possibility of partial dissolution of clots with occult embolization into the systemic venous circulation (simulating clot lysis) could not be assessed. The present study was therefore undertaken in order to evaluate directly the ability of fibrinolysin to dissolve an arterial microthrombus in vivo, with control of the experimental variables mentioned.

## METHOD

Microscopic observations were made in vivo on the effect of fibrinolysin on thrombosis produced in small mesenteric vessels (50 to 100 μ in diameter) of dogs. Mongrel dogs which weighed from 10 to 15 kilograms, were anesthetized intravenously with pentobarbital sodium and subjected to a midline laparotomy. A loop of small bowel with its mesentery was gently brought out and suspended over a porthole in a paraffinized balsa sheet mounted in a hood over the animal's abdomen (Fig. 1). The tissue was continuously moistened with sterile isotonic saline solution at room temperature, and the mesentery was transilluminated with a Knisely quartz-rod apparatus.[3] Observations of the circulation were then made in vivo with a standard binocular dissecting microscope mounted appropriately on a heavy floor stand. Good resolution up to 90 diameters magnification was possible with this instrument.

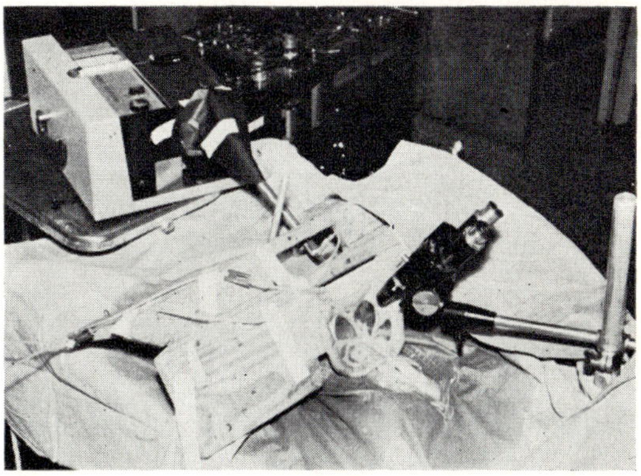

**Fig. 1.** The transillumination apparatus can be simple. Light source here is a standard 500 w. slide projector, and all other parts except the quartz rod are standard laboratory equipment. A later model is more compact, sophisticated, and expensive.

**Series 1.** In a group of 5 dogs, thrombosis was produced in the selected segments of artery and vein by application of a copper microelectrode to the vessels which delivered a 12 v. direct current over a 2- to 5-second period. Duration of the current was determined by the interval necessary to produce complete stasis and agglutination of the blood in the vessel segment. A localized thrombus was uniformly produced without visible microscopic evidence of tissue injury, except a slight degree of turbidity in the alveolar tissue adjacent to the vessels. Fibrinolysin was infused intravenously over a 1-hour period in doses varying from 50,000 to 250,000 units* in 250 ml. of isotonic saline solution. Observations were continued for 3 hours after the infusion was completed.

**Series 2.** Thrombosis was produced as in the first series. A control solution of 250 ml. of isotonic saline was directly perfused into a branch of the mesenteric artery (by cannulation) supplying the clotted segment over a 2-hour period in 10 dogs.

**Series 3.** In 11 dogs thrombosis was produced as in Series 1. Doses of fibrinolysin which varied from 300,000 to 1 million units in 250 ml. of 5 per cent dextrose in distilled water were directly perfused into the mesenteric artery branch supplying the thrombosed segment as before. Observations were continued for 3 hours after the perfusion.

**Series 4.** In 5 dogs no electrical current was used. Thrombosis was produced by injection of a suspension of ground, preformed clot through the intra-arterial cannula into the mesenteric artery vasculature. A clot was formed by withdrawing 2 ml. of blood from the dog and allowing it to clot

*Units as defined by the Ortho Pharmaceutical Corporation for the Actase preparation.

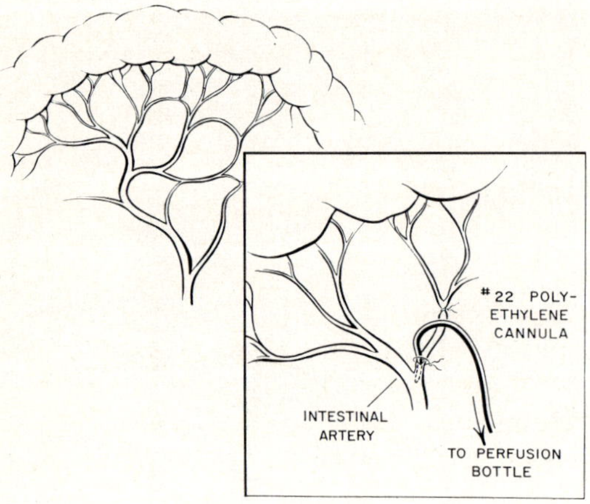


**Fig. 2.** The arterial branch was cannulated through a side limb of a bifurcation to avoid occlusion of the blood flow to the area under study.

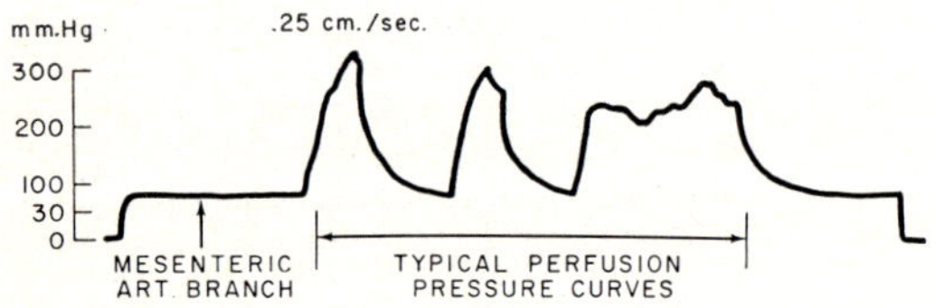


**Fig. 3.** Pressure of perfusion was intermittent. Each cycle lasted 5 to 6 seconds, and reached a peak of approximately 300 mm. Hg.

in a test tube, then adding 3 ml. of isotonic saline solution to the clot and mixing this vigorously with a blunt glass rod. The fragmented, suspended clot was infused through a 22 gauge polyethylene cannula at a transient perfusion pressure of approximately 325 mm. Hg into one proximal limb of a bifurcation of an intestinal artery (Fig. 2). This invariably produced embolization of the other limb of the bifurcation. The route of the embolus was charted by adding 1 to 2 drops of fluorescein to the clot suspension. After the production of thrombosis in this fashion, a control solution of 200 ml. of sterile isotonic saline was perfused into the arterial cannula by intermittent positive pressure ranging from 75 to 300 mm. Hg with a mean perfusion pressure of 160 mm. Hg (Fig. 3). After this control perfusion into the thrombosed area, a solution of 250 ml. of 5 per cent dextrose in water containing 300,000 units of fibrinolysin was perfused into the thrombosed segments of the vessels at a similar perfusion pressure. Three of the 5 dogs were heparinized by the intravenous administration of 3 mg. per kilogram of heparin sodium as the perfusion was begun.

## RESULTS

There was no dissolution of the thrombi in the 5 dogs which received fibrinolysin intravenously in Series 1.

Neither was there any dissolution or flushing of the thrombi produced by electrical current in the dogs which received saline control perfusions intra-arterially in Series 2.

An interesting sequence of events followed the initiation of thrombosis and subsequent intra-arterial infusion of fibrinolysin in 8 of the 11 dogs of Series 3. The electrical stimulus produced complete agglutination of the blood in the vessels, which, prior to perfusion, was quickly replaced by a very sluggish flow of red blood cell aggregates (10 to 50 $\mu$ in diameter) and white clear aggregates believed to be composed of platelets and/or fibrin. These aggregates flowed in a progressively sluggish fashion over approximately a 10-minute period, and then were again replaced by complete agglutination and apparent thrombosis. The subsequent infusion of fibrinolysin resulted in alternate cycles of (1) incomplete dissolution, (2) complete agglutination, and then (3) partial dissolution, and so forth, with the red blood cell and white aggregates breaking off and flowing away from the agglutinated segmental masses. A sluggish flow in the thrombosed vessel would resume, only to be followed again by agglutination. When the fibrinolysin infusion was completed, thrombosis recurred within 15 to 30 minutes and was persistent. Heparinization of 4 dogs in this series during perfusion produced no apparent change in the sequence or ultimate result. In the remaining 3 dogs, there was no demonstrable change in the clotted segment.

In dogs of Series 4, in which thrombosis was initiated with preformed, injected clots to produce an experimental situation in which, theoretically, there was minimal or no vascular endothelial damage, the saline pressure perfusion failed to flush the thrombosed segments or to dissolve the clots. The fibrinolysin pressure perfusion resulted in the same sequence of events that was described for the 8 dogs of Series 3. Partial dissolution of the thrombi was apparently obtained, with flushing of agglutinated masses out of the larger vessels (from 100 $\mu$ up), but many smaller arterioles and venules in a range of size from 15 to 30 $\mu$ remained persistently clotted during the perfusion. The final picture after the perfusion was one of ultimate thrombosis, despite intravenous heparinization of 3 dogs with 3 mg. per kilogram of heparin sodium during the fibrinolysin perfusion.

## DISCUSSION

In order for fibrinolysin to effectively dissolve thrombi in a living organism, 3 factors seem prerequisite. First, the material must possess a sufficiently potent fibrinolytic activity to dissolve the clot before it is itself destroyed by antifibrinolytic materials circulating in the blood of the living organism. Second, the fibrinolytic agent must be placed into the circulation of the organism in such a fashion that it is able to reach the clotted vessel segment and obtain a sufficient concentration in the plasmic fluid which bathes the clot and its fibrin framework. It seems from this that only vessels large enough to possess vasa vasorum could be treated by fibrinolytic dissolution of the thrombi. However, ancillary experiments in this laboratory have demonstrated that the material perfused as in Series 3 and Series 4 reached the interior of the lumens of thrombosed vessels as evidenced by the rapid appearance of perfused fluorescein shown by transilluminated ultraviolet light inside the vessels. Third, effective dissolution of the thrombus should be considered complete dissolution of the thrombus. For example, if a venous thrombus is softened and partially fragmented, it may be swept away from the vessel which it occludes and continue in the systemic venous circulation as unsuspected multiple smaller emboli which may or may not lodge in vessels of circulatory importance, depending upon the size of the clot fragments. In an artery, however, should a clot be incompletely dissolved, the fragments would be swept downstream into a progressively narrowing truncated cone (for such is the physical nature of the shape of arterial vessels[4]), and ultimately occlude many smaller branches of the arteriolar or capillary circulation, depending upon the size of the fragments.

The development of available fibrinolysin preparations represents a significant step toward a successful chemotherapeutic attack upon acute vascular thromboembolic disease. However, the clinical application of this chemotherapeutic concept is limited at the present time by the relative impurity or impotency of the fibrinolysin preparation. A possible exception is the use of fibrinolysin preparation as a chemotherapeutic adjunct to some primarily surgical therapeutic measure, such as arterial thrombectomy with fibrinolysin flushing, or removal of peripheral emboli by retrograde flushing procedures such as have been previously described by Crawford.[2] It is possible and, indeed, probable that the efficiency of such a flush procedure may well be enhanced by the employment of fibrinolysin in the irrigant fluid.

## SUMMARY AND CONCLUSIONS

From the experiments presented and the data available in the literature, the authors have concluded that the fibrinolysin preparation used in these experiments does possess fibrinolytic activity in vivo. This activity, however, is insufficient to dissolve experimental thrombi completely, and in experimental animals venous clots are apparently softened or partially fragmented[1] and swept off in the systemic circulation in the form of multiple emboli, either in liver or lung, depending upon the experimental conditions. (The latter hypothesis is unproved.) In the case of arterial thrombi, the clot is apparently softened and partially lysed, and is swept forward to embolize arteriolar or capillary beds distal to the thrombosed segment. A progressive stasis of blood flow in the total vascular beds supplied by the thrombosed vessel occurs until a point of complete stasis in the vascular bed supplied by this vessel is reached. This ultimately results in recurrent and persistent thrombosis after the perfusion of fibrinolysin.

## REFERENCES


1. Bradham, R. R., and Lee, W. H., Jr.: Dissolution effect of human fibrinolysin on preformed venous thrombi in dogs, Surg. Gynec. & Obst. **112:** 295, 1961.
2. Crawford, E. S., and De Bakey, M. E.: The retrograde flush procedure in embolectomy and thrombectomy, SURGERY **40:** 737, 1956.
3. Knisely, M. H.: An improved fused quartz-rod living tissue illuminator, Anat. Rec. **71:** 503, 1938.
4. Knisely, M. H., Block, E. H., Eliot, T. S., and Warner, L.: Sludged blood, Science **106:** 431, 1947.
5. Wilson, J. S.: Fibrinolysin treatment of induced venous thrombosis in the dog, SURGERY **48:** 469, 1960.

# An attempt at development of agammaglobulinemia in adult rats by treatment with an extract of the fetal thymus

JEREMI CZAPLICKI
ZABRZE, POLAND
*From the Department of Histology and Embryology, Silesian Academy of Medicine*

In animals, intrafetal treatment with an albumin of another individual prevents the recipient from displaying immunologic reactions to the albumin of the donor after birth for a prolonged or permanent period. This phenomenon has been called "acquired tolerance," and the fetal period during which it occurs the "period of tolerance."

To explain tolerance, it has been postulated that a previously unknown hormone arises in the fetal thymus. This idea occurred to me by association of the anergy of fetal life with the condition of status thymicus or lymphatism which arises after birth. I found support of this concept a few years ago in the description by MacLean and associates[1] of agammaglobulinemia and anergy which was observed in a 55-year-old man suffering from a thymic tumor. It is possible that this thymic tumor had caused a functional regression of the thymus back to the fetal state in which the thymus produces the hypothetical hormone.

In order to test the hypothesis, the effect of extracts of the fetal thymus of pigs on the serum gamma globulins of rats was studied. Although these investigations are not yet complete, the preliminary results seem to me to justify this early communication.

Revised by Dr. Richard C. Lillehei, University of Minnesota Medical Center, Minneapolis, Minn.

Received for publication Dec. 15, 1960.

## METHODS AND RESULTS

Nine adult rats have been used in this study so far. The first studies were carried out on 4 of the rats. The first rat was treated subcutaneously with an extract prepared from the thymus of fetal pigs obtained in the first half of fetal life. The second rat was treated in a similar manner. The third was treated with a similarly prepared thymic extract which previously had been frozen. The fourth rat was treated as the first 2, with the exception that the thymus was taken from pigs obtained during the last half of fetal life. The rats were treated thrice weekly for 2 weeks. Five days after the final treatment, the rats were bled out and a blotting-paper electrophoresis of the serum obtained.

The serum gammaglobulin levels in the first 3 rats were low, while in the fourth rat the level was fairly high (Table I).

In the second group of experiments carried out on 3 rats, the first rat was given an extract of the thymus of pigs obtained in the first half of fetal life. The second rat was administered a liver extract from the same fetal pig which was of the same weight and quantity as the thymic extract. The third rat was treated with a splenic extract of the same fetal pig, and again this extract was of the same weight and quantity as the thymic extract. Control blood specimens

**Table I**

| Rat No. | Albumin (%) | Globulin $\alpha_1 + \alpha_2$ (%) | $\beta_1 + \beta_2$ (%) | $\gamma$ (%) |
|---|---|---|---|---|
| 1 | 36.2 | 22.2 | 22.8 | 17.0 |
| 2 | 38.0 | 22.4 | 21.4 | 20.0 |
| 3 | 37.7 | 21.9 | 20.8 | 19.6 |
| 4 | 21.5 | 19.0 | 21.9 | 37.6 |

were obtained from the tail veins of the rats before the start of the injections and again a fortnight after treatment with the various extracts had started. These blood samples were used for blood morphologic studies, total albumin determinations, and blotting-paper electrophoresis of the serum. The results of this second group of experiments are seen in Table II.

**Table II**

| Rat No. | Protein (Gm. %) | | Albumin (%) | | Globulin $\alpha_1 + \alpha_2$ (%) | | $\beta_1 + \beta_2$ (%) | | $\gamma$ (%) | | Erythrocytes (million) | | Leukocytes | |
|---|---|---|---|---|---|---|---|---|---|---|---|---|---|---|
| | Before | After | Before | After | Before | After | Before | After | Before | After | Before | After | Before | After |
| 1 | 7.8 | 8.2 | 27.0 | 27.4 | 25.5 | 19.6 | 23.0 | 27.0 | 24.5 | 26.0 | 6.9 | 3.2 | 11,000 | 12,000 |
| 2 | 7.9 | 14.0 | 33.3 | 18.5 | 23.8 | 13.5 | 22.7 | 15.0 | 27.2 | 53.0 | 5.7 | 17.0 | 14,000 | 19,500 |
| 3 | 7.8 | 17.0 | 27.2 | 13.1 | 23.2 | 13.1 | 22.9 | 12.8 | 26.7 | 61.0 | 7.2 | 13.4 | 10,000 | 21,000 |

**Table III**

| | Before experiment | During experiment After 1 wk. | After 2 wk. | After 3 wk. | After experiment After 1 wk. | After 2 wk. | After 3 wk. | After 4 wk. | After 5 wk. |
|---|---|---|---|---|---|---|---|---|---|
| *Rat No. 1* | | | | | | | | | |
| Protein (mg./100 ml.) | 7.8 | 9.6 | 8.4 | 8.4 | 7.9 | 7.9 | 7.8 | 7.8 | |
| Albumin (%) | 26.3 | 20.5 | 29 | 27.2 | 32.6 | 28.6 | 24.1 | 27.4 | |
| $\alpha$ Globulin (%) | 26.4 | 16.7 | 22.1 | 20.2 | 35.5 | 32.5 | 22.9 | 19.7 | |
| $\beta$ Globulin (%) | 22.9 | 21.2 | 16.8 | 20.2 | 31.9 | 38.9 | 53 | 27 | |
| $\gamma$ Globulin (%) | 24.4 | 41.6 | 32.1 | 32.4 | — | — | — | 25.9 | |
| Erythrocytes (million) | 7.64 | 7.97 | 4.56 | 4.85 | 5.37 | 6.12 | 5.74 | 6.01 | |
| Hemoglobin (%) | 140 | 143 | 99 | 97 | 75 | 73 | 74 | 81 | |
| Index Hb | 0.8 | 0.9 | 1.1 | 1 | 0.7 | 0.6 | 0.6 | 0.7 | |
| Leukocytes | 16,000 | 12,000 | 13,000 | 12,000 | 14,200 | 11,900 | 13,400 | 14,100 | |
| Methamyelocytes (%) | — | 5 | 4 | 1 | 2 | 3 | 1 | 4 | |
| Nonfilamented cells (%) | — | 1 | 3 | — | — | — | — | 1 | |
| Segmented cells (%) | 27 | 23 | 25 | 34 | 17 | 24 | 30 | 23 | |
| Lymphocytes (%) | 71 | 71 | 67 | 65 | 80 | 73 | 69 | 72 | |
| Eosinophils (%) | 1 | — | 1 | — | 1 | — | — | — | |
| Monocytes (%) | 1 | — | — | — | — | — | — | — | |
| *Rat No. 2* | | | | | | | | | |
| Protein (mg./100 ml.) | 7.8 | 9.5 | 9.5 | 8 | 7.8 | 7.9 | | 7.9 | 7.7 |
| Albumin (%) | 32.5 | 31.6 | 29.6 | 30.4 | 30.4 | 29.6 | | 25.1 | 28.4 |
| $\alpha$ Globulin (%) | 22.8 | 22.9 | 23.4 | 22.7 | 37.8 | 31.5 | | 24.9 | 18.7 |
| $\beta$ Globulin (%) | 22.5 | 27.5 | 30.9 | 29 | 31.8 | 38.9 | | 50 | 29.7 |
| $\gamma$ Globulin (%) | 22.2 | 15.4 | 16.1 | 17.9 | — | — | | — | 23.2 |
| Erythrocytes (million) | 5.22 | 4.3 | 3.74 | 3.88 | 5.29 | 5.4 | | 5.75 | 6.42 |
| Hemoglobin (%) | 82 | 73 | 67 | 69 | 76 | 75 | | 74 | 90 |
| Index Hb | 0.7 | 0.6 | 0.9 | 0.9 | 0.7 | 0.7 | | 0.6 | 0.7 |
| Leukocytes | 10,100 | 16,900 | 8,900 | 12,800 | 12,700 | 13,400 | | 14,100 | 18,600 |
| Methamyelocytes (%) | 6 | 7 | 3 | 3 | 2 | 2 | | 4 | 6 |
| Nonfilamented cells (%) | — | — | — | — | 1 | — | | 1 | 1 |
| Segmented cells (%) | 20 | 20 | 20 | 31 | 17 | 19 | | 15 | 21 |
| Lymphocytes (%) | 72 | 73 | 77 | 64 | 80 | 89 | | 80 | 72 |
| Eosinophils (%) | 1 | — | — | 2 | — | — | | — | — |
| Monocytes (%) | 1 | — | — | — | — | — | | — | — |

In the final phase of the experiment, 2 rats were injected intraperitoneally with extract prepared from the thymus of pigs obtained in the first half of fetal life. Morphologic blood analyses and blotting-paper electrophoreses were carried out every week for 2 months. During the period of injections, changes were observed which resembled those in the experiments described. One week after the injections had been stopped, complete agammaglobulinemia occurred which lasted 3 weeks in 1 rat and 4 weeks in the other. These results, as well as erythrocyte counts and hemoglobin indices of the 2 rats in this experiment, are seen in Table III.

## SUMMARY AND CONCLUSIONS

These experiments suggest that the fetal thymus may produce a substance or hormone which inhibits the production of gamma globulins. In the publications at my disposal, no mention of the possibility of achieving total agammaglobulinemia by biologic means has been noted. If the proposed hormone in question can be isolated, this may lead to the achievement of acquired tolerance in postfetal life and to a solution to the problem of organ transplants.

### REFERENCE

1. MacLean, L. D., Zak, S. J., Varco, R. L., and Good, R. A.: Thymic tumor and acquired agammaglobulinemia, SURGERY **40:** 1010, 1956.

# Contribution of functional ablation of the pyloroantral mechanism to malabsorption in gastrectomized dogs

PAUL H. JORDAN, JR., M.D.
GAINESVILLE, FLA., AND LOS ANGELES, CALIF.
*From the Department of Surgery, University of Florida, and the Los Angeles Veterans Administration Hospital*

An increased fecal excretion of fat and protein is a frequent occurrence after operative procedures upon the stomach for treatment of peptic ulcer or gastric carcinoma. Everson[2] has drawn attention to several factors possibly responsible for this phenomenon. Evidence exists that the malabsorption is due to multiple defects created by operation and is not the exclusive result of any one factor.

Ablation or short circuiting of the pyloric sphincter and gastric antrum is common to all operative procedures upon the stomach except segmental resection performed without pyloroplasty. Studies performed upon dogs indicate that the degree of malabsorption associated with the latter operation is less than with any other type of gastric resection.[1] Since the pyloroantral pump, by its muscular action, appears to regulate the rhythmical evacuation of the stomach,[4] it was appropriate to evaluate the contribution made by the loss of this mechanism upon the absorption of fat and protein.

## METHODS

Two groups of mongrel dogs were used and the experiment in each group was divided into 3 phases. Phase 1 in both groups consisted of a control period. The animals of Group I underwent a segmental gastric resection during Phase 2 and subsequently a Heineke-Mikulicz pyloroplasty during Phase 3. The control period in animals of Group II was followed by pyloroplasty during Phase 2 and segmental gastric resection in Phase 3. The animals were allowed a recovery period of 1 month after pyloroplasty and 2 months after gastric resection before studies were performed.

Six dogs in each group completed all phases of the study while 2 dogs in Group I and 1 dog in Group II completed only Phases 1 and 2. Not less than 3 consecutive 6-day metabolic balance studies were made on all dogs during the control periods and after recovery from the operations performed during Phases 2 and 3. In the case of Dog 3 in Group I, alterations in absorption were negligible at the completion of Phase 3. Pyloroplasty was performed, therefore, a second time to insure transection of all the antral musculature. Three additional metabolic periods were performed. Six 6-day metabolic periods were performed after gastric resection during Phase 3 upon Dogs, 4, 5, and 6 of Group II.

The diet during each metabolic period consisted of 80 calories per kilogram of body weight per day based upon the dog's original weight. This included 5 Gm. of protein and 4 Gm. of fat per kilogram. The diet, a commercial dog food supplemented with lard, was analyzed for its fat and protein content. All meals prepared were eaten; thus, no analysis of rejected meals was required.

Each 6-day stool collection was delineated

Supported by United States Public Health Service Grants A-653 and A-2787.

Received for publication Jan. 17, 1961. Resubmitted March 20, 1961.

by carmine markers. Each was homogenized and duplicate aliquots taken for fat and protein analyses which were repeated if they did not agree within 5 per cent. Fat determinations were by the Mojonnier extraction methods.[5] Proteins were measured by the micro-Kjeldahl method and expressed in grams of nitrogen. Because of the analytical accuracy and the meticulous care in the preparation of diets and the collection of stools, it was assumed that the error in the estimated fecal fat and nitrogen levels for any collection period was not greater than 10 per cent. This was equivalent to approximately 1 per cent of the ingested fat and 2 per cent of the ingested nitrogen. Consequently, changes in excretion were considered analytically significant if the differences between periods were in excess of 2 per cent and 4 per cent of the ingested fat and nitrogen, respectively.

The pyloroplasties were constructed by making longitudinal incisions that transected a major portion, if not all, of the musculature of the pylorus and which were extended for an equal distance into the duodenum. The incisions were closed transversely to effectively destroy the function of the pyloroantral pump without compromise of storage capacity. The segmental resections aimed at removal of 75 per cent of the stomach with retention of the cardia, the antrum, and the vagal fibers to the antrum. In order to verify the extent of resection, the mucosa of the resected portion of the stomach was stripped from its muscle and weighed. When the dog was subsequently sacrificed, the remaining mucosa was weighed and the per cent of resection calculated. In Group I the extent of resection ranged from 50 to 89 per cent. In animals of Group II the resection ranged from 48 to 62 per cent. In our opinion this method was not entirely reliable because much of the scar tissue associated with suture lines was included in the remaining mucosal specimen and resulted in underestimation of the magnitude of resection. The weight of mucosa initially removed was a more reliable index of the magnitude of resection and indicated that the gastrectomies were larger in Group I than in Group II.

## RESULTS

**Fat absorption.** Four of the 8 dogs in Group I demonstrated significant increases in fat excretion after gastric resection. Subsequent pyloroplasty was performed upon 6 of the dogs in this group. The excretion of fat was significantly increased in 4 of these animals to an amount above that seen with gastrectomy alone. Comparison of the amounts of fat excreted during Phases 1 and 3 demonstrated that a significant increase in the fecal excretion resulted in 5 of 6 dogs which underwent both operations. The differences between the per cent of ingested fat excreted in the stool by animals of Group I during the 3 phases of this study are tabulated in Table I.

In Group II, fat excretion was significantly increased by pyloroplasty in 2 of 7 dogs. After gastric resection, fat excretion was increased in 5 of 6 dogs above that seen with pyloroplasty alone. The increase was significant in 2. The fecal fat level observed during Phase 3 was increased significantly in 4 dogs above that encountered during the control period (Table II).

**Nitrogen absorption.** All 8 dogs of Group I demonstrated an increased excretion of nitrogen after segmental resection. This increase was significant in 5. In 5 of the 6

**Table I.** *Differences in the per cent of ingested fat in stool during 3 phases of experiment in Group I*

| *Dog No.* | *Sleeve gastric resection–control* | *(Sleeve gastric resection + pyloroplasty)–sleeve gastric resection* | *(Sleeve gastric resection + pyloroplasty)–control* |
|---|---|---|---|
| 1 | 0.8 | 6.0 | 6.8 |
| 2 | 0.5 | 4.7 | 5.2 |
| 3 | −1.1 | 1.3 | 0.2 (−0.3*) |
| 4 | 3.0 | 1.2 | 4.2 |
| 5 | 2.0 | 5.8 | 7.8 |
| 6 | 8.6 | 3.4 | 12.0 |
| 7 | 5.2 | — | — |
| 8 | −0.5 | — | — |

*From second series of metabolic studies performed during Phase 3.

**Table II.** *Differences in the per cent of ingested fat in stool during 3 phases of experiment in Group II*

| Dog No. | *Pyloroplasty – control* | *(Pyloroplasty + sleeve gastric resection)– pyloroplasty* | *(Pyloroplasty + sleeve gastric resection)– control* |
|---|---|---|---|
| 1 | 0.4 | 1.2 | 1.6 |
| 2 | 4.1 | −1.8 | 2.3 |
| 3 | 1.4 | 1.8 | 3.2 |
| 4 | 0.6 | 0.2 | 0.8 (−0.2*) |
| 5 | 0.5 | 6.3 | 6.8 (2.6*) |
| 6 | 0.5 | 8.6 | 9.1 (8.9*) |
| 7 | 2.8 | — | — |

*From second series of metabolic studies performed during Phase 3.

**Table III.** *Differences in the per cent of ingested nitrogen in stool during 3 phases of experiment on dogs in Group I*

| Dog No. | *Sleeve gastric resection– control* | *(Sleeve gastric resection + pyloroplasty)–sleeve gastric resection* | *(Sleeve gastric resection + pyloroplasty)– control* |
|---|---|---|---|
| 1 | 2.3 | 1.7 | 4.0 |
| 2 | 6.5 | .0 | 6.5 |
| 3 | 1.7 | 3.0 | 4.7 (2.9*) |
| 4 | 2.5 | 5.0 | 7.5 |
| 5 | 10.6 | 1.1 | 11.7 |
| 6 | 15.0 | 0.4 | 15.4 |
| 7 | 13.2 | — | — |
| 8 | 6.2 | — | — |

*From second series of metabolic studies performed during Phase 3.

**Table IV.** *Differences in the percent of ingested nitrogen in stool during 3 phases of experiment on dogs in Group II*

| Dog No. | *Pyloroplasty– control* | *(Pyloroplasty + sleeve gastric resection)– pyloroplasty* | *(Pyloroplasty + sleeve gastric resection)–control* |
|---|---|---|---|
| 1 | 3.5 | 4.8 | 8.3 |
| 2 | 1.6 | 9.7 | 11.3 |
| 3 | 5.7 | 4.5 | 10.2 |
| 4 | −2.5 | 1.1 | −1.4 (−3.3*) |
| 5 | 1.6 | −0.2 | 1.4 (2.2*) |
| 6 | 0.4 | 4.8 | 5.2 (4.1*) |
| 7 | 5.7 | — | — |

*From second series of metabolic studies performed during Phase 3.

dogs which underwent subsequent pyloroplasty, nitrogen excretion was increased above that seen with gastrectomy alone and in 1 the increase was significant. In all dogs the excretion of nitrogen observed during Phase 3 was significantly greater than that encountered during the control period. The differences in the per cent of ingested nitrogen excreted in the stool during the 3 phases are tabulated in Table III.

In Group II, nitrogen excretion was significantly increased after pyloroplasty in 2 of the 7 dogs. The addition of gastric resection in 6 dogs significantly increased nitrogen excretion in 4 above that seen with pyloroplasty alone. The fecal nitrogen level observed during Phase 3 was significantly increased in 4 dogs above that encountered during the control period (Table IV).

Ten of the 12 dogs which underwent combined operations in Groups I and II had increased excretion of nitrogen. In 5, this defect was solely attributable to the gastrectomy which was performed as the primary procedure in 3 dogs and the secondary procedure in 2. In 5 dogs, pyloroplasty and gastrectomy appeared equally responsible for the defect in nitrogen absorption. In no dog was the increased fecal nitrogen level attributable to pyloroplasty alone.

The average size of the actual gastrectomies was estimated at 75 per cent in dogs of Group I and 57 per cent in dogs of Group II. The average weight losses during the experiments were 0.6 and 0.2 Kg. in the 2 groups, respectively. It was not possible in this study to correlate the magnitude of gastrectomy with the degree of steatorrhea and azotorrhea. It was also not possible to correlate the amount of fat and nitrogen excreted with changes in body weight.

No time limit was placed upon the dogs for the consumption of their daily rations. It was an impression that the rate with which food was eaten exerted a significant effect upon the animals' nutritional status. This was particularly true for Dog 3 in Group I, which required over 12 hours to eat his daily rations. This dog exhibited nearly normal value for fat and nitrogen excretion during the 3 phases of study and body weight increased during the experiment. A second pyloroplasty in this animal failed to alter the weight or produce any degree of malabsorption.

## DISCUSSION

The importance of the pyloric antrum for the control of gastric emptying was demonstrated by Quigley.[4] Work by Friesen[3] implied that the pylorus, by virtue of its regulation of gastric evacuation, exerts an important influence in the maintenance of body weight in the dog and prevention of the dumping syndrome in man. Everson[2] and others have stated that the loss of fecal fat and protein after segmental gastric resection is less than that which occurs after conventional resections. For these reasons the present study was expected to demonstrate that functional ablation of the pyloroantral pump is a significant factor responsible for malabsorption after gastrectomy. This hypothesis was substantiated; however, the effect was less than that which had been anticipated.

As the primary operation, pyloroplasty appeared to have little effect upon fat and protein absorption. When it was performed as the secondary operation after segmental gastrectomy, absorption of fat was significantly reduced, whereas the absorption of protein was minimally affected. Segmental gastrectomy, on the other hand, had a significant effect upon the absorption of fat and protein when it was performed either as a primary or secondary operation. The malabsorption of fat resulting from segmental resection performed as a secondary operation was not as great, however, as that associated with pyloroplasty performed as a secondary operation. It appears that the magnitude of the segmental resections performed upon dogs of Group II was less than that of the resections performed in Group I and may account for the over-all difference in the absorption of fat after combined operations in the 2 groups. That this is not the complete explanation is suggested by the fact that gastrectomy as the secondary operation in Group II exerted a greater effect upon nitrogen excretion than did pyloroplasty as the secondary operation in Group I. The difference in the effect of segmental gastric resection and pyloroplasty upon the absorption of fat and protein after combined operations suggests that loss of the pyloroantral pump exerts its greatest effect upon absorption of fat while the loss of the stomach's storage capacity exerts its greatest effect upon protein absorption.

## SUMMARY

Conventional subtotal gastrectomy includes ablation of the pyloroantral pump and the storage capacity of the stomach. The effects exerted by the loss of these functions of the stomach upon absorption were evaluated independently and in combination during experimental studies on dogs.

The results suggest that loss of the storage capacity of the stomach exerted a greater effect upon postgastrectomy malabsorption than did interference with the pyloroantral pump. Disruption of the latter mechanism by pyloroplasty when accompanied by segmental gastric resection significantly increased the excretion of fat but had little effect upon excretion of protein. Pyloroplasty unaccompanied by gastrectomy had an insignificant effect upon fecal excretion of fat and protein.

### REFERENCES

1. Everson, T. C.: Experimental comparison of protein and fat assimilation after Billroth II, Billroth I, and segmental types of subtotal gastrectomy, Surgery **36:** 525, 1954.
2. Everson, T. C.: Nutrition following total gastrectomy, with particular reference to fat and protein assimilation, Internat. Abstr. Surg. **95:** 209, 1952.
3. Friesen, S. R., and Rieger, E.: A study of the role of the pylorus in prevention of "dumping syndrome," Ann. Surg. **151:** 517, 1960.
4. Quigley, J. P., and Brody, D. A.: Digestive tract: intralumen pressures: gastrointestinal propulsion, gastric evacuation, pressure-wall tension relationships. *In* Glaser, O., editor: Medical physics, Chicago, 1950, The Year Book Publishers, Inc., vol. 2.
5. Söderhjelm, U., and Söderhjelm, L.: Fat determination in feces using Mojonnier extraction flasks, J. Lab. & Clin. Med. **34:** 1471, 1949.

# Clinical and experimental observations on heterotopic osseous formation in abdominal wall scars

KENNETH L. CLASSEN, M.D.
R. F. WIEDERANDERS, M.D.*
J. LYNWOOD HERRINGTON, JR., M.D.
NASHVILLE, TENN.
*From the Surgical Service, Thayer Veterans Administration Hospital; Department of Surgery, Vanderbilt University School of Medicine; and the Edwards-Eve Clinic*

The occurrence of heterotopic osseous formation in abdominal wall scars has long been regarded as a medical curiosity and represents one of Nature's perplexing whims. The relative infrequency of this clinical finding is evidenced by the paucity of reported cases in the literature.

In a recent report from this institution,[4] 10 clinical cases of bone formation which took place in abdominal wall scars were described. Since the previous publication, 20 additional cases have been discovered on our services. Thus, the present report represents a detailed analysis of the entire group of 30 cases and, in addition, experimental data on our attempts to produce bone growth in laparotomy scars of the experimental animal.

## CLINICAL MATERIAL

The 30 cases of osseous formation in abdominal wall scars occurred entirely in patients of the male sex. The age range extended from 23 to 74 years and the average age at time of discovery of heterotopic bone formation was 56 years. Twelve of the 30 patients were in the seventh decade of life. Each of the patients had originally had a cleanly incised laparotomy which was meticulously closed with a continuous catgut suture for the peritoneum and either interrupted silk sutures, stainless steel wire, or chromic catgut for the fascial layers. The skin was closed routinely with silk.

Among the 30 patients, it is of interest that 23 had laparotomy incisions placed in the supraumbilical area, extending from the ensiform process or the costochondral arch superiorly to the umbilicus or periumbilical area inferiorly. The original operation in the group of 23 patients was vagotomy and gastric resection in 16 cases, repair of esophageal hiatal hernia in 2, resection for gastric carcinoma in 3, exploration for gunshot wound of the upper abdominal viscera in 1, and in 1 instance exploratory laparotomy without definitive intraperitoneal operation. Of the 7 remaining patients, 4 had incisions placed in the low paramedian area of the abdominal wall, while 3 underwent midline incisions extending from the ensiform process to the pubis. The indications for the original operation in this group were carcinoma of the left colon in 4 instances, abdominal aortic aneurysm in 2, and marginal ulcer after inadequate resection in 1. It is to be noted that 3 of the latter 7 incisions extended to or impinged on skeletal structures (Fig. 1). Four of the 30 patients developed postoperative wound infections of mild to moderate severity. In 26 cases the laparotomy wound healed without complications. There was no instance of postoperative hematoma formation, and none of the 4 infected wounds drained for any appreciable length of time (Fig. 2).

The first indication which suggested the

Received for publication Jan. 23, 1961.

*Present address: Department of Surgery, Veterans Administration Hospital, Omaha, Neb.

likelihood of early heterotopic bone formation during the postoperative period was the presence of persistent tenderness in the abdominal wall scar. As a general rule, most tenderness has disappeared in clean wounds after 14 days. In the cases under consideration, persistent and increasing tenderness in the absence of infection was the first sign of early osseous activity in the abdominal wall scar. This was noted in 18 of the 30 patients (60 per cent). Unusual tenderness occurred as early as 2 weeks postoperatively and up to as late as 6 months. As the heterotopic bone developed further, a major portion of the abdominal wall tenderness usually disappeared, as well as abdominal wall hyperesthesia. With further development of bone growth, the patients began to note a "stabbing" sensation in the abdominal wall, usually initiated by flexion of the abdominal wall musculature. The presence of an abdominal wall mass was usually then discovered, as a rule first by the patient and later by the physician. A mass was noted by 25 of the 30 patients (83 per cent). In the remaining 5 patients, a mass was first discovered by the physician on physical examination. Three patients in the group discovered the presence of a mass as early as 2 weeks after operation. In most instances within a few months after operation the mass had grown sufficiently in size to become palpable. In several cases the bone growths were of such length (7 to 15 cm.) as to restrict forward body bending and to limit physical activity. In 6 instances, actual fracture of the bone occurred during exercise. This interesting finding was first demonstrated by roentgen study as a rule, but later, upon careful questioning, the patient could usually recall the exact time and the physical event which resulted in the fracture. Several patients experienced a "grating" sound in the upper abdominal wall at the time of the fracture, after which they no longer experienced discomfort upon flexion of the abdominal wall musculature (Fig. 3).

Routine postoperative gastrointestinal barium studies and scout films of the abdomen were performed on the majority of the 30 patients from 4 to 8 weeks after operation. Approximately one-third of the group examined demonstrated evidence of radiodensity in the abdominal wall within 2

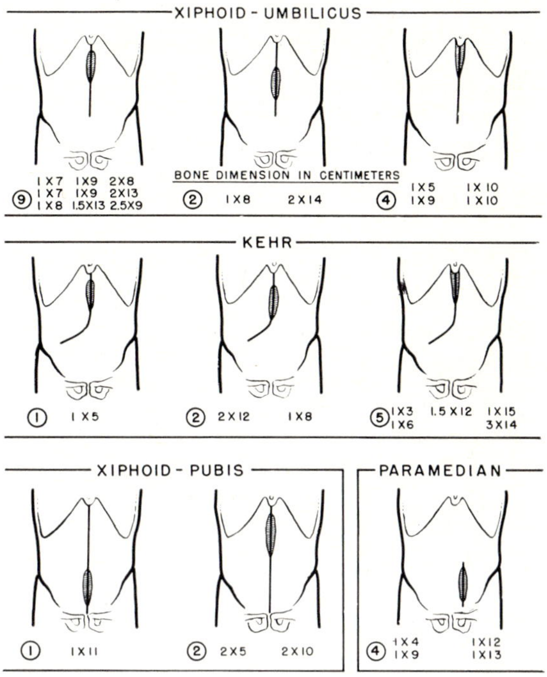


Fig. 1. Site and size of bone formation.

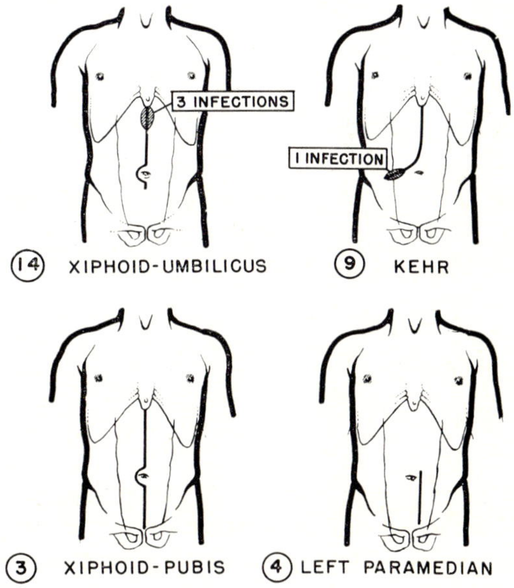


Fig. 2. Original incision.

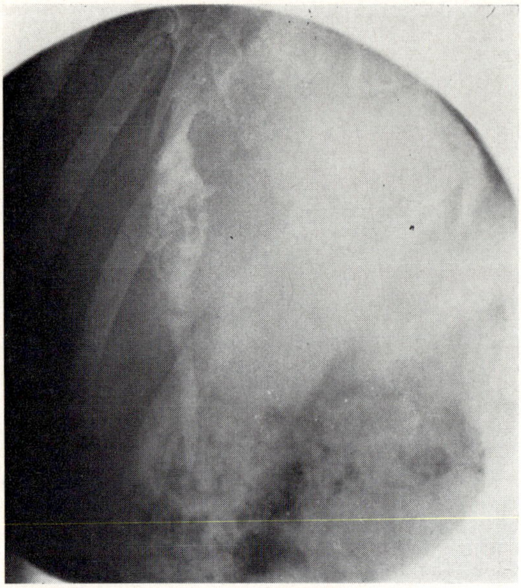

*A*

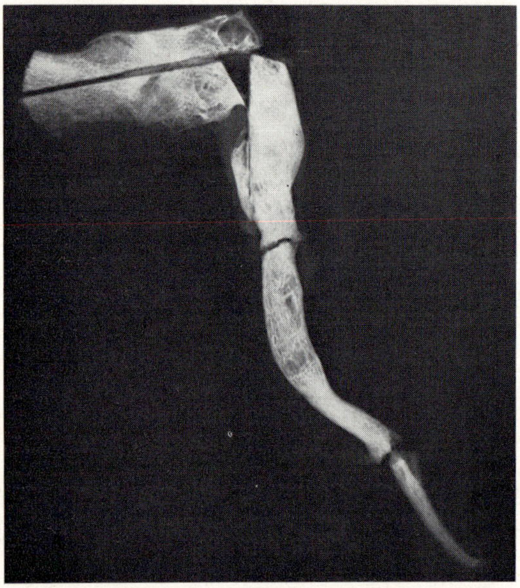

*B*

**Fig. 3.** *A,* Lateral film shows the heterotopic osseous growth. A fracture in the midportion of the bone is demonstrated. (From SURGERY **47:** 918, 1960.) *B,* Excised specimen shows the ensiform process which has been sectioned. The heterotopic bone shows 2 distinct fracture sites.

months after the operative procedure. Presumably this radiodensity represented early deposition of calcium in the soft tissues about the laparotomy scar. This finding was particularly impressive in the patients who had stainless steel wire closure of the abdominal wall, as the sutures were closely invested with radiopaque material. From the fourth to the twelfth month after operation the radiodensity became organized into what appeared by roentgen study to represent true bone formation with anterior and posterior cortices and a medullary canal. The lateral or oblique film taken with soft tissue technique served to bring out the bony detail (Fig. 4). It should be mentioned that among the early cases in which evidence of presumptive calcium formation was shown, the finding was overlooked in several of the roentgen studies. It was only after interest in the problem mounted that the diagnosis was made with increasing accuracy.

Among the group of 30 patients, 25 have shown definite evidence of osseous formation in the soft tissues proved by roentgen study. Three patients recently operated upon show evidence of presumptive calcium formation, but no true bone as yet has appeared in the soft tissues about the abdominal scar. Two patients had bone which was removed at subsequent laparotomy and later verified by microscopic study, but preoperative roentgen studies had not been performed in either case. Twenty-one of the heterotopic bones lay completely free in the soft tissues without attachment to adjacent skeletal structures. In the remaining 9 cases, there was evidence of union between the heterotopic bone and the ensiform process. In several instances, only a fibrous tissue band served to connect the 2 structures. These findings were proved either by roentgen study, palpation, or at subsequent operation. As previously mentioned, all but 4 of the original 30 laparotomy incisons extended to or impinged upon skeletal structures.

Twelve of the 30 patients underwent either complete or partial excision of the heterotopic bone. In 5 cases the symptomatology produced by the bony spicule was of such severity as to warrant excision. In 4 patients, 2 of whom were seen during our early experience, the possibility of recurrent carcinoma in the abdominal wall was thought to exist. At re-exploration, however, only osseous formation was encountered in the abdominal scar. One patient underwent excision of the bone growth during operation for repair of a hiatal hernia. In 2 additional patients operated upon for other reasons, a partial excision of the bone was performed. In the remaining 18 patients, there has been no indication for removal of the heterotopic growth.

Nine of the 12 patients who underwent removal of the heterotopic bone had originally undergone laparotomy through an upper abdominal midline incision or a midline incision with a lateral component (Kehr). In each instance at reoperation heterotopic bone was located in the midline fascia (Fig. 5). In 5 cases the bone was attached to the ensiform process by osseous union, and in removal of the bone the ensiform process was usually excised with the specimen. In 3 patients who had previously undergone low paramedian incisions, the bone was found to lie between the anterior rectus sheath and rectus muscle.

The excised osseous specimens varied in length from 3 to approximately 15 cm. and each was narrow in width, curved in contour, and strongly resembled a rib in gross appearance (Fig. 6). On histologic study, each of the 12 specimens showed the presence of cortical bone with active bone marrow, and 9 of the 12 demonstrated cartilaginous formation. The 12 patients have been followed for a period varying from 12 months to 9 years, and there has been no instance of recurrent or additional bone formation.

The 30 patients who compose the entire series have shown no evidence of heterotopic bone formation elsewhere. Several of the patients have since undergone laparotomy for other conditions through incisions of the longitudinal and transverse types. No patient has shown evidence of parathyroid dysfunction. Twenty-two of the 30 patients have undergone repeated determinations of serum calcium, phosphorus, and alkaline phosphatase levels. Each determination has been within the range of normal. Results of quantitative creatinine and calcium urinary studies have not been abnormal.

## EXPERIMENTAL OBSERVATIONS

An attempt was made to produce heterotopic bone formation in the experimental animal.

Twenty mongrel dogs were divided into 2 groups of 10 each. In the Group I experiments, performed under Surital anesthesia and with aseptic technique, an upper midline and both right and left paramedian incisions were placed in each animal. A strip of perichondrium was then elevated from the ensiform process with care taken to maintain its inferior attachment. The strip was turned down and placed in the midline incision. Thirty milliliters of the animal's blood was injected into the right paramedian wound and a 1 by 0.5 cm. sliver of free ensiform cartilage was placed in the left paramedian incision.

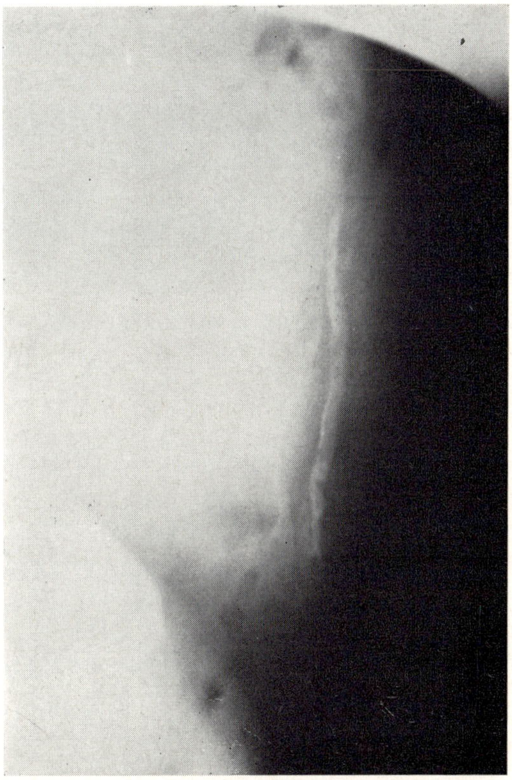

**Fig. 4.** Eight weeks after operation definite evidence of osseous formation is noted.

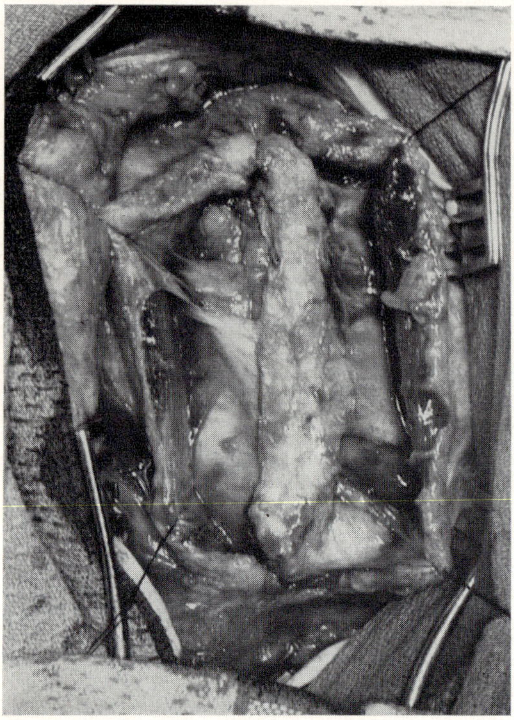

**Fig. 5.** The osseous growth is demonstrated lying in the midline fascia. The superior aspect of the growth has an attachment to the ensiform process.

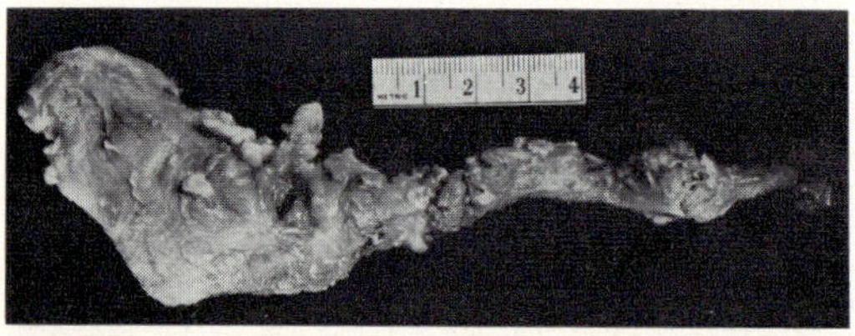


**Fig. 6.** Excised specimen consists of the ensiform cartilage and the heterotopic bone. The bone closely resembles a rib.

In the second group, which consisted of 10 animals, incisions were placed as in the Group I dogs. A sliver of bone and cartilage from the ensiform process was fashioned with the periosteal atachment remaining inferiorly. The sliver was turned down and positioned in the midline incision. A free strip of periosteum was placed in the right paramedian incision and bone chips obtained from a rib were put in the left paramedian incision. All wounds were closed in layers with interrupted silk sutures (Fig. 7).

The animals were sacrificed at the end of 6 months. The wounds were removed en bloc, the tissue carefully dissected, and microscopic sections made. No evidence of heterotopic bone formation was detected on gross examination of the abdominal scars among the 20 animals during the 6-month period of observation.

In the Group I animals at sacrifice, microscopic study of the tissue removed from the midline scar in which an attached strip of perichondrium from the ensiform process had originally been placed showed evidence of actively proliferating cartilage in 8 of the 10 animals. Four of the 8 had islands of cartilage in areas separated from the perichondrium (Fig. 8). The site of previous blood injection in the right paramedian scar showed no evidence of bone or cartilage formation. The left paramedian scar which originally had contained a piece of free ensiform cartilage showed evidence of resorbing cartilage in 8 instances, while in 1 animal a small area of bone formation with active marrow was noted.

In the Group II animals, microscopic study of the midline scar which had contained a sliver of attached bone and cartilage from the ensiform process showed bone resorption and fibrosis in each of the 10 animals. The cartilage was still viable, but was undergoing resorptive changes. The right paramedian scar which had contained a free strip of periosteum showed fibrosis of the periosteum in each case. Studies of the left paramedian scar which had contained free bone chips showed active viable bone in only 1 of the 10 animals.

## DISCUSSION

Heterotopic osseous formation occurring in abdominal wall scars has been an intriguing phenomenon to pathologists and surgeons. Apparently the first collective review of documented cases was published in 1926 by Bouton[2] in a thesis prepared for Le Docteur en Médecine. He gives credit to Askanazy for presenting the first authenticated case before the German Society of Pathology in 1900. Rixford published an account of a case in 1903 and cited the microscopic findings. In 1905 von Eiselsberg, in reporting on 258 gastric operations, mentioned 1 instance of heterotopic osseous formation. Cases were recorded in 1907 by Kopke and Rubesch and by Lecene in 1909. Bouton was able to collect a total of 30 cases of heterotopic osseous formation. He also observed that 20 of the 30 patients had undergone gastric operations and that the bone growths were found in the upper midline area of the abdominal wall. In addition, isolated cases of heterotopic bone were also found in the inguinal area after hernia repair and in appendectomy and umbilical herniorrhaphy scars. In 1 case bone formation occurred after marsupialization of a liver cyst. The vast majority of the patients were men, with an age range extending from 13 to 70 years. Twelve of the 30 patients had wounds which had healed cleanly by first intention, whereas in 18 patients some type of wound complication had taken place. Only 1 instance of postoperative hematoma formation occurred.

Since the report of Bouton, several articles have appeared citing isolated cases of heterotopic osseous formation.[5, 6] Six cases were reported by Sanders[20] in 1955. No doubt the formation of bone growths in laparotomy scars is more common than was formerly thought. The heterotopic growth may at times be small indeed, and when asymptomatic can easily escape clinical detection. Physicians unfamiliar with the occurrence of heterotopic osseous formation may believe that only induration and excessive cicatrix exist in the abdominal wall scar when actually bone is present. In addition, no doubt, cases have been diagnosed and never recorded in the surgical literature.

Several theories have been proposed in attempts to explain the development of heterotopic osseous formation. One concept is that during muscle strain particles of periosteum are avulsed from the bony insertion of the muscle. The particles of periosteum in turn lodge in the muscle fibers and initiate osseous growth. Another theory postulates that bone formation stems from cell metaplasia as a result of muscle, tendon, or soft tissue injury. Leriche and Keith[11] believed that osteoblastic function could be assumed by cells from any part of the body besides the skeletal system. Calcium salts in turn were thought necessary for the production of bone formation, along with possible unknown enzyme mechanisms. Lyall[14] stated that heterotopic bone formation resulted from injury to a bony or cartilaginous structure, presumably through the release of osteoblasts. German observers have emphasized the frequency of pulmonary complications in patients who developed heterotopic bone formation. They believe that coughing and retching during the postoperative period produces increased strain upon the wound with resultant excessive scar tissue deposition and later bone formation.

It is of interest that in all reported cases, heterotopic bone formation has occurred in longitudinal operative scars. In no instance has it been cited in a transverse abdominal

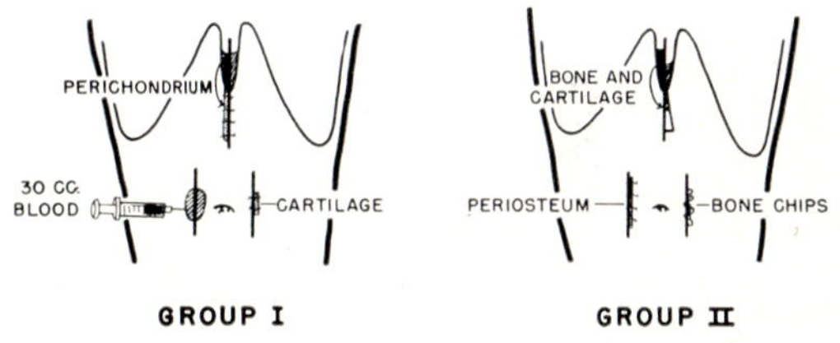


**Fig. 7.** Experimental incisions in 20 dogs.

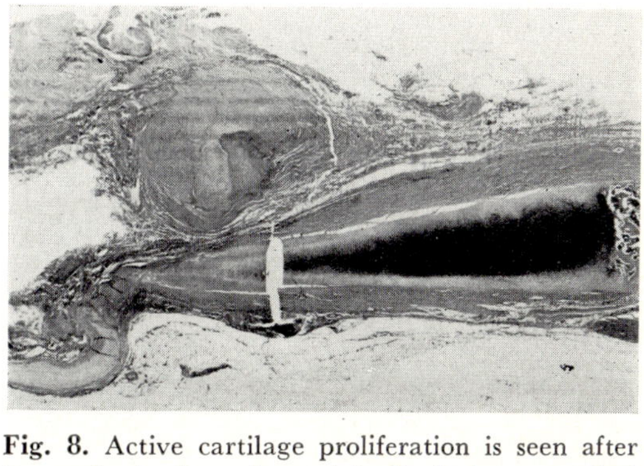

**Fig. 8.** Active cartilage proliferation is seen after 6 months in dogs that originally had an attached flap of perichondrium sutured in the midline wound.

wall scar. In longitudinal wounds the forces of stress are undoubtedly greater and perhaps muscle fibers under tension may be torn from their periosteal insertions and later undergo bone formation.

The presence of bone elsewhere than in the skeleton has long interested students of osteogenesis. Heterotopic bone formation has been frequently encountered in the wall of a sclerotic artery.[3] It also has been observed in pulmonary tissue, in uterine myomas, and in the dura mater.[7] It has also been reported to occur in the eye after a destructive process. Less frequently heterotopic bone has been encountered in areas of squamous-cell carcinoma of the skin,[17] in areas of breast carcinoma, and in lymph nodes. It has also been reported in the Fallopian tube[1] and in tonsillar tissue. Phemister[18] described heterotopic bone in the pedicle attachment of a renal calculus to the kidney pelvis. Bony growths have also been noted in the abdominal wall after operations on the urinary bladder.[12] Experimentally, osteogenic tissue with a well-developed marrow cavity has been produced in the kidney by ligation of its vascular pedicle.

Neuhof[16] apparently was the first to transplant fascia into the urinary bladder and to observe subsequent bone formation in the transplants. In excellently performed experimental studies, Huggins[8, 9] showed that transplants of bladder, ureter, and renal pelvis epithelium, when deposited into certain parietal fascias such as the rectus sheath or fascia lata, developed osteogenic changes. The fibroblasts surrounding the surviving transplants undergo osteoblastic transformation and true bone formation. Strangely, fibroblastic elements in certain other connective tissue areas did not respond to the epithelial stimulus. The urinary tract epithelium was found to possess an osteogenetic power which was not observed in epithelial transplants from other tissues such as stomach or small intestine. Huggins[10] later showed that proliferating gall bladder epithelium in the dog and guinea pig is capable of stimulating bone formation when transplanted into certain connective tissues such as the abdominal wall. Connective tissue areas in other parts of the body did not share in this tissue reaction and resisted the bone stimulus of the transplanted epithelium. He concluded that there was a different physiologic response among connective tissues that were morphologically similar.

Loewi[13] implanted bits of urinary bladder from guinea pigs into the chest wall, belly wall, knee joint, and lip of the same animals. Bone was formed in the granulation tissue surrounding the bladder implants. Rush and Clifton[19] used autogenous bladder mucosa for the reconstruction of tracheal rings in dogs. As a result bone grew actively in the peritracheal tissues. In most experimental studies muscle injury, injection of calcium salts, introduction of synovial fluid into the wound, hematoma production, or combinations thereof have failed to produce true bone formation. Evidence of calcification alone, however, has been produced in many instances.

The experimental findings in the present study were disappointing. In no instance was a sliver of grossly detectable heterotopic bone produced. However, when an attached strip of perichondrium from the ensiform process was placed in the midline fascia, at the end of 6 months there was microscopic evidence of actively proliferating cartilage in 8 of the 10 scars. Also, in 1 case there was microscopic evidence of bone with marrow formation where a free sliver of ensiform cartilage had been placed in the wound. It is possible that a palpable sliver of heterotopic bone might have been produced had these animals been observed for longer time periods. However, heterotopic bone formation developing in the human being has usually been detected grossly in most instances within a 6-month period after operation.

McCurrich[15] observed that with few exceptions all reported instances of heterotopic bone formation had occurred in upper midline abdominal incisions. No associated cartilage formation was present in the cases he reviewed. Nine of the 12 patients who underwent bone removal in the present series showed evidence of active cartilage formation on microscopic study. This may be explained by the fact that the bone growths in our series were excised relatively early. It should be re-emphasized that in 26 of our 30 cases the original laparotomy incision extended to or impinged on skeletal structures, either bone or cartilage. In 21 of the 30 cases it was the clinical and radiographic impression that the bone growth lay free in the soft tissues of the abdominal wall, with no demonstrable attachment to skeletal structures. In the remaining 9 cases there was either fibrous or bony attachment between the heterotopic bone and the ensiform process. Of the 12 patients who underwent removal of the heterotopic bone, 5 were found to have an osseous attachment between the heterotopic bone and the ensiform process. In 9 of the 12 patients the bone was located in the midline fascia. In the remaining 3 patients, who had previously undergone low paramedial incisions, the bone was found to lie between the anterior rectus sheath and rectus muscle.

With the preponderance of the reported cases of heterotopic osseous formation having occurred in upper midline abdominal incisions and usually after operation on the stomach, one cannot help but believe that injury to the ensiform process might play an important role as an etiologic agent. Most of our cases followed operations for duodenal ulcer and the original incision had been purposely extended to the ensiform cartilage, or above and to the left of that structure, to gain added exposure in the performance of vagotomy. On occasion, the authors distinctly remember having actually incised the substance of the ensiform process in entering the abdomen.

It is our present belief that considerable care should be exercised to avoid this technical error. Should the ensiform process be inadvertently injured by incision, partial excision, or trauma from retractors, serious consideration should be given to its removal. Also, it is no doubt important that in closing the upper midline incision care should be taken not to pass the needle point into the periosteum overlying the ensiform process. Should this occur, it is quite possible that the trauma produced could excite osseous proliferation.

The heterotopic bone will necessitate removal only in instances in which symptoms arise from its presence. In all other cases the exact nature of the presenting mass should be explained to the patient and this, along with reassurance, is all that is necessary. Should indication for removal of the bone arise, then complete excision, including removal of the ensiform process, is the method we advise.

The occurrence of heterotopic bone in low midline or low paramedial incisions has rarely been encountered. It has developed in circumstances in which the incision was several centimeters removed from the pubic osseous structures. The development remains even a more perplexing mystery than does the osseous growth which develops in upper abdominal scars.

## SUMMARY

Thirty cases of heterotopic bone formation which occurred in laparotomy scars have been reviewed. The clinical and roentgen findings associated with heterotopic osseous growths have been described. Indication for excision of such growths is stated.

Attempts to produce heterotopic osseous formation in wounds of the experimental animal have been described.

### REFERENCES

1. Asami, G.: Heteroplastic bone formation in the Fallopion tube, Am. J. M. Sc. **160:** 107, 1920.
2. Bouton, M.: L'ossification hétérotypique dans les cicatrices opératoires. Pour le docteur en médecine, faculté de médecine de Paris-Anne, 1926.
3. Buerger, L., and Oppenheimer, A.: Bone formation in sclerotic arteries, J. Exper. Med. **10:** 354, 1908.
4. Classen, K. L., Wiederanders, R. E., and Herrington, J. L., Jr.: Heterotopic bone formation developing in abdominal scars, Surgery **47:** 918, 1960.
5. Cohen, J. H.: Heterotopic bone formation

following suprapubic prostatectomy. Report of a case and review of the literature, Ann. Int. Med. **51:** 166, 1959.
6. Fiddian-Green, W. B.: Case of recurrent duodenal ulcer after pylorectomy and the formation of bone in a laparotomy wound, Brit. J. Surg. **17:** 555, 1930.
7. Halstead, A. E., and Christopher, F.: Calcification and ossification of the meninges, Arch. Surg. **6:** 847, 1923.
8. Huggins, C. B.: Experimental osteogenesis, Proc. Soc. Exper. Biol. & Med. **27:** 349, 1930.
9. Huggins, C. B.: The formation of bone under the influence of epithelium of the urinary tract, Arch. Surg. **22:** 377, 1931.
10. Huggins, C. B., and Sammet, J. F.: Function of the gallbladder epithelium as an osteogenetic stimulus and the physiologic differentiation of connective tissue, J. Exper. Med. **58:** 393, 1933.
11. Keith, A.: Concerning the origin and nature of osteoblasts, Proc. Roy. Soc. Med. **21:** 301, 1927.
12. Lewis, D.: Myositis ossificans, J. A. M. A. **86:** 1281, 1923.
13. Loewi, G.: The stimulation of osteogenesis by urinary bladder tissue, J. Path. & Bact. **68:** 419, 1954.
14. Lyall, A.: Heterotopic bone formation with report of a case, Brit. J. Surg. **31:** 411, 1944.
15. McCurrich, H. J., and Millington, E.: Ossification in abdominal scars, Brit. J. Surg. **31:** 86, 1943.
16. Neuhof, H.: Fascia transplantation into visceral defects, Surg. Gynec. & Obst. **24:** 383, 1917.
17. Nicholson: Ossification in calcified epithelioma, J. Path. & Bact. **21:** 387, 1917.
18. Phemister, D. B.: Ossification in kidney stone attached to the renal pelvis, Ann. Surg. **78:** 239, 1923.
19. Rush, B. F., and Clifton, E. E.: Experimental reconstruction of the trachea with bladder mucosa, SURGERY **40:** 1105, 1956.
20. Sanders, R. L.: Bone formation in upper abdominal scars, Ann. Surg. **141:** 621, 1955.

# Evaluation of portal circulation by percutaneous splenic isotope injection

SEYMOUR I. SCHWARTZ, M.D.*
ROBERT H. GREENLAW, M.D.**
ROCHESTER, N. Y.
*From Departments of Surgery and Radiology, University of Rochester School of Medicine and Dentistry*

Evaluation of the portal circulation has provided the basis for establishing a diagnosis of esophageal varices and determining the patency of a portacaval shunt. This evaluation has been greatly refined by measurements of splenic pulp and hepatic vein wedge pressures and by the more liberal use of percutaneous splenoportography. More recently, techniques of isotopic evaluation have been applied to the portal circulation.

Deterling and associates[3] instilled radioactive sodium into the rectum and, by means of counting over the brachial artery, were able to determine the patency of portacaval shunts. Sigel and coauthors,[16] using $Na^{22}$ injected submucosally into the colon, demonstrated an absence of clearance associated with obstruction of the portal vein. Long and his colleagues[7] injected $Kr^{85}$ into the spleen of dogs and noted that the appearance and peak times of radioactivity measured in the expired air were significantly reduced in the presence of a patent portacaval shunt.

Mena and his group[10, 11] used twin scintillation detectors placed over the heart and liver to record the appearance of radioiodinated serum albumin (RISA), injected intravenously, in an effort to determine cardioportal circulation times. Finally, Iber and associates[5] investigated intrasplenic injection of an isotope with continuous sampling of hepatic and peripheral venous blood as a method of determining portal collateral flow in patients.

Our study with simultaneous external monitoring of the areas over the liver, right heart, and esophagus after percutaneous injection of an isotope into the spleen, has established diagnostic patterns for the normal and for a variety of abnormal types of portal circulation.

## MATERIALS AND METHODS

A Picker dual detection system (Fig. 1) was utilized in all laboratory and clinical studies. The system provided twin scintillation probes, twin rate meters and twin chart recorders. This permitted simultaneous recording of radioactivity in 2 areas of the body. One detector was placed over the right lobe of the liver and directed slightly laterally. The second probe was positioned over the right heart-lung root and included in its field of response the lower half of the esophagus. The rate meters were operated at 0.5 second time constants and the recorders were set at a speed of 12 inches per minute. The recorders were capable of full-scale response in 250 msec. and thus did not add delay to the meter response. Several tracer materials, including Radiorenographin and Hipputope,* were used. The only specification considered was a short biologic half-life. The laboratory and clinical studies were performed with 30 to 100 $\mu c$ of radioiodine in a volume of 1.0 ml. or less.

Received for publication Jan. 20, 1961.

*John and Mary R. Markle Scholar.

**Advanced Clinical Fellow in Radiation Therapy under the American Cancer Society.

*E. R. Squibb & Sons.

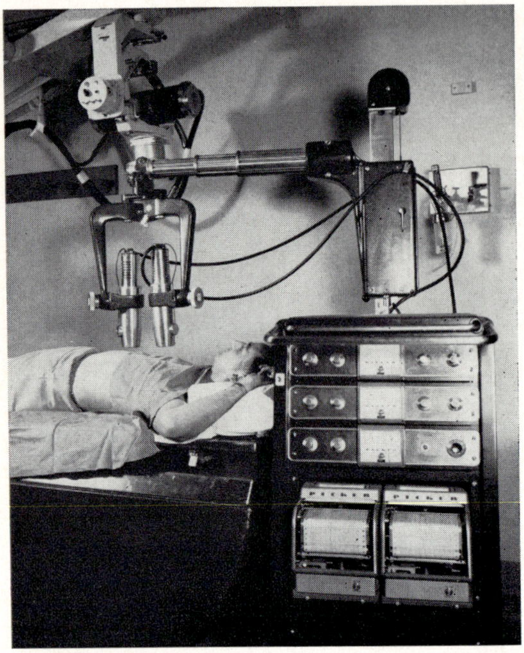

**Fig. 1.** Dual detection system with twin scintillation detectors, twin rate meters, and twin chart recorders.

**Laboratory studies.** Adult mongrel dogs were anesthetized with pentobarbital sodium and a laparotomy was performed. In the control series, after the probes had been positioned over the right lobe of the liver and the right heart-lung root, the isotope was injected into the parenchyma of the spleen under direct vision and simultaneous recordings were made. In other experiments, either the portal vein or splenic vein was occluded prior to splenic injection and, after the initial pattern had been recorded, the occlusion was released and a second pattern demonstrated. The final preparations studied were animals with patent and thrombosed end-to-side portacaval shunts.

**Clinical studies.** All studies were carried out with the patient in the supine position. Percutaneous splenic puncture was performed through the ninth intercostal space in the posterior axillary line after this region had been anesthetized with 3 to 5 ml. of 1 per cent Xylocaine. Measurements of splenic pulp pressure were made in all patients and, in the majority of the patients, concomitant splenoportography was carried out to correlate the findings of this accepted procedure with the results of the isotope curves. The radiologic technique included 3 exposures taken in rapid sequence beginning at the end of injection. In the latter group a No. 18 or 19 needle was used. Patients who were hemorrhaging massively or who for other reasons were studied in the Emergency Department or on the wards, did not undergo roentgenographic studies. In these cases a No. 20 needle was used to measure pressure and inject the isotope.

## RESULTS

**Laboratory studies.** Injection of 30 $\mu$c of $I^{131}$ into the spleens of 3 dogs and into the splenic vein of 1 dog produced similar results (Fig. 2). Radioactivity appeared in the liver in less than 2 seconds. The appearance slopes were steep and the plateau began to decrease after approximately 12 seconds. The isotope gradually appeared in the right heart-lung root 15 to 17 seconds after injection, concomitant with the decrease from the peak of radioactivity in the liver.

In 3 dogs with temporary occlusion of the portal vein, no radioactivity was monitored by either detector after splenic injection of 30 $\mu$c of $I^{131}$. This situation persisted throughout the period of occlusion and, when the occlusion was released in 2 of the dogs, tracings similar to those of the controls resulted. The animal with sustained occlusion continued to show no radioactivity in the liver or right heart-lung root.

Injection of isotope into the spleens of dogs with patent end-to-side portacaval shunts demonstrated a rapid appearance (less than 2 seconds) and a high peak in the right heart-lung root. A minimal temporary rise ("blip") over the liver was noted which reflected the passage of $I^{131}$ through the inferior vena cava as it coursed behind the liver. No radioactivity was monitored over the liver or heart after splenic injection of $I^{131}$ in a dog with an end-to-side portacaval shunt which had been thrombosed several hours prior to study. Direct injection of the isotope into the vena cava caudad to the liver yielded tracings similar to those obtained with splenic injections in dogs with patent portacaval shunts. A high peak of radioactivity appeared over the right heart-lung root in less than 2 seconds and a transient "blip" in the region of the liver which reflected retrohepatic caval flow was also noted.

**Clinical studies.** The patients studied were classified into 5 major groups and a consistently distinctive pattern was demonstrated for each group. The 5 groups included normal patients and patients with portal hypertension without varices, with esophageal varices, with portal vein thrombosis, and with portal-systemic shunts. The individual times for appearance, peak, and plateau of the radioactivity over the liver and the right heart-lung root (esophagus) are listed in Table I. "Appearance time" refers to the number of seconds from initiation of splenic injection until the scintillation detector responded to radioactivity. "Peak time" indicates the duration between isotope injection and maximal radioactivity. In instances in which maximal activity over the liver was temporarily sustained, the interval between the onset of maximal activity and the beginning of decrease from this peak was computed and is defined as "plateau time." This measurement was used to evaluate the rate of flow through the liver.

Twenty-five isotopic evaluations of the portal circulation were performed on 20 patients. Fifteen of these patients were studied in the Radiology Suite to permit correlation of the splenoportography and the remaining investigations were performed at the patient's bedside.

*Normal patients.* The normal patterns of the simultaneous isotope tracings are shown in Fig. 3. As noted in these tracings, the appearance in the liver and the peak occurred early. The hepatic plateau was not prolonged. The detection of radioactivity over the right heart-lung root was delayed, followed the liver peak, and was concomitant with the decrease in liver radioactivity. This isotope evaluation anticipated the patient's normal splenoportogram.

Normal tracings were demonstrated in 5 patients who were studied to determine either the cause of upper gastrointestinal bleeding or splenomegaly. In each instance, the appearance and peak of radioactivity in the liver significantly preceded the appearance and peak times over the right heart root. In all patients the splenic pulp pressures were normal, that is, less than 160 mm. $H_2O$. The 3 patients in whom splenoportography was carried out demonstrated normal hepatic arborization with no evidence of collaterals.

*Patients with portal hypertension without varices.* In this group, the typical tracings demonstrated a delay in the spleen-to-heart circulation coupled with normal spleen-to-liver times. The appearance and peak time for radioactivity over the liver were rapid and similar to those in the normal study. The pertinent diagnostic finding in this group of patients was a prolongation in circulation through the liver as noted in the plateau times (Table I). Four patients with

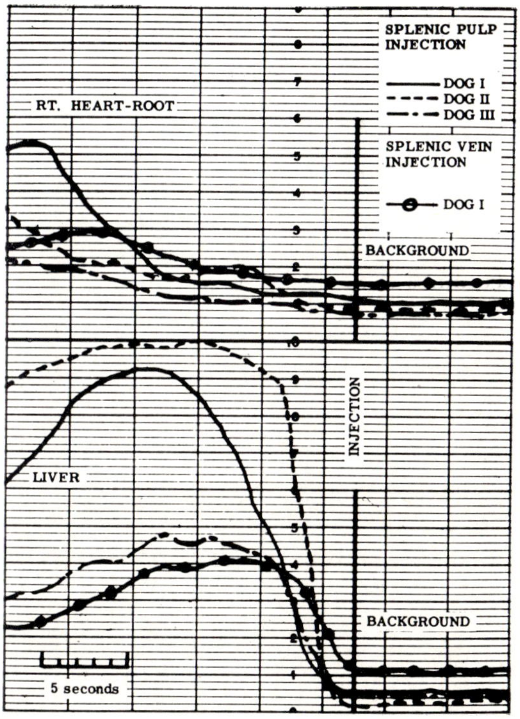


**Fig. 2.** Injection of isotope (30 $\mu c$ of $I^{131}$ as sodium iodide, 0.5 second time constant, 30 K maximum response, 12 inches per minute) into splenic pulp and vein of normal dogs.

**Table I.** *Isotopic evaluation of portal circulation*

| Patient | *Liver* | | | *Right heart root (esophagus)* | |
|---|---|---|---|---|---|
| | *Appearance (sec.)* | *Peak (sec.)* | *Plateau (sec.)* | *Appearance (sec.)* | *Peak (sec.)* |
| *Normal patients* | | | | | |
| E. S. | 0.5 | 3 | 2 | 6 | 21 |
| F. R. | 1 | 5 | 7 | 10 | 22 |
| G. R. | 1 | 4 | 6 | 10 | 17 |
| A. L. | 1 | 3 | 7 | 10 | 12 |
| A. C. | 0.5 | 6 | 6 | 10 | 22 |
| *Patients with portal hypertension without varices* | | | | | |
| A. W. | 0.5 | 3 | 14 | 10 | 17 |
| J. E. | 0.5 | 4 | 30 | 7 | — |
| C. M. | 0.5 | 7 | 10 | 8 | 18 |
| P. B. | 1 | 5 | 8 | 12 | 21 |
| *Patients with esophageal varices* | | | | | |
| W. P. | 2 | 7 | 13 | 0.5 | 7 |
| C. G. | 3 | — | — | 1 | — |
| A. K. | 7 | 12 | 8 | 3 | 10 |
| S. K. | 15 (trace) | — | — | 5 | 11 |
| R. M. | 2 (trace) | — | — | 0.5 | 8 |
| B. M. | 2 | 6 | — | 0.5 | 2 |
| C. A.* | 1 | 5 | — | 0.5 | 7 |
| *Patients with portal vein thrombosis* | | | | | |
| E. K. | No radioactivity | | | 12 second (trace) | |
| *Patients with portal-systemic shunt* | | | | | |
| E. G. | Transient rise (inferior vena cava) | | | 4 | 7 |
| R. M. | Transient rise (inferior vena cava) | | | 4 | 8 |
| C. W. | Transient rise (paraumbilical vein) | | | 7 | 10 |

*Gastric varices seen on portogram. No coronary vein or esophageal varices visualized. Esophagoscopy demonstrated small varices.

cirrhosis confirmed by liver function studies and, in some instances, by needle biopsy were classified in this group. All of these patients had portal hypertension as evidenced by splenic pulp pressures in excess of 220 mm. $H_2O$. In each of these patients no collaterals could be demonstrated on splenoportography.

*Patients with esophageal varices.* Seven patients with esophageal varices secondary to portal hypertension were studied. It is to be stressed that, in the situation of esophageal varices, the probe over the right heart root was essentially monitoring response in the lower half of the esophagus. In each case (Table I), the diagnostic finding of a spleen-to-liver appearance time greater than the spleen-to-esophagus appearance time was apparent. The right heart root (esophageal) peak was also earlier and higher than that detected over the liver area, which indicated preferential flow via the coronary vein and ancillary collateral veins. Representative simultaneous isotope tracings are shown in Fig. 4.

All 7 patients had the diagnosis of esophageal varices substantiated by splenoportography, barium swallow, or esophagoscopy. Patient C. A. was unusual in that although the istotope appeared first over the esophagus, the peak was earlier and higher over the liver. Small gastric varices were seen on the portogram but the coronary vein, esophageal varices, and major collaterals were not visualized. Esophagoscopy showed small varices in the distal end of the esophagus.

One patient was studied at the bedside after a Sengstaken-Blakemore tube had been inserted as treatment for bleeding esophageal varices. The initial tracings were recorded with the esophageal balloon inflated to a pressure of 45 mm. Hg. Fig. 5, *A* shows the tracing with the balloon inflated and demonstrates a gradual slope of radioactivity in the right heart root (esophagus) as contrasted with the steep slope seen when the balloon was deflated (Fig. 5, *B*).

*Patients with portal vein thrombosis.* One patient, E. K., with acute thrombosis of the portal vein, was investigated. This patient had rapid onset of ascites and distended abdominal wall veins 10 days after drainage of an empyema of the gall bladder. Studies performed 3 weeks after the suspected portal vein thrombosis showed no appearance of $I^{131}$ over the liver and a very gradual and minimal evidence of radioactivity in the right heart root (Fig. 6). A splenoportogram recorded the pathologic anatomy.

*Patients with portal-systemic shunt.* Three patients with portal-systemic shunts were included in this category (Table I). In each case, although the $I^{131}$ appeared relatively early in the right heart root, the impressive finding was the occurrence of an early and extremely high peak of radioactivity in this region. It is to be noted that with a portal-systemic shunt the appearance did not occur as rapidly as in the group of patients with esophageal varices. However, the peak was significantly earlier and higher. This difference in appearance time was to be anticipated since, in the case of a portal-systemic shunt, the course of the isotope was from spleen to splenic vein to inferior vena cava and finally to right atrium where it was detected. In comparison, the flow of isotope in patients with esophageal varices was from spleen to splenic vein to coronary vein and esophagus where it was monitored earlier.

Two of the patients were studied subsequent to a surgically created end-to-side portacaval shunt. A set of representative tracings is shown in Fig. 7. In this situation, the transient rise over the region of the liver reflected the flow of isotope through the inferior vena cava as it passed behind the liver. C. W., the third patient in this group, was investigated because of marked meat intoxication associated with minimal abnormalities in the liver function tests. The transient rise in the region of the liver and the rapid and high peak over the right heart root suggested a large pathologic portal-systemic shunt. The splenoportogram con-

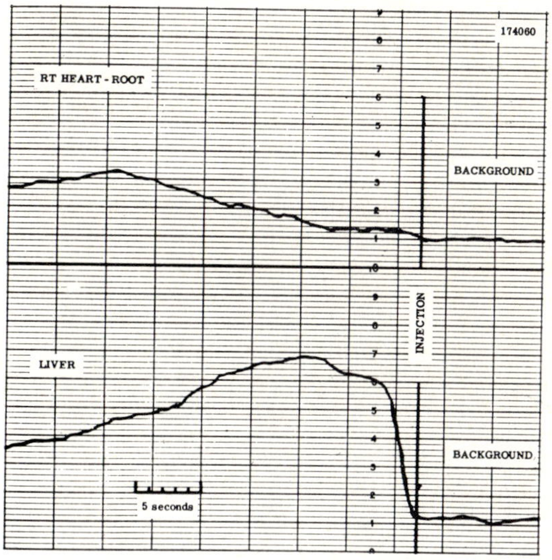


**Fig. 3.** Normal simultaneous tracings (100 $\mu c$ of $I^{131}$ as Renographin, 0.5 second time constant, 100 K maximum response, 12 inches per minute).

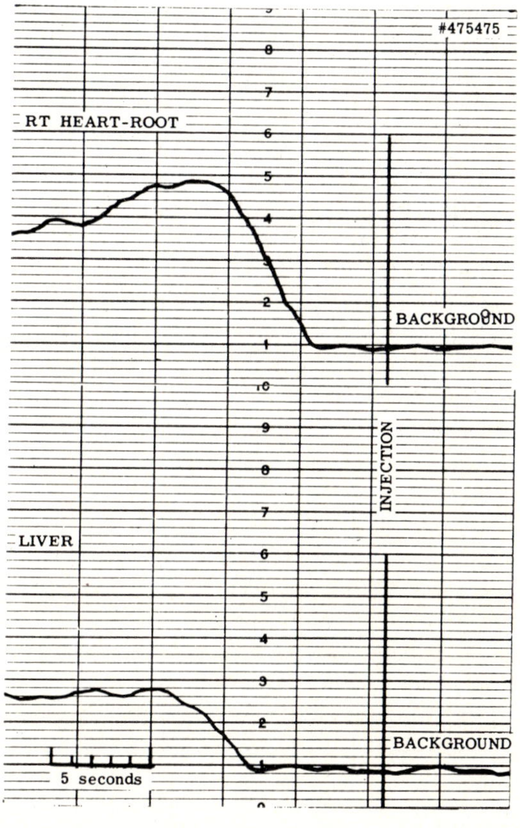


**Fig. 4.** Simultaneous tracings from patient with esophageal varices (100 $\mu c$ of $I^{131}$ as ISA, 0.5 second time constant, 100 K maximum response, 12 inches per minute).

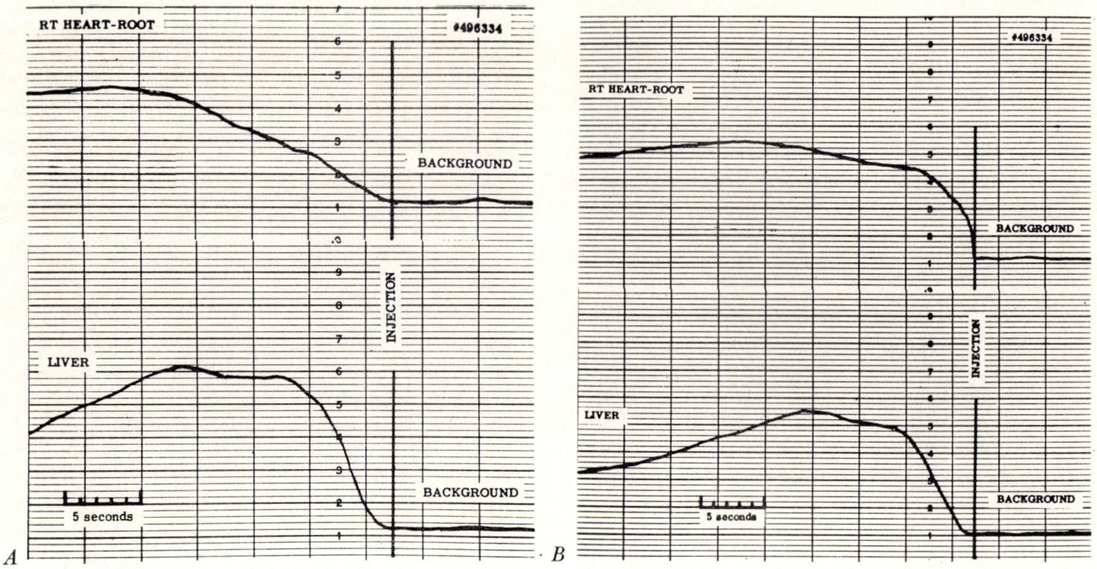


**Fig. 5.** *A,* Esophageal varices (50 μc of $I^{131}$ as Renographin, 0.5 second time constant, 30 K maximum response, 12 inches per minute). Esophageal balloon inflated. *B,* Esophageal balloon deflated.

firmed this pathologic process and demonstrated a large paraumbilical vein and an absence of flow through the liver.

## DISCUSSION

The isotopic evaluation of portal circulation is particularly applicable to the differential diagnosis of acute upper gastrointestinal bleeding. Esophagogastric varices have been implicated as the cause of massive hematemesis in 32 per cent[18] of the patients. Since the management of bleeding varices differs significantly from that of the other causes, it is important to establish a diagnosis on an emergency basis.

Efforts directed at early diagnosis have been suggested. Esophagoscopy requires a skilled endoscopist and interpretation is difficult during the active phase of bleeding. As an elective study, barium swallow has a high percentage of false-negative results which is increased during the acute bleeding episode.[6]

Tests of liver function, such as the Bromsulphalein test, have proved unreliable since they define the presence of liver disease but not necessarily varices.[9] The qualitative test for hyperammoniemia as described by McDermott[9] is more pertinent because the elevation of the ammonia level is due to an extensive portal-systemic collateral circulation and is not indicative of hepatic function. However, as pointed out by the author, pretreatment with antibiotics, glutamic acid, or arginine will negate the value of this test. Also, any large portal-systemic collateral such as a paraumbilical vein or a portarenal shunt will cause a positive result in the absence of esophagogastric varices. Finally, McDermott presented a documented case of hemorrhage from varices with a negative qualitative test result and a quantitative ammonia determination which showed only slight elevation.

Esophageal balloon tamponade has been used but presents certain disadvantages. Reports have indicated failure to control hemorrhage in 25 to 55 per cent of patients with bleeding varices.[4, 8, 12, 14, 15] Also, bleeding from gastric ulcer has been completely arrested by this apparatus.[1] In addition, the hazards associated with tamponade are significant.[2]

Panke and associates[13] proposed splenic pulp manometry as an emergency test. A 90 per cent accuracy was reported, but there was a zone of splenic pulp pressures which included those of patients bleeding from varices and from other causes. In our limited series, we have noted 4 patients (Table I) with portal hypertension unaccompanied by the development of pathways of collateral flow. Furthermore, the admittedly rare situation of esophageal varices associated with normal portal pressures would not be diagnosed by this technique.

Splenoportography affords diagnostic evidence of esophageal varices in a very high percentage of cases but requires an experienced team of technicians. It is rarely used for patients who are actively bleeding since transportation to the Radiology Department and patient cooperation are difficult to achieve.

The technique of isotopic evaluation of portal circulation proposed in this study is simple, can be performed at the patient's bedside, and, therefore, is applicable to patients with massive hematemesis. The dual detector system is run by 1 man and minimal training is required. Diagnosis can be made immediately and interpretation is not dependent upon techniques of exposure and development as in the case of splenoportography. In addition, for the emergency situation when the prothrombin time is not always available, the dangers of splenic rupture and hemorrhage are theoretically reduced since only a small-bore needle and a 1 ml. bolus are introduced into the spleen. Finally, in the patient with acute bleeding to whom balloon tamponade is applied as emergency treatment, the efficacy of the pressure may be determined by comparison of the initial tracing with a second series taken with the balloon inflated.

For elective preoperative studies, isotopic investigation of portal circulation complements splenoportography. While the latter demonstrates the pathologic anatomy, the former permits an evaluation of the dynamic physiologic function of the portal circulation. After insertion of the needle, the injection of the isotope and the monitoring of radioactivity over the liver and heart are used to indicate correct intrasplenic position of the needle. Measurement of the splenic pulp pressure and the splenoportogram are then performed in rapid succession without removal of the needle. Also, by determining the appearance and peak times of radioactivity over the liver, heart, and esophagus, the roentgenograms can be timed for optimum demonstration of the anatomy. Postoperatively, the technique graphically demonstrates the patency or occlusion of a portacaval shunt.

A qualitative determination of the dynamics of flow, rather than a static picture, is particularly appropriate in the investigation of hepatic-portal encephalopathy. This neuropsychiatric syndrome of liver disease is more closely related to the extent of collateral blood flow than to the degree of portal hypertension or to the presence of a specific collateral vessel.[17] The technique of simultaneous isotope detection proposed in this study provides a direct evaluation of relative flows through the liver and along the course of bypassing portal-systemic shunts.

## SUMMARY

After percutaneous injection of isotope tracer compounds into the spleen, circula-

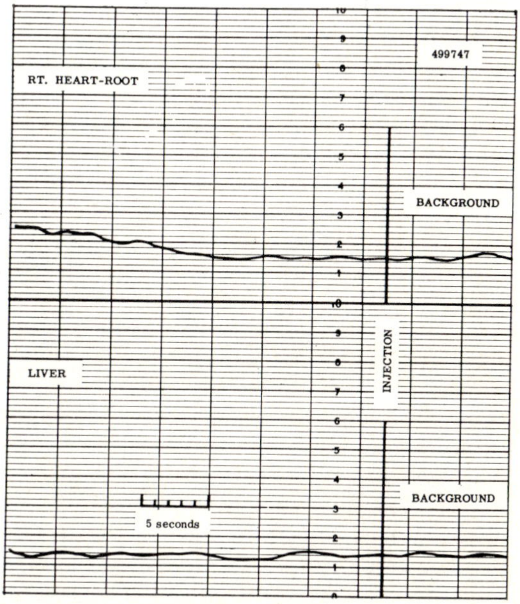


**Fig. 6.** Simultaneous tracings from patients with portal vein thrombosis (40 $\mu$c of $I^{131}$ as Hipputope, 30 K maximum response, 0.5 second time constant, 12 inches per minute).

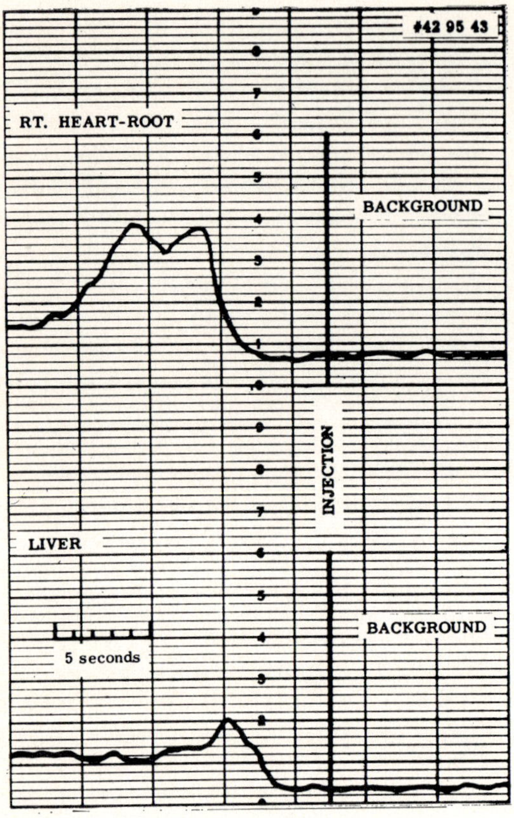


**Fig. 7.** Simultaneous tracings from patients with patent end-to-side portacaval shunts (30 μc of $I^{131}$ as sodium iodide, 0.5 second time constant, 30 K maximum response, 12 inches per minute).

tion times to the liver, right heart, and esophagus are measured simultaneously by means of twin scintillation detectors. The relative appearance times, peaks, and durations of sustained radioactivity over the liver and right heart (esophagus) afford a clear appraisal of portal circulation.

Diagnostic patterns of isotope flow are established for 5 clinical situations—normal, portal hypertension without varices, esophageal varices, portal vein thrombosis, and portal-systemic shunts.

The advantages of the technique are simplicity and adaptability for use at the patient's bedside. Its use in the emergency differential diagnosis of upper gastrointestinal bleeding is emphasized. For elective evaluation, the isotope study complements the splenoportogram and is particularly applicable to the investigation of hepatic-portal encephalopathy.

## REFERENCES

1. Bixby, E. W., Jr.: Correspondence, J. A. M. A. **159:** 1480, 1955.
2. Conn, H. O.: Hazards attending the use of esophageal tamponade, New England J. Med. **259:** 701, 1958.
3. Deterling, R. A., Jr., Powers, S. R., and Bhonslay, S. B.: The use of radioactive sodium in the determination of patency of portacaval shunts, S. Forum **5:** 193, 1954.
4. Hamilton, J. E.: The management of bleeding esophageal varices associated with cirrhosis of the liver, Ann. Surg. **141:** 637, 1955.
5. Iber, F. L., Kerr, Dolle W., and Sherlock, S.: Measurement of blood flow in the collateral vessels of the portal vein: preliminary results of a new method, J. Clin. Invest. **39:** 1201, 1960.
6. Knowles, H. C., Felson, B., Shapiro, N., and Schiff, L.: Emergency diagnosis of upper digestive tract by roentgen examination without palpation (Hampton technic) Radiology **58:** 536, 1952.
7. Long, R. T. L., Lombardo, C. R., and Braunwald, E.: Use of radioactive krypton and cardio-green dilution curves in the detection of experimental portal-systemic shunts, Ann. Surg. **151:** 146, 1960.
8. Ludington, L. G.: A study of 158 cases of esophageal varices, Surg. Gynec. & Obst. **106:** 519, 1958.
9. McDermott, W. V., Jr.: A simple discriminating test for upper gastrointestinal hemorrhage, New England J. Med. **257:** 1161, 1957.
10. Mena, I., Bennett, L. R., and Mellinkoff, S. M.: Hemodynamic patterns in portal cirrhosis determined by external scintillation detection, J. Clin. Invest. **38:** 1025, 1959.
11. Mena, I., Bennett, L. R., Reynolds, T. B., Redeker, A. G., and Mellinkoff, S. M.: Analysis of cardioportal circulation time by means of simultaneous direct hepatic venous counting, New England J. Med. **263:** 940, 1960.
12. Nachlas, M. M., O'Neil, J. E., and Campbell, A. J. A.: The life history of patients with cirrhosis of the liver and bleeding esophageal varices, Ann. Surg. **141:** 10, 1955.
13. Panke, W. F., Rousselot, L. M., and Moreno, A. H.: Splenic pulp manometry as an emergency test in the differential diagnosis of acute upper gastrointestinal bleeding, Surg. Gynec. & Obst. **109:** 270, 1959.
14. Reynolds, T. B., Freedman, T., and Winsor, W.: Results of the treatment of bleeding eso-

phageal varices with balloon tamponage, Am. J. M. Sc. **224:** 500, 1952.

15. Schwartz, S. I.: The management of acute bleeding from esophageal varices, New York J. Med. **59:** 3584, 1959.
16. Sigel, B., Kiernan, T. J., Blum, A. S., and Wolcott, M. W.: Measurement of acute portal obstruction by clearance of radioactive sodium from the colon, SURGERY **47:** 571, 1960.
17. Summerskill, W. H. J., Davidson, E. A., Sherlock, S., and Steiner, R. E.: The neuropsychiatric syndrome associated with hepatic cirrhosis and excessive portal collateral circulation, Quart. J. Med. **25:** 245, 1956.
18. Welch, C. E., Allen, A. W., and Donalson, G. A.: Surgical management of acute upper gastrointestinal hemorrhage, New England J. Med. **252:** 921, 1955.

# Complete homograft replacement of the heart and both lungs

RICHARD R. LOWER, M.D.*
RAYMOND C. STOFER, D.V.M.
EDWARD J. HURLEY, M.D.*
NORMAN E. SHUMWAY, M.D.**
PALO ALTO, CALIF.
*From the Department of Surgery, Stanford University School of Medicine*

The failure of previous attempts at experimental homotransplantation of the heart and both lungs has been attributed to respiratory paralysis.[7, 17] The observations to be reported demonstrate that complete homograft replacement of the heart and lungs is at present technically feasible and that spontaneous respiration resumes which will sustain life until homograft rejection supervenes.

## METHOD

Mongrel dogs which weighed 14 to 17 kilograms were used in these experiments. The donor and recipient animals were anesthetized intravenously with 30 mg. of pentobarbital sodium per kilogram of body weight, intubated, and ventilated with 100 per cent oxygen. The donor was prepared by exposure of the thoracic organs through the right fifth intercostal space. The azygos vein was ligated and divided. The superior and inferior venae cavae were mobilized for division at least 2 cm. from the right atrium. The heart and lungs were further mobilized by division of the pulmonary ligaments, the diaphragmatic reflection of the pericardium, and the anterior mediastinal reflection of the pleura. Tapes were passed about the venae cavae, ascending aorta, and trachea. Two milligrams of heparin per kilogram was injected intravenously.

Supported in part by National Heart Institute, Grant No. H-4658.

Received for publication Jan. 6, 1961.

*Fellow, National Heart Institute, United States Public Health Service.

**Established Investigator, American Heart Association.

A similar thoracotomy incision was made in the recipient animal. The heart and lungs were mobilized and careful hemostasis utilized. The phrenic nerves were dissected free of the pericardium and preserved. Ligation of the bronchial vessels with careful preservation of the vagus nerves required meticulous dissection of the posterior mediastinum. Heparin in a dosage of 2 mg. per kilogram was administered and the animal was prepared for cardiopulmonary bypass. The venous cannulas were inserted peripherally through the right jugular and femoral veins and the catheter tips were advanced to a position approximately 3 cm. from the right atrium. Oxygenated blood was returned to the animal through a cannula in the femoral artery. After institution of cardiac bypass, the venae cavae were occluded with noncrushing clamps just proximal to the venous catheter tips, the ascending aorta was clamped near the bracheocephalic vessels, and the heart and lungs were removed by division of the venae cavae, trachea, and aorta just distal to the coronary ostia. During bypass the animal's temperature was lowered to 28° to 30° C. by priming of the oxygenator initially with cold blood.

Excision of the donor heart and lungs was accomplished rapidly; the vagus and phrenic nerves were not preserved and the bronchial vessels were not ligated. A 1 cm. cuff was left on the venae cavae and on the ascending aorta, and the trachea was divided about 2 cm. above the carina. The donor organs were immediately immersed in normal saline solution at approximately 4° C. for 10 minutes and no saline was allowed to enter the trachea. After being cooled in this manner, the heart and lungs were placed in the recipient thorax and anastomosis of the aorta, trachea, and venae cavae carried out with fine silk sutures. The caval and aortic clamps were removed to restore coronary blood flow and, after rewarming, the animal was electrically defibrillated. After 15 to 20 minutes of support by the pump-oxygenator, bypass was discontinued and the wound closed in layers. A chest catheter was left in place for postoperative drainage and penicillin-streptomycin mixture was administered daily.

## RESULTS

Six recipient dogs resumed spontaneous respirations after the operative procedure. Oxygenation remained adequate but the respiratory pattern was altered in that tidal volume was increased and the respiratory rate was diminished. There was an occasional marked prolongation of the expiratory phase. Four of the animals died of surgical complications 5 to 24 hours after the onset of spontaneous breathing.

The remaining 2 animals recovered fully except for temporary gastrointestinal ileus, presumably due to vagus nerve injury during dissection and ligation of the bronchial vessels. They were ambulatory, active, and eating until they became lethargic on the fourth postoperative day. At this time the arterial oxygen content of 1 animal was 14.21 vol. per cent with an oxygen capacity of 18.19 vol. per cent (78.2 per cent saturation). The arterial carbon dioxide content was 48.8 vol. per cent (method of Van Slyke and Neill). Both animals died on the fifth postoperative day of respiratory insufficiency.

At autopsy the lungs of these 2 dogs were found to be heavy and firm (Fig. 1) and the tracheobronchial tree contained a considerable amount of blood-tinged exudate. The tracheal suture lines appeared to be healing in normal fashion. Microscopically there was considerable atelectasis, but the most striking finding was an extensive infiltration of large mononuclear cells which appeared to be primarily histiocytes (Fig. 2). In some areas there were perivascular infiltrates of typical plasma cells and scattered large unidentified cells resembling Dorothy Reed histiocytes. Except in a few microscopic areas, vascular thrombosis and necrosis of pulmonary tissue were absent. Grossly the heart appeared normal (Fig. 3), but microscopically showed in-

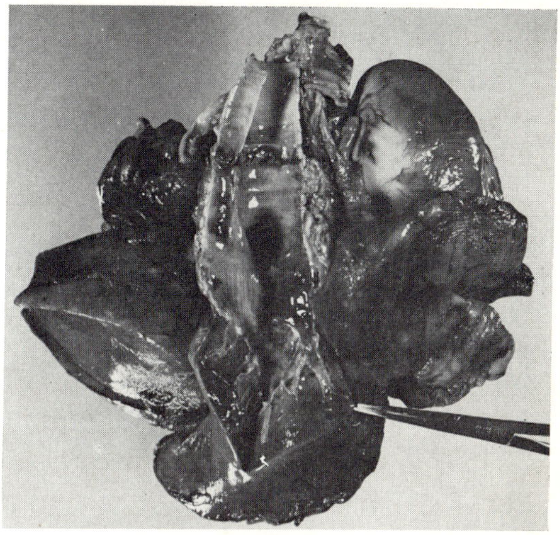

**Fig. 1.** The homograft heart and lungs 5 days after transplantation. The lungs are firm, heavy, and airless.

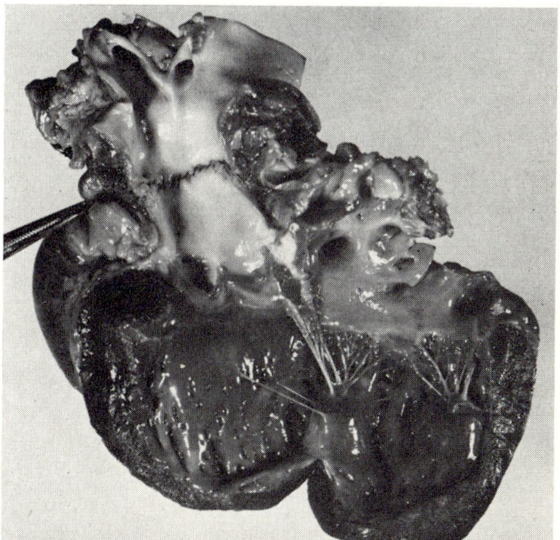

**Fig. 2.** The heart (same specimen as in Fig. 1) appears grossly normal 5 days after homotransplantation.

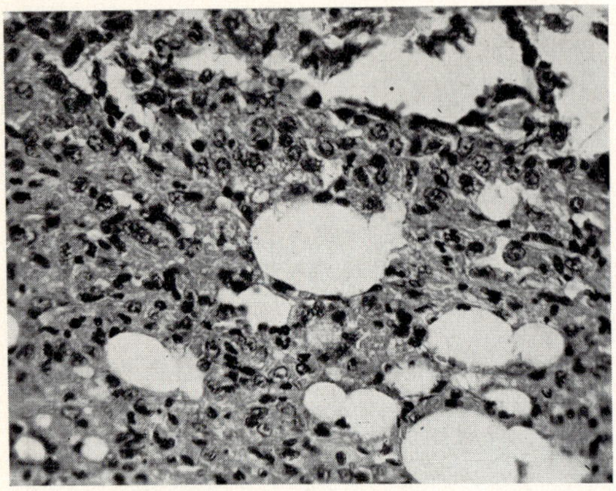

**Fig. 3.** Photomicrograph of the lung parenchyma shows an infiltration of histiocytes. (×525; reduced ⅖.)

filtration of the myocardium with mononuclear cells, primarily the plasma-cell variety, and a few small areas of myocardial necrosis. The changes in the myocardium were much less extensive than those observed with cardiac homografts of longer duration.[13]

## DISCUSSION

Homotransplantation of the heart and lungs as a unit would have obvious clinical application in conditions in which irreparable or irreversible pathologic processes exist in both organs. This experimental study was designed, therefore, to determine the technical feasibility of such a procedure and to elucidate the effects of sacrificing the bronchial arterial supply and the pulmonary nerve supply.

The bronchial arteries were originally thought to be indispensable for nutrition of the mainstem and lobar bronchi.[3] However, experimental reimplantation of the autologous lung with subsequent prolonged observation of viability proved that the bronchial supply can be sacrificed without resulting necrosis.[10, 14, 15] The major problem which the bronchial vessels presented in this study was ligation in the recipient animal without injury to the vagus nerves which are in proximity.

The question of the possibility of prolonged survival after pulmonary denervation remains unanswered. The normal respiratory pattern occurs as a result of both central and peripheral neural control.[4] It is evident that the sacrifice of peripheral innervation which necessarily accompanies pulmonary transplantation results not in respiratory paralysis, but in an altered respiratory pattern which resembles that observed after bilateral cervical vagotomy. The adequacy of this pattern for normal ventilation over prolonged periods and for maintenance of respiratory equilibrium under various stresses remains to be demonstrated. Reimplantation of both autologous lungs or prolongation of homograft acceptance would provide the opportunity for such observations.

The histologic findings in the 2 animals which survived for 5 days are at variance with those described previously in lung homografts. Hume[9] has recently reviewed the prior experience with pulmonary homotransplantation reported by Staudacher,[16] Lanari,[11, 12] and others.[1, 2, 5, 6, 8] The early changes described by these authors were alveolar edema and polymorphonuclear leukocyte infiltration progressing to lymphocytic infiltration, vascular thrombosis, and frank necrosis of parenchymal tissue in the animals which survived for longer periods. None of these conditions was prominent in the pathologic material studied in this experiment. The prominent feature was an extensive infiltration of large mononuclear cells which apparently caused death by interference with respiration at the alveolar level.

## SUMMARY

Complete homograft replacement of the heart and both lungs in the dog has been carried out with survival of 2 animals for 5 days. These animals resumed spontaneous breathing with an altered respiratory pattern. Death from respiratory insufficiency was apparently due to infiltration of mononuclear cells into the lung parenchyma.

### REFERENCES

1. Davis, H. A., O'Connor, J. P., Coloviras, G. J., Jr., and Strawn, D. L.: Homologous transplantation of the lung, A. M. A. Arch. Surg. **64:** 745, 1952.

2. Ellis, E. E., and Richards, V.: The fate of homologous lung transplants in dogs, SURGERY **36:** 1109, 1954.
3. Ellis, F. H., Jr., Grindlay, J. H., and Edwards, J. E.: The bronchial arteries. I. Experimental occlusion, SURGERY **30:** 810, 1951.
4. Gray, J. S.: Pulmonary ventilation and its physiologic regulator, Springfield, 1950, Charles C Thomas, Publisher.
5. Hardin, C. A., and Kittle, C. F.: Experiences with transplantation of the lung, Science **119:** 97, 1954.
6. Hardin, C. A., Kittle, C. F., and Schafer, P. W.: Preliminary observations on homologous lung transplants in dogs, S. Forum **3:** 374, 1952.
7. Howard, H. S., and Webb, W. R.: Respiratory paralysis following pulmonary denervation, S. Forum **8:** 466, 1957.
8. Hughes, F. A., Kehne, J. H., and Fox, J. R.: Replantation and transplantation of pulmonary tissue in dogs, SURGERY **36:** 1101, 1954.
9. Hume, D. M.: Transplantation of lung *in* Peer, L. A.: Transplantation of tissues, Baltimore, 1959, Williams & Wilkins Company, vol. 2, p. 473.
10. Juvenelle, A. A., Citret, C., Wiles, C. E., Jr., and Stewart, J. D.: Pneumonectomy with replantation of the lung in the dog for physiologic study, J. Thoracic Surg. **21:** 111, 1951.
11. Lanari, A., Croxatto, O. C., and Molins, M. E.: Homogreffe et autogreffe du poumon chez le chien, Poumon & coeur **12:** 67, 1956.
12. Lanari, A., Molins, N., and Croxatto, O. C.: Homoinjertos de pulmón en perros. Técnica y resultados funcionales y antómicos, An. Cáted. pat. y clín. tuberc. **12:** 5, 1950.
13. Lower, R. R., and Shumway, N. E.: Studies on orthotopic homotransplantation of the canine heart, S. Forum **11:** 18, 1960.
14. Neptune, W. B., Redondo, H., and Bailey, C. P.: Experimental lung transplantation, S. Forum **3:** 379, 1952.
15. Portin, B. A., Rasmussen, G. L., Stewart, J. D., and Andersen, M. N.: Physiologic and anatomic studies 35 months after successful replantation of the lung, J. Thoracic Surg. **39:** 380, 1960.
16. Staudacher, V. E., Bellinazzo, P., and Pulin, A.: Primi rilievi su tentativi di reimpianti autoplastici e di trapianti omoplastici di lobi polmonari, Chirurgia **5:** 223, 1950.
17. Webb, W. R., Howard, H. S., and Neely, W. A.: Practical methods of homologous cardiac transplantation, J. Thoracic Surg. **37:** 361, 1959.

# Use of the Cheatle-Henry approach in the treatment of cryptorchidism


SIDNEY LIPTON, M.D.

BROOKLYN, N. Y.

*From Maimonides Hospital and State University of New York College of Medicine*


The objective of the surgical treatment of cryptorchidism is to advance the undescended testis into the scrotum. Adequate spermatic cord length must be obtained to permit the testis to reside, without tension, in its new domicile.

The most widely used operations are the Torek[6] and Bevan[1] procedures, with various modifications. Currently, the two-stage Torek technique is in disfavor because fixation of the testis to the thigh can result in vascular impairment of the testis from tension on the cord. The Bevan procedure, which involves tedious dissection of the cord within the inguinal canal, can also lead to damage to the spermatic vessels.

In the operation popularized by Gross,[3] the cord is elongated by retroperitoneal dissection. This method is also advocated by Swenson.[5] To approach the components of the cord in their retroperitoneal position, the deep epigastric vessels are severed and the floor of the inguinal canal is divided. The vas deferens and internal spermatic vessels are then lengthened by stripping adhesive bands and peritoneum by blunt and sharp dissection. The cord is brought through the floor of the inguinal canal just above the pubic tubercle. The floor of the canal is reconstructed by suturing the transversalis fascia over the cord.

Gross' operation has several inherent defects. First, the exposure of the retroperitoneal portion of the cord is not satisfactory and a considerable portion of the dissection is done blindly. Second, the previously ligated sac is frequently torn in the dissection and closure of the thin peritoneum is difficult and frustrating. Third, the division of the inguinal floor and the creation of a new internal ring at a vulnerable site in the floor may contribute to the later development of a direct hernia. Gross[3] acknowledges this possibility, but he stated that he had not seen a direct hernia occurring postoperatively. There has been, however, no report of long-term follow-up studies.

The procedure proposed in this communication is adapted from the Cheatle-Henry[2, 4] approach and is designed to overcome the

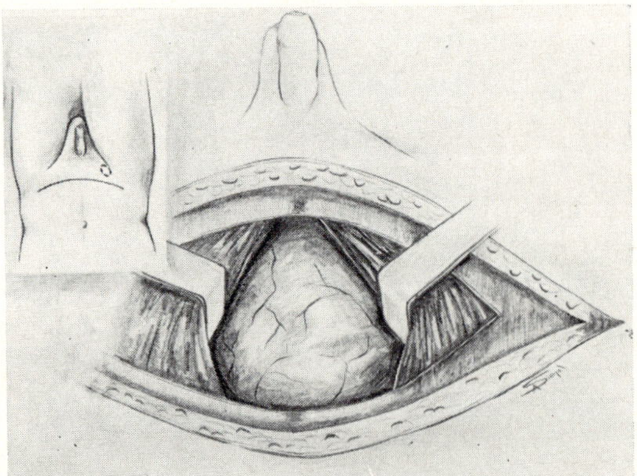

**Fig. 1.** The inset shows the Pfannenstiel incision. The rectus fascia has been divided transversely and dissected off the muscles. The recti are retracted to exposing the preperitoneal space.


Received for publication Dec. 7, 1960.

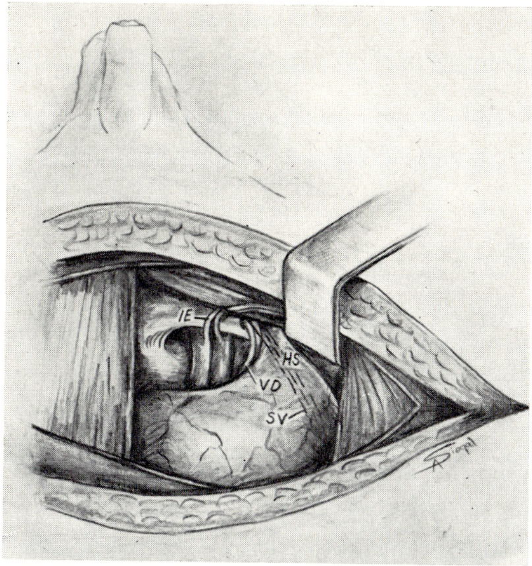


**Fig. 2.** The ipsilateral rectus muscle has been retracted laterally to expose the undersurface of the inguinal floor. The sac (*HS*), vas deferens (*VD*), and spermatic vessels (*SV*) are seen entering the internal inguinal ring. *IE,* internal epigastric vessels.

stated objections. I have been interested in this novel approach to groin hernias and have used the method in 20 cases. In the course of study of this technique, I was impressed with the admirable exposure of the cord structures. This led to the conclusion that the Cheatle-Henry procedure could be applied to the correction of cryptorchidism. The operation has been employed in a case of unilateral cryptorchidism and a case of bilateral cryptorchidism with complete success. A curvilinear suprapubic incision is made extending across both recti (Fig. 1, inset). The rectus fascia is divided transversely from one linea semilunaris to the other. The lower fascial flap is freed down to the pubis. The upper flap is freed for 1 inch from the underlying muscles. The recti are then separated in the midline starting at the pubis and proceeding in a cephalad direction (Fig. 1). The peritoneum is swept away from the overlying rectus and transversalis muscles. The inguinal floor, internal rings, and hernial sac are exposed (Fig. 2). The deep epigastric vessels are divided between ligatures to facilitate dissection about the internal ring. The sac stands out as a taut, funnel-shaped structure. The vessels are on the posterolateral aspect of the sac. The vas enters the internal ring independently. It can be freed and traced down to the base of the bladder. The sac is opened on its anterior aspect. The posterior wall of the sac is incised from within outward. The entire sac, now freed (at one point) from the cord, is stripped upward and a high ligation is performed. The spermatic vessels can now be dissected to the renal pedicle under complete visual control. The peritoneum is intimately adherent to the spermatic vessels. In stripping the peritoneum off the vessels, one can observe the vessels to lengthen and assume a lax position (Fig. 3). If the peritoneum is torn, it can be easily repaired. When, in the judgment of the operator, the vessels and vas have assumed sufficient length, the peritoneum is allowed to fall back. The peritoneum of the opposite side is then stripped off the anterior abdominal wall and the inguinal floor inspected for a hernia. If found, it may be corrected by excision of the sac and repair of the defect.

The skin of the inguinal portion of the incision on the involved side is retracted down-

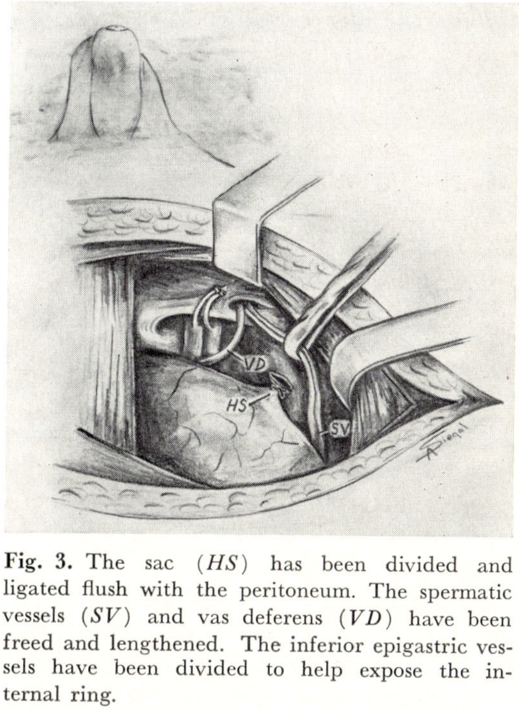


**Fig. 3.** The sac (*HS*) has been divided and ligated flush with the peritoneum. The spermatic vessels (*SV*) and vas deferens (*VD*) have been freed and lengthened. The inferior epigastric vessels have been divided to help expose the internal ring.

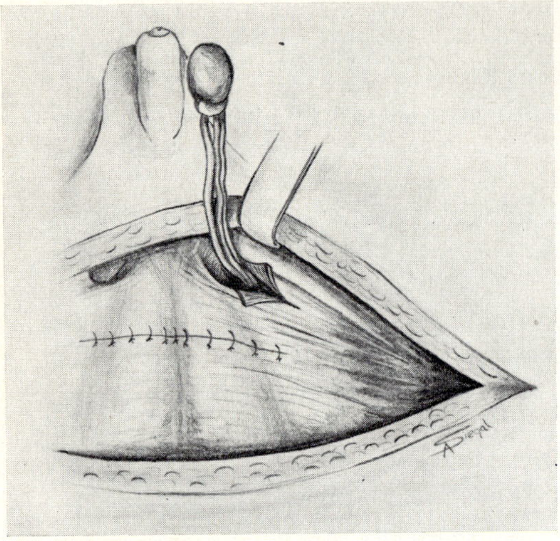

**Fig. 4.** The rectus muscles and fascia have been united. The inferior skin flap is retracted to expose the external ring. The external oblique fascia has been opened and the testicle and cord have been brought out in preparation for insertion into the scrotum.

ward (Fig. 4). The external ring is located and the external oblique fascia divided. The testis and cord are freed from adhesions. The distal remnant of the sac is excised. Gentle traction will bring the freed spermatic vessels and vas into the inguinal canal. If the internal ring is dilated, it is repaired with interrupted No. 3-0 silk sutures. The rectus muscles are then united in the midline with several interrupted No. 3-0 chromic catgut sutures. The rectus fascia is united with interrupted No. 3-0 silk sutures. The scrotum is then prepared for the testis. A silk suture secured to the tunica albuginea is passed through the scrotum and fixed with a rubber band to the thigh. The external oblique fascia is sutured over the cord. The superficial fascia and skin are closed.

## DISCUSSION

This operation permits an unusually extensive exposure of the retroperitoneal portion of the vas deferens and internal spermatic vessels. These structures can be freed under direct vision by sharp dissection. The hernia sac can be ligated at its highest level. The integrity of the inguinal floor is preserved. There is no need for rerouting the spermatic cord. The normal internal inguinal ring and its protective sphincteric mechanism are preserved. Without an additional incision and with minimal trauma, the contralateral side can be inspected for hernia. The contralateral undescended testis may be corrected at the same operation.

## CONCLUSION

The Cheatle-Henry extraperitoneal approach, through a Pfannenstiel type of incision, provides superior exposure for the liberation of the elements of the cords in cryptorchidism, without injury to the inguinal structures. Cases of unilateral and bilateral cryptorchidism were treated by this method with satisfactory results. Bilateral cryptorchidism can be managed through a single incision.

## ADDENDUM

Since this paper was submitted for publication, 4 additional patients have been treated by this method.

J. S., 6 years old, underwent simultaneous correction of right undescended testis, right indirect inguinal hernia, and left indirect inguinal hernia.

B. T., 14 years old, underwent right orchidopexy. The procedure was modified by retraction of the rectus muscle medially.

H. A., 17 years old, had undergone right orchidopexy elsewhere which resulted in complete atrophy of the right testis. The left testis was intra-abdominal. Left orchidopexy was accomplished by preperitoneal dissection of the testis and cord components.

G. E., 8 years old, had bilateral cryptorchidism and hernias. Simultaneous orchidopexy and hernia repair were carried out.

A satisfactory result was obtained in each case.

### REFERENCES

1. Bevan, A. D.: The operation for undescended testis, Ann. Surg. **90:** 847, 1929.
2. Cheatle, G. L.: An operation for inguinal hernia, Brit. M. J. **2:** 1025, 1921.
3. Gross, R. E.: The Surgery of infancy and childhood, Philadelphia, 1953, W. B. Saunders Company, p. 471.
4. Henry, A. K.: Operation for femoral hernia by a midline extra-peritoneal approach, Lancet **1:** 531, 1936.
5. Swenson, O.: Pediatric surgery, New York, 1958, Appleton-Century-Crofts, Inc., pp. 237-239.
6. Torek, E.: Orchiopexy for undescended testicle, Ann. Surg. **94:** 97, 1931.

# The blind-loop syndrome after gastric operations


THOMAS E. STARZL, M.D.*
GEORGE W. BUTZ, JR., M.D.
CHARLES F. HARTMAN, M.D.
CHICAGO, ILL.
*From the Department of Surgery, Northwestern University Medical School*


Since the earliest reports by White[68] and Faber,[19] it has been known that certain mechanical intestinal abnormalities could cause a hematologic syndrome which resembles pernicious anemia, and to date at least 100 examples have been reported. Location and etiology of the intestinal lesion varied, but the end result was stasis and retarded drainage from some portion of the gastrointestinal tract. Cases in which the stagnant loop was associated with certain specific absorption defects have been classified as examples of the blind-loop syndrome.[6, 14, 26] It is probable that only a small number of patients with anatomic blind loops develop the blind-loop syndrome with its metabolically important changes.

Two of the most common operations performed today in which potential stagnant loops are created are Billroth II gastrectomy and gastroenterostomy. The duodenum is converted into a side arm which rejoins the main intestinal tract at the gastrojejunostomy. It is common knowledge that this afferent loop occasionally drains improperly.[15, 30, 32, 37, 41, 42, 44, 46, 48, 53, 57, 58, 66, 67] However, prior to 1953, there were no well-documented reports of the blind-loop syndrome after either operation. Since that time, several examples of the blind-loop syndrome have been described after Billroth II resection or gastroenterostomy. The fact that only a handful of these cases has yet been reported may be due to the subtlety of the clinical manifestations, the difficulty of clearly establishing a diagnosis, and the general unawareness of this complication as a diagnostic possibility. In addition to its immediate clinical application, a consideration of the blind-loop syndrome may cast some light upon the nutritional superiority of the Billroth I over the Billroth II gastrectomy.

## ANATOMIC CONFIGURATION OF BLIND LOOPS

Various examples of gastrointestinal blind loops are shown in Fig. 1 for comparison with the blind loops observed after gastrectomy. These have occurred[6, 26] after creation of dead-end segments by anastomoses (Fig. 1, *A*), with jejunal diverticulosis (Fig. 1, *B*), with intestinal strictures which have most commonly been tuberculous in origin (Fig. 1, *C*), and after enteroenterostomies and fistulas (Fig. 1, *D*).

In experimental studies of the blind-loop syndrome by Tonnis and Brusis,[61] Pearse,[47] Watson and associates,[64] Taylor,[59] and Toon and Wangensteen,[60] a side-arm loop has been employed as in Fig. 1, *A*, in which the loop is arranged so as to be self-filling. The side loop arrangement is the one which most


Aided by United States Public Health Service Grant No. A-3176.

Received for publication May 18, 1961.


*Markle Scholar.

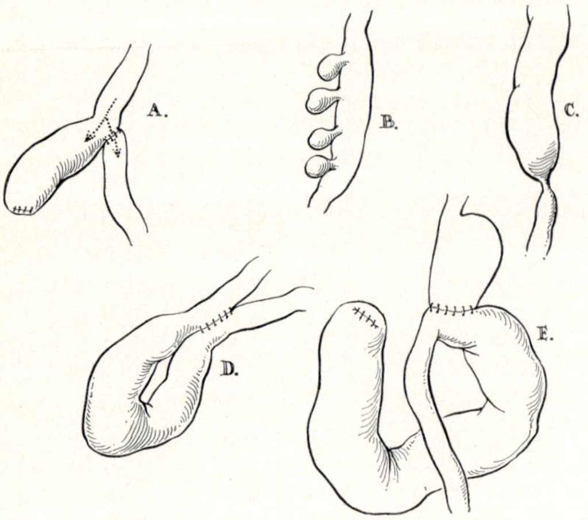


**Fig. 1.** Different types of gastrointestinal blind loops which have caused the blind-loop syndrome. *A,* Anastomosis with formation of a self-filled stagnant loop, *B,* with jejunal diverticulosis, *C,* with intestinal strictures, *D,* after enteroenterostomies or fistulas, and *E,* after gastric operation.

resembles a blind loop which develops after gastrojejunostomy (Fig. 1, *E*).

The structural conditions necessary for the blind-loop syndrome are not present after the Billroth I anastomosis. In all reported cases there has been either a Billroth II resection (8 patients) or a gastroenterostomy (1 patient). The anastomoses (Fig. 2, *A* and *B*) were both antiperistaltic, with the afferent loop to the greater curvature,[25, 45] and isoperistaltic.[13, 30, 45] In 2 cases (Fig. 2, *C* and *D*), an enterostomy had also been performed.[1, 49] Commonly, the afferent loop was excessively long and dilated.[25, 30, 45] The exact site of obstruction was sometimes difficult to define by roentgenogram or even at operation.[13, 45, 49] Usually, the distended loop ended abruptly at the gastrojejunostomy, but in some cases it extended beyond this. Excessively long afferent loops, kinking at the site of anastomosis, and partially obstructing adhesions have all been described as the factor causing blind-loop stasis.[1, 13, 25, 30, 45, 49]

## ABNORMALITIES IN VITAMIN $B_{12}$ METABOLISM IN BLOOD-LOOP SYNDROME

General information concerning the mechanism of the blind-loop syndrome has accumulated from observations on lesions at differing sites in the gastrointestinal tract. The principles involved apply, with variations, to blind loops at all levels. The best-known feature of the blind-loop syndrome is megaloblastic anemia, which is due to disruption of vitamin $B_{12}$ absorption. Normally, dietary vitamin $B_{12}$ (Castle's extrinsic factor) is absorbed after an incompletely understood interaction with intrinsic factor (Fig. 3, *A*), a mucoprotein secreted by the gastric mucosa.[22] In man, the principal site of $B_{12}$ absorption is the ileum.[7, 8]

Vitamin $B_{12}$ deficiency can develop by a number of alternative mechanisms. Rarely is there dietary deficiency of this nutritional factor. Commonly, as in pernicious anemia (Fig. 3, *B*) or after total gastrectomy,[39] there is absent intrinsic factor due to gastric atrophy or the absence of the stomach, respectively. Malabsorption can also occur[4, 23,

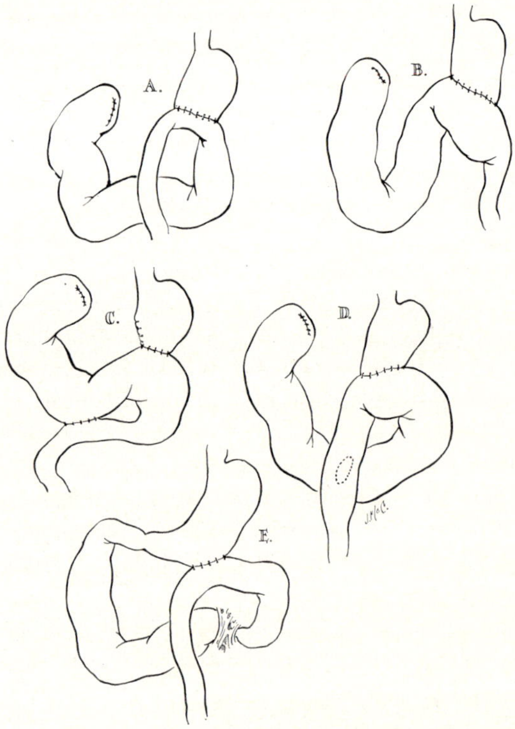


**Fig. 2.** Anatomic conditions after gastric operation which have caused blind-loop syndrome. *A,* 3 cases, *B,* 3 cases, *C,* 1 case, *D,* 1 case, and *E,* 1 case.

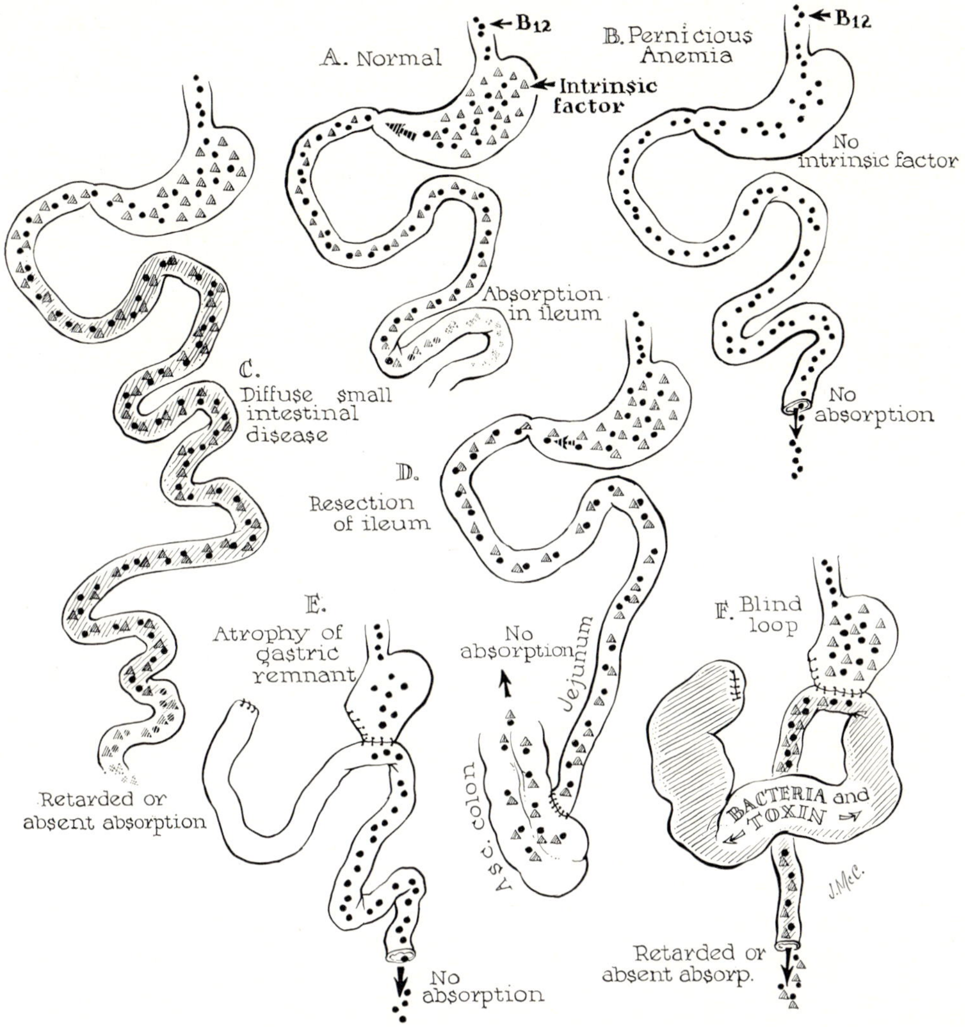


**Fig. 3.** Mechanisms of $B_{12}$ utilization in normal and diseased patients.

[26, 27, 28, 35, 40, 43, 52, 54] with adequate intrinsic factor and dietary vitamin $B_{12}$ in patients who have undergone ileal resection (Fig. 3, *D*) or who have diffuse small bowel disease (Fig. 3, *C*). Here, the malabsorption is due to damage or removal of the normal site of absorption. Vitamin $B_{12}$ deficiency also develops in the blind-loop syndrome despite the presence of intrinsic factor and dietary $B_{12}$ (Fig. 3, *F*). The malabsorption in this circumstance is thought to be due to bacterial overgrowth in a poorly emptying blind loop with consequent interference with $B_{12}$ absorption in the remainder of the intestinal tract.[19, 25, 26, 50, 55, 56, 60, 65, 69] As with pernicious anemia, patients with blind-loop syndrome can proceed to subacute combined degeneration of the spinal cord.[1, 6, 26, 49]

Virtually all authorities agree that a change in the bacterial flora of the torpid loop is responsible for the $B_{12}$ malabsorption. Much of the evidence is based upon clinical impression, but there is solid experimental work to support this opinion. Seyderhelm,[55] employing strictures to study the blind-loop effect in dogs, related the presence or absence of infection above the stenosis to the development or absence of anemia. Watson and Witts[65] have demonstrated in rats that the bacterial flora of small intestinal blind loops resembles that normally found in the colon. They also showed that the bacterial

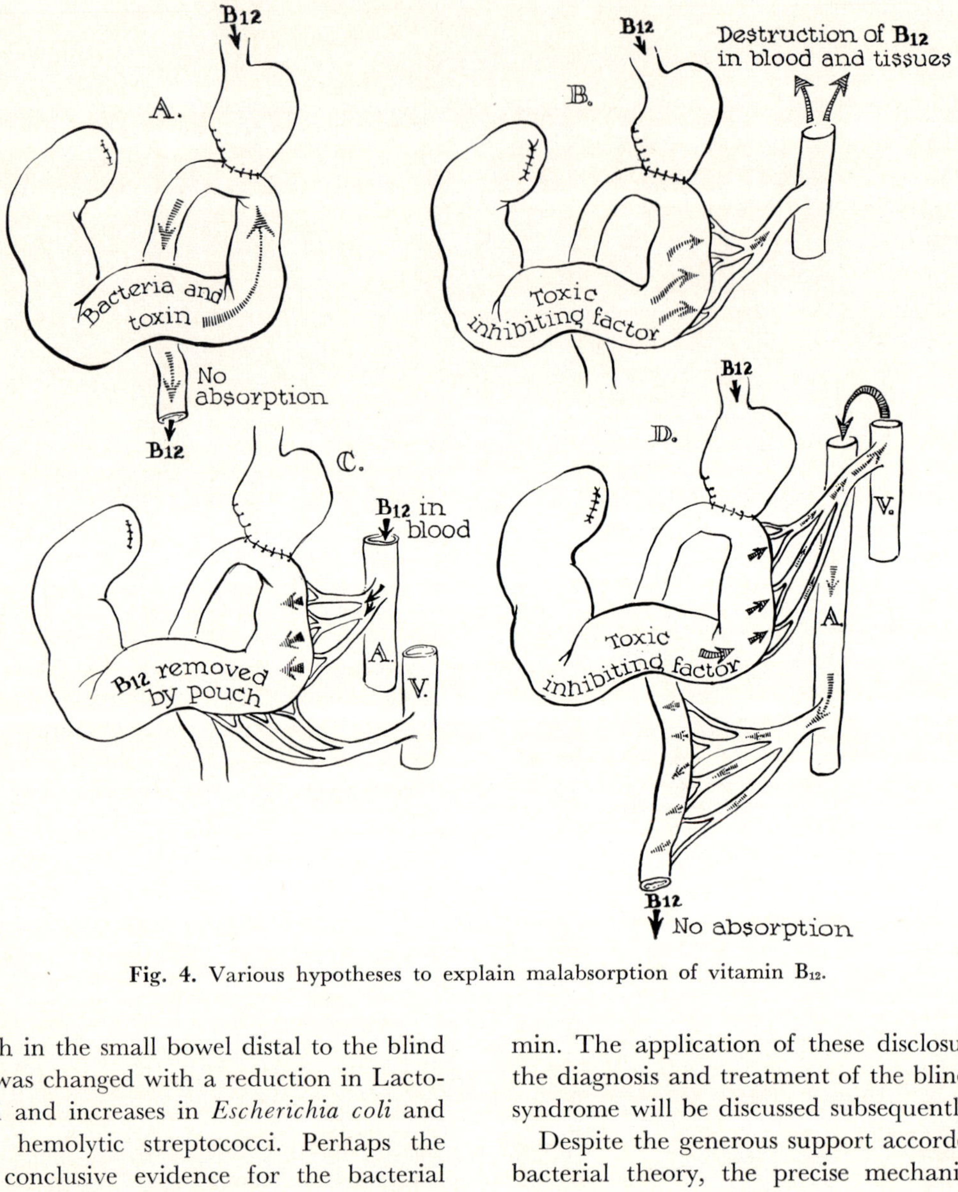


**Fig. 4.** Various hypotheses to explain malabsorption of vitamin $B_{12}$.

growth in the small bowel distal to the blind loop was changed with a reduction in Lactobacilli and increases in *Escherichia coli* and alpha hemolytic streptococci. Perhaps the most conclusive evidence for the bacterial etiology of the malabsorption was provided by Toon and Wangensteen,[60] and later confirmed by Watson and Witts.[65] These authors showed that the anemia of the experimental blind loop syndrome could be prevented by oral administration of chlortetracycline. The therapeutic value of antibiotics in man has been confirmed by Siruala and Kaipainen[56] and numerous other observers,[1, 3, 17, 25, 26, 28, 30, 34, 43, 45, 49, 50, 54] who noted that certain antibiotics could not only prevent the development of, but also reverse, $B_{12}$ deficiency by restoring normal absorption of this vitamin. The application of these disclosures to the diagnosis and treatment of the blind-loop syndrome will be discussed subsequently.

Despite the generous support accorded the bacterial theory, the precise mechanism of vitamin $B_{12}$ malabsorption is not known. One widely accepted theory is that propounded by Witts[69] in which $B_{12}$ metabolism is supposedly affected by direct alimentary contamination of bacteria or their toxic byproducts which spill out of the stagnant loop (Fig. 4, *A*). Since certain strains of *Escherichia coli* and *Streptococcus fecalis* metabolize folic acid or vitamin $B_{12}$,[11, 51] it has been suggested that the anomalously located microorganisms use up the available oral supply. Contrary to this reasoning is the fact that Neomycin and sulphonamides, which are nonabsorbable and which sterilize the nonstagnant intestine are of no therapeutic value[17, 25, 26] despite the fact that they would be expected to come into contact with efflux from the loop. In contrast, oral antibiotics such as chlortetracycline, oxytetracycline, and tetracycline can restore normal absorption of $B_{12}$.

However, if the offending agent were a toxin, its production in a sequestered loop would be suspended only with a systemic antibiotic. Drexler[18] has shown on the basis of in vitro experiments that indole compounds are able to inhibit normal utilization of vitamin $B_{12}$, and he has suggested that indole might be one of the blind-loop "toxins." Recently, Hoffman and Spiro[30] have failed to support either the bacterial or toxin theory of direct intestinal contamination. They instilled into a normal patient's stomach the contents of a resected blind loop with $Co^{60}$-tagged vitamin $B_{12}$. $B_{12}$ absorption was not depressed.

Other theories to explain the $B_{12}$ deficiency involve blood-stream mechanisms. Ungley[62] suggested that a toxin was absorbed from the blind loop which destroyed the vitamin in the blood and tissues (Fig. 4, *B*). He supported this opinion by the demonstration that plasma added from a resected blind loop suspended megaloblastic maturation in bone marrow culture. Card[16] also proposed that $B_{12}$ was actually absorbed, but that increments were returned by enteric recirculation (Fig. 4, *C*) to the blind loop and destroyed. Both theories were weakened by the results of studies of urinary and fecal excretion of radioactive vitamin $B_{12}$ which show that the block in metabolism is primarily at, rather than after, the absorption phase.[1, 3, 17, 25, 26, 28, 30, 34, 40, 43, 45, 49, 50, 54]

An unexplored possibility is that bacterial toxins are picked up from the blind loop and circulated to the uninvolved portion of the small bowel where they alter the absorptive capacity (Fig. 4, *D*). Such a hypothesis is compatible with the evidence obtained from antibiotic therapy, and with present knowledge of the fundamental defect in $B_{12}$ utilization.

## OTHER NUTRITIONAL DEFICIENCIES IN BLIND-LOOP SYNDROME

Absorption of other nutritional substances is often impaired. Fat is probably the most commonly affected. Using experimental midintestinal loops, Aitken and colleagues[2] found that virtually all rats exhibited steatorrhea whether or not the animals became anemic. The development of anemia alone, without steatorrhea, was uncommon.

As with vitamin $B_{12}$ deficiency, it is thought that bacterial overgrowth in the blind loop is the causative factor in the steatorrhea. Specific evidence has been presented by Sammons[51] and by Goldstein and his group[25] that the bacterial growth adversely affects fat utilization. The latter authors have shown that the steatorrhea of the blind-loop syndrome is favorably influenced by antibiotics.

Why some blind loops do and others do not cause steatorrhea is not known. There is some evidence that the location of the blind loop is influential in this respect. Booth[7] has pointed out that a blind loop of the ileum, where normal vitamin $B_{12}$ absorption occurs, may lead to pure $B_{12}$ deficiency. Blind loops of the jejunum, where fat is normally absorbed,[7, 9, 25, 33] usually produce prominent steatorrhea.[4, 54, 63] While such localization is admittedly crude, it may help to explain differences in the malabsorption defect in different cases. Of 9 patients who had blind-loop syndromes after gastric operations, 7 had steatorrhea.

Other nutritional deficiencies are also common. Numerous cases of protein deficiency have been noted with blind loops at various levels, including the blind loops after gastric operations.[13, 25, 45] Usually this is reflected in low plasma protein levels, but 1 example of frank kwashiorkor has been reported in a patient with an intestinal blind loop.[36] Pellagra and vitamin C and vitamin K deficiencies have been recorded. Badenach[3] has warned against the dangerous complication of spontaneous retroperitoneal hemorrhage resulting from vitamin K deficiency.

## INCIDENCE OF BLIND-LOOP SYNDROME AFTER GASTRIC OPERATIONS

The blind-loop syndrome has not been thoroughly evaluated as a cause of poor results after gastric operations. It is probable that this complication is more important than the 9 recorded cases[1, 13, 25, 30, 45, 49] indicate. For example, Kinsella[32] recently reported 7 cases which are probably examples of the blind-loop syndrome, but there is insufficient data to be certain of this. Several factors make the diagnosis an obscure and difficult one which is apt to be overlooked. First, the interval between operation and the onset of symptoms can be prolonged for many years, which tends to minimize the etiologic role of the remote operation in relation to the presenting complaints. In addition, the symptoms often are subtle and nonspecific and resemble psychoneurotic complaints.

Undoubtedly, an additional hindrance has been the preoccupation with macrocytic anemia as a prerequisite for this diagnosis. In point of fact, this feature may be absent as it was in 7 of the 9 cases collected in this review. Macrocytic anemia was frequently masked by prior vitamin $B_{12}$ therapy or by the presence of other and equally important absorption defects of fat, iron, and other materials. Even in the untreated patient, the body stores of vitamin $B_{12}$ are not dissipated for 3 to 4 years in the complete absence of $B_{12}$ intake,[20, 21, 23, 28] so the development of megaloblastic anemia is a late manifestation. However, techniques and knowledge acquired in the past few years allow the blind-loop syndrome to be defined in terms of specific and measurable parameters of malabsorption rather than in terms of their end results. These techniques, outlined in the section on diagnosis, should increase the frequency and accuracy of detection.

It should be emphasized not only that macrocytic anemia is not a prerequisite to the diagnosis of the blind-loop syndrome, but also that most cases of megaloblastic anemia after gastric operations are not due to this cause. McLean[39] has summarized the results of investigations of patients with macrocytic anemia which developed after gastroenterostomy or partial gastrectomy. Almost invariably, these patients have developed atrophy of the gastric remnant with loss of the intrinsic factor (Fig. 3, *E*). Differentiating patients with the blind loop syndrome from those with gastric atrophy is a crucial step in correct diagnosis.

## CLINICAL MANIFESTATIONS OF BLIND-LOOP SYNDROME AFTER GASTRIC OPERATIONS

The clinical features of the blind-loop syndrome are seldom overt. The diagnosis has usually been made only after months or years of disability. Commonly, a gastroenterostomy or Billroth II gastric resection performed as long as 26 years previously had initially been considered to have a good result. When anemia, weight loss, malaise, hypoproteinemia, steatorrhea, or neurologic complaints developed, the possible relation to the previous operation was often overlooked.

Anemia was present in all cases.[1, 13, 25, 30, 45, 49] In only 2, however, was it macrocytic in type.[1, 45] Steatorrhea was the next most common feature and was found in 7 patients.[1, 13, 25, 45] Five of these had diarrhea. Some evidence of malnutrition was always present, and 5 patients had edema or hypoproteinemia.[13, 25, 45] Glossitis, blepharitis, cheilosis, or other signs of vitamin deficiency were seen in 3 patients. Neurologic findings suggestive of subacute combined degeneration of the cord were present in 3 patients with calf pain, changes in deep tendon reflexes, and decreased sense of vibration and proprioception.[1, 13, 49]

Vomiting and abdominal pain were reported in 1[30] and 3[1, 13, 30] cases, respectively. The vomitus consisted of pure bile or foul brown material, and the emesis probably resulted from convulsive emptying of the blind loop. Sporadic bilious vomiting is known to be a characteristic symptom in patients with an obstructed or distended afferent loop,[15, 30, 32, 37, 41, 42, 44, 46, 48, 53, 57, 58, 66, 67] and it is possible that this symptom will prove to be common as more information accumulates concerning the blind-loop syndrome.

## DIAGNOSIS

Radiologic studies may be helpful in establishing the presence of dilatation or stasis in the afferent loop. In some cases, barium entered a dilated, tortuous loop.[25, 30, 45] In others, barium was held up, often for many hours, in an unidentifiable pouch (Fig. 5) near the gastroenterostomy.[13, 49] In some, barium did not enter the afferent loop.[49] In a recent study of afferent loop obstruction, Kinsella and Hennessy[32] reported the various radiologic features of afferent loop obstruction to be (1) absence of barium passage into afferent loop, (2) passage of barium for 1 to 2 cm. into the afferent loop with an abrupt halt at an obstruction, and (3) pendulum effect with passage into the afferent loop and remittent emptying back into the stomach.

During the last 10 years, laboratory techniques have been developed which allow the diagnosis of the blind-loop syndrome to be made with increasing precision. First among these are tests employing $Co^{60}$-tagged vitamin $B_{12}$ either for determination of fecal excretion,[29] hepatic uptake,[24] or urinary excretion.[52] The urinary excretion method, the Schilling test,[52] is the most widely used. The patient is given 0.5 to 1.0 $\mu$g of $Co^{60}$-tagged $B_{12}$ orally, and 2 hours later a flushing dose of 1,000 $\mu$g of nontagged $B_{12}$ is given intramuscularly or subcutaneously. The amount of radioactivity in the ensuing 24-hour urine specimen provides an indirect measure of the amount of oral $Co^{60}$-tagged $B_{12}$ absorbed. Normally 8 to 40 per cent of the $Co^{60}$-tagged $B_{12}$ is excreted in the urine.

When urinary excretion of the $Co^{60}$-tagged $B_{12}$ is subnormal or absent, the test is repeated with concomitant oral administration of intrinsic factor. In cases of pernicious anemia and in postoperative patients in whom gastric atrophy has occurred, urinary excretion will be restored to normal, and the diagnosis of blind-loop syndrome is excluded.[5, 10, 23, 38, 39]

If the combination of $Co^{60}$-tagged $B_{12}$ and intrinsic factor does not increase urinary excretion, the blind-loop syndrome becomes a strong possibility. $Co^{60}$-tagged $B_{12}$ is again given, this time after several days of therapy with tetracycline, chlortetracycline, or oxytetracycline. In many cases, the antibiotics restore absorption and the urinary excretion will become normal. Should this occur, the diagnosis of blind-loop syndrome is virtually established.[1, 3, 17, 25, 26, 28, 30, 34, 43, 45, 49, 50, 54] Failure of the antibiotics may be due to Whipple's disease, sprue, or some other diffuse intestinal disease, or to surgical absence of the ileum. It does not preclude the possibility of the blind-loop syndrome, however, since the bacteria of the blind loop may not be sensitive to the antibiotics used.[13, 17, 25, 43]

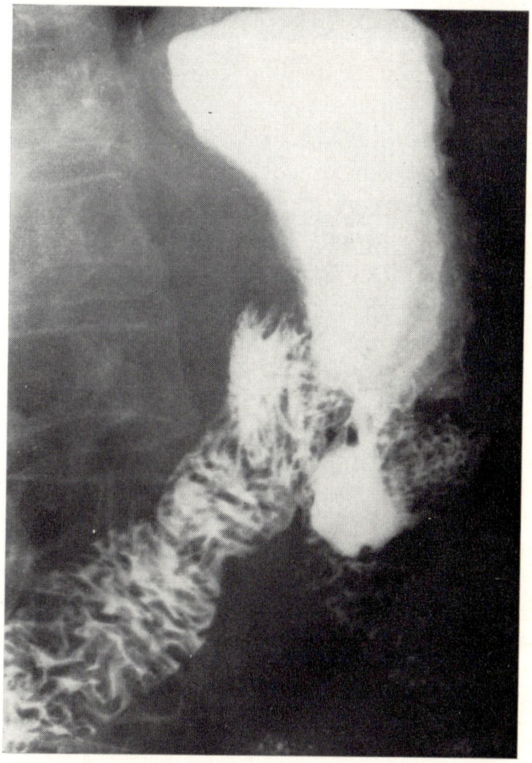

**Fig. 5.** Gastrointestinal series in patient with blind loop syndrome after Billroth II gastrectomy. Note pouch at gastrojejunostomy site and dilated and elongated afferent loop (left). Barium remained in pouch for 6 hours.

Experimental and clinical data previously alluded to emphasize the importance of studying the absorption of other substances, particularly fat. Jackson and Linder[31] and Butler and associates[12] recognized the resemblance of gastroenterostomy and Billroth II gastrectomy to the better-known intestinal blind loops. They speculated that bacterial growth in the afferent limb might account for the higher incidence of steatorrhea after Billroth II than after Billroth I gastrectomy. Recently, Goldstein and his colleagues[25] studied bacterial counts by afferent limb intubation in postoperative patients, and demonstrated a strong correlation between the degree of contamination in the afferent loop and the magnitude of steatorrhea. They also showed that antibiotic therapy reduced steatorrhea, presumably by the same mechanism as $B_{12}$ absorption is improved in other blind loops. This type of testing may prove to be of great value in the study of postgastrectomy malabsorption syndromes and in the detection of afferent blind loops.

Other tests may be useful in individual cases. Gastric analysis for acid should always be carried out, since the presence of free acid excludes gastric atrophy as a cause of $B_{12}$ malabsorption. Badenach[5] has performed endoscopic gastric biopsy and studied urinary uropepsinogen in order to evaluate the secretory capacity of the stomach.

In the diagnosis of the blind-loop syndrome, reliance upon a single symptom, finding, or abnormality of absorption is not wise. The absorption defects are frequently multiple, and other deficiencies may be of greater importance than those which would lead to a specific hematologic picture. Unification of the different aspects presented by the blind-loop syndrome into a well-understood entity would undoubtedly lead to a higher rate of recognition of this complication of gastric operations.

## TREATMENT OF THE BLIND-LOOP SYNDROME AFTER GASTRIC OPERATION

Medical therapy can temporarily improve the health of patients with the blind-loop syndrome. With tetracycline, chlortetracycline, oxytetracycline, chloramphenicol, and possibly other antibiotics, the absorption of vitamin $B_{12}$, fat, and probably other nutrients may be restored toward normal. The improvement may outlast a course of antibiotic therapy by weeks or months,[1, 25, 54] but relapse eventually is expected. Specific vitamin deficiencies, especially of $B_{12}$, should be corrected. High protein, high calorie diet, correction of low blood volume, and restoration of electrolytes are other adjuncts.

Definitive therapy requires surgical correction of the blind afferent loop. In the 9 collected cases, 6 patients had been operated upon at the time of the report.[13, 25, 30, 45, 49] In 4, the Billroth II anastomosis was taken down and converted to a Billroth I,[13, 25, 45, 49] and in a fifth similar reconstruction was carried out with the interposition of a jejunal segment between the stomach and duodenum.[45] A good result was obtained in all with complete or partial correction of the pre-existing absorption defects. In the sixth case, the dilated and elongated afferent loop was resected and a short-loop Billroth II anastomosis performed with a good result.[30] From a mechanical point of view, other operations have been proposed for the treatment of afferent loop obstruction, such as enteroenterostomy, jejunoplasty, support of the afferent loop by suture, and defunctionalization of the afferent loop by Roux Y anastomosis. There are objections to each of these operations, especially in terms of late results, and they probably should not be used.

## REFERENCES

1. Adams, J. F.: Postgastrectomy megaloblastic anemia and the loop syndrome, Gastroenterologia **89:** 326, 1958.
2. Aitken, M. A., Badenoch, J., and Spray, G. H.: Fat excretion in rats with intestinal culs-de-sac, Brit. J. Exper. Path. **31:** 355, 1950.
3. Badenoch, J.: The blind loop syndrome, Proc. Roy. Soc. Med. **53:** 657, 1960.
4. Badenoch, J.: Bedford, P. D., and Evans, J. R.: Massive diverticulosis of the small intestine with steatorrhea and megaloblastic anemia, Quart. J. Med. **24:** 321, 1955.

5. Badenoch, J., Evans, J. R., Richards, W. C. D., and Witts, L. J.: Megaloblastic anemia following partial gastrectomy, Brit. J. Haemat. **1:** 337, 1955.
6. Barker, W. H., and Hummel, L. E.: Macrocytic anemia in association with intestinal strictures and anastomoses, Bull. Johns Hopkins Hosp. **64:** 215, 1939.
7. Booth, C. C., and Mollin, D. L.: The blind loop syndrome, Proc. Roy. Soc. Med. **53:** 658, 1960.
8. Booth, C. C., and Mollin, D. L.: The site of absorption of vitamin $B_{12}$ in man, Lancet **1:** 18, 1959.
9. Borgstrom, B., Dahlquist, A., Lundh, G., and Sjovall, J.: Studies of intestinal digestion and absorption in the human, J. Clin. Invest. **36:** 1521, 1957.
10. Brodine, C., Friedman, B. I., Saenger, E. L., and Will, J. J.: The absorption of $B_{12}$ following subtotal gastrectomy, J. Lab. & Clin. Med. **53:** 220, 1959.
11. Burkholder, P. R.: Microbiological studies on materials which potentiate oral vitamin $B_{12}$ and intrinsic factor activity, Arch. Biochem. **39:** 322, 1952.
12. Butler, T. J., Capper, W. M., and Naish, J. M.: Ileo-jejunal insufficiency following different types of gastrectomy, Gastroenterologia **81:** 104, 1954.
13. Butz, G. W., Jr., Hartman, C. F., and Starzl, T. E.: The blind loop syndrome following subtotal gastrectomy, A. M. A. Arch. Surg. In press.
14. Cameron, D. G., Watson, G. M., and Witts, L. J.: Clinical association of macrocytic anemia with intestinal stricture and anastomosis, Blood **4:** 793, 1949.
15. Capper, W. M., and Welbourne, R. B.: Postcibal symptoms following gastrectomy, Brit. J. Surg. **43:** 24, 1955.
16. Card, W. I.: Blind loop syndrome. Proc. Roy. Soc. Med. **52:** 28, 1959.
17. Doscherholmen, A., and Hagen, P. S.: Absorption of $Co^{60}$ labeled vitamin $B_{12}$ in intestinal blind loop megaloblastic anemia, J. Lab. & Clin. Med. **44:** 790, 1954.
18. Drexler, J.: Effect of indole compounds on vitamin $B_{12}$ utilization, Blood **13:** 239, 1958.
19. Faber, K.: Pernicious anemia following intestinal stricture, Klin. Wchnschr. **34:** 643, 1897.
20. Girdwood, R. H.: Megaloblastic anemia: their investigation and classification, Quart. J. Med. **25:** 87, 1956.
21. Girdwood, R. H.: The occurrence of growth factors for Lactobacillus leichmannii, Streptococcus fecalis, and Leuconostoc citrovorum in the tissues of pernicious anemia patients and controls, Biochem. J. **52:** 58, 1952.
22. Glass, G. B. J.: Hematopoietic activity of glandular mucoprotein of human gastric juice, Gastroenterology **23:** 219, 1953.
23. Glass, G. B. J.: Intestinal absorption and hepatic uptake of vitamin $B_{12}$ in diseases of the gastrointestinal tract, Gastroenterology **30:** 37, 1956.
24. Glass, G. B. J., Boyd, L. J., and Stephanson, L.: Intestinal absorption of vitamin $B_{12}$ in humans as studied by isotope technique, Proc. Soc. Exper. Biol. & Med. **86:** 522, 1954.
25. Goldstein, F., Wirts, C. W., and Kramer, S.: The relationship of afferent limb stasis and bacterial flora to the production of postgastrectomy steatorrhea, Gastroenterology **40:** 47, 1961.
26. Halsted, J. A., Lewis, P. M., and Gasster, M.: Absorption of radioactive vitamin $B_{12}$ in the syndrome of megaloblastic anemia associated with intestinal stricture of anastomosis, Am. J. Med. **20:** 42, 1956.
27. Halsted, J. A., Swendseid, M. E., Gasster, M., and Lewis, P. M.: Absorption of radioactive $B_{12}$ in disease of the small intestine: relation to macrocytic anemia, Tr. Am. Clin. & Climatol. A. **66:** 18, 1954.
28. Halsted, J. A., Swendseid, M. E., Lewis, P. M., and Gasster, M.: Mechanisms involved in the development of vitamin $B_{12}$ deficiency, Gastroenterology **30:** 21, 1956.
29. Heinle, R. W., Welch, A. D., Scharf, V., Meacham, G. C., and Prushoff, W. H.: Studies of excretion (and absorption) of $CO^{60}$ labeled vitamin $B_{12}$ in pernicious anemia, Tr. A. Am. Physicians **65:** 214, 1952.
30. Hoffman, W. A., and Spiro, H. M.: Afferent loop problems, Gastroenterology **40:** 201, 1961.
31. Jackson, W. P. U., and Linder, G. C.: Small gut insufficiency following intestinal surgery, South African J. Clin. Sc. **2:** 205, 1951.
32. Kinsella, V. J., and Hennessy, W. B.: Gastrectomy and the blind loop syndrome, Lancet **2:** 1205, 1960.
33. Kremen, A. J., Linner, J. H., and Nelson, C. H.: An experimental evaluation of the nutritional importance of proximal and distal small intestine, Ann. Surg. **140:** 439, 1954.
34. Krevans, J. R., Conley, C., and Sachs, M.: Influence of certain diseases on the absorption of vitamin $B_{12}$ from the gastrointestinal tract, J. Clin. Invest. **33:** 949, 1954.
35. Krevans, J. R., Conley, C. L., and Sachs, M. V.: Radioactive tracer tests for the recognition and identification of vitamin $B_{12}$ deficiency status, J. Chronic Dis. **3:** 234, 1956.
36. Krikler, D. M., and Schrire, V.: "Kwashiorkor" in an adult due to an intestinal blind loop, Lancet **1:** 510, 1958.

37. Lake, N. C.: The aftermath of gastrectomy, Brit. M. J. **1:** 285, 1948.
38. Lowenstein, F.: Labeled vitamin $B_{12}$ after subtotal gastrectomy, Blood **13:** 339, 1958.
39. MacLean, L. D.: Megaloblastic anemia following total and subtotal gastrectomy, Surg. Gynec. & Obst. **106:** 415, 1958.
40. McIntyre, P. A., Sachs, M. V., and Conley, C. L. J.: Pathogenesis and treatment of macrocytic anemia, A. M. A. Arch. Int. Med. **98:** 541, 1956.
41. McNealy, R. W.: Problems with the duodenal stump in gastric resections, SURGERY **12:** 207, 1942.
42. Mimpriss, T. W., and Birt, St. J. M. C.: Results of partial gastrectomy for peptic ulcer, Brit. M. J. **2:** 1095, 1948.
43. Mollin, D. L., Booth, C. C., and Baker, S. J.: The absorption of vitamin $B_{12}$ in control subjects, in Addisonian pernicious anemia and in malabsorption syndrome, Brit. J. Haemat. **3:** 412, 1957.
44. Muir, A.: Postgastrectomy syndromes, Brit. J. Surg. **37:** 165, 1949.
45. Naish, J., and Capper, W. M.: Intestinal cul-de-sac phenomena in man, Lancet **2:** 597, 1953.
46. Noring, O.: The afferent-loop syndrome elucidated by three cases, Acta chir. scandinav. **115:** 276, 1958.
47. Pearse, A. E.: Experimental chronic intestinal obstruction from blind loops, Surg. Gynec. & Obst. **59:** 726, 1934.
48. Quinn, W. F., and Gifford, J. H.: Syndrome of proximal jejunal loop obstruction following anterior gastric resection, California M. J. **72:** 18, 1950.
49. Ragins, H., and Oberhelman, H. A.: Anemia associated with a stagnant ("blind") jejunal loop, A. M. A. Arch. Surg. **80:** 524, 1960.
50. Reilly, R. W., and Kirsner, J. B.: The blind loop syndrome, Gastroenterology **37:** 491, 1959.
51. Sammons, H. G., Vaughan, D. J., and Frazer, A. C.: Synthesis of long-chain fats by bacteria isolated from human feces, Nature **177:** 237, 1956.
52. Schilling, R. F.: Intrinsic factor studies. II. The effect of gastric juice on the urinary excretion of radioactivity after the oral administration of radioactive vitamin $B_{12}$, J. Lab. & Clin. Med. **42:** 860, 1953.
53. Schofield, J. E., and Anderson, P. St. G.: Postgastrectomy syndrome deviation of the afferent loop from the gastrointestinal anastomosis, Brit. M. J. **2:** 598, 1953.
54. Scudmore, H. H., Hagedorn, A. B., Wollaeger, E. E., and Owen, C. A.: Diverticulosis of the small intestine and macrocytic anemia with report of 2 cases and studies on absorption of radioactive vitamin $B_{12}$, Gastroenterology **34:** 66, 1958.
55. Seyderhelm, R., Lehman, W., and Wichels, P.: Experimental intestinal pernicious anemia in the dog, Klin. Wchnschr. **3:** 1439, 1924.
56. Siurala, M., and Kaipainen, W. J.: Intestinal megaloblastic anemia treated with aureomycin and terramycin, Acta med. scandinav. **147:** 197, 1953.
57. Stammers, F. A. R.: Complications associated with the use of a long afferent loop in the Polya type of partial gastrectomy, Brit. J. Surg. **44:** 358, 1956.
58. Stammers, F. A. R.: Remarks on 15 cases of small bowel obstruction following retrocolic partial gastrectomy, Brit. J. Surg. **42:** 34, 1954.
59. Taylor, D. W.: Absorption from intestine of rats with blind self-filling pouch, Nature **170:** 80, 1952.
60. Toon, R. W., and Wangensteen, O. H.: Anemia associated with blind intestinal segments and its prevention with aureomycin, Proc. Soc. Exper. Biol. & Med. **75:** 762, 1950.
61. Tonnis, and Brusis, A.: Changes of morphological blood picture in acute and chronic intestinal obstruction, Deutsche Ztschr. Chir. **233:** 133, 1931.
62. Ungley, C. C.: Megaloblastic anemia following operations on intestine, Gastroenterologia **79:** 338, 1953.
63. Watkinson, G., Feather, D. B., Marson, F. G. W., and Dossett, J. A.: Massive jejunal diverticulosis with steatorrhea and mealoblastic anemia improved by excision of diverticula, Brit. M. J. **2:** 58, 1959.
64. Watson, G. M., Cameron, D. G., and Witts, L. J.: Experimental macrocytic anemia in the rat, Lancet **2:** 404, 1948.
65. Watson, G. M., and Witts, L. J.: Intestinal macrocytic anemia, Brit. M. J. **1:** 13, 1952.
66. Watson, P. C.: Acute distention of afferent loop after Polya gastrectomy, Brit. M. J. **1:** 1334, 1958.
67. Wells, C. A., and Mac Phee, I. W.: The afferent loop syndrome, bilious regurgitation after subtotal gastrectomy and its relief, Lancet **2:** 1189, 1952.
68. White, W. H.: On the pathology and prognosis of pernicious anemia, Guy's Hosp. Rep. **47:** 149, 1890.
69. Witts, L. J.: Anaemia and the alimentary tract, Edinburgh, 1956, Royal College of Surgeons of Edinburgh, Publication No. 7.

*Conducted by* CLARENCE DENNIS, M.D., AND ALFRED HURWITZ, M.D.

# Pancreaticojejunostomy for chronic relapsing pancreatitis: an evaluation

WILLIAM J. GILLESBY, M.D.
CHARLES B. PUESTOW, M.D.
HINES, ILL.
*From the Hines Veterans Administration Hospital*

It is generally agreed that ductal obstruction is a major etiological factor in the production of pain and the development of chronic relapsing pancreatitis. The literature has been and continues to be plentiful with regard to methods of accomplishing adequate drainage of the pancreas.

The concept[7, 12] that adequate decompression and drainage of the pancreas would relieve the symptoms of chronic relapsing pancreatitis has been supported by the results. Carnevali and associates[3] have experimentally supported the belief that "unroofing" of the pancreatic ducts and anastomosis of the surrounding pancreas to the jejunum is a practical and physiologic procedure.

Bartlett and Nardi[2] have utilized some of these principles with success. They mobilized the pancreas and opened the ducts widely, then performed a vagotomy and gastric division with implantation of the opened pancreas into the isolated antrum of the stomach. Their belief was that by adequate drainage as well as suppression of pancreatic secretion accomplished by means of the vagotomy, they would relieve the symptoms of pancreatitis. They have reported success in a limited number of cases. From our own studies we suspect that the intragastric pancreas is slowly digested and that one of the aims of this treatment, namely, preservation of pancreatic tissue, is thus defeated.[10]

Partington and Rochelle[8] have modified the procedure in an interesting way. They leave the pancreas in situ without removing the spleen and anastomose the opened pancreas to the opened jejunum. In recent cases and as recently reported,[4] we have been performing a somewhat similar procedure by anastomosing the opened pancreas to the opened defunctionalized jejunum, but have not been as successful as Partington and Rochelle in preserving the spleen.

The preservation of the spleen is desirable, but the adhesions between spleen and pancreas in these cases are frequently quite dense and minimal manipulation tears the splenic capsule and makes splenectomy mandatory. The splenic vessels are adherent to the pancreas and must sometimes be ligated to allow mobilization of the spleen. Partington and Rochelle have suggested that splenorenal shunt is to be considered in some of these cases because of the accompanying portal hypertension. We have found that splenorenal shunts in these instances are technically difficult if not impossible, because of the peripancreatic reaction. Preston[11] has treated 2 patients with traumatic splenic rupture in association with chronic relapsing pancreatitis. He believes the rupture occurred because of fixation due to inflammatory reaction and minor trauma to the left side. We have treated 2 such patients and have seen 3 at operation when minimal manipulation of the pancreatic tail resulted

Received for publication July 3, 1961.

in tears in the capsule and hilar pulp which necessitated splenectomy.

Of personal communications[1, 3, 4, 6, 8, 9, 13, 14] with surgeons who have performed retrograde pancreaticojejunostomy (some 25 cases) in the manner we have described, only 2 poor results have been reported.

Twenty-nine patients have been treated by the "opened pancreas" pancreaticojejunostomy method. There was 1 postoperative death. The patient died 30 days postoperatively of peritonitis which was deemed at postmortem examination to be due to a leak in anastomosis. This, we believe, was due to a technical error and could have been avoided by paying more attention to some of the details learned later. Our analysis of these cases places 19 results as excellent, 4 as good, and 2 as fair to poor.Two patients were lost to follow-up. There was one other death. One patient who was lost to follow-up had experienced dramatic relief of pain and had been in excellent condition when last seen 7 months postoperatively. Chronic relapsing pancreatitis had occurred in a paraplegic patient and he was operated on at this institution. Pain was relieved promptly and he was quite well except for numerous urinary tract problems which so often occur in the paraplegic patient. He died 1 year after operation of cirrhosis, chronic brain syndrome, and hemorrhagic cystitis. No postmortem examination was obtained, but the relief of pain had been complete. Two patients showed poor results and no explanation is known. In both of these cases the pancreatic ducts were almost obliterated and the fibrosis and scarring of the pancreas made us wonder if drainage could be accomplished by any procedure. The 4 patients with good results have been well, but occasionally have short bouts of pain which we suspect accompanies alcoholic excess. Of the 19 patients with excellent results, the pain has been relieved in a dramatic fashion. A short description of one of these, an alcoholic individual with chronic relapsing pancreatitis, may be of interest. He had a history of numerous surgical procedures in various institutions. In 1952 he had undergone a gastric resection, later a splanchnicectomy, and later a celiac ganglionectomy. In 1954 a sphincterotomy had been performed without relief. Cholecystectomy was performed 6 months later. In 1956, when he was first seen at this institution, a retrograde pancreaticojejunostomy was performed by our original method,[12] with implantation of the pancreatic tail into a Roux Y jejunal loop and restoration of the intestinal channel performed by a Roux Y anastomosis. The man was relieved of pain and had been well for approximately 9 months when pain recurred. At this time it was decided that a more adequate drainage procedure should be performed and in 1957 reoperation was carried out. The pancreas was opened widely and drained into the defunctionalized jejunal segment. Recovery was uneventful and the man has been well. He has some dumping syndrome symptoms, his weight has increased, and the steatorrhea has markedly improved. Calcifications which

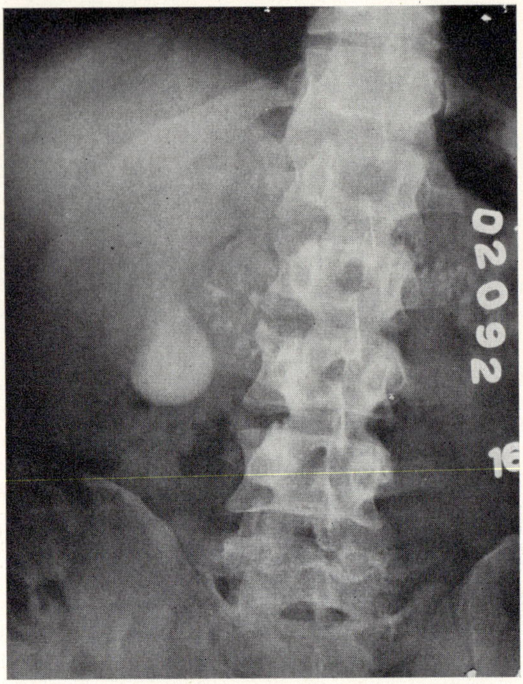


**Fig. 1.** Cholecystogram which shows normally functioning gall bladder with marked calcification throughout the pancreas. These calcifications are not confined to the pancreatic ductal system.

were present in the pancreas over the years have disappeared on roentgenogram.

Most of the patients have been of the alcoholic type and few of those treated have ceased drinking. In reviewing the charts, we noted in most of them the comment that the patient smelled strongly of alcohol. Two operations have been performed when chronic relapsing pancreatitis followed gastric procedures with damage to the pancreatic ducts. One of these operations followed a gastric resection performed elsewhere which had been complicated by postoperative pancreatitis. The patient had a long history of pain and debility which had brought him to the point of psychosis. After observation it was decided to attempt to do something for this unfortunate individual and a reconstruction was carried out. Retrograde pancreaticojejunostomy with Roux Y reconstruction was used. The pain was dramatically relieved, his disposition improved, and he was discharged from the psychiatric section of this institution. Follow-up 6 months postoperatively showed that he was well and believed that he could go back to work soon.

The question has long been in our minds as to whether or not the pancreatic ducts remain open. We have some evidence that they do. A 37-year-old Negro man was first seen in 1956 with intractable pain. He was requiring large doses of narcotics. Medical management failed. Cholecystectomy and common duct exploration were performed with a sphincterotomy. He was not improved and in 1958, a retrograde pancreaticojejunostomy with a Roux Y enteroanastomosis was performed. The patient did well, but had recurrence of pain and in March, 1959, the pancreaticojejunostomy was revised. The dilated duct was opened widely on this occasion and the man recovered well after this procedure. Some 7 months later, he died of an acute myocardial infarction and at postmortem examination the pancreas was markedly constricted and fibrotic, but draining into the jejunal pouch. The postmortem report stated that the pancreaticojejunostomy was

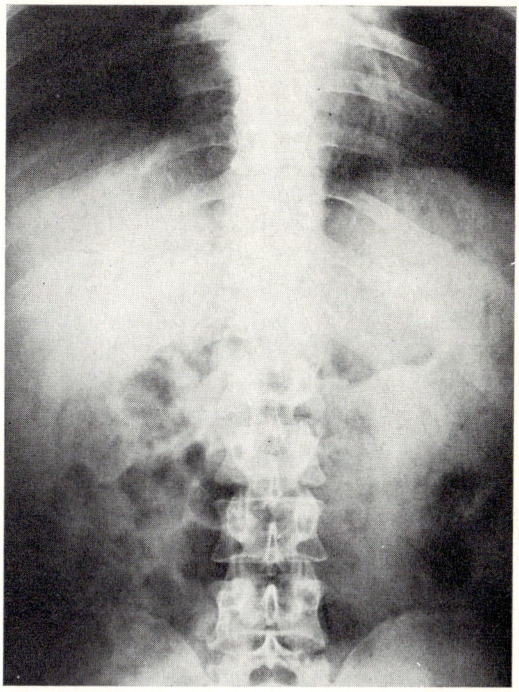

**Fig. 2.** Cholecystogram taken 1 hour after ingestion of a fat meal. There is satisfactory gallbladder emptying.

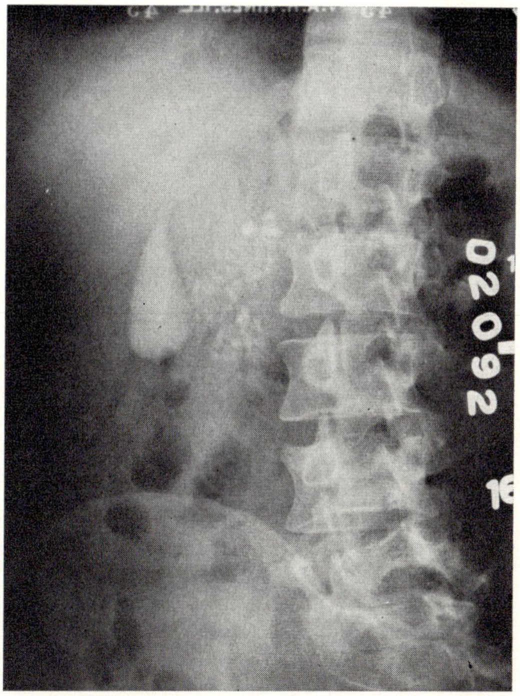

**Fig. 3.** Upright film of abdomen taken 4 years later. Calcifications have disappeared.

functioning well, and we know from the patient's history that the pain had been completely relieved.

Microscopic sections taken preoperatively and 7 months later showed fibrosis and scarring. The preoperative sections showed more leukocytic reaction than the postoperative sections, but we have not as yet found evidence of dramatic glandular regeneration. In view of the studies of Carnevali and associates in dogs, we believe that glandular regeneration may occur.

The pancreatic calcification may be dissolved after pancreaticojejunostomy. Figs. 1 and 2 show calcification throughout the pancreas in a 32-year-old salesman who had a past history of alcoholism. He has been relieved of symptoms after adequate pancreatic drainage by pancreaticojejunostomy. Fig. 3 shows disappearance of the calcifications 4 years later.

## SUMMARY

An analysis of adequate drainage of the pancreas has been presented. We are convinced that pancreatic pain is due to increased pressure within the gland secondary to ductal obstruction and, on clinical grounds, that some recovery of the pancreas occurs after adequate drainage. In these cases the condition has been severe and the alcoholic patients have not been reformed by their disease.

Simplification of the procedure is continuing and we believe that as more surgeons attempt it, new ideas will be developed and the procedure will become standardized. It is our firm belief that the pancreatic duct should be widely opened and adequate drainage provided. No attempt should be made to make a mucosa-to-mucosa anastomosis between the pancreatic duct and the jejunum. The jejunum should be anastomosed to the outer surface of the pancreas some distance from the edges of the pancreatic incision. If this is performed, the results so far are gratifying and well worthwhile.

## ADDENDUM

Three additional surgeons have reported good results in individual cases since preparation of this manuscript.

We would appreciate hearing from surgeons who have performed this procedure.

## REFERENCES

1. Allen, M. J.: Personal communication.
2. Bartlett, M. K., and Nardi, G. L.: Treatment of recurrent pancreatitis by resection, inhibition and retrograde drainage of the pancreas, Ann. Surg. **152:** 861, 1960.
3. Berman, J. K.: Personal communication.
4. Campanale, R. P.: Personal communication.
5. Carnevali, J. F., ReMine, W. H., Dockerty, M. B., Bollman, J. L., and Grindlay, J. H.: An experimental study of side-to-side pancreaticojejunostomy after ductal obstruction, A. M. A. Arch. Surg. **80:** 774, 1960.
6. Garlock, J. H.: Personal communication.
7. Gillesby, W. J., and Puestow, C. B.: Surgery for chronic recurrent pancreatitis, S. Clin. North America **41:** 83, 1961.
8. Maher, R. W.: Personal communication.
9. McEachern, C. G.: Personal communication.
10. Partington, P. F., and Rochelle, R. E. L.: Modified Puestow procedure for retrograde drainage of the pancreatic duct, Ann. Surg. **152:** 1037, 1960.
11. Preston, F. W.: Personal communication.
12. Puestow, C. B., and Gillesby, W. J.: Retrograde surgical drainage of pancreas for chronic relapsing pancreatitis, A. M. A. Arch. Surg. **76:** 898, 1958.
13. Wheeler, J. R.: Personal communication.
14. Zinninger, M. M.: Personal communication.

Volume 50 Number 6 SURGERY

DECEMBER, 1961



Clinical surgery

# Acute perforated peptic ulcer: evaluation of 160 consecutive patients treated by closure

LOUIS T. PALUMBO, M.D.
WENDELL S. SHARPE, M.D.
DES MOINES, IOWA
*From the Department of Surgery, Des Moines Veterans Administration Hospital*

Acute perforation of a peptic ulcer continues to be one of the major life-threatening complications associated with the disease. Early recognition and proper management of this catastrophe save lives and reduce the period of disability.

The method of treatment continues to remain controversial, whether operative or nonoperative. However, a greater swing to operative closure as the method of choice has been apparent again in recent years. There remain a few advocates of the nonoperative method of treatment. Selectivity and a certain percentage of cases in which the diagnosis is incorrect may definitely influence their favorable results and effect the low mortality rate reported.

There are a number of critical reasons against nonoperative management of patients with acute perforations; (1) aspiration rarely is completely successful in stomachs full of either food or liquids, (2) large lesions rarely seal, (3) occasionally the tip of the aspirating tube passes through the perforation, (4) food particles may temporarily plug the perforation and healing will not occur, (5) a number of so-called "successfully treated" ulcers are actually penetrating and not perforated, (6) without operation there is always the danger of a missed diagnosis with involvement of another organ for which operation was necessary, (7) perforation due to malignancy is possible and without operation may go undiagnosed, and (8) bed rest may well delay definitive operation until it cannot safely be performed.

This is a presentation of the results of the surgical management of acute perforations of peptic ulcer in 160 unselected and consecutively treated patients admitted to our hospital from Jan. 1, 1946, to Jan. 1, 1960. A comparison of these results will be made with results in a series of 56 consecutively treated and unselected patients we reported upon in 1953.

It was our opinion then, and still is, that improvement can be expected in the surgical management of these patients by the judicious use of antibiotics, better application of anesthesiology, coordinated and balanced pre- and postoperative care, earlier surgical closure of the perforation and, in a care-

Received for publication Jan. 26, 1961.

**Table I.** *Age incidence*

| Age (yr.) | 1953 report | | Present 14 yr. report | |
|---|---|---|---|---|
| | No. | % | No. | % |
| 20-30 | 8 | 14.0 | 13 | 8 |
| 31-40 | 20 | 36.0 | 48 | 30 |
| 41-50 | 6 | 11.0 | 46 | 29 |
| 51-60 | 15 | 27.0 | 42 | 27 |
| 61-70 | 6 | 10.2 | 7 | 4 |
| Over 70 | 1 | 1.8 | 4 | 2 |
| Totals | 56 | | 160 | |

fully selected group, primary definitive operation at the time of perforation, and finally the establishment of an early "planned definitive resection" at an early date after simple closure. Such planning is accomplished with patient's cooperation and can usually be performed several weeks after preliminary closure. The latter procedure is used to prevent repeated perforations and other serious later complications which cause prolonged periods of disability and life-threatening hazards which lead to greater surgical risks and increased morbidity and mortality rates.

The series of 160 cases* reported represents a controlled group studied under the guidance and direction of one Chief of the Surgical Service (L.T.P.). The rationale of therapy, criteria for operation, and method of management were consistently controlled.

## RESULTS

The patients ranged in age from 21 to 78 years, and the average age was 47.2 years. Approximately 85 per cent of the patients in this series were in the 3 decades after the age of 31 years. Comparison with our earlier paper[1] shows changes, the significance of which may be simply that these decades usually contain the major number of patients with duodenal ulcer and its complications (Table I).

The average time which elapsed from perforation to operation was nearly 9 hours (Table II). The shortest time was less than 3 hours; all of the 5 patients in this group were in the hospital at the time of perforation. All 5 had suffered typical ulcer distress periodically for years. Three had been hospitalized for other complaints when perforation occurred.

The longest time interval was 120 hours and 17 (10.6 per cent) of the entire group showed a total elapsed time from perforation to operation of over 24 hours. There were 98 patients (62.2 per cent) operated upon in less than 6 hours. In a group of 30 (18.75 per cent), operation was delayed more than 6 but less than 12 hours. Finally patients operated upon after 12 and after 18 hours (but before 24 hours) were 9 (5.6 per cent) and 6 (3.75 per cent), respectively.

Table III illustrates a fact of which surgeons have long been aware—that there is a long delay before a patient seeks medical attention and/or is admitted to a hospital for definitive surgical care.

There were 5 patients, not listed in Table III, whom we operated upon within 3 hours from the time of perforation. This is considered an ideal time and represents a reasonable period in which to admit the patient, treat him, and prepare him for operation.

*These patients will be included in a cooperative peptic ulcer study which the Veterans Administration Research in Surgery is conducting.

**Table II.** *Total time interval between perforation and operation*

| Time interval (hr.) | No. of patients | % |
|---|---|---|
| 0- 3 | 5 | 3.1 |
| 0- 6 | 93 | 58.1 |
| 7-12 | 30 | 18.8 |
| 13-18 | 9 | 5.6 |
| 19-24 | 6 | 3.8 |
| Over 24 | 17 | 10.6 |
| Totals | 160 | 100 |

**Table III.** *Time elapsed from perforation to hospitalization*

| Time interval (hr.) | No. of patients | % |
|---|---|---|
| 0- 6 | 93 | 60.0 |
| 7-12 | 30 | 19.4 |
| 13-18 | 9 | 5.8 |
| 19-24 | 6 | 3.8 |
| Over 24 | 17 | 11.0 |

**Table IV.** *Time interval from perforation to operation by age groups*

| Age groups (yr.) | Time interval (hr.) | | |
|---|---|---|---|
| | Average | Longest | Shortest |
| 21-30 | 24.2 | 120.0 | 4 |
| 31-40 | 7.4 | 34.0 | 3 |
| 41-50 | 9.4 | 32.0 | 3 |
| 51-60 | 8.6 | 18.2 | 3 |
| 61-70 | 10.5 | 11.0 | 3 |
| Over 70 | 6.8 | 7.2 | 5 |

Table IV provides a breakdown of patients by age groups and time interval between perforation and operation. The longest period of delay occurs in the youngest age group (21 to 30 years).

The average duration of symptoms in patients in this entire series, from whom a definite history could be obtained, was 6.3 years. In 41 patients (25.6 per cent) a so-called "silent" ulcer was noted. However, by closer evaluation of the patients' records the "silent" ulcer group was only 9.3 per cent. Over 56 per cent of all the patients developed perforation after a spree of immoderate use of alcohol. Bleeding occurred just prior to the perforation in 40 patients (25 per cent). The remaining 14 patients all had undergone a previous operation for perforation.

## PREOPERATIVE STUDIES AND TREATMENT

During the past 4 years no chemicals or antibiotics were introduced into the peritoneal cavity at the time of operation. The use of neomycin was stopped immediately when we observed and read in the literature of the untoward reaction that occurs when curare as an anesthetic agent is used with other anesthetic agents–a depression of respiratory exchange caused by central toxic action in the brain. In fact, in the last 7 years, the usual procedure has been to evacuate as much as possible of the collected fluid and material from the peritoneal cavity. If such soilage was extensive, then saline irrigation or, if believed necessary, irrigation with penicillin and/or streptomycin was employed prior to closure of the wound to lessen the possibility of local collection of irritants and prevent abscess formation.

## ANESTHESIA AND CLOSURE

Practically all the patients were given inhalation anesthesia. A short right transverse incision (154 cases) above the umbilicus, dividing the right anterior and posterior rectus sheaths transversely, was performed. The right rectus muscle was transected.

During the early years, the wound closure was accomplished with catgut in 37 cases, or 23 per cent of the group. In 115 patients (72 per cent) silk was used; wire was used in only 8 patients (5 per cent). There were only 3 wound infections, none of which were severe. This represents an incidence of only 1.8 per cent. One infection (2.7 per cent) occurred in the early group with catgut closure; in the group with silk closure there was only 1 wound infection (0.8 per cent) and in the small group with wire closure there was 1 infection (12.5 per cent).

There were no instances of wound dehiscence or postoperative herniation.

## LOCATION OF ULCER

In the entire series of 160 patients, 119 (74.4 per cent) had perforation of an anterior duodenal ulcer involving the first part of the duodenum. In 26 (16.2 per cent) the perforation was of a gastric ulcer or lesion. There were 15 patients (9.4 per cent) with perforations in the obscure area of the "pyloric canal."

If there existed any question that the perforation might be of gastric origin, a biopsy specimen was taken, as it was in most instances of definite gastric perforation. No evidence of adenocarcinoma of the stomach was found. In only 1 instance was a malignancy found; this finally proved to be a lymphosarcoma. Gastric resection was performed and the patient had no evidence of recurrence of lesion at the time of his accidental death 7 years later.

## CLOSURE

Simple closure of the perforation was performed in 153 patients (95.6 per cent).

This was accomplished by the use of interrupted Lembert sutures, incorporating an omental pedicle as reinforcement. In 2 patients (1.25 per cent) it was necessary to use a purse-string suture of catgut, reinforced by interrupted Lembert sutures, again with an omental pedicle graft. In 2 other patients, the defect was so large and the accompanying edema and friability of the tissue so great that an attempt at the usual closure would have resulted in pyloric obstruction postoperatively. In both instances the round ligaments of the liver and omentum were used as patches.

In the entire 14 years there were only 3 patients (1.9 per cent) for whom we were of the opinion that primary gastric resection was indicated at the time of acute duodenal perforation. In all 3 the operation was performed within 6 hours from the time of perforation and the other conditions were met from the standpoint of pathologic process, ulcer history, obstruction, minimal peritoneal spillage, and chemical peritonitis, and the general condition of the patients was excellent.

## MORTALITY RATE

There were no deaths in the entire series.

## POSTOPERATIVE TREATMENT

The patients treated during the 1946 to 1948 period were ambulatory on the second to the fourth postoperative day. After 1948, all patients were ambulatory on the first day.

Nasogastric suction was continued for from 2 to 3 days postoperatively in the group of patients without complications. Oral feedings were started on the third to the fifth postoperative day. The patient then received a progressive gastric diet.

## EARLY POSTOPERATIVE COMPLICATIONS

Early postoperative complications (Table V) developed in 23 patients (14.3 per cent). This represents a 50 per cent decrease when the current 104 patients were compared. All postoperative gastric hemorrhages were completely controlled by conservative management. Patients with pyloric obstruction did well after planned early definitive resection. The other complications listed in Table V required only treatment ordinarily accorded the specific disease or condition.

## HOSPITAL STAY

In the entire previous group of 56 patients, those without serious complications were discharged from the hospital by the sixteenth postoperative day. They were recalled 28 days later for any necessary study and treatment. Those without complaints or complications were then treated medically.

In the later group, particularly in the last 5 years, definitive surgical treatment for chronic duodenal ulcer was strongly recommended. If the patient did not accept it, he was discharged and recalled for follow-up study at regular intervals. In recent years this recall system has produced a follow-up of over 90 per cent of patients studied.

**Table V.** *Early postoperative complications*

| | *First group (56 patients)* | | *Second group (104 patients)* | | *Total 160 patients* | |
|---|---|---|---|---|---|---|
| *Type* | *No.* | *%* | *No.* | *%* | *No.* | *%* |
| Abscess, pelvic | 1 | 1.8 | 1 | 0.9 | 2 | 1.2 |
| Abscess, subhepatic | 0 | 0 | 1 | 0.9 | 1 | 0.6 |
| Cardiac decompensation | 1 | 1.8 | 1 | 0.9 | 2 | 1.2 |
| Distention, severe | 1 | 1.8 | 1 | 0.9 | 2 | 1.2 |
| Effusion, pleural | 1 | 1.8 | 0 | 0 | 1 | 0.6 |
| Hemorrhage, gastrointestinal | 3 | 5.3 | 2 | 1.9 | 5 | 3.1 |
| Infection, wound | 1 | 1.8 | 2 | 1.9 | 3 | 1.8 |
| Obstruction, pyloric | 3 | 5.3 | 3 | 2.8 | 6 | 3.7 |
| Perforation, esophageal | 1 | 1.8 | 0 | 0 | 1 | 0.6 |
| Totals | 12 | 21.4 | 11 | 10.2 | 23 | 14.0 |

## RESULTS AND RATE OF RETURN FOR FOLLOW-UP

The longest period of follow-up was 13 years and the shortest period was 13 months. The average period of follow-up was 9.5 years with a follow-up rate of 91.3 per cent, or 146 patients. Failure to follow the remaining 14 patients was due to the fact several had moved from our area, and in a few instances no replies could be obtained from our inquiries.

## EVALUATION OF FINAL RESULTS

Of the 143 patients remaining with adequate follow-up studies, 4 classifications of their progress was easily made; (1) patients for whom medical management alone was sufficient, with no symptoms or signs of trouble, and with normal roentgenographic findings (31 patients, 21.7 per cent), (2) patients still under medical management who demonstrated symptoms or signs of recurring ulceration, obstruction, or bleeding in whom the clinical findings were confirmed roentgenographically and for whom further surgical intervention seemed inevitable (23 patients, 16 per cent), (3) patients who already had undergone gastric operation for reasons not associated with the original duodenal ulcer (2 patients, 1.4 per cent), and (4) patients who developed one or more of the classic complications of duodenal ulcer or benign gastric ulcer which necessitated further definitive gastric operations for relief (87 patients, 60.8 per cent).

## COMMENT

Primary early closure of acute peptic ulcer perforation in our hands remains the procedure of choice and results in a minimal morbidity and disability. The advocates of the nonoperative treatment of this type of patient have not met these criteria and our results.

It is our opinion that immediate definitive operation at the time of perforation has its place, but certainly is limited to a select group of patients under rigid indications. The prime tenet is to perform the simplest and safest procedure to save life with the least disablement and to plan a careful and repeated follow-up for selection and preparation of the patient for early "planned definitive gastric operation."

The greatest weakness in the past in most series has been the loss of follow-up and control of the patient who experienced a perforated peptic ulcer. It is difficult to assess accurately the actual number who develop the late serious complications of peptic ulcer disease which necessitate surgical intervention. With the program that we have evolved in the past 5 years, we are able now to predict with some degree of accuracy the number of patients who will need operations after perforation. Therefore, we can anticipate sooner the need for definitive procedures in patients whom we follow and thus recommend to them early elective antrectomy with vagectomy.

The prognosis can be greatly influenced by early surgical closure of a perforation. The interval of time between perforation and closure still remains the most lethal factor. A reduction in this time rests in the hands of both the patient and his physician. Too often, however, the patient himself or his family are responsible for this delay. Frequently the patient is referred for consultation late. Any educational program that will aid in the earlier seeking of medical attention, earlier recognition of the acute emergency, speedier and better preoperative preparation of the patient, coupled with all the advances previously mentioned, will result in continued improvement with further reduction in the morbidity and mortality rates.

The public would benefit even more when realization of the emergency nature of this catastrophe is accepted. Early diagnosis and insistence upon prompt emergency hospitalization regardless of transportation, family, and other conflicts are key factors.

It is important to note that over 60 per cent of the patients in this series, to date, have already undergone definitive gastric operations and that 16 per cent currently are experiencing difficulty from one or more of the complications from chronic ulceration.

## SUMMARY AND CONCLUSIONS

The results of the emergency operative treatment of acute perforated peptic ulcer in 160 consecutively treated male patients are presented. There were no deaths. The patients ranged in age from 21 to 78 years. The average time interval from acute perforation to surgical closure of defect was 9 hours. A small transverse right supraumbilical incision was employed. Silk suture closure of the wound was accomplished. Dehiscence and postoperative herniation did not occur. Neither the peritoneal cavity nor the wound was drained. There were only 3 wound infections (1.8 per cent), and 1 pelvic abscess and 1 subhepatic abscess occurred.

By carefully controlled, early follow-up program, early definitive elective gastric operation was recommended and performed in 60 per cent of the patients in this series to date. This was necessary because of the progressive complications associated with chronic duodenal ulcer. At this time there are an additional 16 per cent who also need definitive operations.

Therefore, in the past several years there has not been an abandonment of our former position that the simple surgical closure procedure is a life-saving emergency measure, that it should be performed early and quickly, that education of the public and members of the profession concerning the harmful effects of delay is mandatory, and that all patients and their families be indoctrinated from the first that very probably 2 procedures requiring 2 separate operations will be necessary. Early planned "definitive gastric operation" in a high per cent of these patients will result in a marked decrease in disability, chronic invalidism, and the many later complications associated with a chronic ulcer diathesis.

### REFERENCE

1. Palumbo, L. T., and Rugtiv, G. M.: Results of operative treatment of acute perforated peptic ulcer, SURGERY **34:** 635, 1953.

# Renal function during and immediately after profound hypothermia

J. TERBLANCHE, M.B., CH.B.
L. C. ISAACSON, B.SC., M.B., CH.B.
L. EALES, M.D.
C. N. BARNARD, M.D., PH.D.
CAPE TOWN, SOUTH AFRICA
*From the Departments of Surgery and Medicine, University of Cape Town and Groote Schuur Hospital*

Although the body is able to make certain adjustments to changing circumstances in order to maintain a satisfactory "milieu interior," such adjustments are not necessarily always favorable. Surgical techniques employed to improve operative conditions in certain organs may evoke responses in others which are perhaps detrimental, and a sound knowledge of such concomitant responses is essential. Only when it is clear that the beneficial effects of these techniques outweigh the dangerous responses can their use be justified.

With the increased use of profound levels of hypothermia in cardiac, brain, and vascular operations, a careful study of the responses of the body to the sudden reduction in temperature that occurs seems justified. This report concerns the changes in certain renal functions observed during and after cardiopulmonary bypass with profound hypothermia.

## METHODS

**Operative and bypass procedure.** Nine healthy adult mongrel dogs which weighed between 15 and 21 kilograms were anesthetized intravenously with thiopental sodium and after intubation anesthesia was maintained with nitrous oxide and oxygen. Polyethylene cannulas were inserted into the left femoral artery and vein and connected to manometers for pressure recordings. One needle was inserted into a vein in one of the forelimbs and a second into a vein in the right hindlimb for intravenous infusions during the experiments.

In 7 of the dogs, profound hypothermia was induced, and in these the heart was approached by a left thoracotomy through the fourth intercostal space. In the 2 control dogs, in which the renal functions were studied under normothermic conditions, the heart was exposed through a right thoracotomy.

After intravenous systemic heparinization with 1.5 mg. of heparin per kilogram of body weight, the right common femoral artery was exposed and catheterized with a stainless steel catheter. The arterial line of the helix reservoir bubble oxygenator,[6, 7, 12] which had been previously assembled[2, 12] and primed[13] with heparinized donor blood, was connected to the arterial catheter. Bennington heat exchange units* were incorporated in the arterial line when hypothermia was to be induced.[25]

In the 7 hypothermic dogs, the venous blood was drained by means of a single No. 32 Bardex catheter introduced into the right atrium through the right atrial appendage; once hypothermic failure of the heart had occurred, a second catheter was introduced into the left atrium through the left atrial appendage, and the blood aspirated from the

Received for publication Feb. 23, 1961.

*Supplied by Westdene Products (Pty) Ltd., Cape Town, South Africa.

left heart was returned to the heart-lung machine in this manner. In the 2 control dogs, the venous blood was drained by means of catheters in the superior and inferior venae cavae.

Flow rates of 70 ml. per kilogram of body weight per minute were maintained throughout the perfusions of all the animals except Dog 1, in which extracorporeal circulation was stopped completely for 30 minutes during the cold phase. No cardiac operation was performed during any of these experiments. Rectal and esophageal temperatures were recorded in the dogs by means of the electric universal thermometer type TE-3, with leads types R-7 and OSG-1.*

At the end of the perfusion, when a normal heartbeat had been established, bypass was discontinued in the conventional manner. The heparin was neutralized with the required amount of protamine sulphate and blood deficit was replaced through the arterial catheter with arterial and venous pressures as monitors.

The wounds were closed and a chest drain was attached to a suction apparatus. The dogs were then returned to a warm recovery cage. No special postoperative care, apart from overnight intravenous administration of fluids and routine antibiotics, was utilized.

**Renal function investigations.** In the hypothermia experiments, the bypass was divided into 4 stages; (1) a period of bypass without active cooling, varying from a few minutes to half an hour, followed by (2) a period of cooling to about 10° C., often in stages, then (3) a static period without active cooling or warming, and finally (4) a period of active rewarming.

Urine collections were obtained from a catheter tied in one or both ureters. The ureters were exposed through a small flank incision and dissected out retroperitoneally. The tip of the catheter was inserted into the renal pelvis and tied firmly in place. Collections were obtained over accurately timed intervals. They were begun at least 20 minutes after the intravenous infusions had been begun and between 7 and 60 minutes before bypass was started to enable prebypass control estimations to be performed. After the completion of the bypass, urinary function was followed in 8 of the 9 dogs for an additional 10 to 79 minutes to enable postbypass control estimations to be made.

Blood samples were taken every 10 to 15 minutes throughout each experiment, usually at the midpoint of each urine collection period.

Each dog received 2 intravenous infusions throughout the experiment. The one which was given into the forelimb consisted of a 10 per cent solution of dextrose in water, and this was run at a rate to ensure a urinary flow of 1 to 6 ml. per minute prior to bypass. No attempt was made to stabilize the urinary flow. The other infusion, which was given through the needle in the vein in the right hindleg, consisted in each case of 1.5 Gm. of creatinine dissolved in 1 L. of 0.9 normal saline solution. This was run at about 4 ml. per minute via a constant rate drip apparatus. Each dog received a priming dose of 0.5 Gm. of creatinine. Twenty minutes was allowed for equilibration before the urine or blood collections were made.

With the institution of bypass, the serum creatinine level was immediately lowered as the dog's creatinized blood was diluted with the fresh donor blood used to prime the bypass machine. Conversely, as hypothermia proceeded and the urinary excretion of creatinine diminished, the serum level tended to rise. Thus the constant infusion of creatinine was not in itself sufficient to ensure a constant serum level. For this reason blood samples were taken every 10 to 15 minutes for the estimation of serum creatinine.

Each urine and blood sample was analyzed for osmolality, creatinine, sodium, and potassium, and each urine sample for protein content. Urine volumes were measured to the nearest 0.1 ml. Osmolality was determined by means of a Fiske osmometer, accurate to 2 per cent. Creatinine and quantitative urinary protein were measured by the methods described by King and Wootton.[11] Sodium

*Manufactured by Elektrolaboratoriet, Copenhagen, Denmark.

**Table I.** *General picture of experiments*

| *Dog No. and weight (Kg.)* | *Experiment* | *Bypass details* | *Total duration of bypass (min.)* | *Plasma Hb. (mg. %)* | *Lowest esophageal temperature (C.)* | *Well 24 hr. after bypass* |
|---|---|---|---|---|---|---|
| 1, 15 | Hypothermic renal function | 30 min. cooling, 30 min. off, 30 min. warming | 60+ 30 off | – | 11 | Yes |
| 2, 21 | Hypothermic renal function | Normothermia, cooling, static, warming | 106 | 54 | 9.3 | Yes |
| 3, 17 | Hypothermic renal function | 10 min. normothermia, 10 min. 25° C., 10 min. 10° C., warming | 89 | 48 | 11 | Yes |
| 4, 20 | Hypothermic renal function | Same | 71 | 112 | 10.2 | No |
| 5, 17 | Hypothermic renal function | Same | 86 | 228 | 11.4 | Yes |
| 6, 20 | Normothermic renal function | 30 min. normothermia | 30 | 40 | – | Yes |
| 7, 20 | Hypothermic renal function | 10 min. normothermia, 62 min. cooling, 20 min. static, 44 min. warming | 136 | – | 11.7 | Sacrificed |
| 8, 17 | Hypothermic renal function | 14 min. normothermia, 37 min. cooling, 8 min. static, 31 min. warming | 90 | 87 | 9.2 | No |
| 9, 16 | Normothermic renal function | 44 min. normothermia | 44 | 35 | – | Yes |

and potassium concentrations were determined by flame photometry. The creatinine clearances, which were calculated for the periods during which each urine sample was collected, were taken to represent glomerular filtration rate. When the appropriate blood sample had not been taken at the midpoint of the urine collection period, the serum creatinine level for this point was calculated by simple proportion. Calculations were made of the percentages of filtered sodium excreted $\frac{U_{Na}\ V}{P_{Na}\ C_{cr}} \times 100$ and filtered water excreted $\frac{U\ V}{C_{cr}} \times 100$.

## RESULTS

Table I represents the general outline of the experiments. The accompanying Figs. 1 through 4 show the results of the renal function studies in graphic form.

**Normothermic perfusion results.** The results obtained in the 2 normothermic dogs were identical and Fig. 1 depicts the events which occurred in Dog 9.

In the period before bypass, there was a fall in urine volume and creatinine clearance, with a rise in the urine osmolality and sodium concentration. This was usually associated with a slight fall in the blood pressure and all these changes can possibly be attributed to the anesthetic and to the fall in cardiac output as a result of operative manipulation of the heart. The reason for the rise in the urinary sodium concentration which occurred in this control period, however, is not clear.

It can be seen that with the institution of normothermic bypass, despite a constant blood pressure, there was a continuation or exaggeration of the prebypass trends, except for the urinary sodium concentration which fell as soon as the bypass was begun.

Calculations show that in this dog the percentage of filtered water excreted fell from 13 to 7 per cent as a result of bypass. The percentage of sodium excreted similarly fell from 5 to 0.2 per cent.

After completion of bypass there was a rapid return of these parameters to normal, except the urinary potassium level, which remained constantly elevated.

**Hypothermic perfusion results.** Fig. 2 presents the findings in Dog 4, which was

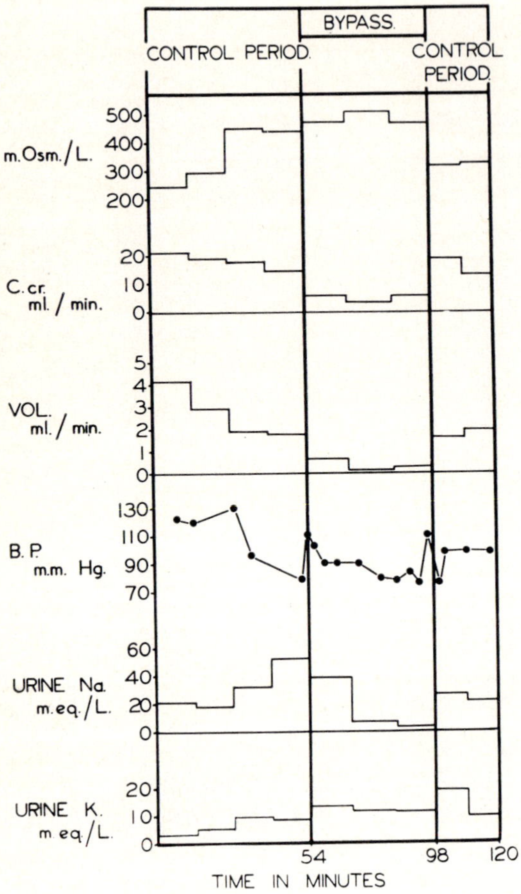


**Fig. 1.** The events which occurred in the normothermic control dogs, as represented by the typical findings in Dog 9.

selected for discussion because the findings were representative of the whole group of hypothermic dogs.

*Changes in blood pressure, creatinine clearance, and urine volume.* With the institution of bypass, prior to cooling, a fall occurred in urine volume and creatinine clearance as it did in the normothermic dogs despite the fact that the blood pressure was well maintained at this stage. Immediately after active cooling was instituted, over the course of the first 3 collection periods, there was a rise in creatinine clearance and urine volume to control levels. This occurred in spite of a steady fall in blood pressure.

As cooling and bypass continued, the blood pressure fell progressively in spite of a constant perfusion flow rate, and with this there was now a fall in creatinine clearance and urine volume.

The changes described were rapidly reversed on rewarming. On discontinuation of bypass after rewarming, creatinine clearance remained unchanged and the urine volume increased to levels exceeding the initial control volume.

*Urinary sodium, potassium, and percentage of filtered water excreted.* With the commencement of active cooling on bypass, the sodium level in the urine rose to approach the serum level. Calculation shows that the percentage of filtered sodium excreted rose from about 1 to 13 per cent at the coldest phase and fell again to about 1 per cent with active rewarming. In addition, the potassium level in the urine fell to approach the serum level.

The percentage of filtered water excreted rose from approximately 6 to 16 per cent and returned to 6 per cent on rewarming.

The urinary sodium and potassium concentrations returned to normal levels with rewarming.

*Urine osmolality.* The urine osmolality fell to approach serum levels with the commencement of active cooling on bypass. This change was reversed with active rewarming. Immediately after the bypass there was a drop in urine osmolality due to diuresis (increase in urinary volume).

**Additional findings in Dog 7.** The findings in Dog 7, as compared with those in the other hypothermic dogs, were similar to those discussed and represented in Fig. 2. In addition, however, as can be seen in Fig. 3, 14 minutes after commencement of active cooling a transient and abrupt rise in arterial pressure was apparent. This appeared to be due to an accidental increase in the perfusion flow rate, which was immediately reflected by a marked rise in both urine volume and glomerular filtration rate (creatinine clearance).

Calculations on this dog showed that the percentage of filtered water which was excreted rose from approximately 23 to 72 per cent when the dog was rendered profoundly hypothermic.

**Proteinuria.** All the dogs except Dog 7 were tested for proteinuria. The concentration of urinary protein during these experiments can be seen in Fig. 4.

In the hypothermic dogs, at 10° C., the urine was protein free, but immediately on commencement of rewarming protein appeared. This reached levels of between 10 and 90 mg. per 100 ml. Only one of the hypothermic dogs tested failed to develop a proteinuria (Dog 3). Dog 1, in which the circulation was stopped during hypothermia and which also developed proteinuria, was not included in Fig. 4. This marked proteinuria did not occur in the 2 normothermic control dogs. In fact, no protein was present in one dog's urine and only a trace was present in that of the other.

## DISCUSSION

A diminution in glomerular filtration rate in the presence of active renal tubular function will lead to a rise in urine osmolality and a fall in the percentage of filtered water and sodium excreted. These changes were a constant finding in the normothermic control dogs and in the control bypass period before active cooling (Figs. 1 through 3). During normothermic bypass with high perfusion flow rate, there is thus a drop in glomerular filtration rate in the presence of unimpaired tubular function. The fall in glomerular filtration in the presence of a relatively well-maintained blood pressure is commensurate with the findings of Corday[5] that one of the earliest mechanisms utilized to maintain systemic blood pressure is renal vasoconstriction.

When, however, profound hypothermia is associated with cardiopulmonary bypass, tubular function is impaired (Figs. 2 and 3). The percentage of excreted sodium and water in the urine increased progressively with cooling (in Dog 7, 72 per cent of the filtered water was excreted as urine), indicating the increasing failure of tubular reabsorption, and this was reflected in the decrease of urine osmolality toward serum levels. Additional evidence of tubular failure was a fall in the urinary potassium level.

The progressive drop in blood pressure, despite the constant high perfusion flow rate and shunt of blood from the heart-lung machine into the dog[19, 20, 23] without a rise in venous pressure, is due at least in part to the impairment of the autonomic nervous function which occurs with cooling,[24] resulting in peripheral vasodilation and an increase in the vascular space.

Glomerular filtration rate and urinary volume promptly rose despite a concomitant fall in blood pressure with the institution of active cooling, and is in accord with Segar's[21, 22] findings that hypothermia induces a marked diuresis in the dog. It appears that at least 2 mechanisms contribute to this phenomenon. One is the transitory increase in glomerular filtration rate, which leads to an immediate and marked increase

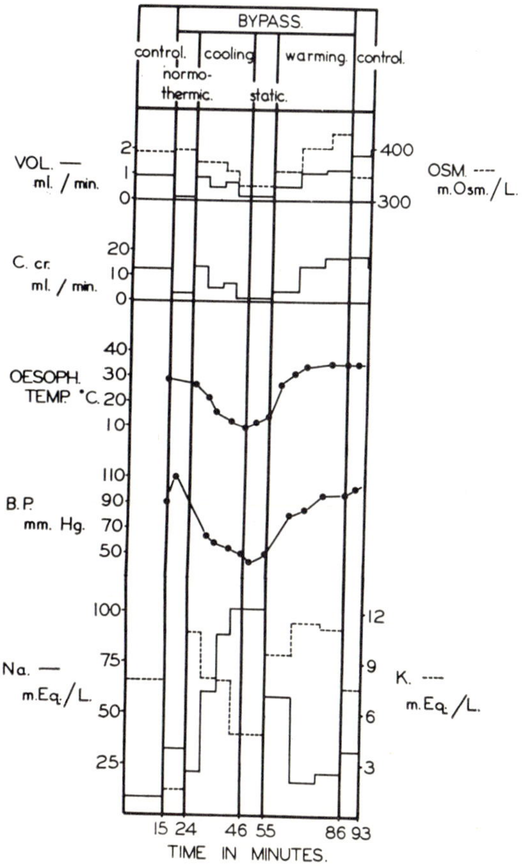


Fig. 2. The events which occurred in the hypothermic dogs, as represented by the typical findings in Dog 4.

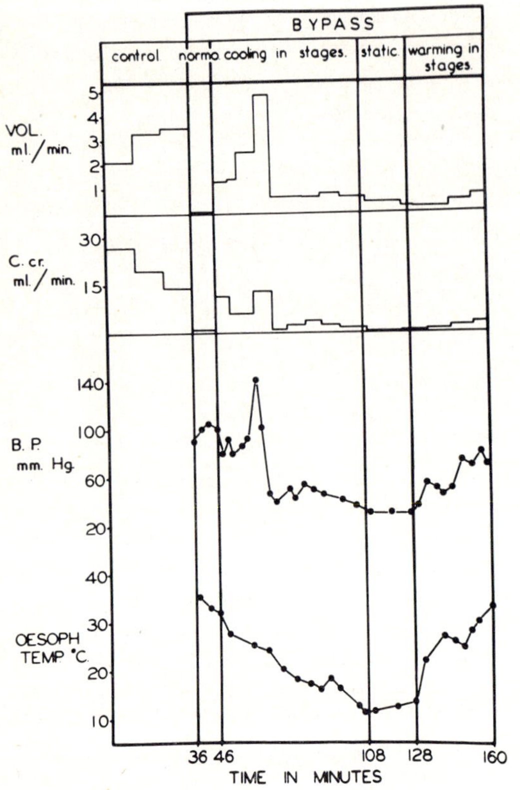


**Fig. 3.** The findings in hypothermic Dog 7, in which the bypass technique differed from the others in this series.

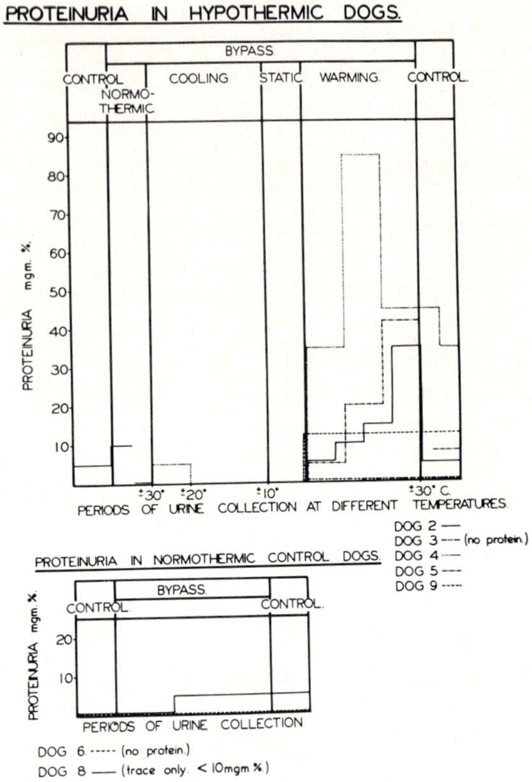


**Fig. 4.** The results of proteinuria tests which were carried out on all the dogs in this series except Dogs 1 and 7.

in urine volume; the other mechanism is the progressive failure of tubular reabsorption of water. The importance of the latter mechanism in hypothermic diuresis has not hitherto been fully appreciated. In the hypothermia experiments there was a closer relationship between glomerular filtration rate, urinary volume, and blood pressure than was observed during normothermic bypass. This phenomenon was clearly shown (1) by the fall and rise which occurred in glomerular filtration rate and urine volume, associated with fall and rise in blood pressure (Figs. 2 and 3), and (2) the accidental increase in perfusion rate, which occurred in Dog 7 and immediately caused a transitory rise in blood pressure, was associated with an immediate rise in glomerular filtration rate and urine volume (Fig. 3).

An important finding in this study was the immediate reversal of all the changes brought about by profound hypothermia on rewarming. If one uses as indices of tubular function the degree of reabsorption of filtered water, sodium, excretion of potassium, and elaboration of concentrated or dilute urine, one can conclude that tubular functions have returned promptly to control levels on rewarming. In only 1 of the 6 hypothermic dogs in which postbypass function was studied did the glomerular filtration rate not return to prebypass level.

In 5 of the 6 hypothermic dogs in which this test was made, proteinuria developed on rewarming. If proteinuria per se is an indication of renal damage, it must be concluded that hypothermia, or the rapid rewarming of the cold organ, can damage the canine kidney in the presence of a high perfusion flow rate. We believe, however, that proteinuria per se is not necessarily an indication of renal damage (as in athletes). It thus seems that the use of profound hypothermia, which is such a useful adjunct in certain branches of modern surgery, is justified, as the extreme changes in renal function which occur during its application are promptly reversed on rewarming.

The effects of cold on the kidney on both dog and in man, usually induced by surface cooling, have been extensively studied.[1, 3, 4, 8-10, 14-18] Even at these temperature levels Segar[21, 22] was able to detect some disturbance of renal tubular function.

In this study, evidence that profound hypothermia affects the tubular transport mechanism was obtained. Further study of this aspect is in progress and will be the subject of another report.

## CONCLUSIONS AND SUMMARY

Seven dogs have been used to observe the variations in renal function which occur during and just after profound hypothermia is induced and maintained by means of an efficient heat exchanger in the arterial line of the bubble oxygenator system. In addition, 2 dogs were subjected to high flow rate normothermic perfusions to act as controls.

Six important points were elicited from these experiments.

1. The changes in renal function which occur during bypass without hypothermia are those associated with a fall in glomerular filtration rate in the presence of normally functioning renal tubules. This fall is apparently out of all proportion to the relatively well-maintained blood pressure. Subsequent to bypass, when the glomerular filtration rate returns to control values, these changes are reversed.

2. The changes in renal function which occur during bypass with profound hypothermia contrast sharply with those which occur with normothermic bypass. Tubular function (as evidenced by the changes in urinary sodium and potassium concentrations, urinary osmolality, and the increase of percentage excretion of filtered water and sodium) becomes progressively impaired, a progressive drop in blood pressure occurs despite the maintenance of a constant high perfusion flow rate, initiation of hypothermia induces a transitory increase of glomerular filtration rate and urine volume, and a more obvious relationship between glomerular filtration rate, urine volume, and blood pressure occurs.

3. Rewarming after profound hypothermia leads to a prompt reversal of the above changes.

4. This reversal is maintained in the immediate postbypass period.

5. During the induction and maintenance of profound hypothermia there is no proteinuria. With rewarming, proteinuria immediately occurs. The significance of this is not certain.

6. In the dog, the prompt reversal of the other abnormal renal functions on rewarming lends support to the continued use of profound hypothermia.

We wish to thank Prof. J. H. Louw of the Department of Surgery, University of Cape Town, for his continued support of our research work and the technical staff, Messrs. C. C. Goosen and C. J. Lockett, and Mrs. V. M. Connell, for their unflagging assistance. Thanks go also to Mrs. P. Kottler for graphs and Mr. G. McManus for photography. Finally, we are indebted to the Council for Scientific and Industrial Research and to the Dr. C. L. Herman Research fund of the University of Cape Town for the financial support of this project.

### REFERENCES

1. Andersen, M., and Nielsen, K. C.: Studies on the renal function under experimental hypothermy in rabbits, Acta med. scandinav. **151:** 191, 1955.
2. Barnard, C. N., McKenzie, M. B., and De Villiers, D. R.: Preparation and assembly of the stainless steel sponge debubbler for use in the helix reservoir bubble oxygenator, Thorax **15:** 268, 1960.
3. Bergstrand, A., and Sterky, G.: Renal function in hypothermia, Acta Physiol. Scandinav. **31:** 13, 1954.
4. Blatters, C. M., and Horvath, S. M.: Renal, cardiovascular and respiratory response and their interrelations during hypothermia, Am. J. Physiol. **192:** 357, 1958.
5. Corday, E., and Williams, J. H., Jr.: Effect of shock and of vasopressor drugs on the regional circulation of the brain, heart, kidney and liver, Am. J. Med. **29:** 228, 1960.

6. DeWall, R. A., Warden, H. E., Read, R. C., Gott, V. L., Ziegler, N., Varco, R. L., and Lillehei, C. W.: A simple, expendable, artificial oxygenator for open-heart surgery, S. Clin. North America **36:** 1025, 1956.
7. DeWall, R. A., Warden, H. E., Varco, R. L., and Lillehei, C. W.: The helix reservoir pump oxygenator, Surg. Gynec. & Obst. **104:** 699, 1957.
8. Hong, S. K.: Renal function during hypothermia and hibernation, Am. J. Physiol. **188:** 137, 1957.
9. Hong, S. K., and Boylan, J. W.: Renal concentrating operation in hypothermic dogs, Am. J. Physiol. **196:** 1150, 1959.
10. Kanter, G. S.: Renal clearance of glucose in hypothermic dogs, Am. J. Physiol. **196:** 866, 1959.
11. King, E. J., and Wootton, I. D. P.: Microanalysis in medical biochemistry, London, 1956, J. & A. Churchill Ltd.
12. McKenzie, M. B., and Barnard, C. N.: Experimental studies in extracorporeal circulation using the helix reservoir bubble oxygenator, South African M. J. **32:** 1145, 1958.
13. McKenzie, M. B., and Barnard, C. N.: A note on priming the DeWall oxygenator, South African M. J. **34:** 108, 1960.
14. Miles, B. E., and Chirchill-Davidson, H. C.: The effect of hypothermia on the renal circulation of the dog, Anesthesiology **16:** 230, 1955.
15. Morales, P., Carbery, W., Morello, A., and Morales, G.: Alteration in renal function during hypothermia in man, Ann. Surg. **145:** 488, 1957.
16. Moyer, J. H.: The effect of hypothermia on renal function and renal damage from ischaemia, Ann. New York Acad. Sc. **80:** 424, 1959.
17. Moyer, J. H., Morris, G., and De Bakey, M. E.: Hypothermia. I. Effect on renal hemodynamics and on excretion of water and electrolytes in dog and man, Ann. Surg. **145:** 26, 1957.
18. Page, L. B.: Effects of hypothermia on renal function, Am. J. Physiol. **181:** 171, 1955.
19. Robard, S., Saiki, H., Malin, A., and Young, C.: Significance of changes in plasma and extracellular volumes in induced hypothermia and hyperthermia, Am. J. Physiol. **167:** 485, 1951.
20. Sanger, P. W., Robicsek, F., Taylor, F. H., Rees, T. T., and Stam, R. E.: Vasomotor regulation during extracorporeal circulation and open-heart surgery, J. Thoracic Surg. **40:** 355, 1960.
21. Segar, W. E.: Effect of hypothermia on tubular transport mechanisms, Am. J. Physiol. **195:** 91, 1958.
22. Segar, W. E., Riley, P. A., Jr., and Barila, T. G.: Urinary composition during hypothermia, Am. J. Physiol. **185:** 528, 1956.
23. Simpson, J. A., Gibson, P., and Bloomfield, D. A.: Profound hypothermia in cardiac surgery, M. J. Australia **47:** 647, 1960.
24. Terblanche, J.: Unpublished data, 1961.
25. Terblanche, J., and Barnard, C. N.: Profound hypothermia using extracorporeal circulation without an artificial oxygenator, South African M. J. **34:** 1003, 1960.

# Retrograde transductal internal drainage of pancreatic pseudocyst

RENÉ MENGUY, M.D., PH.D.*
JOHN C. BLALOCK, M.D.
OKLAHOMA CITY, OKLA.
*From the Department of Surgery, University of Oklahoma Medical Center, and Veterans Administration Hospital*

Recently, we had occasion to treat a patient with a long history of chronic alcoholic pancreatitis complicated by development of a pancreatic pseudocyst associated with obstructive jaundice. It was elected to manage both the chronic pancreatitis and the pseudocyst by internal caudal drainage of the pancreatic duct. To our knowledge, this type of approach had not been described previously. Caudal pancreatic drainage, in our experience, has proved to be a satisfactory method of decompressing the pancreatic duct in patients with chronic pancreatitis. The purpose of this report is to indicate the feasibility of simultaneous drainage of a pseudocyst via this route.

## CASE REPORT

A 43-year-old man was admitted for the first time to the Surgical Service, Veterans Administration Hospital. During the preceding month he had experienced severe epigastric pain, diarrhea, progressively deepening jaundice, and a 30-pound weight loss. Of singular importance in this patient's history was his readily admitted heavy alcoholic intake which dated back to adolescence. The patient had suffered frequent episodes of epigastric pain accompanied by nausea and vomiting over the past 17 years. During the past 8 years these episodes had become more frequent and required 10 admissions to various institutions with diagnoses of acute and chronic pancreatitis. He had obtained moderate relief of symptoms from antispasmodics and dietary measures. The stools gradually became loose and foamy. Five years prior to this admission pancreatic calcification had been recognized. Two years later, a liver biopsy demonstrated portal cirrhosis. One year prior to admission diabetes became evident.

Upon examination jaundice was obvious. The liver was enlarged and the gall bladder was palpable below the liver edge. In the epigastrium a separate smooth, tense mass was palpable. This mass was also readily visible and had all the characteristics of a pancreatic pseudocyst. An upper gastrointestinal series confirmed this impression and also suggested that the cyst was expanding behind the antrum and first portion of the duodenum (Fig. 1, *A*). The significant laboratory findings were an elevated bilirubin level (11.0 mg. per 100 ml.) and hyperglycemia. Results of liver function tests suggested obstructive jaundice. Serum amylase was normal.

The patient underwent abdominal exploration through a bilateral subcostal incision on Oct. 5, 1960. Our preoperative impression was confirmed by the finding of a 15 by 15 by 17 cm. cystic mass overlying the head of the pancreas and bulging behind the antrum and the first portion of the duodenum into the hepatoduodenal ligament. The gall bladder was enlarged, tense, and edematous. A cholangiogram (Fig. 2, *A*) showed obstruction of the distal portion of the common bile duct by extrinsic compression. The tail and head of the pancreas exposed through the gastrocolic ligament had the characteristic diffuse, gritty induration of chronic pancreatitis. The major duct could not be palpated on the surface of the gland. The caudal portion of the pancreas was mobilized and its tip (0.5 cm.) was amputated after removal of the spleen in order to expose the lumen of the major pancreatic duct. A moderate amount of turbid fluid came from the duct as it was opened. This flow could be increased slightly by compression of the cyst. The duct was opened longitudinally up to the level of the mesenteric vessels in the manner described by Puestow.[3] The cephalic portion of the duct was explored and several stones were removed from the lumen. Considerable narrowing of the distal pancreatic duct

Received for publication Feb. 9, 1961.

*John and Mary Markle Scholar in Medical Sciences. Present address: Department of Surgery, University of Kentucky Medical Center, Lexington, Ky.

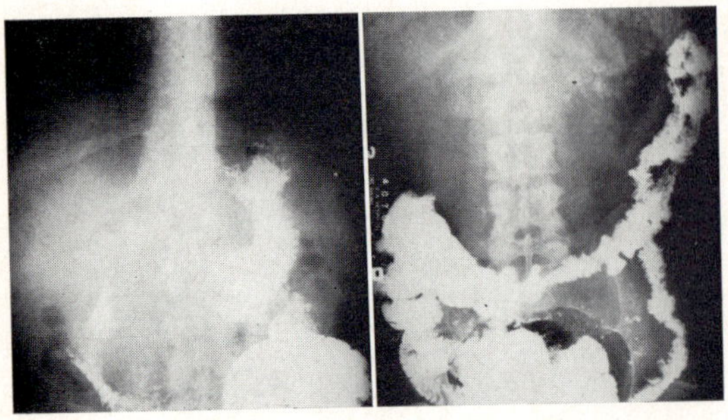

*A* *B*

**Fig. 1.** *A,* Preoperative upper gastrointestinal series demonstrates extrinsic compression of antrum and proximal duodenum by posterior mass. *B,* Preoperative barium enema shows downward displacement of transverse colon. Extensive pancreatic calcification is obvious.

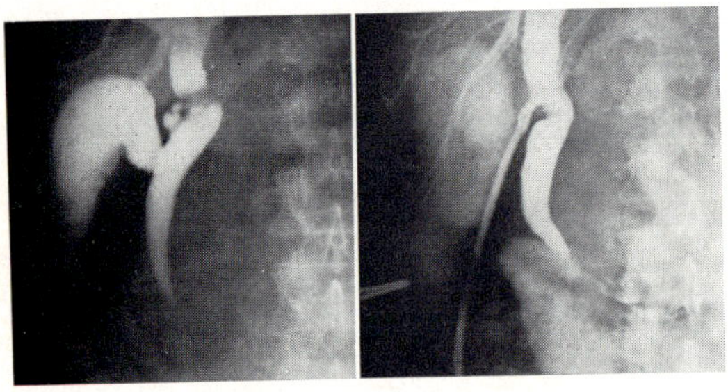

*A* *B*

**Fig. 2.** *A,* Operative cholangiogram taken prior to evacuation of cyst contents demonstrates complete bile duct obstruction due to extrinsic compression of distal bile duct. *B,* Operative cholangiogram taken after evacuation of cyst contents. Note passage of contrast medium into duodenum and absence of cicatricial scarring of the duct.

was obvious upon probing after removal of the stones. A fine-tipped curved clamp was then guided blindly into one of the anterior ramifications of the cephalic portion of the pancreatic duct and with moderate perssure was introduced into the cystic cavity (Fig. 3). There was an immediate gush of dark fluid (1,000 ml.) from the duct as the cyst emptied (Fig. 4). The opening between the cyst and the major pancreatic duct was then enlarged by spreading the jaws of the clamp several times. The tail of the pancreas was anastomosed to a Roux Y jejunal loop (Fig. 3). Another operative cholangiogram taken after drainage of the cyst had been completed (Fig. 2, *B*) showed prompt passage of the dye into the duodenum. In view of the absence of cicatricial scarring of the distal portion of the duct, a cholecystectomy alone was performed.

The patient's postoperative course was uneventful. He was discharged on the thirty-fifth postoperative day after an additional operation for an old traumatic defect of the upper lip. The patient was gaining weight and for the first time in many years was free from abdominal pain and was passing formed, nongreasy stools. He has been seen regularly since and continues to do well.

## DISCUSSION

The principle of internal drainage of pseudocystic lesions of the pancreas is well accepted. Excellent and up-to-date reviews of this problem have been published.[4] There are several methods of internal drainage, but little objective evidence for giving preference to any particular one. We have always preferred to drain pancreatic pseudocysts via a retrocolic Roux Y jejunal loop anastomosed to the cyst in as dependent a position as possible, in order to ensure efficient gravity drainage of the cystic cavity at all times. In our opinion, this is the ideal operation for a large pseudocyst presenting between the stomach and transverse colon behind the gastrocolic ligament. However, there are pseudocysts such as the one in our patient which develop behind the antrum and first portion of the duodenum, compressing these and adjacent structures to the point of pyloric obstruction or obstructive jaundice. Their location may render a cystojejunostomy somewhat impractical. Cystoduodenostomy or cystogastrostomy has been performed for lesions in this location with apparently good results.[4] However, both cystoduodenostomy or cystogastrostomy have the theoretical disadvantage of transforming the pancreatic pseudocyst into a diverticulum of the gastrointestinal tract. Moreover, these operations as well as the other methods of internal drainage do not correct the underlying pancreatic pathologic process. This is unimportant when a pancreatic pseudocyst develops after a first attack of acute pancreatitis or after pancreatic trauma. However, if the patient already has recurrent acute pancreatitis or well-established chronic relapsing pancreatitis, surgical treatment of the underlying pancreatic disease as well as of the pseudocyst should

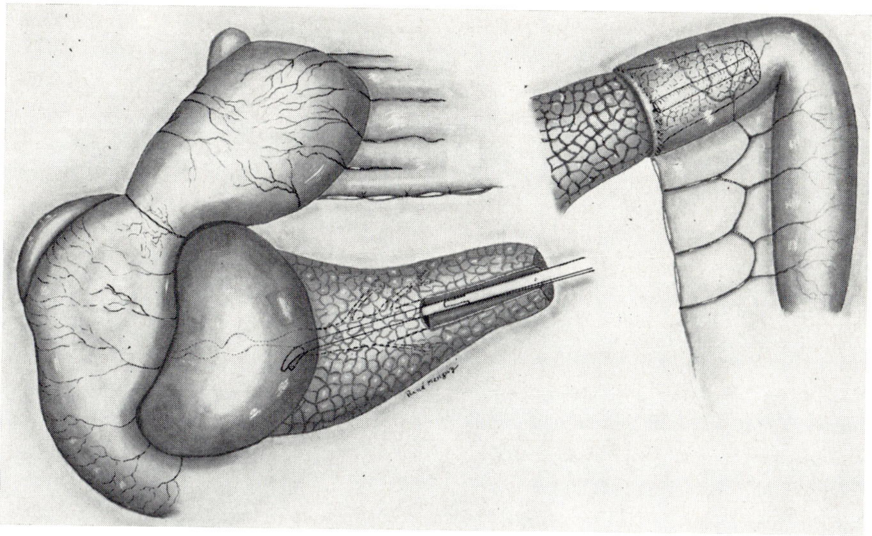

**Fig. 3.** Schematic illustration of operative technique.

be an important consideration. In this regard Doubilet[1] has described a technique of draining pancreatic pseudocysts through the sphincter of Oddi after sphincterotomy via a small plastic tube introduced into the cyst through the pancreatic duct and brought out through the common bile duct with a T tube. Although this method seems appealing, we have always experienced some difficulty in exploring the pancreatic duct through the sphincter of Oddi. On the other hand, we find exploration of the pancreatic duct through its distal end to be technically simple. Furthermore, in our experience as well as that of others,[3] pancreatic ductal obstruction in chronic pancreatitis is a diffuse, stenosing process involving long segments of the cephalic portion of the duct proximal to the sphincter of Oddi. Under these conditions, sphincterotomy is an illogical procedure and cannot be expected to achieve its proposed goal of enhancing drainage of pancreatic secretions into the lumen of the intestine.

Our results with caudal pancreatic drainage in treating chronic pancreatitis have been sufficiently good to warrant use of the principle of caudal drainage to manage both chronic pancreatitis and associated pseudocyst. The purpose of this report is to indicate the feasibility, the technical simplicity, and the satisfactory result of this approach in at least 1 case. The procedure described is certainly not applicable to all pseudocysts. In our opinion, cystic lesions located around the head of the pancreas or occurring in patients with a history either of chronic pancreatitis or suggesting the development of chronic pancreatitis would benefit by this combined technique.

To prevent diabetes or to avoid aggravating diabetes if already present, it is important to remove as little pancreatic tissue as possible. We usually amputate a very short segment (0.5 cm.) of the tip to expose the

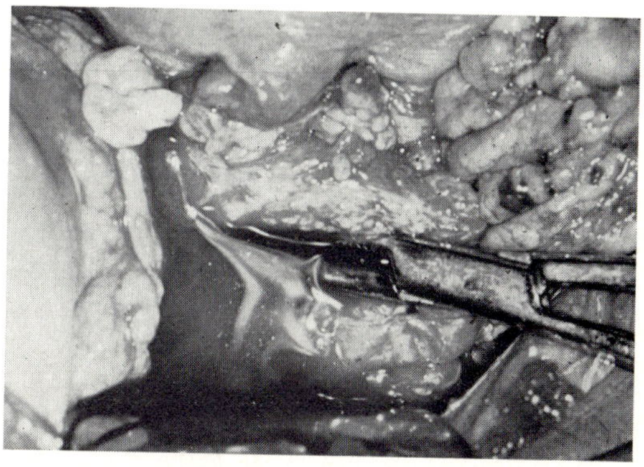

**Fig. 4.** Photograph taken at the moment the clamp was introduced into the cyst on the left. Stomach is retracted above. Clamp lies in the opened duct. Note cyst fluid gushing out of the duct.

ductal lumen. Actually, the tail of the pancreas can be anastomosed to an intestinal loop without prior mobilization.[2] Our only reason for preferring the former method is that we believe that pancreaticojejunostomy is easier and more secure when the body and tail of the pancreas are invaginated into the jejunum.

## SUMMARY

A patient with long-standing pancreatitis complicated by recent development of a large pancreatic pseudocyst was treated successfully by combined retrograde decompression of the pancreatic duct and the pseudocyst via a caudal pancreaticojejunostomy.

The patient was seen in July, 1961. Clinical and radiologic data showed complete cure of the cyst. Symptoms of chronic pancreatitis were considerably improved.

## REFERENCES

1. Doubilet, H., and Mulholland, J. H.: Pancreatic cysts, Surg. Gynec. & Obst. **96:** 683, 1953.
2. Partington, P. F., and Rochelle, R. E. L.: Modified Puestow procedure for retrograde drainage of the pancreatic duct, Ann. Surg. **152:** 1037, 1960.
3. Puestow, C. B., and Gillesby, W. J.: Retrograde surgical drainage of pancreas for chronic relapsing pancreatitis, A. M. A. Arch. Surg. **76:** 898, 1958.
4. Warren, W. D., Marsh, W. H., and Sandusky, W. R.: An appraisal of surgical procedures for pancreatic pseudocyst, Ann. Surg. **147:** 903, 1958.

# An evaluation of actinomycin D and mitomycin C in patients with advanced cancer

EDWARD W. HUMPHREY, M.D.
ALAN C. HYMES, M.D.
ROBERT K. AUSMAN, M.D.
DONALD J. FERGUSON, M.D.
MINNEAPOLIS, MINN.
*From the Surgical Department, Veterans Administration Hospital, and the University of Minnesota*

During the past several years, various antibiotic substances have been tested in the screening program of the Cancer Chemotherapy National Service Center. Those that have shown activity against the animal tumor screens have then been tested against human tumors in an attempt to find an active anticancer agent and also to determine a spectrum of activity for various groups of drugs. At the Minneapolis Veterans Administration Hospital and the University of Minnesota Hospitals, 2 of these substances, antinomycin D and mitomycin C have undergone clinical study.

Actinomycin D is obtained from cultures of *Streptomyces parvullus.* The preparations now available are probably mixtures, with the relative amounts of the different actinomycins varying with each preparation. The mode of action of actinomycin D is not understood. In mice, it produces a decrease in the spleen weight, atrophy of the thymus and lymph nodes, and ulceration of the gastrointestinal tract.[1] It has been inactive when given orally. A very thorough review of the chemical and biological properties of this drug has been published by Moore.[4]

Mitomycin C is obtained from the broth of *Streptomyces casepitosus.* This drug causes a reduction in the size of the thymus and spleen, hemorrhage into the mesenteric lymph nodes, and a bloody diarrhea in mice.[5] It has a pronounced effect upon the bone marrow of dogs. The inhibition of *E. coli* that is caused by this drug may be reversed by guanine or xanthine.[6] In extensive preclinical trials, mitomycin C was found to have one of the widest spectrums of action against animal tumors of any substance screened.

Received for publication Feb. 6, 1961.

## METHODS

The patients treated with these drugs all had a malignancy that was incurable by presently known methods of therapy. The diagnosis in each case was proved by biopsy taken at operation or at the time of autopsy. All of the patients were hospitalized during the entire course of treatment. White blood cell and platelet counts were made in all cases every other day and, in addition, for the first few patients given each drug, liver and kidney function studies were carried out before and at the end of therapy.

Actinomycin D was dissolved in 25 per cent ethanol. The solution given intravenously contained 0.25 mg. of the drug per milliliter. Mitomycin C was diluted to 0.5 mg. per milliliter in 0.01 M phosphate buffer and given intravenously. It was used immediately after dissolving because of evidence that the drug loses its potency in solution.[10]

## RESULTS

Twenty-one patients were treated with actinomycin D. The results of this therapy

**Table I.** *Actinomycin D*

| *Patient* | *Diagnosis* | *Performance status*[3] *(%)* | *Total dose (µg/Kg.)* | *Lowest WBC* | *Day of lowest WBC* | *Other evidence of toxicity* | *Objective improvement* | *Subjective improvement* |
|---|---|---|---|---|---|---|---|---|
| 1 A. K. | Adenocarcinoma of colon | 40 | 75 | No depression | — | Severe ulceration of lips and tongue | None | None |
| 2 A. G. | Adenocarcinoma of colon | 50 | 75 | 1,550 | 15 | Generalized erythema, ulceration of lips and tongue | None | None |
| 3 N. D. | Adenocarcinoma of colon | 50 | 65 | No depression | — | Ulceration of lips, nausea and vomiting | None | None |
| 4 T. T. | Adenocarcinoma of rectum | 40 | 75 | 3,770 | 15 | Fever, generalized erythema | None | None |
| 5 C. V. | Adenocarcinoma of colon | 30 | 65 | No depression | — | Death on day 15 unrelated to drug | None | None |
| 6 L. B. | Adenocarcinoma of rectum | 60 | 65 | No depression | — | None | None | None |
| 7 A. M. | Squamous-cell carcinoma of tongue | 40 | 65 | No depression | — | None | None | None |
| 8 L. D. | Squamous-cell carcinoma of tongue | 50 | 75 | No depression | — | Generalized maculopapular rash, severe oral ulceration, confusion | None | None |
| 9 P. C. | Squamous-cell carcinoma of lip | 80 | 75 | No depression | — | None | None | None |
| 10 P. A. | Squamous-cell carcinoma of pyriform sinus | 70 | 75 | 3,450 | 15 | None | None | None |
| 11 L. F. | Squamous-cell carcinoma of abdominal scar | 30 | 65 | No depression | — | Death on day 15 not related to drug | None | None |
| 12 G. R. | Basal-cell carcinoma of face | 30 | 65 | No depression | — | Died on day 5 | None | None |
| 13 R. B. | Adenocarcinoma of stomach | 60 | 65 | No depression | — | None | None | None |
| 14 A. H. | Adenocarcinoma of pancreas | 40 | 75 | No depression | — | Oral ulceration, ulcer of arytenoids, grand-mal seizures | None | None |
| 15 K. T. | Wilms' tumor | 40 | 65 | No depression | — | None | None | None |
| 16 W. N. | Wilms' tumor | 50 | 70 | No depression | — | None | None | None |
| 17 A. H. | Adenocarcinoma of breast | 80 | 75 | No depression | — | Total alopecia, severe ulceration of mouth | None | None |
| 18 L. R. | Synovioma of arm | 70 | 75 | No depression | — | Oral ulceration | None | None |
| 19 S. L. | Malignant melanoma | 30 | 65 | No depression | — | None | None | None |
| 20 A. C. | Ewing's sarcoma | 40 | 65 | No depression | — | None | None | None |
| 21 J. M. | Hodgkin's disease | 50 | 75 | No depression | — | None | Loss of fever | Weight gain |

are summarized in Table I. Two dosage schedules were employed, the first was 75 μg per kilogram given in divided doses over 5 days and the other was 65 μg per kilogram given in the same manner. The higher dosage level resulted in the development of toxicity in a large percentage of the patients, while at the 65 μg level, toxicity was quite infrequent. Toxicity was manifested most commonly by ulcerations of the lips, tongue, and buccal mucous membrane. Mild nausea was also fairly common, but in no case was it severe. A maculopapular skin eruption occurred in 4 patients. From Table I it is apparent that few patients developed a bone marrow depression and in the cases in which it did occur, it was quite mild. One woman (A. H.) developed a marked alopecia; however, her hair returned during the ensuing 6 months. Three patients died shortly after completing the course of therapy; none of these deaths seemed to be directly related to the drug. In only 1 case did the drug seem to affect favorably the course of the patient's disease; this was in the patient with Hodgkin's disease (J. M.) who developed a remission which lasted for 3 months.

In Table II are listed the patients treated with mitomycin C. The dosage schedule used was 50 μg per kilogram per day for 6 days, and then 50 μg per kilogram every other day until toxicity occurred. In contrast to actinomycin D, the only important manifestation of toxicity to mitomycin C was bone marrow depression. On this dosage schedule, a mild depression of the white blood cell count was quite common, yet severe depression did not occur. Of the 3 deaths which occurred while the effect of the drug was still present, none was thought to be directly related to the therapy. Only 2 patients showed any objective evidence of tumor regression after treatment with mitomycin.

## CASE REPORTS

**Case 15.** A. F. was a 65-year-old man admitted with a 2-month history of weight loss and difficulty in swallowing. An esophagram at that time showed a filling defect in the middle third of the esophagus. The patient refused a thoracotomy and was discharged. Four months later the patient was again admitted with nodular densities in the left lower and right upper lobe of the lung. A biopsy during esophagoscopy was not contributory. The man was discharged. When he was readmitted for the third time 4 months later, he was hoarse and had weakness and numbness of the right hand and the right side of the face. Shortly afterward he developed a complete right hemiplegia with aphasia. Mitomycin C, 50 μg per kilogram, was started and at the end of 2 weeks the aphasia had disappeared and the right hemiplegia had improved. This improvement lasted approximately 1 month after which the patient's condition began to deteriorate. A second course of mitomycin C was ineffective and the patient died 3 months after the first course of mitomycin had been started. An autopsy showed a squamous-cell carcinoma of the esophagus.

**Case 20.** R. E. was a 60-year-old man admitted with a 3-month history of anorexia, weight loss, and epigastric pain. On physical examination, he was found to have a 10 by 10 cm. hard mass in the epigastrium. He underwent exploratory operation and a large carcinoma of the pancreas was found that surrounded the superior mesenteric vessels and involved lymph nodes in the porta hepatis and the mesentery of the small bowel. No resection was performed. The patient was given a total of 116 mg. of mitomycin C beginning 10 days after laparotomy. At the end of 1 month, the epigastric mass had completely disappeared and the patient was essentially free of pain. One month later, however, the pain returned and the liver became progressively larger. His condition deteriorated and he died 3 months after the mitomycin had been started.

## DISCUSSION

Reports of clinical trials of actinomycin D in a wide spectrum of human tumors in both children and adults have been published, but only in Wilms' tumors in children have fairly frequent responses been seen. Farber[2] has reported a 2 to 50 month survival in 35 per cent of the patients with this tumor and Tan and associates[8] found an objective response in 4 of 15 patients with Wilms' tumor. Occasional remissions have been seen in children with neuroblastoma or rhabdomyosarcoma.[7, 8] In adult patients, objective remissions of malignant disease have been few. Of the 20 patients with either a carcinoma or sarcoma in our series, none showed any subjective or objective improvement. It seems that this drug should be considered to have a low therapeutic potential in human tumors.

**Table II.** *Mitomycin C*

| *Patient* | *Diagnosis* | *Performance status*[3] *(%)* | *Total dose (mg.)* | *Lowest WBC* | *Day of lowest WBC* | *Other evidence of toxicity* | *Subjective improvement* | *Objective improvement* |
|---|---|---|---|---|---|---|---|---|
| 1 R. B. | Carcinoma of prostate | 40 | 30.4 | 3,900 | 17 | None | Disappearance of back pain | None |
| 2 C. H. | Carcinoma of prostate | 40 | 41.0 | No depression | — | None | Mild pain relief | None |
| 3 H. H. | Carcinoma of prostate | 30 | 25.8 | 2,750 | 7 | None | Pain relief, decrease in nausea | None |
| 4 O. S. | Carcinoma of prostate | 40 | 18.9 | 3,900 | 16 | None | Pain relief | None |
| 5 W. B. | Squamous cell carcinoma of renal pelvis | 40 | 29.0 | No depression | — | None | None | None |
| 6 S. S. | Adenocarcinoma of rectum | 60 | 23.2 | 4,000 | 7 | None | — | None |
| 7 B. L. | Adenocarcinoma of colon | 30 | 28.0 | 3,500 | 15 | None | None | None |
| 8 G. H. | Squamous-cell carcinoma of esophagus | 30 | 10.0 | | Died on day 4 of therapy | | None | None |
| 9 J. C. | Squamous-cell carcinoma of mouth | 30 | 34.8 | 2,450 | 29 Died on day 32 | None | None | None |
| 10 C. T. | Squamous-cell carcinoma of tongue | 40 | 28.1 | No depression | — | None | None | None |
| 11 C. J. | Squamous-cell carcinoma of tonsil | 40 | 24.8 | 2,000 | 24 | None | None | None |
| 12 L. Q. | Squamous-cell carcinoma of floor of mouth | 60 | 43.5 | 3,350 | 37 | None | None | None |
| 13 F. J. | Adenocarcinoma (primary unknown) | 50 | 30.0 | No depression | — | None | None | None |
| 14 A. J. | Undifferentiated carcinoma (primary unknown) | 70 | 26.4 | No depression | — | None | None | None |
| 15 A. F. | Squamous-cell carcinoma of esophagus | 30 | 35.7 | 4,250 | 14 | None | — | Disappearance of aphasia and hemiplegia |
| 16 J. C. | Carcinoma of thyroid | 50 | 14.4 | 3,850 | 12 | None | None | None |
| 17 W. T. | Glioblastoma multiforme | 30 | 25.8 | No depression | — | None | None | None |
| 18 E. P. | Chondrosarcoma of hip | 80 | 63.9 | 3,150 | 38 | None | None | None |
| 19 G. M. | Adenocarcinoma of pancreas | 40 | 52.5 | No depression | — | None | None | None |
| 20 R. E. | Adenocarcinoma of pancreas | 40 | 116 | 2,400 | 30 | None | Pain relief | Disappearance of abdominal mass |
| 21 R. W. E. | Adenocarcinoma of pancreas | 40 | 20.1 | 3,400 | 15 | None | None | None |
| 22 N. B. | Adenocarcinoma of stomach | 40 | 56.4 | 1,400 | 42 | Dead on day 44 | None | None |

Mitomycin C was first introduced into clinical trial in Japan. Reports from that country indicated that a high degree of antitumor activity could be obtained in man, with an acceptable degree of toxicity. Tasaka and colleagues[9] reported objective improvement in 12 of 36 cases. Yorimae and his group[11] found improvement in carcinoma both of the stomach and of the colon. In contrast to these results, reports from this country have stated the drug to be extremely toxic and of little benefit in the treatment of advanced cancer. Severe bone marrow depression has occurred with doses as low as 0.3 mg. per kilogram. With the dosage schedule reported here, severe leukopenia was not found to be a problem. However, of the 22 patients treated with this drug only 2 showed even a short-term objective response, although admittedly these 2 had tumors which are characteristically refractory to chemotherapy. It does not seem that this drug will be an important addition to our therapeutic measures for human cancer.

## SUMMARY

Twenty-one patients were treated with actinomycin D and 22 with mitomycin C. The principal toxic effects of actinomycin D were ulceration of the mouth and pharynx, nausea, and dermatitis, while the main toxic effect of mitomycin C was bone marrow depression. One patient with Hodgkin's disease improved with actinomycin D. Short improvement was found in a case of carcinoma of the pancreas and carcinoma of the esophagus with mitomycin C. Neither of these drugs is considered to have great value in the treatment of human malignancy.

## REFERENCES

1. DiPaolo, J. A., Moore, G. E., and Niedbala, T. R.: Experimental studies with actinomycin D, Cancer Res. **17:** 1127, 1957.
2. Farber, S.: Actinomycin D, M. News **6:** 11, 1960.
3. Karnofsky, D. A., and Burchenal, H.: The clinical evaluation of chemotherapeutic agents in cancer, Symp. Sect. Microbiol., New York Acad. Med. (1948), No. 2, p. 191, 1949.
4. Moore, G. E., DiPaolo, J. A., and Kondo, T.: The chemotherapeutic effects and complications of actinomycin D in patients with advanced cancer, Cancer **11:** 1204, 1958.
5. Phillips, F. S., Schwartz, H. S., and Sternberg, S. S.: Pharmacology of mitomycin C. I. Toxicity and pathologic effects, Cancer Res. **20:** 1359, 1960.
6. Reilly, H. C., Cappuccino, J. G., and Harrison, D. M.: Studies on mitomycin X, a tumor-inhibiting antibiotic, Proc. Am. A. Cancer Res. **2:** 338, 1958.
7. Shaw, R. K., Moore, E. W., Mueller, P. S., Frei, E., III, and Watkin, D. M.: The effect of actinomycin D on childhood neoplasms, A. M. A. J. Dis. Child. **99:** 628, 1960.
8. Tan, C. C. T., Phillips, R. F., Murphy, M. L., and Burchenal, J. H.: Clinical studies with actinomycin D, Acta Un. Int. Cancer **16:** 927, 1960.
9. Tasaka, S., Mashimo, H., Kusoda, Y., Harada, T., Shimizu, K., Okochi, K., Hatakiyama, M., and Kunii, O.: Basic and clinical studies on mitomycin, Gann No Rinsho **5:** 57, 1959.
10. Wakaki, D., Marumo, H., Tomioka, K., Shimizu, G., Kato, E., Kamoda, H., Kudo, S., and Fujimoto, Y.: Isolation of new fractions of antitumor mitomycins, Antibiot. & Chemother. **8:** 228, 1958.
11. Yorimae, H., Knido, T., Ikada, Y., and Sakakibara, N.: Clinical experience with mitomycin C administration, Shinyaku to Rinsho **8:** 53, 1959.

# Carcinosarcoma of the lung

THOMAS C. MOORE, M.D.
MUNCIE AND INDIANAPOLIS, IND.
*From the Surgical Service, Ball Memorial Hospital, Muncie, and the Department of Surgery, Indiana University Medical Center, Indianapolis*

Carcinosarcoma is one of the rarest types of malignant neoplasm to be found in man. It is encountered most frequently in the uterus. It has been reported as occurring with decreasing frequency in the hypopharynx, the esophagus, and the lung. Bergmann and associates,[1] in 1951, reported 2 cases of carcinosarcoma of the lung from the Barnes Hospital of St. Louis and reviewed in detail 7 cases[5, 6, 8, 12, 15, 16, 18] recorded in the literature prior to 1951. The earliest case reviewed by them was reported in 1914 by Saltykow.[15] The first case report of pulmonary carcinosarcoma generally is attributed to Kika[9] in 1908. However, no information is available concerning this case. All but one of these cases reviewed by Bergmann and his associates were autopsy cases and represented the terminal picture of this condition. They reviewed 3 additional cases[3, 11, 14] and classified the lesions as "collision tumors" to differentiate them from true carcinosarcoma. Since 1951, 4 cases of carcinosarcoma of the lung have been recorded in the literature.[4, 13, 17] A few additional lesions have been labeled carcinosarcoma of the lung. A review of these reports has failed to establish clearly their identity as carcinosarcomas.[10]

The 2 cases reported by Bergmann and his associates are the first recorded instances of successful pulmonary resection for carcinosarcoma of the lung. Both patients were operated upon by Dr. Evarts Graham, and pneumonectomy was carried out in both. The first case reported by Bergmann and his associates had been cited in an earlier publication by Graham and Womack[7] concerning bronchial adenomas. At that time the tumor had been diagnosed as a mixed bronchogenic carcinoma and sarcoma.

The purpose of this paper is to report a case in which lobectomy was performed successfully for endobronchial carcinosarcoma of the lung and to review in some detail the published experience in 7 clinical cases of carcinosarcoma of the lung.

## CASE REPORT

The patient, a 64-year-old white male college professor, was admitted to the Ball Memorial Hospital on March 26, 1960, because of pain in the right side of the chest of 3 weeks' duration. Two days after the onset of the chest pain the patient had been involved in a minor automobile accident and received some exposure to cold and snow. Shortly thereafter, he noticed the onset of coughing and hemoptysis. A roentgenogram of the chest showed evidence of right lower lobe infiltration (Fig. 1). He was treated for 18 days with Achromycin and bed rest. When a second chest roentgenogram showed no evidence of improvement after 18 days of treatment, he was admitted to the hospital for further study. There had been no weight loss.

His past history was essentially negative. He had suffered from psoriasis for many years. Two small skin cancers had been removed in 1959 and had not recurred. He did not drink and had never smoked. His mother was living at 86 years of age and his father had died at 59 years of a heart attack. There was no known family history of malignancy.

The positive findings on physical examination were limited to an expiratory friction rub anteriorly at the base of the right lung. The patient's weight was 166 pounds. His blood pressure was 114/80 mm. Hg. Results of a urine examination on admission to the hospital were within normal limits. The red blood cell count was 4.5 million and the hemoglobin was 14.5 Gm. The white blood

Received for publication Feb. 24, 1961.

cell count was 4,700 with a normal differential. The electrocardiogram was within normal limits. The prothrombin time, the platelet count, and the bleeding and clotting times were normal. The blood urea nitrogen was 13. Tuberculin and histoplasmin skin tests were negative.

Bronchoscopic examination was carried out on March 28 under topical anesthesia. An inflammatory reaction was encountered in the right bronchus intermedius. An edematous-appearing tumor mass was found in the lumen of this bronchus and 2 biopsy specimens were taken. Bronchial washings from this area then were obtained. A catheter was left in the right bronchus and bronchograms were made. Culture of the bronchial washings showed *Staphylococcus aureus.* Repeated cytologic studies on the bronchial washings and on sputum samples thereafter were negative. Evidence only of diffuse submucosal chronic inflammation was found on microscopic examination of the biopsy material. The bronchograms showed bronchiectasis of the basal segments of the right lower lobe (Fig. 2). The bronchus intermedius did not fill well and there was a suggestion of an intraluminal mass. Considerable difficulty was encountered in attempting to fill the right lower lobe segments.

The patient was taken to the operating room on April 1, and the right thoracic cavity was entered through the bed of the resected sixth rib. A mass was encountered in the right lower lobe with evidence of considerable inflammatory change throughout the lobe. Frozen section examination of an adjacent lymph node showed only inflammatory hyperplasia. The artery and vein to the right lower lobe were dissected free and ligated with considerable difficulty due to extensive inflammatory reaction in these areas. An abscess was encountered at the emergence of the inferior pulmonary vein from the pericardial sac. This abscess was opened and evacuated. Because of the abscess and the marked inflammatory reaction about it, it was necessary to open the pericardiac sac and to ligate and divide the inferior pulmonary vein within the sac. The right lower lobe finally was dissected free from all surrounding structures and a bronchus clamp was placed across the lower lobe bronchus immediately distal to the origin of the bronchus to the middle lobe. When the bronchus to the lower lobe had been divided, it was apparent that a portion of an unattached endobronchial tumor had been left behind within the bronchus intermedius. The noncrushing bronchus clamp was momentarily released and a blast of anesthetic gas was delivered through the endotracheal tube by the anesthetist. The residual free endobronchial tumor mass was extruded from the bronchial stump and the bronchus clamp was reapplied. The residual endobronchial tumor mass was cylindrical and measured approximately 3 cm. in length. The excised right lower lobe was opened by the attending pathologists and the tumor was found to be largely a pedunculated endobronchial neoplasm. The diagnosis on frozen section was not clear. The presence of sarcoma was suspected. The tumor did not appear to be a bronchial adenoma as had been thought originally. The bronchial stump was closed with interrupted sutures of fine silk and the thoracotomy incision was closed in layers. A catheter for suction had been left in the right side of the chest and brought out through a stab wound.

Gross pathologic examination of the resected lobe showed the presence of a tumor which was pedunculated with a narrow base and consisted largely of multiple, cylindrical, unattached, fingerlike endobronchial extensions both distally and proximally into the various adjacent segments of the bronchial tree (Fig. 3). The tumor arose by a narrow pedicle from the posterior basal segment bronchus. At the site of the origin of the tumor, there was a 3 cm. mass resulting from extension of the tumor into the adjacent lung. Distal to the tumor there was evidence of considerable infection and bronchiectasis. Abscesses of varying size were encountered in several areas.

On microscopic examination, the tumor was found to be a carcinosarcoma. The carcinomatous and sarcomatous portions were intermingled (Fig. 4). The sarcoma portion appeared to be forming osteoid in areas. It was largely a fibrosarcoma. In a few areas there were cells with cross striations

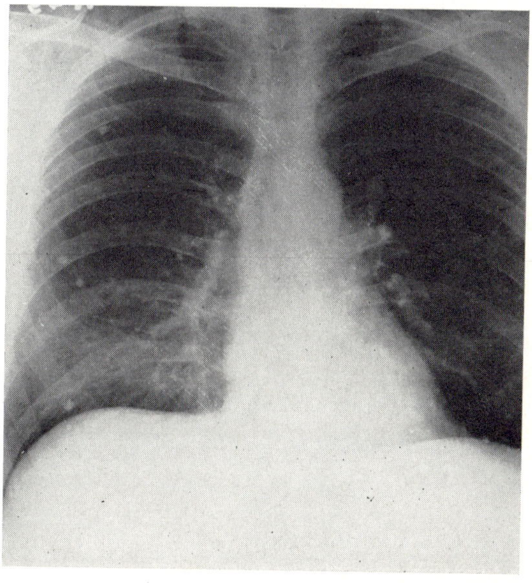

**Fig. 1.** Roentgenogram of the chest shows increased pulmonary markings in the right cardiophrenic area. These findings were interpreted as suggestive of the presence of an acute or chronic pneumonitis.

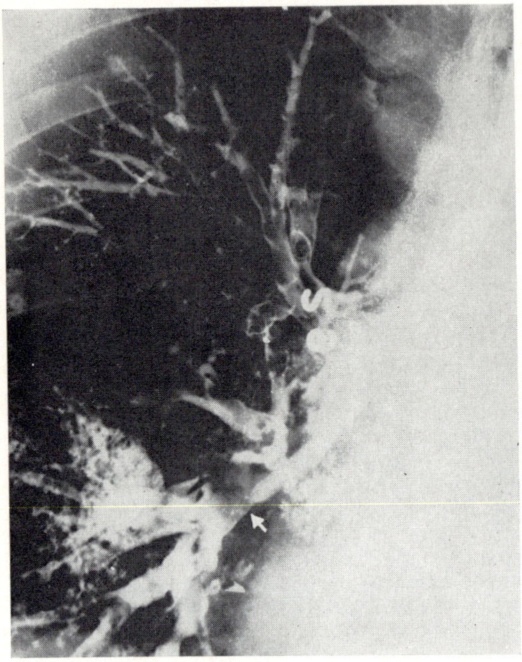

**Fig. 2.** Bronchogram of the right lung demonstrates right lower lobe bronchiectasis. There also appears to be a filling defect in the bronchus *(arrow)*.

which resembled rhabdomyoblasts. The epithelial element was typical of epidermoid carcinoma with good intracellular bridges. In a few areas, small epithelial pearls could be identified. The slides were reviewed by Dr. L. G. Montgomery of the Ball Memorial Hospital, Dr. Edith Parkhill of the Mayo Clinic, Dr. J. B. Hazard of the Cleveland Clinic, Dr. A. A. Liebow of the Grace–New Haven Hospital, and Dr. Frank Vellios of the Indiana University Medical Center. All concurred in the diagnosis of carcinosarcoma of the lung.

The postoperative course was uneventful. Chest suction was discontinued and the tube removed 2 days after operation. The patient received postoperative radiation therapy to the mediastinum. He was given 2,000 r as measured in air through an anterior port and the same amount through a posterior port. He was discharged from the hospital on April 24, 24 days after operation. He has continued to do well since his release from the hospital. When last seen, 19 months after operation, there was no evidence of recurrence of carcinosarcoma, and he was carrying his full work load of college teaching.

## DISCUSSION

The microscopic pathologic characteristics of pulmonary carcinosarcoma and the findings in 6 of the 7 recorded autopsy cases have been discussed in detail in the excellent paper by Bergmann and associates.[1] They emphasized that both the sarcomatous and carcinomatous elements must be intermingled in the microscopic picture of the true carcinosarcoma. The only autopsy case recorded since 1951 was published in 1956 by Cavallero.[4] Distant metastases, generally involving both the sarcomatous and carcinomatous elements of the tumor, were found in 6 of the 7 autopsy cases. Only in the case recorded by Ogawa[12] in 1929 was the patient found to be free of metastases at the time of postmortem examination.

My principal concern is to consider in some detail the interesting features of the cases of 7 patients who have been subjected to clinical analysis and, in all but one instance, to thoracotomy. Even from the limited published experience with this unusual pulmonary neoplasm, it can be seen that some interesting clinical patterns are beginning to emerge.

Two rather distinct clinical types of pulmonary carcinosarcoma appear to exist. One type of tumor is peripheral in location and exists as a solid parenchymal mass which may attain considerable size. These tumors tend to invade the chest wall and the adjacent mediastinal and vascular structures. They also tend to be associated with relatively early distant metastasis. Their prognosis appears to be poor. The second type of tumor is quite different. Its location is more central and it occurs as a pedunculated endobronchial growth with rather limited parenchymal extension in the area of its pedunculated origin from the bronchial wall. Regional lymph node involvement and distant metastasis appear to be infrequent. The symptoms are produced by bronchial obstruction with distal atelectasis, bronchiectasis, and suppuration. The prognosis with this type of tumor appears to be surprisingly good. Two of the clinical cases were of the solid peripheral type and 5 were of the pedunculated endobronchial type.

Both of the patients with the peripheral solid type of carcinosarcoma were dead at the time of the case reports. The patient of

Hochberg and his associates[8] was a 55-year-old woman who had had a chronic cough for 10 years. In the 4 months prior to operation she had experienced an exacerbation of symptoms with production of mucopurulent sputum and hemoptysis. Roentgen study of the chest showed a rather large, well-circumscribed mass in the left upper lobe. Bronchoscopic and cytologic studies had not been carried out. At thoracotomy, a large mass in the left upper lobe was found to be attached to the anterior chest wall and to the aortic arch. A left upper lobectomy was performed and the patient died 17 hours after operation.

The patient with a solid peripheral tumor reported upon by Peabody[13] was a 74-year-old man who had experienced symptoms of chest pain and hemoptysis for 6 weeks. A rather large lobulated mass was seen on roentgen study of the chest in the left upper lobe area. Bronchoscopic examination and cytologic studies were negative. At thoracotomy, a large, smooth, lobulated tumor was found in the anterior segmental portion of the left upper lobe. The tumor appeared to infiltrate the mediastinum, the upper pericardium, and the phrenic nerve. A left upper lobectomy was carried out. The patient recovered from the operation but died 4 months later of a bleeding duodenal ulcer. At autopsy, tumor metastases showing both carcinomatous and sarcomatous elements were found in the retroperitoneal and mesenteric lymph nodes, the liver, the pancreas, the kidneys, and the adrenal glands. The sarcomatous element of the tumor appeared to be a fibrosarcoma. The microscopic appearance of the cells of the epithelial element strongly suggested peripheral (bronchiolar or alveolar) origin.

The published clinical experience with the more centrally located pedunculated endobronchial type of carcinosarcoma of the lung is quite different from that cited for the peripheral type (Table I). There appears to be a remarkable constancy in the clinical picture of the endobronchial type of tumor. All of the patients were men and all were in the fifth and sixth decades of

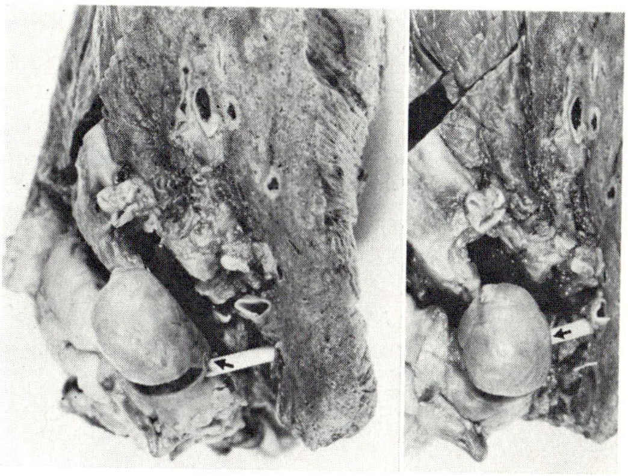

**Fig. 3.** Photographs of the formalin-fixed, cut right lower lobe taken from 2 angles to show the appearance of the terminal portion of one of the cylindrical, finger-like endobronchial growths *(arrow)* which had extended distally from the site of its pedunculated origin from the bronchial wall. Bronchial dilatation in the area of the endobronchial growth and distal bronchiectasis and consolidation also are shown. A section has been taken from the endobronchial growth.

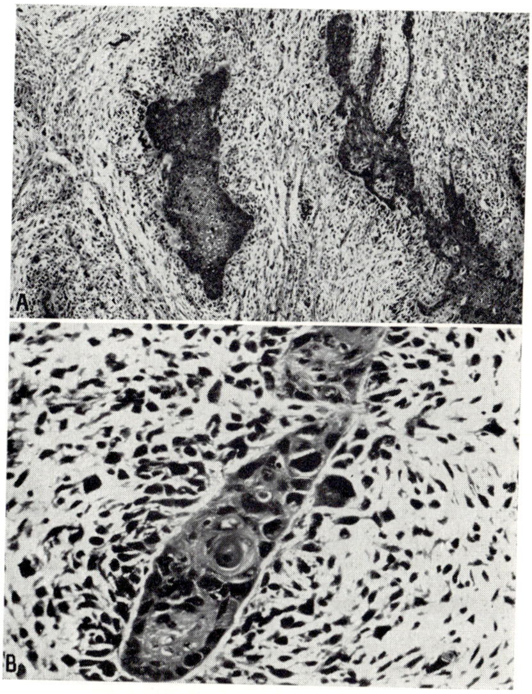


**Fig. 4.** Photomicrographs of the tumor under *A,* relative low power, and *B,* somewhat higher power from another area, illustrate the intermingling of the epithelial and the mesodermal elements of the carcinosarcoma. The epithelial element of the tumor is typical of epidermoid carcinoma. The stroma is fibrosarcoma.

**Table I.** *Summary of published clinical experience with endobronchial carcinosarcoma*

| *Author* | *Age and sex* | *Clinical picture* | *Initial bronchoscopic biopsy* | *Bronchogram* |
|---|---|---|---|---|
| *Bergmann and associates* | | | | |
| Case 1 | 51, M | Nonproductive cough for 1 yr., chest pain, WBC 22,000, lesion on chest roentgenogram, 20-pound weight loss | | Filling defect, right upper lobe bronchus |
| Case 2 | 56, M | Chest pain, fever, malaise and 13-pound weight loss, lesion on chest roentgenogram | Negative for neoplasm | Filling defect, right upper lobe bronchus |
| *Taylor and Rae* | | | | |
| Case 1 | 69, M | Nonproductive cough, fever and malaise, ill 2 mo., right lower lobe and middle lobe atelectasis on roentgenogram | Negative for neoplasm | |
| Case 2 | 57, M | Pain in chest, dyspnea and hemoptysis of 2 mo., 20-pound weight loss, left lung atelectasis on roentgenogram | Negative for neoplasm | |
| *Moore* | 64, M | Pain in chest, cough and hemoptysis of 3 wk., right lower lobe lesion on chest roentgenogram | Negative for neoplasm | Filling defect, left lower lobe bronchus and bronchus intermedius, distal bronchiectasis |

life. The major symptoms were nonproductive cough and chest pain. Fever, malaise, hemoptysis, and weight loss were encountered frequently.

Two of the patients were known to be smokers of cigarettes and 1 had never smoked. The endobronchial tumor mass was seen in all of the 4 cases in which bronchoscopy was carried out. However, the findings on initial bronchoscopic biopsy of the tumor mass proved consistently to be misleading. Initial bronchoscopic biopsy of the tumor mass in all 4 cases was reported as negative for neoplasm. In the first case of Taylor and Rae,[17] a second bronchoscopic biopsy taken 7 days after the initial attempt was reported as positive for malignant neoplasm (suggestive of sarcoma). In the second case of Bergmann and his associates, a positive biopsy for neoplasm was not obtained until the third bronchoscopic examination, 7 months after the initial attempt. In the interim, during which the diagnosis remained in doubt, a second unrewarding bronchoscopic examination and biopsy were undertaken and a thoracotomy was performed at which only drainage of a lung abscess was carried out. There also appears to be a hazard associated with the bronchoscopic biopsy of this type of tumor. The second patient of Taylor and Rae died of massive tracheobronchial hemorrhage 80 hours after bronchoscopic biopsy of the tumor had been performed.

In all of the 3 cases in which bronchograms were made, a filling defect in the bronchus was identified. In the case recorded here, bronchiectasis was demonstrated distal to the partially occluding bronchial mass. The radiopaque material in this case could be forced beyond the bronchial mass into the distal bronchial segments only with considerable difficulty.

Four of the patients with endobronchial carcinosarcoma were operated upon. Pneumonectomy was carried out in 3 and lobectomy in 1. All 4 patients recovered from the operation and all were alive without evidence of recurrence from 1 to 6 years after operation. The case reported here is, to the author's knowledge, the first recorded case of successful lobectomy for endobronchial carcinosarcoma of the lung.

The site of bronchial origin of the pedunculated endobronchial tumor was segmental or lobar in 4 of the 5 reported cases. In the second case reported by Taylor and Rae the tumor originated from the left main bron-

| Cytologic study | Origin of tumor | Regional node metastasis | Operation | Result |
|---|---|---|---|---|
| — | Right upper lobe, apical segment bronchus | None | Pneumonectomy | Living 6 yr. after operation, no recurrence |
| Negative | Right upper lobe, lobar bronchus | None | Pneumonectomy | Living 1.5 yr. after operation, no recurrence |
| Negative | Right lower lobe, lobar bronchus | None | Pneumonectomy | Living 3 yr. after operation, no recurrence, some dyspnea |
| — | Left main bronchus | None | — | Died 80 hr. after bronchoscopic biopsy of tumor, death due to massive tracheobronchial hemorrhage, at necropsy tumor regarded as curable, no metastases found |
| Negative | Right lower lobe, basal segment bronchus | None | Lobectomy | Living 19 mo. after operation, working and asymptomatic, no recurrence |

chus. From these observations, it is apparent the lobectomy was feasible in 4 of the 5 recorded clinical cases of endobronchial carcinosarcoma. Lobectomy is possible even in instances in which the endobronchial growth of the tumor has extended beyond the anatomic limits of the lobe of its pedunculated origin. Removal of the extended endobronchial growth can be achieved by means of the technique employed in the case recorded here; by removing briefly the noncrushing bronchus clamp and forcing out the unattached proximal segment of the endobronchial growth through the open end of the bronchial stump. This can be achieved by pressure exerted through the endotracheal tube by the anesthetist.

It is of interest and of prognostic significance that the regional lymph nodes were free of metastatic tumor involvement in all of the 5 recorded clinical cases of endobronchial carcinosarcoma. The patient of Taylor and Rae who died after bronchoscopic biopsy of the tumor also was found, on postmortem examination, to be free of distant metastases. Additional evidence of the seeming benignancy of these endobronchial tumors is to be found in the second case of Bergmann and his associates. In this case, 7 months elapsed between the initial diagnostic efforts and the final operative removal of the tumor. Nonetheless, this patient survived and had remained free of recurrence for 6 years at the time of their report.

The symptoms encountered in the endobronchial group of cases appear to result largely from the bronchial obstruction produced by the endobronchial tumor growth with distal atelectasis, bronchiectasis, suppuration, and abscess formation. The weight loss so frequently observed in these cases is probably due to acute and chronic pulmonary suppuration. The appearance of the bronchial tree distal to the endobronchial growth was not mentioned in the first case report of Bergmann and his associates. In their second case report, a pulmonary abscess had been found and drained at the time of the initial thoracotomy. Six months later, examination of the resected lung showed an intense acute bronchiectasis distal to the tumor. The bronchi were widely dilated with thinned-out walls and were filled with purulent material. In the first case of Taylor and Rae, bronchiectasis with an accumulation of purulent material was observed distal to the tumor. In their second case, an acute suppurative bronchitis was found distal to the tumor. Pulmonary abscess, bronchiectasis, and considerable inflammatory reaction were encountered in the case recorded here.

Fibrosarcoma and squamous-cell carcinoma were the most frequently encountered cell types in the endobronchial group of carcinosarcomas. It is of interest that the gross appearance of these tumors is somewhat similar to the polypoid character observed in the limited published experience with pure pulmonary fibrosarcoma.[2]

Although reports of only 7 clinical cases of carcinosarcoma of the lung have appeared in the literature, it is probable that the true incidence of these unusual neoplasms is somewhat greater than the limited published experience indicates. Taylor and Rae reported their experience with 2 patients from 2 hospitals in Vancouver. The 2 cases of Bergmann and his associates were encountered in a series of 258 surgically removed bronchopulmonary tumors at the Barnes Hospital in St. Louis. It is hoped that additional case reports may help to establish more clearly the clinical picture and ultimate prognosis of these tumors.

## SUMMARY

1. Thirteen cases of pulmonary carcinosarcoma of the lung have been reported. The literature pertaining to carcinosarcoma of the lung is reviewed. Seven of the cases were seen at autopsy and 6 were seen clinically.

2. A pedunculated endobronchial carcinosarcoma arising from a basal segmental bronchus of the right lower lobe of a 64-year-old white man is reported.

3. From an analysis of the published clinical cases, including the case reported here, it is apparent that there are 2 distinct types of pulmonary carcinosarcoma. In one type, the tumor is peripheral and solid. It may attain considerable size prior to detection and has a tendency toward direct invasion of adjacent chest wall and mediastinal structures. There is also a tendency toward distant metastasis and the prognosis is poor. Two of the clinical cases were of this type. The second type of tumor is more centrally located. It occurs as a pedunculated endobronchial growth with limited parenchymal extension from the site of its pedunculated origin from the bronchial wall. The tumor growth is largely endobronchial. The prognosis with this type of tumor is surprisingly good. Five of the clinical cases were of this type.

4. The symptoms associated with the solid peripheral type of tumor are due to the invasive and metastatic character of the neoplasm. Those of the endobronchial type result from bronchial obstruction with distal atelectasis, bronchiectasis, abscess formation, and acute and chronic suppuration.

5. The principal symptoms reported in cases of endobronchial carcinosarcoma are those of chest pain, cough, fever, malaise, hemoptysis, and weight loss.

6. Bronchoscopic biopsy and cytologic studies in the endobronchial group have proved to be uninformative and misleading. In addition, there appears to be some hazard associated with bronchoscopic biopsy of these tumors.

7. Pulmonary resection was carried out in 4 of the 5 patients with endobronchial carcinosarcoma seen clinically, pneumonectomy in 3 and lobectomy in 1. All 4 patients survived operation and all were reported to be alive and free of tumor recurrence from 1 to 6 years after operation.

8. The regional lymph nodes were free of tumor involvement in all of the 5 clinical cases of endobronchial carcinosarcoma. There was no evidence of tumor metastasis on postmortem examination of the patient who died of hemorrhage after bronchoscopic biopsy of the tumor.

9. The pedunculated origin of the endobronchial tumor was segmental or lobar in 4 of the 5 clinical cases.

10. From the observations described, it is apparent that lobectomy may be regarded not only as feasible, but as the operation of choice in the majority of cases of endobronchial carcinosarcoma of the lung, even when the endobronchial growth has extended beyond the anatomic limits of the lobe of origin.

11. The case reported here is, to the author's knowledge, the first recorded instance of successful lobectomy for endobronchial carcinosarcoma of the lung.

## REFERENCES

1. Bergmann, M., Ackerman, L. V., and Kemler, R. L.: Carcinosarcoma of the lung, Cancer **4:** 919, 1951.
2. Black, H.: Fibrosarcoma of the bronchus, J. Thoracic Surg. **19:** 123, 1950.
3. Bösenberg, M.: Über Carcinosarkome, Ztschr. Krebsforsch. **36:** 416, 1932.
4. Cavallero, G.: Contributo allo studio dei tumori misti maligni del polmone di tipo bidermico (carcinosarcomi), Pathologica (Genova) **48:** 213, 1956.
5. Fischer, W.: Zur Kenntnis des lungenkrebse, Acta Unio internat. contra cancrum **3:** 221, 1938.
6. Frank, A.: Ein Karzinosarkom der Lunge, Schmidt's Jahrb. **322:** 149, 1915.
7. Graham, E. A., and Womack, N. A.: The problem of the so-called bronchial adenoma, J. Thoracic Surg. **14:** 106, 1945.
8. Hochberg, L. A., Grayzel, D., Benson, S. L., and Rosenberg, S.: Multiple primary tumors with fibrosarcoma and co-existing carcinosarcoma of the lung, Arch. Surg. **59:** 166, 1949.
9. Kika: Cited by Herxheimer, G., and Reinke, F., Ergebn. allg. path. Anat. **16:** 281, 1912.
10. Lavnikova, G. A.: Kartsinosarkoma legkogo, Vop. Onkol. **4:** 345, 1958.
11. Nowicki, W.: Carcinom und Sarkom als Kollisionsgeschwulst, Virchows Arch. path. Anat. **289:** 564, 1933.
12. Ogawa, K.: Uber eine Fall vom sehr seltenen primären Karzinosarkom der Lunge mit besonderer Berucksichtigung der histologischen Untersuchungen, J. Orient. Med. **11:** 133, 1929.
13. Peabody, C. N.: Carcinosarcoma of the lung of peripheral origin, J. Thoracic Surg. **6:** 766, 1959.
14. Pée, D.: Über einen Fall von Karzinosarkom der Lunge mit Kalkkugeln. Thesis, Christian-Albrechts Universität zur Kiel, Quakenbrück, 1936.
15. Saltykow, S.: Beiträge zur Kenntnig des Karzinosarkoms, Verhandl. deutsch. path. Gesellsch. **17:** 351, 1914.
16. Selye, H.: Über zwei bemerkenswerte Falle von Karzinosarkom, Med. Klin. **24:** 1197, 1928.
17. Taylor, H. E., and Rae, M. V.: Endobronchial carcinosarcoma, J. Thoracic Surg. **24:** 93, 1952.
18. Weber, F.: Ein Karzinosarkom der Lunge, Zentralbl. allg. Path. Anat. **72:** 113, 1939.

# Subglottic carcinoma with extensive tracheal involvement

WILLIAM S. CALEM, M.D.
H. ROBERT FREUND, M.D.
BROOKLYN, N. Y.
*From the Departments of Surgery, Brooklyn Veterans Administration Hospital and State University of New York Downstate Medical Center*

Carcinoma arising in the subglottic portion of the larynx, especially when the lesion extends below the first tracheal ring, presents special problems in diagnosis and surgical treatment. These are illustrated in the case report that will be presented. A technique devised for the formation of a tracheostomy will be described.

More than 80 years ago, Isambert[5] first differentiated these tumors from other laryngeal carcinomas. In 1881, Delavan[4] was the first to describe a case occurring in this country. Although extension into the trachea is rare, subglottic carcinoma is not uncommon. Thomson[12] classified 26 per cent and Clerf[1] 10 per cent of intrinsic carcinomas in the subglottic category.

These lesions originate on the lower surface of the vocal cord or apart from the cord, sometimes as low as the cricoid ring. The tumor is commonly located in the middle or anterior part of the larynx. It may spread across the midline or through the cricothyroid membrane, and may metastasize to the lymph nodes over this area. The isthmus of the thyroid gland can also be directly invaded. At the onset of symptoms, the only complaints may be difficulty in expelling sputum, weakness of voice, or a sore throat. In other cases, the gradual onset of dyspnea or stridor on exertion may be the first symptom. When the cord becomes secondarily involved by upward extension of the tumor, hoarseness occurs as a late symptom.

The diagnosis is made by direct laryngoscopy and biopsy. Since the subglottic area is often difficult to visualize, the full extent of the lesion may not be appreciated. When immobility of the vocal cord is not justified by the size of the visible growth, subglottic involvement is suggested. Earlier surgeons advocated exploratory thyrotomy prior to resection in order to determine the extent of the lesion. More recently, laryngeal tomography has been used to demonstrate the contours of the subglottic region and when the tumor is large enough to be visualized, this can provide an accurate evaluation of the growth. Knowledge of more superficial extensions, however, is still best provided by direct visualization at operation. It is essential to divide the trachea at a low level in order to insure the widest possible resection. When tracheotomy is indicated prior to operation, it must also be performed at the lowest level.

The incidence of metastases is higher in subglottic malignancy than in cordal carcinoma because of the abundant lymphatics of the subglottic area. Prognosis is, therefore, poor. According to Orton,[9] the possibility of cure diminishes with the extent of the growth away from the vocal cords. The mortality rate reported ranges from 40 to 50 per cent.[2, 9, 12] These figures are considerably higher than those for intrinsic carcinomas. Jackson and Jackson[6] report a sur-

Received for publication Feb. 13, 1961.

vival rate for intrinsic carcinomas of 75 to 80 per cent; in small lesions, the 5-year cure may rise as high as 90 per cent.

Laryngectomy, with the addition of radical neck dissection when indicated, has been the surgical approach to subglottic carcinoma. When the trachea is involved, most authors have believed that the prognosis is hopeless and the lesion inoperable because of extension of the disease between the trachea and the esophagus and invasion of the mediastinal lymphatics. Clerf[3] considers inoperable any lesions which extend below the first tracheal ring. Jackson and Jackson consider operation contraindicated when there is involvement below the second tracheal ring. On the other hand, Thomson records a tumor that necessitated the removal of the first 3 cartilaginous rings; nevertheless the procedure resulted in long-term control of the disease. Thus, it appears that the value of operative procedures in extensive subglottic lesions has not been fully assessed, and that techniques for the management of these lesions should be developed.

## CASE REPORT

**History.** The patient was a 66-year-old white man who was admitted on Dec. 3, 1958, because of hoarseness of 7 months' duration. During that period, there also had been gradually increasing dysphagia, anorexia with occasional vomiting, and a weight loss of 20 pounds. In the last few days prior to admission, only liquids could be swallowed.

**Physical examination.** There was evident cachexia and dehydration. No abnormalities were present in the mouth and pharynx, and there was no cervical lymphadenopathy. The chest was emphysematous with considerable dorsal kyphoscoliosis. On direct and indirect laryngoscopy, a tumor of the entire right vocal cord was seen extending in a subglottic direction. The cord moved only a slight degree. Biopsy showed squamous-cell carcinoma.

Results of urinalysis, blood count, electrocardiogram, and blood chemistry determinations were normal. The chest roentgenograms showed no pleural or pulmonary pathologic process. Soft-tissue films of the neck demonstrated osteoarthritic changes of the cervical spine. Laryngeal tomography revealed a tumor mass in the subglottic region with involvement of the right vocal cord.

**Course in hospital.** Because the patient was unable to swallow, tube feedings were started immediately after admission. It was evident that even if the lesion were operable, long preparation would be required for the operation. Therefore, radiation therapy was given and completed by Jan. 28, 1959. A dosage of 6,400 r was administered in 31 days. Swallowing improved somewhat, but not enough for discontinuation of the tube feedings.

Subsequent laryngoscopy showed fixation of the right vocal cord and a small subglottic nodule 3 to 4 mm. in size was seen below the anterior commissure. Biopsy at this time failed to show residual carcinoma. However, a subsequent biopsy of the subglottic area below the right cord showed squamous-cell carcinoma.

Since the patient's general condition was now adequate, a wide-field laryngectomy was performed on March 20, 1959. The trachea was transected below the third ring, but when the mucosal surface was examined, several discrete, raised, pearly gray, umbilicated plaques, the largest of which was 3 mm. in diameter, were seen on the posterior wall. These lesions extended to the level of the fifth tracheal ring. After removal of the larynx, the remainder of the involved trachea was excised beyond the most distal implant. As a result, the shortened trachea could not be sutured to skin in the usual manner. A skin flap was fashioned into a circular tube and approximated to the trachea.

Pathology confirmed the presence of subglottic carcinoma with tracheal extension and distal tracheal implants. The immediate postoperative course was satisfactory. There was a small area of slough at the sutured corners of the skin tube, but this soon healed. Four weeks after operation the patient was discharged. At that time, he was eating well and the tracheostomy stoma required minimal care. A tracheostomy tube was worn continuously to prevent constriction.

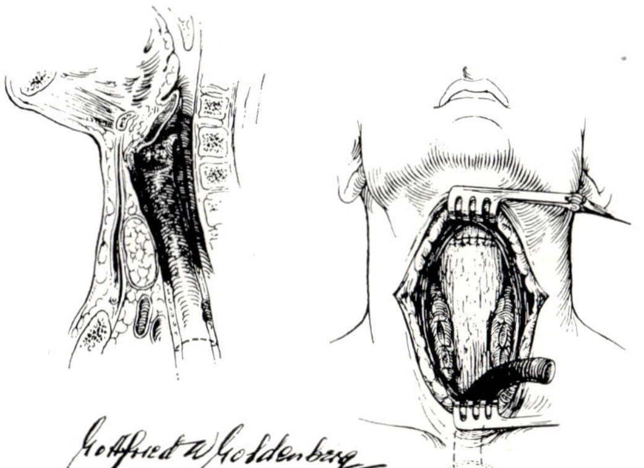


**Fig. 1.** Drawings indicate the extent of the tumor, the level of tracheal amputation, and closure of the pharynx.

**Subsequent course.** At first, there was a gain in weight and apparent good health. However, 4 months after operation, a fixed, firm mass developed on the left side of the neck just beneath the incision. Tumor was also observed within the pharynx at the suture line. There was no recurrence of tumor in the trachea or skin tube. Additional radiation therapy was given, but the patient's condition continued to deteriorate and he died of the disease on Feb. 10, 1960, approximately 10 months after laryngectomy.

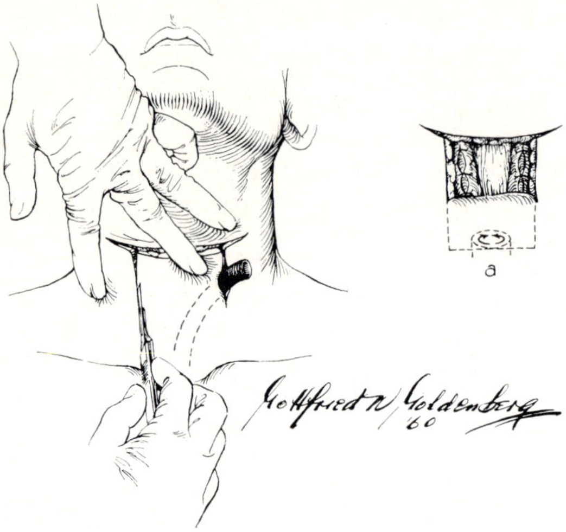


**Fig. 2.** Two parallel vertical incisions are made with utilization of the middle third of the lower skin flap, which is turned down to join the tracheal stump.

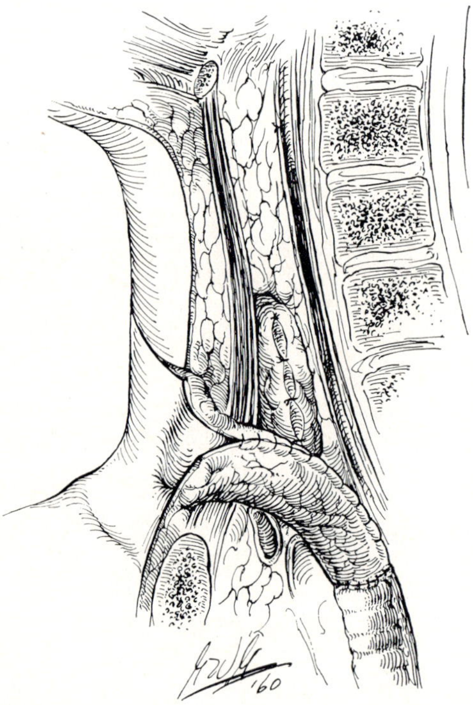

**Fig. 3.** Formation of the skin tube which is sutured to stump of trachea.

## TECHNIQUE

The technique used requires a standard transverse laryngectomy incision and the absence of a previous tracheostomy. In the case reported, skin flaps, including the platysma muscle, were raised and laryngectomy was carried out. The level of the tracheal incision and the level of the remaining tracheal stump are illustrated in Fig. 1. Closure of the pharynx was carried out transversely. A skin tube was then prepared for suture to the trachea. Two parallel vertical incisions were made in the middle third of the lower flap. The distance between the incisions equalled the circumference of the trachea. Their length equalled half the distance between the transverse skin incision and the tracheal stump (Fig. 2). In this case, the incisions were 2 inches long and 2 inches apart, giving the flap a 1 to 1 ratio of length to base, which insured an adequate blood supply. This flap was turned downward and inward, and the distal edge was sutured accurately to the tracheal mucosa with interrupted fine catgut stitches (Fig. 3). The anastomosis was started anteriorly and continued around the trachea until the opposite corners of the skin flap were approximated to each other at the midline posteriorly. The suturing was then continued upward to join the parallel edges of the flap, forming a tube with the suture line in back. After completion of the skin tube, the remainder of the laryngectomy incision was closed in the form of a T. There was no difficulty in approximating the lateral thirds of the lower flaps of this incision because of the defect left by the removal of the larynx. The upper flap was then a third longer than the lower, and this required accurate placement of the sutures to secure an even closure (Fig. 4). The final appearance of the healed tracheostomy is illustrated in Fig. 5.

## DISCUSSION

The method used in this case for construction of a tracheal stoma was not previously described. This technique was made possible by a transverse incision and by the absence of a preoperative tracheostomy. As a solution of the problem presented, it proved quite satisfactory. A method of bringing skin to trachea in the presence of a previous tracheostomy was reported by Watson.[14] In that report, the trachea was resected for a carcinoma which appeared at the point of irritation caused by the continuous use of a tracheostomy tube for 15 years. This procedure also produced a good initial result.

In planning a very low tracheostomy, there are several possible approaches. The best method is to bring the skin down to the undisplaced trachea without resection of the sternum; the other methods involve removal of overlying bone to produce a thoracic tracheostomy. Attempts at the latter approaches have been generally unsatisfactory.

In resection of a carcinoma recurrence at a tracheostomy stoma, Kleitsch[7] transected the manubrium and inserted a polyethylene tube into the trachea just above the innominate artery. Death from hemorrhage occurred in 4 months because of erosion by the tube into the innominate artery. In a similar case, Minor[8] split the sternum and dissected the mediastinal trachea from surrounding structures. The trachea was then angulated forward and secured to the periosteum of the sternum. A skin flap was then used to complete the stoma. Two and one-half months later, this patient also died from massive hemorrhage within the substernal space. Saareste[11] also lost a patient 9 days after a mediastinal tracheostomy because of hemorrhage from the innominate artery. Most recently, Waddel and Cannon[13] revised and extended Minor's technique. They similarly utilized a skin flap from the anterior chest wall which was brought through a hole rongeured at an appropriate site in the sternum. Here, too, it is admitted that the trachea is unavoidably held forward under tension. Two of the 4 patients in which this procedure was carried out died of massive hemorrhage from erosion of one of the great vessels of the chest. In one of these patients, this catastrophe occurred 3 months after discharge from the hospital.

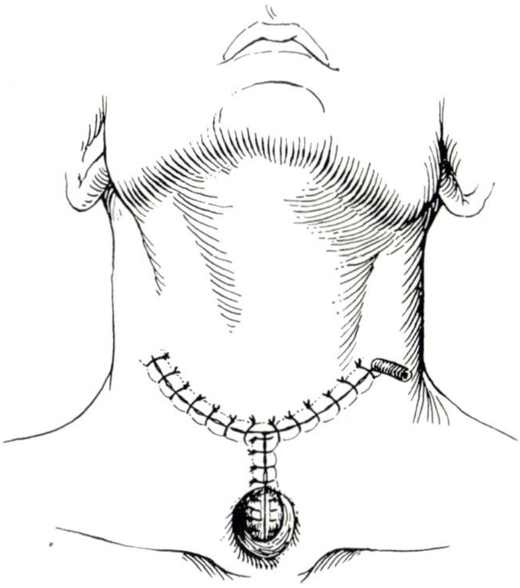

**Fig. 4.** The incision is closed as a T.

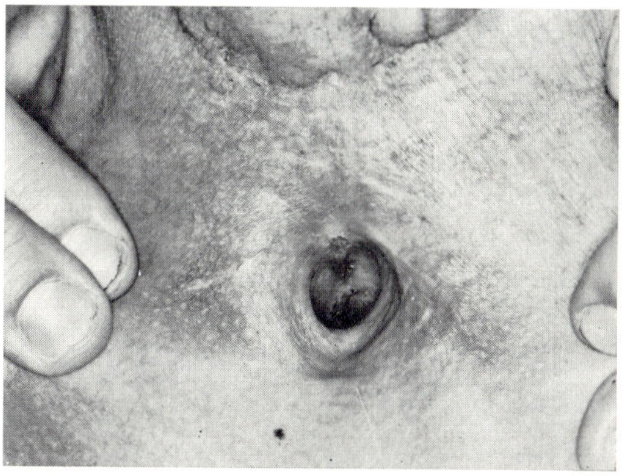

**Fig. 5.** Appearance of skin-tube tracheostomy after healing.

It is evident from these experiences that anterior displacement of the mediastinal trachea or the use of a rigid tube emerging through the sternum is likely to produce pressure on the innominate artery or other great vessels with subsequent erosion and hemorrhage. Therefore, the method of fashioning a skin tube to anastomose to the undisturbed tracheal stump within the thorax is preferable. It produces no tracheal displacement; the tracheostomy tube supported by the manubrium cannot cause pressure on the innominate artery.

## SUMMARY

1. Diagnostic and surgical features of subglottic laryngeal carcinoma are reviewed. A case of extensive tracheal involvement is reported.

2. A technique for the construction of a skin-tube tracheostomy is described and illustrated.

3. The hazard involved in thoracic tracheostomy is discussed.

### REFERENCES

1. Clerf, L. H.: Cancer of the larynx: an analysis of 250 operative cases, Arch. Otolaryng. **32:** 484, 1940.
2. Clerf, Louis H.: Laryngectomy, Surg. Gynec. & Obst. **86:** 197, 1948.
3. Clerf, L. H.: Subglottic carcinoma of the larynx, Pennsylvania M. J. **42:** 527, 1948.
4. Delavan, B.: Primary epithelioma of larynx below vocal cords: unique case, New York M. Rec. **20:** 625, 1881.
5. Isambert, E.: Contributions á l'étude du cancer laryngé, Ann. d. mal. de l'oreille, du larynx **2:** 1, 1876.
6. Jackson, C., and Jackson, C. L.: Cancer of the larynx, Philadelphia, 1939, W. B. Saunders Company.
7. Kleitsch, W. P.: Anterior mediastinal tracheotomy, J. Thoracic Surg. **24:** 38, 1952.
8. Minor, G. R.: Transternal tracheal excision for carcinoma, J. Thoracic Surg. **24:** 88, 1952.
9. Orton, H. B.: Cancer of the larynx, immediate and ultimate results in 102 operative cases, Tr. Am. Laryng. A. **60:** 144, 1938.
10. Orton, H. B.: Surgery of carcinoma of the larynx, A. M. A. Arch. Otolaryng. **64:** 205, 1956.
11. Saareste, F.: Difficult intubation on account of functional laryngeal stenosis after superior tracheostomy for laryngeal diphtheria; death from hemorrhage of the innominate artery nine days after inferior tracheotomy, Monatsschr. Ohrenh. **64:** 1996, 1931.
12. Thomson, St. Clair: Subglottic cancer of the larynx, J. Laryngol. & Otol. **52:** 803, 1937.
13. Waddel, W. R., and Cannon, B.: A technique for subtotal excision of the trachea and establishment of a sternal tracheotomy, Ann. Surg. **149:** 1, 1959.
14. Watson, W. L.: Cancer of the trachea fifteen years after treatment for cancer of the larynx, J. Thoracic Surg. **12:** 142, 1942.

# Surgical treatment of nasal hemorrhage

JOHN A. KIRCHNER, M.D.
NEW HAVEN, CONN.
*From the Section of Otolaryngology, Department of Surgery, Yale University School of Medicine*

Profuse nasal hemorrhage often produces shock and occasionally causes death. Lying deep within the nasal chamber near the origin of the regional artery, the bleeding site is almost impossible to identify because of its inaccessibility to inspection and because of the continued outpouring of blood. Between episodes of bleeding, little or nothing may be found to reveal the source, even on careful examination with the electric nasopharyngoscope.

Any hemorrhage which causes an appreciable fall in blood pressure may produce coronary occlusion in elderly patients. One such case resulting from epistaxis was reported by Bean,[1] whose review of 300 cases of coronary occlusion demonstrated the importance of preventing shock in patients with hypertensive cardiovascular disease. A fatal case of epistaxis from the anterior ethmoid artery was reported by Macbeth.[8]

Most nasal hemorrhages can be controlled by nasal packing combined with the use of sedation, hypnotics, and various medications such as estrogens, vitamin K, and so forth. Particularly effective in posterior nasal hemorrhage are the packs described by Saunders,[12] made of a vaginal tampon, and by Woodruff,[16] who packs cotton tightly under the posterior end of the inferior turbinated bone.

Unfortunately, postnasal packing is not only uncomfortable, but it also frequently causes complications, even though the patient is receiving antibiotics. Purulent sinusitis is not unusual, nor are ear complications such as hemotympanum or, less often, otitis media. Fissures or lacerations may occur where the anchoring silk string contacts the external nares or soft palate.[7] Osteomyelitis of the base of the skull resulting from a tight postnasal pack was reported by Spar and Williams.[15]

In 4 to 8 per cent of hospitalized patients, the packing and medical measures do not control the bleeding, and surgical intervention becomes necessary. This may consist of submucous resection of the nasal septum or of blood-vessel ligation. Removing a deviated portion of the septum allows better inspection, easier packing, and a release of tension over sharp crests or spurs. This procedure alone may allow the bleeding vessel to contract and heal. The operation can quite easily be combined with ligation of the anterior ethmoid artery if necessary.

As in other locations, ligation of the regional artery is the most effective method of controlling hemorrhage. Terminal branches of the internal and external carotid arteries supply the nasal mucosa. The anterior superior portion of the nasal chamber is supplied by the internal carotid through its anterior ethmoid branch of the ophthalmic artery. The posterior inferior portion below the middle turbinated bone is supplied by the sphenopalatine branch of the external carotid artery. Terminal branches of the latter vessel anastomose at Kiesselbach's triangle with branches of the superior labial artery. The posterior ethmoid, also a branch of the ophthalmic artery, is usually ascribed a minor role in epistaxis because of its usual small size. Studies of cadavers, however, show that it is sometimes a sizable vessel, one which might be responsible for continued postnasal bleeding after ligation of the external carotid.[2]

Received for publication Jan. 19, 1961.

**Table I.** *Data on 16 patients who underwent blood-vessel ligation for epistaxis, 1952 through 1959*

| *Case No.* | *Age, race, and sex* | *History and associated conditions* | *Indications* | *Ligation site and date* | *Postoperative course* |
|---|---|---|---|---|---|
| 1. M. S. | 50, WF | Hypertension, nosebleed and cauterization 15 yr. ago | Continued bleeding after 16 transfusions | Right external carotid Jan. 22, 1952<br>Left external carotid Jan. 25, 1952<br>Right anterior ethmoid Jan. 29, 1952 | Left pansinusitis<br>Bleeding recurred 2 yr. later requiring postnasal pack |
| 2. J. D. | 62, WM | Hypertension, arteriosclerosis, liver disease | Shock, continued bleeding for 2 wk. | Right external carotid Mar. 31, 1952<br>Right anterior ethmoid Apr. 3, 1952 | No further bleeding<br>Right pansinusitis |
| 3. M. P. | 57, WF | Rheumatic heart disease, hemiparesis | Shock on admission | Left external carotid Mar. 18, 1953 | No further bleeding |
| 4. J. D. | 52, WM | Alcoholism, hypertension (reserpine) | Pulse 120, Hb. 7.2 Gm., RBC 2.48, Hct. 26 | Left external carotid June 24, 1953<br>Submucous resection and left anterior ethmoid Feb. 28, 1955 | One minor epistaxis in Kiesselbach's area 3 mo. later, none since |
| 5. C. Z. | 32, WM | Smoker (1 pack per day) | 7 pints blood transfused in 9 days, Hb. below 7.5 Gm., pulse 118 | Left external carotid July 10, 1953 | No further bleeding |
| 6. S. S. | 54, WF | Hypertension, smokes 1 pack per day | 6 pints blood transfused in 6 days, Hb. 8 Gm. | Left external carotid Jan. 9, 1954 | No further bleeding |
| 7. W. G. | | Hypertension (reserpine), polypectomies and ethmoidectomies in 1944 | Shock, Hb. 8.2 Gm., bleeding 1 wk. | Right external carotid July 22, 1954 | Epistaxis, right, 2½ yr. later, BP 230/110, controlled by pack |
| 8. S. S. | 49, WM | Ethmoidectomy 24 yr. ago | Hb. 8.6 Gm. after 2 wk. treatment | Left anterior ethmoid Aug. 14, 1954<br>Left posterior ethmoid | None further |
| 9. G. B. | 55, WM | Diabetes, obesity, hypertension, alcoholism | Continued bleeding in spite of packs for 2 wk. and transfusion, Hct. below 28 | Submucous resection Feb. 26, 1955<br>Left external carotid Feb. 28, 1955 | No further bleeding |
| 10. J. D. | 52, WM | Alcoholism, fatty infiltration of liver, congenital heart failure | 1 wk. recurrent bleeding, Hb. 9.5 despite 1,000 ml. blood | Right external carotid Dec. 22, 1955 | None further |
| 11. J. L. | 61, WM | Polyps in right ethmoid area, recurrent nosebleeds for 2 yr. | 6 episodes in past 12 hr. | Right anterior ethmoid June 16, 1958 | Profuse right epistaxis, 1 yr. postoperative, minor epistaxis 15 mo. postoperative, none reported in past year |
| 12. A. S. | 69, WM | Alcoholism, bad septal deviation | Hct. 34 to 27, intermittent epistaxis for 12 days | Right ethmoid<br>Submucous resection Sept. 29, 1958 | No further bleeding |

**Table I.**—*Cont'd*

| *Case No.* | *Age, race, and sex* | *History and associated conditions* | *Indications* | *Ligation site and date* | *Postoperative course* |
|---|---|---|---|---|---|
| 13. T. R. | 37, WM | Hypertension, alcoholism, syphilis, 9 previous admissions for lacerations incurred in falls (drunk) | Hct. 17 despite 1,000 ml. blood in 24 hr. | Right anterior ethmoid Oct. 8, 1958<br>Right exterior carotid Oct. 10, 1958 | No further bleeding |
| 14. A. B. | 56, WM | Smokes 1½ packs per day, septal deviation to left | 2 mo. recurrent epistaxis | Submucous resection<br>Left anterior ethmoid Dec. 22, 1958 | 1 yr. later, left sided hemorrhage, easily controlled by pack 2 days |
| 15. C. C. | 66, WM | Hypertension, alcoholism, smokes 2 packs per day, badly deviated septum, chronic lung disease | 10 days' bleeding, bad septal deflection, Hct. 22 | Submucous resection, right anterior ethmoid Mar. 4, 1960<br>Right external carotid Mar. 11, 1960 | No further bleeding reported |
| 16. A. C. | 47, WF | Hypertension, menopause, Laennec's cirrhosis | Bleeding 1 to 3 times per day for 6 mo., repeated cauterizations | Left anterior ethmoid July 1, 1960 | Palpebral hematomas, bilateral, no further bleeding |

After Flemming's[3] first successful ligation of the common carotid in 1803, this vessel was occasionally ligated for intractable nasal hemorrhage. However, common carotid ligation results in only a 50 per cent decrease in normal flow as a result of the retrograde circulation down the external carotid artery.[14] The more effective and less hazardous ligation of the external carotid for nasal hemorrhage was not reported until 1925 by Hyde,[5] although 2 cases attributed to Jackson were mentioned in McKnight's report of 1926.[9]

Although the regional artery may be ligated in any of 5 locations, the 2 usual sites for ligation are the external carotid above the superior thyroid branch and the anterior ethmoid artery as it enters its foramen in the orbit. Other less common ligation sites are the septal branch of the labial artery, which can be sutured according to Rosenvold's technique as it enters the floor of the nasal vestibule and is used for the rarely intractable anterior septal bleeding[11]; the internal maxillary, which can be ligated after the anterior and posterior walls of the maxillary sinus are opened as described by Seiffert in 1929[13]; and the sphenopalatine artery itself, accessible to ligation by Silverblatt's technique, after the ethmoid cells are exenterated.[14]

## MATERIAL

During the 8 years between January, 1952, and December, 1959, 210 patients were admitted to New Haven Hospital for severe nasal hemorrhage. During this same period 23 blood-vessel ligations were carried out in 16 patients for intractable spontaneous hemorrhage (Table I). Patient 1 was treated at one of our affiliated hospitals, but is not included in the statistical analysis. Other ligations for bleeding associated with injuries, neoplasms, and familial hemorrhagic telangiectasia are not included in this study. Seven per cent of all patients admitted for epistaxis were treated by ligation as compared to 8 per cent in Hallberg's[4] series of 212 and 4.5 per cent of the adults in the series of Ogura and Senturia.[10]

**Age.** Of the 210 patients admitted for epistaxis, 99, or nearly half, were between the ages of 50 and 69. The largest single group was between 50 and 59 years of age (Fig. 1).

**Month.** Nasal hemorrhage appears to be

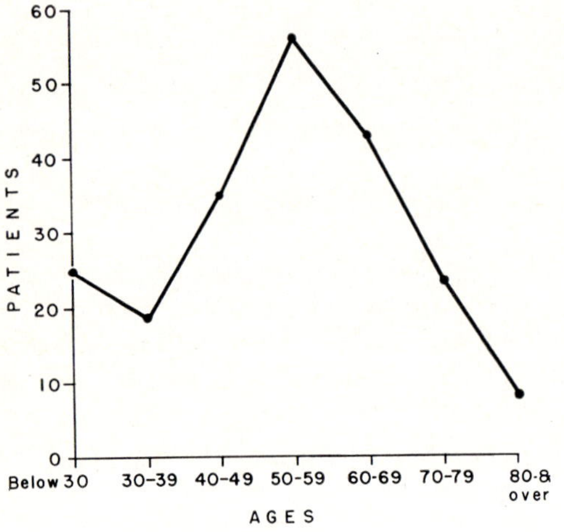


**Fig. 1.** Ages of 210 patients admitted for epistaxis (1952 through 1959).

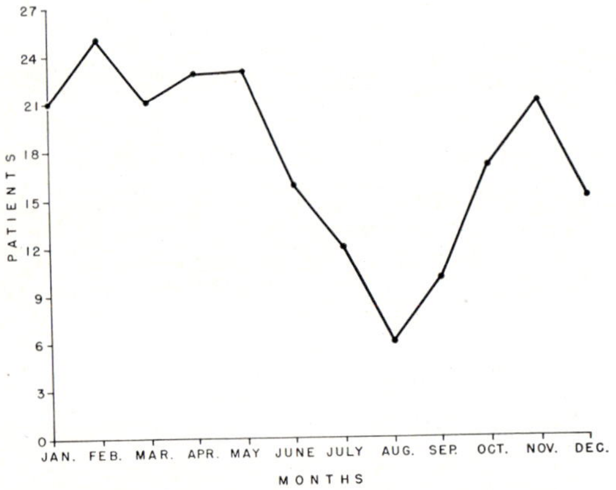


**Fig. 2.** Months in which 210 patients were admitted for epistaxis (1952 through 1959).

a winter condition. Most of our patients were admitted during the months in which artificial heat is necessary in the home. That this is a factor is suggested by the infrequency of nasal hemorrhage in milder climates where central heat is not used (Fig. 2).

**Associated conditions.** Nine of the 16 patients were hypertensive. At least 2 of these were under treatment with reserpine. Whether or not the nasal congestion which frequently results as a side effect of reserpine treatment contributed to the bleeding is an interesting speculation. Six of the 16 patients were alcoholics, either so diagnosed on previous hospital admissions or as estimated by the quantity of daily intake. Two patients had undergone previous ethmoidectomies, one 10 years previously and one 24 years previously.

## INDICATIONS

**Repeated severe hemorrhage.** Most of the 210 patients admitted for epistaxis continued to bleed for from 5 to 7 days in spite of all medical measures. Blood loss, however, was not excessive according to hematocrit and blood pressure determinations. Of the 16 patients who required blood-vessel ligation, 9 had bled for more than 1 week. After this length of time, the patient is usually disheartened by his lack of progress and is extremely reluctant to undergo any further postnasal packing. Repeated transfusions were given in most cases (Patient 1 required 16 pints of whole blood).

**Impending or actual shock.** A hypertensive patient who has suffered a substantial loss of blood may exhibit a blood pressure within normal limits on admission. Such a level may, however, be dangerously low in his case.

## SELECTION OF VESSEL FOR LIGATION

It is important to determine whether the bleeding is from high in the nose or low. The high bleeding vessels generally tend to be located anteriorly and the low ones posteriorly. With profuse hemorrhage, however, it may even be difficult to determine which side of the nose is the source. Five of our patients required ligation of a second vessel within a few days because the wrong arterial system had been tied off. Continued bleeding is almost never due to anastomotic connections.

## TECHNIQUE

Local anesthesia is used because of its simplicity, because of the danger of aspiration of blood under general anesthesia, and because the patients usually present poor risks for general anesthesia.

The external carotid artery is exposed by means of an incision along the anterior border of the sternocleidomastoid muscle extending from the midpoint of the thyroid cartilage to the level of the angle of the mandible. The facial vein and hypoglossal nerve cross the artery and must be identified. The external carotid can be distinguished from the internal by its branches. It should be ligated between the superior thyroid and lingual branches, so that the blood flow through the proximal portion of the external carotid into the superior thyroid will prevent retrograde thrombosis into the internal carotid. With the exception of 1 case in which 3 ligatures were placed on the vessel without dividing it, 1 single ligature has been placed between the superior thyroid and lingual branches of the external carotid artery. While a single ligature carries with it the theoretical risk of necrosis of the vessel wall and subsequent hemorrhage, this has not occurred in our series.

The anterior ethmoid artery is ligated at its foramen where the vessel branches from the ophthalmic artery. An incision is made halfway between the inner canthus of the eye and the midline of the nose, extending slightly into the eyebrow. Incision is carried to the bone through the periosteum, the latter being elevated to expose the frontolacrimal suture. This suture line is followed back by elevation of the orbital periosteum until the anterior ethmoid foramen is seen, where the artery, vein, and nasociliary nerve enter in a common bundle. The foramen is found in the frontal-ethmoid suture line or immediately above it.

Because the anterior ethmoid bundle is short and is located deep within the orbit, there may be considerable difficulty in placing a ligature around it, especially if the usual surgical instruments are used. Therefore, a neurosurgical clip may be applied to the vessel, or a long ligature carrier may be fashioned by wedging the point of a small cutting-edge needle into the end of a spinal needle, crimping it in place with a heavy hemostat, then bending the suture-carrying end into an arc small enough to encompass the artery (Figs. 3 and 4).

If the vessel is ligated, a single tie should be used for several reasons. First, the neurovascular bundle entering the foramen is so short that any effort to expose it sufficiently to allow the placement of 2 ligatures may tear the vessel and result in uncontrollable bleeding. Another reason for a single tie is the possibility of the second ligature's slipping off the vessel's short pedicle. Kulvin reported his experience in dividing the ethmoid artery between ligatures and encountering proptosis of the eye postoperatively as a result of bleeding. Exploration of the orbit revealed that the lateral ligature had slipped off the vessel and the artery had retracted and bled into the orbital cone.[6] If one is unfortunate enough to encounter bleeding from the ethmoid bundle during efforts to expose or ligate it, he can safely control the bleeding by electrocoagulation. However, it is prob-

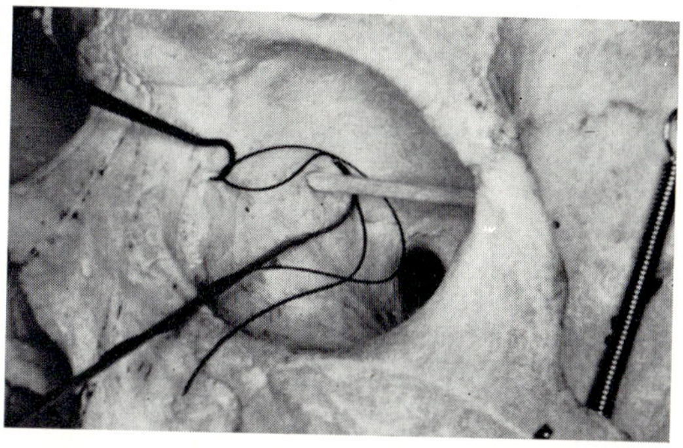

**Fig. 3.** Ligature has been passed around the anterior ethmoid neurovascular bundle, represented by the applicator entering the anterior ethmoid foramen. Ligature is then grasped by hook.

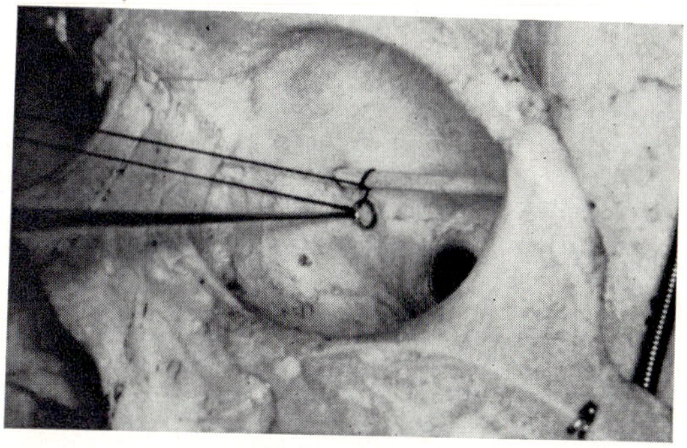

**Fig. 4.** Ligature has been tied and the knot drawn tight by passing the lower silk through a smooth ear curette. Ferris-Smith knot tier is similar and is used in this fashion.

ably well to avoid cauterizing the posterior ethmoid as is sometimes recommended, because of its proximity to the nearby optic nerve (2 to 3 mm.).

## COMPLICATIONS

Except for 1 case of bilateral palpebral hematomas and 1 minor stitch abscess, there were no complications in the 23 blood-vessel ligations. This contrasts sharply with the high incidence of complications in postnasal packing, even though these are usually minor.

## RESULTS

Immediate results were excellent, with prompt control after the proper vessel had been ligated. Late results were of interest in that 2 patients suffered recurrence of bleeding from the same side 2½ years later, 2 patients had a recurrence from the same side 1 year later, and 1 suffered a minor recurrence 1 month after ligation, but has had none in the past 5 years. The recurrences were usually easy to control, either by packing or by electrocautery at the bleeding site.

## DISCUSSION

The low incidence of complications with blood-vessel ligation in this and other series, contrasted with high incidence with postnasal packing, suggests that some of the 93 per cent who recovered on medical management might better have been treated by ligation, so as to spare them unnecessary discomfort and suffering. In this regard, it is interesting that the percentage of ligations among large reported series of patients hospitalized for nasal hemorrhage in various medical centers is relatively similar, 4 to 8 per cent.

## CONCLUSIONS

Profuse bleeding from deep within the nasal cavity may produce shock and endanger life. About 7 per cent of all patients admitted for severe nasal hemorrhage in this series of 210 hospitalizations failed to respond to packing and the usual measures. Ligation of the anterior ethmoid or the external carotid artery in this group controlled the bleeding promptly.

## REFERENCES

1. Bean, W. B.: Infarction of heart: morphological and clinical appraisal of 300 cases: predisposing and precipitating conditions, Am. Heart J. **14:** 684, 1937.
2. Flemming: Quoted by Spar, A. A., and Hallberg, O. E.: Severe epistaxis and its management: report of eleven cases in which the external carotid artery was ligated, Ann. Otol. Rhin. & Laryng. **56:** 141, 1947.
3. Hallberg, O. E.: Severe nosebleed and its treatment, J. A. M. A. **148:** 355, 1952.
4. Hyde, F. T.: Ligation of the external carotid artery for the control of idiopathic nasal hemorrhage, Laryngoscope **35:** 899, 1925.
5. Kirchner, J. A., Yanagisawa, E., and Crelin, E.: Surgical anatomy of the ethmoidal arteries, A. M. A. Arch. Otolaryng. In press.
6. Kulvin, M.: Epistaxis, control by ligation of anterior ethmoid artery, A. M. A. Arch. Otolaryng. **62:** 84, 1955.
7. Kuhn, A. J., and Hallberg, O. E.: Complications of postnasal packing for epistaxis, A. M. A. Arch. Otolaryng. **62:** 62, 1955.
8. MacBeth, R. G.: Anterior ethmoidal hemorrhage, Proc. Roy. Soc. Med. **40:** 280, 1947.
9. McKnight: Quoted by Spar and Hallberg.[3]
10. Ogura, J. H., and Senturia, B. H.: Epistaxis, Laryngoscope **59:** 743, 1949.
11. Rosenvold, L. K.: Intranasal ligation for epistaxis, Arch. Otolaryng. **32:** 1109, 1940.
12. Saunders, W.: Effective control of postnasal hemorrhage, A. M. A. Arch. Otolaryng. **64:** 291, 1956.
13. Seiffert, A.: Unterbindung der Arteria Maxillaris Interna, Ztschr. Hals-Nasen-u. Ohrenh. **22:** 323, 1929.
14. Silverblatt, B. L.: Epistaxis—evaluation of surgical care, Laryngoscope **65:** 431, 1955.
15. Spar, A. A., and Williams, H. L.: Osteomyelitis of the basisphenoid and basiocciput with meningitis and cranial nerve palsies as a complication of nasopharyngeal packing for control of epistaxis, Arch. Otolaryng. **46:** 473, 1947.
16. Woodruff, G. H.: Cardiovascular epistaxis and the naso-nasopharyngeal plexus, Laryngoscope **59:** 1238, 1949.

# The kidney and regional hypothermia

ABRAHAM T. K. COCKETT, M.D.*
LOS ANGELES, CALIF.
*From the Division of Urology, Department of Surgery, University of California Medical Center and the Urology Section, Los Angeles Veterans Administration Hospital*

The search for methods which would permit open-heart operations focused attention on hypothermia induced by surface cooling approximately a decade ago. Because of dangers of cardiac arrhythmias during general hypothermia (26 to 28° C.), regional cooling of isolated organs has recently achieved clinical prominence.

Interest in regional hypothermia of the kidney has been stimulated by the demonstration of a protective effect by hypothermia on the kidney during prolonged ischemia.[7, 16, 26, 27] Recently, emphasis has centered on development of more efficient means of obtaining rapid heat transfer.[7, 8, 28]

## EFFECT OF ISCHEMIA ON RENAL FUNCTION

Numerous studies have confirmed the presence of impaired kidney function after prolonged ischemia. In unilaterally nephrectomized rats,[17] 2-hour occlusion of the renal artery of the remaining solitary kidney is well tolerated. Three hours of ischemia results in a 50 per cent mortality rate. In rabbits with only 1 kidney,[1] renal artery clamping for 2 hours is uniformly fatal. Sheep[18] tolerate 1½ hours of renal ischemia after contralateral nephrectomy.

Controversial findings in dogs are worth mentioning. Friedman and his associates[13] reported negligible depression in renal function after obstruction of the renal artery for 2 hours, which confirms earlier observations of Hamilton and his co-workers.[14] In a small series of dogs, Roof and her associates[24] clamped the renal artery for 2 hours and reported permanent depression in function (50 to 70 per cent of preoperative levels). Birkeland and his group[4] occluded the renal artery of dogs for 3 hours at normal temperature with uniformly fatal results.

Scheibe and associates[25] occluded the renal pedicle and compared this series with one in which the dog's renal artery alone was clamped; less renal damage was noted when the artery alone was clamped.

Data from patients in whom the renal artery was occluded is scanty and inconsistent. Estimates of a safe period of renal artery occlusion vary from 30 minutes to several hours. Bahnson[2] reported the case of a patient who died in uremia 4 days after resection of an aortic aneurysm which had required occlusion of the aorta above the renal arteries for 110 minutes. Another of his patients[3] survived renal artery ischemia for 37 minutes. Semb[27] occluded the renal artery for 90 minutes without evidence of renal damage. Ellis and colleagues[12] resected

Supported by grants-in-aid from the Blalock Foundation and The Garrett Corporation, Los Angeles, Calif.

Presented in part as a preliminary report at the Surgical Forum, Annual Meeting of the American College of Surgeons, San Francisco, Calif., October, 1960.

Received for publication Jan. 26, 1961.

*Present address: Experimental Surgery Branch, School of Aviation Medicine, USAF Aerospace Medical Center (ATC), Brooks Air Force Base, Texas.

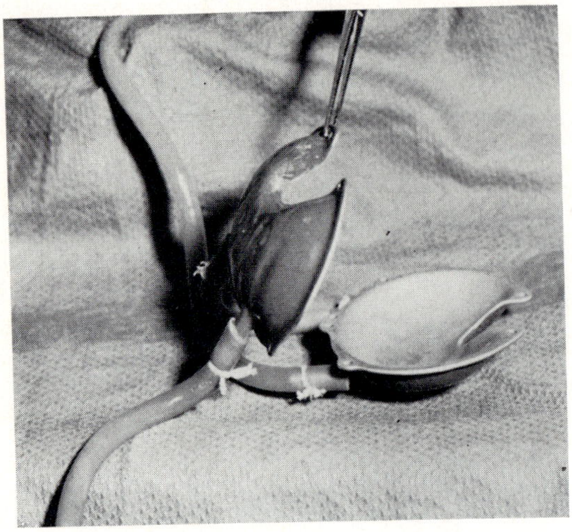

**Fig. 1.** The stainless steel kidney cooler.

an abdominal aortic aneurysm which involved the right renal artery. Ninety-five minute occlusion of the renal artery resulted in temporary loss of function. An intravenous pyelogram was reported as normal 2 weeks after operation. Creech and co-workers[9] resected aneurysms of the upper abdominal and thoracic aorta and occluded the latter vessel for intervals of up to 60 minutes. No significant reduction in renal function was described. In another report by these authors[10] the aorta and renal arteries were occluded for 105 minutes; severe renal depression was observed in this patient, who died from uremia.

## EFFECT OF HYPOTHERMIA ON ISCHEMIC KIDNEY

Bogardus and associates[5] occluded the renal pedicle of dogs for 2 hours and reported a considerable rise in blood creatinine level. Chilling the canine kidney during 2 hours of renal ischemia resulted in a less marked rise in the creatinine level. Schloerb and his group[26] observed the effect of cooling to 3° C. Survival of dogs was apparent during moderate renal ischemia (2 to 4 hours). Steuber and associates[28] confirmed the protective effect of hypothermia on renal function and advocated temperatures in the 0 to 5° C. range. Mitchell and Woodruff[19] observed peripheral cortical infarcts in sheep kidneys when temperatures below 10° C. were obtained. However, at these levels kidney function was protected. Owens and co-workers[22] occluded the upper thoracic aorta of dogs after moderate hypothermia (23 to 26° C). Renal function was not compromised during 3 hours of ischemia. Couch and colleagues[8] excised dog kidneys and perfused them at 25° C. With simple diluents, urine production was maintained for 7 hours, though at slightly reduced levels. Recently Cassie and co-workers[6] perfused excised dog kidneys at normal temperatures. Observed functional impairment was comparable to reduced function found in the excised kidney perfused at 25° C.

## EFFECT OF HYPOTHERMIA ON RENAL FUNCTION

Page and his group[23] reported a linear decrease in glomerular filtration rates and renal plasma flow during decrease in temperature. However, on rewarming of the dogs, renal function returned promptly to normal without evidence of residual damage. Hong[15] confirmed these same results in rats and squirrels. Moyer and associates[21] found a decrease in glomerular filtration rate and renal blood flow in 39 dogs at 27° C. Sodium excretion was not altered. Immediately after return to normothermia, renal function was 75 per cent of normal and return to normal levels was accomplished in 24 hours. Morales and his co-workers[20] treated 11 patients with hypothermia (30° C.). At lower temperatures glomerular filtration rate was reduced to 52 per cent; renal blood flow was 56 per cent of normal.

## METHODS

This study was formulated to evaluate a stainless steel kidney cooler, compact in design and readily adaptable to patients of all age groups. An intrarenal temperature of 18° C. was preselected to determine the effect of 2 hours renal ischemia with this device* (Fig. 1).

Fifteen mongrel dogs which ranged in weight from 11 to 22.5 kilograms were di-

*Manufactured by The Garrett Corporation, Los Angeles, Calif.

vided into 4 groups. All dogs were anesthetized intravenously with pentobarbital sodium, after which laparotomy was performed. Bilateral ureterostomies in situ were performed. The ureters were not divided. Polyethylene catheters were passed from the midureter to the renal pelvis on each side. Urine collections were made from each kidney before and after each procedure. Renal function was measured by standard clearance techniques (creatinine and para-aminohippuric acid infusion). Group I consisted of control dogs (Table I). Experiments were carried out in Groups II, III, and IV. In these 3 groups, the left kidney was cooled to an intrarenal temperature of 16 to 20° C. The right kidney remained at normal body temperature and was used as a control. Temperatures were recorded by small thermocouples imbedded 1 inch into the renal cortex.

In Group II, renal arteries were occluded for ½ hour. After release of the bulldog clamp from the renal artery, urine collections were obtained at hourly intervals for the ensuing 6 hours. In Group III, renal arteries were occluded for 1 hour. The arteries were clamped for 2 hours in Group IV.

After mobilization of the left kidney, 2 stainless steel shells were placed around the kidney before clamping of the renal artery. An inlet from each half shell was connected in series with rubber tubing. The remaining inlet from each shell was connected to a reservoir which supplied the coolant (Fig. 2).

## RESULTS

Effects of intravenous pentobarbital sodium anesthesia on renal function are given in Table I. The data include determinations of kidney function obtained from 3 dogs in the control group.

Fig. 3 represents an experiment which quite generally illustrates the events subsequent to renal ischemia for one-half hour. Five hours after hypothermia the glomerular filtration rate on the left returned to 18.5 ml. per minute, whereas in the right kidney it was 7 ml. per minute. Renal plasma flow followed the same pattern.

**Table I.** *The effect of intravenous pentobarbital sodium on renal function*

| Dog No. | Weight (Kg.) | Glomerular filtration rate (ml./min.) | | Renal plasma flow (ml./min.) | |
|---|---|---|---|---|---|
| | | Left | Right | Left | Right |
| 1 | 12.4 | 21 | 21 | 59 | 59 |
| | | 20.7 | 22 | 57 | 56 |
| 2 | 17.9 | 30 | 31 | 66 | 69 |
| 3 | 22.1 | 38 | 36 | 90 | 95 |
| | | 37 | 35 | 92 | 79 |

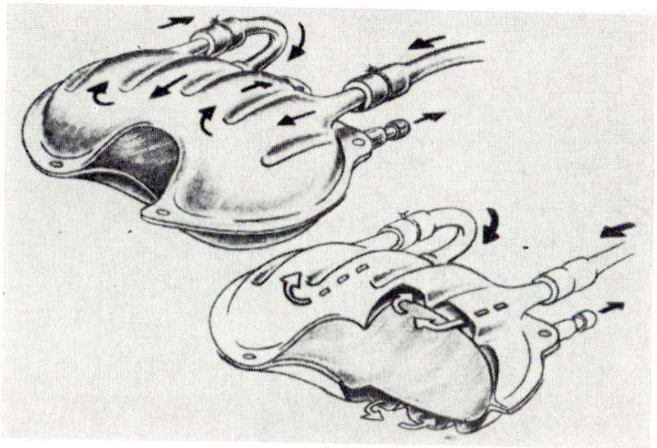

**Fig. 2.** Closed circuit path of coolant.

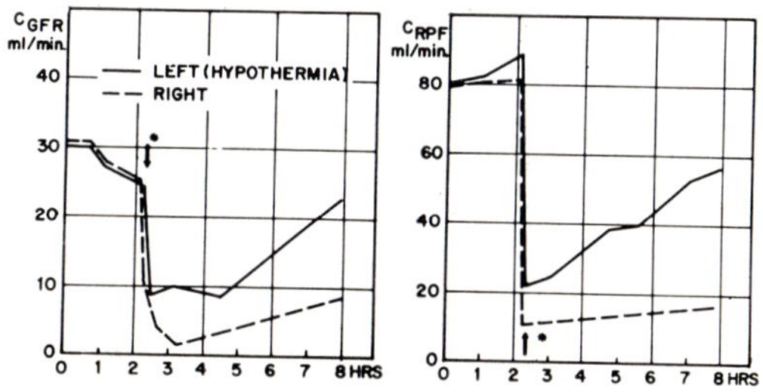


**Fig. 3.** Illustrative experiment from Group II. The effect of 18° C. hypothermia (*) on renal ischemia for one-half hour in a 13.1 kilogram dog.

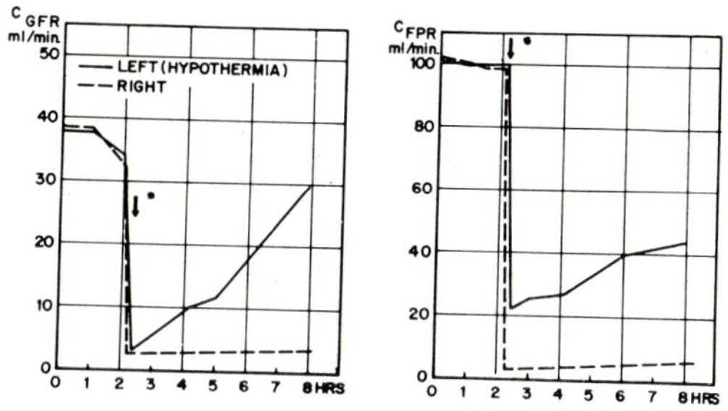


**Fig. 4.** Illustrative experiment from Group III. Effect of 18° C. hypothermia (*) on renal ischemia for 1 hour in a 15.5 kilogram dog.

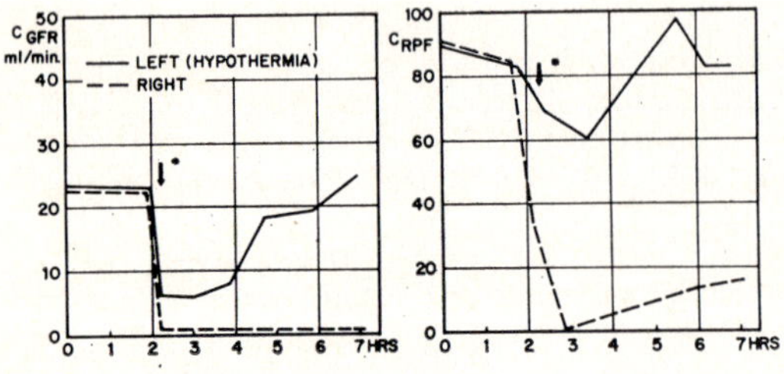


**Fig. 5.** Illustrative experiment from Group IV. Effect of 18° C. hypothermia (*) on renal ischemia for 2 hours in an 11.2 kilogram dog.

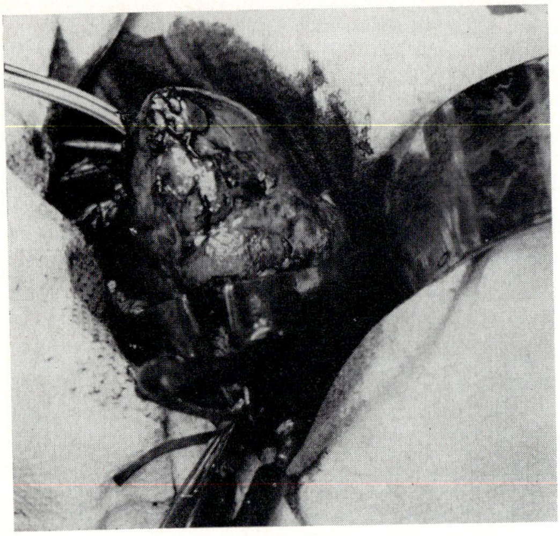

**Fig. 6.** Two quarter shells of the cooler in place on half of kidney prior to heminephrectomy.

Fig. 4 depicts the effects of hypothermia which are more marked 5 hours after the renal artery clamps are removed. Renal function in the right kidney remains depressed (less than 5 ml. per minute).

The events found after 2 hours of ischemia are plotted in Fig. 5. The differences observed are quite pronounced; return to normal on the hypothermic side is seen.

The kidney cooler has been employed in 6 clinical cases. Fig. 6 is a photograph of the cooler prior to heminephrectomy for a solitary calculus in the lower pole.

In Fig. 7 the apparatus is in position prior to a renal bivalving procedure. Temperatures of 12 to 18° C. were obtained in each instance. The renal artery was clamped 55 to 92 minutes in the 6 patients. An intravenous pyelogram obtained 5 days after renal bivalving for removal of a staghorn calculus showed prompt function.

Rate of cooling is graphically illustrated in Fig. 8. Kidney core and surface temperatures were monitored. Five minutes after occlusion of the renal artery, core temperature was 27° C., whereas surface temperature was 22° C. Within 15 minutes temperatures of 16 to 19° C. were obtained.

## DISCUSSION

These findings add to evidence already available that regional kidney hypothermia protects renal function during ischemia. At temperatures of 18° C., 2 hours of renal ischemia is well tolerated by the experimental animal. In the 6 clinical cases hypothermia was tolerated without apparent loss of renal function. Heminephrectomies were performed with use of 2 mirror-image quarter shells which encased half of the kidney.

These studies give additional support to views previously expressed that regional kidney hypothermia is indicated in situations which demand prolonged clamping of the renal vessels or the adjacent aorta. Renal endarterectomies and bypass operations may be handled in this manner in the future. In many instances, renal function is at a reduced level prior to operation.

Because renal homotransplantations may soon be carried out on a wide scale, the cooler may prove useful during the interval before the donor kidney is transplanted.

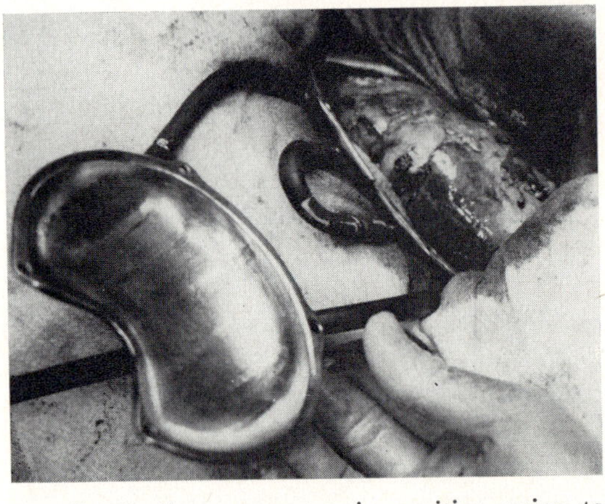

**Fig. 7.** Cooling apparatus in position prior to renal bivalving procedure.

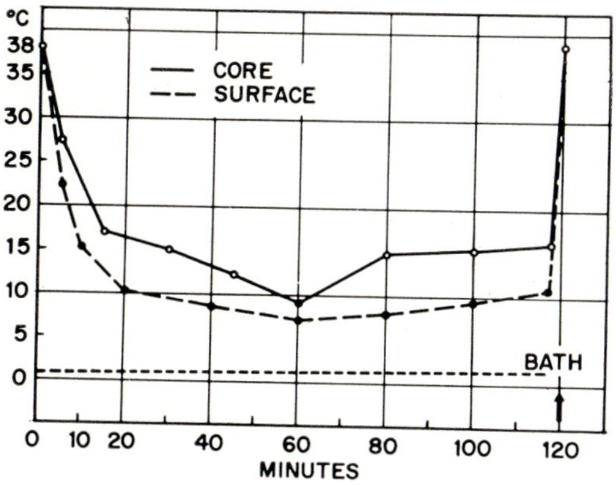


**Fig. 8.** Rate of cooling with regional kidney hypothermia.

Often, heminephrectomies or bivalving operations on the kidney require occlusion of the renal artery. Regional hypothermia can be beneficial in these instances.

## SUMMARY

Previous reports have demonstrated depression of kidney function when renal ischemia was prolonged. This study presents additional evidence of a protective effect when regional renal hypothermia is utilized.

A device is described which rapidly attains hypothermic levels (12 to 18° C.) and maintains kidney core temperature at this lower level, thus allowing several hours of operating time.

The new method for cooling has been used in 6 clinical cases without apparent deleterious effects. Renal flow was temporarily interrupted in these patients for from 55 to 92 minutes.

The author is indebted to Dr. Willard E. Goodwin, Professor of Surgery/Urology, for his encouragement and kind support. Technical assistance of Shelley Johnson is gratefully acknowledged.

## REFERENCES

1. Badenoch, A. W., and Darmady, E. M.: The effect of temporary occlusion of the renal artery in rabbits and its relationship to traumatic uremia, J. Path. & Bact. **59:** 79, 1947.
2. Bahnson, H. T.: Definitive treatment of saccular aneurysms of the aorta with excision of sac and aortic suture, Surg. Gynec. & Obst. **96:** 383, 1953.
3. Bahnson, H. T.: Treatment of abdominal aortic aneurysm by excision and replacement by homograft, Circulation **9:** 494, 1954.
4. Birkeland, S., Vogt, A., Krog, J., and Semb, C.: Renal circulatory occlusion and local cooling, J. Appl. Physiol. **14:** 227, 1959.
5. Bogardus, G. M., and Schlosser, R. J.: The influence of temperature upon ischemic renal damage, Surgery **39:** 970, 1956.
6. Cassie, G. F., Couch, N. P., Dammin, G. J., and Murray, J. E.: Normothermic perfusion and replantation of the excised dog kidney, Surg. Gynec. & Obst. **109:** 721, 1959.
7. Cockett, A. T. K.: An experimental study: an apparatus for regional kidney hypothermia, S. Forum, Annual Meeting of the American College of Surgeons, San Francisco, Calif., 1960.
8. Couch, N. P., Cassie, G. F., and Murray, J. E.: Survival of the excised dog kidney perfused in a pump-oxygenator system, Surgery **44:** 666, 1958.
9. Creech, O. Jr., De Bakey, M. E., Morris, G. C., and Moyer, H.: Experimental and clinical observations on the effects of renal ischemia, Surgery **40:** 129, 1956.
10. De Bakey, M. E., Creech, O., Jr., and Morris, G. C.: Aneurysm of thoracoabdominal aorta involving celiac, superior mesenteric, and renal arteries. Report of four cases treated by resection and homograft replacement, Ann. Surg. **144:** 549, 1956.
11. Deterling, R. A., Jr., Nelson, E., Bhonslay, S., and Howland, L.: Study of basic physiologic changes associated with hypothermia, A. M. A. Arch. Surg. **70:** 87, 1955.
12. Ellis, F. H., Jr., Helden, R. A., and Hines, E. A., Jr.: Aneurysm of the abdominal aorta involving the right renal artery, Ann. Surg. **142:** 992, 1955.
13. Friedman, S. M., Johnson, R. L., and Friedman, C. L.: The pattern of recovery of renal function following renal artery occlusion in the dog, Circulation Res. **2:** 231, 1954.
14. Hamilton, P. B., Phillips, R. A., and Hiller, A.: Duration of renal ischemia required to produce uremia, Am. J. Physiol. **152:** 517, 1948.
15. Hong, Suk Ki: Renal function during hypothermia and hibernation, Am. J. Physiol. **188:** 137, 1957.
16. Kerr, W. K., Kyle, V. N., Keresteci, A. C., and Smythe, C. A.: Renal hypothermia, J. Urol. **84:** 236, 1960.
17. Koletsky, S.: Effects of temporary interruption of renal circulation in rats, A. M. A. Arch. Path. **58:** 592, 1954.

18. Mitchell, R. M.: Studies on renal transplantation in sheep, Australian & New Zealand J. Surg. **28:** 263, 1959.
19. Mitchell, R. M., and Woodruff, M. F. A.: The effects of local hypothermia in increasing tolerance of the kidney to ischemia, Transplantation Bull. **4:** 15, 1957.
20. Morales, P., Carbery, W., Morello, A., and Morales, G.: Alterations in renal function during hypothermia in man, Ann. Surg. **145:** 488, 1957.
21. Moyer, J. H., Morris, G., and De Bakey, M. E.: Hypothermia. I. Effect on renal hemodynamics and on excretion of water and electrolytes in dog and man, Ann. Surg. **145:** 26, 1957.
22. Owens, J. C., Prevedel, A. E., and Swan, H.: Prolonged experimental occlusion of thoracic aorta during hypothermia, A. M. A. Arch. Surg. **70:** 95, 1955.
23. Page, L. B.: Effects of hypothermia on renal function, Am. J. Physiol. **181:** 171, 1955.
24. Roof, B. S., Lauson, H. D., Bella, S. T., and Eder, H. A.: Recovery of glomerular and tubular function, including p-aminohippurate extraction, following two hours of renal artery occlusion in the dog, Am. J. Physiol. **166:** 666, 1951.
25. Scheibe, J. R., Giraldi, E., and Vermeulen, C. W.: The effect of temporary renal vascular occlusion on kidney function, SURGERY **25:** 724, 1949.
26. Schloerb, P. R., Waldorf, R. D., and Welsh, J. S.: The protective effect of kidney hypothermia on total renal ischemia, S. Forum **8:** 633, 1957.
27. Semb, C.: Partial resection of the kidney: anatomical, physiological and clinical aspects, Ann. Roy. Coll. Surg. **19:** 137, 1956.
28. Steuber, P. J., Jr., Kovacs, S., Koletsky, S., and Persky, L.: Regional hypothermia in acute renal ischemia, J. Urol. **79:** 793, 1958.

# Studies in balanced hypothermic perfusion

WILLIAM F. BERNHARD, M.D.
HANS F. SCHWARZ, M.D.*
PAUL M. LEAND, B.A.**
JAMES G. CARR
BOSTON, MASS.
*From the Laboratory for Surgical Research, Children's Hospital, and the Department of Surgery, Harvard Medical School*

In the laboratory and on the cardiovascular service of the Children's Hospital, profound hypothermia is induced by the incorporation of a heat exchange mechanism in a siphon-drainage pump-oxygenator system.[2, 7] Prior to initiation of cardiopulmonary bypass, the temperature of the priming blood volume is reduced to 5° to 10° C. by recirculation through the heat exchanger for a 10-minute period. Commencement of perfusion with this precooled blood results in a rapid reduction of temperatures recorded from the heart, brain, liver, esophagus, and rectum. Cardiac asystole becomes evident within the first minute of cold perfusion which permits immediate cardiotomy.

During the cooling phase (at approximately 20° C.), a reduction in perfusion blood flow occurs secondary to increments in peripheral vascular resistance and blood viscosity. This physiologic decrease in total flow diminishes bronchial return to the arrested heart and facilitates visualization of many intracardiac defects. If more adequate exposure becomes a necessity, the combination of profound hypothermia and extracorporeal circulation permits periods of total circulatory arrest with interruption of the coronary arterial circulation alone.

Hypothermic perfusions of long duration (60 to 120 minutes) have been accomplished without difficulty in animals and in patients who weighed more than 10.0 kilograms.[3] However, in small animals (4.0 to 9.0 kilograms body weight), the usual methods of maintaining an equilibrium between venous return to the oxygenator and arterial outflow are not entirely satisfactory. In the experiments to be described, all perfusions were carried out with the oxygenator and venous reservoir mounted on a sensitive scale mechanism. This permitted an accurate quantitation of blood flow in and out of the animal, and eliminated complications due to hypervolemia.

The metabolic and hemodynamic studies also included in this investigation were (1) determination of changes in total body oxygen consumption which occur during cooling to 10° C. and throughout the rewarming phase and (2) evaluation of left ventricular work capacity after periods of total circulatory arrest (15 to 45 minutes in duration) at 10° C.

## METHODS AND MATERIALS

**Experimental procedure.** Thirty-six mongrel dogs of either sex which weighed 4.0 to 18 kilograms were used. The animals were anesthetized intravenously with pentobarbital sodium, 30 mg. per kilogram, and intu-

Supported by research grants from the National Heart Institute, National Institutes of Health, United States Public Health Service, and the American Heart Association.

Received for publication Jan. 30, 1961.

*Research Fellow in Surgery, Children's Hospital, and Research Fellow in Surgery, Harvard Medical School.

**Research Fellow in Surgery, Children's Hospital.

bated. Respirations were controlled with a Bennett automatic respirator. A polyethylene catheter was placed in the left femoral artery, and mean blood pressure measured by means of a Statham pressure transducer and recorded with a Sanborn direct writer. Cannulation of the left femoral vein was also carried out to permit the intravenous administration of heparin, an antiheparin compound (hexadimethrine bromide), and a muscle relaxant (succinylcholine chloride). Serial electrocardiograms were obtained in all animals and recorded with a Sanborn Viso-Cardiette.

Simultaneous myocardial, brain, hepatic, and muscle temperatures were measured with thermocouples mounted on 22 gauge needles. The brain needle was inserted through a temporal burr hole created prior to thoracotomy. Individual thermistor probes were also placed in the midesophagus and rectum and connected to a multiple-channel telethermometer for recording purposes.

A bilateral anterior thoracotomy was performed in all animals. The pleura was entered through the fifth intercostal space. Sodium heparin (1 mg. per kilogram of body weight) was administered intravenously after completion of the thoracotomy. In preparation for bypass, cannulation of the superior and inferior venae cavae was carried out in addition to insertion of sump drains through the atria into the right and left ventricles. This provided the return of systemic venous blood, coronary sinus blood, and bronchial collateral flow to a siphon-drainage Gross model pump-oxygenator system. A gas mixture containing 98 per cent oxygen and 2 per cent carbon dioxide (at a flow rate of 6 L. per minute) was used routinely in the oxygenator. Oxygenated blood was pumped through a stainless steel cannula in the right femoral artery.

The cooling phase of each experiment was accomplished in an average of 24 minutes, at which time the brain temperature was reduced to 10° C. After an interval of total circulatory arrest (15 to 45 minutes), rewarming of the blood was begun by circulation of warm fluid (40° to 42° C.) through the heat exchanger. Electrical defibrillation of the ventricles was accomplished with ease when the cardiac temperature reached 30° C., and decannulation of the cavae was carried out at a rectal temperature of 32° to 35° C. The mean duration of the rewarming period was 40 minutes.

For purposes of obtaining an accurate balance of perfusion blood flow, the disc oxygenator, motor, and venous reservoir were mounted directly on a Toledo scale (model 4020).* The connecting plastic tubing was suspended from a single vertical post fixed to the pump chassis (Fig. 1). Standardization of the scale with weights (1.0 to 100 Gm.) before each experiment permitted determination of changes in extracorporeal blood volume in increments of 2.5 Gm. A "zero" balance of the system was obtained after priming of the pump-oxygenator system with blood (2,800 ml.), and coupling of the caval and arterial perfusion lines to the animal.

**Metabolic determinations.** The changes in oxygen utilization which occurred during the intervals of cooling and rewarming were quantitated in 24 of the 36 dogs (Group I). To permit calculation of the oxygen consumption at 37° C., arteriovenous blood samples were obtained in 6 animals prior to thoracotomy. Simultaneous cardiac output determinations were carried out with a Gilford cuvette densitometer and indocyanine green dye.[10] During the reduction of body temperature, additional arteriovenous specimens were drawn anaerobically from the aorta and inferior vena cava at intervals of 5° C. (using brain temperature as reference). Blood samples were procured in a similar fashion throughout the rewarming phase beginning 2 minutes after the onset of warm perfusion. The oxygen capacity and percentage saturation of all specimens were measured by a spectrophotometric method.[8]

In 5 of the 24 animals (Group I), a muscle relaxant was administered intravenously throughout rewarming. This eliminated the effects of shivering and spontaneous muscular activity upon the oxygen consumption.

*Toledo Scale Corporation, Brighton, Mass.

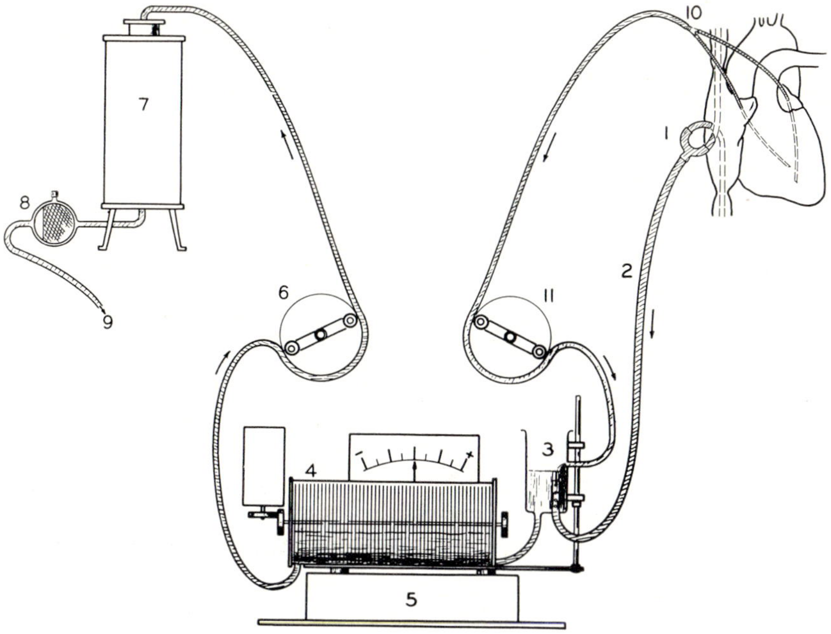


**Fig. 1.** Schematic representation of hypothermic perfusion with pump-oxygenator mounted on a Toledo scale. *1,* Y-tube with cannulas from both cavae. *2,* Caval drainage line. *3,* Venous reservoir. *4,* Kay-Cross oxygenator. *5,* Toledo scale. *6,* Pump returning blood to animal. *7,* Heat exchanger. *8,* Filter. *9,* Infusion into femoral artery. *10,* Coronary sinus and left ventricular sump drains. *11,* Pump for sump drains.

**Evaluation of left ventricular function after varying periods of total circulatory arrest.** In a separate group of 12 dogs (Group II), left ventricular stroke work (gram-meters) was calculated from the formula:

$$\text{left ventricular stroke work} = \frac{\text{stroke volume in cubic centimeters} \times \left(\text{mean arterial pressure (cm. } H_2O) - \text{mean left atrial pressure (cm. } H_2O)\right)}{100}$$

Left atrial pressure, mean arterial pressure, and cardiac rate (electrocardiogram) were monitored continuously on a 4 channel Poly-Viso recorder. The left atrial pressure was varied between 10 and 30 cm. $H_2O$ by infusion of whole blood through a polyethylene cannula secured in the left auricular appendage. Cardiac output determinations (with indocyanine green dye, a constant-speed withdrawal pump, and a cuvette densitometer) were performed after stabilization of the atrial pressure. Left ventricular function curves were constructed from these data by plotting stroke work (gram-meters) against left atrial filling pressure.[9] A composite "normal" curve containing the mean stroke work data from 8 animals (37° C.) was used for comparison with the posthypothermic stroke work data. The latter values were obtained in dogs which survived total circulatory arrest for periods of 15 to 45 minutes at 10° C. (heart, brain, liver, and esophagus), and rewarmed to 35° to 37° C. During the interval of circulatory arrest, the application of cold saline solution to the epicardial surface of the heart was necessary to prevent spontaneous cardiac rewarming.

## RESULTS

**Balanced hypothermic perfusion.** In 24 animals (Group I) utilized for the oxygen consumption study, the rapidity of cooling and rewarming was directly proportional to the existing blood flow and perfusion pressure (Figs. 2 and 3). Throughout the cooling phase (mean duration 24 minutes), temperatures recorded in the esophagus, heart, brain, rectum, and muscle decreased at rates varying from 1.2° C. per minute to 0.6° C. per minute. These changes were associated with a decline in the average perfusion blood flow (70 ml. per kilogram per minute to 50 ml. per kilogram per minute) and mean arterial pressure (136 to 100 mm. Hg).

Rewarming required an average of 40 minutes. At the conclusion of this period, the rectal and brain temperatures were elevated to the range of 32° to 35° C. Termination of the warm perfusion (40° C.) prior to this time resulted in a hazardous downward drift of cardiac, brain, liver, and esophageal temperatures toward the level of the existing rectal temperature.

An accurate balance of the extracorporeal blood volume (venous return and arterial outflow) was maintained by observation of the "zero" indicator on the scale chart. When variations in the rate of perfusion were noted, compensation was accomplished by adjustment of the speed (revolutions per minute) of the rotary arterial pump. This

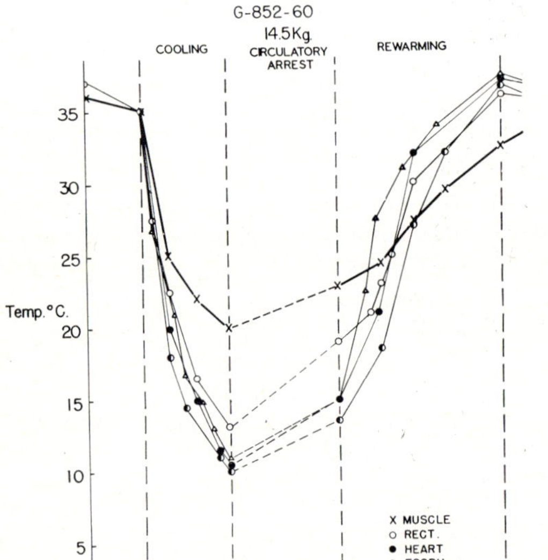


**Fig. 2.** Graphic presentation of changes in body temperature during cooling, a 20-minute period of total circulatory arrest, and throughout the rewarming phase. An upward drift in temperature occurs during interruption of perfusion.

system of perfusion control proved to be of maximal value in 5 small animals of Group I which weighed 4.0 to 9.0 kilograms (Table I). In these dogs, perfusion flows during cooling ranged from a maximum of 60 ml. per kilogram per minute to a minimum of 39 ml. per kilogram per minute, and increased slightly during the return to normothermia (41 to 68 ml. per kilogram per minute). The mean duration of each phase was similar to that recorded for animals which weighed over 10.0 kilogram (Fig. 3).

The 5 puppies in Group I survived for intervals of 3 to 14 days, and will be included in a larger series of small animal perfusions to be reported separately in a more comprehensive study. The remaining 19 larger dogs were sacrificed at the conclusion of rewarming to provide a source of donor blood.

**Oxygen consumption during profound hypothermia.** The effects of temperature and a 40-minute period of total circulatory arrest upon oxygen consumption are graphically presented in Fig. 4. The mean uptake of oxygen by 19 of 24 dogs (Group I) was found to be 5.0 c.c. per kilogram body weight per minute at 37° C., 3.0 ± 0.59* c.c. per kilogram per minute at 30° C., 1.8 ± 0.28* c.c. per kilogram per minute at 20° C., and 0.8 ± 0.16* c.c. per kilogram per minute at 10° C. The perfusion flow rate in all animals during cooling ranged between 50 and 70 ml. per kilogram per minute.

A 5 degree upward drift in temperature (using brain temperature as reference) occurred during the 40-minute interval of circulatory arrest. Therefore, active rewarming was begun at 15° C. The data collected at intervals of 5° C. disclosed a mean oxygen utilization of 3.4 c.c. per kilogram body weight per minute at 15° C., 3.9 c.c. per kilogram per minute at 20° C., 3.9 c.c. per kilogram per minute at 25° C., 4.6 c.c. per kilogram per minute at 30° C., and 4.7 c.c. per kilogram per minute at 37° C. In 5 additional animals (Group I), succinylcholine chloride was administered intravenously throughout rewarming. The mean

*Standard error of the mean.

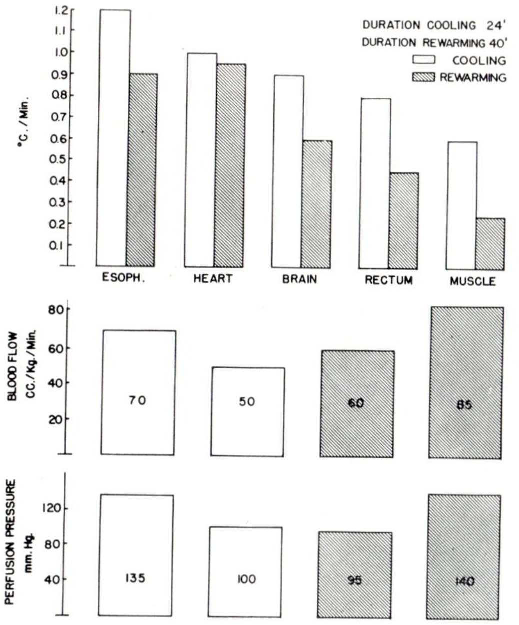


**Fig. 3.** Rapid rates of temperature change are noted in the esophagus, heart, and brain throughout cooling and rewarming, while temperature from the rectum and muscle mass lag behind. During the cooling phase, an increase in blood viscosity is the predominant factor responsible for the decrease in blood flow and mean perfusion pressure. All data represent mean values from 10 animal experiments.

oxygen uptake in these animals was 4.0 c.c. per kilogram per minute at 20° C., 4.0 c.c. per kilogram per minute at 25° C., and 4.1 c.c. per kilogram per minute at 37° C.

**Left ventricular function studies.** Each animal of Group II was subjected to a single period of total circulatory arrest (15, 30, or 45 minutes in duration) at 10° C. Post-arrest left ventricular function studies were performed 30 minutes after termination of rewarming, when the rectal, brain, and cardiac temperatures were in the range of 35° to 37° C. Representative curves before and after interruption of the circulation for the maximum period (45 minutes) are presented in Fig. 5. They demonstrate a mean stroke work capacity equivalent to 90 per cent of the control values.

## DISCUSSION

Profound hypothermia in conjunction with cardiopulmonary bypass facilitates the surgical correction of many complex cardiac defects. The method used in this center incorporates a heat exchanger with a siphon-drainage pump-oxygenator system, and includes the initiation of perfusion with a precooled (5° to 10° C.) extracorporeal blood volume. This preliminary step accelerates the rate of total body cooling and produces a precipitous reduction in myocardial temperature. Cessation of rhythmic cardiac contractions occurs during the first minute of perfusion which permits prompt cardiotomy.

The versatility of this method is evident from the fact that several of the more common congenital defects (tetralogy of Fallot and ventricular septal defect) can be repaired in the cold arrested heart during continuous perfusion. In other cases (valvular or supravalvular aortic stenosis, for example), interruption of the coronary circulation alone or total circulatory arrest can be employed to enhance intracardiac visibility.

**Table I.** *Balanced hypothermic perfusion in 5 small animals (4.0 to 9.0 kilograms)*

| | | *Perfusion flow (ml./min.)* | | | | *Perfusion pressure (mm. Hg)* | | | | *Lowest temperatures (C.)* | | |
|---|---|---|---|---|---|---|---|---|---|---|---|---|
| | | *Cooling* | | *Rewarming* | | *Cooling* | | *Rewarming* | | *Prior to circulatory arrest* | | |
| *Animal No.* | *Weight (Kg.)* | *Maximum* | *Minimum* | *Maximum* | *Minimum* | *Maximum* | *Minimum* | *Maximum* | *Minimum* | *Rectum* | *Esophagus* | *Heart* |
| G-216-60 | 9.0 | 600 | 450 | 600 | 450 | 135 | 125 | 145 | 120 | 14 | 9 | 9 |
| G-678-60 | 8.0 | 450 | 300 | 500 | 300 | 145 | 70 | 130 | 100 | 17 | 9 | 9 |
| G-M55-60 | 6.5 | 360 | 240 | 600 | 300 | 100 | 70 | 110 | 80 | 17 | 11 | 10 |
| G-M136-60 | 4.5 | 300 | 150 | 360 | 180 | 100 | 75 | 150 | 75 | 15 | 10 | 10 |
| G-M134-60 | 4.0 | 240 | 150 | 300 | 180 | 140 | 85 | 75 | 130 | 13 | 13 | 12 |

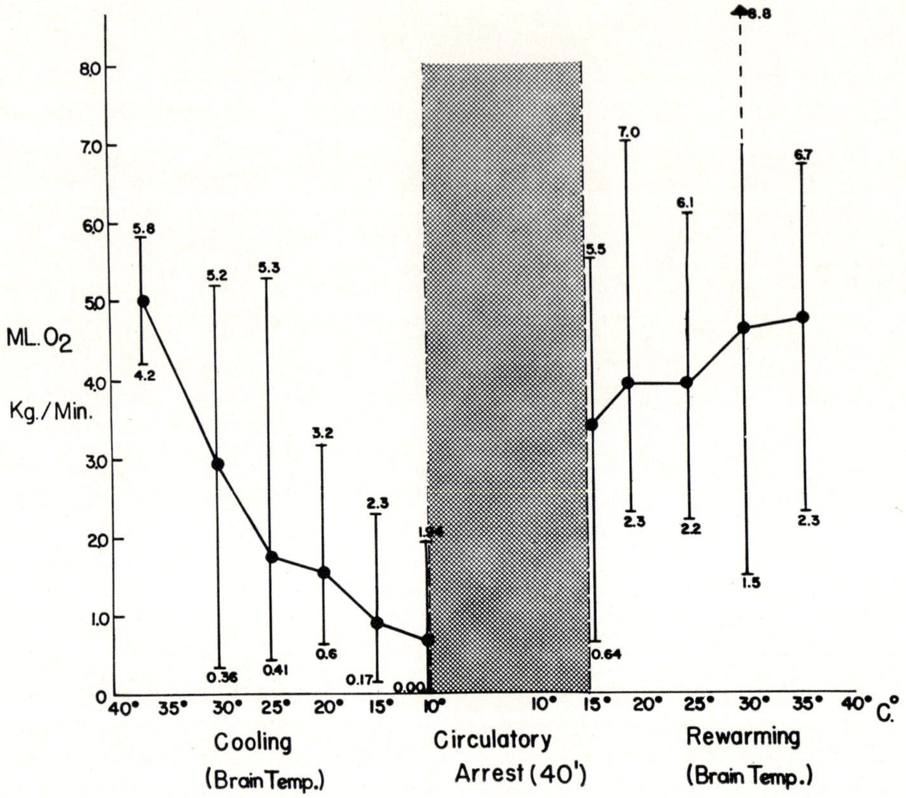


**Fig. 4.** Mean oxygen utilization data (and range of the mean) from the animals of Group I during the phases of cooling and rewarming. The rewarming values indicate the existence of an oxygen debt, incurred mainly within the interval of total circulatory arrest.

A comparison seems warranted between this technique for the production of profound hypothermia and that developed by Drew.[5] The most salient feature of the latter method is the use of autologous lung as the oxygenator. Although a more physiologic gas exchange may be accomplished in this manner, certain disadvantages appear evident. First, 2 separate propulsion circuits are required to pump venous blood through the lungs and to return oxygenated blood to the arterial tree. Second, the necessity of maintaining pulmonary blood flow during cooling delays the beginning of cardiotomy (20 to 30 minutes). Third, pulmonary perfusion under sufficient pressure to overcome varying degrees of vascular obstruction (pulmonary hypertension) may result in irreversible pulmonary parenchymal damage. Fourth, cardiac operations may be carried out only during periods of total circulatory arrest, an unnecessary risk in many instances.

The establishment of an equilibrium between venous return to the oxygenator and arterial outflow to the experimental animal is essential for a successful bypass. Although this is accomplished in the majority of instances, present techniques do not eliminate transient errors in the balance of perfusion flow (100 to 300 ml.). In the immediate postperfusion period, discrepancies of this magnitude are tolerated by dogs with an initial blood volume of 1,000 ml. or greater. However, errors of similar degree in smaller animals (blood volumes of 500 ml. or less) result in severe hypervolemia and right heart failure.

The quantitative type of hypothermic perfusion utilized in these experiments offers 1 solution to the problem. In this method, an oxygenator and venous reservoir are mounted on 1 side of a double-pan Toledo scale. After priming with donor blood, all of the apparatus is counterbalanced with approximately 30 Kg. of standard weights. Thereafter, equilibration between caval return and arterial outflow (measured in grams) is maintained by varying the speed (r.p.m.) of a rotary arterial pump. Throughout each perfusion, the single objective of the pump operator is to maintain the scale indicator arm on the "zero" mark. Accomplishment of this objective guarantees an accurate, balanced perfusion.

The change in left ventricular function after periods of total circulatory arrest (10° C.) permits a critical evaluation of the protective effect of reduced temperature upon the myocardium.[4] The data obtained from the animals of Group II demonstrate a 10 per cent reduction in work capacity after cessation of blood flow for a maximum of 45 minutes. No reduction was noted after total arrest for intervals of 15 and 30 minutes. These results are in general agreement with those given in another published report and indicate that a cardiac temperature of 10° C. provides a substantial degree of protection from the degenerative effects of hypoxia.[6]

In vitro studies of tissue homogenates and oxidizing enzyme systems (cytochrome oxidases) indicate that neither oxygen uptake nor electron transfer are limited at temperatures near 0° C.[1] Therefore, the decrease in oxygen consumption which accompanies a reduction in body temperature is dictated only by a lessened demand for oxygen in each metabolically active cell.

Quantitation of this reduction in utilization is presented in the data obtained from the animals of Group I. A 40 per cent decrease (from the control value, 37° C.) is evident at 30° C. and this progresses to 64 per cent at 20° C. and 84 per cent at 10° C. These data tend to confirm the impression that no physiologic end point exists above 0° C. at which the demand for oxygen completely ceases.

The mean oxygen uptake during the rewarming phase (after 40 minutes of total circulatory arrest) indicates the occurrence of an oxygen debt. Substantiation of this fact is provided by the presence of similar increases in utilization (at 15°, 20°, and 25° C.) noted in the animals which received succinylcholine. Since the oxygen uptake at the end of rewarming (37° C.) never exceeds the precooling control values, the existing debt must be satisfied during the period of warm perfusion.

## SUMMARY

1. A method of balanced hypothermic perfusion is described which permits quantitation of changes in total blood flow in increments as small as 2.5 Gm.

2. The practicality of this technique is demonstrated for cardiopulmonary bypass in small animals (4.0 to 9.0 kilograms body weight).

3. The total body oxygen consumption was determined during cooling to 10° C., after a 40-minute period of total circulatory arrest, and throughout rewarming.

4. An oxygen debt was detected during the rewarming phase of all experiments.

5. The administration of succinylcholine

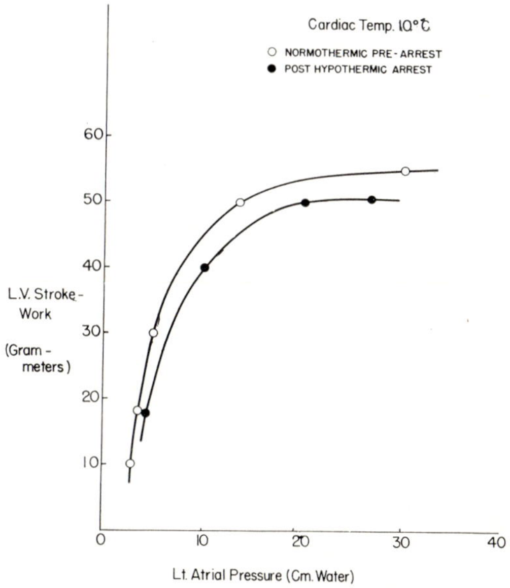


**Fig. 5.** Comparison of a left ventricular function curve after hypothermic arrest with precooling values. The study was performed 30 minutes after rewarming and indicated a slight decrease in stroke work ability.

chloride throughout this period failed to alter the dimensions of the debt.

6. Since the oxygen utilization during return to normothermia never exceeded the precooling (control) rate, a rapid satisfaction of this deficiency must have occurred.

7. Evaluation of left ventricular stroke work was performed before and after varying periods of total circulatory arrest at 10° C. The postarrest studies (carried out 30 minutes after rewarming) disclosed a 10 per cent reduction in left ventricular function after 45 minutes of cardiac ischemia.

## REFERENCES

1. Adolph, E. F.: Effects of low body temperature on tissue oxygen utilization. The physiology of induced hypothermia, National Research Council, Pub. No. 451, p. 44, 1956.
2. Bernhard, W. F., and Gross, R. E.: Extracorporeal circulation and profound hypothermia. A new surgical technique, Proc. New England Cardiovasc. Soc., vol. XIX, 1960-1961.
3. Bernhard, W. F., Schwarz, H. F., and Mallick, N. P.: Intermittent cold coronary perfusion as an adjunct to open heart surgery, Surg. Gynec. & Obst. **111:** 744, 1960.
4. Bernhard, W. F., Schwarz, H. F., and Mallick, N. P.: Profound hypothermia as an adjunct to cardiovascular surgery, J. Thoracic Surg. **42:** 263, 1961.
5. Drew, C. E., Keen, G., and Benazon, D. B.: Profound hypothermia, Lancet **1:** 745, 1959.
6. Greenberg, J. J., Edmunds, H. L., and Brown, R. B.: Myocardial metabolism and postarrest function in the cold and chemically arrested heart, SURGERY **48:** 31, 1960.
7. Gross, R. E., Sauvage, L. R., Pontius, R. G., and Watkins, E.: Experimental and clinical studies of siphon-filling disc oxygenator system for complete cardiopulmonary by-pass, Ann. Surg. **151:** 285, 1960.
9. Stainby, W. W., Fales, J. T., and Lilienthal, J. L.: A rapid spectrophotometric method for determining oxygen content of dog's blood, J. Appl. Physiol. **7:** 577, 1955.
8. Sarnoff, S. J., and Berglund, E.: Ventricular function. I. Starling's law of the heart studied by means of simultaneous right and left ventricular function curves in the dog, Circulation **9:** 706, 1954.
10. Wood, E. H., Swan, H. J., and Helmholz, H. F.: Symposium on diagnostic applications of indicator-dilution techniques, Proc. Staff Meet. Mayo Clin. **32:** 463, 1957.

# The influence of hypothermia on experimental bacteremia in dogs

GEORGE F. GOWEN, M.D.
GEORGE J. FRIOU, M.D.
WEST HAVEN, CONN.
*From the Yale University School of Medicine and West Haven Veterans Administration Hospital*

General hypothermia alters many physiologic mechanisms, but its influence on the response to infection and bacteremia at 30° C. (86° F.) is not clearly understood. Recently Allen[1] reported on a small group of patients thought to be in profound septic shock who improved promptly after the induction of hypothermia. It is difficult to define the sites at which hypothermia may have exerted its beneficial effects, but it seems probable that clinical improvement attended the use of hypothermia. A search of the literature yielded few reports on this subject and much of the evidence was conflicting.[1, 4, 5, 10, 11] In studying this problem, we noted that in hypothermic dogs the removal of bacteria from the blood was slower than normal. This report describes a controlled series of experiments intended to test this initial observation.

## METHOD

A pair of dogs of approximately equal weight was studied in each experiment. Each animal was used in 1 experiment only. After intravenous induction of anesthesia with pentobarbital sodium, 25 mg. per kilogram, 1 member of the pair was immersed in ice water until the temperature in the distal esophagus was 33.5° C. The dog was then removed and dried, and an endotracheal tube was inserted to which a respirator was connected. When the temperature had stabilized between 29° and 31° C., the pulse rate was found to have fallen from the normal rate of over 160 beats per minute to 80 beats per minute or less. Under sterile conditions a polyethylene catheter was inserted through the femoral vein into the iliac vein. Through this catheter a control specimen for blood culture was taken. Equal aliquots of *E. coli* in saline suspension (50 to 200 million colonies per milliliter) were injected into the 2 animals and the catheter then replaced with a longer one which extended into the inferior vena cava.

The infecting dose varied from experiment to experiment, but each animal of a pair received a volume of a uniformly dispersed suspension proportional to its body weight. The patency of the catheter was maintained by a continuous infusion of 5 per cent dextrose in distilled water at 60 drops per minute. Blood samples were taken in acid citrate dextrose solution at 10-minute intervals for 40 minutes after injection. Pour plates, with appropriate dilutions, were made immediately. In Experiments 1, 7, and 8 more frequent specimens were taken. The plates were incubated at 37° C. and inspected on the next day. Colony counts were made over a lighted grid. After the last specimen had been obtained the catheter was removed, the vein ligated, and the wound closed. The hypothermic dog was rewarmed with a Therm-O-Rite blanket until the esophageal temperature was 34.5° C. and spontaneous respirations were adequate. The rewarming process required 1½ to 2 hours. The animals were returned to their

Received for publication Jan. 30, 1961.

cages and observed. No antibiotics were given. Food and water were made available.

## RESULTS

**Bacteremia.** In 7 out of 8 experiments the hypothermic dog showed a delay in clearing the blood of injected bacteria as compared to the clearing in the normothermic control dog (Fig. 1). This delay was most evident at 10 minutes, but the same tendency was present at 20 minutes. After 30 and 40 minutes, the colony counts were approximately equal. The statistical significance of this early variation is indicated by a p value between 0.03 and 0.04.

**Mortality rate.** Five of the 8 hypothermic dogs died after rewarming, whereas there were no deaths among the control animals. There were no late deaths in either group. In 1 experiment it was possible to perform an autopsy immediately after death, 5 hours after the experiment had been completed. Blood taken from the heart in this animal was sterile on culture. All viscera were found to be markedly congested and sections of the liver, spleen, kidney, and lung did not show evidence of inflammation or bacteria. The p value for deaths lies between 0.01 and 0.02.

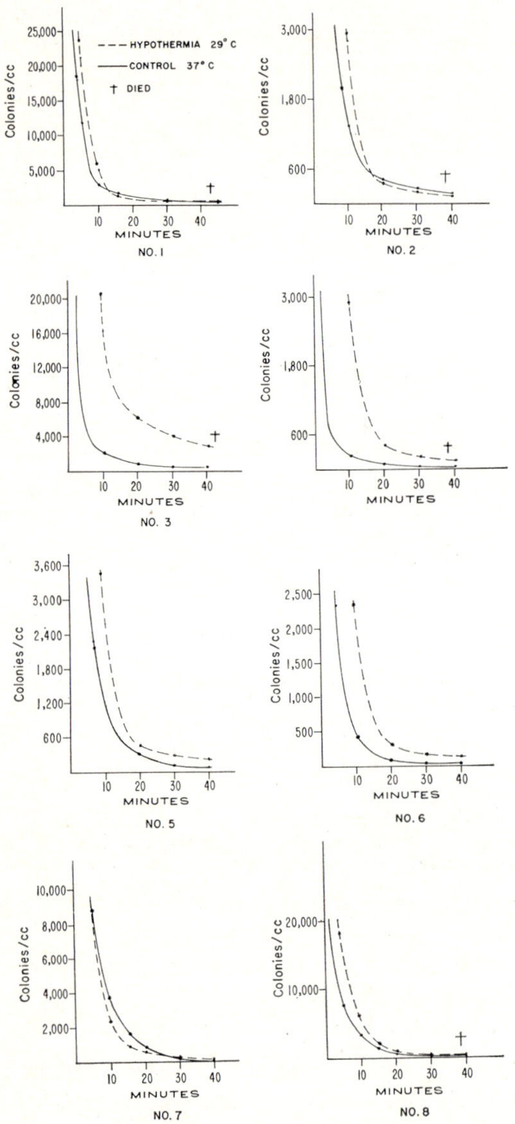


**Fig. 1.** Clearing of bacteria in 8 experiments. Dotted lines represent hypothermic animals and solid lines represent controls. In 7 of the 8 experiments removal of injected bacteria was slower in the hypothermic dog than in the control. In Experiments 1, 2, 3, 4, and 8, the hypothermic dog died after rewarming. There were no deaths among the controls.

## COMMENT

In 1943 Muschenheim,[9] using Goodner's[7, 8] standard pneumococcic dermal infection in rabbits, found that nonfatal infections became fatal if hypothermia were used. On the other hand, Wotkyns and associates,[11] in 1956, studied experimental pneumococcic peritonitis in mice and found that survival was prolonged when a fatal dose was given while the animals were hypothermic. Moreover, they found that with smaller doses the survival rates were improved by hypothermia. Also in 1956, Fedor and associates[5] induced a coliform bacteremia in dogs and found that the number of bacteria in the peripheral blood was reduced by 99 per cent 6 hours later. The cultures remained positive during the 12 to 18 hour periods of hypothermia, but became negative with rewarming. It is of interest that 7 out of their 13 animals died, a mortality rate consistent with our observations. Frank and colleagues[6] found a high mortality rate when bacteremia was induced in dogs under hemorrhagic shock, but when hypothermia was used, the mortality rate was reduced. However, Sanders and co-workers[10] repeated the work of Muschenheim[9] and confirmed the observation that hypothermia increased the mortality rate in pneumococcic infections in rabbits.

The present study demonstrated that in a hypothermic dog the blood stream is not cleared of injected viable bacteria as quickly as in a normothermic dog. Although the mechanism of delay has not been defined, the removal of particulate matter from the blood is known to occur in the reticuloendothelial system, principally the liver.[2] In hypothermia the blood flow to the liver is reduced[3] along with a decrease in cardiac output. Phagocytic activity was not studied in this experiment, but there is conflicting experimental evidence[4] on the in vivo influence of hypothermia on this function.

The second point of interest is the high mortality rate in the hypothermic dogs and absence of deaths in the control group. In Fedor's[4] experiment as stated previously, 7 out of 13 hypothermic dogs with induced bacteremia died. In the 5 deaths among our animals, 4 occurred between the sixth and twentieth hours after rewarming. Postmortem heart blood culture and histologic examination, performed in 1 animal, failed to show evidence of residual viable organisms. This finding may indicate that susceptibility to the lethal effect of gram-negative endotoxins is increased in the hypothermic state.

A direct comparison of our results with those of others is made difficult by the differences in experimental design. Despite the variations in animals used, the type and dosage of organism, and the duration of hypothermia, the evidence indicates an impairment of resistance due to hypothermia. Further investigation will be necessary to clarify the effects of hypothermia on the humoral and cellular responses to infection.

## SUMMARY

In order to test the effect of hypothermia on the removal of gram-negative bacteria from the blood, a series of controlled experiments was made in dogs. Blood cultures obtained at intervals of up to 40 minutes demonstrated a delay in removal of the bacteria by the hypothermic dog as compared with a normothermic control animal. In the hypothermic groups there was a 62 per cent mortality rate. No deaths occurred among the controls. It is concluded that under the conditions of these experiments hypothermic dogs have an impaired ability to cope with bacteria injected into the blood stream.

### REFERENCES

1. Allen, J. M., Estes, J. T., and Mansburger, A. R.: The use of hypothermia in septic shock, Am. Surgeon **26:** 1, 1960.
2. Beeson, P. B., Brannon, E. S., and Warren, J. V.: Observations on the sites of removal of bacteria from the blood in patients with bacterial endocarditis, J. Exper. Med. **81:** 9, 1945.
3. Dripps, R.: The physiology of hypothermia, National Research Council, Pub. No. 451, 1956.
4. Fedor, E. J., Fisher, B., and Fisher, E. R.: Observations on the bacterial defense mechanisms during hypothermia, SURGERY **43:** 807, 1958.
5. Fedor, E. J., Fisher, E. R., Lee, S. H., Weitzel, W. K., and Fisher, B.: The effect of hypothermia upon induced bacteremia, Proc. Soc. Exper. Biol. & Med. **93:** 510, 1956.
6. Frank, E. D., Davidoff, D., Friedman, E. W., and Fine, J.: Host resistance to bacteremia in hemorrhagic shock. IV. Effect of hypothermia on intravenously injected bacteria, Proc. Soc. Exper. Biol. & Med. **91:** 188, 1956.
7. Goodner, K.: The effect of pneumococcic autolysates upon pneumococcic dermal infection in the rabbit, J. Exper. Med. **58:** 153, 1933.
8. Goodner, K.: Experimental intradermal pneumococcic infection in rabbits, J. Exper. Med. **48:** 1, 413, 1928.
9. Muschenheim, C., Duerachner, D. R., Hardy, J. D., and Stoll, A. M.: Hypothermia in experimental infections, J. Infect. Dis. **72:** 187, 1943.
10. Sanders, F., Crawford, E. S., and De Bakey, M. E.: Effects of hypothermia on experimental intracutaneous pneumococcic infection in rabbits, S. Forum **8:** 92, 1957.
11. Wotkyns, R. S., Hirose, H., and Eiseman, B.: Prolonged hypothermia in experimental pneumococcic peritonitis, S. Forum **8:** 89, 1957.

# Reconstruction after total gastrectomy

P. CHRYSOSPATHIS, M.D.
H. LOUIS, M.D.
N. CAMPANIS, M.D.
ATHENS, GREECE
*From the Second Surgical Department, University of Athens, School of Medicine*

Although indications for total gastrectomy in patients with cancer of the stomach have been fairly well established and the immediate postoperative mortality rate for this operation has been reduced to acceptable levels, an important problem remains, namely, the type of reconstruction of the alimentary tract which is to be utilized. This consideration is important because it is well known that total excision of the stomach is frequently followed by a complex of symptoms known as the "agastric syndrome" which consists of bilious regurgitation, esophagitis, anemia, steatorrhea, and the dumping syndrome. Since a number of these sequelae may be due to technical factors, many improvements in technique have been suggested to avoid them.

To the more simple methods of reconstruction, such as the Roux Y or end-to-side esophagojejunostomy combined with a side-to-side Braun anastomosis, have been added other more complex methods of reconstruction. The aim of the latter is to create an interposed artificial stomach with a segment of either the small or large intestine. For example, Hunt[3] improved the Roux Y method by constructing a pouch from the upper part of the mobilized jejunal loop by a side-to-side anastomosis. Nakayama[8] utilized a loop of jejunum joined to itself by an end-to-side anastomosis which he interposed between esophagus and duodenum. Engel,[1] Tomoda,[11] Longmire,[5, 6] and others have interposed the small intestine in various ways. Hunnicult,[2] Lee,[4] and McClone[7] have utilized the cecum for this purpose, while State[10] utilized the transverse colon as a substitute stomach pouch.

During the decade from 1951 through 1960 we have had the opportunity to perform 79 total gastrectomies for gastric cancer. In the first 14 of the patients a simple technique was employed for reconstruction of the alimentary tract; in 7 the Roux Y anastomosis was performed, and in 7 an end-to-side esophagojejunostomy with a Braun anastomosis was carried out. In the next 23 patients the method of Nakayama was utilized. In the final 42 patients of this series, the technique to be described was carried out. This reconstruction consists of transection of the jejunum 7 to 10 cm. distal to the ligament of Treitz. The free end of jejunum is folded over and joined end-to-side to itself. To the loop thus formed the esophagus is anastomosed above, and distal to the loop the transected duodenum is anastomosed to the side of jejunum. Finally, an end-to-side anastomosis between the cut proximal end of the jejunum and the mobilized segment is performed (Fig. 1).

## CLINICAL MATERIAL

During the decade from 1951 through 1960, 221 patients were operated upon in

Revised for publication by Dr. John F. Perry, Jr., Department of Surgery, University of Minnesota Hospitals, Minneapolis 14, Minn.

Received for publication Feb. 8, 1961.

this clinic for gastric cancer. Table I shows the type of operation performed and the immediate postoperative mortality rate.

The type of operation to be employed was decided upon only after consideration of the patient's general condition and age, the situation of the tumor, and the presence or absence of metastases. Unresectable tumors were considered to be those in which diffuse spread or multiple metastases were present. Gastroenterostomy was performed for aged and debilitated patients with large pyloric tumors, usually with metastases in the liver and elsewhere. Wide subtotal gastrectomy was performed for localized pyloric tumor and was always combined with resection of the greater omentum. In a small number of patients this was a palliative procedure. Total gastrectomy was utilized for patients with cancer of the body or cardia or for those with very large tumors in the pylorus with metastases to the local lymph nodes. In Table II is shown the location of tumors for which total gastrectomy was performed.

Usually a midline incision was used which extended from the xiphoid process to a few centimeters below the umbilicus. This proved to be sufficient for any tumor of the body or pylorus. However, for cancers in the cardiac region a thoracoabdominal incision was utilized.

**Table I.** *Type of operation and mortality rate*

| *Type of operation* | *No. of cases* | *Deaths* | *Mortality rates (%)* |
|---|---|---|---|
| Unresectable tumor | 53 | 2 | 3.8 |
| Gastroenterostomy | 28 | 3 | 10.7 |
| Subtotal gastrectomy | 61 | 16 | 26.2 |
| Total gastrectomy | 79 | 10 | 12.6 |
| Totals | 221 | 31 | 14.03 |

**Table II.** *Location of tumors*

| *Situation of tumor* | *No. of cases* |
|---|---|
| Cardiac region | 11 |
| Body of the stomach | 42 |
| Pylorus | 26 |
| Total | 79 |

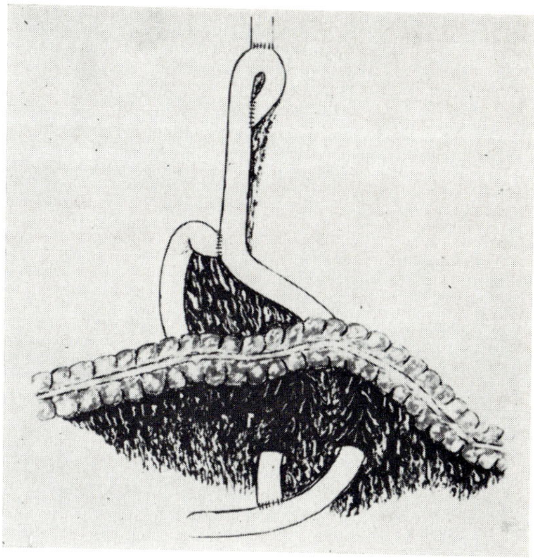

**Fig. 1**

Extent of the operation depended upon the findings at the time of laparotomy. If it was decided to perform a total gastrectomy, the lower 2 to 3 cm. of esophagus, the stomach and first part of the duodenum, the omenta, the tail of the pancreas, and the spleen were included in the resection. On 4 occasions we have resected the left lobe of the liver and in another 3 patients the operation was combined with resection of the transverse colon for spread of the tumor. Follow-up of patients has shown that resection of the left lobe of the liver was well tolerated, whereas results were less gratifying when resection of the transverse colon was added to the operation of total gastrectomy.

## MORTALITY RATES

Table I shows the immediate postoperative mortality rates encountered. Twenty six and seven-tenths per cent of 61 patients who were treated by subtotal gastrectomy died, whereas 10 of 79 (12.6 per cent) patients treated by total gastrectomy died. The higher mortality rate encountered after subtotal gastrectomy is probably explicable by the fact that in many of the patients this operation was a palliative procedure.

In Table III are shown the mortality rates encountered after the various types of reconstruction utilized after total gastrectomy.

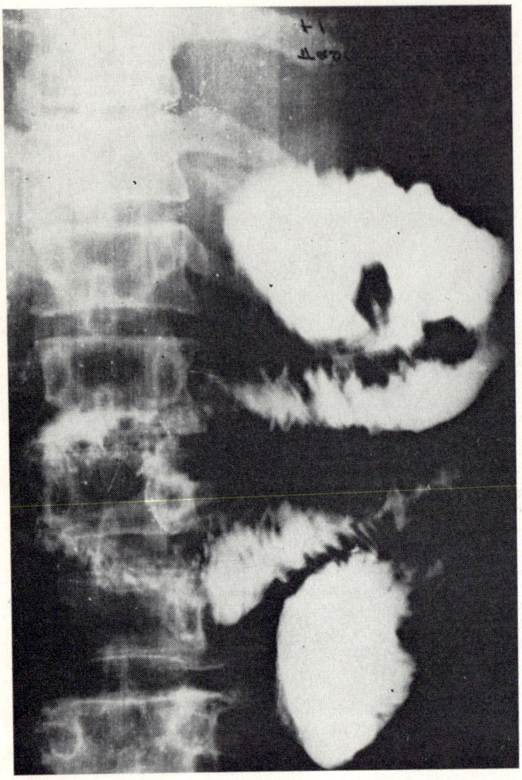

**Fig. 2**

Both patients who died after simple esophagoenterostomy Roux Y died because of disruption of the anastomosis followed by peritonitis. This complication was also responsible for 1 of the 2 deaths of patients operated upon by the Nakayama technique. In this instance peritonitis was caused by rupture of the end-to-end anastomosis of the mobilized distal end of the jejunum to the duodenum. The second death in this group was that of a patient with a cancer of the cardia for which a thoracoabdominal incision had been used. Six patients of a total of 42 operated upon by the technique described herein died. One died from irreversible postoperative shock, 2 from uremia, 1 from staphylococcal enterocolitis, and 2 from pneumonia. In 2 of the patients resection of the transverse colon which had been infiltrated by tumor was combined with total gastrectomy. Five of the 42 patients treated by this technique had carcinoma of the cardia which was removed with use of a thoracoabdominal incision. Four of the patients had neoplastic infiltration of the left lobe of the liver and another 3 had infiltration extended to the transverse colon. It is obvious that all the latter patients were operated upon in advanced stages of their disease. However, none of the deaths in the series were due to disruption of the anastomoses.

## SURVIVAL RATES

Of the total of 69 patients who underwent a total gastrectomy and survived the operation, 12 died within 1 year, 7 died before the end of the second year, and 16 died before the end of the third year. Two patients are still alive 7 years, 2 are alive 5 years, and 6 are alive 3 years after the operative procedure. Fifteen patients are alive and well 1 year after the operation. The fate of the remaining 9 patients is unknown because they have been lost to follow-up.

## DISCUSSION

Comparison of the results with the method described in 42 patients with cancer of the stomach with results of other methods which we have utilized in the past led us to conclude that this method has certain advantages over the other techniques. There have been no deaths from peritonitis due to disruption of an anastomosis and this, we believe, is due to the fact that the technique offers a double isoperistaltic outlet for food to the jejunum. The majority of food appears to pass through the duodenum. This has been verified by postoperative radiographs (Figs. 2 and 3).

Necrosis of the jejunal loop appears to be avoided in that a completely isolated loop is not utilized to join esophagus to duodenum.

**Table III.** *Technique of total gastrectomy and mortality rate*

| *Method used* | *No. of cases* | Deaths | *Mortality rates (%)* |
|---|---|---|---|
| Simple technique | 14 | 2 | 14.3 |
| Nakayama's method | 23 | 2 | 8.7 |
| Our method | 42 | 6 | 14.3 |

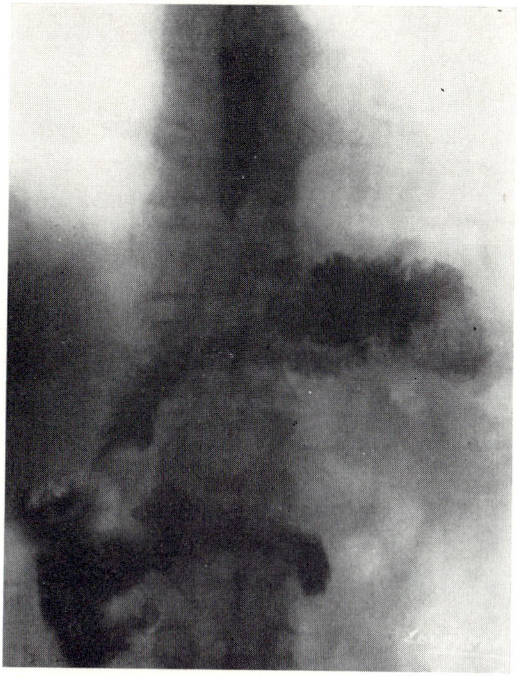

Fig. 3

In none of the patients treated by this technique was regurgitation of bile noted, whereas in 5 patients operated upon by other methods this distressing symptom was encountered and 3 of them developed severe esophagitis.

## SUMMARY

1. Experiences with operative treatment of gastric cancer by total gastrectomy in 79 patients are reported.

2. A new technique for reconstruction of the alimentary tract after total gastrectomy is described.

## REFERENCES

1. Engel, G. C.: The creation of a gastric pouch following total gastrectomy, SURGERY **17:** 512, 1945.
2. Hunnicult, A. J.: Replacing stomach after total gastrectomy with right ileocolon, A. M. A. Arch. Surg. **65:** 1, 1952.
3. Hunt, C. J.: Construction of food pouch from segment of jejunum as substitute for stomach in total gastrectomy, A. M. A. Arch. Surg. **64:** 601, 1952.
4. Lee, M.: Transplantation of a colon segment as a gastric reservoir after total gastrectomy, Surg. Gynec. & Obst. **92:** 456, 1951.
5. Longmire, W. P., Jr.: Total gastrectomy for carcinoma of the stomach, Surg. Gynec. & Obst. **84:** 21, 1947.
6. Longmire, W. P., Jr., and Beel, J. M.: Construction of a substitute gastric reservoir following total gastrectomy, Ann. Surg. **135:** 637, 1952.
7. McClone, F. B.: Total gastrectomy with replacement of stomach by ileocolic segment, J. A. M. A. **151:** 622, 1953.
8. Nakayama, K.: Evaluation of the various operative methods for total gastrectomy, SURGERY **40:** 488, 1956.
9. Paulson, M. H.: Hematological alteration after total gastrectomy, J. A. M. A. **156:** 1956, 1954.
10. State, D., Barkley, T. H. C., and Kelly, W. D.: Total gastrectomy with utilization of a segment of transverse colon to replace the excised stomach, Ann. Surg. **134:** 1035, 1951.
11. Tomoda, M.: Über den Stoffwechsel nach totalen Magenexstirpation, Chirurg. **23:** 545, 1952.

# Prolonged functional survival of a secondary renal homotransplant in the dog

C. F. ZUKOSKI, M.D.*
H. M. LEE, M.D.
D. H. HUME, M.D.
RICHMOND, VA.
*From the Medical College of Virginia*

Since Medawar[15] first convincingly demonstrated the occurrence of accelerated rejection in secondary skin transplant, it has been generally accepted that all types of secondary grafts will endure for shorter periods of time than the corresponding primary grafts, provided that the time interval between the implantation of the two is not too great.

In our laboratories, primary renal homografts in mongrel dogs were shown to have an average functional survival of 5.9 days, with a range of 2 to 14 days.[10] Dempster[6] reported a functional period of 4.4 days (range 1 to 10 days) in purebred greyhounds. The secondary transplants reported by Dempster[6] were performed 5 to 18 days after the primary transplants, at a time when the primary ones had ceased to function, and had an average functional period of 1.3 days (1 to 3 days) in 11 dogs. In another series of 10 secondary transplants, Dempster[5] removed the primary transplants on the first to fourth day, usually the fourth, while they were still secreting. The secondary transplants were placed 8 to 28 days after the primary ones. Seven of them functioned for 4 to 5 days. Egdahl and Hume[8] found an average functional period of 1.8 days (0 to 5 days) in 15 secondary renal transplants in mongrel dogs. The primary grafts in this same group had shown an average functional period of 6.2 days, and the secondary transplants had been performed 14 to 133 days after the first.

In none of the 26 instances in which functional periods were measured for both primary and secondary transplants did the secondary graft function for a longer period than the primary,[7] though there was a tendency for the secondary graft to function somewhat longer in animals in which the primary grafts had functioned longest. In the present report, a secondary renal transplant is described which functioned for a much longer time than any secondary transplant previously reported, and for a longer time than the primary or any other canine renal primary homotransplant reported.

The 2 dogs were obtained from our usual sources for mongrel dogs, but showed recognizable characteristics of relatively pure boxer ancestry. The dogs bore no more than a superficial resemblance to each other, however. The right kidney of Dog 1 was removed and a transplant from Dog 2 was placed in the renal fossa with the ureter brought to the skin by methods previously described.[10] A prolonged survival of the primary transplant was noted, with a 24-hour output of 500 ml. of clear urine on the twenty-first day and a continuous secretion for 39 days. Collections after the twenty-first day were incomplete because the suture holding the catheter in place cut through the ureter at this time, and the tip of the ureter retracted back to the skin. On the fifty-first day after transplanta-

*Special trainee, National Institute of Neurological Diseases and Blindness, BT-538(01). Present address: Nashville Veterans Administration Hospital and Vanderbilt University School of Medicine, Nashville, Tenn.

Supported in part by grant from the Beaumont Foundation.

Received for publication Feb. 7, 1961.

tion, the primary transplant was removed. Both artery and vein were patent. A secondary transplant from Dog 2 was placed in the pelvic fossa, and the remaining kidney of Dog 1 was transferred in the same manner to Dog 2. The ureter of each kidney was anastomosed to the bladder. Both animals were thus bilaterally nephrectomized. Dog 1 was maintained solely by a secondary transplant from Dog 2, and Dog 2 solely by a primary transplant from Dog 1.

Both animals continued to eat ravenously, had intestinal worms and diarrhea, lost weight, and had dependent edema and generalized eczema which tended to clear as the blood urea nitrogen (BUN) approached a more normal level.

Dog 2 (primary transplant from Dog 1) survived 60 days and died from an acute gastrointestinal hemorrhage from an undiscovered site. At the time of death, there was 80 ml. of urine in the bladder.

Dog 1 survived 88 days, during all of which time the secondary transplant continued to function. The cause of death was volvulus of the small intestine which was due to an adhesive band. The blood pressure was 100/60 on day 57. The general condition of the animal appeared better than that of Dog 2 and the eczema cleared more as the BUN level came down. The BUN levels during the course of the experiment are shown in Fig. 1. It is apparent that there was a progressive decline in the BUN level in both dogs after the peak levels were noted by the third week. Both dogs showed an elevation of the BUN to over 180 mg. per 100 ml. by the third week, which declined to 70 mg. per 100 ml. by the fifty-eighth day in Dog 2 and to 40 mg. per 100 ml. on the eighty-sixth day in Dog 1. Table I shows the blood and urine chemistry determinations for Dog 1 on day 56 after the secondary transplantation.

The microscopic appearance of the renal homograft is shown in Figs. 2 through 5. The primary transplant in Dog 1 showed a moderate homograft reaction on day 27 (Fig. 2) and by day 45 (Fig. 3) the kidney was nearly destroyed. The secondary transplant in Dog 1 showed a homograft rejection pattern when biopsied on day 8 (Fig. 4) and this was still present at death on the eighty-eighth day, but there was considerably less round-cell infiltration at this time than had been seen at the earlier biopsy (Fig. 5).

The primary transplant in Dog 2 showed a typical homograft reaction on day 13, which appeared more intense than that seen at

**Table I.** *Urine and blood values, Dog 1, day 56*

| | *Urine* | *Blood* |
|---|---|---|
| Sodium (mEq.) | 26 | 144 |
| Potassium (mEq.) | 86 | 5.3 |
| Chloride (mg.%) | 45 | 106 |
| Creatinine (mg.%) | 53 | 1.3 |
| Urea nitrogen (mg.%) | 1,100 | — |
| BUN (mg.%) | — | 57 |

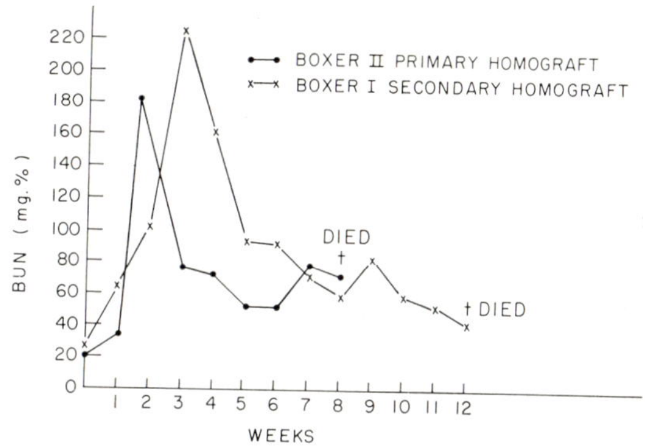


**Fig. 1.** The BUN levels during the course of the experiment.

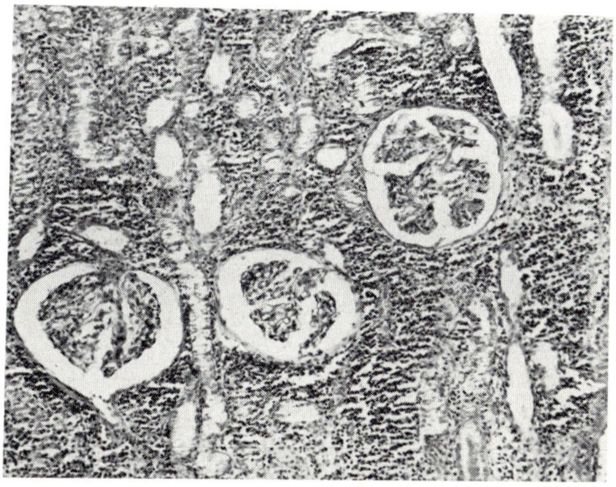

**Fig. 2.** Dog 1. Biopsy specimen of primary kidney transplant on twenty-seventh day. (Hematoxylin and eosin; × 100; reduced 3/7.)

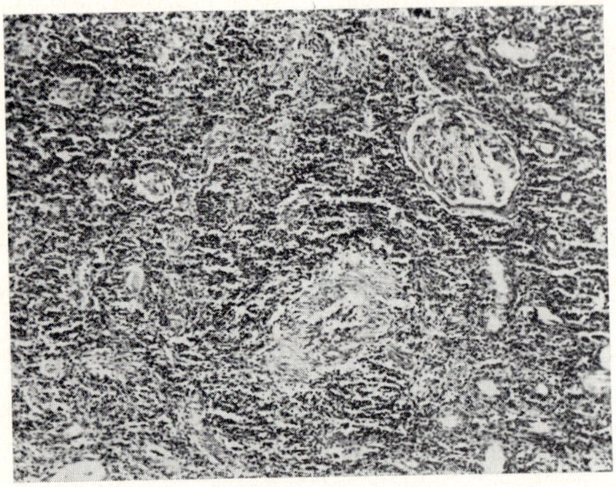

**Fig. 3.** Dog 1. Biopsy specimen of primary kidney transplant on the forty-fifth day. (Hematoxylin and eosin; × 100; reduced ¾.)

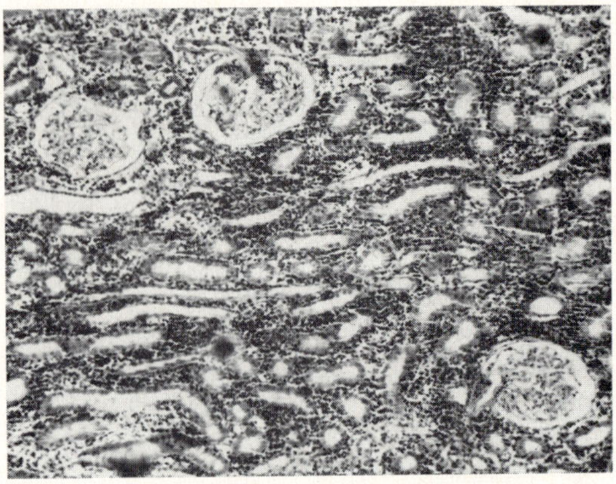

**Fig. 4.** Biopsy specimen on eighth day of secondary renal transplant in Dog 1. (Hematoxylin and eosin; × 100; reduced ¾.)

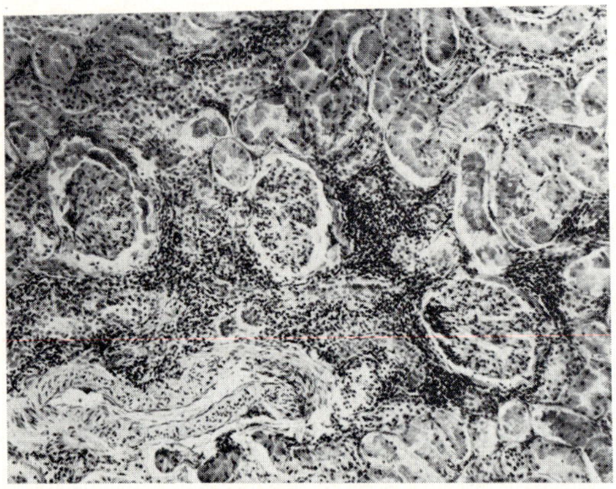

**Fig. 5.** The secondary renal homograft at eighty-eighth day. (Hematoxylin and eosin, × 100; reduced ¾.)

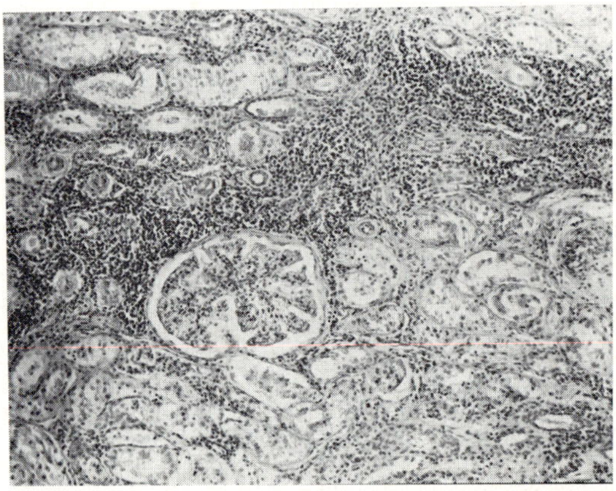

**Fig. 6.** Dog 2. The primary renal homograft on the sixtieth day. (Hematoxylin and eosin; × 100; reduced ¾.)

death on day 60. At death (Fig. 6) there was infarcation and hyalinization of some glomeruli, while others appeared hypertrophied. There was relatively little round-cell infiltration, and tubular damage, while present, was not complete.

## DISCUSSION

The production of acquired immunologic tolerance to homografts has been demonstrated in several species of animals by exposing them to antigens during immunologic immaturity. Tolerance has also apparently been achieved under some circumstances in the adult animal by prolonged antigenic exposure, or prior antigenic exposure with a prolonged interval before grafting. Werder and Hardin[18] showed that in the mouse, repeated homografts of skin from different donors to the same host permit prolonged survival of the later transplants provided that the interval between transplants was long enough. Billingham and Sparrow[2] showed that prolonged "take" of rabbit skin homografts followed pretreatment of the host with epidermal cells from the prospective donor. A secondary transplant from the same donor also showed prolonged survival, sometimes longer than that of the primary. Billingham and associates[1] performed secondary grafts in 16 mice in which the primary graft "take" had been prolonged and noted that the secondary grafts survived longer than would ordinarily be expected, but not as long as the primary grafts in the same animal. Martinez and colleagues[14] have demonstrated tolerance to a skin graft transferred between mice in parabiosis. The skin graft placed during the parabiotic union persisted after the termination of this union, and future grafts from the same donor were not rejected. A secondary homotransplant between dogs placed in cross-circulation has persisted without evidences of rejection for 4 days.[9] It appears, therefore, that the dose of the antigen and the time of the exposure to the primary graft may influence the survival of the secondary transplant. In the experiment reported here, the primary renal homograft in Dog 1 remained in place for 51 days and during this entire time both artery and vein were patent in spite of the fact that the kidney had been completely destroyed by a typical homograft reaction. It is possible that this prolonged intravenous exposure to the antigens of the transplant may have induced a state of partial tolerance somewhat like that seen by Martinez[14] in parabiotic mice.

It is also of interest that the primary transplant from Dog 1 into Dog 2 appeared to have had a prolonged survival, although its function was not as good as that of the secondary transplant and its ultimate destruction seems to have been more complete. It is possible that the prolonged survival of this graft may have simply reflected the state of partial compatibility that must have existed between the 2 animals, though it is possible that its exposure during the time that it resided in Dog 1 to the antigens from the renal homotransplant from Dog 2 may in some way have conditioned its response to the subsequent transplantation into Dog 2.

In other experiments in our laboratory, it was found that bilaterally nephrectomized dogs survived an average of 7.5 days.[19] This corresponds well to the figure of 7.8 days found by Dempster.[6] Ten bilaterally nephrectomized dogs with a pelvic renal homotransplant survived an average time of 15 days, with a range from 9 to 25 days.[19] Not only did the 88-day survival period for the secondary transplant reported greatly exceed these survival times, but it was noteworthy that there was a continued rise of the BUN level during the lifespan of the bilaterally nephrectomized animals with transplants, while in the experiment reported here the BUN level fell progressively after the third week. Although the prolonged survival of human renal[11] or skin[3] homotransplants, or dog[12] renal homotransplants may be related to a state of chronic uremia, this mechanism was not operative in the present experiments because the animals were not uremic at the time of transplantation and the progressive uremia in the dogs which had pelvic renal homotransplants without prolonged survival was much greater than in this pair.

In general, the closer the genetic relationship between 2 animals, the longer the survival of the graft.[17] Skin grafts between human fraternal twins will survive 3 times as long as those between unrelated human donors, and a renal transplant between 1 pair of dizygotic human twins appears to have been permanently accepted.[4] This is not always true in the human being, however, because in at least 1 instance a renal transplant between a mother and her son was very rapidly rejected[16] while a markedly prolonged survival was achieved for a renal transplant from a completely unrelated person.[11] Furthermore, in animals no prolongation of survival of renal homotransplants was noted when purebred greyhounds[6] or purebred beagles[13] were used. We cannot absolutely rule out the possibility that the 2 animals used by us were related, although this is extremely unlikely. We have failed to achieve prolonged primary renal homograft function in transplants between 2 other pairs of boxer dogs. Other workers have performed renal homotransplants between litter-mate dogs and have shown that prolonged functional survival does not occur.[12] Therefore, it is unlikely that genetic similarity due to closeness of breeding was a factor in the results described here.

## SUMMARY AND CONCLUSIONS

1. Rejection of a secondary renal homotransplant is not always more rapid or more severe than the rejection of the corresponding primary graft.

2. A secondary canine renal homotransplant is reported which maintained a bilateral nephrectomized dog for 88 days, at which time the animal died from causes unrelated to renal failure. There was functional and anatomic evidence of continued survival of the homograft at this time. Microscopically, the homograft reaction was less prominent on the eighty-eighth day than it had been in the biopsy specimen taken on the eighth day after secondary homotransplantation.

3. Although the primary transplant between these 2 animals showed a prolonged survival, it had been completely destroyed by the fifty-first day. The crossed primary transplant from the recipient of the secondary transplant back into the donor also showed a prolonged survival, but not as long and with less adequate function than that seen for the secondary transplant.

4. It is suggested that a state of partial immunologic tolerance of the recipient may have occurred in this experiment as a consequence, perhaps, of prolonged survival of the primary homotransplant.

### REFERENCES

1. Billingham, R. E., Brent, L., and Medawar, P. B.: Quantitative studies on tissue transplantation immunity, Phil. Tr. Bull. **239:** 357, 1956.
2. Billingham, R. E., and Sparrow, E.: The effect of prior intravenous injections of dissociated epidermal cells and blood on the survival of skin homografts in rabbits, J. Embryol. & Exper. Morphol. **3:** 265, 1955.
3. Dammin, G. J., Couch, N. P., and Murray, J. E.: Prolonged survival of skin homografts in uremic patients, Ann. New York Acad. Sc. **64:** 967, 1957.
4. Dealy, J. B., Jr., Dammin, G. J., Murray, J. E., and Merrill, J. P.: Total body irradiation in man: tissue patterns observed in attempts to increase the receptivity of renal homografts, Ann. New York Acad. Sc. **87:** 572, 1960.
5. Dempster, W. J.: A consideration of the cause of functional arrest of homotransplanted kidneys, Brit. J. Urol. **27:** 66, 1955.
6. Dempster, W. J.: Kidney homotransplantation, Brit. J. Surg. **40:** 447, 1953.
7. Egdahl, R. H., and Hume, D. M.: Immunological studies in renal homotransplantation, Surg. Gynec. & Obst. **102:** 450, 1956.
8. Egdahl, R. H., and Hume, D. M.: Secondary kidney homotransplantation, S. Forum **6:** 423, 1955.
9. Egdahl, R. H., and Hume, D. M.: Studies on kidney homotransplant rejection using a cross-circulation technique, Ann. New York Acad. Sc. **64:** 950, 1957.
10. Hume, D. M., and Egdahl, R. H.: Progressive destruction of renal homografts isolated from the regional lymphatics of the host, SURGERY **38:** 194, 1955.
11. Hume, D. M., Merrill, J. P., Miller, B. F., and Thron, G. W.: Experiences with renal homotransplantation in the human: report of nine cases, J. Clin. Invest. **34:** 327, 1955.
12. Mannick, J. A.: Personal communication.
13. Mannick, J. A., Lochte, H. L., Ashley, C. A., Thomas, E. D., and Ferrebee, J.: A functioning kidney homotransplant in the dog, SURGERY **46:** 821, 1959.
14. Martinez, C., Shapiro, F., and Good, R. A.: Essential duration of parabiosis and development of tolerance to skin homografts in mice, Proc. Soc. Exper. Biol. & Med. **104:** 256, 1960.
15. Medawar, P. B.: The behavior and fate of skin autografts and skin homografts in rabbits, J. Anat. **78:** 176, 1944.
16. Oeconomos, N., Hamburger, J., Delinotte, P., Voysse, J., and others: Attempted homograft (maternal kidney) after nephrectomy because of trauma to a solitary kidney, Internat. Abst. Surg. **98:** 570, 1954.
17. Rogers, B. O.: The genetics of skin homotransplantation in the human, Ann. New York Acad. Sc. **64:** 741, 1957.
18. Werder, A. A., and Hardin, C. A.: A study of consecutively homografted skin on CFW mice, SURGERY **36:** 371, 1954.
19. Zukoski, C. F., Lee, H. M., and Hume, D. M.: The effect of 6-mercaptopurine on renal homograft survival in the dog, Surg. Gynec. & Obst. **112:** 707, 1961.

# Theme and variations on blood oxygenators
# I. Bubble oxygenators

RICHARD A. DEWALL, M.D.*
THEODOR B. GRAGE, M.D.
ARTHUR S. MCFEE, M.D.
MICHELE A. CHIECHI, M.D.
MINNEAPOLIS, MINN.
*From the Department of Surgery, University of Minnesota Medical School.*

There are no new ideas in medicine, just new applications of old themes—at least this study seems to suggest that this is true. Extracorporeal circulation is now a routine procedure in the operating room, but it took 150 years to make it so. What were the important steps in this transition? The idea had to be conceived and the methods for accomplishment of this objective had to be developed. This initially was the role of physiologists who were interested in the study of isolated organs. Probably the most important single factor which made extracorporeal circulation feasible clinically was the discovery and isolation of the natural anticoagulant, heparin. A receptive and talented surgeon with foresight was then necessary who could envision an intact, surviving patient beyond the isolated organ studies. The development of modern blood banking methods was the final step in the evolution of successful extracorporeal circulation.

Good historical references on oxygenators

Supported by Research Grants from the American Heart Association and Minnesota Heart Association.
Received for publication Feb. 23, 1961.
*Established Investigator, American Heart Association.

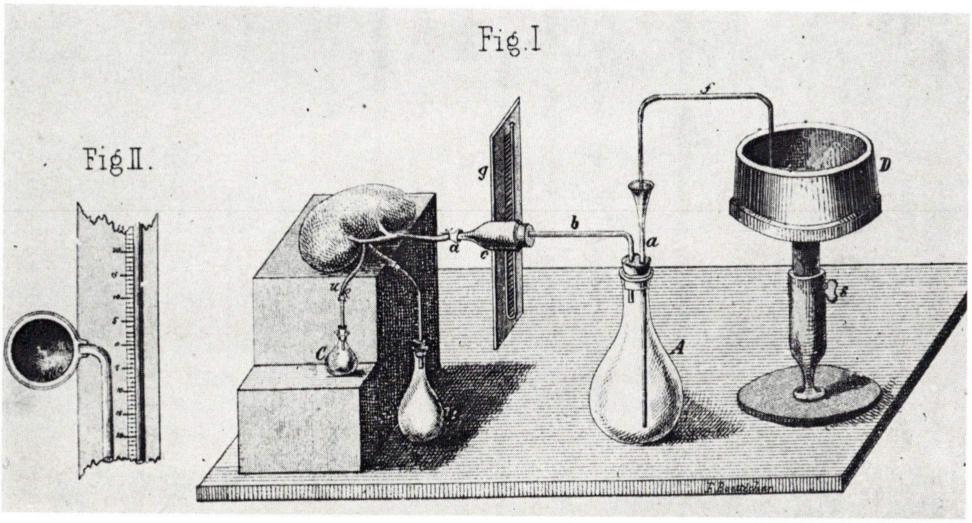


**Fig. 1.** Bidder used defibrinated blood removed from an artery of a donor animal and placed in a closed vessel marked *A*. Mercury was then introduced from vessel *D* to *A* by means of a siphon, draining the blood through tube *B-C* and *A* to perfuse the isolated organ. A manometer marked *G* measured perfusion pressures. (From E. Bidder.[1])

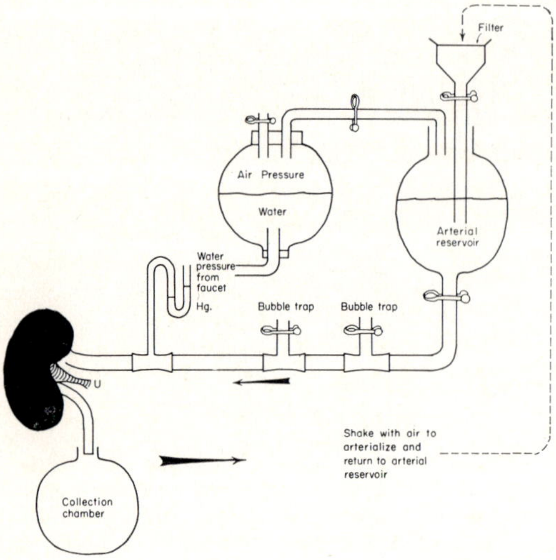


**Fig. 2.** The apparatus of Bunge. Oxygenation of the blood was accomplished by shaking the venous blood in a large vessel and returning it to an arterial reservoir from which it was forced to the isolated organ.

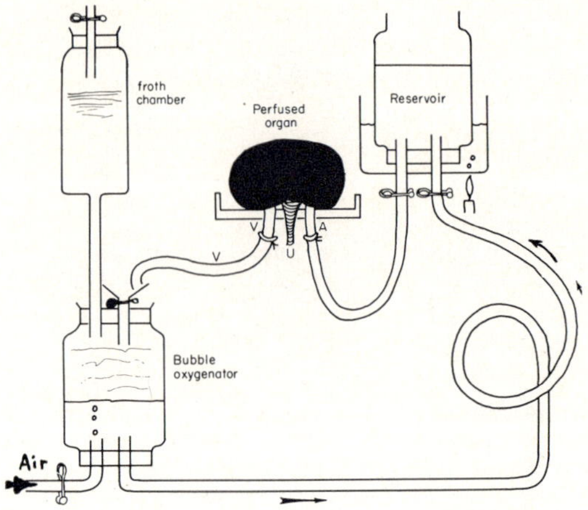


**Fig. 3.** In Schröder's system, gas was bubbled into venous blood and the oxygenated blood was then driven to a reservoir from which it was perfused to an isolated organ by means of hydrostatic pressure.

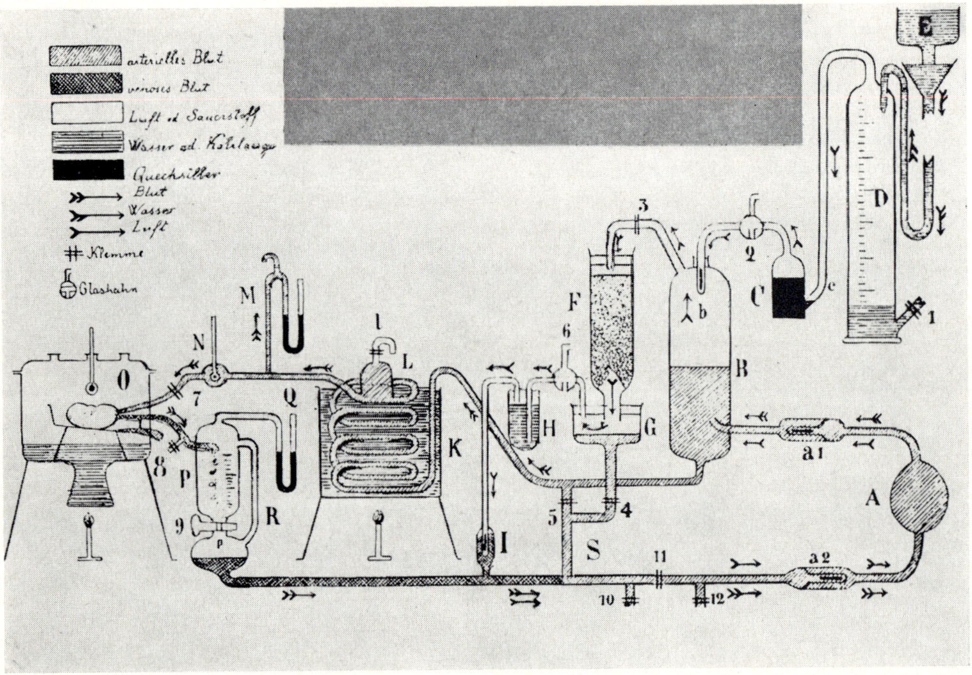


**Fig. 4.** Jacobi's apparatus. Beginning at upper right, *E,* water pressure system to drive the oxygenating gas by displacing it from vessel *D; D,* graduate to measure the quantity of gas; *C,* mercury valve; *B,* air and blood reservoir; *F,* sand-filled chamber to coalesce foam which passes from *b; H,* alkali chamber to absorb carbon dioxide; *I,* oxygen introduced into the venous blood; *A,* bladder pump for the oxygenated blood; *K,* water bath and coil to maintain blood temperature; *O,* chamber for isolated organ, and *P,* flowmeter. (From C. Jacobj.[15])

were gathered by Skatul,[25] Skramlik,[24] Björk,[2] and Karlson.[16] However there is no available collection of the original diagrams which illustrate the transition of the ideas concerning the extracorporeal oxygenation of blood. We have included these original diagrams when possible.

Our study is concerned with bubble and film oxygenators, excluding the biologic (homologous lung and so forth), chemical, and membrane systems. No attempt is to be made to show all of the variations, especially those of more recent years, but only to indicate the different patterns which have been conceived.

## FACTORS CONSIDERED IN CONSTRUCTION OF AN OXYGENATOR

All oxygenators subscribed more or less to a single theme—a respiratory gas mixture must be placed in close relationship to blood. The reaction time between hemoglobin and oxygen is less than one-tenth of a second and for practical purposes less than one-hundredth of a second.[11, 12] Consequently this is not a limiting factor in the construction of an efficient oxygenator. The gas diffusion coefficient is the quantity of that gas that will diffuse across the plane of unit dimensions in unit time under unit concentration gradient. Oxygen must pass through the plasma and the red blood cell membrane in order to react with hemoglobin (excluding the pulmonary membrane; this is not a problem with these oxygenators). An oxygenator must therefore create a film of blood of maximal area and minimal thickness and expose it to an oxygen-containing gas phase under pressure of from 0.2 to 3 atmospheres.

Carbon dioxide is eliminated from the systems by one of two means. One method which is not currently used in oxygenators is passage of the gas through a carbon dioxide–absorbing solution, usually an alkali. The currently preferred method is to allow its escape from the blood by simple diffusion into an atmosphere which contains a concentration of carbon dioxide lower than that of the blood.

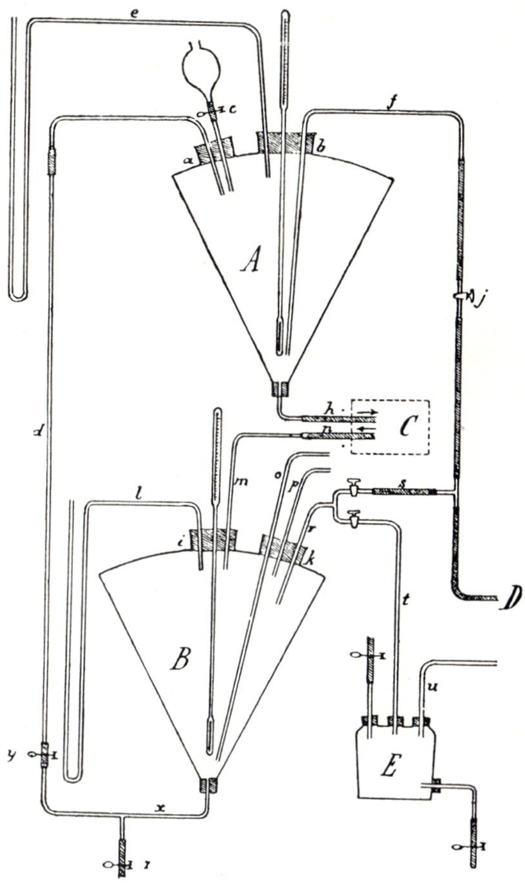


**Fig. 5.** Salaskin's oxygenator. *A,* Arterial reservoir; *C,* chamber for isolated organ; *D,* gas inlet to create a perfusion pressure; *E,* overflow chamber; *B,* venous reservoir; and *o,* gas inlet to oxygenate blood. (From S. Salaskin.[21])

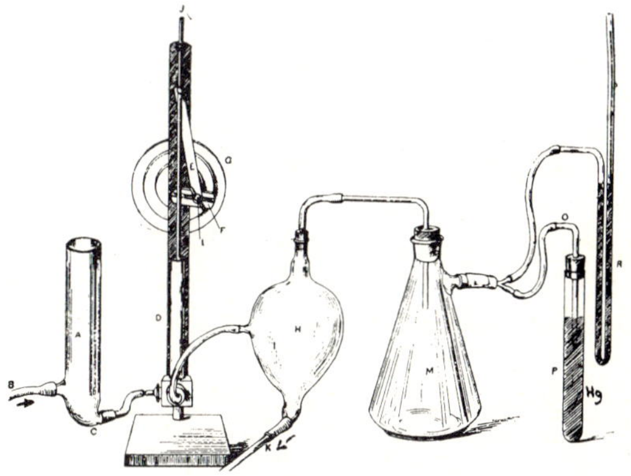


**Fig. 6.** Brodie's system. *A,* Venous reservoir; *B,* venous inlet; *D,* pump aspirating venous blood and air from *A* and propelling it to *H,* the arterial reservoir; *K,* arterial cannula; and *M,* overflow system for froth. (From T. G. Brodie.[3])

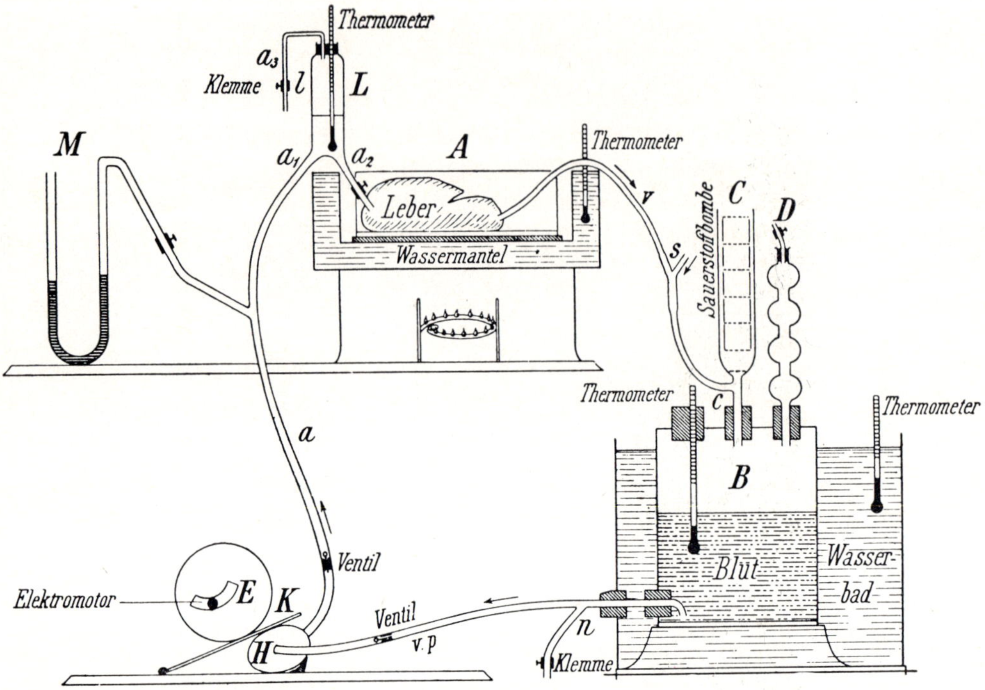


**Fig. 7.** The Neubauer system. *A,* Chamber for isolated organs; *v,* venous blood; *s,* oxygen inlet; *C,* bubbling chamber containing perforated, paraffin-coated porcelain plates; *D,* froth overflow chamber; and *B,* arterial reservoir. (From O. Neubauer and W. Gross.[20])

Two methods for creating a blood film predominate, the planar or bidimensional methods (film types) and the spherical or 3-dimensional methods (bubble formations). These two methods will be discussed separately.

## HISTORICAL REVIEW

The first suggestion of extracorporeal circulation may well be attributed to LaGallois[17] in 1812. However, the work of Loebell[18] in 1849 seems to be the starting point of more active investigations relating to perfusions. Loebell, whose paper was written in Latin, employed isolated kidney perfusion with defibrinated blood to study the formation of urine and the concentration of solids in renal blood and in urine. He also was one of the first investigators to attempt renal homotransplantation; however, because of his inability to control the clotting of blood in the renal vessels, the transplants failed. He included no diagram of his perfusion system. It may well have been much like that described by Bidder[1] in 1862.

The apparatus of Bidder (Fig. 1) consisted of a reservoir of oxygenated, defibri-

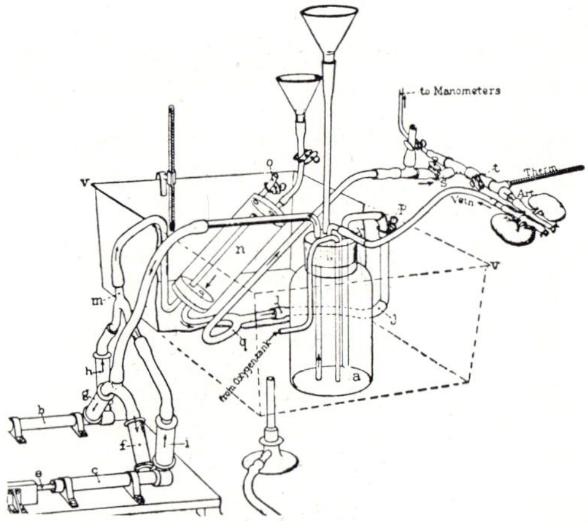


**Fig. 8.** The oxygenator of Hooker. *a,* Venous reservoir into which oxygen was introduced; *f, g, h,* pumping system; and *n,* arterial reservoir and debubbling chamber. (From D. R. Hooker.[13])

nated, and filtered blood connected by tubes to an isolated kidney. To obtain oxygenated blood, Bidder bled a donor animal from the carotid artery. The perfusion pressure was created by means of mercury which was transferred from vessel *D* through a siphon *(F)*, displacing the blood from vessel *A*. At a perfusion pressure of 160 to 200 mm. Hg, he obtained a flow rate of approximately 500 ml. one-half hour later. Bidder's work was inspired by that of Loebell in spite of the fact that he did not speak kindly of Loebell's Latin grammar. The low perfusion rates that were observed disturbed him, as did the high pressures necessary for the perfusion.

In 1868, Ludwig and Schmidt,[19] studying metabolism of isolated muscles, also used a mercury displacement method for perfusions as described by Bidder, but added extracorporeal oxygenation of defibrinated blood. This was accomplished by shaking the blood in air.

Bunge and Schmiedeberg[4] published their studies on renal perfusions in 1876, but did not include a diagram of their apparatus. Fig. 2 was created from their word picture. Oxygenation was accomplished by shaking the defibrinated filtered blood in a large glass chamber. The arterialized blood was then deposited in a reservoir from which it flowed to the isolated organ by means of water pressure. Flow rates up to 100 ml. per minute were obtained.

The direct introduction of air into a venous reservoir was described in 1882 by Schröder,[22] and thus the first bubbler came into existence (Fig. 3). By manipulation of the proper clamps, air pressure could be built up in the venous reservoir forcing the bubbled blood into an arterial reservoir from which the isolated organ was perfused.

A rather sophisticated bubble oxygenator was described by Jacobj[15] in 1890 which had a great many attractive features, even by

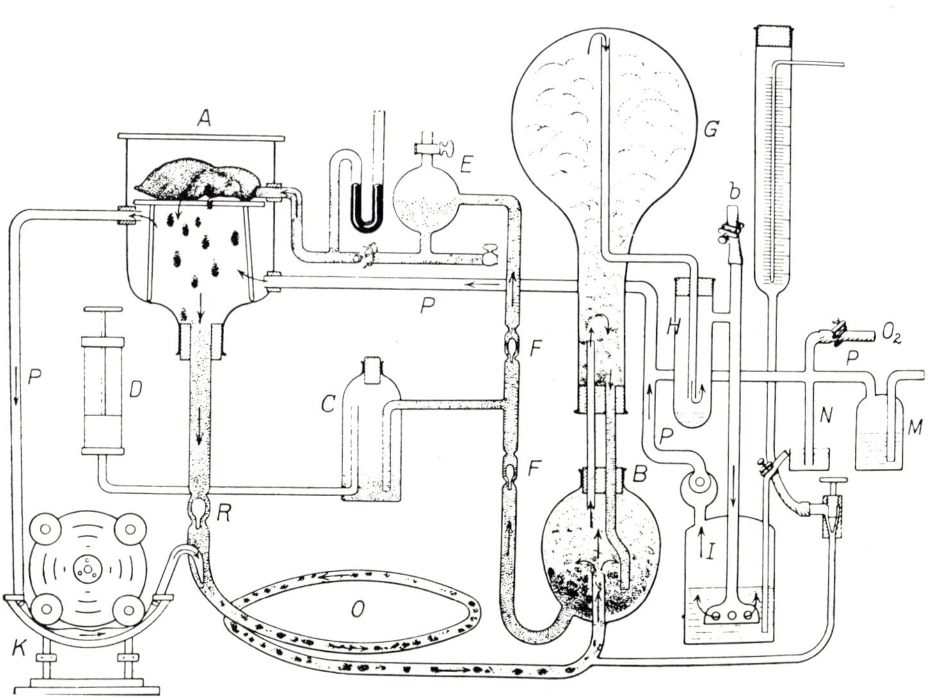


**Fig. 9.** The Issekutz system. *A,* Chamber for isolated organs; *R,* venous reservoir; *K,* roller pump adding gas to the venous line; *B,* coalescence chamber; *G,* froth chamber; *I,* carbon dioxide–absorbing chamber containing sodium hydroxide; and *E,* bubble separator. The blood flow is maintained by the pressure of the oxygenating gases introduced at point marked $O_2$. (From B. v. Issekutz.[14])

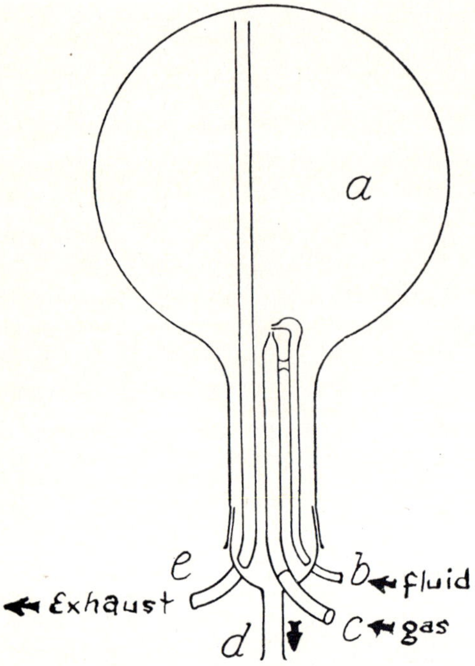


**Fig. 10.** *A,* Collection chamber for the "atomized" blood; *B,* venous blood inlet and arterialized blood outlet; *C,* gas inlet; *D,* arterial outlet; and *E,* gas exhaust. (From U. S. von Euler and C. Heymans.[27])

present-day standards (Fig. 4). A helical reservoir was used in this system at point *L* both as a debubbling chamber and a heating chamber. Oxygen was directly introduced into venous blood at point *I.* This bubbled blood was then passed through the debubbling system by a bladder pump at point *A.* Point *H* marks a vessel containing sodium hydroxide for the absorption of carbon dioxide. *D* is an air-flow meter. The isolated organ is contained in vessel *O,* and the blood flow is measured by cylinder *P.*

An inverted conical bubble oxygenator was used by Salaskin[21] in 1898 (Fig. 5), but he attributed the design to an associate with whom he had previously worked (Dr. S. Dzierzgowski, *Archives des sciences biologigues de St. Petersburg,* 1897, vol. 41). It was used for metabolism studies of isolated livers contained in vessel *C.* Venous blood was drained into chamber *B* and air or oxygen could be introduced through tube *O.* By means of a hand pump at *D,* air was injected into *B* to raise the pressure sufficiently to move the blood from *B* to *A* and to the isolated organ.

Brodie[3] developed his own modifications of a bubble oxygenator which he described in 1903. This apparatus mixed air with the venous blood by means of a pump as shown in Fig. 6. The pump also served to drive the blood into the isolated organ. The temperature of the blood was maintained at a constant level by placing the apparatus in a water bath. Filtered defibrinated blood was used to prime this apparatus. Because there was some froth formation, a separate foam chamber was connected to the main arterial reservoir, bottle *H.* Heterologous blood was used which did not prove to be satisfactory. Brodie made note of the difficulty in achieving adequate perfusion rates and believed that it was due to persistence of tonus in the arterioles. However, he apparently did not recognize existence of vasotonins in the blood. As an anticoagulant, he used either the Leech extract, hirudin, or blood collected into a sodium citrate solution. The citrated blood, which he thought gave better performance than defibrinated blood, allowed a good flow for several hours. This apparatus at times did not oxygenate adequately.

A model of a well-written scientific paper was presented by Neubauer and Gross[20] in 1910. It described a simple but complete bubble oxygenator as shown in Fig. 7, which provided a perfusion rate of 75 ml. of blood per minute per 100 Gm. of liver. Blood passed from the pump to a bubble trap (*L*) which contained a thermometer and a small glass tube for the escape of air emboli. From *L* it passed to the isolated organ (liver) in a hermetically sealed container kept at a constant temperature by a water bath. The blood left the liver through tube *V,* at which point a controlled source of oxygen was interposed. Aerated and debubbled blood flowed into *B,* after having passed the first debubbling chamber *C* which consisted of a cylinder with several perforated paraffin-coated porcelain plates. Any excess bubbles were allowed to escape into a second debubbler, bottle *D.*

Hooker[13] also used a system which bubbled oxygen directly into the venous blood, vessel *a*, as it left the isolated organ (Fig. 8). A large-bore inclined tube (*n*) was used for a debubbling vessel. The heavier blood sank to the bottom of the vessel and escaped as indicated by the arrow, while the lighter, bubble-containing blood would rise to the top and be evacuated.

Issekutz[14] investigated liver metabolism by an isolated organ perfusion system described in 1927 (Fig. 9). He stated that his work was greatly influenced by Skramlik.[24] This apparatus incorporated another pump to control the introduction of oxygen into the venous blood, and a vessel (*I*) containing sodium hydroxide for the absorption of carbon dioxide.

An "atomizer oxygenator" was described in 1932 by von Euler[27] (Fig. 10). A jet of oxygen or air was directed at a 90 degree angle into a stream of venous blood which was then blown to the walls of a large glass balloon. Von Euler used defibrinated blood after it had been allowed to stand in an icebox for 24 hours in order to inactivate the vasotonins, a precaution described by Bornstein in 1926 for use with his film oxygenator. The capacity of von Euler's oxygenator was 250 ml. per minute. Drying of the finely dispersed blood was encountered which he avoided by saturating the oxygen with water vapor prior to its use. He observed that with the upper degrees of oxygen saturation, small bubbles were liberated from the arterialized blood. This bubble formation could be avoided by keeping the oxygenator at the same temperature as that of the blood.

The apparatus of Thomas[25, 26] created a blood-gas interphase within a layer of quartz sand. The diagram, Fig. 11, is somewhat

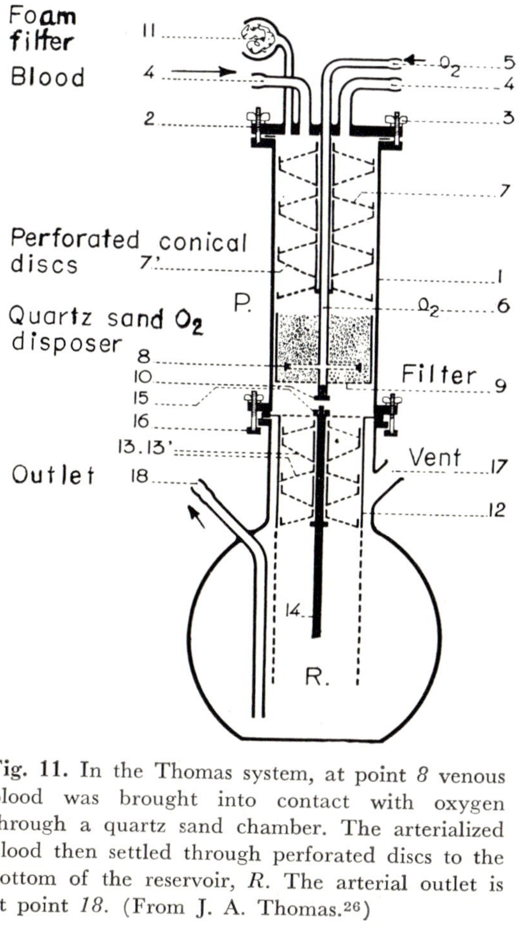


**Fig. 11.** In the Thomas system, at point *8* venous blood was brought into contact with oxygen through a quartz sand chamber. The arterialized blood then settled through perforated discs to the bottom of the reservoir, *R*. The arterial outlet is at point *18*. (From J. A. Thomas.[26])

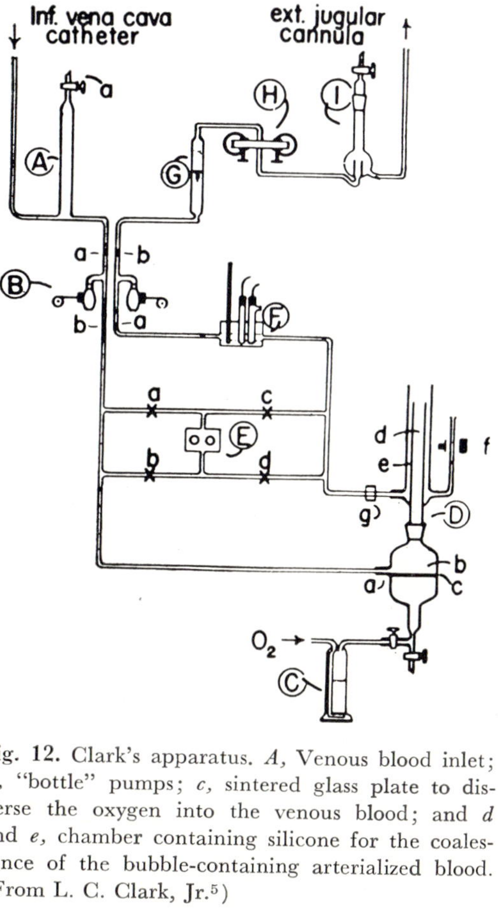


**Fig. 12.** Clark's apparatus. *A*, Venous blood inlet; *B*, "bottle" pumps; *c*, sintered glass plate to disperse the oxygen into the venous blood; and *d* and *e*, chamber containing silicone for the coalescence of the bubble-containing arterialized blood. (From L. C. Clark, Jr.[5])

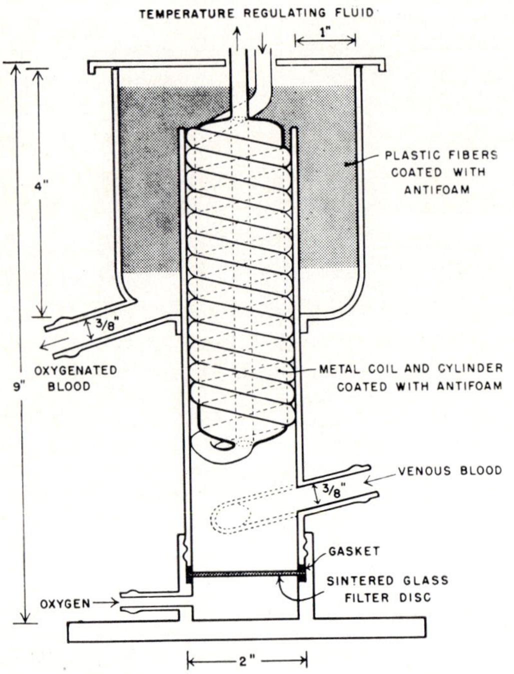


**Fig. 13.** The perfusion hypothermia bubble oxygenator of Gollan.[11]

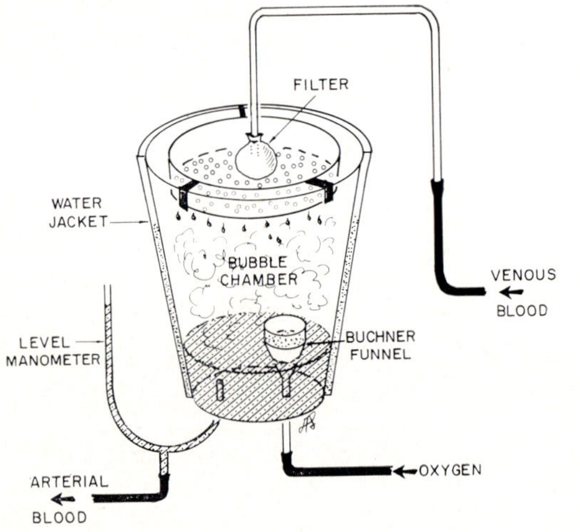


**Fig. 14.** In Waud's system, the venous blood filters down through the bubble chamber and is collected at the base of the chamber to be evacuated as arterialized blood. (Diagram adapted from original in R. A. Waud.[28])

self-explanatory. Its main application was for isolated organ perfusions.

A paper by Clark and associates[5] in 1950 could certainly be said to have marked the opening of the modern era of the bubble oxygenator. Fig. 12 is a diagram of this system in which oxygen was dispersed through sintered glass filter (*a-c*) to transmit fine bubbles into the venous blood. The major contribution of this paper was the introduction of the silicone defoaming agents. The defoaming agent was used to coat the collection chamber, marked at points *D* and *E* of their system.

The first human application of a pump-oxygenator was in August of 1951, at which time Dogliotte[8] performed a partial bypass on a patient with mediastinal tumor. The blood was removed from the brachial vein and returned to the brachial artery after passing through the oxygenator. The apparatus of Dogliotte was similar to Clark's.

Gollan[10] let his imagination go in 1952 to produce some fascinating experiments which anticipated clinical surgery by at least 5 years. His experiments demonstrated that perfusion hypothermia was practical with the aid of a pump-oxygenator. Fig. 13 illustrates the Gollan oxygenator.

The experiments of Waud[28] and Gimbel,[9] both writing in 1952, produced oxygenators which were similar in principle and which

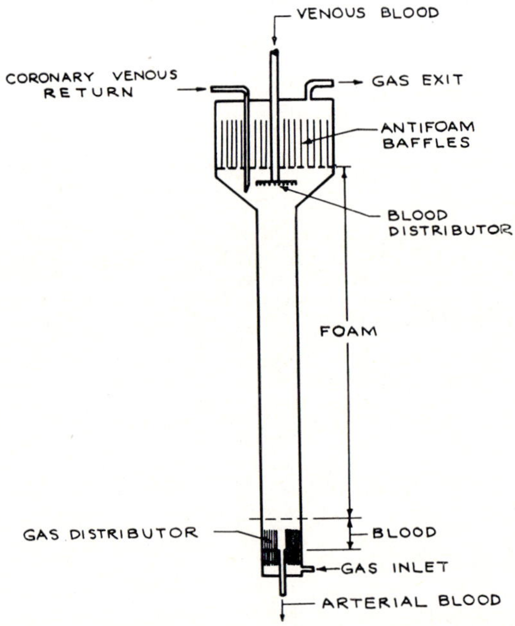


**Fig. 15.** In Gimbel's oxygenator, venous blood passes through a foam chamber to be evacuated at the base of the oxygenator as arterialized blood. (From S. Gimbel and J. Engelberg.[9])

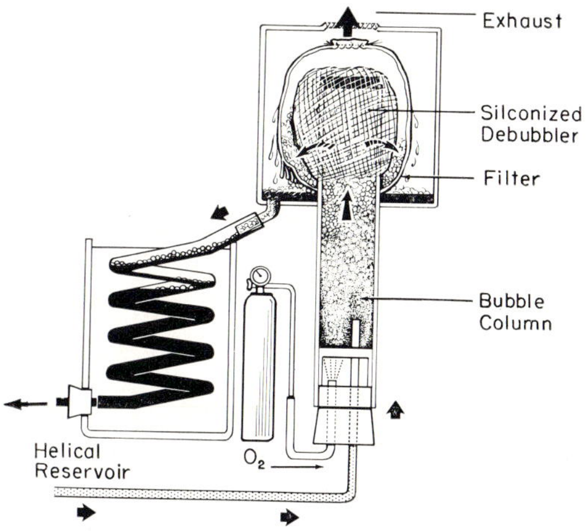


**Fig. 16.** Perfusion hypothermia system of Zuhdi[29] which employs 5 per cent dextrose to prime the oxygenator in a quantity equivalent to one-third of the patient's daily fluid requirement. No blood is required for operation of the perfusion apparatus as described by Zuhdi.

greatly influenced experimentors that followed. Fig. 14 is a diagram of the Waud apparatus and Fig. 15 is the system described by Gimbel.

The helical reservoir bubble oxygenator[7] (Fig. 16) has been in use at the University of Minnesota since May of 1955 and has been applied to over 1,500 patients for successful perfusions, some of which lasted for over 3 hours. A silicone debubbling chamber is used to disperse the bubbles. A helical reservoir serves to clear the blood of any free gas before it reaches the arterial pump at the base of the helix. Hydrostatic pressure equivalent to the height of blood in the coils causes any free gas to rise upward. Several coils of the helix are maintained full of blood during its operation. The inclined plane of the coil causes the arterialized blood to flow in a laminar fashion down the tube forming a trap for any gas not in solution or in combination with hemoglobin.

Cooley,[6] in 1958, incorporated a helical trough joining the bubbling chamber to the reservoir which served to prevent the free fall of blood from the upper to the lower reservoir (Fig. 17).

Zuhdi[29] described a double helical bubble oxygenator in 1959 (Fig. 18). The inner metal helix carried a thermostatically controlled fluid which allowed simply controlled hypothermia of the blood carried in the outer helix. With this technique he was able

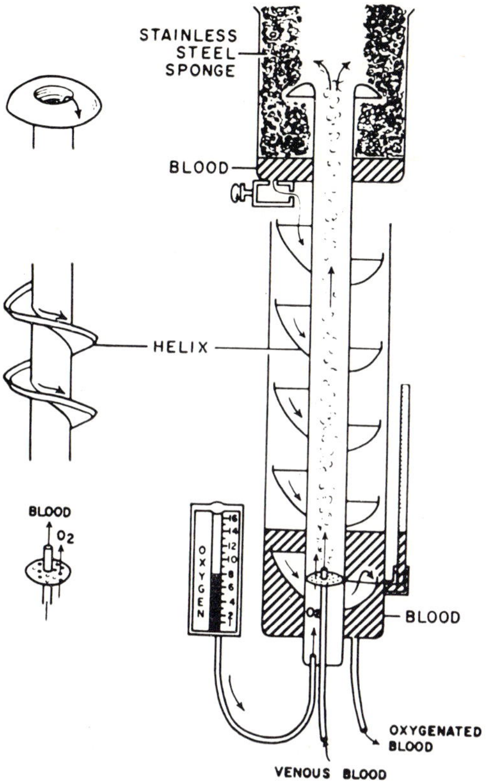


**Fig. 17.** The helical trough oxygenator of Cooley.[6]

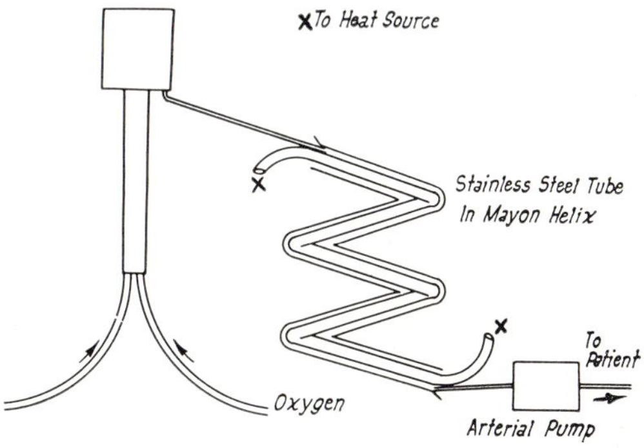


**Fig. 18.** The oxygenator used at the University of Minnesota. Oxygen and venous blood are introduced at the base of a vertical plastic column. The silicone-coated chamber coalesces the oxygenated blood and releases the excess carbon dioxide through its top. The arterialized blood then passes to a helical reservoir which serves as a final bubble separator, reservoir, and temperature control chamber.

to prime his system with 5 per cent dextrose and utilize only the patient's own blood volume which reduced blood requirements to a minimum.

## CONCLUSION

Bubble oxygenators are currently in use at many centers here and abroad. The bubble oxygenator has attained a youthful maturity. However, it is apparent that changes have evolved periodically over the last 100 years. In the future one can only expect a continuing metamorphosis of the designs.

### REFERENCES


1. Bidder, E.: Beiträge zur Lehre von der Function der Nieren. Inaugural dissertation, Dorpat, 1862.
2. Björk, V. O.: Brain perfusions with artificially oxygenated blood, Acta chir. scandinav. **96:** 1, 1948.
3. Brodie, T. G.: The perfusion of surviving organs, J. Physiol. 29: 266, 1903.
4. Bunge, G., and Schmiedeberg,, O.: Über die Bildung der Hippursaure, Arch. exper. Path. Pharmakol. **6:** 233, 1876.
5. Clark, L. C., Jr., Gollan, F., and Vishwa, B.: The oxygenation of blood by gas dispersion, Science **111:** 85, 1950.
6. Cooley, D. A., Belmonte, B. A., Latson, J. R., and Pierce, J. F.: Bubble diffusion oxygenator for cardiopulmonary bypass, J. Thoracic Surg. **35:** 131, 1958.
7. DeWall, R. A., Warden, H., Varco, R. L., and Lillehei, C. W.: The Helix reservoir pump oxygenator, Surg. Gynec. & Obst. **104:** 699, 710, 1957.
8. Dogliotti, A. M., and Costantini, A.: Primo caso di applicazione all'uomo un apparecchio di circolazione sanguigna extracorporea, Minerva Chir. **6:** 657, 1951.
9. Gimbel, N. S., and Engelberg, J.: An oxygenator for use in a heart-lung apparatus, S. Forum (1952) pp. 154-157, 1953.
10. Gollan, F., Blos, P., and Schuman, H.: Exclusion of heart and lungs from circulation in the hypothermic closed chest dog by means of a pump-oxygenator, J. Appl. Physiol. **5:** 180, 1952.
11. Hartridge, H., and Roughton, F. J. W.: The kinetics of haemoglobin. II. The velocity with which oxygen dissociates from its combination with haemoglobin, Proc. Roy. Soc. **104:** 395, 1923.
12. Hartridge, H., and Roughton, F. J. W.: The rate of distribution of dissolved gases between the red blood corpuscle and its fluid environment, J. Physiol. **62:** 232, 1927.
13. Hooker, D. R.: A study of the isolated kidney—the influence of pulse pressure upon renal function, Am. J. Physiol. **27:** 24, 1910.
14. Issekutz, v. B.: Beiträge zur Wirkung des Insulins, Biochem. Ztschr. **183:** 283, 1927.
15. Jacobj, C.: Apparat zur Durchblutung isolirter Uberlebender Organe, Arch. exper. Path. Pharmakol. **26:** 388, 1890.
16. Karlson, K. E., Dennis, C., Westover, D., and Sanderson, D.: Pump-oxygenator to supplant the heart and lungs for brief periods, SURGERY **29:** 678, 1951.
17. LaGallois, J. J. C.: Quoted by Griffenhagen, G. B., and Hughes, C. H.: The history of the mechanical heart, Smithsonian Report for 1955. Publication No. 4241, pp. 339-356.
18. Loebell, C. E.: De conditionibus quibus secretiones in glandulis perficiuntur, Diss. Marburg., 1849.
19. Ludwig, C., and Schmidt, A.: Das Verhalten der Gase, Welche mit dem Blut durch dem reizbaren Saugethiermuskel strömen, Leipz. Ges. Wissen. Berisht. **20:** 12, 1868.
20. Neubauer, O., and Gross, W.: Zur Kenntniss des Tyrosinabbaus in der kunstlich durchbluteten Leber, Ztschr. physiol. Chem. **67:** 219, 1910.
21. Salaskin, S.: Über die Bildung von Harnstoff in der leber der Saugethiere aus Amidosauren der Frettreihe, Ztschr. physiol. Chem. **25:** 128, 1898.
22. Schröder, W. v.: Über die Bildungsstatte des Harnstoffs, Arch. exper. Path. Pharmakol. **15:** 364, 1882.
23. Skutul, K.: Über Durchstromungsapparate, Arch. ges. Physiol. **123:** 249, 1908.
24. Skramlik, E.: Ein Apparat zur Durchströmung der Leber, Arch. ges. Physiol. **180:** 1, 1920.
25. Thomas, J. A.: Un appareil pour la perfusion steríle et automatique de gros organes ou de parties d' organismes, Ann. Physiol. Physiocochem. Biol. **15:** 432, 1939.
26. Thomas, J. A.: Nouveaux procédés de perfusion physiologique et aseptique permettant la survie prolongée d'organes ou d'organismes pesant plusieurs kilogrammes, J. Physiol. **40:** 123, 1948.
27. Von Euler, U. S., and Heymans, C.: An oxgenator for perfusion experiments, J. Physiol. **74:** 2p, 1932.
28. Waud, R. A.: A mechanical heart and lung, Canad. J. M. Sc. **30:** 130, 1952.
29. Zuhdi, N., Greer, A., Kimmell, G. M., Redmond, R., Donnell, J., Carey, J., Geigerman, D., and Krieger, C.: Clinical study of hypothermic perfusion, J. Oklahoma M. A. **52:** 671, 1959.

# The measurement of the pulmonary venous cross-circulation through the conjugated heart of thoracopagous twins with radioactive $O^{15}$

JOHN S. SPRATT, JR., M.D.*
MICHEL TER-POGOSSIAN, PH.D.
SANFORD RUDMAN, B.A.
ANDREW SPENCER, M.D.
ST. LOUIS, MO.
*From the Department of Surgery and the Mallinckrodt Institute of Radiology, Washington University School of Medicine*

The purpose of this article is to report the development of a new technique for measuring the distribution of oxygenated blood coming from the lungs and to report the measurement of the cross-circulation of pulmonarily oxygenated blood through the conjugated heart of thoracopagous twins. The technique for measuring the distribution of oxygenated blood is one developed at the Washington University cyclotron with radioactive $O^{15}$ administered by inhalation to tag the unsaturated hemoglobin circulating through the pulmonary alveoli. The circulation time between the lung and the periphery and the relative concentration of pulmonarily oxygenated blood in the peripheral tissue can be measured with external scintillation counters.

Previously, $I^{131}$-labeled human serum albumin[3] and tagged red blood cells[1] have been used to measure the cross-circulation between thoracopagous twins. These techniques have proved useful in the estimation of the rates of hemic mixing between the twins, but the use of $O^{15}$ has 2 peculiar advantages. First is the simplicity of the technique. Second, the measurements obtained can be used to assess the cross-circulation of pulmonary venous drainage.

Supported by United States Public Health Service Grants CS-9741 and H-4390(R1) and Atomic Energy Commission Grant AT(11-1)-782.

Received for publication Jan. 19, 1961.

*Advanced Clinical Fellow, American Cancer Society.

## THE THORACOPAGUS

At birth on Sept. 8, 1960, the thoracopagus, subsequently designated V1 and V2, weighed 4,600 grams. The combined weight on Nov. 18, 1960 (2 days before death), was 4,400 grams, and the maximum weight ever attained was 4,900 grams on Nov. 5, 1960.

During life, physical examination and various radiographic studies determined that the twins possessed separate nervous systems, genitourinary tracts, esophagi, gall bladders, stomachs, duodenums, rectums, colons, tracheobronchial trees, and skeletal systems. A small congenital omphalocele in V2 became covered with skin without surgical intervention (Fig. 1). The crossing of swallowed barium and carmine red into the colon of the second infant established that an enteroenteric communication existed but the extent of the connection was not known with certainty.

The electrocardiographic tracings obtained on each infant are shown in Fig. 2. The anatomic union of the twins precluded an accurate placement of the V leads. These routine tracings did not establish with absolute certainty that a common conduction system existed in the conjoined heart, but the rates and conduction intervals were the same. Furthermore, if the $L_1$, $L_2$, $aV_R$, and $aV_L$ tracings are rotated 90 degrees from the long axis of the tracing, and if the tracings from one infant are faced toward a mirror and the tracings from the other infant are

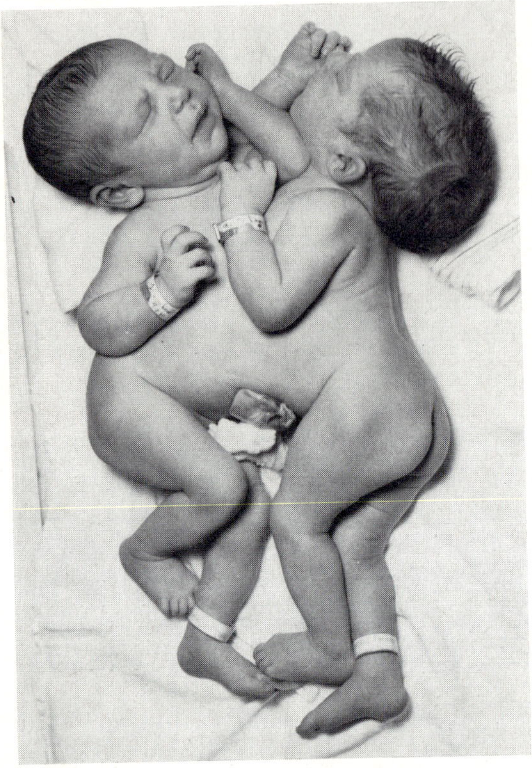

**Fig. 1.** Appearance of the conjoined thoracopagous twins on Sept. 9, 1960. The omphalocele of V2 closed without surgical repair.

placed beside the mirror image, the observation that the complete tracings in these leads are almost perfect mirror images of one another can be appreciated. This is very strong evidence for the presence of a single conduction system within the conjugated heart.

On Oct. 29, 1960, an angiocardiogram was performed by the injection of 11 ml. of Hypaque through a polyethylene catheter threaded from a leg vein of V2 through the vena cava of V2 into an auricle of V2. The serial angiograms established that a large communication existed between the hearts of V1 and V2, that a large patent ductus arteriosus existed in V2, that contrast media appeared in the aortae of both infants simultaneously, and that there were at least 2 ventricles. Other minor variations of the arterial outflow tract were noted. No information on the pulmonary venous drainage was obtained.

Cyanosis had been absent at birth but was evident in V2 with straining or crying by the second week of life. Oxygen saturation in the ear lobes of V1 and V2 on Oct. 3, 1960, was 77.5 and 78 per cent, respectively. By Oct. 22, 1960, the twin V2 became distinctly more cyanotic upon crying. By Nov. 15, 1960, the cyanosis of V2 was deeper and continuous. The breathing of nasal oxygen by V2 did not reduce the cyanosis of V2. The twins received digoxin according to their combined weight (0.045 mg. times 4.8 Kg. equals 0.2160 mg. over 48 hours) on November 15 without diminution of the cyanosis. Physical signs of pulmonary edema never developed during life and none were present at necropsy. On Nov. 18, 1960, V2 had a complete but temporary respiratory arrest. On Nov. 19, 1960, V2 passed a tarry stool and some blood was present also in the stool of V1. On Nov. 20, 1960, both twins died of a sudden, simultaneous respiratory and cardiac arrest.

At necropsy the ante mortem observations were confirmed and in addition several anatomic anomalies were noted. First, the splenic veins drained into a common portal vein, which then arborized into each liver at the porta hepatis. Second, the livers were joined only over an area of less than 6 $cm.^2$ and no major blood vessels traversed the parenchymatous junction. Third, the hepatic venous drainage consisted of a large vessel from each liver that joined to form a common channel into the inferior vena cava of V2 draining into auricle 1 (Fig. 3). Fourth, the common bile ducts of each twin joined in a single ampulla of Vater. Fifth, the twins shared a common small intestine from the ampulla of Vater to the ileum and just distal to the ileal bifurcation, twin V2 possessed a Meckel's diverticulum that contained both aberrant pancreatic tissue and gastric mucosa but no demonstrable ulceration. For several days before death the stools of both infants contained blood and at necropsy both colons were found to contain old blood. However, the mucosal surface of the entire intestine appeared normal and no source of bleeding was evident. Each twin had 2 adrenal glands and each gland weighed approximately 1.5 grams. Atrophy of the adrenal glands in 1 twin had not occurred. The hearts were conjugated in a most complex and obviously inseparable manner (Fig. 3).

## MEASUREMENT OF THE CROSS-CIRCULATION OF BLOOD OXYGENATED BY THE BREATHING OF RADIOACTIVE $O^{15}$

$O^{15}$ is a radioactive isotope of oxygen which has a half-life of 2.25 minutes and decays by the emission of 1.68 mev positrons. The radioactivity from its decay is measurable by externally situated scintillation counters. The measurable radiation counted is 0.51 mev photons arising from the interaction of the positrons with matter. The isotope is produced, purified, and used at the Washington University cyclotron in the form of circulating tagged air. The radioactivity in the tagged air behaves as molecular oxygen with a purity of over 99.4 per cent. The $O^{15}$ is bound proportionally to hemoglobin, enters into oxidative metabolism, and is incorporated rapidly into water of metabolism.[4]

The total irradiation received by the infants during the cross-circulation studies did not exceed 1.0 rad, an amount considerably less than the estimated 10 rads received during the various radiographic studies.

The cross-circulation studies were conducted by placing one of a pair of shielded, balanced scintillation counters over the greater trochanter of each infant. The counting rates were fed through a count rate meter into a 2-channel recorder. Then, 1 infant (V1) breathed flowing air tagged with $O^{15}$ through a standard infant-size anesthetic face mask for several breaths and a continual recording of circulation times from the lungs to the pelves and the relative accumulation of $O^{15}$ in the pelves was made with the scintillation counters. Then, the administration of $O^{15}$ was discontinued, but the recording of the radioactivity in the pelves was continued until radioactivity in each pelvis was in equilibrium. Within 10 half-lives of the isotope (10 times 2.25 minute half-life of oxygen equals 22.5 minutes) all detectable radioactivity disappeared from the infants. Subsequently, the procedure was repeated identically but with the second twin (V2) breathing the tagged air.

Figs. 4 and 5 and Table I contain the data derived from the $O^{15}$ studies performed on Oct. 27, 1960. The conclusions from these data were (1) the pulmonary venous blood from V1 went entirely to the body of infant V1 and entered the body of V2 only after completion of a circulation through the body of V1, (2) one-half of the pulmonary venous drainage from the lungs of V2 entered the peripheral circulation of V1 at the same rate and concentration that the other half entered the body of V2, (3) the cross circulation between the 2 infants was of such great magnitude that complete mixing occurred in 20.5 seconds, and (4) V1

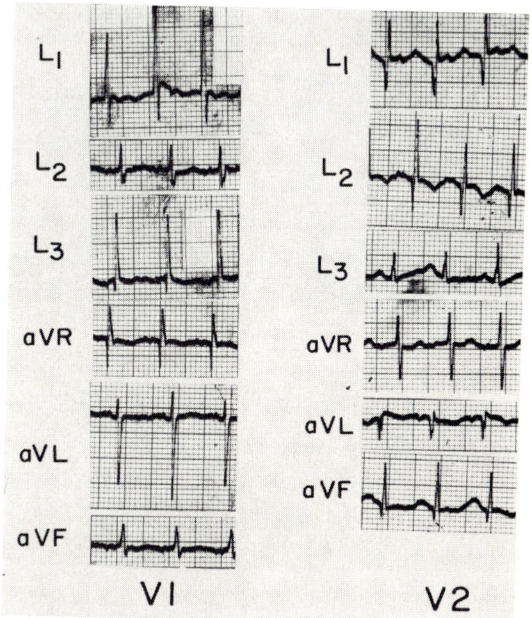


**Fig. 2.** Admission electrocardiograms. In each twin the P-R interval was 0.11 seconds; the QRS complex, 0.06 seconds, and the ventricular rate, 150 per minute. The direction of all deflections in the alternate leads from each twin are practically mirror images about the longitudinal axes of the tracings. There is some variation in the wave amplitudes of the deflections in the mirror images.

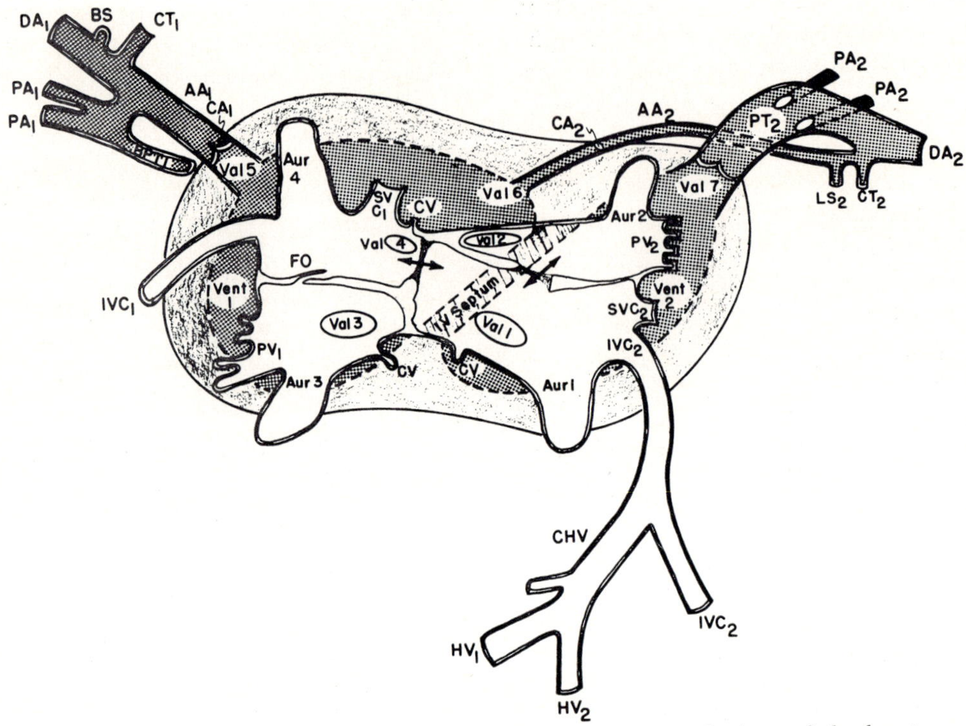


**Fig. 3.** Anatomic drawing of the conjugated heart viewed from the base of the heart.

was obviously favored over V2 by the cross-circulation of the oxygenated blood.

## DISCUSSION

The picture was one of the progressive circulatory dominance of V1 over V2. At birth the infants had been acyanotic and on Oct. 3, 1960, no significant difference existed in the ear-lobe oxygen saturation of either infant. Both had the same degree of anoxia, although by this time V2 became "dusky" with crying. However, by Oct. 27, 1960, V2 became distinctly cyanotic with effort and on this date the $O^{15}$ studies, showing the preferential oxygenation of V1, were performed. Obviously, the hemic mixing was very great in the portal circulations but there must also have been significant mixing of blood among the intercommunicating auricular chambers and in ventricle 1. Had the interauricular septal defects not been present, it is doubtful that V2 would have survived birth. The reason for the latter statement can be seen in the arrangement of the auriculoventricular valves in Fig. 3. Peculiarly, 3 of the 4 auriculoventricular valves, including the auriculoventricular valve from auricle 2 which received the pulmonary venous drainage from infant V2, communicated with ventricle 1. Only 1 auriculoventricular valve *(Val 1)* entered

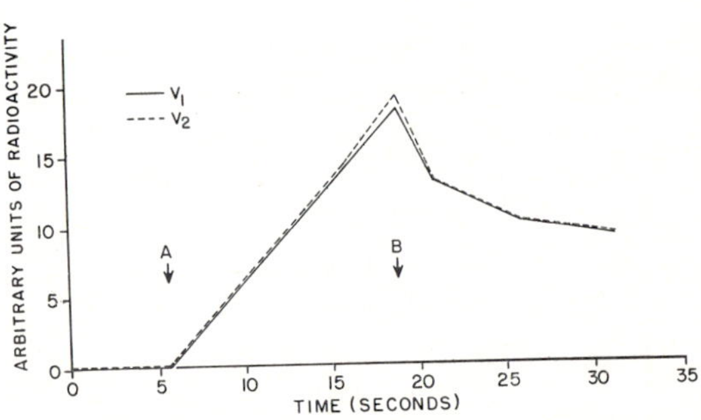


**Fig. 4.** Measurement of cross-circulation of oxygenated blood from V2. The lines record the relative number of counts per second above background recorded by balanced scintillation counters externally situated over the greater trochanter of each infant. At *0* time V2 began breathing tagged air. At *A* the radioactivity began to accumulate in the pelves. At *B* V2 stopped breathing tagged air.

ventricle 2, and the auricle of origin *(Aur 1)* received only vena caval blood. All of the peripheral arterial blood to twin V1 came from ventricle 1 with partial recirculation into the pulmonary arteries of V1 through the patent ductus arteriosus, and all peripheral arterial blood to twin V2 came from ventricle 2 via the patent ductus from the large pulmonary truncus. The blood going to twin V2 via the atretic aorta (diameter 1 to 2 mm.) from ventricle 1 must have been inconsequential. However, the coronary arterial supply to ventricle 2 did come from this atretic aorta. The ventricular walls and the interventricular septum were hypertrophied and the degree of hypertrophy seemed to compromise further the smaller chamber of ventricle 2.

As a result of the favored status of twin V1 in the cross-circulation, she was receiving all of the pulmonary venous drainage from her own lungs and one-half of the pulmonary venous drainage from twin V2. Twin V2 was receiving only one-half of her own pulmonary venous blood on October 27, and from the progressive deepening of the cyanosis in V2 there is reason to believe that the percentage of pulmonary venous blood received by V2 steadily decreased, ultimately causing a unilateral anoxic respiratory arrest in V2 2 days before the simultaneous infant death from cardiac arrest occurred. That either twin could have been saved even by the surgical sacrifice of the second twin is most unlikely.

Chang Bunker, the alcoholic twin in P. T. Barnum's Siamese twins, inadvertently conducted the first known cross-circulation studies between conjoined twins. In spite of Chang's frequently excessive intake of alcoholic beverages, he never affected the sobriety of his brother Eng, and the physicians of the day concluded that the cross-circulation through the bridge could not be great. The necropsy studies of Chang and Eng seemingly supported this conclusion.[2] The complete mixing of tagged red blood cells between Aird's conjoined twins required 29 minutes,[1] the complete mixing of iodinated serum albumin between the conjoined twins

**Table I.** *The circulation and equilibration times of $O^{15}$ in thoracopagous twins*

| *Circulation time* | *Ratio of maximum radio-activity in pelves* | *Equilibration time* |
|---|---|---|
| *V1 breathing $O^{15}$* | | |
| Lung of V1 to pelvis of V1, 6.6 sec.; lung of V1 to pelvis of V2, 15.6 sec. | V1:V2 = 2.32:1* | Time required for equilibration of radioactivity in pelves of V1 and V2 after discontinuation of $O^{15}$ inhalation by V1 equals 20.5 sec. |
| *V2 breathing $O^{15}$* | | |
| Lung of V2 to pelvis of V2, 5.7 sec.; lung of V2 to pelvis of V1, 5.7 sec. | V1:V2 = unity at all times | |

*Recorded 25.6 seconds after V1 began breathing $O^{15}$.

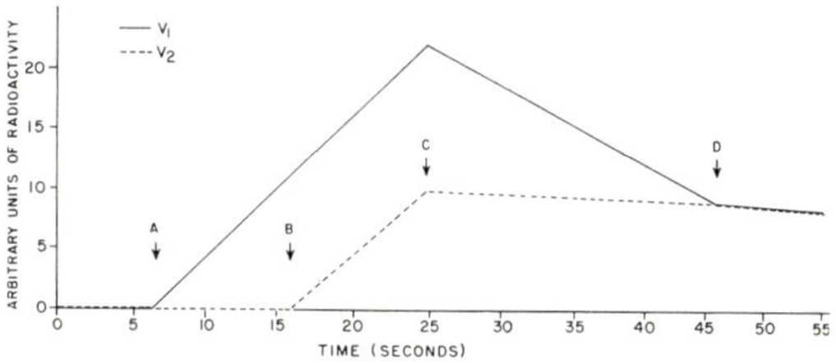


**Fig. 5.** Measurement of cross-circulation of oxygenated blood from V1. At *0* time V1 began breathing tagged air. At *A* radioactivity began to accumulate in the pelvis of V1 and at *B* in the pelvis of V2. At *C* V1 stopped breathing tagged air. At *D* the activity in the pelves of V1 and V2 became equal.

of Peterson and Hill required 10 minutes,[3] and the equilibration of $O^{15}$ in this set of conjoined twins required only 20.5 seconds.

## CONCLUSION

The anatomic detail of the complex cardiac conjugation between conjoined thoracopagous twins is described. Radioactive $O^{15}$ administered by inhalation was used to evaluate the flow and distribution of oxygenated pulmonary venous blood through the conjugated heart and into the periphery of the twins.

The authors wish to acknowledge the assistance of Dr. William S. Medart of the Department of Pathology and of Miss Marilyn Harris of the Department of Medical Illustration. The extensive ante mortem radiographic studies were performed by Drs. William H. McAlister and Håkan Arvidsson of the Mallinckrodt Institute of Radiology and the details and interpretation of their studies will be reported elsewhere.

## REFERENCES

1. Aird, I.: The conjoined twins of Kano, Brit. M. J. **1:** 831, 1954.
2. Luckhardt, A. B.: Report of the autopsy of the Siamese twins together with interesting information covering their life, Surg. Gynec. & Obst. **72:** 116, 1941.
3. Peterson, C. G., and Hill, A. J.: Separation of conjoined thoracopagus twins, Ann. Surg. **152:** 717, 1960.
4. Ter-Pogossian, M., Spratt, J. S., Jr., Rudman, S., and Spencer, A.: Radioactive oxygen-15 for the study of the kinetics of the oxygen of respiration, Am. J. Physiol. In press.

# Arterial prosthesis of collagen-impregnated Dacron tulle

ALFRED W. HUMPHRIES, M.D.
WILLIAM A. HAWK, M.D.
ALAN M. CUTHBERTSON, M.D.*
CLEVELAND, OHIO
*From The Cleveland Clinic Foundation and The Frank E. Bunts Educational Institute*

Arterial surgery has earned a secure, if still poorly defined, niche in the armamentarium of surgical procedures. The scope of arterial replacement within the field of arterial surgery is also poorly defined. In some conditions, the question of arterial replacement does not apply; in others, it is obligatory; in still others, it is elective. For example, in the treatment of most emboli and most traumatic arteriovenous fistulas, the question of arterial replacement does not arise since the patient's own vessel is still employed. When an arterial wall is hopelessly diseased, as in the case of aneurysms, its replacement is mandatory. When an artery is occluded by disease, it may be possible merely to remove the occlusion by endarterectomy or it may be necessary to replace the artery or to bypass the occlusion.

The search for a durable, trustworthy arterial substitute has resulted in extensive programs of laboratory experimentation by many investigators in the past decade. That the ideal prosthesis has not yet been found is testimony to the many technical, biologic, and immunologic difficulties involved. Many materials have been tested. Equine, bovine, and porcine heterografts, autogenous skin, bowel, peritoneum-lined rectus sheath, chamois, silicone, polyvinyl sponge, nylon, Orlon, Dacron, Vinyon-N, and Teflon are among the materials which have been fashioned into conduits and investigated in experimental animals.[1, 4, 5, 14, 16-22, 25-27, 29] Arterial homografts have been extensively studied.[3, 19, 22] Equine heterografts have functioned well in dogs for as long as 2 years,[21] but have disadvantages similar to those of the homograft in man, that is, the formation of aneurysms.[16] The use of skin, bowel, and peritoneum-lined rectus sheath has not proved successful experimentally.[19] Chamois functioned satisfactorily in dogs and was well organized 115 days after implantation.[14] Silicone, because of its elastic properties, seemed attractive but was abandoned because of the prohibitively high incidence of thrombosis.[29] Polyvinyl sponge and Ivalon sponge appeared to be well tolerated by dogs and to organize well, but they lacked the necessary strength for clinical application.[10, 11, 19, 26] Nylon was one of the first materials employed in plastic prostheses. Much experimentation was carried out on types of weave and structure,[7, 10, 11, 19, 23, 25] but nylon has been clinically unsatisfactory because of its great loss of tensile strength after implantation.[12] Orlon at first seemed favorable,[18, 22, 27, 28] but the inelasticity and the high porosity with resultant hemorrhage made this prosthesis unacceptable. Dacron and Teflon have emerged as the most satisfactory plastic prostheses now available. Both have displayed excellent retention of tensile strength over long periods of time and both are essentially in-

Received for publication Jan. 31, 1961.

*Formerly Special Fellow in the Department of Vascular Surgery, The Cleveland Clinic Foundation, and The Frank E. Bunts Educational Institute. Present address: 2 Ranfurlie Crescent, Glen Iris S. E. 6, Victoria, Australia.

ert,[10, 11] although Teflon is slightly more inert and slightly stronger than Dacron.

## GRAFT MATERIAL IN CURRENT CLINICAL USE

**Dacron and Teflon.** Of the many experimental substitutes, Dacron and Teflon are virtually alone in their clinical use today. In general, the complications associated with each are the same.

Failure of the host tissue to grow to the graft across an anastomotic line leaves the patient dependent to a large degree upon the strength of the suture material used at the anastomosis. Silk, which loses much of its strength in 6 to 12 months, has failed many times, resulting in false aneurysms in the groin and popliteal space and death when disruption occurred in the abdomen. The current availability of Dacron suture material has obviated this problem to a great extent.

Failure of the fibrin lining to organize in the human being makes continuing appositional deposition of blood elements possible with resultant thickening, particularly at an anastomotic line, and final occlusion of the graft. Thickening of the intima frequently occurs at the host side of anastomotic lines, perhaps because of the increased metabolism secondary to an attempt at healing after operation, but the unorganized lining of the present plastic materials adds further to the postoperative stenosis. This is most critical in the smaller femoropopliteal grafts—so much so that femoral grafting, except for emergent need, has been given up by many clinicians in the field. Also, cracking or splitting of the unorganized lining because of such trauma as acute flexion may lead to dissection of the lining and acute occlusion of the lumen.

The fibrous envelope surrounding the graft does not become adherent to the graft and a periprosthetic space persists indefinitely. In more than 40 grafts in the lower extremity, either of Dacron or of Teflon, which for one reason or another we have replaced over periods of time of up to 2½ years, no graft has failed to show this surrounding space. The graft has always been easily removed merely by cutting it at both ends and pulling it through the submuscular or subcutaneous tunnel. The only graft in this group which we found adherent was one which had been thrombosed and therefore nonfunctional for 6 months. Because the periprosthetic space is present, infection at any point may spread rapidly throughout the length of the graft and an infection at a groin insertion of an aortofemoral graft may readily spread and cause rupture at the aortic anastomosis.

All of these problems stem from a common cause—failure of the host tissue to grow to, into, and through the prosthetic replacement. This failure is in contrast to the response of the experimental animal (dog) to these same materials (Fig. 1)[9] and indicates that although the results of canine experimentation are suggestive, there are species differences involved and absolute prediction of human response cannot be made from animal experimentation.

**Homograft.** The homograft has the advantage of being accepted by the host with ingrowth of host tissue to one-fourth or one-third of its external coat as time goes on. This obviates the first problem of suture-line rupture, since the host tissue grows en-

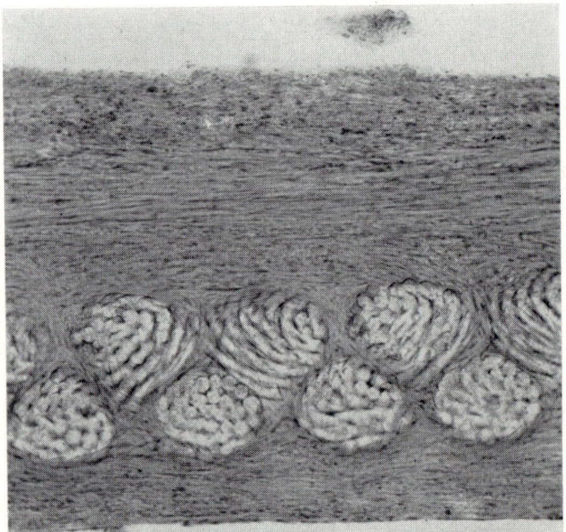

**Fig. 1.** Longitudinal section of "close-weave" Dacron graft in the dog at 6 months. (From J. Harold Harrison.[9])

tirely around and into the anastomotic line unless the graft is infected before such growth can occur.

However, the inner lining of the graft is nonliving and consists of the internal elastic lamina. There is, then, nothing to prevent appositional thickening, particularly at anastomotic lines, and occlusions occur in small grafts with this material also. Finally, the nonviable state of the homograft wall makes it particularly vulnerable to local infection.

In a small percentage of homografts (less than 2 per cent) aneurysm formation develops either through the use of a graft that has an inherently weak point at the time of implantation, or through weakening resulting from low-grade subclinical infection or tissue degeneration.

Vein grafts are usually autogenous and will not be considered here as a "foreign" substitution material.

## THEORETICAL AND PRACTICAL CONSIDERATIONS FOR AN IDEAL PROSTHESIS

It has been an opinion that preservation of the elastica was desirable for continued strength of a homograft or a heterograft. This is open to question. In 1942, Hass[13] extracted aortic rings with formic acid and obtained an intact, purified network of elastic fibers. These showed a high degree of extensibility on stress with almost perfect elastic recoil upon relief of stress. However, these rings were weak and ruptured under loads averaging 80 Gm. Untreated aortic rings did not rupture until many pounds were applied. Krafka,[15] in 1939, showed that the calculation of Young's modulus obtained for the collagen component of the arterial wall was very high when compared with that determined for the musculoelastic portion. The difference was of the order of several hundred times. Burton[2] in 1954, undertook to explain the independent roles of elastica and collagen, and believed that the elastica elongated under minimal load but that arterial expansion was limited by the collagen rather than by the elastica at a predesigned safe point of stretch. Although it is desirable to have an elastic artery to cushion the systolic pressure upon ventricular contraction, this is not a necessity as shown by the many senile sclerotic aortas with nonfunctional elastica and high collagen content. Patients with these vessels usually get along quite well for many years with nothing more than a systolic hypertension. It seems, therefore, that strength is of more importance than elasticity.

The physical requirements of pliability without collapse, maintenance of integrity upon cutting, the possibility of fashioning side arms, suturability, ease of storage, availability, and reasonable cost must all be met. The homograft has the tremendous advantage of being integrated into the patient; the plastic prosthesis has the advantages of continuance of strength and ready availability. The first is partially living; the second is completely inert. Theoretically, one might suppose that a graft made of an inert, permanently strong material, which becomes at least partially viable (the viability consisting of living host tissue) might best approximate a normal vessel. Such a graft might have no inherent problems within itself, and the only problems then facing the clinician would be the quality and size of the host vessel and the sometimes relentless advancement of the original disease. One might imagine such a graft to consist of a framework of plastic of a very wide mesh, but still strong enough to prevent aneurysm formation. The interstices between the fibers should be large enough to permit easy invasion by the host, but would be initially filled by an inert, nonreactive, blood-tight, inherently strong material that is readily replaceable by the host and which, during the phase of replacement, does not involve periods of loss of strength.

## DACRON-COLLAGEN GRAFT

Such a graft has been under investigation in our institution for the past 10 months. It consists of a Dacron tulle impregnated with a coating of bovine collagen and has been prepared by Ethicon, Inc. The work has been performed on mongrel dogs which averaged 15 kilograms in weight. In each instance replacement segments were placed in the abdominal aorta. The animals were sacrificed at varying periods of time of up to 8 months.

In the hope that this work could be compared with similar experimental work performed on other materials, the literature was reviewed. However, it is almost impossible to make a direct comparison of our material with any of the others since the early chronologic achievements with these has not been specifically stated. Many of the arterial prostheses made from various plastics are well tolerated by dogs and appear to have organized well.[7, 9, 18, 22, 23, 25, 26, 28, 29] In some photomicrographs, this organization is seen to represent an ingrowth of fibrous tissue through the interstices of the prosthesis, so that a well-defined fibrous tissue lining is produced (Fig. 1). An adherent fibrous envelope surrounds the prosthesis and fibrous tissue has grown in over the anastomosis so that the prosthesis and host artery are continuous. The actual lining of the prosthesis is variously reported as being endothelial or a compressed layer of fibroblasts. Generally it has been accomplished in the dog at the end of 6 months. Shumway and associates[26] report an endothelial lining in their prosthesis at 2 months and Schumacher's[24] photomicrographs show apparently excellent organization with a nylon polythene graft in 92 days. Unfortunately, this type of response, as has been mentioned, has not been seen by us in the human being with Dacron and Teflon, and it may well be that the results given here for the new Dacron-collagen prosthesis in dogs may not be achieved in the human being. Nevertheless, the theoretical advantages of this type of prosthesis are such that we believe it advisable to present a preliminary report in the hope that further work along these lines will be stimulated. Parenthetically, it is of interest that recently Halpert[6] has theorized along these same lines, stating that the ideal prosthesis still to be found will consist of a synthetic material, the fibers of which are interspersed with absorbable hemostatic fibers woven or knitted tightly enough to prevent blood loss at the time of insertion and of sufficient porosity to allow satisfactory ingrowth of fibroblasts and endothelial cells, resulting in attachment of the prosthesis to the host tissues.

Grossly, the Dacron-collagen prosthesis shows an orderly pattern of organization at varying periods of time after insertion of the graft. The prostheses were all 5 cm. long. divided into 2 types, thick and thin, according to the amount of impregnating collagen. No significant response difference could be detected in the 2 types. However, there was a significant difference, particularly in regard to initial hemorrhage, between the untreated collagen and the collagen that had been tanned.

**One week.**

*Gross specimen.* The 1 week specimens were contained in a fibrous envelope which was not in any way adherent to the prosthesis (Fig. 2). The interstices of the graft were still occluded by the impregnating collagen and the lumen lined by a red, granular coagulum.

*Microscopic section.* Sections of the proximal portion showed an artefactual separation of the Dacron prosthesis from the surrounding fibroadipose tissue (Fig. 3).

The fibroadipose tissue showed active fibroplasia and a minimal inflammatory infiltrate comprised of polymorphonuclear leukocytes, a few lymphocytes, and some plasma cells. The prosthesis itself showed the open meshwork with the interstices filled

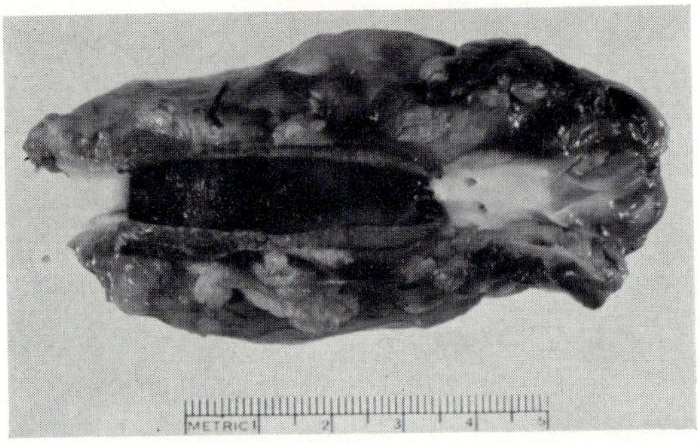


**Fig. 2.** One-week gross specimen.

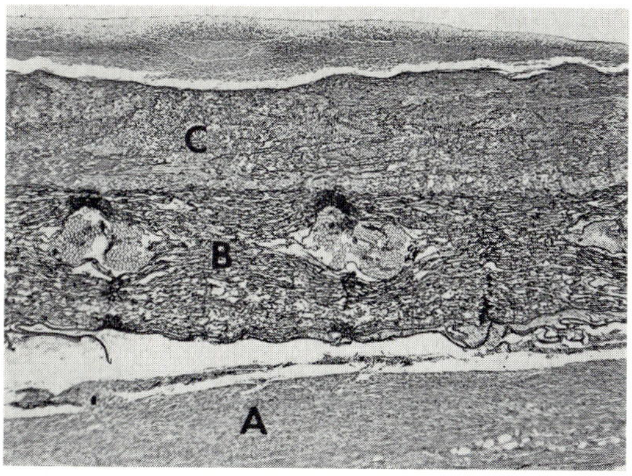


**Fig. 3.** One-week microscopic section. *A,* Fibroadipose tissue. *B,* The prosthesis. *C,* Fibrin clot covering surface of prosthesis.

by a series of haphazardly arranged, tangled fibrils of bovine collagen with irregular interstices containing small numbers of erythrocytes. The surface of the prosthesis was covered by fibrin clot containing a few histiocytes, erythrocytes, and neutrophils. There was no tonguelike extension of fibroplasia extending from the severed end of the aorta out into the graft, although there was a focal zone of reactive hyperplasia with capillaries and occasional inflammatory elements present at the anastomotic line. The lining consisted of a thin fibrin layer, maximally 1 mm. in thickness.

**Two weeks.**

*Gross specimen.* By 2 weeks the fibrous envelope was partially adherent but could be readily dissected free by lysis of delicate fibrous and fibrinous bands (Fig. 4). The wall of the prosthesis and the lining were similar to those of the 1-week specimen.

*Microscopic section.* The 2-week specimen showed a lack of inflammatory reaction similar to that in the specimen at 1 week (Fig. 5). The zone of fibrosis and fibroplasia in the fibroadipose tissue adjoining the prosthesis was more mature but, as yet, there had been no extension of fibroblasts into the prosthesis except at microscopic points. At the anastomosis a well-developed zone of fibroplasia extended across the anastomotic line onto the surface of the prosthesis and this tongue, in turn, was covered in part by endothelium. The prosthesis itself appeared quite similar to the 1-week specimen. The impregnating collagen appeared well retained. The lining surface of the prosthesis now appeared to be of more dense fibrin with enmeshed erythrocytes and was somewhat thinner than the fibrin lining of the 1-week specimen.

**Three weeks.**

*Gross specimen.* At 3 weeks the fibrous envelope was more adherent than earlier, but still could be separated by forceful dissection. The lining was smoother and averaged approximately 1 mm. in thickness.

*Microscopic section.* The peripheral enveloping zone of fibrosis was wider than previously and there was extension of fibroblasts into the interstices of the prosthesis at numerous points. Foreign-body reaction to the Dacron of the prosthesis was present but still remained minimal. The inflammatory reaction was largely composed of histiocytes containing hemosiderin, plasma cells, and lymphocytes. A mural fibrin thrombus was present and was focally organized, particularly at the anastomotic line. This organization was part of the tongue of advancing fibroblasts.

**Four weeks.**

*Gross specimen.* The 4-week specimen was firmly adherent to the fibrous envelope (Fig. 6). A thin, semitransparent membrane covered the anastomotic lines.

*Microscopic section.* A dense surrounding fibrous envelope of mature collagenous connective tissue stained bright green in a Masson trichrome stain. The prosthesis adhered densely to this envelope and there were irregular extensions of this material into the

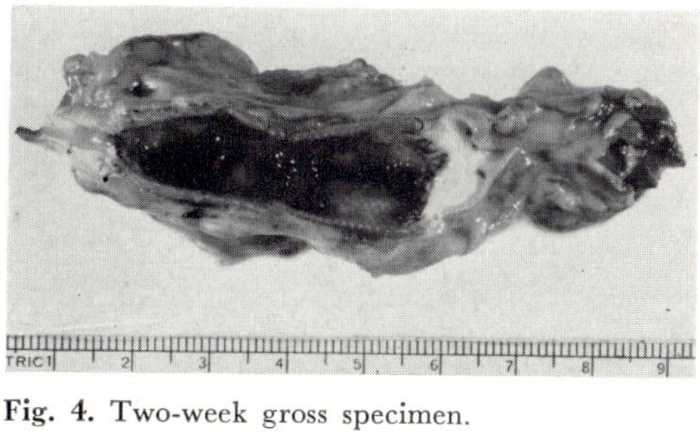


**Fig. 4.** Two-week gross specimen.

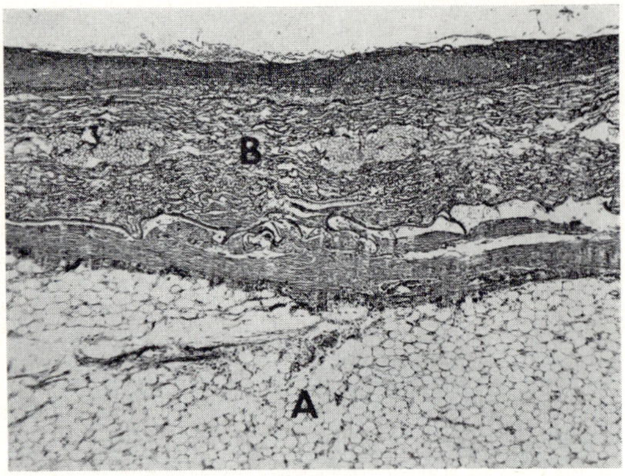


**Fig. 5.** Two-week microscopic section. *A,* Fibro-adipose tissue. *B,* The prosthesis.

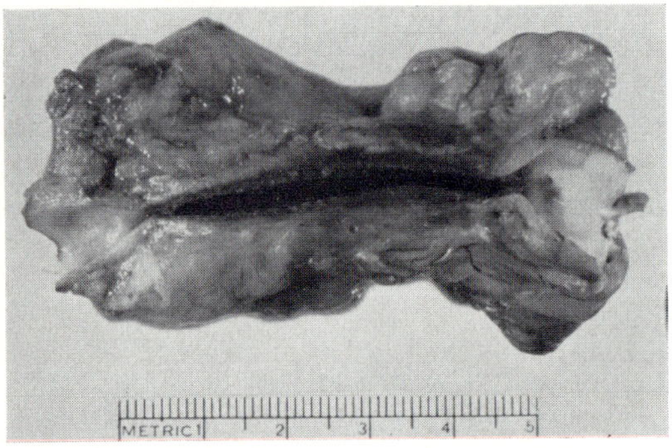


**Fig. 6.** Four-week gross specimen.

interstitial areas of the prosthesis, most particularly between the Dacron meshwork (Fig. 7). The interstices of the bovine collagen were now partially filled with green-staining collagenous connective tissue from the host. Inflammatory reaction was meager. The lining of the prosthesis consisted of a zone of fibrous tissue apparently covered by endothelium that ranged in thickness from about 1 mm. to less than 0.1 mm., being thinnest in the more central extent. This lining was continuous with the lining of the dog's aorta.

**Five weeks.**

*Gross specimen.* The 5-week specimen was essentially the same as the 4-week specimen.

*Microscopic section.* The appearance was substantially the same as that of the 4-week specimen, although there was slightly less of the bovine collagen remaining and more of green-staining collagen contributed by the host, particularly at the anastomosis.

**Two and one-half months.**

*Gross specimen.* The organization was almost complete. The fibrous envelope was firmly adherent and the lumen lined by a thin, well-defined, smooth, semitransparent, grayish membrane.

*Microscopic section.* There was notable progress of the fibrous-tissue ingrowth into the prosthesis. Only an occasional, longitudinally oriented wavy thread of the original prosthetic impregnation remained.

**Eight months.**

*Gross specimen.* The prosthesis was solidly united to the fibrous envelope (Fig. 8). In cross section, the entire thickness of the prosthetic wall was slightly less than 2 mm. The lumen was covered by a smooth, glistening, grayish membrane that appeared continuous with the intima of the host artery.

*Microscopic section.* The prosthesis was completely organized by mature collagen that filled all of the interstices and had replaced all but a few of the original bovine collagen fibrils (Fig. 9). The luminal aspect of the prosthesis was smooth and continuous with the dog's aorta. There was virtually no inflammatory reaction. The Dacron material of the prosthetic meshwork appeared embedded in a continuous, rather uniform collagen mass. Externally, the prosthesis blended with the adjoining fibroadipose tissue.

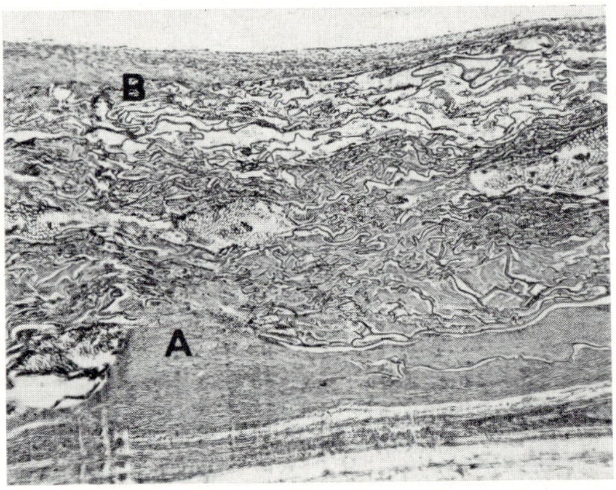


**Fig. 7.** Four-week microscopic section. *A,* Dense surrounding envelope of mature collagenous connective tissue. *B,* Fibrous tissue apparently covered by endothelium which lines the prosthesis.

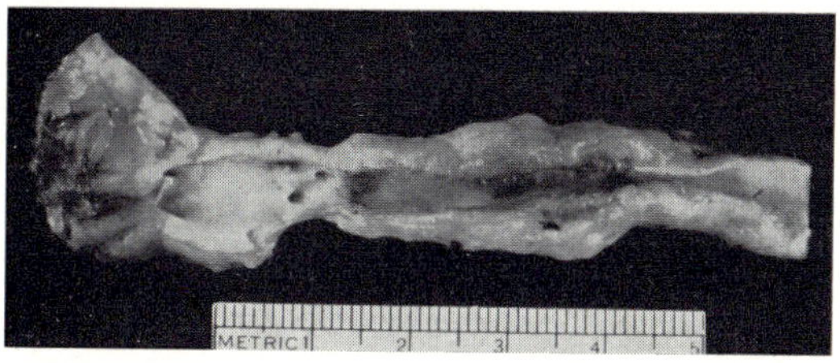

**Fig. 8.** Eight-month gross specimen.

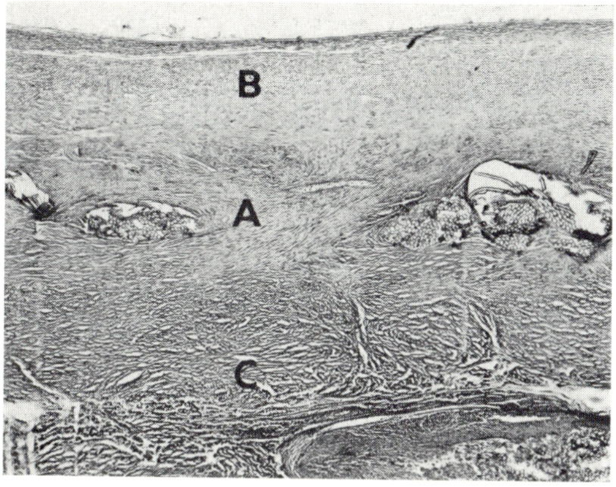

**Fig. 9.** Eight-month microscopic section. *A,* Mature collagen which fills all of the interstices. *B,* Smooth luminal aspect of prosthesis. *C,* Adjoining fibroadipose tissue which blends into prosthesis.

## COMMENT

Our early enthusiasm for the Dacron-colagen graft is tempered by the knowledge that the results of work in the experimental animal are not necessarily the results to be obtained in the human being. However, we believe that the concept of a graft that is not protein, nor yet all plastic, but which retains the better elements of both substances and that encourages the eventual replacement of most of the graft by the host's own living tissue may offer a key to better arterial surgery in the future.

### REFERENCES

1. Barnett, W. O.: Experimental nylon aortic substitutes, A. M. A. Arch. Surg. **76:** 1, 1958.
2. Burton, A. C.: Relation of structure to function of the tissues of the wall of blood vessels, Physiol. Rev. **34:** 619, 1954.
3. Denman, F. R., Brown, W. G., Skinner, S. J., Fitch, E. A., and Glass, H. G.: Fate of human aortic homografts—ten, twenty-four, and twenty-seven months after transplantation, A. M. A. Arch. Surg. **76:** 944, 1958.
4. Egdahl, R. H.: Silicone rubber as aortic grafting material, A. M. A. Arch. Surg. **71:** 694, 1956.
5. Girvin, G. W., Wilhelm, M. C., and Merendino, K. A.: The use of Teflon fabric as arterial grafts, Am. J. Surg. **92:** 240, 1956.
6. Halpert, B., De Bakey, M. E., Jordan, G. L., Jr., and Henly, W. S.: The fate of homografts and prostheses of the human aorta, Surg. Gynec. & Obst. **111:** 659, 1960.
7. Harris, E. J., Schumacker, H. B., Jr., Siderys, H., Moore, T. C., and Grice, P. F.: Pliable plastic aortic grafts: experimental comparison of a number of materials, A. M. A. Arch. Surg. **71:** 449, 1955.
8. Harrison, J. H.: Limitation to knitted synthetic tubes as vascular prostheses, A. M. A. Arch. Surg. **74:** 557, 1957.
9. Harrison, J. H.: Personal communication, 1961.
10. Harrison, J. H.: Synthetic materials as vascular prostheses. I. A comparative study in small vessels of nylon, Dacron, Orlon, Ivalon sponge and Teflon, Am. J. Surg. **95:** 3, 1958.
11. Harrison, J. H.: Synthetic materials as vascular prostheses. II. A comparative study of nylon, Dacron, Orlon, Ivalon sponge and Teflon in large blood vessels with tensile strength studies, Am. J. Surg. **95:** 16, 1958.
12. Harrison, J. H., and Adler, R. A.: Nylon as a vascular prosthesis in experimental animals with tensile strength studies, Surg. Gynec. & Obst. **103:** 613, 1956.
13. Hass, G. M.: Elastic tissue: study of elasticity and tensile strength of elastic tissue isolated from human aorta, Arch. Path. **34:** 971, 1942.
14. Kittle, F., and Taquechel, C.: A preliminary investigation of dermal heterografts (leather) as vascular prostheses for vascular defects, A. M. A. Arch. Surg. **74:** 96, 1957.
15. Krafka, J., Jr.: Comparative study of histophysics of the aorta, Am. J. Physiol. **125:** 1, 1939.
16. Newton, W. T., Weichselbaum, T. E., and Butcher, H. R.: Equine arterial heterografts altered by controlled enzymatic digestion, A. M. A. Arch. Surg. **73:** 432, 1956.
17. Ouzounian, G. S.: Arterial grafting with yardgoods, nylon cloth, A. M. A. Arch. Surg. **73:** 192, 1956.
18. Poppe, J. C., Miller, D., and Thatcher, B.: Selection and preparation of fabric for blood vessel grafts, Am. J. Surg. **92:** 248, 1956.
19. Pratt, G. H.: Replacement arterial grafts, A. M. A. Arch. Surg. **76:** 271, 1958.

20. Rosenberg, N., Henderson, J., Douglas, J. F., Lord, G. H., and Gaughran, E. R. L.: The use of arterial implants prepared by enzymatic modification of arterial heterografts, A. M. A. Arch. Surg. **74:** 89, 1957.
21. Rosenberg, N., Henderson, J., Lord, G. H., Gaughran, E. R. L., and Douglas, J. F.: Use of enzyme-digested heterografts as segmental arterial substitutes, A. M. A. Arch. Surg. **76:** 275, 1958.
22. Sanger, P. W., Taylor, F. H., Matsuba, T., and Salomone, F.: The use of artificial fiber as an artery substitute, Ann. Surg. **143:** 862, 1956.
23. Sanger, P. W., Taylor, F. H., McCall, R. E., Duchesne, R., and Lepage, G.: Seamless Synthetic arterial grafts, J. A. M. A. **160:** 1403, 1956.
24. Schumacker, H. B., Jr., Harris, E. J., and Siderys, H.: Pliable plastic tubes as aortic substitutes, SURGERY **37:** 80, 1955.
25. Self, M. M., Cooley, D. A., De Bakey, M. E., and Creech, O., Jr.: The use of braided nylon tubes for aortic replacement, Ann. Surg. **142:** 836, 1955.
26. Shumway, N. E., Gliedman, M. L., and Lewis, F. J.: Experimental study of the use of polyvinyl sponge for aortic grafts, Surg. Gynec. & Obst. **100:** 703, 1955.
27. Voorhees, A. B., Jr., Jaretzki, A., III, and Blakemore, A. H.: Use of tubes constructed from Vinyon "N" cloth in bridging arterial defects: preliminary report, Ann. Surg. **135:** 332, 1952.
28. Wesolowski, S. A., and Sauvage, L. R.: Comparison of the fate of Orlon mesh prosthetic replacement of the thoracic aorta and aortic bifurcation, Ann. Surg. **143:** 65, 1956.
29. Whittlesey, R. H., Sekerak, N. W., Blunt, J. W., and Hudack, S. S.: Observations of elastic synthetic fabric sleeves as vascular prostheses, A. M. A. Arch. Surg. **73:** 440, 1956.

# The vascular pattern of intestinal villi in rats after partial gastrectomy

G. NYLANDER, M.D.
S. OLERUD, M.D.
UPPSALA, SWEDEN
*From the Department of Surgery, University Hospital*

The gastrointestinal function after partial gastrectomy—either by the technique of bringing the gastric remnant into continuity with the duodenum (Billroth I) or by creation of an upper jejunal loop (Billroth II)—has been a frequent subject of experimental as well as clinical investigation. Recent literature on this topic has been thoroughly reviewed and critically evaluated by several Scandinavian authors.[1, 4, 8]

Today, every surgeon is aware of the fact that signs of nutritional disorder (loss of weight, anemia, sideropenia, avitaminosis, and so forth) often appear after gastric resections. Since various manifestations of malnutrition are found also in the presence of a normal caloric intake, metabolic studies have been focused on other possible causes such as increased intestinal motility and defective digestion and/or absorption. Recenty a critical analysis of some of these postoperative complications has been presented.[4]

The particular intestinal function of absorption is intimately linked with the capillary blood flow in the vascular unit of the intestinal villus. If the arterial blood flow is directed away from this capillary area and is shunted directly into the veins, the functional capacity of the intestinal villus is completely eliminated as to its contribution to the passage of water and nutrient solutes from the intestinal lumen into the blood stream.

During recent years the vascular microanatomy of the gastrointestinal wall has been a subject of primary research in our laboratory. Using the rat, we have been able to visualize microangiographically the arteriovenous anastomoses in the intestinal villi of an isolated jejunal loop. These arteriovenous communications were essentially the same as those previously demonstrated by us in the gastric mucosa after vagotomy.[6, 7] The arterial component was a precapillary vessel. We previously proposed the term "arcade arteries" to describe these 2 precapillary vessels which ordinarily supply the dense capillary network of the intestinal villus. The drainage of the anastomosis was via the main venous components of the villus.

In consideration of the nutritional disorders which follow gastric resections, we have thought it perhaps applicable to analyze microangiographically the vascular and especially the capillary patterns of the intestinal villus in rats after Billroth I and II resections. To facilitate a comparative analysis, experimental studies of this type were conducted on animals with an operative anastomosis between the intact stomach and an upper loop of the jejunum.

## MATERIAL AND METHODS

Fifteen white laboratory rats which weighed initially 200 to 280 grams were used. With open ether anesthesia gastric resections were performed which invariably sacrificed two-thirds of the secretory part of the rat stomach. Gastrointestinal continuity was restored by anastomosis of the gas-

Received for publication Jan. 25, 1961.

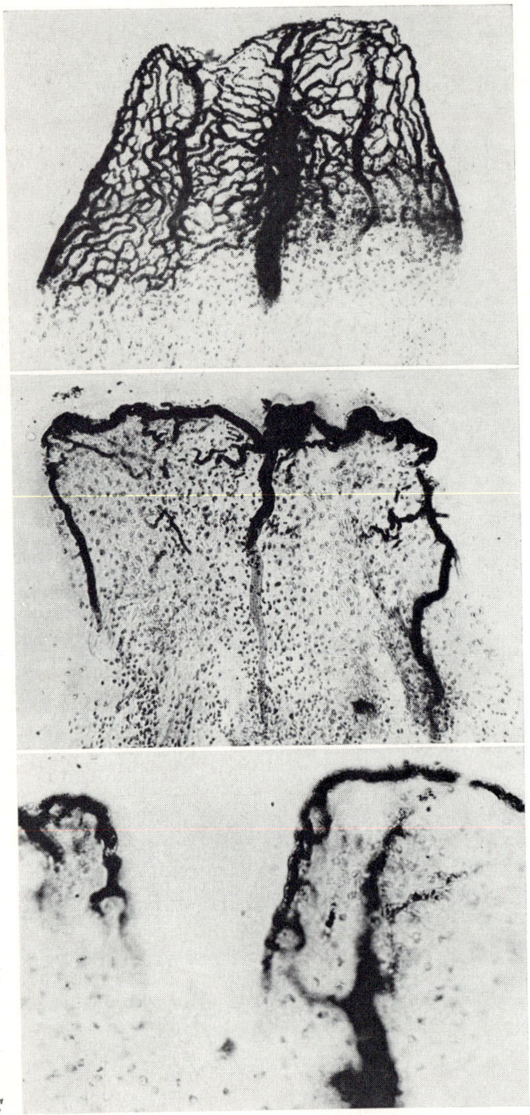

A

B

C

**Fig. 1.** *A,* Completely normal vascular unit of duodenal villus. *B,* Duodenal villus from region of anastomosis (Billroth I). Note the complete blocking of the capillary area. The central artery divides in the shape of a T into the arcade arteries. *C,* Detail of such a villus which shows the precapillary arcade artery draining directly into the stem vein.

tric remnant with the duodenum (Billroth I group) or an upper jejunal loop (Billroth II group). In every case one-third of the transverse section of the gastric remnant corresponding to the greater curvature was used to accomplish the gastrointestinal anastomosis. The Billroth I and II groups were represented by 5 animals, respectively. A simple gastroenterostomy was performed in 5 additional rats. The diameter of the anastomosis and the level of the jejunal loop corresponded to those in the rats of the Billroth II group.

During the first 2 or 3 postoperative days the animals received 15 ml. of physiologic salt solution daily by subcutaneous injection. Water and food were allowed orally beginning on the fourth postoperative day.

The immediate postoperative course was often complicated and the mortality rate considerable. The most frequent cause of death was leakage from the anastomotic site. The 15 animals included in this study, however, experienced uneventful recoveries during the experimental period of 4 to 8 weeks.

Laparotomy was then performed under open ether anesthesia. The anatomy of the operating field was carefully surveyed with special attention to the gastrointestinal anastomosis. Satisfactory integrity of the gastrointestinal anastomosis was present in all cases.

Microangiography was then performed according to the principles previously recommended by us which included a hemoglobin staining method.[5] For this purpose representative sections of the small intestinal wall were always taken from the same area of the duodenum and the jejunum, including the gastrointestinal anastomoses. For a detailed description of the technique used to visualize the vascular system of isolated intestinal villi, the reader is referred to the aforementioned paper.

## OBSERVATIONS

**Billroth I group.** Intestinal villi were completely devoid of capillary vessels at the site of the anastomosis as well as in the proximal part of the duodenum. The striking difference between the normal vascular pattern of duodenal villi, dominated by the finely meshed capillary net, and that of duodenal villi obtained from these experimental animals is evident from Fig. 1. The central artery is clearly seen in the empty villus running upward to the subepithelial region. No branches are given off during its course through the villus, although it terminates in a T-shape and gives rise to the 2 arcade arteries. A capillary net is not visualized and the precapillary arcade arteries eventually drain into the stem veins of the villus. This vascular picture corresponds to that of an arteriovenous anastomosis established by a precapillary artery and a stem vein.

Distalward, the capillary area of the duodenal villi gradually opens. At upper levels of the section there is a sparse anastomosing and the capillary net is of wider mesh as illustrated by Fig. 2. Approaching the duodenojejunal flexure, the capillary area becomes more nearly normal. In the jejunum the vascular pattern of intestinal villi is completely normal (Fig. 3).

**Billroth II group.** In the proximally closed duodenal loop intestinal villi have a rather normal vascular pattern. There is a minimal reduction of the capillary network in contrast to the almost nonexistant capillary arrangement in the Billroth I group (Fig. 4). The jejunal section of the gastrojejunal anastomosis demonstrates intestinal villi with good capillary visualization even though there is a definite quantitative reduction of the capillary unit. The relative sparseness of anastomoses between the capillary vessels is a characteristic feature. The capillaries derived from the arcade arteries divide in a fan shape and empty into the stem vein (Fig. 4). More distally the vascular pattern of the jejunal villi becomes quite normal with a dense capillary system filling the villus.

**Gastroenterostomy group.** Intestinal villi from the duodenum, the afferent and efferent jejunal loops, and the jejunal section of the gastrojejunal anastomosis had vascular units of normal appearance. At every level of the small intestine thus investigated the capillary area was completely outlined as a finely meshed net dominating the vascular architecture of the villus. No deviation from the normal, either qualitative or quantitative, could be observed. This is fully demonstrated in Fig. 5.

## DISCUSSION

After gastric resection with Billroth I anastomosis some significant circulatory changes could be visualized microangiographically. In intestinal villi from the proximal half of the duodenum it was possible to demonstrate a complete blocking of the capillary area. The arterial blood was accordingly shunted directly into the stem veins without entering the capillary bed. A capillary area of normal extent and density was gradually encountered in the distal por-

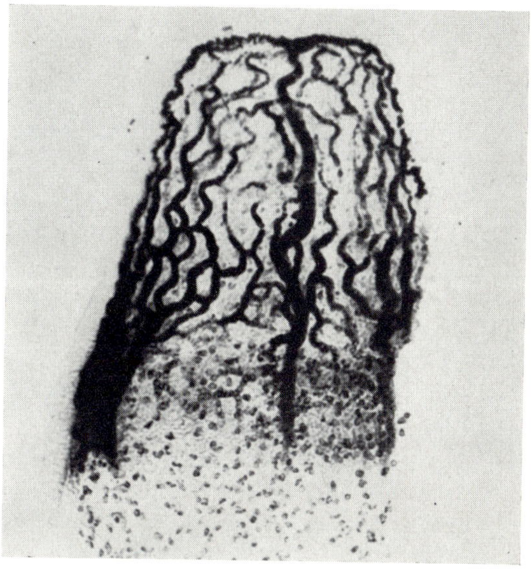

**Fig. 2.** Villus from distal portion of the duodenum (Billroth I). The capillary unit is relatively sparse.

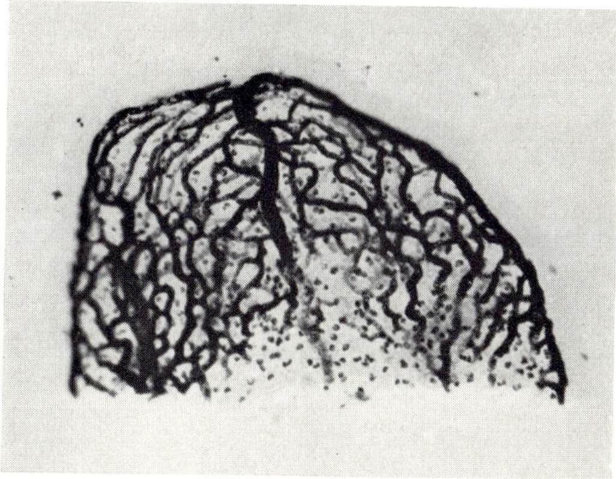

**Fig. 3.** Jejunal villus (Billroth I) with normal density of capillary pattern.

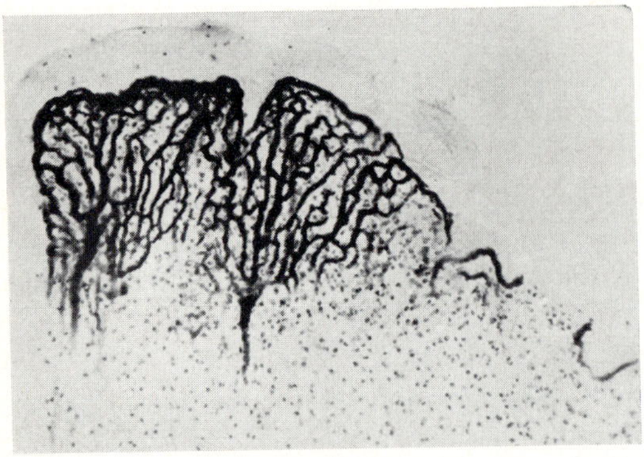

**Fig. 4.** Jejunal villus from region of anastomosis (Billroth II) showing somewhat reduced capillary area. The capillaries are seen to converge toward the stem veins in a fan shape.

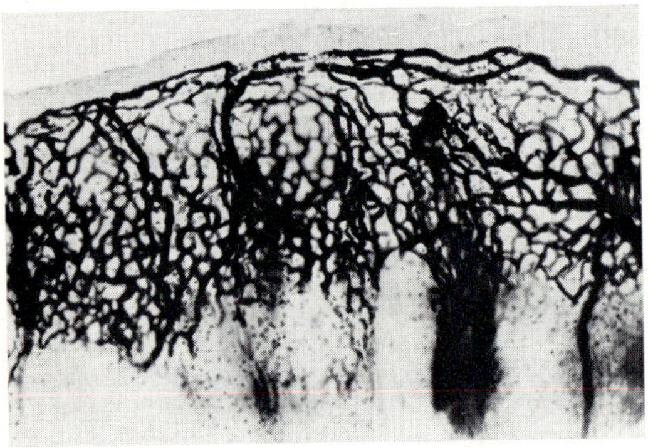

**Fig. 5.** Jejunal villus from region of anastomosis (gastroenterostomy). A dense capillary pattern is visualized.

tions of the duodenum. These findings are in obvious contrast to the sparsely reduced capillary unit found in the duodenal and, in particular, the jejunal villi from animals operated upon with the Billroth II technique. Furthermore, these findings and those from the Billroth I group especially are significantly different when compared to the completely normal capillary filling observed in villi from different intestinal portions of animals subjected to only gastroenterostomy.

Investigators of the nutritional disorders which follow partial gastrectomy generally agree that these complications are more frequent and pronounced after use of the Billroth II technique.[3, 4, 8] Furthermore, it has been demonstrated conclusively that digestion as well as absorption is most active in the upper parts of the small intestine.[2]

In view of these studies, our observations appear somewhat contradictory.

The absence of capillary circulation in the intestinal villi should completely abolish the absorptive function of these structures in at least the upper half of the duodenum of the Billroth I group animals. In the Billroth II group, however, only a slight reduction of corresponding capillary filling (absorptive capacity) was noted in the duodenum and the upper jejunal loop.

In the rat, and under the given experimental conditions, it seems that the proximal half of the duodenum after Billroth I gastric resection loses much of its absorptive capacity. Its primary function might instead be one of food transport and digestion.

The absorptive activity of the upper jejunum after a Billroth II resection does not seem to be influenced by the direct flow of gastric contents. This activity might be such a predominating function of this portion of the intestine that it is not decisively altered by the changed anatomic conditions.

The results demonstrated in this experimental study with rats indicate further investigation focusing on activities such as digestion and intestinal motility. An alteration of these functions rather than of absorption might explain the nutritional disorders which follow partial gastrectomy in man.

Another point of interest suggested by the experimental observations might be discussed and, if applicable to man, may aid us in understanding the comparative frequency of recurrence of ulcers after Billroth I operations. The defective capillary circulation noted in the villi of the upper half of the duodenum should in all probability impair the mucosal nutrition in this intestinal section. This might decrease its resistance to the digestive effects of the gastric secretions.

## SUMMARY

The vascular patterns of duodenal and jejunal villi have been visualized microangiographically in rats operated upon with partial gastrectomies. The gastrointestinal continuity was restored by anastomosis of the gastric remnant to the duodenum (Billroth I group, 5 animals) and an upper jejunal loop (Billroth II group, 5 animals). To permit a comparative analysis 5 additional rats were operated upon with gastroenterostomy only (gastroenterostomy group, 5 animals).

In the Billroth I group arteriovenous anastomoses were constantly found in the intestinal villi of the proximal half of the duodenum. Accordingly, the capillary area was completely shunted off in this intestinal portion. A gradual transition to the normal occurred in the distal portion of the duodenum.

In the Billroth II group only a slight reduction of the capillary area was noted in the intestinal villi of the duodenum and especially in the jejunal section included in the anastomosis.

The gastroenterostomy group demonstrated normal capillary filling in villi obtained from all portions of the small intestine investigated.

The experimental results are briefly discussed with special reference to the nutritional disorders known to appear after gastrectomies.

A theoretical explanation is suggested for the higher tendency for anastomotic ulcer development in patients operated on according to the Billroth I technique.

## REFERENCES

1. Borg, I.: Gastric flow and acidity before and after Billroth II and Billroth I for gastroduodenal ulcer, Acta chir. scandinav., suppl. 256, 1959.
2. Borgström, B., Dahlquist, A., Lund, G., and Sjövall, J.: Studies on intestinal digestion and absorption in the human, J. Clin. Invest. **36:** 1521, 1957.
3. Harkins, H. N., and Nyhus, L. M.: A comparison of the Billroth I and Billroth II procedures: clinical and experimental studies, Bull. Soc. internat. chir. **15:** 111, 1956.
4. Lund, G.: Intestinal digestion and absorption after gastrectomy, Acta chir. scandinav., suppl. 231, 1958.
5. Nylander, G., and Olerud, S.: A simple microangiographic procedure for study of the vascular pattern in the alimentary canal, Acta Soc. med. upsal. **65:** 374, 1960.
6. Nylander, G., and Olerud, S.: The vascular pattern of the gastric mucosa of the rat following vagotomy, Surg. Gynec. & Obst. **112:** 475, 1961.
7. Nylander, G., and Olerud, S.: The vascular pattern of an isolated jejunal loop—a microangiographic study in the rat, Acta chir. scandinav. **121:** 39, 1961.
8. Wallensten, S.: Results of the surgical treatment of peptic ulcer by partial gastrectomy according to Billroth I and Billroth II methods, Acta chir. scandinav., suppl. 191, 1954.

# Iliac osteoclast: a new instrument which facilitates operation for exstrophy of the bladder


CHRIS T. OECONOMOPOULOS, M.D.*
MONTREAL, CANADA
*From The Royal Victoria Hospital*


Exstrophy of the bladder has attracted the interest of surgeons for many years. Recently several authors[1, 2, 3, 4] have recommended the turn-in procedure with plastic reconstruction of the urethra and abdominal wall. This can more easily be accomplished after restoration of the anatomic configuration of the infant's pelvis by bringing the greatly separated pubic bones together (Fig. 1). Bilateral iliac osteoclasis, which was first recommended by Trendelenburg[5] in 1906 and was recently emphasized by Shultz,[2] has been accepted in most centers as a routine procedure. The dotted lines in Fig. 2, *A* show the location of the osteoclasis.

Considering the difficulties which this procedure involves, I came to the conclusion that the usual available osteotomes are not very satisfactory or safe instruments for this kind of operation, even in the most experienced hands. Laceration of the superior gluteal artery has occurred with dangerous hemorrhage. Control of the bleeding is a problem because of the location of the artery in the sciatic notch and the position of the patient during the procedure. Accidental penetration of structures underlying the iliac bones may also occur.

## THE INSTRUMENT

An instrument especially designed for bilateral iliac osteoclasis may help the pediatric surgeon to overcome the difficulties that have been pointed out. The instrument is actually a combination of a periosteal elevator and a lateral osteotome, so that 2 instruments are made into a single one.

The iliac osteoclast* is of stainless steel and measures 21 cm. in length (Fig. 3). The instrument consists of a head and handle united at an angle of 130 degrees. This angulation facilitates the cutting of the iliac bone without exertion of significant pressure on the underlying exstrophic bladder.

The tip of the head acts as a periosteal elevator and pushes the strip of periosteum


Received for publication May 9, 1961.



*Present address: 14 Stournara Street, Athens, Greece.


*The instrument is manufactured by the V. Mueller and Company, 320 South Honore Street, Chicago 12, Ill.

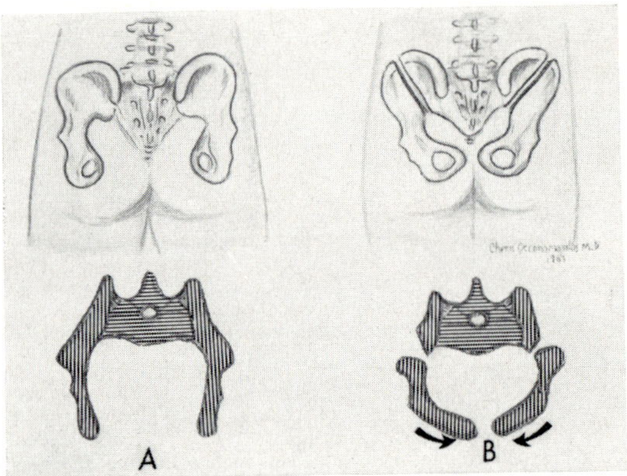


**Fig. 1.** Semischematic drawing of the pelvis of an infant with exstrophy of the bladder. *A,* Note the greatly separated pubic bones. *B,* The pubic bones have been approximated after bilateral iliac osteoclasis.

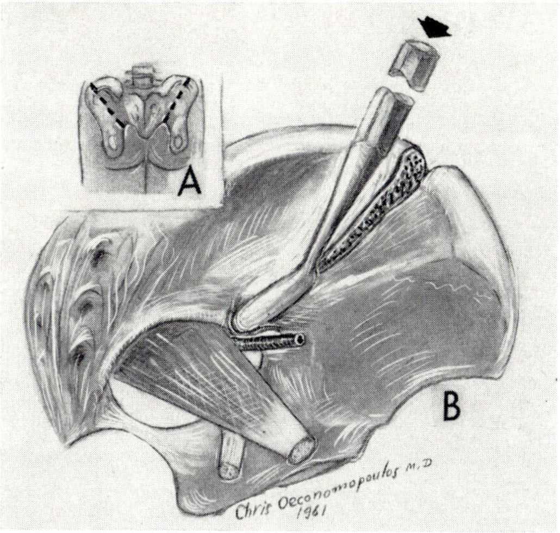


**Fig. 2.** An outline of the iliac osteoclasis. *A,* The dotted lines indicate the location of the osteoclasis. *B,* The instrument elevating the periosteum which then acts as a protector of the superior gluteal artery when the bone is subsequently cut.

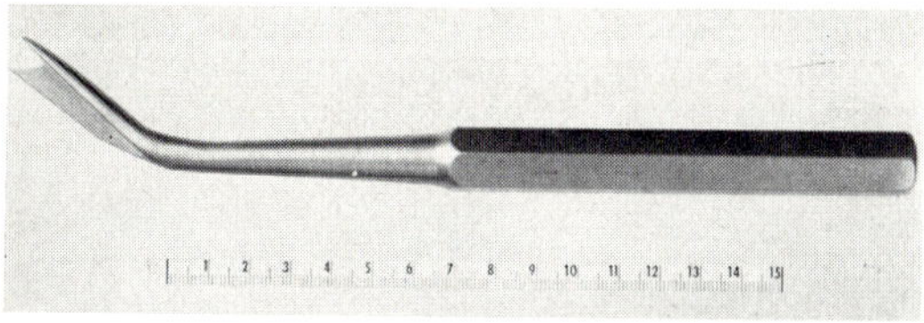

**Fig. 3.** View of the iliac osteoclast for infants.

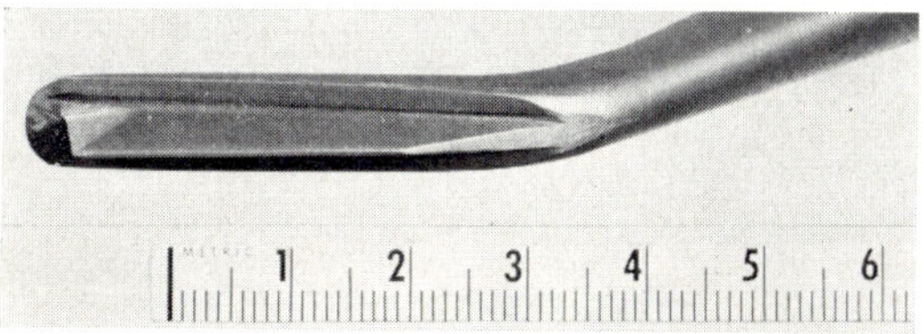


**Fig. 4.** Close-up of the head of the instrument.

which protects the superior gluteal artery, while the lower tip cuts the iliac bone completely (Fig. 2, *B*). The cutting edge of the head is 8 mm. in depth. This size is adequate for complete division of the iliac bone in children from 2 weeks to 3 years of age. This figure was obtained after measurements of the thickness of the iliac bone in 20 infants at autopsy.

An important feature of the instrument is the protective edge which does not permit accidental penetration and injury to the underlying structures (Fig. 4).

The iliac osteoclast has been tested on 11 cadavers and on 4 patients with exstrophy of the bladder and was found effective and satisfactory.

## CONCLUSIONS AND SUMMARY

Some of the practical features of the iliac osteoclast for infants are (1) simplicity of instrument–it does the work of 2 instruments with minimal injury to tissues, (2) acceleration of the operation–the procedure can be performed within 15 minutes by 2 teams simultaneously, (3) safety and suitability for small infants in whom exposure is limited, (4) elimination of the problem of injury to the superior gluteal artery, (5) protection from penetration of and accidental injury to the underlying vital structures, (6) small size, simplicity, and inexpensiveness.

### REFERENCES

1. Lattimer, J. K., Dean, A. L., Jr., Dougherty, L. J., Ju, D., Ryder, C., and Uson, A.: Functional closure of the bladder in children with exstrophy: a report of twenty-eight cases, J. Urol. **83:** 647, 1960.
2. Shultz, G. W.: Plastic repair of exstrophy of bladder combined with bilateral osteotomy of ilia, J. Urol. **79:** 453, 1958.
3. Sweetser, T. H.: Plastic reconstruction for exstrophy of the urinary bladder, South. M. J. **53:** 1519, 1960.
4. Swenson, O.: Changing trends in the management of exstrophy of the bladder, Surgery **42:** 61, 1957.
5. Trendelenburg, F.: The treatment of ectopia vesicae, Ann. Surg. **44:** 281, 1906.

# Exsanguinating gastric hemorrhage in the newborn infant and observations on the "ulcer problem" in children

ALBAN H. LALONDE, M.D.
EDWARD J. BERMAN, M.D.
INDIANAPOLIS, IND.

Massive bleeding from the upper intestinal tract is rare in the newborn infant. Of approximately 500 cases of peptic ulcer reported in infants and children, about 10 per cent occurred in the neonatal period (1 to 14 days).[1, 2, 6] Most of the cases detected in the first year of life manifest themselves through melena, hematemesis, perforation, or obstruction.[2] The association of gastric bleeding and Ritter's disease has been reported only once previously. The child suffered hematemesis at the age of 2 days and Ritter's disease at 6 days, and died on the seventh day. Although the hematemesis persisted until the child's death, he was not operated upon.

The purpose of this paper is to investigate the cause, surgical treatment, and prognosis of gastric and duodenal hemorrhage (loosely ascribed to "peptic ulceration") and to report an interesting case pertinent to our observations.

## CASE REPORT

D. F., a full-term white female infant, weighed 6 pounds, 12 ounces, at birth and was the product of a normal pregnancy and delivery. She seemed normal until she was 13 hours old, at which time she vomited 3 ounces of bright red blood. Hemoglobin concentration, determined immediately thereafter, was 23.4 Gm. per 100 ml. During the next few hours hematemesis recurred 4 times and it was decided to perform esophagoscopy. Blood clots were seen in the stomach. It was the endoscopist's impression that the bleeding did not originate in the esophagus. Shortly after this examination the hemoglobin concentration was 17.2 Gm. per 100 ml. A small French catheter was anchored and continuous nasogastric suction begun. The stomach was washed with saline solution to help determine the amount of bleeding. Frequent hemoglobin determinations showed a fall to 7 Gm. per 100 ml., at which time blood transfusion was begun. Because bleeding continued, laparotomy was performed. (At this time, at the age of 29 hours, the hemoglobin concentration was about 10 Gm. per 100 ml.) Complete examination of the large and small bowel showed the presence of blood throughout the gastrointestinal tract, although there seemed to be a particular concentration toward the stomach and duodenum. The gastric antrum was incised longitudinally and found to be full of clotted blood. This was evacuated, but a bleeding point could not be visualized. At this point a guaze pack was inserted into the distal half of the stomach, isolating it from the field. A spotlight was focused on the upper half of the stomach into which saline solution was instilled. A crimson jet could then be seen pulsating across the pool of saline solution, permitting identification of a pin-point bleeding vessel. It must be emphasized that no ulcer was seen. Without the crimson jet the entire pathologic process would have been absolutely undetectable. One suture ligature of No. 4-0 silk stopped the bleeding. The stomach was closed and a gastrostomy performed.

Convalescence was satisfactory until the second postoperative day, at which time exfoliation of the skin about the face was noted. The picture was that of a second degree burn after blistered skin has been removed. The process soon involved the trunk and extremities. A diagnosis of exfoliative dermatitis neonatorum, "Ritter's disease," was

Received for publication March 10, 1961.

made. Administration of hydrocortisone, penicillin, and achromycin was begun. The baby was wrapped in gauze saturated with normal saline solution. Oral alimentation was begun on the second postoperative day. Temperature never exceeded 100.8° F. The gastrostomy tube was removed on the tenth postoperative day. Hydrocortisone and antibiotics were discontinued on the seventh postoperative day. After healing of a superficial wound infection, recovery was considered complete. The child was released from the hospital on the twenty-fifth postoperative day and has since remained well.

## DISCUSSION

From 1945 to 1959, among 135,386 pediatric patients admitted at Methodist Hospital of Indianapolis (of which 81,766 were newborn) the diagnosis of peptic ulcer was made in 5 instances, not including the case we are reporting. Uncertain roentgenographic evidence was the basis of diagnosis in 4 of these. The fifth patient, age 2 months, died of hemorrhage and perforation of a duodenal ulcer proved at autopsy.

The Mayo Clinic has had about 110 cases of duodenal ulcer in infants and children, of which 92 cases were recently reported.[6] Only 3 of the patients were newborn. One infant died of gastrointestinal hemorrhage and is not included in the group of 92. The other 2 babies survived, but there is no indication as to the severity of the bleeding and "presumptive diagnosis of duodenal ulcer was made from the clinical history and physical examination—without x-ray examination." In all, 53 had no difficulty beyond the initial episode; 39 had persistent symptoms or recurrence in adult life. In 7 of 9 children operated upon (youngest 6 years), an apparently correct diagnosis had been made at least 2 years prior to operation, which perhaps indicates some reliability of diagnosis. Notwithstanding this, however, it can readily be seen that statistical analysis of the incidence of peptic ulceration in infants and children is almost impossible. The symptoms are unreliable; the roentgenographic diagnoses are often unverified. It is often difficult to make an accurate diagnosis at laparotomy,[3] and even at postmortem examination the ulcer may be difficult to detect.[2] Until diagnostic techniques are refined, therefore, we may quite possibly correctly identify only a small group of the ulcer patients and it is possible that much of the upper gastrointestinal bleeding ascribed to peptic ulcer will ultimately prove to be due to another cause.

It seems probable that the newborn infant suffering massive blood loss will deteriorate more rapidly than the adult in spite of blood transfusions. This is hypothesized on the basis of immature kidneys plus the altered levels of blood pH and electrolytes present in stored blood,[5] and the considerable difficulties of accurate estimation of blood loss. For these reasons we favor early intervention (24 to 36 hours) in cases of massive gastrointestinal bleeding in the newborn infant.

## SUMMARY

1. A newborn infant with gastric hemorrhage postoperatively complicated by Ritter's disease is presented.

2. Filling part of the stomach with saline solution and looking for a "crimson jet" is a good way for the surgeon to identify the bleeding point.

3. It may be that exsanguinating gastroduodenal hemorrhage in the newborn infant should be treated operatively if it does not abate within 24 to 36 hours.

4. How often infants have peptic ulcer and the best treatment for the infant with massive gastroduodenal bleeding has not yet been determined.

### REFERENCES

1. Bird, C. E., Limper, M. A., and Mayer, J. M.: Surgery in peptic ulceration of stomach and duodenum in infants and children, Ann. Surg. **114:** 526, 1941.
2. Hollander, M. H., and Stark, M. W.: Duodenal ulcer in infancy with presentation of a case, Pediatrics **6:** 676, 1950.
3. Karelitz, S., and Kahn, J. L.: Bleeding peptic ulcer, J. Pediat. **34:** 98, 1949.
4. Kendall, N., and Aegerter, E. E.: Ritter's disease, review of literature with report of a case, J. Pediat. **15:** 733, 1939.

5. McLaughlin, E. D., Nealon, T. F., Jr., and Gibbon, J. H., Jr.: Treatment of bank blood by resins, J. Thoracic Surg. **40:** 602, 1960.
6. Michener, W. M., Kennedy, R. L., and DuShane, J. W.: Duodenal ulcer in childhood, Am. J. Dis. Child. **100:** 814, 1960.
7. Williams, H., Guynn, V. L., and Reynolds, T. T.: Diagnostic procedures in bleeding of the gastrointestinal tract, S. Clin. North America, 1956.

# The surgical treatment of chronic pancreatitis by pancreaticojejunostomy: an 8-year reappraisal

MERLIN K. DuVAL, JR., M.D.
IRVING F. ENQUIST, M.D.
OKLAHOMA CITY, OKLA., and
BROOKLYN, N. Y.
*From the Departments of Surgery, University of Oklahoma School of Medicine and the State University of New York College of Medicine*

In 1954, it was reported that decompression of the pancreatic duct brought symptomatic relief to selected patients with chronic pancreatitis. Although Longmire[10] and Jordan[9] have subsequently described situations in which good results were not achieved, others have substantiated the validity of the basic concept. Indeed, the scope of the original pancreaticojejunostomy, whether accomplished by a jejunal loop[14] or by caudal anastomosis,[5] has been greatly extended by the modifications introduced by Puestow,[12] Doubilet,[3] Bartlett,[1] Partington,[11] Gillesby,[8] and Carnevali.[2]

Although an earlier report reviewed our experience over the first 3 years,[7] the current reappraisal summarizes our cumulative experience with a single, unmodified operative approach, namely; caudal pancreaticojejunostomy, as used consecutively between 1953 and 1958, thus providing follow-up information for from 3 to 8 years since operation.

## PATIENT MATERIAL

Twenty-eight patients have been studied. The pertinent data for all are summarized in Table I. The specific criteria by which these patients were selected for operation have been adequately described earlier.[7] Their ages varied from 26 to 53 years. All had a history of recurrent abdominal pain of from 1 to 10 years' duration (mean 4.9 years), and all but one had lost weight in amounts from 10 to 100 pounds (mean 26.9 pounds). Twenty-three (82 per cent) admitted to either current or prior excessive intake of alcohol, 8 (30 per cent) were diabetic, and 16 (57 per cent) had evidence of calcification in the pancreas. Many of the patients had disturbed personalities, generally of the psychopathic variety, including both criminal tendencies and drug addiction. None had pancreatitis as a complication of biliary tract disease, mumps, trauma, surgical operation, or other of the entities with which secondary pancreatitis has been described.

An identical clinical evaluation was conducted on all patients, including oral cholecystography and fluoroscopic examination of the upper gastrointestinal tract with barium.

At operation, 22 (78.6 per cent) had a pancreatic duct in excess of 3.0 mm. in diameter at the point of transection in the tail of the pancreas. Organic obstruction of the duct was demonstrated at the time of operation in 16 of the 20 patients so investigated (80 per cent).

All underwent resection of the distal 3 to 4 cm. of the tail of the pancreas, followed by end-to-end anastomosis of the remaining gland to a Roux Y limb of proximal jejunum in the retrocolic position. Details of the operative technique have been described elsewhere.[4]

Received for publication July 3, 1961.

## RESULTS

There were no operative deaths after pancreaticojejunostomy in this series. One patient (with known treatment failure) was lost to follow-up 9 months after operation and 5 others are currently not traceable, although follow-up information is available for from 2 to 4 years after their operations. One patient died 3 months after operation with diabetic acidosis incident to an abscessed tooth. Table I summarizes these data, although certain observations concerning the operation and the disease process itself seem warranted.

**The operation.** Decompression of the pancreatic duct by pancreaticojejunostomy was frequently successful in bringing symptomatic relief of pain. In 18 patients the relief was immediate and complete from the time of operation. In 2 others, only a single attack of pain, at 5 and seven months, respectively, interrupted an otherwise excellent course of over 4 years' duration. When failure did occur, it was readily apparent within a few months of operation in most instances, although 1 patient had been relieved of pain for 23 months before relapse. This indicates that decompression of the pancreatic duct successfully eliminated the abdominal pain in 71 per cent of the patients in this series.

**The disease.** Relief of pain was not necessarily of prognostic significance with regard to the course of events after pancreaticojejunostomy. Indeed, a review of the clinical

**Table I.** *Summary of data on 28 patients with chronic pancreatitis*

| *Preoperative data* | | | | | | | *Operative findings* | | *Results* | | | |
|---|---|---|---|---|---|---|---|---|---|---|---|---|
| *Patient No.* | *Age and sex* | *Duration (yr.)* | *Weight loss (lb.)* | *Alcoholism* | *Diabetes* | *Calcification* | *Pancreatic duct size (mm.)* | *Duct obstruction* | *Since operation* | *Last follow-up* | *Free of pain* | *Time of recurrence (mo.)* |
| 1 | 40, M | 1 | 15 | + | 0 | + | 4 | + | 91 | 82 | + | — |
| 2 | 45, M | 9 | 20 | + | + | + | 8 | + | 86 | 78 | + | — |
| 3 | 37, M | 1 | 100 | + | + | + | 7 | + | 85 | 69 | + | — |
| 4 | 33, M | 1 | 35 | + | 0 | + | 6 | + | 78 | 38 | + | — |
| 5 | 53, M | 2 | 10 | + | 0 | 0 | 2 | + | 76 | 61 | + | — |
| 6 | 28, F | 6 | 20 | 0 | + | 0 | 4 | + | 72 | 3 | + | — |
| 7 | 35, F | 6 | 15 | 0 | 0 | + | 9 | + | 72 | 63 | + | — |
| 8 | 46, M | 5 | 30 | + | 0 | + | 7 | + | 70 | 55 | + | — |
| 9 | 26, M | 5 | 12 | + | 0 | 0 | 3 | + | 67 | 57 | 0 | 23 |
| 10 | 41, F | 4 | 20 | 0 | + | + | 7 | + | 65 | 63 | 0 | 12 |
| 11 | 52, M | 2 | 30 | 0 | 0 | 0 | 3 | 0 | 64 | 32 | + | — |
| 12 | 31. M | 7 | 25 | + | 0 | 0 | 6 | ? | 63 | 48 | + | — |
| 13 | 39, M | 10 | 21 | + | + | + | 8 | + | 63 | 32 | + | — |
| 14 | 39, M | 5 | 0 | + | 0 | 0 | 4 | + | 63 | 54 | + | — |
| 15 | 31, M | 3 | 30 | + | 0 | 0 | 8 | + | 62 | 47 | 0 | 3 |
| 16 | 36, F | 9 | 20 | + | 0 | + | 8 | ? | 61 | 52 | + | — |
| 17 | 36, M | 8 | 39 | + | 0 | + | 8 | + | 60 | 24 | 0 | 1 |
| 18 | 44, M | 8 | 40 | + | + | + | 4 | + | 59 | 53 | + | — |
| 19 | 44, M | 4 | 25 | + | 0 | 0 | 3 | 0 | 58 | 25 | 0 | 13 |
| 20 | 39, M | 7 | 25 | + | + | + | 5 | 0 | 58 | 39 | + | — |
| 21 | 36, M | 4 | 30 | + | ? | + | 8 | + | 56 | 19 | 0 | 3 |
| 22 | 28, M | 2 | 30 | + | 0 | 0 | 3 | 0 | 56 | 54 | 0 | 2 |
| 23 | 29, F | 7 | 20 | + | 0 | 0 | 4 | ? | 55 | 40 | + | — |
| 24 | 38, M | 6 | 15 | + | 0 | 0 | 2 | ? | 55 | 9 | 0 | 7 |
| 25 | 32, F | 8 | 30 | + | 0 | + | 4 | ? | 51 | 39 | + | — |
| 26 | 27, F | 1 | 20 | + | 0 | 0 | 4 | ? | 50 | 36 | + | — |
| 27 | 46, M | 5 | 40 | + | + | + | 8 | ? | 41 | 36 | + | — |
| 28 | 50, F | 1 | 10 | 0 | 0 | + | 7 | ? | 37 | 36 | + | — |
| Mean | | 4.9 | 26.9 | 23 | 8 | 16 | 5.5 | 16/20 | 63.2 | 51.8 | 20 | 8 |
| Per cent | | | | 82 | 29.7 | 57 | | 80 | | | 71.4 | |

Key: ? signifies information not available, + signifies present, 0 signifies absent.

**Table II.** *Follow-up information on 8 patients whose pain was not relieved by pancreaticojejunostomy*

| | *Subsequent treatment* | | | | *Late complications* | | | | | |
|---|---|---|---|---|---|---|---|---|---|---|
| *Patient No.* | *Thoraco-lumbar sympathec-tomy* | *Im-proved* | *Total pancre-atectomy* | *Im-proved* | *Dia-betes* | *Tubercu-losis* | *Ulcer* | *Jaundice* | *Death* | *Lost* |
| 9 | + | 0 | | | | | + | | | |
| 10 | + | 0 | + | + | | | | + | | |
| 15 | | | | | | | | | | + |
| 17 | + | 0 | + | 0 | + | + | | | + | |
| 19 | + | ? | | | | | | | | + |
| 21 | + | 0 | | | + | | | | + | |
| 22 | | | + | + | | | | + | | |
| 24 | + | ? | | | | | | | | + |
| Totals | 6 | 0 | 3 | 2 | 2 | 1 | 1 | 2 | 2 | 3 |

**Table III.** *Follow-up information on 20 patients relieved of pain by pancreaticojejunostomy*

| *Patient No.* | *Diabetes* | *Tuberculosis* | *Ulcer* | *Jaundice** | *Death* | *Lost* |
|---|---|---|---|---|---|---|
| 1 | | | | | | |
| 2 | | + | | | | |
| 3 | | + | | | + | |
| 4 | + | + | | | | + |
| 5 | | | | | | |
| 6 | | | | | + | |
| 7 | | | | | | |
| 8 | | | | | | |
| 11 | | | | | | + |
| 12 | + | | | + | + | |
| 13 | | | | | | + |
| 14 | + | | | | | |
| 16 | | | | | | |
| 18 | | | | | | |
| 20 | | | | + | + | |
| 23 | | | | | | |
| 25 | | | | | | |
| 26 | + | | + | | + | |
| 27 | | | | | | |
| 28 | | | | | | |
| Totals | 4 | 3 | 1 | 2 | 5 | 3 |

*Both patients who developed jaundice died after total pancreatectomy.

course of each patient after operation shows, with disturbing clarity, the vicious nature of this form of pancreatitis.

Table II summarizes the experience with 8 patients in whom pancreaticojejunostomy failed to relieve the abdominal pain. One refused further treatment and has since been lost to follow-up. Another subsequently underwent total pancreatectomy and is greatly improved. The remaining 6 were subjected to thoracolumbar sympathectomy. Two have since been lost to follow-up, the other 4 were not relieved. Two of these then underwent total pancreatectomy. One was improved while the other was not. In other words, the ultimate salvage rate among the 8 who failed to respond to pancreaticojejunostomy was only 25 per cent. Among the others, 2 later developed diabetes, 1 developed pulmonary tuberculosis, and 1 an active duodenal ulcer. Two of them are known to have died.

Table III summarizes the clinical course of patients who were relieved of pain by the operation. Five are known to be dead, 4 have developed diabetes (which was not present prior to operation), and 3 have developed pulmonary tuberculosis. Two developed obstructive jaundice which mimicked carcinoma of the pancreas and required total pancreatectomy. One patient has developed an active duodenal ulcer, and another is bed-ridden with progressive peripheral vascular disease which has already required amputation of the foot. In other words, in spite of relief of pain in 20 patients who underwent pancreaticojejunostomy, only 9 are known to be living and apparently well without evidence of continued destruction of the pancreas or severe intercurrent disease.

## DISCUSSION

The results observed in the carefully followed series of 28 patients seem to warrant discussion from 2 viewpoints.

First, it is apparent that operative decompression of the pancreatic duct is rewarded with success in approximately 70 per cent of selected patients with chronic pancreatitis. The improvement is manifested in 2 ways, by relief of the severe abdominal pain and by improvement in the patients' demeanor and sense of well-being. The latter are often present even when complete relief of pain is not achieved. It should be emphasized that the proper selection of patients for duct decompression requires a basic appreciation of the clinical variations of pancreatitis,[6] since neither acute pancreatitis nor recurrent acute pancreatitis would be expected to yield to pancreaticojejunostomy.

The presence of certain criteria preoperatively was of some prognostic value relative to relief of pain by pancreaticojejunostomy in this series. The most important of these were chronic alcoholism, diabetes, and calcification of the pancreas. For example, among 11 patients in whom neither diabetes nor calcification was present preoperatively, there were 5 failures (45 per cent). Meanwhile, of 10 patients in whom at least one or the other was present before operation, there were only 2 failures (10 per cent). Among patients who were diabetic, chronic alcoholics, and with pancreatic calcification, there were no failures. An analysis of the 8 patients who failed to respond to pancreaticojejunostomy showed no factors in common. Thal[13] has reported that pancreatic duct obstruction may occur at different sites and the description of multiple simultaneous points of duct obstruction by Puestow[12] may explain many failures after operations in which the duct is decompressed at a single point.

Second, our experience has greatly enhanced our appreciation of, and respect for, the ruthless impact of the disease process itself. Indeed, the overwhelming evidence in our series indicates that surgical relief of pain by no means arrests some of the other manifestations of chronic pancreatitis in the patient as a whole. Consider, for example, that in spite of a 70 per cent "success" rate in the 28 cases reviewed, 25 per cent of the patients are already dead, 21 per cent developed diabetes, 14 per cent acquired far-advanced pulmonary tuberculosis, and 18 per cent developed either severe jaundice, duodenal ulcer, or other disabling intercurrent disease.

## CONCLUSIONS

1. Twenty-eight patients with chronic pancreatitis treated by caudal pancreaticojejunostomy between 1953 and 1958 have been studied.

2. Seventy per cent were relieved of the abdominal pain by this operation, and the success rate was highest in patients with the most severe forms of the disease, especially when diabetes, alcoholism, and pancreatic calcification were already present.

3. Relief of pain by pancreaticojejunostomy did not (of and by itself) protect the patient against the subsequent appearance of other manifestations of the underlying chronic disease, such as diabetes, jaundice, and tuberculosis.

## REFERENCES

1. Bartlett, M. K., and Nardi, G. L.: Treatment of recurrent pancreatitis by resection inhibition and retrograde drainage of the pancreas, Ann. Surg. **152:** 861, 1960.
2. Carnevali, J. F., Remine, W. H., Dockerty, M. B., Bollman, J. L., and Grindlay, J. H.:

An experimental study of side-to-side pancreaticojejunostomy after ductal obstruction, A. M. A. Arch. Surg. **80:** 774, 1960.
3. Doubilet, H.: The physiological basis for the surgical management of acute and chronic pancreatitis, S. Clin. North America **38:** 505, 1958.
4. DuVal, M. K.: Caudal pancreatico-jejunostomy for chronic pancreatitis. Operative technique, S. Clin. North America **36:** 831, 1956.
5. DuVal, M. K.: Caudal pancreatico-jejunostomy for chronic relapsing pancreatis, Ann. Surg. **140:** 775, 1954.
6. DuVal, M. K.: Chronic pancreatitis. A review, Quart. Rev. Surg. Obst. & Gynec. **16:** 77, 1959.
7. DuVal, M. K.: Pancreatico-jejunostomy for chronic pancreatitis. A reappraisal, SURGERY **41:** 1019, 1957.
8. Gillesby, W. J., and Puestow, C. B.: Surgery for chronic recurrent pancreatitis, S. Clin. North America **41:** 831, 1961.
9. Jordan, G. L., Jr., and Howard, J. M.: Caudal pancreaticojejunostomy in the management of chronic relapsing pancreatitis, SURGERY **44:** 303, 1958.
10. Longmire, W. P., Jordan, P. H., Jr., and Briggs, J. D.: Experience with resection of the pancreas in the treatment of chronic relapsing pancreatitis, Ann. Surg. **144:** 681, 1956.
11. Partington, P. F., and Rochelle, R. E.: Modified Puestow procedure for retrograde drainage of the pancreatic duct, Ann. Surg. **152:** 1037, 1960.
12. Puestow, C. B., and Gillesby, W. J.: Retrograde surgical drainage of the pancreas for chronic relapsing pancreatitis, A. M. A. Arch. Surg. **76:** 898, 1958.
13. Thal, A. P., Goott, B., and Margulis, A. R.: Sites of pancreatic duct obstruction in chronic pancreatitis, Ann. Surg. **150:** 49, 1959.
14. Tollinger, R. M., Keith, L. M., Jr., and Ellison, E. H.: Pancreatitis, New England J. Med. **251:** 497, 1954.

# Surgical history

*Conducted by* JOHN R. PAINE, M.D.

# Andreas Vesalius, surgeon

DAVID CHAS. SCHECHTER, M.D., M.S.
HENRY SWAN, M.D. D.SC.
DENVER, COLO.
*From the Department of Surgery, University of Colorado School of Medicine*

As December 1914 approached, my friend Dr. E. C. Streeter, who had a far better collection of books than I, proposed that we call attention to the date by an exhibit of Vesaliana for the Spring meeting of the American Medical Association in Atlantic City. For this purpose we were allotted a booth and had a small pamphlet printed with a description of the books we had selected for display. It aroused little if any interest. We had arranged to alternate as showmen, Streeter in the morning hours, I in the afternoon. We met at lunch after the first morning, and on my enquiring "How did it go?" he replied, "Well, only one old codger stopped long enough to read the sign VESALIAN EXHIBIT and said, 'Got any samples?'" Streeter asked "Samples of what?" He pointed to the sign and said, "Samples of Vaseline, of course." Sadder and wiser we returned to Boston with our "samples" at the end of the week.

Harvey Cushing
*A Bio-Bibliography of Andreas Vesalius,* 1943

The Ionian Islands consist of jutting, sun-burnished mounds of rock which stud the blue Aegian west of Greece. It was on one of these, the Isle of Zante, that perhaps the brightest flame in medical history was extinguished on Oct. 15, 1564. So much score has been placed on the monumental work of Andreas Vesalius as the Father of Anatomy that even his most enthusiastic hierographers, such as Osler, Roth, Cushing, Fulton, and Singer, allude only in the briefest terms to his role as a practicing surgeon. Because Vesalius laid the foundations of modern medicine, perhaps no single specialty may truly claim him as its own; and yet, that he started and ended his career in the practice of surgery is incontestable.

Received for publication Sept. 14, 1961.

## EARLY DAYS

Vesalius was born on Dec. 13, 1514, in the town of Brussels, a fourth generation physician of a distinguished Belgian family named Witing. His father, who served and accompanied Emperior Charles V on his journeys and campaigns, chose to call himself Andreas of Wesalia in designation of his high office. The young Andreas rebelled against this status-symbolism and became known simply as Vesalius. Trained at the University of Louvain, which he had entered at the age of 14, he manifested an early keen interest in zoology and slaked his thirst for knowledge by performing dissections on small animals. In 1533, he migrated to Paris, then the best of medical teaching centers, and had as preceptors 2 Galenist doctrinarians of great renown, Sylvius and

Guinterius. One of his fellow-prosectors was Michael Servetus, the ill-fated martyr of science. While in Paris, his ardent preoccupation with the structure and function of the body was frustrated by inept instruction and paucity of material. "My study of anatomy," he wrote later, "would never have succeeded had I, when working in Medicine at Paris, been willing that the viscera should be merely shown to me and to my fellow-students at one or another public dissection by wholly unskilled barbers, and that in the most superficial way. I had to put my own hand to the business."

He "put his hand" by surreptitiously raiding cemeteries and gibbets for bones, usually at great risk to his person. Discouraged and dissatisfied, he returned to Louvain, and in February, 1537, published his thesis, a translation and paraphrase of the ninth tome of Rhazes.

Unsatisfied and restless, he joined the Hospital at Venice, where he met Ignatius Loyola, another revolutionary figure marked for immortality. The fiery-eyed Flemish prodigy was quickly noticed. On Dec. 6, 1537, the day after he was awarded his medical degree ("with highest distinction") and when he was but 23 years of age, Andreas Vesalius was appointed by the Venetian Senate to the Chair of Surgery at the University of Padua. He was to lecture mainly on fractures and tumors, but was entrusted with the incidental added responsibility of conducting demonstrations in anatomy. Thus, initially an avocation, the latter discipline was destined to receive his all-consuming attention.

## THE *TABULAE*

In 1538, Vesalius published the *Tabulae Anatomicae Sex*, a series of 6 anatomic sheets with captions simultaneously in Latin, Hebrew, and Greek. In the dedication to Narcissus Parthenopeus, Chief Physician of the Imperial Court, Vesalius explained his reasons for the plates:

> Not so long ago, most learned Narcissus, when I was chosen to lecture on Surgical Medicine at Padua, and was occupied with the treatment of inflammations, having in mind to explain the statements of the divine Hippocrates and Galen concerning revulsion and derivation, I made on a sheet of paper a hasty sketch of the veins, thinking that I might be able easily in this manner to explain what Hippocrates had meant to say. . . . You know what a tempest of dissentions and contentions this expression was the case of, even among erudite men, with regard to venesection; some say Hippocrates had meant by this expression the correct arrangement of the fibers. Others say he meant, I don't know what else. That delineation of the veins, however, proved so pleasing to all the professors and students of Medicine, that they strenuously urged me to supply a description of the arteries and nerves also. Since my teaching included the field of anatomy, I had no right to refuse them, particularly as I knew that such outlines would be of no little help to those attending dissections. . . .

The work was an overwhelming success, and was promptly pirated and counterfeited by publishers throughout Europe. It provided a more accurate depiction of anatomic structures than, for example, those drawn by Mundinus. It was deemed a visual teaching aid proffered by a naturalist, not an unorthodox pamphlet against established canons; so that the wrath of the Galenists was not excited, and there was nothing for the ecclesiastical censorship to expunge. Vesalius was in his heyday. He was much sought for lecturing, and journeyed to Pisa, Bologna, and other university cities for this purpose. In 1538, he and his former professor, Guinterius, published the *Institutiones*, a compendium of the anatomicophysiologic views of Galen, intended as a companion synopsis to the *Tabulae*.

## THE *VENESECTION EPISTLE*

Vesalius' first joust with the dogmatists was an indirect product of his prefatory remarks in the *Tabulae*, as a result of which his opinion was asked on a surgical problem. A vituperative controversy already existed regarding the choice site for phlebotomy. The Arabian school had long taught that blood-letting should be "revulsive," that is, as distant as possible from the seat of disease. Pierre Brissot, a distinguished member of the Paris Faculty, had maintained in 1525 that this was in contradiction to Hippocrates' instructions that blood should be drawn in a "derivative" fashion, near the sick part. Brissot was perfunctorily banished for his heresy, but the polemic he had issued was propagated with fury. With due respect to Cushing, who has labeled the whole argument "a tempest in a bleeding bowl," we must remember that disease in those days was thought to be caused by noxious humors, and that consequently the optimal region for evacuating these humors was of pressing concern. In inflammatory lesions, should bloodletting be performed in one or the other manner, depending on whether the accumulated humors were still in a state of flux, or whether they had already settled in tissues and undergone corruption? In the latter circumstance, would bleeding by "revulsion" not tend to disseminate the humors by reversing their flow? Thus, should phlebotomy by "derivation" be reserved for early stages of sickness only ("prophylactically") before the humors had become firmly anchored in some locality?

The Prince of Piedmont, a kinsman of the Emperior, died of pleuritis, and the canard was disseminated that he had been bled after the fashion of the Arabs during the agonal phase of the disease. Nicolaus Florenas, Vesalius' former professor of medicine at Louvain, requested his advice on which method of lancing was the correct one. Vesalius responded with a massive illustrated letter, dated Jan. 1, 1539, which was published in brochure form as the *Venesection Epistle*. Although he took a stand with the Hippocrates-Brissot camp, Vesalius insinuated that the raging dispute was ridiculous and irrelevant, since pleurisy occurred in a region drained by the vena cava. Mocking statements such as the following, however, served to throw his gauntlet into an arena from which he was never thereafter to extirpate himself fully:

> . . . . you know with what open variance, with what excited feelings and with what array of argument all the most learned authorities combat one another with regard to the particular vein to be opened in pleurisy—to such a degree that few doctors of any reputation can be found who have not undertaken to publish upon that subject some sample or other of their erudition, arousing against themselves very fierce rebukes from their opponents and very serious storms of ill-will. But let me pass over for the moment those argumentative persons who reject everything new, and, being eager to defend the heresy they have once imbibed, attack with the severest insults and abuse those who think a vein should be opened on the same side as that affected.
>
> I imagine that what I wrote some time ago about the Louvain doctors has not yet dropped out of your recollection. Among them was one, remarkably learned in his own opinion and self-satisfied because of his private wealth, who in a crowded assemblage was not ashamed to call Manardus, Fuchs, Curtius and Brissot the Luthers of Medicine. . . . Of course this reverend gentleman thought that those who were reclaiming Hippocrates' ancient system of healing . . . ought to be thus derided . . . while he, wise to himself alone . . . accuses them of heresy. . . .
>
> . . . if distance or nearness were the sole consideration of our discussion of cutting the elbow vein in cases of pleurisy, I should not consider it of the slightest importance whether I lanced a vein in one or the other elbow, no matter what part of the chest the inflammation attacked. Don't they then seem to you to be having a fine wrangle and to be barking like dogs at each other, while they reject that noble principle of Hippocrates regarding the alignment and continuity of the fibers? In fact, it has gone so far that in a public edict to those practising Medicine in Spain, venesection on the same side as that affected has been forbidden; for after long discussion held at Salamanca regarding this point, those who yielded complained to "the most illustrious Spanish Senate" (as you call it) that venesection on the same side causes not less harm to the human body than the Lutheran heresies to the human soul. . . .

The latter ukase was not surprising in Spain, where the dagger of the Inquisition was at the throat of all engaged in social and professional activities. Since Vesalius had inadvertently entered the fray, it might seem paradoxical that he would then consent, during 1541 and 1542, to editing the massive *Opera Galeni* being readied for publication by the famous printing firm of Giunta and Froben. Actually, this task enabled him to acquaint himself even more thoroughly with Galen's dogmas before launching his stupendous attack, in 1543, with the publication of his crowning achievement, the *Fabrica*. At the end of the introduction to the *Tabulae,* Vesalius had remarked, "If I shall find this work acceptable to you and to students, some day I hope to add something greater." Few, if any, had foreseen what the "something greater" was to be, as the indefatigable Vesalius labored incessantly for 5 years in the preparation of his opus magnum.

## PUBLICATION OF THE *FABRICA* AND *EPITOME*

Many consider that the *De Humani Corporis Fabrica* of Andreas Vesalius ushered in the era of modern medical science, and is the most momentous single contribution of the Christian era. In Osler's words, "The worth of a book, as of a man, must be judged by results, and so judged, the *Fabrica* is one of the great books of the world." It was to medical illustration what Da Vinci's "La Gioconda" represented to painting—an unexcelled masterpiece. In fact, the mystery of the identity of its artist has not been solved to this day. Its exquisite format and design and the creative artistry of its woodcuts have been ascribed variously to Campagnola, Vesalius himself, the celebrated Titian, or to one of his pupils, Kalkar.

The *Fabrica* was accompanied by an *Epitome* which, Vesalius explained, was "prepared as a pathway to these books and as an index of the things demonstrated in them." In other words, it was a small volume written in simpler style, and was intended to help orient readers before they sought to cope with the more advanced work. The 2 texts came as a peal of thunder heralding the Renaissance in medical science.

*The Fabric of the Human Body* was dedicated to Charles V. In the lengthy preface, which is partly autobiographical and gives insight into his masterful command of medicosociologic problems, Vesalius deplored the current state of decadence of the profession of surgery. He made it clear that his book was an attempt to rectify this lamentable condition by providing proper instruction to "those who practise medicine with the hands." Several passages in the introduction are indicative of this goal. The following one, of much historical interest, has seldom appeared in print:

> . . . . Although once upon a time three schools of doctors existed, namely the Logical, the Empirical and the Methodic, nevertheless the founders of these schools directed the aim of the art as a whole to the preservation of health and the elimination of diseases. In short, they referred to this end all the things which the individual men in their schools deemed necessary to their art, and they were accustomed to make use of three aids. Of these, the first was a rational plan of diet; the second, all the uses of drugs; the third, Surgery. The last shows with particular aptness that Medicine consists in the supplying of deficiencies and the removal of superfluities; and it ever stands ready for the cure of affections. Time and use have shown that, as often as we engage in medical work, Surgery is very helpful to the human race in its benefit to these affections.
>
> This three-fold scheme of doctoring was equally familiar to the doctors of each sect. The doctors themselves accommodated their own hands to curing in accordance with the nature of the affections; and they expended no less energy in training their hands than in the business of arranging the diet or of knowing and compounding drugs. For instance, over and above his other books, the volumes which the divine Hippocrates wrote on the Role of the Doctor, on the Fractures of Bones, on the Dislocations of Joints, and evils of this type—the best written of all his works—shows this clearly. . . .
>
> But no one of the ancients seems to have handed down to posterity with equal care the curing which is wrought by the hand and that which is accomplished by diet and medicines. After the devastation of the Goths particularly, when all the sciences, which had previously been so flourishing and had been properly practised, went to the dogs, the more elegant doctors at first in Italy in imitation of the ancient Romans began to be ashamed of working with their hands, and began to prescribe to their servants what operations they should perform upon the sick, and they merely stood alongside after the fashion of architects. When, soon, others also began to refuse the inconveniences of those practising true Medicine, meanwhile subtracting nothing from their profit and honor, they promptly fell away from the standards of the early doctors. They left the manner of cooking, and in fact the whole preparation, of the diet for the sick, to their attendants, and they left the composition of drugs to the vendors of medicines, and Surgery to the barbers. And so in the course of time the technique of curing was so wretchedly torn apart that the doctors, prostituting themselves under the names of "Physicians," appropriated to them-

selves simply the prescription of drugs and diets for unusual affections; but the rest of Medicine they relegated to those whom they call "Chirurgians" and deem as if they were mere servants. They shamefully reject that which is the principal and the most ancient branch of Medicine, the one which rests primarily upon the observation of Nature (if indeed it is anything else!). Yet this branch of Medicine even the kings in India practise today; and by the law of heredity in Persia they pass it all on to their children, as once the families of the Asclepiades did. The Thracians, along with many other peoples cultivate and venerate it. Although this art accomplishes absolutely nothing without the help of Nature, but rather desires to aid her as she works to free herself from disease; when a part of the art, which the Romans in times past have proscribed from the State as if designed to deceive and destroy men, has been almost wholly neglected, the result is that the utility of the art as a whole is removed and destroyed. To this primarily we owe the fact that this most sacred art is ridiculed, although many censures are normally cast at doctors anyway, since that part of the art which those educated in the liberal arts have shamefully allowed to be torn away is the part which permanently illuminates Medicine with its especial glory.

When Homer, the fount of talents, affirms that the medical man is more pre-eminent than many, and when he and the other Greek poets celebrate Podalirius and Machaon, these sons of the divine Aesculapius are not lauded because they did away with a little fever—which Nature alone cures more easily without the aid of a doctor than when the aid is applied—or because they humored the palate of men in peculiar and lamentable affections. They were celebrated because they were especially pre-eminent in the cure of hemorrhages, dislocations, fractures, contusions, wounds, and the other breaks in the continuity of the body. They freed the most noble soldiers of Agamemnon from arrow points, javelins, and other evils of this sort which are principally caused by wars and which demand the careful attention of the doctor.

But . . . I have in no manner proposed to exalt any one instrument of Medicine above the others, since the aforesaid three-fold method of help absolutely can not be disjoined and taken apart. The whole method belongs to one workman. To effect this synthesis properly, all the parts of Medicine should be constituted and prepared equally so that all the individual elements can be put to use more advantageously, and each element in turn unites all together more perfectly. . . . Therefore tyros in the art should be encouraged in all the methods, and, if it please the gods, scorning the whisperings of the "physicians," they should apply their hands likewise to curing in whatever manner the nature of the art and reason really demand, as the Greeks did. This they should do lest they turn mutilated Medicine to the destruction of the common life of man. And they must be encouraged in this more diligently in proportion as we see today that the men who are more thoroughly grounded in the art abstain from Surgery as from the plague. They are afraid that they will be traduced by the fanatics of the medical profession before the unlettered populace as "barbers." They also fear that afterwards they may not get half the profit, honor, or reputation in the eyes of either the unlearned mob or the leaders. This detestable opinion of many people in the first place keeps us from taking up the whole craft of healing; and when we arrogate to our selves only the cure of internal affections, we desire to be doctors only in a small way (to tell the truth for once!). The ensuing damage to mortals is great. . . .

One of the chapters of the *Fabrica* dealt with vivisection. In it may be found classical descriptions. There is a paragraph entitled "Examination of the recurrent nerves and the loss of voice from the cutting of them." Collapse of the lungs when the chest is punctured was discussed, together with the possibility of prolonging life for awhile by artificial respiration when the thorax is opened. That a heart which had almost stopped beating could be revived by the timely use of bellows was indicated, as well as the fact that an animal could live after removal of the spleen. Vesalius also demonstrated that it was the brain which governed motor activity of the trunk and limbs, and that the spinal cord served to relay this control.

Concerning the physiology of circulation, Vesalius might have conceivably anteceded Servetus and Harvey had he gone further than being content with casting this sarcastic barb at current dogma:

> The septum of the ventricles, composed as I have said of the thickest substance of the heart, abounds on both sides with little pits impressed in it. Of these pits, none, so far at least as can be perceived by the senses, penetrate through from the right into the left ventricle; so that we are driven to wonder at the handiwork of the Almighty, by means of which the blood sweats from the right into the left ventricle through passages which escape human vision.

The *Fabrica* was calculated to be a clarion

call freeing medicine from the fetters of Galenism, and Vesalius was unsparing in the use of vitriolic language. It was generally believed that an obscure bone in the body named "Luz" was the pivot point from which the human race was regenerated. Vesalius ground the mythical bone of Luz into dust with this acrimonious salvo:

> The dogma which asserts that man will be regenerated from this bone, of which we have just narrated the immense fiction, may be left for elucidation to those philosophers who reserve to themselves alone the right to free discussion and pronouncement on the resurrection and immortality of the soul. And even on their account we should attach no importance whatever to the miraculous and occult powers ascribed to the internal ossicle of the right great toe, however much one may be concerned about it. At our public dissections and even as an amateur, we have often obtained a better supply of these bones than those truculent male strumpets of the Venetian horde, who, to obtain the bone for purposes of comparison, as also the heart of an unpolluted male infant, lately killed a child, cut the heart from its living body, and were punished, as they richly deserved for the foulest of crimes. Moreover, this ossicle, called Albadaran by the Arabs and the truly occult and obscure philosophers alluded to, is less known to actual students of anatomy than to certain superstitious men who are capable of likening the fourth carpal bone to a chickpea.

Vesalius was also unflinching in acknowledging no authority except what his senses perceived. He dismissed Galen with acerbity, stating that his predecessor "was cheated by his monkeys in the manifold divergence of the human body from that of monkeys. He hardly noticed anything different except in the fingers and the bend at the knee."

All this was not only phenomenal audacity, coming from a 29-year-old youth, but was tantamount to overt sacrilege. In those days, the appropriate theocratic penalties for blasphemers were blazing faggots or the rack. Servetus had already been immolated at the stake. Vesalius was spared this fate, however, just as Paré was to escape the St. Bartholomew's Eve massacre, only because of royal patronage and intercession. Repercussions of other sorts, nevertheless, were not long in coming fast and furiously.

## SEQUELAE OF THE *FABRICA*

Sylvius, Vesalius' former teacher at Paris, soon unleashed a tirade of vilification. His tract was entitled "A repudiation of the calumnies of a certain madman, Vaesanus, concerning Hippocratic and Galenic anatomy, by Jacobus Sylvius, the Royal Interpreter of things medical at Paris." The play on the name "Vaesanus," similar to "Vesalius," was deliberate invective, and no typographical error. "Vaesanus" is a Latin word signifying "a two-legged ass." Sylvius was appalled at the use of illustrations which went so far as to reveal unmentionable portions of the human body. After all, he argued, "Galen did not allow even plants to be depicted." He petitioned Charles V to either castigate Vesalius or have him recant:

> I implore his Majesty the Emperor to punish severely, as he deserves, this monster born and reared in his own home, this most pernicious exemplar of ignorance, ingratitude, and impiety; and to suppress him completely, lest he poison the rest of Europe with his pestilential breath. With his deadly spume, he has already infected certain Frenchmen, Germans, and Italians; but they, I believe, are ignorant of anatomy and of the other branches of Medicine. . . .

The above, multiplied severalfold, is a sample of the barrage of opposition which Vesalius faced from certain quarters until almost the closing years of his life. A brief respite from his detractors occurred with the declaration of hostilities against France in 1544. During this short-lived foray, Vesalius served in the field in the capacity of Imperial Surgeon. As in the case of many other illustrious surgeons, war supplied a proving-ground for his teachings, and honed his skill in applying them to the razor edge of experience. It also marked the end of his academic career as an anatomist.

At the Siege of Saint-Dizier, in the Marne Valley, Vesalius operated on the Prince of Orange-Chalon, who had a fatal wound of the shoulder. Outside the walls of Vitry, he treated the Lord of Aluhin and several other officers who had been mortally injured by flaming cannon-balls. By a remarkable coincidence, the Royal Physician attached to the opposition forces was Ambroise Paré, who was rapidly gaining stature as the most ingenious surgeon in Europe. These two surgical peers, foes only through military exigency, nevertheless displayed professional gallantry. Paré introduced and popularized the *Fabrica* among the French intelligentsia by abstracting it in the vernacular. Vesalius, in turn, attempted on a certain Captain Solis disarticulation at the elbow, an operation developed originally by Paré. However, in this campaign, Vesalius still employed boiling oil, while Paré was already discarding this barbaric practice after disproving that gunshot wounds were poisonous. In September, 1544, the Peace of Crespy was signed, and Vesalius, not yet 30, returned to Court as personal physician and surgeon to the Emperor and his entourage.

## VESALIUS BURNS HIS NOTES

While at Court, Vesalius also conducted postmortem examinations and embalmings on members of the nobility as a prelude to burial with pomp. His acumen in surgical pathology, then a neglected study, was brought into the open by the publication in 1546 of a series of communications under the title, *The China-Root Epistle,* after one section dealing with the use of a variety of sarsaparilla against diverse afflictions. In the very last chapter of this publication, Vesalius gave indication of the immense despondency and chagrin which had befallen him after the initial adverse reception and spoliation of the *Fabrica.* In utter disgust and anguish, he had impulsively made a sacrificial pyre of his accumulated documents!

> As to my notes, which had grown into a huge volume, they were all destroyed by me; and on the same day there similarly perished the whole of my paraphrase of the ten books of Rhazes to King Almansor, composed by me with far more care than the "Paraphrasis" which I published on the ninth book. With these also went the books of some author or other on the formula and preparation of medicines, to which I had added much matter of my own that I judged to be not without utility; and the same fate overtook all the books of Galen which I had used in learning anatomy, and which I had liberally disfigured in the usual fashion. I was on the point of leaving Italy and going to Court; those physicians of whom you know had given the Emperor and the nobles a most unfavorable report of my books and of all that is published nowadays for the promotion of study; I therefore burnt all these works mentioned, thinking at the same time it would be an easy matter to abstain from writing for the future. I have since repented more than once of my impatience, and regretted that I did not take the advice of the friends who were then with me.

## WAR, AGAIN, AND THE *CONSILIA*

In the cockpit of Europe, battles were ignited for the slightest real or imagined wrong. In 1546, a civil war against the Lutheran princes of the Smalkaldic League was sparked, and flared into the conflagration that Luther had prophesied on his deathbed. Vesalius' skill in surgical operations was augmented by a wealth of material. Descriptions of his procedures have survived through the writings of eyewitnesses or professional contemporaries such as Daza Chacon and Ingrassia.

Vesalius was the first to perform a deliberate operation for osteomyelitis of the distal part of the femur, and was duly censured for this unheard-of temerity. He modified and reintroduced with success the long-abandoned Hippocratic operation of thoracentesis for empyema. He was called on to incise the foot of the Cardinal of Trent, a very particular distinction for one who had clashed with established theologic tenets. He caused an immense sensation by correctly diagnosing, and predicting the exact hour of death and autopsy findings, of the Count Maximilian of Buren, who perished as a result of an extensive mediastinal abscess from quinsy. He cured the Marquis of Velena of a chronic fistula of the chest wall ensuing from a poorly-treated empyema.

It was customary then, as now, to seek in consultation prominent surgeons for difficult cases. Written consultations, or "consilia" as they were called, were not infrequently published. Only 6 of Vesalius' *Consilia* have been preserved. The third consilium was a retort to an enquiry regarding the treatment to be employed in the case of Don Carlos of Aragon, the Duke of

Terranova, who, during a tournament, had incurred a broken rib with penetration of the left hemithorax. Vesalius' detailed description of the operation for empyema is a remarkably lucid piece of thoracic surgical literature. He quoted 4 recent instances in which he had performed the operation; 3 of the patients had recovered completely. In 1 case, he pointed out, the scapula had been perforated by the weapon, so that a different approach to the abscess had had to be employed. The fifth consilium consisted of an aggregate of letters on the surgical management of phlegmons and ulcers. In it is reported a successful operation on Chancellor Granvelle, a Knight of the Golden Fleece and the most powerful personage at Court next to the Emperor, which reveals what favor Vesalius' surgical prowess must have enjoyed.

In 1555, Charles V, who was ill of health, abdicated. He was replaced by the supercilious and insipid Philip II of Spain, whose only fame rested on his marriage to the daughter of the King of France which terminated Franco-Hispanic hostilities. The royal betrothal took place in 1559 with great éclat, including royal jousting. Henry II, the French monarch, participated in a tourney, and was struck above the right eye by a broken lance. The most important doctors of the realm were summoned immediately. In this retinue were Vesalius and the now celebrated Ambroise Paré, neither of whom was able to forestall the eventual fatal outcome. As foreseen by Vesalius, death resulted from subdural hemorrhage, the possibility of which had been discounted by the other physicians because of the absence of obvious skull fracture.

## THE ROAD TO ZANTE

In 1562, the pathetic Infante Don Carlos struck the back of his head in a fall. Vesalius advised trephining, but was repulsed as a meddling alien by the royal surgeons of Spain, to which Philip had transferred his court. Instead, all sorts of religious relics and amulets, including the disintegrated corpse of a monk who had been idolized for

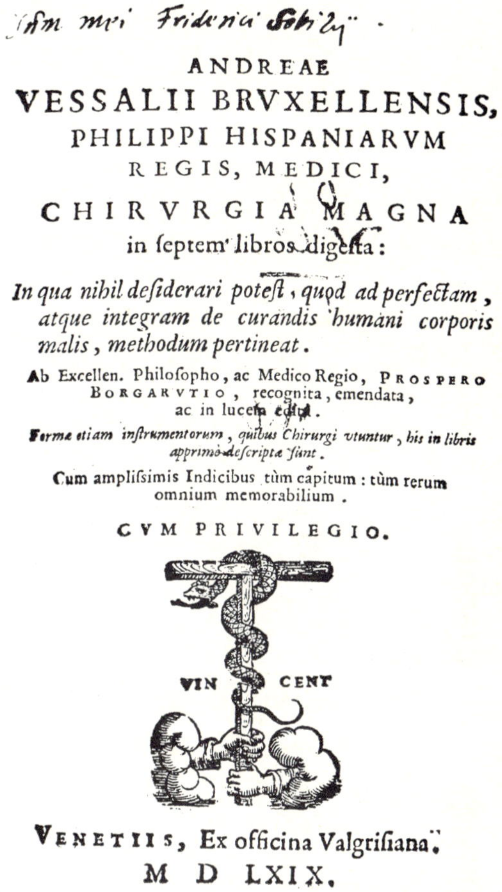
ANDREAE
VESSALII BRVXELLENSIS,
PHILIPPI HISPANIARVM
REGIS, MEDICI,
CHIRVRGIA MAGNA
in septem libros digesta:

*In qua nihil desiderari potest, quod ad perfectam, atque integram de curandis humani corporis malis, methodum pertineat.*

Ab Excellen. Philosopho, ac Medico Regio, PROSPERO BORGARVTIO, recognita, emendata, ac in lucem edita.

*Formæ etiam instrumentorum, quibus Chirurgi utuntur, his in libris apprimè descriptæ sunt.*

Cum amplissimis Indicibus tùm capitum: tùm rerum omnium memorabilium.

CVM PRIVILEGIO.

VIN [illegible] CENT

VENETIIS, Ex officina Valgrisiana.
M D LXIX.

Fig. 1. Title page of the original *Surgery* of Vesalius, published in 1569, 5 years after his death, by a student, Prospero Borgarutius.

his holiness, were placed on the bed of the gravely sick prince. Finally, at the insistence of Vesalius, these grisly proceedings were discontinued, and incisions were made into the scalp to evacuate considerable amounts of pus. The boy recovered, and later shed a sequestrum from the diseased bone.

Because he had unavoidably humbled the bigoted and fanatical coterie of Iberian physicians, Vesalius' life in cleric-ridden Spain was thereafter made unbearable, and he was snubbed and rebuffed at every excuse. But in other more enlightened parts of the Continent, Vesalius was gaining staunch supporters every day. The last work he authored before his death was a reply to the *Observationes Anatomicae* of Gabriel Fallopius, one of his most zealous adherents,

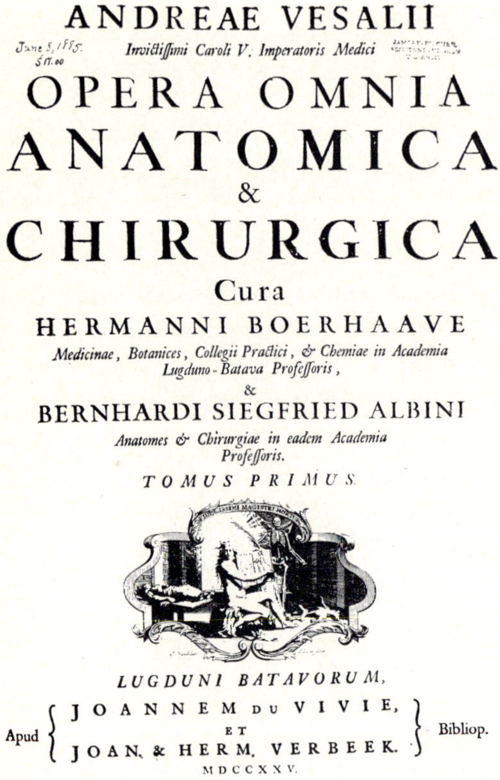
ANDREAE VESALII

*Invictissimi Caroli V. Imperatoris Medici*

OPERA OMNIA

ANATOMICA

&

CHIRURGICA

Cura

HERMANNI BOERHAAVE

*Medicinae, Botanices, Collegii Practici, & Chemiae in Academia Lugduno-Batava Professoris,*

&

BERNHARDI SIEGFRIED ALBINI

*Anatomes & Chirurgiae in eadem Academia Professoris.*

*TOMUS PRIMUS.*

*LUGDUNI BATAVORUM,*

Apud { JOANNEM DU VIVIE, ET JOAN. & HERM. VERBEEK. } Bibliop.

MDCCXXV.

**Fig. 2.** Edition of 1725 by Boerhaave, combining the *Fabrica* and *Chirurgia.* Observe the notation indicating that this 1156-page tome was purchased in 1885 for $17.00.

who made reference in his book about "the divine Vesalius." To this kindred spirit, Vesalius imparted his deep learning to be rid of the intolerable life in Spain, and to return to an academic atmosphere:

> I sincerely hope that you may long maintain this purpose in that sweet leisure of letters which is yours, and in that throng of learned men whose studies are dear to their hearts and with whom you can daily compare the concepts of your mind. For I feel that the ornaments of our art originate in that arena from which as a young man I was diverted to the mechanical practice of Medicine, to numerous wars, and to continuous travels . . . therefore continue to embellish with the fruits of your talents and industry our common school, whose memory is most dear to me.

Shortly after writing this commentary, which he was never to see in print, Vesalius left Madrid, ostensibly for a pilgrimage to the Holy Land. The circumstances of his voyage and death have been the objects of analysis and conjecture for centuries. None appears to be fully reliable, and the reader may draw his own conclusions as he sees fit from the bulky literature on this final facet of Vesalius' life. In any case, the road ended at Zante, in a lonely and unbefitting grave.

## THE *CHIRURGIA*

The largest of Vesalius' surgical works was published posthumously under the heading *Chirurgia Magna in Septum Libros Digesta.* The manuscript of notes on surgery by Vesalius for a book he was apparently meditating fell into the hands of a Parisian bookseller. A student and devotee of Vesalius, one Prospero Borgarutius, obtained possession of the manuscript, appended notes which he had taken during lectures by his professor, and published the book at his own expense in 1569. There is a recital of this story in the preface, in which Borgarutius also explains rather eloquently the reasons why he keenly believed the surgical teachings of Vesalius should be preserved:

> Because of this factor it happened that after Hippocrates, Galen, Avicenna, Celsus, and many others of the same type, Andreas Vesalius of Brussels, at one time physician to the King, and a Caesarine, had shown many new things. Some of these are known. Others, because of his untimely death, would be therefore buried, unless they should be published by the industry of someone, especially one of the number that had the greatest opportunity of study with him. Since I, especially, am of this number, and since I understand that he was the personification of a kindly heart (and if anyone loves such a one let him desire his immortality), and as I have realized how much I have been forwarded by the great name of Vesalius whom I have always obeyed as if there were the power of God in this human; therefore, I have always avowed this by the immortal gods, that should the opportunity at any time offer itself to me by which I might show the incredible benevolence of that great man, I would follow him by that opportunity most diligently.

Borgarutius' gesture of gratitude was admirable; but, in his reverence for Vesalius, he seemingly deemed it unbecoming to make any changes whatsoever in the manuscript. The lack of conscientious editing, a task at which Vesalius was expert, is glaring in the text. It is more of an uncut precious stone than the finished polished jewel. These imperfections have led some Vesalian venerators to dismiss the book as spurious, so that it has received negligible study compared to the other works. Such an a priori judgment has been, in our opinion, too hasty, because many portions of the book bear the unmistakable stamp of Vesalius. To question its authenticity would be the equivalent of rejecting the notes on surgery of John Hunter merely because they were compiled by Everard Home and others.

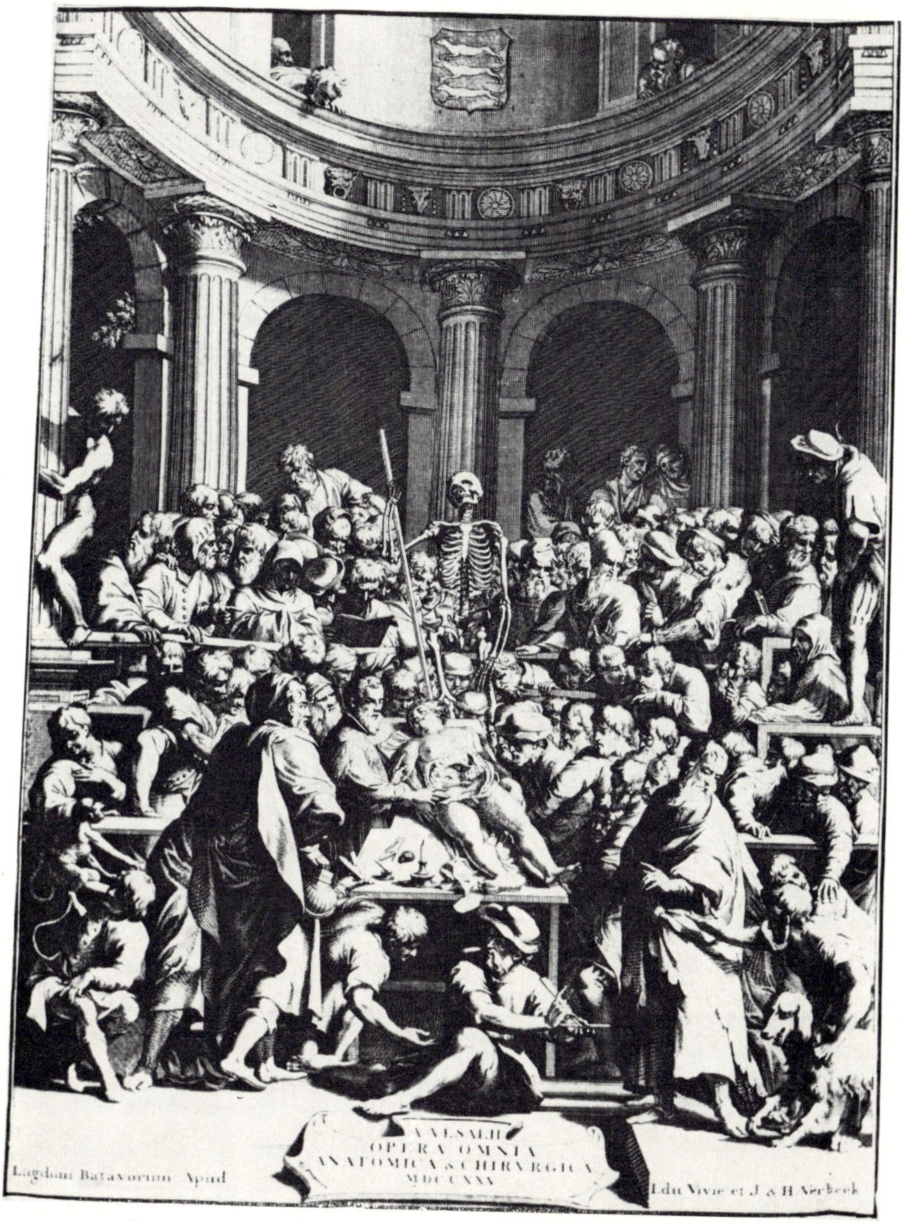


**Fig. 3.** Frontispiece of the 1725 edition is a facsimile of the one in the original *Fabrica* except for a few minor changes. The shield at the top is replaced by the Vesalian coat of arms depicting 3 weasels, a pun Vesalius employed regarding the sources of his name. The colophon at the bottom of the page has been modified to indicate inclusion of the *Chirurgia*.

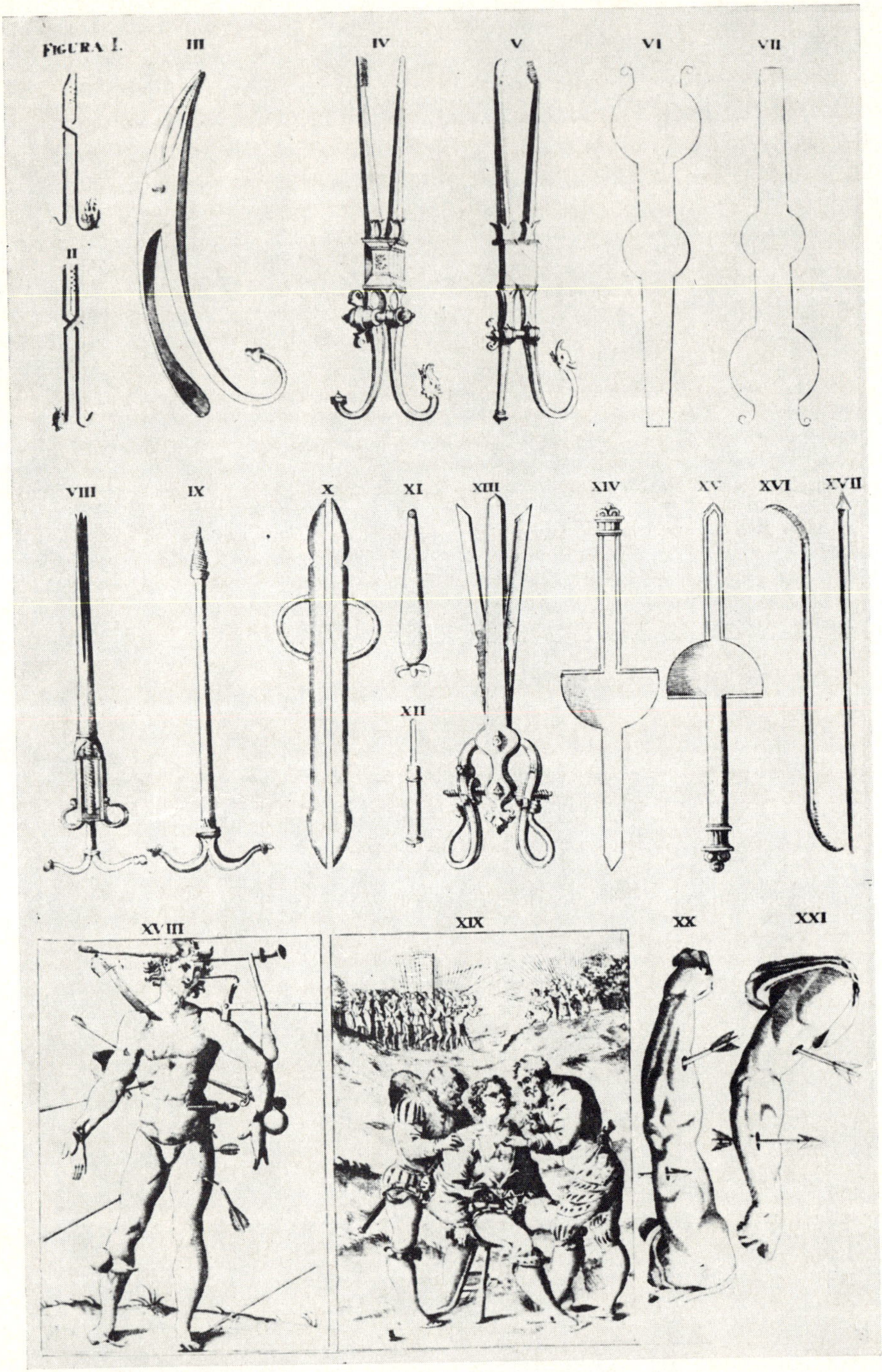


**Fig. 4.** Illustrations in the *Chirurgia* are reproductions from other contemporary surgical texts. Fig. XVIII is from Gerssdorff, and depicts the zodiacal "wound man." Fig. XIX, after Brunschiwig, shows extraction of a bullet ("quomodo plumbeus globus immissus extrahatur").

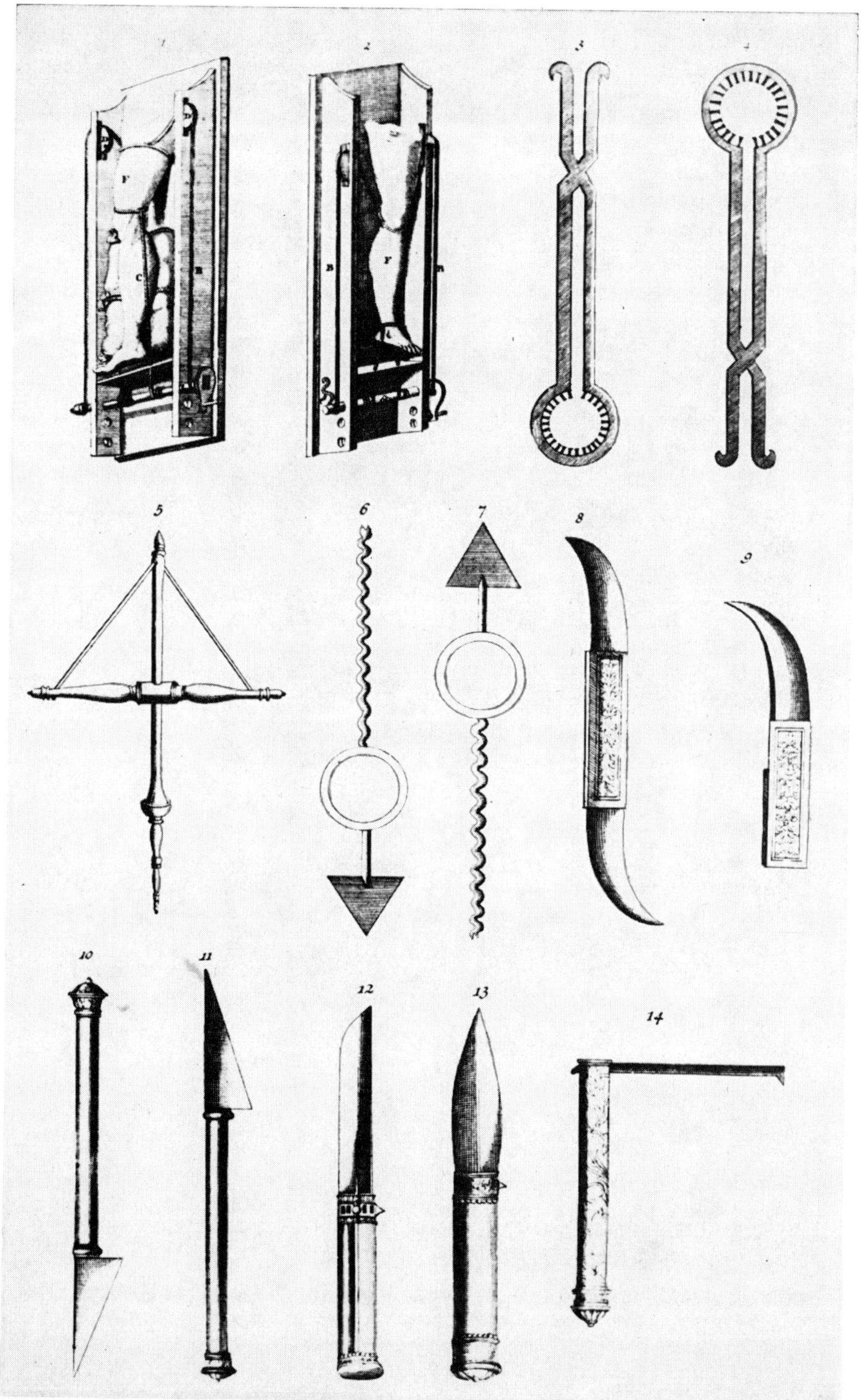


**Fig. 5.** More illustration replicas in the *Chirurgia*. Figs. 1 and 2 are copied from Tagault. The others show trephine apparatus, forceps, scalpels, lancets, and an instrument used for phlebotomy.

The book, 475 pages long, is divided into 7 parts, as its title indicates; first, dislocations; second, fractures; third, wounds; fourth, ulcers; fifth, neoplasms; sixth, an antidotary; and seventh, the manner of use of medicaments in surgical conditions. Before each of the surgical maladies, properly called, there is an anatomic résumé of each region. ("No anatomist, no surgeon." Vesalius was adamant on this point.) There is a paucity of illustrations, and the ones included are all facsimilies from the surgical texts of other authors. Since the printing press of Valgrisius, which produced this volume, was the same one which printed one of the editions of Tagault's *De Chirurg Institutione,* it is not surprising that the works of the 2 surgeons are typographically twin books. Of interest in the chapter on tumors is Vesalius' differentiation between "occult" and surface scirrhi, and his advocacy of surgical excision in mammary carcinoma, a truly avant-garde position at a time when the cautery was in vogue for this disease.

In the introduction to the *Chirurgia,* there is a discussion of the Art of Healing in general, its end, its means, and distinctions between the role of surgeons and that of other members of the profession. In the second chapter, Vesalius traces a portrait of the ideal surgeon, the words of which have the same cogency as when they were put on paper:

> It is necessary that the surgeon should have practised for a long time upon the cadaver; that he should be a profound observer; that he should follow the precepts of the best masters; that he should be patient and laborious; above all the friend of truth; upright and conscientious; that he should refrain from touching incurable cases which present no chance of healing; that he should be temperate, disinterested, affable, and of easy access with his colleagues; and, finally, that he should be young or of age of virile force when the hand is firm and light, the eye quick; that he should be bold and pitiless when the well-being or safety of his patient is involved.

One of the illustrations in the *Fabrica* bears the legend, "Vivitur ingenio, caetera mortis erunt" ("Genius endures. All else is mortal.") Carved in bold letters on the rock at Zante, this would be an appropriate epitaph for the great surgeon named Andreas Vesalius.

The authors are indebted to Miss Eleanor Safstorm, Chief Librarian of the Denver Medical Society, for her loan of the priceless old manuscripts employed in the preparation of this essay.

# Index to volume 50

## Author index

A


ABBOTT, A. C., GOODHAND, T. K., McCORD, W. J., AND MACDOUGALL, J. T. Observations on the isolated ileal loop as a substitute in urinary tract operations, 467
ABSOLON, KAREL B. The surgical school of Theodor Billroth, 697
AFFIFI, RASHEED. (*See* Welch et al.), 390
AGOSTINO, DOMENICO. (*See* Cliffton and Agostino), 395
ALICAN, FIKRI. (*See* Hardy and Alican), 107
ANYLAN, WILLIAM G. (*See* Weaver et al.), 207
APPLEN, JOHN E., LERMAN, GEORGE S., AND WALKER, PAUL E. Measurement of arterial flow in the lower extremities with radioisotopes, 315
ARHELGER, STUART W. (*See* Griffen et al.), 458
AUSMAN, ROBERT K. (*See* Humphrey et al.), 881


B


BAIRD, R. J. (*See* Mustard et al.), 301
BAPTISTA, A. M. (*See* Clode et al.), 725
BARNARD, C. N. (*See* Terblanche et al.), 869
BARRY, KEVIN G., COHEN, ARTHUR, AND LEBLANC, PRESTON. Mannitolization. I. The prevention and therapy of oliguria associated with cross-clamping of the abdominal aorta, 335
BASCOM, JOHN U. Gelatin sealing to prevent blood loss from knitted arterial grafts, 504
BASTO, E. LIMA. (*See* Clode et al.), 725
BEAL, JOHN M. (*See* Moody et al.), 540
BEARDSLEY, J. MURRAY. Technique in resection of esophageal diverticulum, 747
BELL, J. W. (*See* Strandness et al.), 488
BERMAN, EDWARD J. (*See* Lalonde and Berman), 962
BERNHARD, WILLIAM F., SCHWARZ, HANS F., LEAND, PAUL M., AND CARR, JAMES G. Studies in balanced hypothermic perfusion, 911



July, pp. 1-300; August, pp. 301-436; September, pp. 437-578; October, pp. 579-724; November, pp. 725-862; December, pp. 863-1004.



BESSMAN, SAMUEL P., RUDO, FRIEDA, AND COWLEY, R ADAMS. The relation of blood pH to the movement of ammonia into cerebral and peripheral tissues during hypothermia, 478
BILISOLY, FRANK N. (*See* Devine et al.), 419
BLAISDELL, F. WILLIAM, AND GAUDER, PETER J. Paradoxical variation of the femoral pulse in occlusion of the iliac artery, 529
BLALOCK, JOHN C. (*See* Menguy and Blalock), 877
BOLEY, SCOTT J., McKINNON, WILLIAM M. P., AND MARZULLI, VINCENT F. The management of familial gastrointestinal polyposis involving stomach and colon, 691
—, —, AND WRIGHT, ARTHUR R. Surgical fact or fancy. I. Fate of cholecystojejunostomy in the absence of common bile duct obstruction, 676
BORMES, WILLIAM A., GORMAN, WILLIAM C., KAYSER, KENNETH L., AND LEPLEY, DERWARD, JR. The identification of the conduction system of the heart by audiofrequency conductimetry, 50
BRADHAM, R. R. (*See* Lee et al.), 812
BRENNAN, TIMOTHY A. (*See* McCarthy et al.), 740
BURKE, JOHN F. The effective period of preventive antibiotic action in experimental incisions and dermal lesions, 161
BUTZ, GEORGE W., JR. (*See* Starzl et al.), 849


C


CALEM, WILLIAM S., AND FREUND, H. ROBERT. Subglottic carcinoma with extensive tracheal involvement, 894
CAMPANALE, RALPH P., AND GARDNER, BERNARD. "Fore and aft" split pancreaticojejunostomy for chronic pancreatitis, 618
CAMPANIS, N. (*See* Chrysospathis et al.), 922
CARR, JAMES G. (*See* Bernhard et al.), 911
CHANG, K. H. RONALD, AND NIGUIDULA, FAUSTINO N. Metastatic malignant schwannoma with bilateral pulmonary resection, 749
CHEUNG, CHE-SUN. (*See* Rush et al), 359
CHIECHI, MICHELE A. (*See* DeWall et al.), 931
CHILD, CHARLES G., III. (*See* Wolfman et al.), 231

Chrysospathis, P., Louis, H., and Campanis, N. Reconstruction after total gastrectomy, 922
Chung, W., and Šima, V. Renal tubular necrosis: its relation to norepinephrine administration, 328
Clagett, O. Theron. (*See* Engel et al.), 593
—. (*See* Moersch and Clagett), 579
Clarke, R. L. (*See* Cliffton et al.), 644
Clarkson, Bayard. (*See* Lawrence et al.), 248
Classen, Kenneth L., Wiederanders, R. F., and Herrington, J. Lynwood, Jr. Clinical and experimental observations on heterotopic osseous formation in abdominal wall scars, 824
Cliffton, Eugene E., and Agostino, Domenico. Cancer cells in the blood in simulated colon cancer, resectable and unresectable: effect of fibrinolysin and heparin on growth potential, 395
—, Clarke, R. L., and Murphy, J. Studies on fibrinolytic activity with venous occlusion: treatment of thrombophlebitis, 644
—, Grossi, Carlo E., and Esakof, Ernest R. Management of pulmonary complications of surgical operations (primarily atelectasis) with pancreatic dornase inhalations, 176
Clode, W. H., Sobral, J. M. V., Basto, E. Lima, and Baptista, A. M. Elective uptake of radioiodine by cancer of the stomach, 725
Cockett, Abraham T. K. The kidney and regional hypothermia, 905
Cohen, Arthur. (*See* Barry et al.), 335
Coil, James A. (*See* Davis and Coil), 169
Cole, Donald R. (*See* Rousselot and Cole), 639
Condie, John D., and Ferguson, Donald J. Experimental wound infections: contamination versus surgical technique, 367
Connaughton, Peter J., Holt, Gordon, and Lewis, F. John. Prolonged hypothermia below 25° C. for periods over 20 hours: influence of therapy and technique on survival, 372
Cook, Galen B., and Margulis, Alexander R. The silicone-foam diagnostic enema. I. An assessment with surgical specimens of human sigmoid colon, 513
— and —. The silicone-foam diagnostic enema. II. An experimental evaluation in dogs, 519
Cooper, Philip. Duodenal closure after gastrectomy for duodenal ulcer, 425
Cooper, Theodore, Morrow, Andrew G., Roberts, William C., and Herman, Lloyd G. Postoperative endocarditis due to Candida: clinical observations and the experimental production of the lesion, 341
Cowley, R Adams. (*See* Bessman et al.), 478
Cuthbertson, Alan M. (*See* Humphries et al.), 947
Czaplicki, Jeremi. An attempt at development of agammaglobulinemia in adult rats by treatment with an extract of the fetal thymus, 817

D

Daggett, Ronald L. (*See* Gott et al.), 382
Dahl, Elmer V., Edwards, Eric C., Grindlay, John H., and Edwards, Jesse E. Effect of removal of adventitia from arteries: an experimental study, 533
Davenport, C. (*See* Lee et al.), 812
Daviglus, George F. (*See* Rush et al.), 359
Davis, John H., and Coil, James A. Studies of surgically induced pyelonephritis, 169
De Bakey, Michael. (*See* Wesolowski et al.), 91
De Castro Silva, Luciano, São Thiago, João Baptista, Ferrarini, Ermettis, and Goffi, Fábio Schmidt. The percutaneous transhepatic approach of the portal vein in man in the determination of patency of splenorenal shunts, 473
De Forest, Margie. (*See* Weatherley-White et al.), 784
Degenshein, George A., and Hurwitz, Alfred. An intimate view of the Letheon controversy, 716
Del Guercio, Louis R. M. (*See* Sabga et al.), 547
DeLuca, Frank G., and Swenson, Orvar. The use of fascial grafts in experimental bladder wall defects: preliminary report on application in the repair of exstrophy of the bladder, 404
Dennis, Clarence, and Karlson, Karl E. Cancer risk in ulcerative colitis: formidability per patient-year of late disease, 568
Derrick, John R. A technique of attaching a synthetic graft to the side of a severely arteriosclerotic aorta, 782
Deterling, Ralph A., Jr. Review of Meeting of Society of University Surgeons, 299
—. (*See* Nabseth and Deterling), 347
Devine, Patrick C., Bilisoly, Frank N., and Smith, E. Ide. Surgical treatment of bowel and bladder dysfunction in a case of spina bifida with meningomyelocele, 419
Devloo, Robert A. (*See* Kirklin et al.), 58
DeWall, Richard A., Grage, Theodor B., McFee, Arthur S., and Chiechi, Michele A. Theme and variations on blood oxygenators. I. Bubble oxygenators, 931

DRAPANAS, THEODORE, AND McDONALD, JOHN. Peritoneal tap in abdominal trauma, 742
DUVAL, MERLIN K., JR., AND ENQUIST, IRVING F. The surgical treatment of chronic pancreatitis by pancreaticojejunostomy: an 8-year reappraisal, 965
DYSON, BURTON C. Periductal mastitis associated with reticulum-cell sarcoma in the breast, 634

E

EALES, L. (*See* Terblanche et al.), 869
EDWARDS, ERIC C. (*See* Dahl et al.), 533
EDWARDS, JESSE E. (*See* Dahl et al.), 533
EGERTON, WILLIAM S. (*See* Kay et al.), 67
EISEMAN, BEN. (*See* Silen and Eiseman), 213
ELLIOTT, DAN W., TAFT, DAVID A., PASSARO, EDWARD, JR., AND ZOLLINGER, ROBERT M. Pancreatic influences on gastric secretions, 126
ELLIS, F. HENRY, JR. (*See* Payne et al.), 731
EMERY, J. L., AND HILTON, H. B. Lung and heart complications of the treatment of hydrocephalus by ventriculoauriculostomy, 309
ENGEL, STEPHEN, CLAGETT, O. THERON, AND HARRISON, EDGAR G., JR. Chylous cysts of the abdomen, 593
ENQUIST, IRVING F. (*See* DuVal and Enquist), 965
—. (*See* Rosen and Enquist), 525
ERICSSON, N. O., RUDHE, ULF, AND LIVADITIS, ALEX. Hydronephrosis associated with aberrant renal vessels in infants and children, 687
ESAKOF, ERNEST R. (*See* Cliffton et al.), 176

F

FEDOR, E. J. (*See* Fisher et al.), 758
FEKETE, F. (*See* Lortat-Jacob et al.), 600
FELTS, JOHN H. (*See* Whitley et al.), 673
FERGUSON, DONALD J. (*See* Condie and Ferguson), 367
—. (*See* Humphrey et al.), 881
FERRARINI, ERMETTIS. (*See* De Castro Silva et al.), 473
FINBERG, LAURENCE (*See* Rush et al.), 359
FISHBEIN, RONALD. (*See* Rush et al.), 40
FISHER, BERNARD. (*See* Lee and Fisher), 668
—, FEDOR, E. J., AND SMITH, J. W. Temperature gradients associated with extracorporeal perfusion and profound hypothermia, 758
—, AND FISHER, EDWIN R. Experimental studies of factors which influence hepatic metastases. VIII. Effect of anticoagulants, 240
FISHER, EDWIN R. (*See* Fisher and Fisher), 240
FONKALSRUD, ERIC W. (*See* Lee et al.), 29
—, AND LONGMIRE, WILLIAM P., JR. The occurrence of pancreatic antibodies and the experimental production of pancreatitis with pancreatic antiserum, 134
FOSTER, J. H. (*See* Symbas et al.), 97
FRANCIS, G. J. (*See* Harrison et al.), 151
FRAWLEY, THOMAS F. (*See* Hernandez et al.), 143
FREUND, H. ROBERT. (*See* Calem and Freund), 894
FRICK, M. H., VIRKKULA, L., AND PAASONEN, M. K. 5-Hydroxytryptamine and antidiuresis after operation, 447
FRIES, CHARLES C. (*See* Wesolowski et al.), 91
FRIOU, GEORGE J. (*See* Gowen and Friou), 919

G

GAGNER, PHILIP L. (*See* McCarthy et al.), 740
GARDNER, BERNARD. (*See* Campanale and Gardner), 618
GAUDER, PETER J. (*See* Blaisdell and Gauder), 529
GILLESBY, WILLIAM J., AND PUESTOW, CHARLES B. Pancreaticojejunostomy for chronic relapsing pancreatitis: an evaluation, 859
GOFFI, FÁBIO SCHMIDT. (*See* De Castro Silva et al.), 473
GOOD, ROBERT A. (*See* Pierce et al.), 186
GOODHAND, T. K. (*See* Abbott et al.), 467
GORMAN, WILLIAM C. (*See* Bormes et al.), 50
GOTT, VINCENT L., KOEPKE, DONALD E., DAGGETT, RONALD L., ZARNSTORFF, WILLIAM, AND YOUNG, WILLIAM P. The coating of intravascular plastic prostheses with colloidal graphite, 382
GOWEN, GEORGE F., AND FRIOU, GEORGE J. The influence of hypothermia on experimental bacteremia in dogs, 919
GRAGE, THEODOR B. (*See* DeWall et al.), 931
—, LOBER, PAUL H., AND SHAHON, DONALD B. Benign tumors of the major salivary glands, 625
GRANT, RICHARD L. Antyllus, the elusive surgical genius of antiquity: an analysis of his writings, 572
GREENLAW, ROBERT H. (*See* Schwartz and Greenlaw), 833
GREGG, DONALD E. (*See* Hall et al.), 560
GRIFFEN, WARD O., JR., JENSON, CONRAD B., ARHELGER, STUART W., AND WANGENSTEEN, OWEN H. Treatment of malignant retroperitoneal sarcomas with use of the second-look approach, 458
—. (*See* Santoro et al.), 354
GRINDLAY, JOHN H. (*See* Dahl et al.), 533
GROSSI, CARLO E. (*See* Cliffton et al.), 176

H

HALL, ROBERT J., KHOURI, EDWARD M., AND GREGG, DONALD E. Coronary–internal mammary artery anastomosis in dogs, 560
HARDY, JAMES D., AND ALICAN, FIKRI. Ischemic gangrene without major organic vascular occlusion: an enlarging concept, 107
HARRISON, EDGAR G., JR. (*See* Engel et al.), 593
HARRISON, R. C., WILLIAMS, H. T. G., PISESKY, W., HUSAIN, S., SILBERMANN, O. H., FRANCIS, G. J., AND IRVINE, J. W. The relative importance of the vagus nerve, antrum, and acid-secreting mucosa in the prevention of experimental peptic ulceration, 151
HARTMAN, CHARLES F. (*See* Starzl et al.), 849
HAWK, WILLIAM A. (*See* Humphries et al.), 947
HAYS, DANIEL M., AND POWELL, TRACY, O. Vesicoileosigmoidostomy in the treatment of exstrophy of the bladder, 411
HEALEY, WILLIAM V. (*See* Wangensteen et al.), 651
HENRY, JAMES W. (*See* Nelson et al.), 115
HERMAN, LLOYD G. (*See* Cooper et al.), 341
HERINGMAN, E. CRAIG. (*See* Shore and Heringman), 612
HERNANDEZ, IVAN A., POWERS, SAMUEL R., JR., AND FRAWLEY, THOMAS F. The role of the parathyroid glands in calcium and magnesium metabolism in acute hemorrhagic pancreatitis, 143
HERRINGTON, J. LYNWOOD, JR. (*See* Classen et al.), 824
HILAL, SADEK. (*See* Longerbeam et al.), 274
HILTON, H. B. (*See* Emery and Hilton), 309
HINDBERG, JÖRGEN, NAKAMOTO, SATORU, AND KOLFF, WILLEM J. Anuria after operation for abdominal aortic aneurysm treated by hemodialysis with complete recovery, 755
HOLT, GORDON. (*See* Connaughton et al.), 372
HOLT, MARSH H. A simple cooling device for treatment of upper gastrointestinal bleeding, 728
HOVNANIAN, H. PHILIP. (*See* McCarthy et al.), 740
HUDSON, THOMAS L. (*See* Spencer and Hudson), 678
HUME, D. H. (*See* Zukoski et al.), 926
HUMPHREY, EDWARD W., HYMES, ALAN C., AUSMAN, ROBERT K., AND FERGUSON, DONALD J. An evaluation of actinomycin D and mitomycin C in patients with advanced cancer, 881
HUMPHRIES, ALFRED W., HAWK, WILLIAM A., AND CUTHBERTSON, ALAN M. Arterial prosthesis of collagen-impregnated Dacron tulle, 947
HURLEY, EDWARD J. (*See* Lower et al.), 842
HURWITZ, ALFRED. (*See* Degenshein and Hurwitz), 716
HUSAIN, S. (*See* Harrison et al.), 151
HYMES, ALAN C. (*See* Humphrey et al.), 881

I

INOKUCHI, KIYOSHI, KONISHI, TETSURO, YAGI, HIROSHI, NAKAMURA, TERUSHISA, SAKAGUCHI, MASAAKI, AND NAKAMURA, NOZOMU. Thrombogenic properties at the site of vascular anastomoses studied by a new technique for measuring platelet adherence, 493
IRVINE, J. W. (*See* Harrison et al.), 151
ISAACSON, L. C. (*See* Terblanche et al.), 869

J

JACKSON, BENJAMIN B. Venous occlusion of the terminal ileum: an experimental study, 322
JASCALEVICH, MARIO E. The 2-limb temporary gastrostomy tube, 736
JENSON, CONRAD B. (*See* Griffen et al.), 458
JORDAN, PAUL H., JR. Contribution of functional ablation of the pyloroantral mechanism to malabsorption in gastrectomized dogs, 820

K

KARLSON, KARL E. (*See* Dennis and Karlson), 568
—. (*See* Wesolowski et al.), 91
—, AND LERNER, BERNARD. Coagulation studies on bleeding surgical patients, 798
KAY, JEROME HAROLD, EGERTON, WILLIAM S., AND ZUBIATE, PABLO. The surgical treatment of mitral insufficiency and combined mitral stenosis and insufficiency with use of the heart-lung machine, 67
KAYSER, KENNETH L. (*See* Bormes et al.), 50
KESTENS, PAUL J., AND MCDERMOTT, WILLIAM V., JR. Perfusion and replacement of the canine liver, 196
KHOURI, EDWARD M. (*See* Hall et al.), 560
KIRCHNER, JOHN A. Surgical treatment of nasal hemorrhage, 899
KIRKLIN, JOHN W., DEVLOO, ROBERT A., AND WEIDMAN, WILLIAM H. Open intracardiac repair for transposition of the great vessels: 11 cases, 58
KLEINSASSER, LEROY J. The removal of a wire lodged in the interventricular septum of the heart, 500
KNUDSON, LYNN. (*See* Krementz and Knudson), 266
KOEPKE, DONALD E. (*See* Gott et al.), 382
KOLFF, WILLEM J. (*See* Hindberg et al.), 755

KONISHI, TETSURO. (*See* Inokuchi et al.), 493
KOWALCZYK, R. (*See* Wolfman et al.), 231
KREMENTZ, EDWARD T., AND KNUDSON, LYNN. The effect of increased oxygen tension on the tumoricidal effect of nitrogen mustard, 266
KRUMHAAR, DIETER. (*See* Lee et al.), 29
KUEHN, PAUL. (*See* Lawrence et al.), 248

L

LALONDE, ALBAN H., AND BERMAN, EDWARD J. Exsanguinating gastric hemorrhage in the newborn infant and observations on the "ulcer problem" in children, 962
LAWRENCE, WALTER, JR., KUEHN, PAUL, MORI, SHYUNIGHI, POPPELL, J. W., AND CLARKSON, BAYARD. Regional perfusion of the pelvis: consideration of the "leakage" problem, 248
LEAND, PAUL M. (*See* Bernhard et al.), 911
LEBLANC, PRESTON. (*See* Barry et al.), 335
LEE, H. M. (*See* Zukoski et al.), 926
LEE, S. H., AND FISHER, BERNARD. Portacaval shunt in the rat, 668
LEE, W. H., JR., BRADHAM, R. R., THREAT, B., AND DAVENPORT, C. Evaluation of the dissolution effect of fibrinolysin (plasmin) on induced vascular microthrombi, 812
—, KRUMHAAR, DIETER, FONKALSRUD, ERIC W., SCHJEIDE, OLE A., AND MALONEY, JAMES V., JR. Denaturation of plasma proteins as a cause of morbidity and death after intracardiac operations, 29
LEPLEY, DERWARD, JR. (*See* Bormes et al.), 50
LERMAN, GEORGE S. (*See* Applen et al.), 315
LERNER, BERNARD. (*See* Karlson and Lerner), 798
LEWIS, F. JOHN. (*See* Connaughton et al.), 372
LILLEHEI, C. WALTON. (*See* Long et al.), 12
LILLEHEI, RICHARD C. (*See* Longerbeam et al.), 274
LIPTON, SIDNEY. Use of the Cheatle-Henry approach in the treatment of cryptorchidism, 846
LIVADITIS, ALEX. (*See* Ericsson et al.), 687
LOBER, PAUL H. (*See* Grage et al.), 625
LONG, DAVID M., JR., SANCHEZ, LUIS, VARCO, RICHARD L., AND LILLEHEI, C. WALTON. The use of low molecular weight dextran and serum albumin as plasma expanders in extracorporeal circulation, 12
LONGERBEAM, JERROLD K., LILLEHEI, RICHARD C., YUNIS, EDMUND, AND HILAL, SADEK. Techniques of obtaining and preparing suspensions of spleen and bone marrow for the treatment of supralethally irradiated dogs, 274
LONGMIRE, WILLIAM P., JR. (*See* Fonkalsrud and Longmire), 134
—. (*See* Rochlin and Longmire), 586
LORTAT-JACOB, J. L., MAILLARD, J. N., AND FEKETE, F. A procedure to prevent reflux after esophagogastric resection: experience with 17 patients, 600
LOUIS, H. (*See* Chrysospathis et al.), 922
LOWER, RICHARD R., STOFER, RAYMOND C., HURLEY, EDWARD J., AND SHUMWAY, NORMAN E. Complete homograft replacement of the heart and both lungs, 842
LUKE, WALLACE K. (*See* Orahood et al.), 656
—. (*See* Wangensteen et al.), 651
LYMAN, JAMES H. (*See* Nelson et al.), 115

M

MACDOUGALL, J. T. (*See* Abbott et al.), 467
MAHALEY, STEPHEN. (*See* Shingleton et al.), 260
MAILLARD, J. N. (*See* Lortat-Jacob et al.), 600
MALONEY, JAMES V., JR. (*See* Lee et al.), 29
—. (*See* Schmutzer et al.), 452
MARGULIS, ALEXANDER R. (*See* Cook and Margulis), 513, 519
MARZULLI, VINCENT F. (*See* Boley et al.), 691
MCCARTHY, H. FRANK, HOVNANIAN, H. PHILIP, BRENNAN, TIMOTHY A., AND GAGNER, PHILIP L. Magnetic intubation, 740
MCCORD, W. J. (*See* Abbott et al.), 467
MCDERMOTT, WILLIAM V., JR. (*See* Kestens and McDermott), 196
MCDONALD, JOHN (*See* Drapanas and McDonald), 742
MCFEE, ARTHUR S. (*See* DeWall et al.), 931
MCKINNON, WILLIAM M. P. (*See* Boley et al.), 676, 691
MCPEAK, CHARLES J. Resection of inferior vena cava and graft replacement (aortic homograft) for retroperitoneal sarcoma, 778
MCSHERRY, CHARLES K. (*See* Moody et al.), 540
MENGUY, RENÉ, AND BLALOCK, JOHN C. Retrograde transductal internal drainage of pancreatic pseudocyst, 877
—, AND MINGS, HAROLD. Role of pancreatic and biliary juices in regulation of gastric secretion: pathogenesis of the Mann-Williamson ulcer, 662
MENNO, ALBERT D., AND SCHENK, WORTHINGTON G., JR. Dynamics of coronary arterial flow: flow alterations resulting from certain surgical procedures and drugs of surgical importance, 82
MESCHAN, I. (See Whitley et al.), 673
MINGS, HAROLD. (*See* Menguy and Mings), 662
MOERSCH, RICHARD N., AND CLAGETT, O. THERON. Pulmonary resection for metastatic tumors of the lungs, 579
MOODY, FRANK G., MCSHERRY, CHARLES K., AND BEAL, JOHN M. Mucosal replacement of gastric explants by free autogenous grafts, 540

MOORE, THOMAS C. Carcinosarcoma of the lung, 886
MORI, SHYUNIGHI. (*See* Lawrence et al.), 248
MORROW, ANDREW G. (*See* Cooper et al.), 341
MURPHY, J. (*See* Cliffton et al.), 644
MUSTARD, W. T., BAIRD, R. J., AND TRUSLER, G. A. The use of hypothermia in the closure of atrial septal defects in children, 301

N

NABSETH, DONALD C., AND DETERLING, RALPH A., JR. Surgical management of mycotic aneurysms, 347
NAKAMOTO, SATORU. (*See* Hindberg et al.), 755
NAKAMURA, NOZOMU. (*See* Inokuchi et al.), 493
NAKAMURA, TERUHISA. (*See* Inokuchi et al.) 493
NELSON, RUSSELL M., HENRY, JAMES W., AND LYMAN, JAMES H. Influence of l-norepinephrine on renal blood flow, renal vascular resistance, and urine flow in hemorrhagic shock, 115
NEVILLE, WILLIAM E. (*See* Sabga et al.), 547
NIGUIDULA, FAUSTINO N. (*See* Chang and Niguidula), 749
NYLANDER, G., AND OLERUD, S. The vascular pattern of intestinal villi in rats after partial gastrectomy, 955

O

OECONOMOPOULOS, CHRIS T. Iliac osteoclast: a new instrument which facilitates operation for exstrophy of the bladder, 960
OLERUD, S. (*See* Nylander and Olerud), 955
OLSEN, ARTHUR M. (*See* Payne et al.), 731
ONEAL, R. M. (*See* Wolfman et al.), 231
ORAHOOD, RICHARD C. (*See* Wangensteen et al.), 651
—, WANGENSTEEN, STEPHEN L., AND LUKE, WALLACE K. Physiologic effects of gastric hypothermia. II. The effect on renal blood flow, renal plasma flow, and glomerular filtration rate in the normal anesthetized dog, 656
ORLOFF, MARSHALL J., AND SNYDER, GILBERT B. Experimental ascites. I. Production of ascites by gradual occlusion of the hepatic veins with an internal vena caval cannula, 789
— AND —. Experimental ascites. II. The effects of portacaval shunts on ascites produced with an internal vena cava cannula, 220

P

PAASONEN, M. K. (*See* Frick et al.), 447
PACE, WILLIAM G. A venous cannula for use in experimental animals, 402
PALUMBO, LOUIS T., AND SHARPE, WENDELL S. Acute perforated peptic ulcer: evaluation of 160 consecutive patients treated by closure, 863
PARKER, ROY T. (*See* Shingleton et al.), 260
PARRISH, D. G. (*See* Strandness et al.), 488
PASSARO, EDWARD, JR. (*See* Elliott et al.), 126
PAYNE, W. SPENCER, ELLIS, F. HENRY, JR., AND OLSEN, ARTHUR M. Treatment of cardiospasm (achalasia of the esophagus) in children, 731
PERSIDSKY, MAXIM. (*See* Richards and Persidsky), 288
PIERCE, J. C., VARCO, R. L., AND GOOD, ROBERT A. Prolonged survival of a renal homograft in a dog treated with 6-mercaptopurine, 186
PISESKY, W. (*See* Harrison et al.), 151
POPPELL, J. W. (*See* Lawrence et al.), 248
POSTLETHWAIT, R. W. (*See* Weaver et al.), 207
POWELL, TRACY O. (*See* Hays and Powell), 411
POWERS, SAMUEL R., JR. (*See* Hernandez et al.), 143
PUESTOW, CHARLES B. (*See* Gillesby and Puestow), 859

R

RASCHKE, EKKEHART. (*See* Schmutzer et al.), 452
RAVITCH, MARK M. (*See* Rush et al.), 40
RICHARDS, VICTOR, AND PERSIDSKY, MAXIM. Studies in the preservation of bone marrow, 288
ROBERTS, WILLIAM C. (*See* Cooper et al.), 341
ROCHLIN, DONALD B., AND LONGMIRE, WILLIAM P., JR. Primary tumors of the small intestine, 586
ROSANO, CARMEN L. (*See* Welch et al.), 390
ROSEN, RICHARD G., AND ENQUIST, IRVING F. The healing wound in experimental diabetes, 525
ROTH, LOREN. (*See* Weidner et al.), 75
ROUSSELOT, LOUIS M., AND COLE, DONALD R. Intravisceral (topical) use of chemotherapeutic (radiomimetic) agents, 639
RUDMAN, SANFORD. (*See* Spratt et al.), 941
RUDO, FRIEDA. (*See* Bessman et al.), 478
RUHDE, ULF. (*See* Ericsson et al.), 687
RUSH, BENJAMIN F., JR., FINBERG, LAURENCE, DAVIGLUS, GEORGE F., AND CHEUNG, CHE-SUN. Pathologic lesions in experimental hypernatremia induced by extracorporeal dialysis, 359
—, WILDER, ROBERT J., FISHBEIN, RONALD, AND RAVITCH, MARK M. Effects of total circulatory standstill in profound hypothermia, 40

S

SABGA, GABRIEL A., NEVILLE, WILLIAM E., AND DEL GUERCIO, LOUIS R. M. Anomalies of the lungs associated with congenital diaphragmatic hernia, 547
SAKAGUCHI, NASAAKI. (*See* Inokuchi et al.), 493
SAKATA, MITSUAKI. (*See* Sunada et al.), 437
SANCHEZ, LUIS. (*See* Long et al.), 12
SANTORO, BENJAMIN T., GRIFFEN, WARD O., JR., AND WANGENSTEEN, OWEN H. The second-look procedure in the management of ovarian malignancies and pseudomyxoma peritonei, 354
SÃO THIAGO, JOÃO BAPTISTA. (*See* De Castro Silva et al.), 473
SATO, KUNSO. (*See* Sunada et al.), 437
SATO, TORU. (*See* Sunada et al.), 437
SAWYER, PHILIP N. (*See* Wesolowski et al.), 91
SCHECHTER, DAVID CHAS., AND SWAN, HENRY. Andreas Vesalius, surgeon, 970
— AND —. Historical views of the ideal surgeon, 427
SCHEEL, KONRAD W. Artificial respirator for dogs, 544
SCHENK, WORTHINGTON G., JR. (*See* Menno and Shenk), 82
SCHJEIDE, OLE A. (*See* Lee et al.), 29
SCHMUTZER, KARL J., RASCHKE, EKKEHART, AND MALONEY, JAMES V., JR. Intravenous l-norepinephrine as a cause of reduced plasma volume, 452
SCHOBINGER, ROBERT A. Percutaneous iliofemoral arteriography, 765
SCHWARTZ, SEYMOUR I., AND GREENLAW, ROBERT H. Evaluation of portal circulation by percutaneous splenic isotope injection, 833
SCHWARZ, HANS F. (*See* Bernhard et al.), 911
SCOTT, H. WILLIAM, JR. Basic surgical education, 1
—. (*See* Symbas et al.), 97
SHAHON, DONALD B. (*See* Grage et al.), 625
SHARPE, WENDELL S. (*See* Palumbo and Sharpe), 863
SHINGLETON, WILLIAM W., PARKER, ROY T., AND MAHALEY, STEPHEN. Abdominal perfusion for cancer chemotherapy with hypothermia and hyperthermia, 260
SHORE, J. MANNY, AND HERINGMAN, E. CRAIG. Successful inferior vena cava–superior mesenteric vein shunt in an unusual case of portal hypertension, 612
SHUMACKER, HARRIS B., JR. A new operation for transposition of the great vessels, 773
SHUMWAY, NORMAN E. (See Lower et al.), 842
SILBERMANN, O. H. (See Harrison et al.), 151
SILEN, WILLIAM, AND EISEMAN, BEN. Evidence for histamine as the agent responsible for gastric hypersecretion after portacaval shunt, 213
ŠIMA, V. (*See* Chung and Šima), 328
SIMEONE, F. A. (*See* Weidner et al.), 75
SLACK, W. W. Paper electrophoresis of extracts from normal and malignant human breast tissue, 464
SMITH, E. IDE. (*See* Devine et al.), 419
SMITH, J. W. (*See* Fisher et al.), 758
SNYDER, GILBERT B. (*See* Orloff and Snyder), 220, 789
SOBRAL, J. M. V. (*See* Clode et al.), 725
SOPER, R. T. Management of recurrent or metastatic Wilms' tumor, 555
SPENCER, ANDREW. (*See* Spratt et al.), 941
SPENCER, ROWENA, AND HUDSON, THOMAS L. Idiopathic muscular hypertrophy of the gastrointestinal tract in a child, 678
SPRATT, JOHN S., JR., TER-POGOSSIAN, MICHEL, RUDMAN, SANFORD, AND SPENCER, ANDREW. The measurement of the pulmonary venous cross-circulation through the conjugated heart of thoracopagous twins with radioactive $O^{15}$, 941
STARK, RICHARD B. (*See* Weatherley-White et al.), 784
STARZL, THOMAS E., BUTZ, GEORGE W., JR., AND HARTMAN, CHARLES F. The blind-loop syndrome after gastric operations, 849
STOFER, RAYMOND C. (*See* Lower et al.), 842
STRANDNESS, D. E., JR., PARRISH, D. G., AND BELL, J. W. Mechanism of declamping shock in operations on the abdominal aorta, 488
SUGIHARA, HIROSHI. (*See* Sunada et al.), 437
SUNADA, TERUTAKE, SUGIHARA, HIROSHI, SATO, KUNSO, SAKATA, MITSUAKI, AND SATO, TORU. Hemorrhagic tendency after massive transfusion of preserved blood, 437
SWAN, HENRY. (*See* Schechter and Swan), 427, 970
SWENSON, ORVAR. (*See* DeLuca and Swenson), 404
SYMBAS, P. N., FOSTER, J. H., AND SCOTT, H. W., JR. Experimental vein grafting in the portal venous system, 97

T

TAFT, DAVID A. (*See* Elliott et al.), 126
TERBLANCHE, J., ISAACSON, L. C., EALES, L., AND BARNARD, C. N. Renal function during and immediately after profound hypothermia, 869
TER-POGOSSIAN, MICHEL. (*See* Spratt et al.), 941
THREAT, B. (*See* Lee et al.), 812
TRUSLER, G. A. (*See* Mustard et al.), 301
TURCOTTE, J. (*See* Wolfman et al.), 231

V

VARCO, RICHARD L. (*See* Long et al.), 12
—. (*See* Pierce et al.), 186
VIRKKULA, L. (*See* Frick et al.), 447

W

Walker, Paul E. (*See* Applen et al.), 315
Wangensteen, Owen H. (*See* Griffen et al.), 458
—. (*See* Santoro et al.), 354
Wangensteen, Stephen L. (*See* Orahood et al.), 656
—, Orahood, Richard C., Luke, Wallace K., and Healey, William V. Physiologic effects of gastric hypothermia. I. The effect on estimated hepatic blood flow in the normal anesthetized dog, 651
Weatherley-White, R. C. A., Stark, Richard B., and De Forest, Margie. Physiologic evidence of lymphatic repair after skin homotransplantation, 784
Weaver, William T., Anlyan, William G., and Postlethwait, R. W. Blood coagulation factors in liver disease, 207
Weidman, William H. (*See* Kirklin et al.), 58
Weidnerk, M. G., Jr., Roth, Loren, and Simeone, F. A. Myocardial response to prolonged acute oligemic hypotension, 75
Welch, Harold F., Affifi, Rasheed, and Rosano, Carmen L. Effect of hypothermia on blood ammonia formation, 390
Wesolowski, Sigmund A., Fries, Charles C., Karlson, Karl E., De Bakey, Michael, and Sawyer, Philip N. Porosity: primary determinant of ultimate fate of synthetic vascular grafts, 91
Whitley, Joseph E., Witcofski, Richard L., Felts, John H., and Meschan, I. The investigation of renal complications of aortic clamping, 673
Wiederanders, R. F. (*See* Classen et al.), 824
Wilder, Robert J. (*See* Rush et al.), 40
Williams, H. T. G. (*See* Harrison et al.), 151
Witcofski, Richard L. (*See* Whitley et al.), 673
Wolfman, Earl F., Jr., Zuidema, G. D., Oneal, R. M., Turcotte, J., Kowalczyk, R., and Child, Charles G., III. Sodium excretion after intrasplenic and systemic injections of sodium chloride in normal dogs and after portacaval shunt, 231
Wright, Arthur R. (*See* Boley et al.), 676

Y

Yagi, Hiroshi. (*See* Inokuchi et al.), 493
Young, William P. (*See* Gott et al.), 382
Yunis, Edmund. (*See* Longerbeam et al.), 274

Z

Zarnstorff, William. (*See* Gott et al.), 382
Zollinger, Robert M. (*See* Elliott et al.), 126
Zubiate, Pablo. (*See* Kay et al.), 67
Zuidema, G. D. (*See* Wolfman et al.), 231
Zukoski, C. F., Lee, H. M., and Hume, D. H. Prolonged functional survival of a secondary renal homotransplant in the dog, 926

# Subject index


A

Abdomen, chylous cysts of (Engel et al.), 593
Abdominal aorta, cross-clamping, oliguria associated with, prevention and therapy (Barry et al.), 335
 operation on, mechanism of declamping shock in (Strandness et al.), 488
 aortic aneurysm, operation for, anuria after, treated by hemodialysis with complete recovery (Hindberg et al.), 755
 perfusion for cancer chemotherapy with hypothermia and hyperthermia (Shingleton et al.), 260
 trauma, peritoneal tap in (Drapanas and McDonald), 742
 wall scars, heterotopic osseous formation in, clinical and experimental observations on (Classen et al.), 824
Achalasia of esophagus (cardiospasm) in children, treatment (Payne et al.), 731
Acid-secreting mucosa, vagus nerve, and antrum, relative importance in prevention of experimental peptic ulceration (Harrison et al.), 151
Actinomycin D and mitomycin C in patients with advanced cancer, evaluation (Humphrey et al.), 881
Adventitia, effect of removal from arteries (Dahl et al.), 533
Agammaglobulinemia, attempt at development in adult rats by treatment with extract of fetal thymus (Czaplicki), 817
Albumin, serum, and low molecular weight dextran, use as plasma expanders in extracorporeal circulation (Long et al.), 12
Ammonia formation, blood, effect of hypothermia on (Welch et al.), 390
 movement into cerebral and peripheral tissues during hypothermia, relation of blood pH to (Bessman et al.), 478
Anastomoses, vascular, thrombogenic properties at site of, studies by new technique for measuring platelet adherence (Inokuchi et al.), 493
Anastomosis, coronary–internal mammary artery, in dogs (Hall et al.), 560
Anesthesia, discovery of (Degenshein and Hurwitz), 716



July, pp. 1-300; August, pp. 301-436; September, pp. 437-578; October, pp. 579-724; November, pp. 725-862; December, pp. 863-1004.



Aneurysm, aortic, abdominal, operation for, anuria after, treated by hemodialysis with complete recovery (Hindberg et al.), 755
Aneurysms, mycotic, surgical management (Nabseth and Deterling), 347
Antibiotic action, preventive, effective period of, in experimental incisions and dermal lesions (Burke), 161
Antibodies, pancreatic, occurrence, and experimental production of pancreatitis with pancreatic antiserum (Fonkalsrud and Longmire), 134
Anticoagulants, effect on hepatic metastases (Fisher and Fisher), 240
Antidiuresis, 5-hydroxytryptamine and, after operation (Frick et al.), 447
Antiserum, pancreatic, experimental production of pancreatitis with, and occurrence of pancreatic antibodies (Fonkalsrud and Longmire), 134
Antrum, vagus nerve, and acid-secreting mucosa, relative importance in prevention of experimental peptic ulceration (Harrison et al.), 151
Antyllus, elusive surgical genius of antiquity: analysis of his writings (Grant), 572
Anuria after operation for abdominal aortic aneurysm treated by hemodialysis with complete recovery (Hindberg et al.), 755
Aorta, abdominal, cross-clamping, oliguria associated with, prevention and therapy (Barry et al.), 335
 operations on, mechanism of declamping shock in (Strandness et al.), 488
 severely arteriosclerotic, technique of attaching synthetic graft to side of (Derrick), 782
Aortic aneurysm, abdominal, operation for, anuria after, treated by hemodialysis with complete recovery (Hindberg et al.), 755
 clamping, renal complications of, investigations of (Whitley et al.), 673
 homograft replacement, resection of inferior vena cava and, for retroperitoneal sarcoma (McPeak), 778
Arterial flow, coronary, dynamics: flow alterations resulting from certain surgical procedures and drugs of surgical importance (Menno and Schenk), 82
 in lower extremities, measurement with radioisotopes (Applen et al.), 315
 grafts, knitted, blood loss from, gelatin sealing to prevent (Bascom), 504
 prosthesis of collagen impregnated Dacron tulle (Humphries et al.), 947

Arteries, effect of removal of adventitia from (Dahl et al.), 533
Arteriography, iliofemoral, percutaneous (Schobinger), 765
Arteriosclerotic aorta, technique of attaching synthetic graft to side of (Derrick), 782
Artificial respirator for dogs (Scheel), 544
Ascites, experimental. II. Effects of portacaval shunts on ascites produced with internal vena caval cannula (Orloff and Snyder), 220
production by gradual occlusion of hepatic veins with internal vena caval catheter (Orloff and Snyder), 789
Atelectasis, management with pancreatic dornase inhalations (Cliffton et al.), 176
Atrial septal defects in children, use of hypothermia in closure (Mustard et al.), 301
Audiofrequency conductimetry, identification of conduction system of heart by (Bormes et al.), 50
Autogenous grafts, free, mucosal replacement of gastric explants by (Moody at al.), 540

B

Bacteremia, experimental, in dogs, influence of hypothermia on (Gowen and Friou), 919
Biliary and pancreatic juices, role in regulation of gastric secretion: pathogenesis of Mann-Williamson ulcer (Menguy and Mings), 662
Billroth, Theodor, surgical school of (Absolon), 697
Bladder and bowel dysfunction in case of spina bifida with meningomyelocele, surgical treatment (Devine et al.), 419
exstrophy, iliac osteoclast which facilitates operation for (Oeconomopoulos), 960
repair, preliminary report on use of fascial grafts in (DeLuca and Swenson), 404
treatment, vesicoileosigmoidostomy in (Hays and Powell), 411
wall defects, experimental, use of fascial grafts in: preliminary report on application in repair of exstrophy of bladder (DeLuca and Swenson), 404
Bleeding surgical patients, coagulation studies on (Karlson and Lerner), 798
upper gastrointestinal, simple cooling device for treatment (Holt), 728
Blind-loop syndrome after gastric operations (Starzl et al.), 849
Blood ammonia formation, effect of hypothermia on (Welch et al.), 390
coagulation factors in liver disease (Weaver et al.), 207
flow, hepatic, estimated, in normal anesthetized dog, effect of gastric hypothermia on (Wangensteen et al.), 651

Blood flow—Cont'd
renal, effect of gastric hypothermia on, in normal anesthetized dog (Orahood et al.), 656
influence of l-norepinephrine on, in hemorrhagic shock (Nelson et al.), 115
loss from knitted arterial grafts, gelatin sealing to prevent (Bascom), 504
oxygenators, theme and variations on. I. Bubble oxygenators (DeWall et al.), 931
pH, relation to movement of ammonia into cerebral and peripheral tissues during hypothermia (Bessman et al.), 478
preserved, massive transfusion of, hemorrhagic tendency after (Sunada et al.), 437
Bone marrow, preservation, studies in (Richards and Persidsky), 288
and spleen, suspensions of, techniques of obtaining and preparing, for treatment of supralethally irradiated dogs (Longerbeam et al.), 274
Bowel and bladder dysfunction in case of spina bifida with meningomyelocele, surgical treatment (Devinc et al.), 419
Breast, reticulum-cell sarcoma in, periductal mastitis associated with (Dyson), 634
tissue, human, normal and malignant, paper electrophoresis of extracts from (Slack), 464

C

Calcium and magnesium metabolism in acute hemorrhagic pancreatitis, role of parathyroid glands in (Hernandez et al.), 143
Cancer, advanced, patients with, evaluation of actinomycin D and mitomycin C in (Humphrey et al.), 881
cells in blood in simulated colon cancer, resectable and unresectable: effect of fibrinolysin and heparin on growth potential (Cliffton and Agostino), 395
chemotherapy, abdominal perfusion for, with hypothermia and hyperthermia (Shingleton et al.), 260
colon, simulated, resectable and unresectable, cancer cells in blood in: effect of fibrinolysin and heparin on growth potential (Cliffton and Agostino), 395
risk in ulcerative colitis: formidability per patient-year of late disease (Dennis and Karlson), 568
of stomach, elective uptake of radioiodine by (Clode et al.), 725
Candida, postoperative endocarditis due to (Cooper et al.), 341
Canine liver, perfusion and replacement (Kestens and McDermott), 196
Cannula, venous, for use in experimental animals (Pace), 402

Carcinoma, subglottic, with extensive tracheal involvement (Calem and Freund), 894
Carcinosarcoma of lung (Moore), 886
Cardiopulmonary bypass, treatment of mitral insufficiency and combined mitral stenosis and insufficiency with use of (Kay et al.), 67
Cardiospasm (achalasia of esophagus) in children, treatment (Payne et al.), 731
Cells, cancer, in blood in simulated colon cancer, resectable and unresectable: effect of fibrinolysin and heparin on growth potential (Cliffton and Agostino), 395
Cerebral and peripheral tissues, movement of ammonia into during hypothermia, relation of blood pH to (Bessman et al.), 478
Cheatle-Henry approach, use in treatment of cryptorchidism (Lipton), 846
Chemotherapeutic (radiomimetic) agents, intravisceral (topical) use of (Rousselot and Cole), 639
Chemotherapy, cancer, abdominal perfusion for, with hypothermia and hyperthermia (Lawrence et al.), 260
Cholecystojejunostomy, fate of, in absence of common bile duct obstruction (Boley et al.), 676
Chylous cysts of abdomen (Engel et al.), 593
Circulation, extracorporeal, plasma expanders in, use of low molecular weight dextran and serum albumin as (Long et al.), 12
  portal, evaluation by percutaneous splenic isotope injection (Schwartz and Greenlaw), 833
Circulatory standstill, total, effects in profound hypothermia (Rush et al.), 40
Clamping, aortic, renal complications, investigation of (Whitley et al.), 673
Coagulation factors, blood, in liver disease (Weaver et al.), 207
  studies on bleeding surgical patients (Karlson and Lerner), 798
Coating of intravascular plastic prostheses with colloidal graphite (Gott et al.), 382
Colitis, ulcerative, cancer risk in: formidability per patient-year of late disease (Dennis and Karlson), 568
Collagen-impregnated Dacron tulle, arterial prosthesis of (Humphries et al.), 947
Colon cancer, simulated, resectable and unresectable, cancer cells in blood in, effect of fibrinolysin and heparin on growth potential (Cliffton and Agostino), 395
  and stomach, familial gastrointestinal polyposis involving, management (Boley et al.), 691
Cooling device, simple, for treatment of upper gastrointestinal bleeding (Holt), 728
Conductimetry, audiofrequency, identification of conduction system of heart by (Bormes et al.), 50
Conduction system of heart, identification by audiofrequency conductimetry (Bormes et al.), 50
Congenital diaphragmatic hernia, anomalies of lungs associated with (Sabga et al.), 547
Coronary arterial flow, dynamics: flow alterations resulting from certain surgical procedures and drugs of surgical importance (Menno and Schenk), 82
  –internal mammary artery anastomosis in dogs (Hall et al.), 560
Cross-circulation, venous, pulmonary, measurement through conjugated heart of thoracopagous twins with radioactive $O^{15}$ (Spratt et al.), 941
Cryptorchidism, use of Cheatle-Henry approach in treatment (Lipton), 846
Cysts, chylous, of abdomen (Engel et al.), 593

D

Dacron tulle, collagen impregnated, arterial prosthesis of (Humphries et al.), 947
Declamping shock, mechanism, in operations on abdominal aorta (Strandness et al.), 488
Denaturation of plasma proteins as cause of morbidity and death after intracardiac operations (Lee et al.), 29
Dermal lesions and incisions, experimental, effective period of preventive antibiotic action in (Burke), 161
Dextran, low molecular weight, and serum albumin, use as plasma expanders in extracorporeal circulation (Long et al.), 12
Diabetes, experimental, healing wound in (Rosen and Enquist), 525
Diagnostic enema, silicone-foam. I. Assessment with surgical specimens of human sigmoid colon (Cook and Margulis), 513
  II. Experimental evaluation in dogs, (Cook and Margulis), 519
Dialysis, extracorporeal, experimental hypernatremia induced by, pathologic lesions in (Rush et al.), 359
Diaphragmatic hernia, congenital, anomalies of lungs associated with (Sabga et al.), 547
Dissolution effect of fibrinolysin (plasmin) on induced vascular microthrombi (Lee et al.), 812
Diverticulum, esophageal, technique in resection (McDonald), 747
Dornase, pancreatic, inhalations, management of pulmonary complications of surgical operations (primarily atelectasis) with (Cliffton et al.), 176
Drainage, internal, retrograde transductal, of pancreatic pseudocyst (Menguy and Blalock), 877

Drugs of surgical importance and certain surgical procedures, alterations in coronary arterial flow resulting from (Menno and Schenk), 82
Duodenal closure after gastrectomy for duodenal ulcer (Cooper), 425
  ulcer, gastrectomy for, duodenal closure after (Cooper), 425
Dynamics of coronary arterial flow: flow alterations resulting from certain surgical procedures and drugs of surgical importance (Menno and Schenk), 82

E

Education, surgical, basic (Scott), 1
Electrophoresis, paper, of extracts from normal and malignant human breast tissue (Slack), 464
Endocarditis, postoperative, due to Candida (Cooper et al.), 341
Enema, diagnostic, silicone-foam. I. Assessment with surgical specimens of human sigmoid colon (Cook and Margulis), 513
  II. Experimental evaluation in dogs (Cook and Margulis), 519
Esophageal diverticulum, technique in resection (Beardsley), 747
Esophagogastric resection, procedure to prevent reflux after (Lortat-Jacob et al.), 600
Esophagus, achalasia of (cardiospasm) in children, treatment (Payne et al.), 731
Excretion, sodium, after intrasplenic and systemic injections of sodium chloride in normal dogs and after portacaval shunt (Wolfman et al.), 231
Expanders, plasma, in extracorporeal circulation, use of low molecular weight dextran and serum albumin as (Long et al.), 12
Explants, gastric, mucosal replacement by free autogenous grafts (Moody et al.), 540
Exstrophy of bladder, iliac osteoclast which facilitates operation for (Oeconomopoulos), 960
  repair, preliminary report of use of fascial grafts in (DeLuca and Swenson), 404
  treatment, vesicoileosigmoidostomy in (Hays and Powell), 411
Extracorporeal circulation, plasma expanders in, use of low molecular weight dextran and serum albumin as (Long et al.), 12
  dialysis, experimental hypernatremia induced by, pathologic lesions in (Rush et al.), 359
  perfusion and profound hypothermia, temperature gradients associated with (Fisher et al.), 758
Extremities, lower, arterial flow in, measurement with radioisotopes (Applen et al.), 315

F

Familial gastrointestinal polyposis involving stomach and colon, management of (Boley et al.), 691
Fascial grafts, use in experimental bladder wall defects: preliminary report on application in repair of exstrophy of bladder (DeLuca and Swenson), 404
Femoral pulse, paradoxical variation in occlusion of iliac artery (Blaisdell and Gauder), 529
Fetal thymus, extract of, attempt at development of agammaglobulinemia in adult rats by treatment with (Czaplicki), 817
Fibrinolysin and heparin, effect on growth potential of cancer cells in blood in simulated colon cancer, resectable and unresectable (Cliffton and Agostino), 395
  (plasmin), dissolution effect on induced vascular microthrombi, evaluation of (Lee et al.), 812
Fibrinolytic activity, studies on with venous occlusion: treatment of thrombophlebitis (Cliffton et al.), 644
Filtration rate, glomerular, effect of gastric hypothermia on, in normal anesthetized dog (Orahood et al.), 656
Flow, arterial, in lower extremities, measurement with radioisotopes (Applen et al.), 315

G

Gangrene, ischemic, without major organic vascular occlusion (Hardy and Alican), 107
Gastrectomized dogs, malabsorption in, contribution of functional ablation of pyloroantral mechanism to (Jordan), 820
Gastrectomy for duodenal ulcer, duodenal closure after (Cooper), 425
  partial, vascular pattern of intestinal villi in rats after (Nylander and Olerud), 955
  total, reconstruction after (Chrysospathis et al.), 922
Gastric explants, mucosal replacement by free autogenous grafts (Moody et al.), 540
  hemorrhage, exsanguinating, in newborn infant and observations on "ulcer problem" in children (Lalonde and Berman), 962
  hypersecretion after portacaval shunt, evidence for histamine as agent responsible for (Silen and Eiseman), 213
  hypothermia, physiologic effects. I. Effect on estimated hepatic blood flow in normal anesthetized dog (Wangensteen et al.), 651
    II. Effect on renal blood flow, renal plasma flow, and glomerular filtration rate in normal anesthetized dog (Orahood et al.), 656

Gastric—Cont'd
operations, blind-loop syndrome after (Starzl et al.), 849
secretion, role of pancreatic and biliary juices in regulation of: pathogenesis of Mann-Williamson ulcer (Menguy and Mings), 662
secretions, pancreatic influences on (Elliott et al.), 126
Gastrointestinal bleeding, upper, simple cooling device for treatment (Holt), 728
polyposis familial, involving stomach and colon, management of (Boley et al.), 691
tract, idiopathic muscular hypertrophy of, in child (Spencer and Hudson), 678
Gastrostomy tube, temporary, 2-limb (Jascalevich), 736
Gelatin sealing to prevent blood loss from knitted arterial grafts (Bascom), 504
Glands, parathyroid, role in calcium and magnesium metabolism in acute hemorrhagic pancreatitis (Hernandez et al.), 143
salivary, major, benign tumors of (Grage et al.), 625
Glomerular filtration rate, effect of gastric hypothermia on, in normal anesthetized dog (Orahood et al.), 656
Graft replacement (aortic homograft), resection of inferior vena cava and, for retroperitoneal sarcoma (McPeak), 778
synthetic, technique of attaching to side of severely arteriosclerotic aorta (Derrick), 782
Grafting, vein, experimental, in portal venous system (Symbas et al.), 97
Grafts, arterial, knitted, blood loss from, gelatin sealing to prevent (Bascom), 504
autogenous, free, mucosal replacement of gastric explants by (Moody et al.), 540
fascial, use in experimental bladder wall defects: preliminary report on application in repair of exstrophy of bladder (DeLuca and Swenson), 404
vascular, synthetic, ultimate fate of, porosity as primary determinant (Wesolowski et al.), 91
Graphite, colloidal, coating of intravascular plastic prostheses with (Gott et al.), 382
Growth potential of cancer cells in blood in simulated colon cancer, resectable and unresectable, effect of fibrinolysin and heparin on (Cliffton and Agostino), 395

H

Healing wound in experimental diabetes (Rosen and Enquist), 525
Heart and both lungs, complete homograft replacement (Lower et al.), 842
Heart—Cont'd
conduction system of, identification by audio-frequency conductimetry (Bormes et al.), 50
conjugated, of thoracopagous twins, measurement of pulmonary venous cross-circulation through, with radioactive $O^{15}$ (Spratt et al.), 941
interventricular septum of, removal of wire lodged in (Kleinsasser), 500
and lung complications of treatment of hydrocephalus by ventriculoauriculostomy (Emery and Hilton), 309
-lung machine, surgical treatment of mitral insufficiency and combined mitral stenosis and insufficiency with use of (Kay et al.), 67
Hemodialysis, anuria after operation for abdominal aortic aneurysm treated by, with complete recovery (Hindberg et al.), 755
Hemorrhage, gastric, exsanguinating, in newborn infant and observations on "ulcer problem" in children (Lalonde and Berman), 962
nasal, surgical treatment (Kirchner), 899
Hemorrhagic pancreatitis, acute, role of parathyroid glands in calcium and magnesium metabolism in (Hernandez et al.), 143
shock, influence of 1-norepinephrine on renal blood flow, renal vascular resistance, and urine flow in (Nelson et al.), 115
tendency after massive transfusion of preserved blood (Sunada et al.), 437
Heparin and fibrinolysin, effect on growth potential of cancer cells in blood in simulated colon cancer, resectable and unresectable (Cliffton and Agostino), 395
Hepatic blood flow, estimated, in normal anesthetized dog, effect of gastric hypothermia on (Wangensteen et al.), 651
metastases, experimental studies of factors which influence. VIII. Effect of anticoagulants (Fisher and Fisher), 240
veins, gradual occlusion with internal vena caval cannula, production of ascites by (Orloff and Snyder), 789
Hernia, diaphragmatic, congenital, anomalies of lungs associated with (Sagba et al.), 547
Heterotopic osseous formation in abdominal wall scars, clinical and experimental observations on (Classen et al.), 824
Histamine as agent responsible for gastric hypersecretion after portacaval shunt, evidence for (Silen and Eiseman), 213
Historical views of ideal surgeon (Schechter and Swan), 427
Homograft, aortic, replacement, resection of inferior vena cava and, for retroperitoneal sarcoma (McPeak), 778

Homograft—Cont'd
renal, prolonged survival of, in dog treated with 6-mercaptopurine (Pierce et al.), 186
replacement, complete, of heart and both lungs (Lower et al.), 842
Homotransplant, renal, prolonged functional survival, in dog (Zukoski et al.), 926
Homotransplantation, skin, lymphatic repair after, physiologic evidence of (Weatherley-White et al.), 784
Hydrocephalus, treatment by ventriculoauriculostomy, lung and heart complications of (Emery and Hilton), 309
Hydronephrosis associated with aberrant renal vessels in infants and children (Ericsson et al.), 687
5-Hydroxytryptamine and antidiuresis after operation (Frick et al.), 447
Hypernatremia, experimental induced by extracorporeal dialysis, pathologic lesions in (Rush et al.), 359
Hypersecretion, gastric, after portacaval shunt, evidence for histamine as agent responsible for (Silen and Eiseman), 213
Hypertension, portal, unusual case, successful inferior vena cava–superior mesenteric vein shunt in (Shore and Heringman), 612
Hyperthermia and hypothermia, abdominal perfusion for cancer chemotherapy with (Shingleton et al.), 260
Hypertrophy, muscular, idiopathic, of gastrointestinal tract in child (Spencer and Hudson), 678
Hypotension, oligemic, prolonged, acute, myocardial response to (Weidner et al.), 75
Hypothermia, effect on blood ammonia formation (Welch et al.), 390
gastric, physiologic effects. I. Effect on estimated hepatic blood flow in normal anesthetized dog (Wangensteen et al.), 651
II. Effect on renal blood flow, renal plasma flow, and glomerular filtration rate in normal anesthetized dog (Orahood et al.), 656
and hyperthermia, abdominal perfusion for cancer chemotherapy with (Shingleton et al.), 260
influence on experimental bacteremia in dogs (Gowen and Friou), 919
movement of ammonia into cerebral and peripheral tissues during, relation of blood pH to (Bessman et al.), 478
profound, effects of total circulatory standstill in (Rush et al.), 40
and extracorporeal perfusion, temperature gradients associated with (Fisher et al.), 758
renal function during and immediately after (Terblanche et al.), 869

Hypothermia—Cont'd
prolonged, below 25° C. for periods over 20 hours: influence of therapy and technique on survival (Connaughton et al.), 372
regional, kidney and (Cockett), 905
use in closure of atrial septal defects in children (Mustard et al.), 301
Hypothermic perfusion, studies in (Bernhard et al.), 911

I

Ideal surgeon, historical views of (Schechter and Swan), 427
Ileal loop, isolated, as substitute in urinary tract operations, observations on (Abbott et al.), 467
Ileum, terminal, venous occlusion (Jackson), 322
Iliac artery, occlusion, paradoxical variation of femoral pulse in (Blaisdell and Gauder), 529
osteoclast: new instrument which facilitates operation for exstrophy of bladder (Oeconomopoulos), 960
Iliofemoral arteriography, percutaneous (Schobinger), 765
Incisions and dermal lesions, experimental, effective period of preventive antibiotic action in (Burke), 161
Infections, wound, experimental: contamination versus surgical technique (Condie and Ferguson), 367
Inferior vena cava–superior mesenteric vein shunt, successful, in unusual case of portal hypertension (Shore and Heringman), 612
Inhalations, pancreatic dornase, management of pulmonary complications of surgical operations (primarily atelectasis) with (Cliffton et al.), 176
Injections, intrasplenic and systemic, of sodium chloride in normal dogs and after portacaval shunt, sodium excretion after (Wolfman et al.), 231
Insufficiency, mitral, and combined mitral stenosis and insufficiency, surgical treatment with use of heart-lung machine (Kay et al.), 67
Interventricular septum of heart, removal of wire lodged in (Kleinsasser), 500
Intestinal villi, vascular pattern of, in rats after partial gastrectomy (Nylander and Olerud), 955
Intestine, small, primary tumors of (Rochlin and Longmire), 586
Intracardiac operations, denaturation of plasma proteins as cause of morbidity and death after (Lee et al.), 29
repair, open, for transposition of great vessels (Kirklin et al.), 58

Intravascular plastic prostheses, coating with colloidal graphite (Gott et al.), 382
Intravenous l-norepinephrine as cause of reduced plasma flow (Schmutzer et al.), 452
Intravisceral (topical) use of chemotherapeutic (radiomimetic) agents (Rousselot and Cole), 639
Intubation, magnetic (McCarthy et al.), 740
Irradiation, supralethal, in dogs, suspensions of spleen and bone marrow for treatment, techniques of obtaining and preparing (Longerbeam et al.), 274
Ischemic gangrene without major organic vascular occlusion (Hardy and Alican), 107
Isotope injection, splenic, percutaneous, evaluation of portal circulation by (Schwartz and Greenlaw), 833

J

Juices, pancreatic and biliary, role in regulation of gastric secretion: pathogenesis of Mann-Williamson ulcer (Menguy and Mings), 662

K

Kidney and regional hypothermia (Cockett), 905

L

"Leakage" problem, consideration of: regional perfusion of pelvis (Lawrence et al.), 248
Letheon controversy, intimate view of (Degenshein and Hurwitz), 716
Liver, canine, perfusion and replacement (Kestens and McDermott), 196
  disease, blood coagulation factors in (Weaver et al.), 207
Loop, ileal, isolated, as substitute in urinary tract operations, observations on (Abbott et al.), 467
Lung, carcinosarcoma (Moore), 886
  and heart complications of treatment of hydrocephalus by ventriculoauriculostomy (Emery and Hilton), 309
Lungs, anomalies, associated with congenital diaphragmatic hernia (Sabga et al.), 547
  both, and heart, complete homograft replacement (Lower et al.), 842
  metastatic tumors of, pulmonary resection for (Moersch and Clagett), 579
Lymphatic repair after skin homotransplantation, physiologic evidence of (Weatherley-White et al.), 784

M

Magnesium and calcium metabolism in acute hemorrhagic pancreatitis, role of parathyroid glands in (Hernandez et al.), 143
Magnetic intubation (McCarthy et al.), 740
Malabsorption in gastrectomized dogs, contribution of functional ablation of pyloroantral mechanism to (Jordan), 820
Malignancies, ovarian, and pseudomyxoma peritonei, second-look procedure in management (Santoro et al.), 354
Malignant retroperitoneal sarcomas, treatment with use of second-look approach (Griffen et al.), 458
  schwannoma, metastatic, with bilateral pulmonary resection (Chang and Niguidula), 749
Mann-Williamson ulcer, pathogenesis of: role of pancreatic and biliary juices in regulation of gastric secretion (Menguy and Mings), 662
Mannitolization. I. Prevention and therapy of oliguria associated with cross-clamping of abdominal aorta (Barry et al.), 335
Mastitis, periductal, associated with reticulum-cell sarcoma in breast (Dyson), 634
Measurement of arterial flow in lower extremities with radioisotopes (Applen et al.), 315
  of pulmonary venous cross-circulation through conjugated heart of thoracopagous twins with radioactive $O^{15}$ (Spratt et al.), 941
Meeting of Society of University Surgeons, review of (Deterling), 299
Meningomyelocele, spina bifida with, bowel and bladder dysfunction in case of, surgical treatment (Devine et al.), 419
6-Mercaptopurine, dog treated with, prolonged survival of renal homograft in (Pierce et al.), 186
Metabolism, calcium and magnesium, in acute hemorrhagic pancreatitis, role of parathyroid glands in (Hernandez et al.), 143
Metastases, hepatic, experimental studies of factors which influence. VIII. Effect of anticoagulants (Fisher and Fisher), 240
Microthrombi, vascular, induced, dissolution effect of fibrinolysin (plasmin) on evaluation of (Lee et al.), 812
Mitomycin C and actinomycin D in patients with advanced cancer, evaluation (Humphrey et al.), 881
Mitral insufficiency and combined mitral stenosis and insufficiency, surgical treatment with use of heart-lung machine (Kay et al.), 67
  stenosis and insufficiency, combined, and mitral insufficiency, surgical treatment with use of heart-lung machine (Kay et al.), 67
Mucosa, acid-secreting, vagus nerve, and antrum, relative importance in prevention of experimental peptic ulceration (Harrison et al.), 151

Mucosal replacement of gastric explants by free autogenous grafts (Moody et al.), 540
Muscular hypertrophy, idiopathic, of gastrointestinal tract in child (Spencer and Hudson), 678
Mycotic aneurysms, surgical management (Nabseth and Deterling), 347
Myocardial response to prolonged acute oligemic hypotension (Weidner et al.), 75

N

Nasal hemorrhage, surgical treatment (Kirchner), 899
Necrosis, renal tubular: its relation to norepinephrine administration (Chung and Šima), 328
Nerve, vagus, antrum, and acid-secreting mucosa, relative importance in prevention of experimental peptic ulceration (Harrison et al.), 151
Nitrogen mustard, tumoricidal effect, effect of increased oxygen tension on (Krementz and Knudson), 266
Norepinephrine administration, relation of renal tubular necrosis to (Chung and Šima), 328
l-Norepinephrine, influence on renal blood flow, renal vascular resistance, and urine flow in hemorrhagic shock (Nelson et al.), 115
  intravenous, as cause of reduced plasma volume (Schmutzer et al.), 452

O

$O^{15}$, radioactive, measurement of pulmonary venous cross-circulation through conjugated heart of thoracopagous twins with (Spratt et al.), 941
Occlusion, gradual, of hepatic veins with internal vena caval cannula, production of ascites by (Orloff and Snyder), 789
  of iliac artery, paradoxical variation of femoral pulse in (Blaisdell and Gauder), 529
  venous, studies on fibrinolytic activity with: treatment of thrombophlebitis (Cliffton et al.), 644
    of terminal ileum (Jackson), 322
Oligemic hypotension, prolonged acute, myocardial response to (Weidner et al.), 75
Oliguria associated with cross-clamping of abdominal aorta, prevention and therapy Barry et al.), 335
Osseous formation, heterotopic, in abdominal wall scars, clinical and experimental observations on (Classen et al.), 824
Osteoclast, iliac: new instrument which facilitates operation for exstrophy of bladder (Oeconomopoulos), 960
Ovarian malignancies and pseudomyxoma peritonei, second-look procedure in management (Santoro et al.), 354
Oxygen tension, increased effect on tumoricidal effect of nitrogen mustard (Krementz and Knudson), 266
Oxygenators, blood, theme and variations on. I. Bubble oxygenators (DeWall et al.), 931
  bubble (DeWall et al.), 931

P

Pancreatic antibodies, occurrence, and experimental production of pancreatitis with pancreatic antiserum (Fonkalsrud and Longmire), 134
  antiserum, experimental production of pancreatitis with, and occurrence of pancreatic antibodies (Fonkalsrud and Longmire), 134
  and biliary juices, role in regulation of gastric secretion: pathogenesis of Mann-Williamson ulcer (Menguy and Mings), 662
  dornase inhalations, management of pulmonary complications of surgical operations (primarily atelectasis) with (Cliffton et al.), 176
  influences on gastric secretion (Elliott et al.), 126
  pseudocyst, retrograde transductal internal drainage (Menguy and Blalock), 877
Pancreaticojejunostomy for chronic relapsing pancreatitis: an evaluation (Gillesby and Puestow), 859
  "fore and aft" split, for chronic pancreatitis (Campanale and Gardner), 618
  surgical treatment of chronic pancreatitis by: 8-year reappraisal (DuVal and Enquist), 965
Pancreatitis, chronic, "fore and aft" split pancreaticojejunostomy for (Campanale and Gardner), 618
    relapsing, pancreaticojejunostomy for (Gillesby and Puestow), 859
    surgical treatment by pancreaticojejunostomy: 8-year reappraisal (DuVal and Enquist), 965
  experimental production with pancreatic antiserum, and occurrence of pancreatic antibodies (Fonkalsrud and Longmire), 134
  hemorrhagic, acute, role of parathyroid glands in calcium and magnesium metabolism in (Hernandez et al.), 143
Paper electrophoresis of extracts from normal and malignant human breast tissue (Slack), 464
Parathyroid glands, role in calcium and magnesium metabolism in acute hemorrhagic pancreatitis (Hernandez et al.), 143

Pelvis, regional perfusion: consideration of "leakage" problem (Lawrence et al.), 248
Peptic ulcer, perforated, acute: evaluation of 160 consecutive patients treated by closure (Palumbo and Sharpe), 863
ulceration, experimental, prevention of, relative importance of vagus nerve, antrum, and acid-secreting mucosa in (Harrison et al.), 151
Percutaneous ileofemoral arteriography (Schobinger), 765
transhepatic approach of portal vein in man in determination of patency of splenorenal shunts (De Castro Silva et al.), 473
Perfusion, abdominal, for cancer chemotherapy with hypothermia and hyperthermia (Shingleton et al.), 260
extracorporeal, and profound hypothermia, temperature gradients associated with (Fisher et al.), 758
hypothermic, studies in (Bernhard et al.), 911
regional, of pelvis: consideration of "leakage" problem (Lawrence et al.), 248
and replacement of canine liver (Kestens and McDermott), 196
Periductal mastitis associated with reticulum-cell sarcoma in breast (Dyson), 634
Peripheral and cerebral tissues, movement of ammonia into during hypothermia, relation of blood pH to (Bessman et al.), 478
Peritoneal tap in abdominal trauma (Drapanas and McDonald), 742
pH, blood, relation to movement of ammonia into cerebral and peripheral tissues during hypothermia (Bessman et al.), 478
Plasma expanders in extracorporeal circulation, use of low molecular weight dextran and serum albumin as (Long et al.), 12
flow, renal, effect of gastric hypothermia on, in normal anesthetized dog (Orahood et al.), 656
proteins, denaturation of, as cause of morbidity and death after intracardiac operations (Lee et al.), 29
volume, reduced, intravenous l-norepinephrine as cause (Schmutzer et al.), 452
Plasmin, dissolution effect on induced vascular microthrombi, evaluation of (Lee et al.), 812
Platelet adherence, new technique for measuring, thrombogenic properties at site of vascular anastomoses studied by (Inokuchi et al.), 493
Polyposis, gastrointestinal, familial, involving stomach and colon, management of (Boley et al.), 691
Porosity: primary determinant of ultimate fate of synthetic vascular grafts (Wesolowski et al.), 91
Portacaval shunt, gastric hypersecretion after, evidence for histamine as agent responsible for (Silen and Eiseman), 213
in rat (Lee and Fisher), 668
sodium excretion after intrasplenic and systemic injections of sodium chloride after (Wolfman et al.), 231
shunts, effects on ascites produced with internal vena cava cannula (Orloff and Snyder), 220
Portal circulation, evaluation by percutaneous splenic isotope injection (Schwartz and Greenlaw), 833
hypertension, unusual case, successful inferior vena cava–superior mesenteric vein shunt in (Shore and Heringman), 612
vein in man, percutaneous transhepatic approach in determination of patency of splenorenal shunts (De Castro Silva et al.), 473
venous system, experimental vein grafting in (Symbas et al.), 97
Preservation of bone marrow, studies in (Richards and Persidsky), 288
Prostheses, plastic, intravascular coating with colloidal graphite (Gott et al.), 382
Prosthesis, arterial, of collagen-impregnated Dacron tulle (Humphries et al.), 949
Protein, plasma, denaturation of, as cause of morbidity and death after intracardiac operations (Lee et al.), 29
Pseudocyst, pancreatic, retrograde transductal internal drainage (Menguy and Blalock), 877
Pseudomyxoma peritonei, and ovarian malignancies, second-look procedure in management (Santoro et al.), 354
Pulmonary complications of surgical operations (primarily atelectasis), management with pancreatic dornase inhalations (Cliffton et al.), 176
resection, bilateral, metastatic malignant schwannoma with (Chang and Niguidula), 749
for metastatic tumors of lungs (Moersch and Clagett), 579
venous cross-circulation through conjugated heart of thoracopagous twins, measurement with radioactive $O^{15}$ (Spratt et al.), 941
Pulse, femoral, paradoxical variation, in occlusion of iliac artery (Blaisdell and Gauder), 529
Pyelonephritis, surgically induced, studies of (Davis and Coil), 169
Pyloroantral mechanism, functional ablation, contribution of, to malabsorption in gastrectomized dogs (Jordan), 820

R

Radioactive $O^{15}$, measurement of pulmonary cross-circulation through conjugated heart of thoracopagous twins with (Spratt et al.), 941
Radioiodine, elective uptake by cancer of stomach (Clode et al.), 725
Radioisotopes, measurement of arterial flow in lower extremities with (Applen et al.), 315
Reflux after esophagogastric resection, procedure to prevent (Lortat-Jacob et al.), 600
Regional perfusion of pelvis: consideration of "leakage" problem (Lawrence et al.), 248
Renal blood flow, effect of gastric hypothermia on, in normal anesthetized dog (Orahood et al.), 656
  renal vascular resistance, and urine flow, influence of l-norepinephrine on, in hemorrhagic shock (Nelson et al.), 115
 complications of aortic clamping, investigation of (Whitley et al.), 673
 function during and immediately after profound hypothermia (Terblanche et al.), 869
 homograft, prolonged survival of, in dog treated with 6-mercaptopurine (Pierce et al.), 186
 homotransplant, prolonged functional survival, in dog (Zukoski et al.), 926
 plasma flow, effect of gastric hypothermia on, in normal anesthetized dog (Orahood et al.), 656
 tubular necrosis: its relation to norepinephrine administration (Chung and Šima), 328
 vascular resistance, renal blood flow, and urine flow, influence of l-norepinephrine on, in hemorrhagic shock (Nelson et al.), 115
 vessels, aberrant, hydronephrosis associated with, in infants and children (Ericsson et al.), 687
Replacement, mucosal, of gastric explants by free autogenous grafts (Moody et al.), 540
Respirator, artificial, for dogs (Scheel), 544
Reticulum-cell sarcoma in breast, periductal mastitis associated with (Dyson), 634
Retrograde transductal internal drainage of pancreatic pseudocyst (Menguy and Blalock), 877
Retroperitoneal sarcoma, resection of inferior vena cava and graft replacement (aortic homograft) for (McPeak), 778
 sarcomas, malignant, treatment with use of second-look approach (Griffen et al.), 458
Review of meeting of Society of University Surgeons (Deterling), 299
Risk, cancer, in ulcerative colitis: formidability per patient-year of late disease (Dennis and Karlson), 568

S

Salivary glands, major, benign tumors of (Grage et al.), 625
Sarcoma, reticulum-cell, in breast, periductal mastitis associated with (Dyson), 634
 retroperitoneal, resection of inferior vena cava and graft replacement for (McPeak), 778
Sarcomas, retroperitoneal, malignant, treatment with use of second-look approach (Griffen et al.), 458
Scars, abdominal wall, heterotopic osseous formation in, clinical and experimental observations on (Classen et al.), 824
School, surgical, of Theodor Billroth (Absolon), 697
Schwannoma, malignant, metastatic, with bilateral pulmonary resection (Chang and Niguidula), 749
Sealing, gelatin, to prevent blood loss from knitted arterial grafts (Bascom), 504
Second-look approach, treatment of malignant retroperitoneal sarcomas with use of (Griffen et al.), 458
 procedure in management of ovarian malignancies and pseudomyxoma peritonei, (Santoro et al.), 354
Secretion, gastric, role of pancreatic and biliary juices in regulation of: pathogenesis of Mann-Williamson ulcer (Menguy and Mings), 662
Secretions, gastric, pancreatic influences on (Elliott et al.), 126
Septal defects, atrial, in children, use of hypothermia in closure (Mustard et al.), 301
Septum, interventricular, of heart, removal of wire lodged in (Kleinsasser), 500
Shock, declamping, mechanism, in operations on abdominal aorta (Strandness et al.), 488
 hemorrhagic, influence of l-norepinephrine on renal blood flow, renal vascular resistance, and urine flow in (Nelson et al.), 115
Shunt, inferior vena cava–superior mesenteric vein, successful, in unusual case of portal hypertension (Shore and Heringman), 612
 portacaval, gastric hypersecretion after, evidence for histamine as agent responsible for (Silen and Eiseman), 213
  in rat (Lee and Fisher), 668
  sodium excretion after intrasplenic and systemic injections of sodium chloride after (Wolfman et al.), 231
Shunts, portacaval, effects on ascites produced with internal vena cava cannula (Orloff and Snyder), 220
 splenorenal, determination of patency of, percutaneous transhepatic approach of portal vein in man in (De Castro Silva et al.), 473

Silicone-foam diagnostic enema. I. Assessment with surgical specimens of human sigmoid colon (Cook and Margulis), 513
II. Experimental evaluation in dogs (Cook and Margulis), 519
Skin homotronsplantation, lymphatic repair after, physiologic evidence of (Weatherley-White et al.), 784
Society of University Surgeons issue, 1-300
review of meeting of (Deterling), 299
Sodium chloride, intrasplenic and systemic injections in normal dogs and after portacaval shunt, sodium excretion after (Wolfman et al.), 231
excretion after intrasplenic and systemic injections of sodium chloride in normal dogs and after portocaval shunt (Wolfman et al.), 231
Spina bifida with meningomyelocele, bowel and bladder dysfunction in case of, surgical treatment (Devine et al.), 419
Spleen and bone marrow, suspensions of, techniques of obtaining and preparing, for treatment of supralethally irradiated dogs (Longerbeam et al.), 274
Splenic isotope injection, percutaneous, evaluation of portal circulation by (Schwartz and Greenlaw), 833
Splenorenal shunts, determination of patency of, percutaneous transhepatic approach of portal vein in man in (De Castro Silva et al.), 473
Standstill, circulatory, total, effects in profound hypothermia (Rush et al.), 40
Stenosis, mitral, and insufficiency, combined, and mitral insufficiency, surgical treatment with use of heart-lung machine (Kay et al.), 67
Stomach, cancer of, elective uptake of radioiodine by (Clode et al.), 725
and colon, familial gastrointestinal polyposis involving, management of (Boley et al.), 691
Subglottic carcinoma with extensive tracheal involvement (Calem and Freund), 894
Surgeon, ideal, historical views of (Schechter and Swan), 427
Surgeons, University, Society of, issue, 1-300
review of meeting of (Deterling), 299
Surgical education, basic (Scott), 1
Synthetic vascular grafts, ultimate fate of, porosity as primary determinant (Wesolowski et al.), 91

T

Tap, peritoneal, in abdominal trauma (Drapanas and McDonald), 742
Temperature gradients associated with extracorporeal perfusion and profound hypothermia (Fisher et al.), 758
Terminal ileum, venous occlusion (Jackson), 322
Thoracopagous twins, conjugated heart of, measurement of pulmonary venous cross-circulation through, with radioactive $O^{15}$ (Spratt et al.), 941
Thrombogenic properties at site of vascular anastomoses studied by new technique for measuring platelet adherence (Inokuchi et al.), 493
Thrombophlebitis, treatment of (Cliffton et al.), 644
Thymus, fetal, extract of, attempt at development of agammaglobulinemia in adult rats by treatment with (Czaplicki), 817
Tissue, breast, human, normal and malignant, paper electrophoresis of extracts from (Slack), 464
Tissues, cerebral and peripheral, movement of ammonia into during hypothermia, relation of blood pH to (Bessman et al.), 478
Tracheal involvement, extensive subglottic carcinoma with (Calem and Freund), 894
Transfusion, massive, of preserved blood, hemorrhagic tendency after (Sunada et al.), 437
Transhepatic approach, percutaneous, of portal vein in man in determination of patency of splenorenal shunts (De Castro Silva et al.), 473
Transposition of great vessels, new operation for (Shumacker), 773
open intracardiac repair for (Kirklin et al.), 58
Tube, gastrostomy, temporary, 2-limb (Jascalevich), 736
Tubular necrosis, renal: its relation to norepinephrine administration (Chung and Šima), 328
Tumor, Wilms', recurrent or metastatic, management of (Soper), 555
Tumoricidal effect of nitrogen mustard, effect of increased oxygen tension on (Krementz and Knudson), 266
Tumors, benign, of major salivary glands (Grage et al.), 625
metastatic, of lungs, pulmonary resection for (Moersch and Clagett), 579
primary, of small intestine (Rochlin and Longmire), 586
Twins, thoracopagous, conjugated heart of, measurement of pulmonary venous cross-circulation through, with radioactive $O^{15}$ (Spratt et al.), 941

U

Ulcer, duodenal, gastrectomy for, duodenal closure after (Cooper), 425
Mann-Williamson, pathogenesis of: role of pancreatic and biliary juices in regulation of gastric secretion (Menguy and Mings), 662
peptic, perforated, acute: evaluation of 160 consecutive patients treated by closure (Palumbo and Sharpe), 863
problem in children, observations on exsanguinating gastric hemorrhage in newborn infant and (Lalonde and Berman), 962
Ulceration, peptic, experimental, prevention of, relative importance of vagus nerve, antrum, and acid-secreting mucosa in (Harrison et al.), 151
Ulcerative colitis, cancer risk in: formidability per patient-year of late disease (Dennis and Karlson), 568
University Surgeons, Society of, issue, 1-300
review of meeting of (Deterling), 299
Urinary tract operations, isolated ileal loop as substitute in, observations on (Abbott et al.), 467
Urine flow, renal blood flow, and renal vascular resistance, influence of l-norepinephrine on, in hemorrhagic shock (Nelson et al.), 115

V

Vagus nerve, antrum, and acid-secreting mucosa, relative importance in prevention of experimental peptic ulceration (Harrison et al.), 151
Variation, paradoxical, of femoral pulse in occlusion of iliac artery (Blaisdell and Gauder), 529
Vascular anastomoses, thrombogenic properties at site of, studied by new technique for measuring platelet adherence (Inokuchi et al.), 493
grafts, synthetic, ultimate fate of, porosity as primary determinant (Wesolowski et al.), 91
pattern of intestinal villi in rats after partial gastrectomy (Nylander and Olerud), 955
resistance, renal, influence of l-norepinephrine on, in hemorrhagic shock (Nelson et al.), 115
Vein grafting, experimental, in portal venous system (Symbas et al.), 97
portal, in man, percutaneous transhepatic approach in determination of patency of splenorenal shunts (De Castro Silva et al.), 473
Veins, hepatic, gradual occlusion with internal vena caval cannula, production of ascites by (Orloff and Snyder), 789
Vena cava cannula, internal, ascites produced with, effects of portacaval shunts on (Orloff and Snyder), 220
inferior, resection, and graft replacement (aortic homograft) for retroperitoneal sarcoma (McPeak), 778
Venous cannula for use in experimental animals (Pace), 402
occlusion, studies on fibrinolytic activity with: treatment of thrombophlebitis (Cliffton et al.), 644
of terminal ileum (Jackson), 322
system, portal, experimental vein grafting in (Symbas et al.), 97
Ventriculoauriculostomy, treatment of hydrocephalus by, lung and heart complications of (Emery and Hilton), 309
Vesalius, Andreas, surgeon (Schechter and Swan), 970
Vesicoileosigmoidostomy in treatment of exstrophy of bladder (Hays and Powell), 411
Vessels, great, transposition, new operation for (Shumacker), 773
open intracardiac repair for (Kirklin et al.), 58
renal, aberrant, hydronephrosis associated with, in infants and children (Ericsson et al.), 687
Villi, intestinal, vascular pattern of, in rats after partial gastrectomy (Nylander and Olerud), 955

W

Wilms' tumor, recurrent or metastatic, management of (Soper), 555
Wire lodged in interventricular septum of heart, removal (Kleinsasser), 500
Wound, healing, in experimental diabetes (Rosen and Enquist), 525
infections, experimental: contamination versus surgical technique (Condie and Ferguson), 367